Advanced Practice
Nursing in the
Care of Older Adults

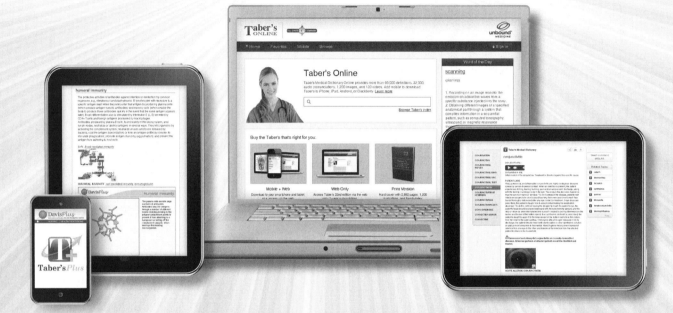

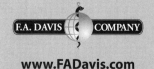

Advanced Practice **Nursing** in the Care of Older Adults

Laurie Kennedy-Malone, PhD, GNP-BC, FAANP, FGSA
Professor of Nursing, School of Nursing
University of North Carolina at Greensboro
Greensboro, North Carolina

Kathleen Ryan Fletcher, RN, DNP, GNP-BC, FAAN
Geriatric Director
Riverside Health System
Newport News, Virginia
Clinical Assistant Professor of Nursing
University of Virginia School of Nursing
Charlottesville, Virginia

Lori Martin-Plank, PhD, FNP-BC, NP-C, GNP-BC, FAANP
Clinical Assistant Professor, College of Nursing
University of Arizona
Tucson, Arizona

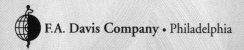
F.A. Davis Company • Philadelphia

F. A. Davis Company
1915 Arch Street
Philadelphia, PA 19103
www.fadavis.com

Printed in the United States of America

Last digit indicates print number: 10 9 8 7 6 5 4 3 2 1

Publisher, Nursing: Joanne P. DaCunha, RN, MSN
Director of Content Development: Darlene D. Pedersen
Project Editor: Elizabeth Hart
Electronic Project Editor: Sandra Glennie
Design & Illustration Manager: Carolyn O'Brien

As new scientific information becomes available through basic and clinical research, recommended treatments and drug therapies undergo changes. The author(s) and publisher have done everything possible to make this book accurate, up to date, and in accord with accepted standards at the time of publication. The author(s), editors, and publisher are not responsible for errors or omissions or for consequences from application of the book, and make no warranty, expressed or implied, in regard to the contents of the book. Any practice described in this book should be applied by the reader in accordance with professional standards of care used in regard to the unique circumstances that may apply in each situation. The reader is advised always to check product information (package inserts) for changes and new information regarding dose and contraindications before administering any drug. Caution is especially urged when using new or infrequently ordered drugs.

Library of Congress Cataloging-in-Publication Data

Kennedy-Malone, Laurie, 1957- author.
  Advanced practice nursing in the care of older adults / Laurie Kennedy-Malone, Kathleen Ryan Fletcher, Lori Martin-Plank.
    p. ; cm.
  Includes bibliographical references and index.
  ISBN 978-0-8036-2491-7
  I. Fletcher, Kathleen Ryan, 1951- author. II. Plank, Lori Martin, author. III. Title.
  [DNLM: 1. Advanced Practice Nursing. 2. Geriatric Nursing. 3. Geriatric Assessment. WY 152]
  RC954
  618.97'0231—dc23
                            2013039204

I dedicate this book to my husband Chris and to my son Brendan for their unwavering support during the writing of this book. To my parents, Nancy and Edward Kennedy, you continue to be models of successful aging that motivate me to continue to be passionate about advanced practice gerontological nursing.

—L.K.-M.

I dedicate this book to my husband Steve and my son Ian, who have always been present and supportive of all my professional pursuits. I am most appreciative of my mother, Eleanor Ryan, who has always been a role model for persistence, determination, and risk-taking.

—K.R.F.

To my husband Rick and daughter Erin, thank you both for your patience and encouragement throughout the writing of this book. I also would like to acknowledge the mentorship of Dr. Priscilla (Patt) O'Connor, PhD, and the inspiration provided by two dear friends and colleagues now deceased, Joan Zieja, RN, MPH, and Cecelia Jarek, PA-C. Finally, to my patients, who are also my teachers, thank you for entrusting your health to me; it has been my honor and privilege to serve you and to learn from you.

—L.M.-P.

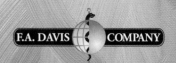

With the continued rapid growth of the older adult population, there remains an increased demand for healthcare providers to deliver age-specific care and direct disease management. *Advanced Practice Nursing in the Care of Older Adults* will serve as a guide for advanced practice nurses who are privileged to provide care to older adults. Designed as a text for students as well as a reliable source of evidence-based practice for advanced practice nurses, this book contains information on healthy aging, comprehensive geriatric assessment, and common symptoms and illnesses that present in older adults. The book concludes with a chapter on care delivery for patients with chronic illnesses who face end-of-life care. In addition, case studies are included throughout the text to provide further practice and review. An important feature of this book is the use of the Strength of Recommendation Taxonomy (S.O.R.T) (Ebell, M.H., Siwek, J., Weiss, B.D., Woolf, S.H., Susman, J., Ewigman, B., & Bowman, M. [2004]. Strength of Recommendation Taxonomy (SORT): a patient-centered approach to grading evidence in medical literature. *American Family Physician, 69*[3], 548–556.), which provides a direct reference to evidence-based practice recommendations for clinicians to consider in the care of older adults.

In Unit I: "The Healthy Older Adult," the first chapter, "Changes with Aging," addresses the normal changes of aging, expected laboratory values in older adults, pharmacokinetic and pharmacodynamic changes, presentation of illness, and the impact of chronic illness on functional capacity. In the second chapter, "Health Promotion," updated information pertaining to health promotion and disease prevention strategies for older adults from *Healthy People 2020* and the U.S. Preventive Services Task Force (USPSTF) is provided, including an immunization schedule and information on the Welcome to Medicare Visit. Also covered is an overview of physical activity, sexual behavior, dental health, and substance use as well as a section pertaining to the older traveler. Recommendations for exercise and safe physical activity are provided in this unit.

Unit II, "Assessment," opens with a detailed chapter on comprehensive geriatric assessment. Information on physical, functional, and psychological health is delineated, and information on quality of life measures is included. Next is the fifth chapter, "Symptoms and Syndromes," which provides the clinician with a concise description of more than 20 symptoms prevalent in older adults. A rapid reference detailing common contributing factors and associated symptoms and clinical signs that should be worked up for each presenting condition is included. Recommendations for diagnostic tests with accompanying results are used to form a differential diagnosis.

Unit III, "Treating Disorders," provides 11 chapters of concise, updated information pertaining to disease management of illnesses common in older adults, presented by body systems. Each chapter opens with an assessment section that provides the reader with a focused review of systems and the physical examinations needed to obtain pertinent information for diagnosis and treatment of the older adult. Signal symptoms indicating atypical presentation of illness are highlighted at the beginning of each condition. The discussion of each problem and disorder follows a consistent monograph format:

- Signal symptoms
- Definitions
- Etiology
- Occurrence
- Age
- Ethnicity
- Gender
- Contributing factors
- Signs and symptoms
- Diagnostic tests
- Differential diagnosis
- Treatment
- Follow-up
- Sequelae
- Prevention/prophylaxis
- Referral
- Education

Unit IV, "Complex Illness," addresses complex management of patients requiring nutritional support, chronic illness management, palliative care, and supportive care at end of life. The text concludes with two appendices—"Physiological Influences of the Aging Process" and "Laboratory Values in the Older Adult"—both of which are ready references for the busy practitioner.

In addition to the content of the book, online resources to aid the user in practice and review of the key concepts are available at DavisPlus. **Case studies** are provided in an interactive format that offers the user suggested answers for each discussion question. A **question bank** of multiple-choice questions for each chapter tests knowledge and understanding of the content. Online **learning activities** to support critical thinking are available for users to complete on their own or for educators to incorporate into their course requirements. Lists of **Web links and resources** for important Web sites and organizations related to the care of the older adult are consolidated in one place for easy reference.

This book is written by and for advanced practice nurses involved in the care of older adults across multiple settings of care. While intended as a guide for the management of care for older adults, clinicians are encouraged to deliver individualized, patient-centered care considering the latest clinical practice guidelines on prevention and management of conditions common in older adults.

Contributors

Tracey Ballard, MSN, GNP-BC
Gerontological Nurse Practitioner
OptumHealth
Greensboro, North Carolina
Gastroenteritis

Norma Branham, RN, MSN, GNP-BC, CWCN
Gerontological Nurse Practitioner
Senior Services at UVA Health System
Orange, Virginia
Diarrhea; Dizziness; Hematuria; Hemoptysis; Palliative End-of-Life Care

Peggy Brewer, DNP, GNP-BC
Gerontological Nurse Practitioner
Chatham Medical Specialists
Siler City, North Carolina
Colorectal Cancer

Helen Brooks, DNP, ANP-BC, ACNP-BC
Zach Hall MD
Reidsville, North Carolina
Hyperlipidemia

Charisse Buchert, MSN, CRNP
Adult-Gerontological Nurse Practitioner
Lake Erie Obstetrics & Gynecology
Erie, Pennsylvania
Cystitis

Karen L. Beard Byrd, MSN, GNP-BC
Gerontological Nurse Practitioner
Commonwealth Community Care
Women of Means Medical Home Without Walls
Boston, Massachusetts
Brain Cancer

Kristin R. Curcio, AGPCNP-BC
Adult-Gerontological Nurse Practitioner
Cone Health Cancer Center
Greensboro, North Carolina
Bladder Cancer; Liver Cancer

Margaret Dean, RN, CS-BC, GNP-BC, MSN
Geriatric Nurse Practitioner/Faculty Associate
Texas Tech University Health Sciences Center at Amarillo
Amarillo, Texas
Elder Abuse; Wandering

Nancy E. Dirubbo, FNP-C, Certificate in Travel Health, FAANP
Nurse Practitioner, Owner
Travel Health of New Hampshire
Laconia, New Hampshire
Travel and Leisure

John W. Distler, DPA, MBA, MS, FNP-C, FAANP
Dean, NP Tracks, Specialty Tracks
Chamberlain College of Nursing
Chicago, Illinois
Rhinitis

Kenyon Draper, APRN, ANP-C, MSPH
Adult-Gerontology Primary Care Nurse Practitioner
Lincolnton Medical Group
Lincolnton, North Carolina
Gout

Evelyn G. Duffy, DNP, G/ANP-BC, FAANP
Associate Professor
Director of the Adult-Gerontological Nurse Practitioner Program
Associate Director of the University Center on Aging and Health
Frances Payne Bolton School of Nursing
Case Western Reserve University
Cleveland, Ohio
Fungal Infection; Diabetes Mellitus; Osteoporosis; Psoriasis

Renee E. Edkins, MA, MSN, ANP-C
Nurse Practitioner, Burn Reconstruction
UNC Division of Plastic & Reconstructive Surgery
North Carolina Jaycee Burn Center
Chapel Hill, North Carolina
  Burns

Sheree L. Loftus Fader, PhD, GNP-BC
Gerontologist/Nurse Scientist
Beth Israel Medical Center
New York, New York
  Parkinson's Disease and related movement disorder;
  Restless Legs Syndrome

Carrie Fernald, ANP-BC, GNP-BC, FCN
HouseCalls Care Improvement Plus Provider
United Health Care
Greensboro, North Carolina
  Arthritis; Bursitis, Tendinitis, Soft Tissue Syndromes;
  Herniated Nucleus Pulposus; Rheumatoid Arthritis

Windy Forch, RN, MSN, GNP-BC
Study Coordinator
University of Virginia School of Nursing
Charlottesville, Virginia
  Bowel Incontinence; Chest Pain

M. Jane Griffith, RN, MSN, GNP-BC, ACHPN
Geriatric Nurse Practitioner
Mercy Care, Hospice Care and Palliative Care
  Partners Program
Myrtle Beach, South Carolina
  Palliative and End-of-Life Care

Candace Harrington, DNP, A/GNP-BC
Clinical Assistant Professor
East Carolina University College of Nursing
Greenville, North Carolina
  Heart Failure

Jeanette C. Hartshorn, PhD, RN, FAAN
Professor, Nursing Education
South University College of Nursing
Savannah, Georgia
  Headache; Seizure Disorders

Theresa Hollander, PhD, CRNP
Coordinator, Cardiac Assist Device Program
Temple University Hospital
Philadelphia, Pennsylvania
  Ischemic Heart Disease

Ellen Jones, DNP, FNP-C, FAANP
Clinical Professor of Nursing
UNC Greensboro School of Nursing
Greensboro, North Carolina
Nurse Practitioner, TargetCare
Charlotte, North Carolina
  Diabetes Mellitus; Obesity

Heejung Kim, PhD, RN
Assistant Professor
University of Kansas Medical Center School of
  Nursing
Kansas City, Kansas
  Constipation; Dehydration

Pam Koenig, MSN, APRN, FNP-BC
Family Nurse Practitioner
Eastport Health Care (FQHC)
Eastport, Maine
  Delirium; Dementia; Depression

Nanette Lavoie-Vaughan, MSN, APRN-C, DNP, ANP-BC
Clinical Assistant Professor
East Carolina University, College of Nursing
Greenville, North Carolina
  Agitation; Chronic Constipation; Clostridium difficile
  Colitis; Failure to Thrive

Kathy Long Lewis, MSN, ANP-BC
Adult Nurse Practitioner
Wilmington Health Associates
Wilmington, North Carolina
  Skin Cancer

Denise Lucas, PhD, RN, CRNP
Assistant Professor of Nursing
Duquesne University
Pittsburgh, Pennsylvania
  Prostate Cancer; Prostatitis

Laurie Lovejoy McNichol, MSN, GNP, CWOCN
Clinical Nurse Specialty/WOC
Cone Health
Greensboro, North Carolina
  Pressure Ulcers

Christine R. Moran, MSN, FNP-BC
Family Nurse Practitioner
Holy Redeemer Hospital and Medical Center
Meadowbrook, Pennsylvania
  Anemia of Chronic Disease; Iron Deficiency Anemia

LaTroy Navaroli, DNP, FNP-BC, CWS
Nurse Practitioner Wound Specialist
Navaroli Medical
Warren, Pennsylvania
  Oral Nutritional Supplementation

Rose Nieves, PhD, ARNP-C, FNP
Doctor of Nursing Practice Program Director
South University, Tampa Campus
Tampa, Florida
  Breast Cancer

Loretta J. Phillips, RN, MSN, NP-C, APRN-BC
Adult Nurse Practitioner
Capital Nephrology Associates
Raleigh, North Carolina
  Acute Kidney Injury; Chronic Renal Failure

Catherine Ratliff, PhD, APRN-BC, GNP-BC, CWOCN
Clinical Associate Professor of Nursing
Program Director of the Wound, Ostomy, and
  Continence Graduate Program
University of Virginia School of Nursing
Charlottesville, Virginia
  Peripheral Vascular Disease

Lauren Robbins, MSN, RN, GNP-BC
Gerontological Nurse Practitioner
OptumHealth
Norcross, Georgia
  Bowel Obstruction

Barbara Barnes Rogers, CRNP, MN, AOCN, ANP-BC
Nurse Practitioner
Fox Chase Cancer Center
Philadelphia, Pennsylvania
  Leukemias

Susan Sanner, PhD, APRN, FNP-BC, CNE
Clinical Coordinator and Associate Professor
South University Online
Morrow, Georgia
  Hypertension

Lorna Schumann, PhD, NP-C, ACNP-BC, ACNS-BC, CCRN, FAANP
Associate Professor of Nursing
Washington State University, College of Nursing
Yakima, Washington
  HIV

Terri Williams Setzer, MSN, ANP-BC
Adult Nurse Practitioner, Gastroenterology
Cone Health
Reidsville, North Carolina
  Nonalcoholic Fatty Liver Disease

Marianne Shaughnessy, PhD, CRNP
Program Analyst
Veterans Health Administration
Office of Geriatrics and Extended Care Services
Baltimore, Maryland
  Stroke; Transient Ischemic Attack

Tracey Parker Sherrod, MSN, ANP-C, GNP-BC
Adult-Gerontological Nurse Practitioner
MD Health Care
Wilson, North Carolina
  Nephrolithiasis

Lynn Simpkins, RN, MSN, FNP-BC, GNP-BC, CDE
Family and Geriatric Nurse Practitioner
Adaptive Geriatrics
Richmond, Virginia
  Involuntary Weight Loss; Peripheral Edema

DarLene Stevens, PhD, ARNP, FNP-BC
Lead Nurse Practitioner, Cardiology/Nuclear
  Medicine
North Texas VA Medical Center
Dallas, Texas
  Myocardial Infarction

David V. Strider, RN, MSN, CCRN, ACNP, DNP
Nurse Practitioner for Vascular Surgery
University of Virginia Medical Center
Charlottesville, Virginia
  Peripheral Vascular Disorders

Cristy Glover Stumb, DNP, MBA, APRN-BC
Assistant Professor
South University College of Nursing
Savannah, Georgia
  Arrhythmias

Ladsine Taylor, MSN, GNP-BC
Nurse Practitioner in the Community Living Center
Bill Hefner V.A. Medical Center
Salisbury, North Carolina
Peripheral Neuropathy

Cynthia M. Turner, DNP, FNPC
Adjunct Faculty
South University School of Nursing
Savannah, Georgia
Valvular Heart Disease

Lois Von Cannon, MSN, APN-BC
Clinical Associate Professor
UNC Greensboro School of Nursing
Greensboro, North Carolina
Acute Pancreatitis; Chronic Pancreatitis; Pancreatic Cancer

Steven Weiss, CRNP, MSN, BSN, BA
Psychiatric Nurse Practitioner
Lenape Valley Foundation
Doylestown, Pennsylvania
Anxiety

Eileen Weston, MSN, A/GNP-C
Adult-Gerontology Primary Care Nurse Practitioner
Cornerstone Care Outreach Clinic
High Point, North Carolina
Malnutrition

Suzann Williams-Rosenthal, RN, MSN, GNP, CWOCN
Geriatric Nurse Practitioner, Colonnades Medical Associates
University of Virginia Health System
Charlottesville, Virginia
Urinary Incontinence

Colleen T. Wojciechowski, MSN, GNP-BC
Nurse Practitioner
Durham Veterans Affairs Medical Center
Community Living Center
Durham, North Carolina
Cough

M. Catherine Wollman, DNP, RN, CRNP
Gerontological Nurse Practitioner
M. Catherine Wollman Consulting
West Chester, Pennsylvania
Chronic Illness and the APRN

Reviewers

Kathleen Anderson, MS, RNP-C
Assistant Clinical Professor
Binghamton University
Binghamton, New York

Carolyn Auerhahn, EdD, ANP, GNP-BC, FAANP
Consultant, Adult-Gerontology APRN Education
North Cape May, New Jersey

Susan Barnason, PhD, RN, APRN-CNS, CEN, CCRN, FAHA
Professor of Nursing
University of Nebraska Medical Center
Lincoln, Nebraska

Mary P. Cadogan, DrPH, RN, GNP-BC
Professor, Adjunct Series
Lead Faculty, Adult/Gerontology Primary
    Care Nurse Practitioner Program
UCLA School of Nursing
Los Angeles, California

Bonni Cohen, MSN, APRN, ANP-BC, FNP-BC
Instructor/ANP Coordinator
Valdosta State University
Valdosta, Georgia

Jaclyn Conelius, PhD, FNP-BC
Assistant Professor
Fairfield University
Fairfield, Connecticut

Carolynn A. DeSandre, MSN, CNM, FNP-BC
Assistant Professor of Nursing
North Georgia College & State University
Dahlonega, Georgia

Karen Dick, PhD, GNP-BC, FAANP
Graduate Program Director & Clinical Associate
    Professor
University of Massachusetts, Boston
Boston, Massachusetts

Jill F. Diede, DNP, FNP-C
Chief, Disease Management Clinic
Evans Army Hospital
Ft. Carson, Colorado

Shirley Dinkel, PhD, APRN-BC
Associate Professor
Washburn University
Topeka, Kansas

Mary Elesha-Adams, RN, MSN, FNP-BC
Clinical Assistant Professor
East Carolina University
Greenville, North Carolina

Jane Flanagan, PhD, ANO-BC, ANP-BC
Associate Professor
Boston College
Chestnut Hill, Massachusetts

Donna Freeborn, PhD, FNP-BC, CNM
Director, FNP program
Brigham Young University
Provo, Utah

Constance H. Glenn, RN, MSN, APRN, FNP-BC
Clinical Assistant Professor
Sacred Heart University
Fairfield, Connecticut

Imani C. Goodwin, PhD, RN, FNP-BC
Assistant Professor
Troy University School of Nursing
Troy, Alabama

Debra J. Hain, PhD, ARNP, GNP-BC
Assistant Professor/Nurse Practitioner
Florida Atlantic University, Christine E. Lynn College
    of Nursing
Cleveland Clinic Florida, Department of Nephrology
Boca Raton, Florida

Mellisa Hall, DNP, ANP-BC, FNP-BC, GNP-BC
Assistant Professor of Nursing
University of Southern Indiana
Evansville, Indiana

Mary Blaszko Helming, PhD, APRN, FNP-BC, AHN-BC
Professor of Nursing and FNP Track Coordinator for
    MSN and DNP Tracks
Quinnipiac University
Hamden, Connecticut

Laima Karosas, PhD, APRN
Clinical Associate Professor
Quinnipiac University
Hamden, Connecticut

Linda J. Keilman, DNP, GNP-BC
Assistant Professor, Gerontological Nurse
    Practitioner
Michigan State University, College of Nursing
East Lansing, Michigan

Katherine Kenny, DNP, RN, ANP-BC, CCRN
Director, DNP Program
Arizona State University
Phoenix, Arizona

Cathy R. Kessenich, DSN, ARNP, FAANP
Professor of Nursing, MSN Program Director
University of Tampa
Tampa, Florida

Jan Kimble, RN, MSN, EdD
Associate Professor
Troy University
Montgomery, Alabama

Pamela L. King, PhD, MSN, FNP
MSN Program Director
Spalding University
Louisville, Kentucky

Rose Knapp, DNP, RN, APN-BC
Assistant Graduate Professor, Assistant Director of
    the DNP Program
Monmouth University
West Long Branch, New Jersey

Greta M. Kostac, DNP, APRN
Associate Professor, Program Director-NP Program
Marian University
Fond du Lac, Wisconsin

Laura LaRue, DNP, FNP-BC
Assistant Professor, FNP Coordinator
Radford University
Radford, Virginia

Eileen McCann, DNP, FNP
Director, FNP Program
St Xavier University
Chicago, Illinois

Dana Roe, DNS, WHNP-BC
Director of Graduate Studies and Research
    in Nursing
Northwestern State University College of Nursing
    and Allied Health
Shreveport, Louisiana

Gloria M. Rose, PhD, RN, NP-C, FNP-C
Assistant Professor, Coordinator FNP Program
Prairie View A&M University
Houston, Texas

Amy L. Silva-Smith, PhD, ANP-BC
Associate Professor, A/GNP Program Coordinator
University of Colorado, Colorado Springs
Colorado Springs, Colorado

Jennifer K. Sofie, MSN, FNP-C, ANP-BC
Assistant Teaching Professor, MSU
Primary Care Provider, Three Rivers Clinic
Montana State University
Bozeman, Montana

Joyce McCullers Varner, DNP, ANP/GNP-BC, GCNS
Associate Professor and Director of the BSN-DNP
    Adult-Gerontology NP with Palliative Care
    Specialty Program
University of South Alabama
Mobile, Alabama

Mary L. Wilby, MSN, CRNP
Assistant Professor, Adult NP Track Coordinator
La Salle University School of Nursing and Health
    Sciences
Philadelphia, Pennsylvania

Acknowledgments

This book would not have become a reality if not for the kind assistance and gentle persistence of some wonderful people whom we would like to thank. To Joanne DaCunha, our acquisitions editor, who believed in the importance of the book given the changes mandated by the APRN consensus model for the required inclusion of gerontology and geriatrics for all advanced practice nurses taking care of older adults. To Elizabeth Hart, our project editor, who kept us on track and provided us order; to Jennifer Schmidt for patience and creative editing, without which we would not have completed the task; to Rhonda Lucas, who assisted with information retrieval; and to our dedicated contributors, who believe in the importance of creating a reference specific to the care of older adults written by advanced practice registered nurses. We also would like to acknowledge those who contributed to our previous books. Their contributions helped to make this brand new book possible.

L.K.-M.
K.F.
L.M.-P

Contents in Brief

Contents

unit I

The Healthy Older Adult

chapter 1

Changes With Aging

Kathleen Fletcher

FUNDAMENTAL CONSIDERATIONS

The aged population continues to be incredibly diverse; it includes some individuals who are nearly twice as old as others and is reflective of growing cultural diversity as well. Knowing what is expected in aging, what is disease in aging, and what constitutes successful aging is an immense challenge even for the most skillful advanced clinician. When assessing the aged individual, the advanced practice nurse should be familiar with the range of normal and expected changes associated with aging so that older persons falling outside this range may be identified and interventions taken appropriately and expeditiously.

In the past, wellness was considered the mere absence of disease, but with more information from longitudinal studies of aging, we are learning a great deal about the characteristics of successful physiological and psychosocial agers. A profile of what constitutes successful aging is beginning to emerge, and the illness-health continuum continues to expand to include agers. This chapter focuses on familiarizing the advanced practice nurse with fundamental underpinnings that serve to guide the approach to assessment and management of the older adult. In addition to appreciating the physiological changes that come with aging, the advanced practice nurse needs to understand how aging changes influence pharmacokinetics, pharmacodynamics, and reference laboratory values. Recognizing that presenting features of disease/illness may be different and having a greater awareness of the impact of chronic illness on functional capacity and quality of life provide the advanced practice nurse with a perspective in approaching the older adult that is different from that of younger adults.

PHYSIOLOGICAL CHANGES WITH AGING

The physiological changes associated with the usual aging process have been detailed by system, and the impact of these changes has been described. (These can be found in Appendix A.) Although Appendix A uses a single-system approach, the clinician must be aware that all the systems interact and, in doing so, can increase the older person's vulnerability to illness/disease. For example, the risk of respiratory infection in the geriatric population is considerable, and the physiological influences may include limited chest wall expansion, cilia atrophy, and alterations in the immune system. During the clinical decision-making process, the clinician knowledgeable about physiological changes with aging will be less likely to undertreat a treatable condition. For example, the astute clinician will use the diagnostic process to differentiate the more benign seborrheic keratosis from the more serious actinic keratosis in the aged individual. While educating the older patient, the informed professional will be less likely to attribute a finding to the aging process alone. When clinicians attribute findings to aging alone, the older person may conclude that there is no point in changing behavior, because the process is inevitable.

The major impact of all of these physiological changes can be highlighted with three primary points. First, there is a reduced physiological reserve of most body systems, particularly cardiac, respiratory, and renal. Second, there are reduced homeostatic mechanisms that fail to adjust regulatory systems such as temperature control and fluid and electrolyte balance. Third, there is impaired immunological function: infection risk is greater, and autoimmune diseases are more prevalent. The clinician is advised not to be complacent in that some processes previously considered normal, age-related changes are now being refuted. Historically, normal aging studies were conducted using a cross-sectional study method. Today, results are becoming increasingly available from longitudinal studies of aged populations, some of which began in the 1930s. This more reliable methodology provides some challenges to previously held conclusions. The clinician is encouraged to keep informed regarding the research in the area of expected and successful aging so that this information may be carefully considered, interpreted, and translated quickly into the clinical setting.

LABORATORY VALUES IN OLDER ADULTS

Healthy individuals of all ages often have asymmetrical distribution of test results. Normality in a statistical sense may be extrapolated incorrectly to normality in terms of health. In addition, the standards previously available to the health-care worker with which to compare normal laboratory values have been based on randomly collected samples of younger healthy adults. Many factors can influence laboratory value interpretation in the elderly, including the physiological changes with aging, the prevalence of chronic disease, changes in nutritional and fluid intake, lifestyle (including activity), and the medications taken (Brigden & Heathcote, 2000). Reference ranges therefore may be preferable. Reference ranges or intervals, such as age, sex, or race, can be defined demographically. For example, the reference range for older adults might be the intervals within which 95% of persons over age 70 fall. These may be further defined physiologically (e.g., fasting or activity status) or pharmacologically (e.g., medication, tobacco or alcohol use). Even this more precise method does not ensure a healthy sampled population as the standard, and using the reference range method may not differentiate normal aging from

disease. The reference values presented for the older adult cohort (see Appendix B) are not necessarily desirable ones. Longitudinal chemical studies support the concept of biochemical individuality; that is, each individual's variation is often much smaller than that of the larger group as a whole. Biochemical individuality is of particular importance in detecting asymptomatic abnormalities in older adults. Significant homeostatic disturbances in the same individual may be detected through serial laboratory tests, even though all individual test results may lie within normal limits of the reference interval for the entire group.

The clinician must determine whether a value obtained reflects a normal aging change, a disease, or the potential for disease. Although abnormal laboratory findings are often attributed to old age, rarely are they true aging changes. Misinterpretation of an abnormal laboratory value as an aging change can lead to underdiagnosis and undertreatment in some situations (e.g., anemia or urinary tract infection) and overdiagnosis and overtreatment in others (e.g., hyperglycemia or asymptomatic bacteriuria). At times, the result of a laboratory value may be within the appropriate reference range yet indicate pathology for the older adult. The serum creatinine level may be within the normal range yet indicate renal impairment in a patient with inadequate protein stores, and different measures might need to be considered. One value of particular significance to the practitioner with prescriptive privileges is the calculation of creatinine clearance in the estimation of renal function.

Reduced renal function, particularly the glomerular filtration rate (GFR), affects the clearance of many drugs, and creatinine clearance provides an index of renal function for use in choosing doses of renally eliminated or nephrotoxic drugs (such as digoxin, H_2 blockers, lithium, and water-soluble antibiotics). The Modification of Diet in Renal Disease (MDRD) and the Cockcroft-Gault equations both provide useful estimates of the GFR (Boparai & Korc-Grodzicki, 2011). The performance of these two formulas was compared in an elderly population, and the Cockcroft-Gault formula was found to be inferior to the MDRD equation; however, the MDRD is not as practical and is more complex to use (Fliser, 2008). The use of serum drug concentration measurements (where these are available) or timed urine specimens is recommended until more acceptable methods of calculating renal function in this population become available.

Finally, when considering which laboratory tests to order, it is worth remembering the doctrine *primum non nocere,* to do no harm. Excessive blood sampling may lower the hematocrit; repeated fasting tests may provoke nutritional compromise; and extensive use of tests often requires drugs that may cause adverse reactions. Any risks involved in laboratory testing must be considered with respect to the patient's clinical condition and weighed against the test's expected benefits. The clinician should plan in advance the use for each test result value obtained, especially for less specific or less sensitive tests such as sedimentation rate and serum alkaline phosphatase levels.

PHARMACOKINETIC/ PHARMACODYNAMIC CHANGES

Polypharmacy and the potential for an adverse drug reaction (ADR) remain major concerns in geriatric health care. Although older adults represent 12% of the population, they are the biggest consumers of medications. One-third of community-dwelling elderly take more than 5 prescribed medications, and nearly 20% take more than 10 prescribed medications. Forty-two percent of older adults take more than one over-the-counter drug, and 49% take more than one nutritional supplement (Slone Epidemiology Center at Boston University, 2006). Polypharmacy is a primary predictor for an ADR, which is any undesired or unwanted consequence that occurs as a result of taking medications.

The magnitude of the problem is reflected in some current statistics. ADRs account for approximately 10% of all emergency department visits and up to 17% of all hospital admissions (Hanlon, Sloane, Pieper, & Schmader, 2011; Hohl, Dankoff, Colacone, & Afilalo, 2001). The most significant factor contributing to the risk of an ADR in older individuals is the number of drugs taken. Factors contributing to the increased ADR risk in elderly people include not only polypharmacy but also pharmacokinetics and pharmacodynamics that are altered with aging, adherence problems, and inappropriate health-care provider prescribing and self-prescribing. In general, the therapeutic window narrows with age, so the potential for benefiting the patient measured against the risk of doing harm becomes more significant for the prescribing professional.

Certain changes occurring with the aging process alter the dynamic processes that drugs undergo to produce therapeutic effects. These changes involve the processes of pharmacokinetics (what the body does to the drug) and pharmacodynamics (what the drug does to the body).

Absorption

Drug absorption is generally thought to have a less significant impact on pharmacokinetics than do drug distribution, metabolism, or excretion. Gastric acidity declines with age because of decreased intestinal blood flow and fewer absorbing cells in the gastrointestinal tract. These changes appear to be offset, however, by the longer contact time that occurs as transit time slows (in aging, this slowing is more functional than physiological). Another factor that affects drug absorption is the presence of food and other drugs in the stomach at the same time. Antacids and iron, for example, inhibit the absorption of tetracycline; antacids can significantly decrease the bioavailability of digoxin. Anticholinergic medications cause a slowing of colonic motility and can result in greater absorption rates. Metabolic diseases, such as thyroid disease or diabetes, can cause an increase or decrease in transit time and therefore can cause either increased or decreased drug absorption.

Another consideration is whether an oral medication actually passes through the esophagus before it is absorbed. Many older adults take medications without adequate fluid, increasing the potential for esophageal damage from the dissolution of drugs in the esophagus. Esophageal erosions have been noted with caustic drugs such as alendronate potassium and tetracycline. Drug–drug, drug–disease, and drug–food interactions are likely to influence drug absorption (Boparai & Korc-Grodzicki, 2011).

Distribution

Drug distribution is affected by aging, particularly in individuals of smaller body size, those who have decreased body water, and those with higher body fat. Drugs distributed in water (e.g., alcohol and lithium) have a higher concentration in elderly persons, thereby exerting a more profound effect. Drugs distributed in fat (e.g., most psychoactive drugs) have a wider distribution and a less intense effect but a more prolonged action, particularly in those individuals with more adipose tissue. Medications with a higher protein-binding rate (e.g., phenytoin, warfarin, salicylates) have a greater potential to cause an ADR in those with less lean body mass. Because these individuals have fewer receptor sites and less albumin for binding, plasma concentration is greater, and more free drug is available for tissue distribution, pharmacological activity, and elimination. Protein-bound drugs in particular may reach toxic levels if the patient is not monitored closely. Distribution influences are marked in the patient who is malnourished and dehydrated.

Drug distribution also relies on the bioavailability of the drug. The amount of the drug that reaches the systemic circulation may be increased or decreased, depending on certain influencing factors: (1) route of administration is important to consider, because inhalants and drugs given intravenously and topically are usually more readily available than drugs administered intramuscularly, subcutaneously, orally, or rectally; (2) solubility of the drug is influential, because aqueous solutions are available more quickly than oily ones; and (3) general circulation to the site of drug administration has an impact, because blood flow increases with massage or heat or in the presence of an occlusive dressing and decreases during shock or during the administration of vasoconstrictors.

Metabolism

Biotransformation occurs in all body tissues but primarily in the liver, where enzymatic activity (cytochrome P [CYP] system) alters and detoxifies the drug and prepares it for excretion. With advancing age, the ability of the liver to metabolize drugs does not decline similarly for all pharmacological agents. Although liver size and blood flow do decline with age, routine liver function test results are typically normal when no disease exists. Decreased liver size and blood flow can result in decreased first-pass metabolism; drug activity for some medications is prolonged, because drugs are metabolized and eliminated more slowly.

Being familiar with the age-related pharmacokinetics of drugs is of the utmost importance when determining the initial and maintenance dosages. When prescribing for an elderly patient, it is critical to understand whether the drug inhibits or induces the CYP enzymes. Other factors influence biotransformation also. For example, smoking may slow it. Men have faster and more efficient biotransformation, presumably because of serum testosterone. Conditions of increased or decreased liver perfusion alter the overall level of the drug that is absorbed and how it is metabolized.

Elimination

The most profound pharmacokinetic change is reduced elimination of drugs. Most drugs are excreted in the urine via the renal system, although some are excreted in the feces via the biliary system. Water-soluble drugs are excreted directly by the kidneys, and fat-soluble drugs are converted to water-soluble drugs by the liver first. Changes in kidney function begin in the fourth decade of life and continue to decline with each subsequent decade (Coresh et al., 2005). Therefore, by age 70, an individual might reasonably have a 40% to 50% decrease in renal function, even in the absence of disease. These kidney function changes may prolong the half-lives of drugs. This is particularly important for drugs that are excreted unchanged in the urine and for drug categories known to be particularly nephrotoxic in older persons (e.g., radiocontrast materials, aminoglycosides, angiotensin-converting enzyme inhibitors, and NSAIDs).

Pharmacodynamics

It is important to know the pharmacodynamic influences of the drug (what the drug does to the body). A drug's pharmacodynamics describe the effect at the site of action and the time and intensity of the drug effect. A good example is that the older adult tends to exhibit enhanced responses to drugs affecting the central nervous system (e.g., benzodiazepines), and this is attributed to greater tissue sensitivity caused by aging. Older adults often experience more sedation from central nervous system drugs than younger persons at the same concentration. Older adults given opiates are more likely to experience ataxia, and those taking haloperidol are more likely to experience extrapyramidal symptoms. Some studies demonstrate that older individuals may have increased tissue sensitivity for oral anticoagulants. In certain instances, patients may exhibit a decreased, rather than an exaggerated, response at this tissue level; this appears to be the case with beta blockers in which an increased dosage may be required to have a desired effect. Drug responsiveness may vary depending on the patient's activity and stress levels and on the environment. These factors have not yet been adequately studied. There is a general trend of assuming greater pharmacodynamic sensitivity in the elderly; however, this sensitivity is not universal, and age-related changes need to be investigated agent by agent until further research yields greater understanding of the aging process (Bowie & Slattum, 2007). In addition to understanding the fundamental changes that accompany aging and their influence on interpreting laboratory values and medication management, the advanced practice nurse needs to understand the presenting features of illness/disease in older adults.

PRESENTING FEATURES OF ILLNESS/DISEASE IN THE ELDERLY

The manifestations of illness and disease in the elderly can be very different even if the underlying pathological process is the same as in younger individuals. The advanced practice nurse should be aware of what can influence the presentation. Four factors are discussed here: nonpresentation of illness, multiple complaints, an altered pattern of illness, and atypical, nonspecific, or vague symptoms or signs.

Underreporting of symptoms by older adults may occur if they attribute the new sign or symptom to age itself. This represents a form of ageism that older adults, their families, and sometimes health-care providers demonstrate. By erroneously associating aging with disease, disuse, and disability, older adults perceive this change as inevitable and either fail to present to the health-care provider or, if they do, fail to challenge the assumption that this represents normal aging. At times an acute symptom, such as pain or dyspnea, is superimposed on a chronic symptom, and the older adult may not recognize that it represents a new or exacerbated pathology. The advanced practice nurse is well advised to never attribute something to normal aging without doing a careful and methodical search for a treatable condition.

Older adults do sometimes present with multiple complaints, and the first inclination of the provider may be to think that they are hypochondriacal. Because of the prevalence of chronic disease in this population, the clinician is advised to explore the possibility of a constellation of symptoms and signs that when analyzed may represent more than one condition/problem. Another consideration might be an underlying depression. Depression often manifests atypically in older adults, and somatic symptoms are not uncommon.

The pattern of disease progress may be different for the elderly. Certain diseases are more common in the elderly, and an understanding of the epidemiology is critical in the interpretation. Illustrative examples include jaundice, which is suggestive of viral hepatitis in younger individuals but may represent gallbladder disease or a malignancy in the elderly, and delusions or hallucinations, which are suggestive of bipolar disorder in younger individuals but may represent dementia or medication side effects in the elderly (Williams, 2008).

Altered presentation is another common feature in older adults. The patient with a urinary tract infection may not present with a fever, elevated white blood cell count, or tachycardia, and the primary symptom may be confusion. The patient with depression may not present with a dysphoric mood but rather agitation and psychotic features. The older adult may present with cardiac manifestations of thyroid disease. Because the symptoms or signs of illness or disease may be vague and nonspecific, even a modest change in a functional level or behavior should alert the clinician to carefully explore the potential for a treatable condition.

CHRONIC ILLNESS AND FUNCTIONAL CAPACITY

Approximately 80% of those 65 or older have one chronic disease, and 50% have two or more (Centers for Disease Control and Prevention [CDC], 2003). The most common of these are related to heart disease, arthritis, respiratory problems, cancer, diabetes, and stroke (U.S. Department of Health and Human Services [USDHHS], CDC, 2007). These conditions often impair functional capacity and limit the person's ability to perform activities of daily living (ADLs), such as bathing and dressing, and instrumental activities of daily living (IADLs) such as managing medications and traveling. More than 25% of community-dwelling Medicare beneficiaries report difficulties performing ADLs, and 14% report difficulties performing IADLs (USDHHS, Administration on Aging [AOA], 2010).

SUMMARY

Assessment and management of older adults is different from that of younger adults, and it is of critical importance that the advanced practice nurse working with the elderly has the knowledge, skill, and ability to recognize these differences and take them into consideration. This chapter highlighted how the approach of the clinician might be different based on an understanding of the physiological changes of aging and the impact of these changes on medication management and laboratory interpretation; how the presenting features of disease and illness may be different in the elderly; and how the elderly are disproportionately affected with chronic disease and functional impairments.

REFERENCES

Boparai, M. K., & Korc-Grodzicki, B. (2011). Prescribing for older adults. *Mount Sinai Journal of Medicine, 78*(4), 613–626.

Bowie, M. W., & Slattum, P. W. (2007). Pharmacodynamics in older adults: a review. *American Journal of Geriatric Pharmacotherapy, 5*(3), 263–303.

Brigden, M., & Heathcote, J. C. (2002). Problems in interpreting laboratory tests. *Postgraduate Medicine, 107*(7), 145–158.

Centers for Disease Control and Prevention. (2003). Public health and aging: trends in aging—United States and world-wide. *Morbidity and Mortality Weekly Report (MMWR), 52*(6), 101–106.

Coresh, J., Byrd-Holt, D., Astor, B. C., Briggs, J. P., Eggers, P. W., Lacher, D. A., & Hostetter, T. H. (2005). Chronic kidney disease awareness, prevalence, and trends among U. S. adults, 1999–2000. *Journal of the American Society of Nephrology, 16*(1), 180–188.

Fliser, D. (2008). Assessment of renal function in elderly patients. *Current Opinion in Nephrology and Hypertension, 17*(6), 604–608.

Hanlon, J. T., Sloane, R. J., Pieper, C. F., & Schmader, K. E. (2011). Association of adverse drug reactions with drug–drug and drug–disease interactions in frail older outpatients. *Age and Ageing, 40*(2), 274–277.

Hohl, C. M., Dankoff, J., Colacone, A., & Afilalo, M. (2001). Polypharmacy, adverse drug-related events, and potential adverse drug interactions in elderly patients presenting to an emergency department. *Annals of Emergency Medicine, 38*(6), 666–671.

Slone Epidemiology Center at Boston University. (2006). Patterns of medication use in the United States, 2006. Retrieved October 2, 2011, from www.bu.edu/slone/files/2012/11/SloneSurveyReport2006.pdf

U.S. Department of Health and Human Services, Administration on Aging. (2010). A profile of older Americans: 2010. Retrieved October 2, 2011, from www.aoa.gov/aoaroot/aging_statistics/Profile/index.aspx

U.S. Department of Health and Human Services, Centers for Disease Control and Prevention. (2007). The state of aging and health in America 2007. Retrieved October 2, 2011, from www.cdc.gov/aging/pdf/saha_2007.pdf

Williams, M. E. (2008). Geriatric physical diagnosis: a guide to observation and assessment. Jefferson, NC: McFarland & Company.

chapter 2

Health Promotion

Lori Martin-Plank

The concept of health promotion includes activities to which an individual is committed and performs proactively to further his or her health and well-being. This includes not only preventive and health-protective measures but also actualization of one's health potential. The broadest definition, identified by the World Health Organization (WHO), includes healthy lifestyle promotion, creation of supportive environments for health, community action, redirection of health services, and healthy public policy formulation. In 2006, WHO incorporated the need for research to create an evidence base for health promotion (Smith, Tang, & Nutbeam, 2007).

All these measures are within the scope of practice for the nurse practitioner (NP) and enhance the visibility of the role while advancing the needs of patients. Additionally, NPs are in a unique and pivotal position to guide and encourage health-promotion programs and individual efforts. From our nursing background, we bring a holistic orientation to health and wellness as well as knowledge of developmental tasks and the wellness-illness continuum. Our advanced practice education helps us to diagnose and treat patients in a way that supports their return to optimal level of function and/or maximizes their coping abilities within the limits of their existing function. This particular blend of NP competencies is especially valuable in working with older patients. Heterogeneity increases with aging, presenting the NP with the challenge of individualizing health-promotion recommendations for each patient.

Because older adults have not been included in studies on health promotion (Richardson, 2006) and because single-focused interventions for health promotion often do not "fit" with the interrelatedness of older adult health-promotion challenges, clear age-specific preventive health guidelines for the older population are scarce. Many disorders in older adults encompass multiple risk factors that involve several systems and interventions to achieve outcomes; this presents a challenge when measuring and synthesizing evidence and reporting outcomes (Leipzig, 2010). Medicare will only pay for A and B level recommendations that meet the U.S. Preventive Services Task Force (USPSTF) stringent evidence guidelines, leaving other beneficial interventions without coverage. Another confounding factor is the way that outcomes for screening are measured in terms of years of life saved; for older adults, quality of life or functional life is a more realistic goal (Leipzig, 2010). The USPSTF Older Adult group is working on a blueprint for developing health-promotion guidelines for older adults (Leipzig, 2010), with a model depicted in Figure 2-1.

The Healthy People 2020 program has also set specific objectives for prevention in older adults; these include increased use of the Welcome to Medicare visit, an increased percentage of older adults who are up to date on all preventive services, and decreased use of the emergency department for falls by older adults, among others. Because of the focus on chronic disease management and the complexities of multiple comorbidities in older adults, many primary health-care providers are not oriented toward the potential of healthy aging and discount the importance of health promotion in this age group.

Current life expectancy is 78.7 years (Murphy, Xu, & Kochanek, 2012), with many people living to 100 years and beyond. It behooves us to focus on prevention and health promotion in our older patients to maximize

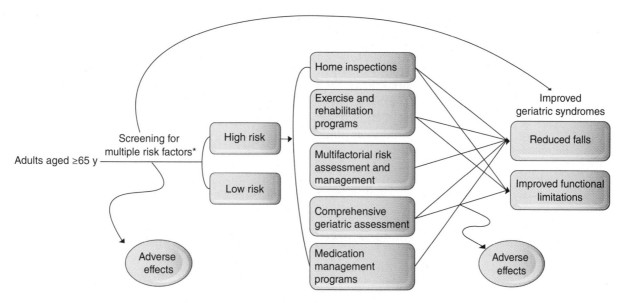

* Risk factors include increasing age, baseline functional impairment and limitations, incontinence, polypharmacy, medical risks, or sensory and cognitive deficits.

FIGURE 2-1. Ideal analytic framework. (*Source: Leipzig, R. M., Whitlock, E. P., Wolff, T. A., Barton, M. B., Michael, Y. L., Harris, R., . . . Siu, A.; U.S. Preventive Services Task Force Geriatric Workgroup. [2010]. Reconsidering the approach to prevention recommendations for older adults. Annals of Internal Medicine, 153, 809–814.*)

the quality of these years. A collaborative plan should include consideration of the patient's health beliefs and goals, present and anticipated levels of function, risks and benefits of proposed interventions, and effectiveness of specific preventive interventions for older adults. The Welcome to Medicare visit provides a good opportunity to focus solely on preventive services and health promotion; this is followed by the Medicare-supported annual prevention visit. Health-promotion activities should be incorporated into every patient encounter, as opposed to being addressed selectively, and should be individualized to the patient. Recent efforts are being focused on partnering population-based, community-centered programs with personal health initiatives in older adults to make interventions more available and more economical and to increase socialization opportunities and harness the power of group support (Centers for Disease Control and Prevention [CDC], 2011; Ogden, Richards, & Shenson, 2012).

PRIMARY, SECONDARY, AND TERTIARY PREVENTION

Preventive services are typically divided into the categories of primary, secondary, and tertiary. Primary prevention refers to those activities undertaken to prevent the occurrence of a disease or adverse health condition, including mental health. Health counseling and immunization are examples of primary prevention.

Secondary prevention refers to those tasks directed toward detection of a disease or adverse health condition in an asymptomatic individual who has risk factors but no detectable disease. Screening tests are examples of secondary prevention. The screening test must detect the condition at a stage where it is treatable and a positive outcome is expected as a result of treatment. Mammography for breast cancer screening is an example of secondary prevention.

Tertiary prevention refers to management of existing conditions to prevent disability and minimize complications, striving for optimal level of function and quality of life. Pulmonary rehabilitation for a chronic obstructive pulmonary disease (COPD) patient is an example of tertiary prevention.

HEALTHY LIFESTYLE COUNSELING

The Welcome to Medicare visit (Centers for Medicare and Medicaid, 2011) provides an ideal opportunity for healthy lifestyle counseling. In addition to a thorough history (including some risk assessment, physical activity, diet, and tobacco and alcohol use), home safety and depression assessment are included. The Medicare MedLearn network has a link to guide providers covering all areas (www.cms.gov/Outreach-and-Education/Medicare-Learning-Network-MLN/MLN Products/downloads//MPS_QRI_IPPE001a.pdf). Healthy lifestyle counseling should be addressed at each visit, using brief motivational interviewing (Green, Cifuentes, Glasgow, & Stange, 2008; Shenson, Adams, Bolen, & Anderson, 2011).

Physical Activity

Older adults are the least active age group, although recent trends show an increase in physical activity in older adults. The American College of Sports Medicine and the American Heart Association (Nelson et al., 2007) recently issued updated recommendations for physical activity in all adults, with additional recommendations tailored to adults over age 65 and adults ages 50 to 64 with chronic conditions that are clinically significant or result in functional limitations. Counseling on physical activity should include any type of activity that the patient is able and willing to do. The health benefits of regular physical activity are well documented and include flexibility, increased muscle mass, maintenance of desirable weight, decreased insulin resistance, decreased peripheral vascular resistance, lower blood pressure, and a sense of well-being. Whenever possible, the components of aerobic activity (low to moderate), flexibility, balance, and strengthening (weight training) should be included, and the physical activity prescription should be individualized to the patient. Active hobbies, such as gardening, golfing, tennis, dancing, bowling, hiking, and swimming, are beneficial. Tai chi and yoga are helpful for stretching and balance. Frail elderly or older adults with impaired mobility can benefit from armchair exercises and modified ambulation (U.S. Preventive Services Task Force, 2010). Patients need to be reassured that expensive equipment or fitness memberships are not necessary to increase physical activity; motivation is the key. There are also many community exercise programs targeted to older adults as well as Web sites that can be shared if the patient has access to the Internet (Etz et al., 2008; Hall & Bernhardt, 2012; Ogden et al., 2012; Shenson, Benson, & Harris, 2008). Several government and community group programs have handouts for patients. Before embarking on an exercise program, all patients should have an evaluation of health history, including medications, present physical activity and functional level, potential barriers to exercise, and a physical examination. Older adults with known or suspected cardiac risk factors should have a stress test before engaging in vigorous exercise. All participants should be reminded of the need for adequate hydration and use of caution during extreme weather conditions.

Nutrition

The heterogeneity of older adults is evident in the wide range of nutritional issues affecting them. Before initiating counseling on diet, obtain baseline information on current dietary intake and activity pattern and combine this with height and weight data and other health status information. For patients in the long-term-care setting, this information is obtained easily from chart documentation. For community-dwelling older adults, a brief nutrition screening tool such as the Mini Nutritional Assessment (MNA) can be helpful. The abbreviated MNA consists of six questions, and there is a patient self-questionnaire that can be downloaded or mailed in advance of the visit. The MNA Web site contains a section on tools for clinicians, including a user guide and streaming video (www.mna-elderly.com/tools_for_clinicians.html). It is available in multiple languages as well.

The importance of a healthy, balanced diet to the overall health of older adults cannot be overemphasized. Chronic illness and disability can interfere with the activities of daily living such as shopping or preparing meals. Financial hardship can limit food choices. Prescribed medications can affect absorption of nutrients, sense of taste, or appetite. Depression or social isolation can contribute to poor nutrition. Another problem commonly seen in community-dwelling older adults is obesity. Close to one-half of U.S. older adults are overweight or obese (Fakhouri, Ogden, Carroll, Kit, & Flegal, 2012). Overweight and obesity are associated with heart disease, certain types of cancer, type 2 diabetes, breathing difficulties, stroke, arthritis, and psychological problems. Although there is a decline in the prevalence of overweight and obesity after age 60 years, it remains a problem for many older adults. It is a major risk factor for decreased mobility and functional impairment as well as a cardiovascular risk. General guidelines for dietary counseling include the following.

- Limit fat and cholesterol.
- Maintain a balanced caloric intake.
- Emphasize the inclusion of grains, fruits, and vegetables daily.

- Ensure an adequate calcium intake, especially for women.
- Limit alcohol, if used, to one drink daily for women and two drinks daily for men: one drink = 12 oz beer, 5 oz wine, or 1.5 oz of 80-proof distilled spirits.

Tufts University Friedman Center for Nutrition has adapted the governmental nutrition initiative "MyPlate" for older adults; this can be used as a teaching tool and a handout for patients (see Chapter 4). Their Nutrition Navigator also rates nutrition Web sites for patients who are computer savvy.

Safety

Prevention of injury in the older adult is of paramount importance to continuing functionality and quality of life. Part of this counseling involves reinforcement of extant recommendations, including wearing lap and shoulder seat belts in a motor vehicle, avoiding drinking and driving, having working smoke detectors in the residence, and keeping hot water set below 120°F. For older adults who drive a motor vehicle, periodic assessment of their ongoing ability to drive safely is vital to the older adult and the public at large. Most motor vehicle accidents involve young drivers and old drivers.

Two recommendations are especially important for ensuring the safety of the older adult. The first involves the safe storage and removal of firearms. Possession of a firearm combined with depression, caregiver stress, irreversible illness, or decline in functional abilities can invite self-inflicted injury, suicide pacts, or other acts of violence. Counsel patients to avoid firearms in the home and to use alternative means for self-protection such as alarm systems and pepper mace spray. The second recommendation involves the prevention of falls, the leading cause of nonfatal injuries and unintentional death from injury in older persons. Certain combinations of physiological and environmental factors place some patients at increased risk. About 85% of falls occur at home, in the later part of the day. Office-based providers can assess for falls by asking if there is a history of falling and by performing the Get Up and Go test in the office. If indicated, evaluation of risk factors and a home safety assessment by a home health nurse or a geriatric assessment team can provide direction for preventive intervention and education. Potential recommendations include exercise programs to build strength, modification of environmental hazards, monitoring and adjusting of medications, external protection against falling on hard surfaces, and measures to increase bone density. If urinary incontinence is a contributing factor, a urological work-up may be indicated. Falls are often alarming to patients and families; in some cases, family members may desire nursing home placement for the patient because of a fall. In other cases, patients may be fearful of ambulation as a result of a fall. Falls also pose a challenge in the long-term-care environment. Education and counseling combined with an assessment of the patient's environment are helpful. Keeping water, call bell, telephone, and other necessities available and toileting regularly can minimize the potential for falling. Several home safety checklists are available on the Internet and can be given to patients for self-assessment.

Sexual Behavior

Assumptions regarding lack of sexual expression in the healthy older adult are unfounded. With the possibility of pregnancy eliminated, many mature adults feel less restraint. As a result of divorce or widowhood, they may seek satisfaction with new partners yet lack the knowledge to protect themselves from sexually transmitted diseases, especially HIV. More than 10% of HIV cases diagnosed in the United States are in people more than 50 years old (CDC, 2013). Older adults need to be taught methods for safe sex with use of a barrier to avoid sexually transmitted diseases, including HIV and hepatitis B. Using the patient's sexual history, explore patient needs, preferences, and medical or psychological obstacles to sexual expression. This exploration facilitates counseling and interventions to promote healthy sexual behavior.

Dental Health

Counseling regarding dental health in the older adult includes the need for regular visits to the dental-care provider, daily flossing, and brushing with fluoride toothpaste. Many elders have dentures or dental implants and assume that dental checkups are no longer necessary. Oral screening for cancer is still indicated, as is periodic assessment of denture fit and functionality. Another concern is for the condition of the remaining teeth of some older adults. Periodontal disease, erosion of dentin, or other problems may render the teeth nonfunctional for chewing and a potential source for infection. Dependence on others for transportation or lack of available dental resources for patients in long-term care settings further complicates the problem. Caregivers simply may overlook this aspect of preventive health, or financial considerations may preclude treatment. Patient and family education regarding dental health is essential.

Substance Use

Counseling about substance use (tobacco, alcohol, and drugs) and injury prevention can be combined naturally within the issue of safety. Smoking is the leading preventable cause of death in the United States. Smoking cessation yields many benefits to former smokers in terms of reduction of risk for several chronic illnesses and stabilization of pulmonary status. Clear and specific guidelines are available to help health-care providers advise tobacco users to quit and to provide them with follow-up encouragement and relapse prevention management. Quitting smoking may not be a choice for the institutionalized older adult but rather dictated by the policy of the institution. Health-care providers can offer support and encouragement, emphasizing the positive health changes that will result.

Counseling regarding alcohol or other drug use can be preventive or interventional, depending on the initial assessment. Use the Michigan Alcohol Screening Test (MAST), the CAGE questionnaire, or the Alcohol Use Disorders Identification Test (AUDIT) to assess risk. Emphasize the dangers of drinking and driving and the increased risk of falling while under the influence of alcohol or any drug that acts on the central nervous system. Teach patients about the coincidental interactions between alcohol and many prescription drugs, over-the-counter preparations such as acetaminophen, and herbal remedies. The contribution of alcohol abuse to problems, such as insomnia, depression, aggressive behaviors, and deteriorating social relationships, should be addressed. Likewise, the problem of dependence on prescription drugs, such as analgesics, hypnotics, tranquilizers, and anxiolytics, should be assessed and addressed. Counseling in the form of individual follow-up sessions, group support, or outpatient or inpatient rehabilitation may be indicated. In a group-living situation, the governing body (i.e., resident council) may become involved if the patient's behavior threatens the safety or well-being of the other group members.

SCREENING AND PREVENTION

The following table contains the areas of screening and prevention that are covered by Medicare for older adults and the relevant evidence to support these initiatives.

CLINICAL RECOMMENDATION	EVIDENCE RATING	REFERENCE
Hearing loss is common in the elderly, and good-quality evidence suggests that common screening tests can identify patients at higher risk for hearing loss.	A	Chou, Dana, Bougatsos, Fleming, & Beil (2011)
Screen for HIV in all adolescents and adults at increased risk for HIV infection.	A	Chou, Huffman, Fu, Smits, & Korthuis (2005)
Screen and offer behavioral counseling interventions to reduce alcohol misuse by adults in primary care settings.	B	Whitlock, Polen, Green, Orleans, & Klein (2004)
Screen adults for tobacco use and provide tobacco cessation intervention.	A	Agency for Healthcare Research and Quality (2005)
Screen adults for depression when staff-assisted depression care supports are in place to ensure accurate diagnosis, effective treatment, and follow-up.	B	O'Connor, Whitlock, Bell, & Gaynes (2009)

CLINICAL RECOMMENDATION	EVIDENCE RATING	REFERENCE
Screen for high blood pressure in adults ages ≥18 years every 2 years or more frequently in those with higher blood pressure.	A	Sheridan, Pignone, & Donahue (2003) Wolff & Miller (2007)
Screen for type 2 diabetes in asymptomatic adults with sustained blood pressure (either treated or untreated) >135/80 mm Hg.	B	U.S. Preventive Services Task Force (2008)
Screen men ages ≥35 years and women ages ≥45 years for lipid disorders. An age to stop screening has not been established. Screening may be appropriate in older people who have never been screened; optimal interval for rescreening has not been established; 5 years is suggested.	A	U.S. Preventive Services Task Force/Agency for Healthcare Research and Quality (2008)
The U.S. Preventive Services Task Force (USPSTF) recommends one-time screening for abdominal aortic aneurysm (AAA) by ultrasonography in men ages 65–75 who have ever smoked.	B	Fleming, Whitlock, Beil, & Lederle (2005)
The USPSTF recommends that clinicians screen all adult patients for obesity and offer intensive counseling and behavioral interventions to promote sustained weight loss for obese adults.	B	LeBlanc, O'Connor, Whitlock, Patnode, & Kapka (2011)
Although mammography screening has been a major advance and reduces breast cancer mortality in women ages 39–49, there is insufficient evidence that mammography screening reduces breast cancer mortality for women ≥70 years. No benefit has been shown for clinical breast examination or breast self-examination.	C	Nelson et al. (2009)
Though visual impairments are common and effective treatments are available, direct evidence shows that screening for vision impairment in older adults is not associated with improved visual or other clinical outcomes and may cause harm (such as falls).	C	Chou & Bougatsos (2009)
Routine screening of women ≥65 years for osteoporosis with dual-energy x-ray absorptiometry of the femoral neck is recommended.	A	Nelson et al. (2002)

Continued

CLINICAL RECOMMENDATION	EVIDENCE RATING	REFERENCE
Prostate cancer is common in older men. Prostate-specific antigen screening benefits remain uncertain and may be associated with psychological harm.	C	Lin et al. (2008)
Dementia is a common concern. Brief screening tools can detect early undiagnosed dementia; however, no randomized, controlled trials have been done.	B	Boustani et al. (2003)
Colorectal cancer is common and preventable in adults >50 years. The USPSTF recommends screening for colorectal cancer using fecal occult blood testing, sigmoidoscopy, or colonoscopy, in adults, beginning at age 50 years and continuing until age 75 years. The risks and benefits of these screening methods vary.	A	Whitlock, Lin, Liles, Beil, & Fu (2008)
Recommend the use of aspirin for men ages 45–79 years when the potential benefit of a reduction in myocardial infarctions outweighs the potential harm of an increase in gastrointestinal hemorrhage. Recommend the use of aspirin for women ages 55–79 years when the potential benefit of a reduction in ischemic strokes outweighs the potential harm of an increase in gastrointestinal hemorrhage.	A	Wolff, Miller, & Ko (2009)

A = consistent, good-quality, patient-oriented evidence; B = inconsistent or limited-quality, patient-oriented evidence; C = consensus, disease-oriented evidence, usual practice, expert opinion, or case series. For information about the SORT evidence rating system, go to www.aafp.org/afpsort.xml.

IMMUNIZATIONS

Influenza vaccine is now recommended annually for all adults over 50 years old, unless contraindicated (Table 2-1). Residents of long-term care facilities that house persons with chronic medical conditions are at especially high risk for developing the disease. Health-care workers also should receive the vaccine. Patients with a severe egg allergy or severe reaction to the influenza vaccine in the past and patients with a prior history of Guillain-Barré syndrome should talk with their health-care provider before getting the vaccine.

Tetanus-diphtheria pertussis (Td) vaccine is administered as a once-in-a-lifetime booster to every adult. Following this, a tetanus-diphtheria booster is recommended every 10 years or at least once in later adulthood. For acute, traumatic wound management, a booster may be given if more than 5 years have elapsed since the previous tetanus immunization.

Pneumococcal vaccine usually is administered once to adults 65 years of age or older. Younger persons with severe chronic health conditions, including

TABLE 2-1	2012 Adult Immunization Schedule for Older Adults	
VACCINE	**AGE GROUP**	**DOSING**
Pneumococcal polysaccharide	65	Single dose; for those with chronic health conditions may administer a dose before age 65 and boost with a second dose after age 65
Zoster	60	Single dose
	Contraindicated in HIV with CD4 <200 or other immunocompromise	
Diphtheria-tetanus-pertussis (DTaP)	Any adult—one time substitute for Td	Single dose
Tetanus diphtheria (Td)	Every 10 years after single dose of DTaP	Single dose every 10 years
Influenza; >50 give inactivated	All adults; anaphylactic reaction to eggs is a contraindication	Annual
Hepatitis B	All with risk factors due to lifestyle	Three doses

Source: Recommended adult immunization schedule—2012. Retrieved from www.cdc.gov/vaccines/recs/images/adult-schedule-chart-1.jpg

hemoglobinopathies, renal disease, diabetes, heart disease, lung disease, or immunodeficiency or immunosuppressive disorders, also should receive the vaccine. A repeat dose may be given 5 years after the initial dose for adults at highest risk or adults vaccinated before 65 years of age.

Hepatitis A vaccine is recommended for persons traveling to countries where the disease is common. It is given in two doses; the initial dose should be administered at least 4 weeks before departure. The second dose should be given 6 to 12 months later. *Hepatitis B vaccine* is recommended for high-risk persons such as IV drug users or persons who are sexually active with multiple partners. The initial dose is given, followed 1 month later by the second dose, then the third dose is given 4 to 6 months after the second dose. *Zostavax* is recommended for all persons over age 60 as a single dose. Persons who have had a prior episode of zoster can be vaccinated.

TRAVEL AND LEISURE

Travel can be one of the most enjoyable experiences one can have. People travel to see new things, to understand the world and themselves better, to visit friends and family, to return to the land of their ancestors, to volunteer, to challenge themselves, and because it is fun. They travel alone, in groups, and with their families. They go on cruises, and they go on safari. They stay in five-star resorts and in host family homes. They take planes, buses, trains, jeeps, and rickshaws. They scuba dive, hike the Himalayas, and bicycle in Tuscany. They teach and learn. They volunteer in Haiti, Ghana, and Honduras. But travel can pose some unique health risks for the older traveler. The gerontology NP in primary care can provide pretrip advice to help ensure safer travel.

Travel Health and Nursing

National and international travel is on the rise. Tourism is now the largest industry in the world. Thirty-six percent of all leisure travelers and 30% of all business travelers are people over the age of 50 (U.S. Travel Association, n.d.).

Travel health and medicine is a new interdisciplinary specialty that has grown out of the need to protect travelers from illness and injury. It developed in the 1970s as infectious disease and tropical medicine clinicians treating returned travelers recognized that many of the problems they encountered could be prevented by pretravel evaluations, immunizations, chemoprophylaxis, and counseling about safety, food and water, and insect precautions.

In 1991 the International Society of Travel Medicine (ISTM) (www.istm.org) was formed and established an international body of knowledge to define travel medicine. It is the only body offering an examination to demonstrate competences for physicians, NPs, registered nurses (RNs), physician assistants (PAs), and pharmacists. Those who pass are awarded a Certificate in Travel Health (CTH).

The American Travel Health Nurses Association (ATHNA) (www.athna.org) was formed in 2004 to promote and support travel health nursing in North America. ATHNA provides many resources, policies and procedures, standing orders, and continuing education for nurses and NPs who specialize in travel health as well as for those in primary care.

Travel health is rapidly evolving and growing as a specialty but is also growing as a part of primary care. NPs will need to know how to evaluate older travelers, develop a plan of care to keep them healthy while they travel by means of pretravel counseling, and provide interventions and self-treatment plans. They need to know how, when, and where to refer to a travel health specialist. Currently, the majority of travelers who could benefit from pretravel consultations do not receive them (Keystone, Kozarsky, & Freedman, 2008). NPs are in a unique position to educate patients and the public about the benefits of this service.

The Older Traveler

Some of the physiological and psychosocial changes that can occur with aging pose special risks during travel. How a patient functions at home may not be indicative of how well he or she will function in an unfamiliar environment.

Diminished musculoskeletal strength, agility, mobility, and endurance can affect a person's ability to navigate safely. Travel often involves more walking and standing than an elder may be accustomed to. Whereas most places in the United States are handicapped accessible, many places abroad are not. Uneven stairs and walkways, lack of handrails, and lack of elevators can be challenging.

Cardiopulmonary function can decrease with age and contribute to fatigue. Long flights in low humidity and lowered oxygen, in cramped seats, can increase risk of thromboembolic events. The elderly are at increased risk of altitude illness, which affects cardiac and cerebral functioning. Increased air pollution is a significant problem in many countries and affects pulmonary function.

The ability to tolerate temperature changes affects the older traveler. Heat and humidity can aggravate underlying conditions, and older travelers will become dehydrated more easily. They are more prone to thermal damage in colder climates.

Central nervous system changes affect the older traveler's ability to deal with the stresses of travel. It can be anxiety inducing to be in a place where everything is so different—the language, food, customs, and climate. Jet lag is harder to cope with as one ages. Any traveler can experience unexpected delays and be without food and sleep for hours. This can take an even greater toll on the older traveler.

Sensory changes may result in decreased hearing, which is especially difficult on airplanes or trains with background engine noise. Decreased vision can result in greater risk of injuries. Decreased night vision, longer reaction time, and driving on unfamiliar, poorly lit roads increase the risk of accidents.

Bathroom facilities vary around the world. Bathroom stops may be at longer intervals than needed for an older traveler with diminished bladder capacity or any degree of incontinence. Some facilities may consist only of holes in the floor that the elder may have to balance over to use.

Older travelers have less robust immune systems. Fever is not always a reliable indicator of illness in the elderly. Seroconversion rates decrease with age, rendering some vaccines less effective for older travelers. People over the age of 60 have higher rates of serious side effects from yellow fever vaccine. The rate increases even more for those over the age of 80 (Brunette, Kozarsky, Magill, Shlim, & Amanda, 2012). Although many older travelers are very healthy, many have comorbidities that contribute to the development of health problems abroad. Patients with chronic disease that is well managed at home may decompensate in foreign environments because of heat, humidity, altitude, fatigue, changes in diet, and exposure to infectious diseases. It is very important that older travelers know what to do if they become ill or injured away from home. Because this can be very expensive, advise the traveler to obtain travel health insurance that includes emergency medical evacuation. This is frequently offered by tour groups and travel agents when booking trips. Medicare does not cover the cost of health care outside the United States.

Taking a document on paper or electronically with a patient's complete medical history, medication list, allergies, and copies of pertinent imaging studies or electrocardiograms (ECGs) is prudent. There are USB devices (flash drives) designed for this purpose (Keystone et al., 2008). Patients can e-mail themselves an electronic document with these data that they can retrieve later, if needed. Internet and cell phone access exist in many underdeveloped countries.

The NP with expertise in gerontology can provide pretravel care that will not only reduce the morbidity and mortality risks associated with travel but also enhance the elder's travel experience. When destinations or itineraries are complicated or when a patient's condition poses special risks, a visit to or a consultation with a travel health specialist is warranted.

Preparing the Elder in a Primary Care Setting for Travel

To develop an individualized pretravel plan of care, the NP needs to evaluate the traveler, the destination, and the itinerary. Assessing the traveler consists of reviewing the following areas:

- Current health status—stability of preexisting conditions
- Past medical history
- Medications and allergies
- Diet
- Mental status
- Immunization status

CURRENT MEDICAL STATUS

Ideally, the traveler should be seen at least 6 to 8 weeks before the trip to allow for time to optimize preexisting chronic disease and adequate immune response to vaccine-preventable diseases. Evaluate the patient's current medications. Simplifying medication schedules enhances compliance. Are there any that do not need to be taken on this trip? Are there any factors that will affect your patient's ability to take any medications during travel? Does the patient know how to adjust medication schedules to accommodate air travel and time zone changes? All prescription medications should be brought in original bottles and not in unlabeled pill containers. If your patient gets his or her prescriptions in 90-day supplies, give the patient new prescriptions for smaller amounts for travel, including a few extra in case of delays. Does the patient need to take any medical equipment with him or her such as a wheelchair, walker, glucometer, hearing aids, or nebulizer? Remind the patient to check all batteries and bring extras. Is adequate electricity reliably available at a current that will work with the equipment? Will adapters be needed, and will they work properly?

MEDICATIONS AND ALLERGIES

- Is the patient taking any medication that could prove life threatening if lost or stolen? If so, is it accessible at the patient's destination?
- Does the patient have any life-threatening allergies?

- Does the patient take any medications that require refrigeration? Decompose from heat and humidity? Require syringes? A nebulizer?
- Is the patient on oxygen? If so, he or she must notify the airline well in advance of travel.

All medications should be packed in carry-on luggage, not in checked bags. Certain countries restrict bringing in any controlled substances and some psychotropic drugs whether legally prescribed in the United States or not.

DIET

Does the patient have any special dietary restrictions? Airlines offer diabetic and vegetarian options but may not offer gluten-free or sodium-restricted comestibles. These must be ordered in advance. Cruise ships accommodate many specialty diets but also offer many temptations. Restaurant menus in many countries do not list all the ingredients in the dishes offered.

MENTAL STATUS

Short-term memory decreases with age. Many elders cope with these changes by adhering to routines that travel may disrupt. Misplacing passports, room keys, or wallets or not remembering hotel names or addresses can be distressing. Family members or travel companions may need to offer additional assistance. Advise that elders carry a hotel's business card that includes the hotel's name, address, and phone number.

IMMUNIZATION STATUS

All *routine* immunizations should be current. This includes influenza, pneumococcal, Td/Tdap (tetanus, diphtheria, and acellular pertussis), zoster, and for some, hepatitis B vaccination (CDC, 2012). Certain vaccines may be *recommended* based on destination, and some vaccines are *required* for entry into some African and South American countries (Brunette et al., 2012) (Table 2-2).

Yellow fever vaccinations can only be given by certified yellow fever centers. If the patient is seeing a primary care provider before getting a yellow fever vaccine, be aware of the live virus vaccine rule (Brunette et al., 2012).

Yellow fever and herpes zoster vaccine are the only live virus vaccines that people over age 50 receive. Immune response can be impaired if live virus vaccines are given within a 28- to 30-day interval of each other. Yellow fever vaccine is not effective until 10 days after administration. If the NP gives a patient a herpes

TABLE 2-2 Adult Vaccinations for Travel	
RECOMMENDED ADULT VACCINATIONS FOR TRAVEL	**REQUIRED ADULT VACCINATIONS FOR TRAVEL**
Hepatitis A	Yellow fever for some African and South American countries
Hepatitis B	
Typhoid	Meningococcal for Saudi Arabia during the Hajj
Polio	
Meningococcal	
Japanese encephalitis	
Rabies	

zoster vaccine, that patient cannot receive a yellow fever vaccine for 30 days. If the patient is required to have a yellow fever vaccine for travel, he or she cannot enter a yellow fever country until 10 days after receiving the yellow fever vaccine (or 40 days after receiving a herpes zoster vaccine). If the administration of a herpes zoster vaccine precludes the administration of a time-sensitive yellow fever vaccine, travel plans could be interrupted, with serious financial consequences for the traveler. If the NP has any questions about when to vaccinate a patient whose trip is imminent, discuss this with a travel health specialist. If a patient receives a yellow fever vaccine, he or she cannot receive a herpes zoster vaccine for 28 days. The patient may receive both vaccines on the same day with no decrease in immune response (Brunette et al., 2012). Typhoid oral vaccine is a live *bacterial* vaccine and will not interfere with live viral vaccine administration.

After assessing the destination and itinerary (see the following section), decide which vaccines to recommend for this specific patient for this specific trip. The most common vaccines used for protecting travelers are hepatitis A, hepatitis B, typhoid fever, adult booster polio, Japanese encephalitis, meningococcal, and rabies. If the NP does not have access to these vaccines, referral to a travel health specialist will be needed. To help the patient make an informed decision about which recommended vaccines to receive, consider the indications, contraindications, side effects, timing of doses for immune response, and costs. Medicare will cover hepatitis B in very limited patient populations and will not cover the cost of the other recommended vaccines (Official U.S. Government Web site for Medicare, n.d.). Many third-party insurance carriers and supplemental plans do not cover vaccines

for travel. The patient should inquire about this directly with his or her insurer. Federal regulations require the NP to give patients Vaccine Information Statements (VISs), which are available in many different languages at www.cdc.gov/vaccines/pubs/vis/default.htm.

All patients should have a copy of their immunization record. If a patient has an incomplete vaccine series, continue the series but do not restart it. For example, if a patient received one dose of hepatitis A several years ago but never received the second, final injection, give the next and final dose now. If the patient received only one dose of hepatitis B years ago, give the second dose now and the third dose 5 months from now, and the series will be complete.

If a patient cannot complete a series before travel, partial immunization may confer enough protection. Some vaccines can be given on an accelerated schedule; otherwise, do not give a vaccine sooner than the recommended interval between doses. One dose of hepatitis A given just before travel will confer enough protection to make it worth giving to the last-minute traveler. For adults over age 40 leaving in less than 2 weeks to a hepatitis A-endemic area, the CDC recommends giving the hepatitis A vaccine and immune globulin (IG), 0.02 mL/kg, in a separate injection site (Brunette et al., 2012).

Hepatitis A and B vaccines are also available as a combined vaccine given at 0, 1, and 6 months. If there are at least 21 days before the patient's departure, the vaccine can be given in an accelerated schedule of 0, 7, and 21 to 30 days with a booster at 12 months (Brunette et al., 2012). Typhoid fever vaccine is available in two forms, a single-dose injectable and orally as a series of 4 capsules given every other day for 1 week. The oral vaccine then takes a week to be effective. The injectable vaccine needs to be boostered every 2 years and the oral vaccine at 5 years, if needed. Before prescribing the oral form, be sure the patient can comply with the proper administration (Brunette et al., 2012).

Because of worldwide efforts to eradicate polio, only a few countries require adults to get a polio booster for travel. Consult the CDC Web site for the most current recommendations (wwwnc.cdc.gov/travel/notices/in-the-news/polio-outbreaks.htm). If your patient has had polio in the past, he or she does not need vaccination. If your patient has been fully vaccinated for polio, a single booster dose as an adult will protect.

If your patient is unvaccinated or incompletely vaccinated or his or her vaccine status is unknown for polio, give injectable polio vaccine (IPV) at 0, 1, and 6 months. If you have 8 weeks or more before travel, give three doses at 4-week intervals. If you have between 4 and 8 weeks before travel, give two doses 4 weeks apart. If you have less than 4 weeks before travel, give one dose of IPV (Brunette et al., 2012). Japanese encephalitis, meningococcal vaccine, and rabies pre-exposure vaccine are not usually given to elders for travel in a primary care setting. Japanese encephalitis vaccine is only advised for long-term stays in high-risk areas of Southeast Asia, Australia, and Western Pacific Islands.

Meningococcal vaccine is only licensed for people ages 2 to 55. Depending on the country visited, length of stay, and potential exposure to rabid animals, decisions regarding rabies pre-exposure vaccine are usually made with a travel health specialist. Cost and vaccine availability play a role in deciding pre-exposure vaccination (Brunette et al., 2012). It is important to warn travelers of the risk of rabies and to educate them in animal bite prevention strategies, especially concerning dogs.

The CDC Yellow Book is an invaluable resource for vaccine administration and is available in paperback and online in its entirety for free. The Advisory Council on Immunization Practice (ACIP) has a section on its Web site (www.immunize.org) called Ask the Expert that can be searched for answers to immunization questions. Listings for travel health specialists and clinics can be found at the ISTM Web site (www.istm.org) and the CDC Web site (wwwnc.cdc.gov/travel/page/travel-clinics.htm).

Assessing the Destination and Itinerary

The gerontology NP needs to know where the traveler is going and what he or she will do there to provide anticipatory guidance for risk reduction. The NP may decide to refer to a travel clinic for the remainder of the pretrip evaluation. Either way, the following overview will help the NP to understand what comprises a comprehensive pretravel evaluation.

Mexico, China, India, Peru, Kenya, Australia, Europe, and the Caribbean all pose different risks for the elder traveler. The time of year, duration of the trip, type of accommodations, modes of transportation, and purpose of the trip all influence travel risk. A 70-year-old couple going to the Dominican Republic who plan to stay at an all-inclusive resort will need different advice than a 70-year-old couple traveling to build an orphanage and staying in a host family home. There are Web sites that offer current advice about destinations that the NP can use. Some are free, such as the CDC Web site and MDtravelhealth.com,

and some are subscription based, such as Shoreland (www.travax.com) and Tropimed (www.tropimed.com).

The most common risks for travel to tropical, subtropical, and underdeveloped countries are trauma and food-, water-, and insect-borne diseases. Because so much information is relayed at the pretravel visit, it is important to provide written information for review at home. Handouts for insect, food, and water precautions are found on the CDC Web site (wwwnc.cdc.gov/travel/yellowbook/2012/chapter-2-the-pre-travel-consultation/self-treatable-conditions.htmwww.cdc.gov) and the ATHNA Web site (http://www.athna.org).

SAFETY

Accidents and injuries are the most common cause of preventable death and disability for travelers. Tourists are 10 times more likely to die from trauma than infectious disease (Brunette et al., 2012). The most common risks travelers face from trauma result from motor vehicle, pedestrian, and water accidents; personal safety/crime; natural disasters and environmental hazards; and animal-related injuries.

In many parts of the world, roads and vehicles are poorly maintained. Seat belts and helmets are typically unavailable. Roads are shared by pedestrians, animals, motorbikes, bicycles, trucks, buses, and rickshaws. Traffic accidents are more common because the traveler is unfamiliar with the roads, may be driving on the opposite side of the road, and may need to drive to the left on roundabouts. Road signs and lighting are suboptimal. To help prevent accidents, always take the following precautions.

■ Wear seat belts when available.
■ Avoid driving or riding at night in underdeveloped countries.
■ Avoid motorcycles and mopeds altogether.
■ Do not drive impaired by alcohol or fatigue or drive with someone who is.
■ Do not use cell phones or text or type on GPS systems while driving.
■ Avoid overcrowded buses and vans.
■ Be alert when crossing the street.

The Association for International Road Travel (ASIRT) has a very helpful web site with patient handouts for accident prevention (www.asirt.org).

Drowning is the leading cause of accidental death for U.S. travelers visiting countries where water recreation is a major activity (Brunette et al., 2012). Warn travelers to avoid diving into shallow water or swimming or boating under the influence of alcohol, and remind them to use life vests. Boating in unfamiliar waters, and in unfamiliar boats, increases risk of accidents. Many countries do not have laws and regulations concerning public safety to the same extent as the United States. Outfitters may not be as careful about safety. Divers Alert Network (DAN) (www.DAN.org) provides education, support, and travel and health insurance worldwide for scuba divers. They staff a 24-hour hotline for divers and health-care providers for medical support at 1-919-684-9111.

Personal crime rates vary from country to country. The U.S. Department of State Web site provides current information about worldwide safety and security (http://travel.state.gov/travel/travel_1744.html). Homicide was the second leading cause of death from injuries for U.S. citizens. In Honduras, Columbia, Guatemala, and Haiti, 38% to 52% of all deaths from injuries for U.S. travelers were homicides (Brunette et al., 2012). Elderly travelers are seen as wealthy, vulnerable targets, and travel in high-poverty, high-crime areas; travel during civil unrest; or travel at night in unfamiliar places increases the risk of assault.

FOOD- AND WATER-BORNE ILLNESSES

It is not safe to drink the water in many places in the world. Food and water precautions must be carefully adhered to for preventing disease. The easiest way for travelers to remember this is to tell them to boil it, peel it, cook it, or forget it. Bottled water, carbonated beverages without ice, coffee, tea, and alcohol are safe to drink. Do not brush teeth or soak dentures in tap water. Some travelers tie a ribbon or small rope around the faucet to remind them not to drink the water. Despite best efforts, traveler's diarrhea is common, and often the health-care provider will prescribe drugs for the traveler to take with him or her in the event that this occurs. Ninety percent of the cases are bacterial and can be treated very effectively with ciprofloxacin, 500 mg twice a day for 1 day, or azithromycin, 500 mg once daily for 1 to 3 days (Brunette et al., 2012). Oral rehydration solution (ORS) packets help prevent dehydration and are more palatable flavored with sugar-free lemonade packets.

INSECT-BORNE DISEASES

When traveling to areas where insect-borne diseases are a risk, the older traveler should be advised to avoid bites day and night by using insect repellents, wearing appropriate clothing, and using bed nets when air conditioning or screens are not available. Prevention of malaria is essential for any traveler going to a malaria-endemic area regardless of age. Malaria is more severe in the elderly, and mortality risk from malaria increases with age (Keystone et al., 2008). When traveling to malaria-endemic areas, travelers should always practice bite avoidance and consider chemoprophylaxis depending on their specific itinerary and season of travel. Mosquitoes that transmit malaria bite from sunset to sunrise. If a traveler is taking a cruise and spends the day in port in a malaria-endemic area but returns to the ship before sunset, insect repellent and protective clothing may suffice.

Malaria chemoprophylaxis is generally well tolerated in the elderly. Drug choice depends on the destination, side effects, drug interactions, and cost. All medications are started before travel, taken during travel, and taken for a period of time after travel. The CDC provides maps of malaria-endemic areas and guidelines for prescribing (Brunette et al., 2012).

There is no prevention, vaccine, or treatment for dengue fever, so it is imperative to be aware of destinations at risk and avoid being bitten by mosquitoes. Maps of dengue-endemic countries are updated on the CDC Web site (Brunette et al., 2012). The National Institute of Allergy and Infectious Disease is an excellent resource for dengue fever prevention, diagnosis, and treatment (www.niaid.nih.gov/topics/denguefever/pages/default.aspx).

It is important for patients who are being evaluated for fever or flu-like symptoms, especially with myalgia, to tell their health-care providers that they have traveled to a dengue- or malaria-endemic area for up to a year after the trip.

Motion Sickness

Motion sickness can be prevented with pharmacological and nonpharmacological methods. Many large, modern cruise ships are designed to greatly reduce motion sickness. Commonly used medications for motion sickness include dimenhydrinate, diphenhydramine, and anticholinergic agents such as scopolamine. Review possible side effects and drug and alcohol interactions carefully. Methods, such as closing your eyes, focusing on the horizon line, and acupressure wrist bands, can also be helpful.

Jet Lag

Jet lag can be mitigated by getting proper rest before travel and maintaining proper hydration during flight. Zolpidem has been shown to be more effective in the treatment of jet lag than melatonin (Suhner, Schlagenhauf, & Hofer, 2001). The patient should try a dose of zolpidem at bedtime at home before travel to test tolerance. Confusion, ataxia, and falls are potential side effects of zolpidem.

Heat and Humidity

Hyperthermia occurs more frequently in the elderly. Acclimatization to heat and humidity may take several days. Many of the drugs frequently used by the elderly, such as antihistamines, anticholinergics, calcium channel blockers and beta blockers, diuretics, and anti-Parkinson's medications, impair thermoregulation. The elder traveler should use caution in hot and humid environments, drink adequate fluids, and avoid caffeine and alcohol and overexertion. Self-treatment measures may also include using ORS packets in clean bottled water.

Altitude Illness

Altitude illness can range from mild shortness of breath to life-threatening acute mountain sickness (AMS). Prior tolerance of altitude does not predict future tolerance. Those with underlying cardiopulmonary disease may experience greater hypoxia. Since the body's normal response to lowered oxygen is to increase the pulse rate, beta blockers can reduce the body's compensatory response. Acetazolamide is used to prevent AMS but needs to be started 24 to 48 hours before ascent, and side effects versus benefits need to be carefully evaluated. If symptoms of AMS develop, descent, if possible, is the best treatment. Many areas, such as Cusco, Peru, are experienced in treating AMS in tourists, because it is such a common occurrence.

Respiratory Infections

Low humidity from airline travel and exposure to crowds and air pollution will make the elderly more prone to respiratory infections during travel. If your patient has chronic pulmonary disease, consider giving him or her an antibiotic to self-treat, if infection occurs.

Sexually Transmitted Infections

Older people may be at increased danger from sexually transmitted infections (STIs) because of the decreased perception of risk by both health-care providers and patients, resulting in less screening and treatment. Older adults are less likely to practice safe sex. The rate of casual sex increases with travel (Jong & Sanford, 2008). Encounters may be with fellow travelers, locals, or commercial sex workers. Many older women are told they do not need Pap smears based on their age

alone. Current sexual history may determine the need for continued screening for human papillomavirus (HPV) and cervical cancer.

Fitness for Travel

Travel can be strenuous. Airports and cruise ships are huge. If a trip involves a higher level of activity than what travelers are accustomed to, they need to be sure they are fit for that trip. Tour operators will often give specific suggestions for fitness for walking, hiking, or bicycling trips but not for sightseeing tours. Each traveler should bring a first aid kit and an emergency dental kit and have a plan for getting health care abroad if needed.

National and international travel by the elderly will continue to increase. A knowledgeable NP, either alone or in conjunction with a travel health specialist, can prepare the older patient to safely enjoy travel to many destinations around the world (Table 2-3).

TABLE 2-3	Online Resources for Travel Health
Travel Clinic Locator and Certified Yellow Fever Centers	CDC: wwwnc.cdc.gov/travel
	ISTM: www.istm.org
Practice Protocols and Standing Orders	ATHNA: www.athna.org
	ISTM: www.istm.org
	ACIP: www.immunize.org
Immunizations	CDC: wwwnc.cdc.gov/travel
	ACIP: www.immunize.org
Safety and Accident Prevention	Association for International Road Travel: www.asirt.org
	U.S. Department of State: http://travel.state.gov/travel/travel_1744.html
Continuing Education in Travel Health	ATHNA, nursing: www.athna.org
	ISTM, general: www.istm.org
Vaccine Information Statements	CDC: www.cdc.gov/vaccines/pubs/vis
Journals	*Journal of Travel Medicine:* www.istm.org
Destination Information—subscription	Tropimed: www.tropimed.com
	Shoreland—Travax: www.shoreland.com
Destination Information—free	MD Travel Health: www.MDtravelhealth.com
	CDC: wwwnc.cdc.gov/travel/#25

SUMMARY

Evidence-based health promotion for older adults is an evolving science. As the population of older adults increases, lifestyle management for prevention of chronic illness, self-management of chronic conditions, safety, and quality-of-life issues will be more at the forefront. NPs are well positioned to advance health-promotion efforts and keep older adults healthy and functional.

CASE STUDY

J. S. is a 66-year-old African American woman who presents to your practice for a well-adult physical checkup. She is widowed and works part-time as a mental health technician to support herself. Family history includes father deceased from a stroke at age 50 years, mother living with hypertension and type 2 diabetes mellitus, a half-sister deceased with breast cancer, and a brother with pancreatic cancer and coronary artery disease and end-stage renal disease secondary to type 2 diabetes mellitus.

J. S. has not seen a health-care provider for several years, because she had no health insurance. Now she has Medicare, so she is coming in for care. She is a former smoker who quit 5 years ago after smoking 1 pack per day since age 20 years. She has four grown children, all of whom live nearby, and she has eight grandchildren. Vital signs are blood pressure (BP) 150/92, heart rate (HR) 76 (reg), respiratory rate 18 breaths per minute (afebrile), and body mass index (BMI) 32.1.

1. What additional subjective data are you seeking?

2. What additional objective data will you be assessing for?

3. What national guidelines are appropriate to consider?

4. What tests will you order?

5. Are there any screening tools that you want to use?

6. What are the priorities for primary, secondary, and tertiary prevention?

7. What is your plan of care?

8. Are there any Healthy People 2020 objectives that you should consider?

9. What additional patient teaching may be needed?

10. Will you be looking for a consultation?

REFERENCES

Blanc, E. S., O'Connor, E., Whitlock, E. P., Patnode, C. D., & Kapka, T. (2011). Effectiveness of primary care-relevant treatments for obesity in adults: a systematic evidence review for the USPSTF. *Annals of Internal Medicine, 155*(7), 434–447.

Boustani, M., Peterson, B., Hanson, L., Harris, R., Lohr, K. N., & U. S. Preventive Services Task Force. (2003) Screening for dementia in primary care: a summary of the evidence for the U. S. Preventive Services Task Force. *Annals of Internal Medicine, 138*(11), 160.

Centers for Disease Control and Prevention. (2013). HIV surveillance report, 2011, vol. 23. Retrieved from www.cdc.gov/hiv/topics/surveillance/resources/reports/

Centers for Disease Control and Prevention, Administration on Aging, Agency for Healthcare Research and Quality, and Centers for Medicare and Medicaid Services. (2011). Enhancing use of clinical preventive services among older adults. Washington, DC: AARP. Retrieved from www.cdc.gov/aging/services/index.htm

Centers for Medicare and Medicaid. (2011). Staying healthy: what Medicare pays for. Retrieved from www.medicare.gov/Publications/Pubs/pdf/11100.pdf

Chou, R., & Bougatsos, C. (2009). Screening older adults for impaired visual acuity: a review of the evidence for the U. S. Preventive Services Task Force. *Annals of Internal Medicine, 151*(1), 44–58.

Chou, R., Dana, T., Bougatsos, C. Fleming, C., Beil, T. (2011). Screening adults aged 50 or older for hearing loss: a review of the evidence for the U.S. Preventive Services Task Force. *Annals of Internal Medicine, 154*(5), 347–355.

Chou, R., Huffman, L. H., Fu, R., Smits, A. K., & Korthuis, P. T. (2005). Screening for HIV: a review of the evidence for the U.S. Preventive Services Task Force. *Annals of Internal Medicine, 143*(1), 55–73.

Etz, R. S., Cohen, D. J., Woolf, S. H., Holtrop, J. S., Donahue, K. E., Isaacson, N. F., . . . Olson, A. L. (2008). Bridging primary care practices and communities to promote healthy behaviors. *American Journal of Preventive Medicine, 35*(5, Suppl), S390–S397.

Fakhouri, T. H. I., Ogden, C. L., Carroll, M. D., Kit, B. K., & Flegal, K. M. (2012). Prevalence of obesity among older adults in the United States, 2007–2010. NCHS data brief, no 106. Hyattsville, MD: National Center for Health Statistics.

Fleming, C., Whitlock, E. P., Beil, T. L., & Lederle, F. A. (2005). Screening for abdominal aortic aneurysm: a best-evidence systematic review for the US Preventive Services Task Force. *Annals of Internal Medicine, 142*(3), 203–211.

Green, L. A., Cifuentes, M., Glasgow, R. E., & Stange, K. C. (2008). Redesigning primary care practice to incorporate health behavior change: prescription for health round-2 results. *American Journal of Preventive Medicine, 35*(5 Suppl), S347–S349.

Hall, A. K., Stellefson, M., & Bernhardt, J. M. (2012). Healthy aging 2.0: the potential of new media and technology. *Preventing Chronic Disease, 9*(E67) doi: 10.5888/pcd9.110241.

Leipzig, R. (2010). Preventive healthcare for older adults: framing the issue. USPSTF Prevention and Chronic Care Program: improving primary care improving preventive health care for older Americans. Retrieved from www.ahrq.gov/clinic/uspstfix.htm

Lin, K., Lipsitz, R., Miller, T., & Janakiraman, S. (2008). Benefits and harms of prostate-specific antigen screening for prostate cancer: an evidence update for the U. S. Preventive Services Task Force. *Annals of Internal Medicine, 149*(3), 137.

Mini Nutritional Assessment. Retrieved from http://www.mna-elderly.com/

Murphy, S. L., Xu, J. Q., & Kochanek, K. D. (2012). Deaths: preliminary data for 2010. National vital statistics reports. National Center for Health Statistics, *60*(4). http://www.cdc.gov/nchs/data/nvsr/nvsr60/nvsr60_04.pdf

Nelson, H. D., Helfand, M., Woolf, S. H., & Allan, J. D. (2002). Screening for postmenopausal osteoporosis: a review of the evidence for the U. S. Preventive Services Task Force. *Annals of Internal Medicine, 137*(6), 529–541.

Nelson, H. D., Tyne, K., Naik, A., Bougatsos, C., Chan, B. K., Humphrey, L., U.S. Preventive Services Task Force. (2009). Screening for breast cancer: an update for the U.S. Preventive Services Task Force. *Annals of Internal Medicine, 15*(10), 727–737.

Nelson, M. E., Rejeski, W. J., Blair, S. N., Duncan, P. W., Judge, J. O., King, A. C., . . . Castaneda-Sceppa, C. (2007). Physical activity and public health in older adults: recommendation from the American College of Sports Medicine and the American Heart Association. *Medicine and Science in Sports and Exercise, 39*(8), 1435–1445.

O'Connor, E. A., Whitlock, E. P., Bell, T. L., & Gaynes, B. N. (2009). Screening for depression in adult patients in primary care settings: a systematic evidence review. *Annals of Internal Medicine, 151*(11), 793–803.

Ogden, L. I., Richards, C. L., & Shenson, D. (2012). Clinical preventive services for older adults: the interface between personal health care and public health services. *American Journal of Public Health, 102*(3), 419–425.

Richardson, J. P. (2006). Considerations for health promotion and disease prevention in older adults. *Medscape.* Retrieved from www.medscape.com/viewarticle/531942

Shenson, D., Adams, M., Bolen, J., & Anderson, L. (2011). Routine checkups don't ensure that seniors get preventive services. *Journal of Family Practice, 60*(1), E1–E10.

Shenson, D., Benson, B., & Harris, A. (2008). Expanding the delivery of preventive services through community collaboration: the SPARC model. *Preventing Chronic Disease, 5*(1), A20.

Sheridan, S., Pignone, M., & Donahue, K. (2003). Screening for high blood pressure: a review of the evidence for the U.S. Preventive Services Task Force. *American Journal of Preventice Medicine, 25*(2), 151–158.

Smith, J. B., Tang, K. C., & Nutbeam, D. (2007). WHO health promotion glossary: new terms. *Health Promotion International, 21,* 340–345. doi:10.1093/heapro/dal033

U.S. Department of Health and Human Services. Healthy people 2020. Retrieved from www.healthypeople.gov/2020/topicsobjectives2020/objectiveslist.aspx?topicid=31

U.S. Preventive Services Task Force. (2008). Screening for lipid disorders in adults: U.S. Preventive Services Task Force recommendation statement. Retrieved from: www.uspreventiveservicestaskforce.org/uspstf/uspschol.htm

U.S. Preventive Services Task Force. (2008). Screening for type 2 diabetes mellitus in adults: U.S. Preventive Services Task Force recommendation statement. *Annals of Internal Medicine, 148*(11), 846–854.

U.S. Preventive Services Task Force, Prevention and Chronic Care Program. (2010). Improving primary care improving preventive health care for older Americans 2010. Retrieved from http://www.ahrq.gov/clinic/uspstfix.htm

Whitlock, E. P., Lin, J. S., Liles, E., Beil, T. L., & Fu, R. (2008). Screening for colorectal cancer: a targeted updated systematic review for the U.S. Preventive Services Task Force. *Annals of Internal Medicine, 149*(9), 638–658.

Whitlock, E. P., Polen, M. R., Green, C. A., Orleans, T., Klein, J, & U.S. Preventive Services Task Force. (2004). Behavioral counseling interventions in primary care to reduce risky/harmful alcohol use by adults: a review of the evidence for the US Preventive Services Task Force. *Annals of Internal Medicine, 140*(7), 557–568.

Wolff, T., & Miller, T. (2007). Evidence for the reaffirmation of the U.S. Preventive Services Task Force recommendation on screening for high blood pressure. *Annals of Internal Medicine, 147*(11), 787–791.

Wolff, T., Miller, T., & Ko, S. (2009). Aspirin for the primary prevention of cardiovascular events: an update of the evidence for the U.S. Preventive Services Task Force. *Annals of Internal Medicine. 150*(6), 405–410.

Travel and Leisure

Brunette, G., Kozarsky, P., Magill, A., Shlim, W., & Amanda, D. (2012). *CDC health information for the international traveler. The yellow book 2012.* Oxford: The Oxford Press. Retrieved from wwwnc.cdc.gov/travel/yellowbook/2012

Centers for Disease Control and Prevention. (2012). *MMWR weekly: immunization guide for adults, US 2012,* 61(4).

Jong, E., & Sanford, C. (2008). *The travel and tropical medicine manual* (4th ed.). Philadelphia, PA: Saunders Elsevier.

Keystone, J., Kozarsky, P., & Freedman, D. (2008). *Travel medicine* (2nd ed.). Philadelphia, PA: Mosby Elsevier.

Official U.S. Government Web site for Medicare. Retrieved from www.medicare.gov/navigation/manage-your-health/preventive-services/hepititis-b-shots.aspx

Suhner, A., Schlagenhauf, P., & Hofer, I. (2001). Effectiveness and tolerability of melatonin and zolpidem for the alleviation of jet lag. *Aviation Space Environmental Medicine, 727,* 638–646.

U.S. Travel Association. (n.d.). Travel facts and statistics. Retrieved from www.ustravel.org/news/press-kit/travel-facts-and-statistics

chapter 3

Exercise in Older Adults

Lori Martin-Plank

Current population statistics (Administration on Aging [AOA], 2010) indicate that Americans more than 65 years of age now represent the most rapidly growing segment of the U.S. population. As those born from 1946 to 1964 enter the over-65 age group, these numbers will increase exponentially (AOA, 2011), and with that growth is an anticipated skyrocketing of medical costs for chronic health conditions. Lifestyle interventions at any stage can mitigate the effects of chronic illness (King, 2001; Liu et al., 2011), but they are usually given short shrift during patient encounters (Conn, Minor, Burks, Rantz, & Pomeroy, 2003; Cyarto, Moorhead, & Brown, 2004; Forbes et al., 2008; Hamer, Ingle, Carroll, & Stamatakis, 2012; Howe, Rochester, Neil, Skelton, & Ballinger, 2011; Liu & Latham, 2009; Marcus et al., 2006; Mishra et al., 2012; Montgomery & Dennis, 2002; van der Bij, Laurant, & Wensing, 2002; White, Wójcicki, & McAuley, 2009). A recent survey showed that there is a steady decline in exercise counseling of patients aged 45 years or older by primary care providers (Centers for Disease Control and Prevention [CDC], 2007). Many providers feel inadequately prepared to initiate realistic discussions about lifestyle changes with older adult patients (Artinian et al., 2010). According to one report, less than 30% of all adults who are in a program of exercise were initially charged with increasing their physical activity by their primary care provider (Young & Dinan, 2005). Recent statistics related to exercise in older adults (Federal Interagency Forum on Aging Statistics, 2010) show that 11% of adults over age 65 had an exercise program that met federal physical activity guidelines in 2010, compared to 6% in

1998. This report (Older Americans, 2012) also reveals an increase in obesity in older adults, from 22% in 1988 to 1994 to 38% in 2009 to 2010. These facts underscore the need for a new paradigm to promote increased physical activity in older adults as part of a program of lifestyle intervention for wellness and quality of life. According to Burman et al. (2009), nurse practitioners are uniquely positioned to assume the primary role in health promotion of both healthy persons and those with chronic illness.

AVAILABLE RESOURCES

Guidelines and position statements for increasing physical activity in adults and older adults have been issued by several authorities, including the American College of Sports Medicine (ACSM) (Chodzo-Zajko et al., 2009; Nelson et al., 2007), American Heart Association (Artinian et al., 2010; Marcus et al., 2006), U.S. Preventive Services Task Force (Moyer, 2012), U.S. Department of Health and Human Services (USDHHS) (Physical Activity Guidelines Advisory Committee, 2008), and American Geriatrics Society (Christmas & Andersen, 2000). The White House Conference on Aging in 2005 focused on Screening and Physical Activity in older adults, and the Healthy People 2020 initiative has several sections dedicated to health promotion in older adults. Numerous agencies, such as the CDC, AOA, National Institute on Aging, and Centers for Medicare and Medicaid, have programs to promote wellness and quality of life in older adults, including physical activity projects. The ACSM has a

Web site, Exercise is Medicine, with extensive resources for providers and the public (http://exerciseismedicine.org), and the Preventive Cardiovascular Nurses Association has a Heart Healthy Toolbox (http://pcna.net/clinical-tools/tools-for-healthcare-providers/heart-healthytoolbox?utm_source=webinar&utm_medium=webinarresources&utm_campaign=toolbox) with a variety of free tools for use by clinicians. Despite the availability of these tools, they are largely unknown to most health-care providers, who are focused on the day-to-day activities of disease management.

BARRIERS AND FACILITATORS TO EXERCISE FOR OLDER ADULTS

In 2006, a subcommittee of the American Heart Association Council on Nutrition, Physical Activity, and Metabolism undertook a review of existing physical activity intervention studies, focusing on subpopulations and settings to gain perspective on the state of the science and to help identify future goals (Marcus et al., 2006). Studies that focused on older adults and exercise found that short-term interventions, both individual and group, face-to-face and by phone, were effective in increasing physical activity when delivered as part of a multifaceted program of educational and cognitive-behavioral participation. Health education alone was ineffective in this population. Both individual, home-based exercise programs and group programs were effective in the short term (Ashworth, Chad, Harrison, Reeder, & Marshall, 2005). Health-care personnel–recommended physical activity and an exercise prescription were effective in the short term. None of the studies reviewed had a long enough duration to measure persistence of effort (Marcus et al., 2006).

Patient Barriers

- Lack of time
- Perceived need for equipment
- Perceived barrier to beginning exercise/physical activity
- Disability or functional limitation
- Unsafe neighborhood or weather conditions
- No parks or walking trails
- Depression
- High body mass index (BMI)
- Lack of motivation
- Interpersonal loss or significant life event
- Ignorance of what to do

Patient Facilitators

- Social support
- Positive self-efficacy
- Motivation to engage in physical activity
- Good health, no functional limitations
- Frequent contact with prescriber
- Regular schedule, planned program
- Satisfaction with program
- Insurance incentive
- Improvement in mobility or health condition
- Staff (of exercise facility) support

Medical Contraindications for Exercise Therapy (Chodzko-Zajko et al., 2007)

- Unstable angina
- Uncompensated heart failure
- Severe anemia
- Uncontrolled blood glucose
- Unstable aortic aneurysm
- Uncontrolled hypertension or tachycardia
- Severe dehydration or heat stroke
- Low oxygen saturation

PLAN FOR INCORPORATING EXERCISE INTO PATIENT ENCOUNTER

The ACSM has designed a program for primary care providers called "Exercise is Medicine." The goal of this program is to counsel the patient at every visit to increase physical activity. In conjunction with the American Heart Association, the ACSM has also issued guidelines for physical activity in older adults (Nelson et al., 2007). These guidelines can be used to incorporate physical activity and exercise recommendations into patient encounters.

All authorities agree that whenever possible, older adults should engage in physical activities that strengthen muscles, maintain flexibility, promote good balance, and are aerobic in nature; further qualifications include the development of a plan incorporating both preventive and therapeutic goals and risk management and reducing sedentary lifestyle (Artinian et al., 2010; Chodzko-Zajko et al., 2009; Christmas & Andersen, 2000; Elsawy & Higgins, 2010; Garber et al., 2011; Koeneman, Verheijden, Chinapaw, & Hopman-Rock, 2011; National Institute on Aging, 2011; Nelson et al., 2007; Physical Activity Guidelines Advisory Committee, 2008). The preferred amount of exercise is 30 minutes per day for 5 days a week of moderate exercise; if weight management is part of this, 60 minutes per day is advised. This can be broken up into as little as 10-minute intervals throughout the day; any increase in physical activity is desirable and has some value over sedentary behavior (Garber et al., 2011; Nelson et al., 2007). If older adults with chronic health conditions cannot achieve the 150 minutes per week of aerobic activity recommended, they should be as physically active as possible within the constraints of their conditions and abilities (Chodzko-Zajko et al., 2009; Physical Activity Guidelines Advisory Committee, 2008).

The initial Welcome to Medicare visit can focus on healthy lifestyle counseling, including assessment of current physical activity level and specific guidance or exercise prescription for the patient. In the case of a patient with disabilities or functional limitations, referral to physical therapy or a community-based program targeting those with physical restrictions is appropriate. For those who are already very active, an exercise physiologist or ACSM-certified personal fitness trainer can help them to maximize their program benefits. Following up at each visit will emphasize the importance of ongoing exercise in maintaining or promoting healthy aging. Health coaches from the insurance carrier can also be used to keep the patient engaged. Strategies, such as using the Transtheoretical Model of Change (Prochaska & DiClemente, 1982; Prochaska, Norcross, & DiClemente, 1994) or Motivational Interviewing (Miller & Rollnick, 2002; Rollnick, Heather, & Bell, 1992), can be helpful in persuading the patient to adopt a new behavior. The annual Medicare wellness visit can also be used to reinforce or expand on the importance of lifestyle changes. Exercise prescriptions that are individualized to fit the patient's abilities and preferences are most likely to be implemented (Conn et al., 2003; Weiss, Wolfson, Yaffe, Shrier, & Puts, 2012). Actually handing the patient a program or exercise prescription is more effective than just speaking about it. Knowing resources that are available in the community for group exercise or individual walking programs is a valuable adjunct to counseling. Knowledge of Internet resources for computer-savvy patients is also helpful. Goal setting and self-monitoring by the patient are very effective. A clinician who is aware of some common excuses (e.g., lack of time, no equipment) can counter these with positive suggestions such as acknowledging the 10-minute benefit, using stairs in the home, or walking around the block (Conn, Hafdahl, & Mehr, 2011; Koeneman et al., 2011).

Clinician judgment should be exercised in assessing the patient and prescribing an exercise routine. Major authorities agree that all adults who do not have symptoms and have no diagnosed chronic health condition, such as osteoarthritis, heart disease, or diabetes mellitus, do not need to consult with a health-care professional about increasing physical activity (Office of Disease Prevention and Health Promotion, 2008). Patients with chronic conditions should consult a health-care provider for physical activity goals that are realistic and safe (Physical Activity Guidelines Advisory Committee, 2008). Healthy adult men older than 45 years and healthy women of more than 55 years who are considering a *vigorous* exercise program need health-care provider screening and routine stress testing. Sedentary older adults and all adults with cardiac disease or strong risk factors should undergo screening and stress test if they are undertaking a *vigorous* exercise program (Gibbons et al., 2002).

KEY GUIDELINES FOR SAFE PHYSICAL ACTIVITY (PHYSICAL ACTIVITY GUIDELINES ADVISORY COMMITTEE, 2008)

To perform physical activity safely and reduce risk of injuries and other adverse events, people should do the following:

- Understand the risks and yet be confident that physical activity is safe for almost everyone.
- Choose to do types of physical activities that are appropriate for their current fitness level and health goals, because some activities are safer than others.
- Increase physical activity gradually over time whenever more activity is necessary to meet guidelines or health goals. Inactive people should "start low and go slow" by gradually increasing how often and how long activities are done.
- Protect themselves by using appropriate gear and sports equipment, looking for safe environments, following rules and policies, and making sensible choices about when, where, and how to be active.
- Be under the care of a health-care provider if they have chronic conditions or symptoms. People with chronic conditions and symptoms should consult their health-care provider about the types and amounts of activity appropriate for them.

Examples of Common Health Conditions in Older Adults With Exercise Recommendations

HEALTH CONDITION: CONSIDER COMORBIDITIES FOR ALL	RECOMMENDED ACTIVITIES: START LOW INTENSITY, GO SLOW	COMMENTS: CONSIDER COMORBIDITIES FOR ALL
Osteoarthritis	Walking, aquatic activities, tai chi, resistance exercises, cycling	Vary type and intensity to avoid overstressing joints; heated pool
Coronary artery disease	Walking, treadmill walking, cycle ergometry	Supervised program with BP and heart rate monitoring
Congestive heart failure	Walking, treadmill walking, cycle ergometry	Individualize to client; supervised program
Type 2 diabetes mellitus	Resistive, aerobic, aquatic, recreational activities	Proper shoe fit; may need insulin reduction if insulin dependent
Anxiety disorders	Walking, biking, weight lifting	If able to do high-intensity exercise, this benefits anxiety
Depression	Walking, cycling, recreational activities	Group participation helpful to keep patient engaged
Fibromyalgia	Aerobic, aquatic therapy, strengthening, tai chi, Pilates	Heated pool, gentle stretches, counsel about possible increased pain initially
Chronic obstructive pulmonary disease	Cycle ergometer, treadmill walking; individualize	Supervised program—consider pulmonary rehabilitation program
Chronic venous insufficiency	Walking, standing exercises	Supervised program
Osteoporosis	Weight-bearing exercises, weight training	Assess balance and risk for falls before beginning
Parkinson's disease	Walking, treadmill walking, stationary bike, dancing, tai chi, Pilates	Assess balance and risk for falls before beginning; American Parkinson's Disease Association resources
Peripheral arterial disease	Lower extremity exercises, treadmill walking, walking	Very short intervals initially, progress as tolerated
Age-related sleep disorders	Tai chi, walking, aquatherapy, biking	Assess balance and risk for falls before beginning
Dementia	Walking, recreational activities	Provide safe environment, assess fall risk and ability to participate

Source: Adapted from Goodman, C., & Helgeson, K. (2011). *Exercise prescriptions for medical conditions.* Philadelphia: F. A. Davis.

CLINICAL RECOMMENDATION	EVIDENCE RATING	REFERENCE
To promote and maintain health, older adults need moderate-intensity aerobic activity for a minimum of 30 min on 5 days each week or vigorous-intensity aerobic activity for a minimum of 20 min on 3 days each week.	A	Nelson et al. (2007)
To promote and maintain health and physical independence, older adults will benefit from performing activities that maintain or increase muscular strength and endurance for a minimum of 2 days each week. It is recommended that 8–10 exercises be performed on 2 or more nonconsecutive days per week using the major muscle groups.	A	Nelson et al. (2007)

Continued

CLINICAL RECOMMENDATION	EVIDENCE RATING	REFERENCE
Participation in aerobic and muscle-strengthening activities above minimum recommended amounts provides additional health benefits and results in higher levels of physical fitness.	A	Nelson et al. (2007)
To maintain the flexibility necessary for regular physical activity and daily life, older adults should perform activities that maintain or increase flexibility on at least 2 days each week for at least 10 min each day.	A	Nelson et al. (2007)
To reduce risk of injury from falls, community-dwelling older adults with substantial risk of falls (e.g., with frequent falls or mobility problems) should perform exercises that maintain or improve balance.	A	Nelson et al. (2007)
Older adults with one or more medical conditions for which physical activity is therapeutic should perform physical activity in the manner that effectively and safely treats the condition(s).	A	Nelson et al. (2007)
Older adults should have a plan for obtaining sufficient physical activity that addresses each recommended type of activity. Those with chronic conditions for which activity is therapeutic should have a single plan that integrates prevention and treatment. For older adults who are not active at recommended levels, plans should include a gradual (or stepwise) approach to increase physical activity over time. Many months of activity at less than recommended levels is appropriate for some older adults (e.g., those with low fitness), because they increase activity in a stepwise manner. Older adults should also be encouraged to self-monitor their physical activity on a regular basis and to reevaluate plans as their abilities improve or as their health status changes.	C	Nelson et al. (2007)

A = consistent, good-quality, patient-oriented evidence; B = inconsistent or limited-quality, patient-oriented evidence; C = consensus, disease-oriented evidence, usual practice, expert opinion, or case series. For information about SORT evidence rating system, go to www.aafp.org/afpsort.xml.

SUMMARY

There is strong evidence from a variety of sources that increasing physical activity in older adults will improve health and quality of life in both healthy adults and those with chronic health conditions (Conn et al., 2003; Cyarto et al., 2004; Forbes et al., 2008; Hamer et al., 2012; Howe et al., 2011; Liu & Latham, 2009; Marcus et al., 2006; Mishra et al., 2012; Montgomery & Dennis, 2002; van der Bij et al., 2002; White et al., 2009). Primary care practitioners can play an important role in promoting physical activity for all older adult patients at every visit. Resources are available to assist with this effort; further research is needed regarding effective counseling methods and outcomes.

CASE STUDY

A. G., a 72-year-old man, comes in for follow-up of laboratory test results. He has coronary artery disease (CAD), hypertension (controlled), impaired fasting glucose (IFG), benign prostatic hyperplasia, and mild degenerative joint disease (DJD). Since being diagnosed with IFG he has cut back on soda consumption and is also seeing a dietitian for counseling. He is a former smoker (last use 12 years ago) and admits to being a "couch potato." Current medications: Lisinopril 20 mg orally (PO) daily, hydrochlorothiazide 12.5 mg PO daily, simvastatin 20 mg PO daily in the evening, and tamulosin 0.4 mg PO daily. He has a prescription for nitroglycerin 0.4 mg sublingually as needed for chest pain but has never needed to use it. He occasionally takes Tylenol Arthritis Pain or Aleve if DJD bothers him. Vital signs are blood pressure (BP) 134/72, heart rate (HR) 70 (reg), respiratory rate 18 breaths per minute (afebrile), and body mass index (BMI) 34.2. Laboratory test results are unremarkable except for high-density lipoprotein (HDL) 32 and fasting blood sugar (FBS) 125. Mr. G expresses frustration at the lack of change in his fasting glucose despite cutting back on soda. He asks you, "What else can I do? I don't want to get diabetes." You encourage him to increase his physical activity level gradually, beginning with walking.

1. What strategies will you use to promote increased physical activity in this patient?

2. What additional objective data will you be assessing for?

3. What national guidelines are appropriate to consider?

4. Will you need to order any tests before he begins this program? If so, what tests?

5. Are there any screening tools that you want to use?

6. What is your plan of care?

7. Are there any Healthy People 2020 objectives that you should consider?

8. What additional patient teaching may be needed?

9. How will you follow up on the planned increase in physical activity?

REFERENCES

Administration on Aging, U.S. Department of Health and Human Services. (2010). *A profile of older Americans: 2010*. Retrieved from www.aoa.gov/AoAroot/Aging_Statistics/Profile/2010/docs/2010profile.pdf

Administration on Aging, U.S. Department of Health and Human Services. (2011). *A profile of older Americans: 2011*. Retrieved from www.aoa.gov/AoAroot/Aging_Statistics/Profile/2011/docs/2011profile.pdf

Artinian, N. T., Fletcher, G. F., Mozaffarian, D., Kris-Etherton, P., Van Horn, L., Lichtenstein, A. H., . . . Burke, L. E.; on behalf of the American Heart Association Prevention Committee of the Council on Cardiovascular Nursing. (2010). Interventions to promote physical activity and dietary lifestyle changes for cardiovascular risk factor reduction in adults: a scientific statement from the American Heart Association. *Circulation, 122*(4), 406–441. doi:10.1161/CIR.0b013e3181e8edf1

Ashworth, N. L., Chad, K. E., Harrison, E. L., Reeder, B. A., & Marshall, S. C. (2005). Home versus center based physical activity programs in older adults. *Cochrane Database of Systematic Reviews*, Issue 1. Art. No.: CD004017. doi:10.1002/14651858.CD004017.pub2

Burman, M. E., Hart, A. M., Conley, V., Brown, J., Sherard, P., & Clarke, P. N. (2009). Reconceptualizing the core of nurse practitioner education and practice. *Journal of the American Association of Nurse Practitioners (JAANP), 21*(1), 11–17. doi:10.1111/j.1745-7599.2008.00365.x

Centers for Disease Control and Prevention. (2007). QuickStats: estimated percentage of patients aged >45 years who received exercise counseling from their primary-care physicians, by sex and age group—National Ambulatory Medical Care Survey and National Hospital Ambulatory Medical Care Survey, United States, 2003–2005. *Morbidity and Mortality Weekly Report (MMWR), 56*(43), 1142.

Chodzko-Zajko, W. J., Proctor, D. N., Fiatarone Singh, M. A., Minson, C. T., Nigg, C. R., Salem, G. J., & Skinner, J. S. (2009). American College of Sports Medicine position stand: exercise and physical activity for older adults. *Medicine & Science in Sports & Exercise, 41*(7), 1510–1530. doi:10.1249/MSS.0b013e3181a0c95c

Christmas, C., & Andersen, R. A. (2000). Exercise and older patients: guidelines for the clinician. *Journal of the American Geriatrics Society, 48*(3), 318–324.

Conn, V. S., Hafdahl, A. R., & Mehr, D. R. (2011). Interventions to increase physical activity among healthy adults: meta-analysis of outcomes. *American Journal of Public Health, 101*(4), 751–758. doi:10.2105/AJPH.2010.194381

Conn, V. S., Minor, M. A., Burks, K. J., Rantz, M. J., & Pomeroy, S. H. (2003). Integrative review of physical activity intervention research with aging adults. *Journal of the American Geriatrics Society, 51*(8), 1159–1168.

Cyarto, E. V., Moorhead, G. E., & Brown, W. J. (2004). Updating the evidence relating to physical activity intervention studies in older people. *Journal of Science and Medicine in Sport, 7*(Suppl), 30–38.

Elsawy, B., & Higgins, K. E. (2010). Physical activity guidelines for older adults. *American Family Physician, 81*(1), 55–59, 60–62.

Federal Interagency Forum on Aging Statistics. (2010). *Older Americans: 2010.* Retrieved from www.agingstats.gov/agingstatsdotnet/Main_Site/Data/Data_2010.aspx

Forbes, D., Forbes, S., Morgan, D. G., Markle-Reid, M., Wood, J., & Culum, I. (2008). Physical activity programs for persons with dementia. *Cochrane Database of Systematic Reviews,* Issue 3. Art. No.: CD006489. doi:10.1002/14651858.CD006489.pub2

Garber, C. E., Blissmer, B., Deschenes, M. R., Franklin, B. A., Lamonte, M. J., Lee, I. -M., . . . Swain, D. P. (2011). American College of Sports Medicine position stand. Quantity and quality of exercise for developing and maintaining cardiorespiratory, musculoskeletal, and neuromotor fitness in apparently healthy adults: guidance for prescribing exercise. *Medicine & Science in Sports & Exercise, 43*(7), 1334–1359. doi:10.1249/MSS.0b013e318213fefb

Gibbons, R. J., Balady, G. J., Bricker, J. T., Chaitman, B. R., Fletcher, G. F., Froelicher, V. F., . . . Smith, S. C., Jr. (2002). ACC/AHA 2002 guideline update for exercise testing: summary article: a report of the American College of Cardiology/American Heart Association Task Force on Practice Guidelines (Committee to Update the 1997 Exercise Testing Guidelines). *Circulation, 106*(14), 1883–1892.

Goodman, C., & Helgeson, K. (2011). *Exercise prescriptions for medical conditions.* Philadelphia, PA: F. A. Davis.

Hamer, M., Ingle, L., Carroll, S., & Stamatakis, E. (2012). Physical activity and cardiovascular mortality risk: possible protective mechanisms? *Medicine & Science in Sports & Exercise, 44*(1), 84–88. doi:10.1249/MSS.0b013e3182251077

Howe, T. E., Rochester, L., Neil, F., Skelton, D. A., & Ballinger, C. (2011). Exercise for improving balance in older people. *Cochrane Database of Systematic Reviews,* Issue 11. Art. No.: CD004963. doi:10.1002/14651858.CD004963.pub3

King, A. C. (2001). Interventions to promote physical activity by older adults. *Journals of Gerontology Series A: Biological Sciences and Medical Sciences, 56*(Spec No 2), 36–46.

Koeneman, M. A., Verheijden, M. W., Chinapaw, M. J. M., & Hopman-Rock, M. (2011). Determinants of physical activity and exercise in healthy older adults: a systematic review. *International Journal of Behavioral Nutrition and Physical Activity, 8,* 142. Retrieved from www.ijbnpa.org/content/8/1/142

Liu, C. J., & Latham, N. K. (2009). Progressive resistance strength training for improving physical function in older adults. *Cochrane Database of Systematic Reviews,* Issue 3. Art. No.: CD002759. doi:10.1002/14651858.CD002759.pub2

Liu, R., Sui, X., Laditka, J. N., Church, T. S., Colabianchi, N., Hussey, J., & Blair, S. N. (2011). Cardiorespiratory fitness as a predictor of dementia mortality in men and women. *Medicine & Science in Sports & Exercise, 44*(2), 253–259. doi:10.1249/MSS.0b013e31822cf717253

Marcus, B. H., Williams, D. M., Dubbert, P. M., Sallis, J. F., King, A. C., Yancey, A. K., & Claytor, R. P. (2006). Physical activity intervention studies: what we know and what we need to know. A scientific statement from the American Heart Association Council on Nutrition, Physical Activity, and Metabolism (Subcommittee on Physical Activity); Council on Cardiovascular Disease in the Young; and the Interdisciplinary Working Group on Quality of Care and Outcomes Research. *Circulation, 114*(24), 2739–2752.

Miller, W. D., & Rollnick, S. (2002). *Motivational interviewing: preparing people for change.* New York City, NY: Guildford Press.

Mishra, S. I., Scherer, R. W., Snyder, C., Geigle, P. M., Berlanstein, D. R., & Topaloglu, O. (2012). Exercise interventions on health-related quality of life for people with cancer during active treatment. *Cochrane Database of Systematic Reviews, 8,* CD008465. doi:10.1002/14651858.CD008465.pub2

Montgomery, P., & Dennis, J. A. (2002). Physical exercise for sleep problems in adults aged 60+. *Cochrane Database of Systematic Reviews,* Issue 4. Art. No.: CD003404. doi:10.1002/14651858.CD003404

Moyer, V. A.; on behalf of the U.S. Preventive Services Task Force. (2012). Prevention of falls in community-dwelling older adults: U.S. Preventive Services Task Force recommendation statement. *Annals of Internal Medicine, 157*(3), 197–204.

National Institute on Aging of the National Institutes of Health. (2011, December 19). *Go4Life Program.* Retrieved from http://go4life.nia.nih.gov

Nelson, M. E., Rejeski, W. J., Blair, S. N., Duncan, P. W., Judge, J. O., King, A. C., . . . Castenada-Sceppa, C. (2007). Physical activity and public health in older adults: recommendation from the American College of Sports Medicine and the American Heart Association. *Circulation, 116,* 1094–1105. doi:10.1161/CIRCULATIONAHA.107.185650

Office of Disease Prevention and Health Promotion, U.S. Department of Health and Human Services. (2008). *2008 Physical Activity Guidelines for Americans.* Retrieved from www.health.gov/paguidelines/pdf/paguide.pdf

Physical Activity Guidelines Advisory Committee. (2008). *Physical Activity Guidelines Advisory Committee Report, 2008.* Washington, DC: U.S. Department of Health and Human Services.

Prochaska, J. O., & DiClemente, C. C. (1982). Transtheoretical theory: toward a more integrative model of change. *Psychotherapy, 20,* 161–173.

Prochaska, J. O., Norcross, J. C., & DiClemente, C. C. (1994). *Changing for good: a revolutionary six-stage program for overcoming bad habits and moving your life positively forward.* New York City, NY: Quill.

Rollnick, S., Heather, N., & Bell, A. (1992). Negotiating behaviour change in medical settings. The development of brief motivational interviewing. *Journal of Mental Health, 1*(1), 25–37. doi:10.1249/MSS.0b013e3181a0c95c

van der Bij, A. K., Laurant, M. G., & Wensing, M. (2002). Effectiveness of physical activity interventions for older adults: a review. *American Journal of Preventive Medicine, 22*(2), 120–133.

Weiss, D. R., Wolfson, C., Yaffe, M. J., Shrier, I., & Puts, M. T. E. (2012). Physician counseling of older adults about physical activity: the importance of context. *American Journal of Health Promotion, 27*(2), 71–74.

White, S. W., Wójcicki, T. R., & McAuley, E. (2009, Feb 6). Physical activity and quality of life in community dwelling older adults. *Health and Quality of Life Outcomes, 7,* 10. doi:10.1186/1477-7525-7-10. Retrieved from www.hqlo.com/content/7/1/10

Young, A., & Dinan, S. (2005). Activity in later life. *British Medical Journal, 330*(7484), 189–191.

unit II

Assessment

chapter 4

Comprehensive Geriatric Assessment

Kathleen Fletcher

Because older individuals represent a richly diverse population, the components of assessment may vary from person to person. We all age at different rates, and body organ failure, psychosocial adaptations, environmental supports, and functional ability evident over time can differ dramatically among individuals of the same chronological age. Because the physical health of the older adult is inextricably related to functional ability, psychosocial health, and a safe and enabling environment, a comprehensive approach to geriatric assessment is recommended. Older individuals in most need of this approach are the vulnerable elderly (those at risk for decline) and the frail elderly (those already demonstrating decline). Comprehensive geriatric assessment (CGA) helps not only to diagnose treatable conditions and improve patient outcomes, but also helps to identify potentially preventable conditions.

CGA has been defined as a multidimensional, interdisciplinary, diagnostic process to identify care needs, plan care, and improve outcomes for older people (Rubenstein, 2004). It is important to note, however, that a screening approach to CGA may be undertaken by an individual clinician with the interdisciplinary team called in only for selected patients. Broadly, the domains of CGA might be grouped into five different categories: physical health, functional status, psychological health, socioenvironmental supports, and measure of quality of life. A number of geriatric assessment instruments are focused on these domains. Some are screening instruments (detecting conditions), some are evaluation instruments (confirming a condition), and others are measurement instruments (following a condition over time) (Arseven, Chang, Arseven, & Emanuel, 2005). These tools can facilitate the assessment, diagnosis, and evaluation processes, and those with the most clinical utility are highlighted in this chapter. Randomized, controlled trials on the value of CGA have provided inconsistent results on the influence on hospitalization and functional status; however, CGA has led to effective strategies in fall prevention, appropriate use of pharmacotherapy, and reduction of in-hospital delirium in the elderly (Scanlan, 2005). Suggested dimensions within each CGA domain are identified in Table 4-1. Each of these domains is described in greater detail below.

PHYSICAL HEALTH

The physical assessment of the older adult includes all the components of a conventional medical history (chief complaint, history of present illness, past history, family and social history, and a review of systems), the conventional physical examination (system by system and measurements), and appropriate diagnostics based on the findings. The approach to the physical assessment process, however, needs to be tailored to the older adult. Before beginning the assessment, consider the physical space and determine a suitable environment.

TABLE 4-1 Comprehensive Geriatric Assessment	
DOMAINS OF COMPREHENSIVE GERIATRIC ASSESSMENT	**DIMENSIONS OF COMPREHENSIVE GERIATRIC ASSESSMENT**
Physical health	History taking
	Physical examination
	Diagnostics
	Nutritional assessment
	Medication review
Functional health	Activities of daily living
	Instrumental activities of daily living
	Sensory assessment (hearing, vision)
	Gait and balance
Psychological health	Cognitive disorders (delirium, dementia, mild cognitive impairment)
	Affective disorders (depression)
	Spiritual well-being
Socioenvironmental supports	Social network and support
	Living situation
	Environmental safety
	Economic resources
Quality of life measures	Environmental conditions
	Social conditions
	Physical conditions
	Personal resources (mental health, life perspective)
	Preferences for care

Pay attention to privacy, comfort, and quiet, and ask permission to turn off the TV or radio, pull the curtain, and/or close the door. Allow for uninterrupted time for the examination. Turn beepers to vibration mode or hold calls; staff should be alert to the importance of minimizing disruption of the examiner and the patient. Ask the geriatric patient specifically whether he or she needs to void, so he or she may be more comfortable and undisturbed during the examination. Finally, the preparations should include a check to ensure that all the equipment is available and in working order. The methods of data collection include observation, interviewing, examination, measurements, and diagnostic testing.

Observation

Observation begins at the time the clinician first sees the patient and continues throughout the encounter. Important components of observation include the older patient's appearance, language, and behaviors. Does the individual look the stated age? Is there evidence of neglect in self-care? Is he or she dressed appropriately? What is the manner and content of his or her speech? What behaviors are observed, including facial expressions, eye contact, gestures, or abnormal movements?

Interviewing

Interviewing begins before the physical examination and typically continues throughout the examination. If this is the first encounter with a new patient, there may be less time spent on a chief complaint and history of present illness and more on assessing multiple diseases and symptoms in order to generate a comprehensive problem list and on creating a database for the future. A comprehensive health history provides the best data, but it is quite time consuming, frequently requiring several lengthy visits to complete. To save time, some professionals send a geriatric history-taking form to the able patient in advance so that the completed details may be reviewed and expanded on during the visit. For older persons, the format for history taking (with certain modifications) is similar to that for younger adults. Less emphasis may be placed on family medical history and more on family support; little time is spent on childhood illness, but greater attention is given to chronic illness and functional impairment. Too often, without a comprehensive health history, abbreviated versions of the history and sketchy details of past illnesses are all that is available to the clinician during episodic patient evaluations.

Most encounters between the geriatric patient and the practitioner are triggered by an episodic change in health status, in which the patient has experienced new or changed symptoms of illness or has developed some physical signs of disease. During the evaluation of a complaint, it helps to put the complaint into the context of the patient's previous health and illness. Older adults are likely to experience vision, hearing, speech, and cognition deficits, impairing their ability to communicate. These impairments must be recognized and measures taken to maximally correct or accommodate for them at the onset of the visit. Although the mental status examination, if performed early in the history-taking process, may reveal the unreliable historian, it may also pose a threat to the patient with early-onset dementia. When feeling threatened, the patient might be reluctant to answer further questions or might resort to cover-up strategies in attempts to hide a cognitive deficit. The clinician should not underestimate the patient's abilities to give relevant information. This low expectation of abilities can be avoided by eliciting details of the symptom from the patient first and then supplementing the information with contributions from the caregiver. The clinician should use short, one-dimensional questions and recognize nonverbal signs of discomfort so as not to provoke an anxiety response common in cognitively impaired individuals when excess demand is placed on them. The caregiver can provide valuable information about the patient's behavioral or functional changes, which may reflect a change in the patient's overall health status.

A record of the history of present illness should begin with the current experience, followed by its chronological evolution. The chief complaint is always stated in the patient's own terms and written in quotes. The history of present illness is recorded using the seven dimensions of symptomatology as a guide (location and radiation, quantity and quality, aggravating and alleviating factors, associated symptoms and signs, absence of associated symptoms and signs, evolution and course of the symptom, and effect of the symptom on normal daily activities). These parameters can be applied to any symptom, placing greater emphasis on selected components in the presentation. Relevant past medical history and family history is important to capture. The review of systems is conducted as it would be in younger individuals with a focus on eliciting some of the more common signs and symptoms of disease/illness seen in the elderly.

Taking the health history of an older adult poses some challenges because of an expectation that the significant elements of the patient's prior health status can be obtained in an unrealistically short time. This is because what the patient considers significant often differs from what the clinician considers significant. A good strategy is to begin with an open-ended question and then target the relevant data by asking the patient specific questions. The narrative should be directed without risking the therapeutic relationship by interrupting the patient's discourse.

After taking the history of an older adult, the clinician should summarize for the patient what was heard. This gives the patient the opportunity to clarify or deny any parts of the discussion. Summarization is an important step in the history-taking process, particularly when the interview has been conducted very quickly. It also helps to establish the trusting relationship that is necessary to the assessment process. This is the time when the patient may reveal any hidden agenda: the chief complaint is not always the reason the patient is seeking help. After a more trusting relationship has been established, the patient is more likely to reveal any underlying concerns.

Examination

Because of time constraints, there is a need to be both efficient and effective in the evaluation of the older adult. The examination should be conducted in an organized fashion; once a suitable sequencing has been established, the examiner is encouraged to follow this method each time. Once committed to memory, the examination sequence flows better and saves time. A new clinician often spends an hour conducting a complete examination, whereas a more experienced one can complete the same examination in approximately half the time. In the office practice, the first visit is often scheduled for 1 hour and follow-up visits are approximately 15 to 20 minutes, although the frail geriatric patient may need longer. There is no standardized way of organizing the examination. The most important considerations are patient comfort and the efficiency and effectiveness of the examination. Always consider the efficiency of motion of both yourself and the patient. When performing a physical examination on an older adult, the advanced practice nurse should be alert for some of the common signs and symptoms. The U.S. Preventive Services Task Force has evaluated the evidence on age-appropriate screening, and the following levels of evidence table identifies selected screening and the strength of some of the evidence.

CLINICAL RECOMMENDATION	EVIDENCE RATING	REFERENCE
Hearing loss is common in the elderly, and good-quality evidence suggests that common screening tests can identify patients at higher risk for hearing loss.	A	Chou, Dana, Bougatsos, Fleming, & Beil (2011)

CLINICAL RECOMMENDATION	EVIDENCE RATING	REFERENCE
Although mammography screening has been a major advance and reduces breast cancer mortality in women ages 39–49, there is insufficient evidence that mammography screening reduces breast cancer mortality for women ≥70 years. No benefit has been shown for clinical breast examination or breast self-examination.	C	Nelson et al. (2009)
Though visual impairments are common and effective treatments are available, direct evidence shows that screening for vision impairment in older adults is not associated with improved visual or other clinical outcomes and may cause harm (such as falls).	C	Chou, Dana, & Bougatsos (2009)
Routine screening of women ≥65 for osteoporosis with dual-energy x-ray absorptiometry of the femoral neck is recommended.	A	Nelson, Helfand, Woolf, & Allan (2002)
Prostate cancer is common in older men. Prostate-specific antigen screening benefits remain uncertain and may be associated with psychological harm.	C	Lin, Lipsitz, Miller, & Janakiraman (2008)
Dementia is a common concern. Brief screening tools can detect early undiagnosed dementia; however, no randomized, controlled trials have been done.	B	Boustani, Peterson, Hanson, Harris, & Lohr (2003)

A = consistent, good-quality, patient-oriented evidence; B = inconsistent or limited-quality, patient-oriented evidence; C = consensus, disease-oriented evidence, usual practice, expert opinion, or case series. For information about the SORT evidence rating system, go to www.aafp.org/afpsort.xml.

A focused comprehensive physical examination of the older adult is recommended, and a sample focused examination is identified in Table 4-2. After completing the examination, discuss the general findings with the patient. The patient might be commended for positive behaviors taken to improve or maintain health. This is also an opportune time to teach the patient self-assessment and self-care management strategies.

Measurements

Assessment of vital signs remains unchanged in the elderly. Because vital signs are taken often and routinely, we sometimes become complacent and cut corners or delegate the responsibility to others. Clinicians working with the elderly are advised to collect the vital signs attentively, accurately, carefully, and completely (Williams, 2008). Because of changes in thermoregulation, older adults may have a lower core body temperature at baseline and are less likely to have much of a febrile response during infection (even 2°F above baseline may be significant). Because of the prevalence of cardiovascular disease and arrhythmias in older adults, attention to the pulse rate and rhythm and careful measurement of the blood pressure are essential. A pulse deficit (difference between heartbeat at the apex of the heart and pulsations into the periphery) is checked by auscultating at the aorta while simultaneously checking radial pulsations. Common errors in blood pressure measurement include placing the cuff over clothing, using the wrong sized cuff, not having the cuff at heart level, not pumping the cuff up high enough, and lowering the pressure too rapidly (Williams, 2008). Because of the prevalence of orthostatic hypotension in older adults due to volume depletion and medication effects, it is

TABLE 4-2	Sample Focused Geriatric Physical Examination	
SIGNS	**PHYSICAL SIGN OR SYMPTOM**	**DIFFERENTIAL DIAGNOSES**
Vital signs — Blood pressure	Hypertension	Adverse effects from medication, autonomic dysfunction
	Orthostatic hypotension	Adverse effects from medication, atherosclerosis, coronary artery disease
Heart rate	Bradycardia	Adverse effects from medication, heart block
	Irregularly irregular heart rate	Atrial fibrillation
Respiratory rate	Increased respiratory rate >24 breaths per min	Chronic obstructive pulmonary disease, congestive heart failure, pneumonia
Temperature	Hyperthermia, hypothermia	Hyperthyroidism and hypothyroidism, infection
General	Unintentional weight loss	Cancer, depression
	Weight gain	Adverse effects from congestive heart failure, medication
Head	Asymmetrical facial or extraocular muscle weakness or paralysis	Bell's palsy, stroke, transient ischemic attack
	Frontal bossing	Paget disease
	Temporal artery tenderness	Temporal arteritis
Eyes	Eye pain	Glaucoma, temporal arteritis
	Impaired visual acuity	Presbyopia
	Loss of central vision	Age-related macular degeneration
	Loss of peripheral vision	Glaucoma, stroke
	Ocular lens opacification	Cataracts
Ears	Hearing loss	Acoustic neuroma, adverse effects from medication, cerumen impaction, faulty or ill-fitting hearing aids, Paget disease
Mouth, throat	Gum or mouth sores	Dental or periodontal disease, ill-fitting dentures
	Leukoplakia	Cancerous and precancerous lesions
	Xerostomia	Age-related, Sjögren syndrome
Neck	Carotid bruits	Aortic stenosis, cerebrovascular disease
	Thyroid enlargement and nodularity	Hyperthyroidism and hypothyroidism
Cardiac	Fourth heart sound (S4)	Left ventricular thickening
	Systolic ejection, regurgitant murmurs	Valvular arteriosclerosis
Pulmonary	Barrel chest	Emphysema
	Shortness of breath	Asthma, cardiomyopathy, chronic obstructive pulmonary disease, congestive heart failure
Breasts	Masses	Cancer, fibroadenoma
Abdomen	Pulsatile mass	Aortic aneurysm
Gastrointestinal, genital/rectal	Atrophy of the vaginal mucosa	Estrogen deficiency
	Constipation	Adverse effects from medication, colorectal cancer, dehydration, hypothyroidism, inactivity, inadequate fiber intake

TABLE 4-2	Sample Focused Geriatric Physical Examination—cont'd	
SIGNS	**PHYSICAL SIGN OR SYMPTOM**	**DIFFERENTIAL DIAGNOSES**
	Fecal incontinence	Fecal impaction, rectal cancer, rectal prolapse
	Prostate enlargement	Benign prostatic hypertrophy
	Prostate nodules	Prostate cancer
	Rectal mass, occult blood	Colorectal cancer
	Urinary incontinence	Bladder or uterine prolapse, detrusor instability, estrogen deficiency
Extremities	Abnormalities of the feet	Bunions, onychomycosis
	Diminished or absent lower extremity pulses	Peripheral vascular disease, venous insufficiency
	Heberden nodes	Osteoarthritis
	Pedal edema	Adverse effects from medication, congestive heart failure
Muscular/skeletal	Diminished range of motion, pain	Arthritis, fracture
	Dorsal kyphosis, vertebral tenderness, back pain	Cancer, compression fracture, osteoporosis
	Gait disturbances	Adverse effects from medication, arthritis, deconditioning, foot abnormalities, Parkinson's disease, stroke
	Leg pain	Intermittent claudication, neuropathy, osteoarthritis, radiculopathy, venous insufficiency
	Muscle wasting	Atrophy, malnutrition
	Proximal muscle pain and weakness	Polymyalgia rheumatica
Skin	Erythema, ulceration over pressure points, unexplained bruises	Anticoagulant use, elder abuse, idiopathic thrombocytopenic purpura
	Premalignant or malignant lesions	Actinic keratoses, basal cell carcinoma, malignant melanoma, pressure ulcer, squamous cell carcinoma
Neurologic	Tremor with rigidity	Parkinson's disease

Source: From Elsay, B., & Higgins, K. E. (2011). The geriatric assessment. *American Family Physician, 83*(1), 48–56.

recommended the blood pressure be checked positionally with each encounter.

The respiratory rate and rhythm should be measured with care. Pulse oximetry is now readily available in practice settings, and this gives a measure of oxygen saturation. Tachypnea is a sign of infection and often sepsis or may be a reflection of lung disease, heart failure, or a metabolic disorder. Weight is another measurement in which accuracy is important, because it is a good marker for both nutritional and fluid status. Some would suggest that pain is the fifth vital sign in the elderly. Quantifying pain can be accomplished in various ways, although older adults may prefer verbally descriptive scales.

Diagnostics

Chapter 1 discusses the changes associated with aging that are reflected in laboratory values. This section provides some general guidelines on when to order testing. The reader is referred to the disease sections of this text for more specific guidelines. Tests used to screen geriatric patients and tests used to aid in diagnosis have different objectives. Screening can be defined as the presumptive identification of unrecognized disease or defect by the application of tests, examinations, or other procedures. The screening parameters for those over age 65, which include laboratory and diagnostic testing, are covered in Chapter 2, Health Promotion. One of the considerations in ordering tests for diagnostic purposes is whether the test result will alter the diagnosis, prognosis, or management of a condition. Some guidelines for use of diagnostics in decision making include the following: What is the prevalence of the disease being screened for with the test? Is the test necessary to make the diagnosis? Will the test be accepted and tolerated by the patient? Does the benefit of the test outweigh the risk? Is it the least invasive test available? Can the results be interpreted? Will the results change the treatment of the patient? For example, will the positive Pap smear in the 78-year-old woman affect the plan of care? If the answer is "no," then the risk (i.e., cost and discomfort of the procedure) outweighs the benefits and testing is not indicated. What is the sensitivity and specificity of the test? To be of diagnostic value, a test for a given disease must produce patient results that differ substantially from normal results, as well as from results in patients with other diseases that may be mistaken for that disease. Even highly accurate tests produce false results when applied inappropriately and without a firm understanding of the concepts.

Another consideration is cost and risk. Are there simpler, less-expensive, less-invasive ways to make the same diagnosis? Will computed tomography (CT) give adequate information, or is magnetic resonance imaging (MRI) essential? For example, endoscopy and biopsy are not cost-effective first steps in managing a suspected peptic ulcer. Empirical antisecretory therapy, along with antibiotics for those who test serologically positive for *Helicobacter pylori,* is more cost effective than more invasive and costly procedures. Most important, consider the test's acceptability to the patient. This is perhaps most significant in the patient who cannot make a choice and give consent. In such individuals, a proxy is needed to gain permission to give the test. Although some patients may be unable to express themselves verbally, their behavior may give nonverbal expression to their feelings toward the test's acceptability.

Nutritional Assessment

Several age-associated changes influence the nutritional status of older adults. These primarily include the loss of lean body mass, a decrease in the basal metabolic rate, the loss of body matter, and an increase in body fat. Although overall caloric intake should decrease due to decreased metabolism and often decreased physical activity, certain nutrient needs may change as one ages. A nutritional assessment needs to be a part of the CGA, because inadequate intake is common in older adults. An estimated 5% to 10% of elderly people living in the community setting are malnourished; about 60% of hospitalized older adults (age 65 or older) and 35% to 85% of those in long-term care facilities experience malnutrition (Furman, 2006). There are four components of nutritional assessment: (1) nutritional history using a validated tool; (2) food intake diary of 1 to 3 days; (3) physical assessment, including anthropometric measurements and signs of nutritional deficiencies; and (4) biochemical markers, if applicable.

Obesity is the most common nutritional disorder in the elderly living in the community, and undernutrition is most common in those institutionalized (acute and long-term care facilities). There is no uniformly accepted definition of malnutrition in the elderly, although abnormal weight loss (more than 10 pounds in 6 months), body mass index (of more than 27 or less than 22), and abnormal biomarker or micronutrient levels have been suggested to be indicators of malnutrition (Arseven et al., 2005).

The nutritional history can be facilitated using a standardized tool. Several assessment instruments have clinical utility in the nutritional evaluation of older adults. The two most commonly used are the Nutrition Health Checklist, part of the Nutritional Screening Initiative project by the American Academy of Family Medicine, the American Dietetic Society, and the National Council on Aging for healthy older adults, and the Mini Nutritional Assessment Instrument, a tool that can identify older adults who have or are at risk for malnutrition, both available online. A food diary completed by the patient and reviewed by the clinician can help to identify both the quantity and the quality of food and fluid intake. MyPlate for Older Adults serves as a guide for evaluation (Fig. 4-1). The physical examination may reveal some indicators of malnutrition, including weight loss, muscle wasting, dry and dull hair, mental impairments, and poor wound healing. The body mass index (BMI) may be calculated using the following formula: BMI = weight in kilograms/height in meters, and anthropometric measurements may be taken. These are noninvasive, quantitative techniques for determining an individual's body fat composition by measuring, recording, and analyzing specific dimensions of the body (height and weight, skinfold thickness, and bodily

MyPlate for Older Adults

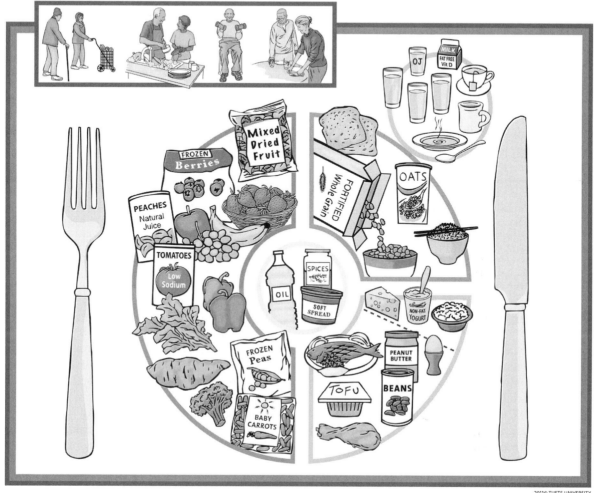

FIGURE 4-1. MyPlate for Older Adults. *(©2011 Tufts University.)*

circumference). There is no gold standard for biomarkers of nutritional deficiencies in the elderly, but some indicators include pre-albumin, transferrin, albumin, chemistries, complete blood count (CBC), vitamin B_{12}, folate, 25(OH) vitamin D, and thyroid panel.

Medication Assessment

It is imperative that each older adult is assessed at every encounter in the use of prescribed and over-the-counter medications. Polypharmacy can be the cause of many adverse effects, and suspected failure of treatment may be related to medication nonadherence. The Medication Appropriateness Index (Hanlon et al., 1997; Hanlon, Sloane, Pieper, & Schmader, 2011;

Table 4-3) is a validated tool that can be used to determine the appropriateness of prescribed medications for elderly patients (Lund, Carnahan, Egge, Chrischilles, & Kaboli, 2010).

The most frequently used criteria for inappropriate drug use in the elderly are the Beers criteria, first published in 1991 and most recently updated in 2012 (Beers, 1997; AGS, 2012). Limitations of the Beers criteria have led to the development of more explicit criteria, including the Screening Tool of Older Persons' Prescriptions (STOPP) and Screening Tool to Alert Doctors to Right Treatment (START) (Gallagher & O'Mahoney, 2008; Gallagher, Ryan, Byrne, Kennedy, & O'Mahoney, 2008).

TABLE 4-3	Medication Appropriateness Index Criteria

Is there an indication for the drug?
Is the medication effective for the condition?
Is the dosage correct?
Are the directions correct?
Are the directions practical?
Are there clinically significant drug–drug interactions?
Are there clinically significant drug–disease interactions?
Is there unnecessary duplication with other drugs?
Is the duration of therapy acceptable?
Is this drug the least expensive alternative compared with others of equal usefulness?

TABLE 4-4	Selected Elements of Functional Independence/Dependence	
ADLs	**IADLs**	
Bathing	Traveling	
Dressing	Managing finances	
Toileting	Managing medications	
Feeding	Shopping	
Mobility	Household chores	

The physical assessment is of critical significance in comprehensive geriatric assessment, though many would argue that functional assessment is of even more importance.

FUNCTIONAL HEALTH

Although functional decline is common with advanced aging, the two are not synonymous. Although functional decline occurs in every system, the distinction between functional usual aging and functional successful aging remains unclear. Older individuals aging successfully somehow seem to escape disease and truly die of "old age," maintaining an active and healthy lifestyle until the very end (Rowe & Kahn, 1998). More recently, other terms such as *healthy* or *optimal aging* are being preferred, the thinking being that successful aging implies that those in less than perfect health are not successful (Brummel-Smith, 2007). The goal in geriatric care is always to improve function if at all possible; if not, to prevent functional decline; and if that is not possible, to slow down the process of functional deterioration. The parameters of function include both activities of daily living (ADLs) and instrumental activities of daily living (IADLs). Basically, ADLs primarily involve physical function and IADLs involve both physical and cognitive function (see examples in Table 4-4).

Two well-established tools used to evaluate function in older adults are the Katz Activities of Daily Living Scale (Katz et al., 1963) and the Lawton and Brody scale for Instrumental Activities of Daily Living (Lawton & Brody, 1969). It is important to be cautious about self-report of function (rather than direct observation of function) and to ask, "Do you . . . ?" instead of "Can you . . . ?" in order to determine if patients actually perform the activity. Bathing is often the first ADL that poses problems for older adults. Mobility, toileting, dressing, transferring, and feeding, respectively, follow (Jagger, Arthur, Spiers, & Clarke, 2001). A scale combining a few of the ADL and IADL items has been shown to capture 93% variation of complete scales in a study in the Medicare population (Saliba, Orlando, Wenger, Hays, & Rubenstein, 2000).

Sensory loss often precludes the ability of the older adult to live independently, and visual and hearing acuity is part of the functional assessment. Measured visual acuity (corrected with lenses) equal to or worse than 20/40 constitutes a visual impairment. The Jaeger pocket card and the Snellen wall-mounted card are performance-based assessment instruments used in clinical practice. Hearing screening can be accomplished using a handheld audiometer, which is more accurate than the whispered voice test (Lichtenstein, Bess, & Logan, 1988).

Falls are a leading cause of death and disability in the elderly, and assessment of both intrinsic and extrinsic factors contributing to falls is important (Zecevic, Salmoni, Speechley, & Vandervoort, 2006). There are several fall risk assessment tools, and one of the most widely used clinically is the Morse scale, which is a valid and sensitive tool that identifies at-risk elderly (Morse, 2006). Patients should be screened with the Timed Get Up and Go Test. This test involves observing for unsteadiness as the patient gets up from a chair without using the arms, walks 10 feet, turns around, walks back, and resumes a seated position. Timing the process, which should take less than 16 seconds, enhances the sensitivity of this test (Rao, 2005). Patient difficulties performing this test indicate mobility issues, weakness of the extremities, and an increased risk for falling.

Tinetti's Performance Oriented Mobility Assessment is a task-oriented test that measures gait and balance abilities (Tinetti, 1986).

PSYCHOLOGICAL HEALTH

Cognitive and affective disorders, specifically dementia, delirium, and depression, are common in the elderly. There are a number of validated tools used to screen for cognitive dysfunction; however, only two have been used primarily in the clinical setting, the Mini Mental Status Examination (MMSE) and the Mini-Cog. The Mini-Cog has been demonstrated to have comparable psychometric properties to the MMSE (Borson, Scanlan, Chen, & Ganguli, 2003). The primary advantage of the Mini-Cog is that it is shorter than the MMSE and measures executive function. It is composed of a three-item recall and the Clock Drawing Test (CDT) and takes about 3 minutes to administer (Doerflinger, 2007). The Montreal Cognitive Assessment (MoCA) is another comprehensive tool that is available online; unlike the MMSE, which is copyrighted, the MoCA is free to use.

Delirium is common in acutely ill older adults and is underrecognized and underdiagnosed. There are a number of screening instruments designed to screen for delirium; however, the best evidence supports the use of the Confusion Assessment Method (CAM), which takes 5 minutes to administer (Wong, Holroyd-Leduc, Simel, & Straus, 2010). The CAM diagnostic algorithm is based on four cardinal features of delirium: (1) acute onset and fluctuating course, (2) inattention, (3) disorganized thinking, and (4) altered level of consciousness (Wei, Fearing, Sternberg, & Inouye, 2008).

Depression is also underrecognized in older adults. There are several screening tools for depression, though the most widely used in the clinical practice setting is the Geriatric Depression Scale: Short Form (GDS:SF). It consists of 15 questions requiring a "yes" or "no" response so it can be completed quickly in any setting (Greenberg, 2007). It has been suggested that a single question sensitive to depression such as "Do you ever feel sad or depressed?" be the first step in screening (Arseven et al., 2005). The PHQ-9 is a nine-item depression scale of the Patient Health Questionnaire that assesses depressive symptoms and functional impairment and screens for symptom severity (Kroenke & Spitzer, 2002).

A spiritual assessment may be done in order to determine the older patient's spiritual beliefs and the comfort associated with these beliefs. One tool that has been used in spiritual assessment is the HOPE. Additional tools that have proven useful in spiritual assessment include the FICA and SPIRIT tools. FICA is an acronym that represents components of the spiritual history (Puchalski & Romer, 2000):

- Faith or belief
- Importance or influence
- Community
- Address

SPIRIT is also an acronym (Ambuel, 2005):

- Spiritual belief system
- Personal spirituality
- Integration with a spiritual community
- Ritualized practice and restrictions
- Implications for medical care
- Terminal event planning

The four interview questions include sources of hope, participation in organized religion or spiritual activities, personal beliefs and practices, and the effects of the interviewee's personal beliefs relating to medical care up to and including end-of-life care (Anandarajah & Hight, 2001). Social factors are influential in health status, and understanding the older adult's social network and support system is also part of the CGA.

SOCIOENVIRONMENTAL SUPPORTS

Although there are a plethora of research instruments to measure social support and social interactions, there is no consensus on an appropriate clinical screening tool. To determine social isolation, a few questions might be useful (Kane, 1995):

- Is there any one special person you could call or contact if you need help? (If yes, identify.)
- In general, other than your children, how many relatives do you feel close to and have contact with at least once a month? (Number.)
- In general, how many friends do you feel close to and have contact with at least once a month? (Number.)

A brief screen for social support can be accomplished with the following questions (Arseven et al., 2005):

- In the past 2 weeks, how often would you say someone let you know they care about you?

▪ In the past 2 weeks, how often has someone provided you with help such as giving you a ride somewhere, helping around the house, or assisting with some other kind of activity?

Additional social and economic resources are assessed by exploring the following:

▪ Living situation
▪ Housing
▪ Transportation
▪ Income
▪ Assets
▪ Degree of financial burden resulting from health concerns

Although triggering questions may be helpful, the assessment of the living environment is best accomplished by an on-site visit by a clinician trained in evaluating environmental safety.

QUALITY OF LIFE MEASURES

Quality of life in aging individuals involves identifying the person's general satisfaction with life in a number of the domains identified in the CGA. The Medical Outcomes Study—Short-Form 36 (Stewart & Ware, 1992) is a tool that looks at three of these: the physical, the mental, and the social domains. Although not specifically designed for the elderly, it remains the gold standard of quality of life instruments because of its longevity, applicability, and ease of administration and analysis. A final assessment involves having a frank discussion with the older adult about preferences for care at present and at end of life and encouraging the patient to complete an advance directive so these preferences are documented.

SUMMARY

Comprehensive geriatric assessment (CGA) is a multidimensional process designed to identify care needs, plan care, and improve outcomes for older adults. The domains of CGA include, but are not limited to, physical health, functional status, psychological health, socioenvironmental supports, and measures of quality of life. This chapter covered both the tools and techniques that can be used to conduct a CGA and also highlighted the supportive research where it exists. The evidence of the value of CGA in general has been inconsistent. The evidence is clear that parts of the CGA do improve certain outcomes in older patients, but continued rigorous research is indicated.

REFERENCES

Ambuel, B. (2005). Taking a spiritual history (2nd ed.). Retrieved from http://www.eperc.mcw.edu/EPERC/FastFactsIndex/ff_019.htm

American Geriatrics Society 2012 Beers Criteria Update Expert Panel. (2012). American Geriatrics Society updated beers criteria for potentially inappropriate medication use in older adults. *Journal of the American Geriatrics Society, 60*(4), 616–631. doi: 10.1111/j.1532-5415.2012.03923.x

Anandarajah, G., & Hight, E. (2001). Spiritual and medical practice: using the HOPE questions as a practical tool for spiritual assessment. *American Family Physician, 63*(1), 81–89.

Arseven, A., Chang, C. H., Arseven, O. K., & Emanuel, L. L. (2005). Assessment instruments. *Clinics in Geriatric Medicine, 21*(1), 121–146.

Beers, M. H. (1997). Explicit criteria for determining potentially inappropriate medication use by the elderly: an update. *Archives of Internal Medicine, 157*(14), 1531–1536.

Borson, S., Scanlan, J. M., Chen, P., & Ganguli, M. (2003). The Mini-Cog as a screen for dementia: validation in a population-based sample. *Journal of the American Geriatrics Society, 51*(10), 1451–1454.

Boustani, M., Peterson, B., Hanson, L., Harris, R., & Lohr, K. N. (2003). Screening for dementia in primary care: a summary of the evidence for the U.S. Preventive Services Task Force. *Annals of Internal Medicine, 138*(11), 927–937.

Brummel-Smith, K. (2007). Optimal aging, part 1: demographics and definitions. *Annals of Long Term Care, 15*(1), 26.

Chou, R., Dana, T., & Bougatsos, C. (2009). Screening older adults for impaired visual acuity: a review of the evidence for the U.S. Preventive Services Task Force. *Annals of Internal Medicine, 151*(1), 44–58.

Chou, R., Dana, T., Bougatsos, C., Fleming, C., & Beil, T. (2011). Screening adults aged 50 or older for hearing loss: a review of the evidence for the U.S. Preventive Services Task Force. *Annals of Internal Medicine, 154*(5), 347–355.

Doerflinger, C. (2007). How to try this: the Mini-Cog. *American Journal of Nursing, 107*(12), 71–72.

Fick, D. M., Cooper, J. W., Wade, W. E., Waller, J. L., Maclean, J. R., & Beers, M. H. (2003). Updating the Beers criteria for potentially inappropriate medication use in older adults: results of a U.S. Consensus Panel of Experts. *Archives of Internal Medicine, 163*(22), 2716–2724.

Furman, E. F. (2006). Undernutrition in older adults across the continuum. *Journal of Gerontological Nursing, 32*(1), 22–27.

Gallagher, P., & O'Mahony, D. (2008). STOPP (Screening Tool of Older Persons' potentially inappropriate Prescriptions): application to acutely ill elderly patients and comparison with Beers criteria. *Age and Ageing, 37*(6), 673–679.

Gallagher, P., Ryan, C., Byrne, S., Kennedy, J., & O'Mahoney, D. (2008). STOPP (Screening Tool of Older Persons' Prescriptions) and START (Screening Tool to Alert doctors to Right Treatment): consensus validation. *International Journal of Clinical Pharmacology and Therapeutics, 46*(2), 72–83.

Greenberg, S.A. (2007). How to try this: the geriatric depression scale: short form. *American Journal of Nursing, 107*(10), 60–69.

Hanlon, J. T., Schmader, K. E., Koronkowski, M. J., Weinberger, M., Landsman, P. B., Samsa, G. P., & Lewis, I. K. (1997). Adverse drug events in high risk older outpatients. *Journal of the American Geriatrics Society, 45*(8), 945–948.

Hanlon, J. T., Sloane, R. J., Pieper, C. F., & Schmader, K. E. (2011). Association of adverse drug reactions with drug–drug and drug–disease interactions in frail older outpatients. *Age and Ageing, 40*(2), 274–277.

Jagger, C., Arthur, A. J., Spiers, N. A., & Clarke, M. (2001). Patterns of onset of disability in activities of daily living with age. *Journal of the American Geriatrics Society, 49*(40), 404–409.

Kane, R. A. (1995). Assessment of social functioning: recommendation for comprehensive geriatric assessment. In L. Z. Rubenstein, D. Wieland, & R. Bernabei (Eds.), *Geriatric assessment technology: the state of the art* (pp. 91–110). New York City, NY: Springer.

Katz, S., Ford, A. B., Moskowitz, R. W., Jackson, B. A., Jaffe, M. W., & Cleveland, M. A. (1963). Studies of illness in the aged. *Journal of the American Medical Association, 185*(12), 914–919.

Kroenke, K., & Spitzer, R. L. (2002). The PHQ-9: a new depression and diagnostic severity measure. *Psychiatric Annals, 32*(9), 509–521.

Lawton, M. P., & Brody, E. M. (1969). Assessment of older people: self-maintaining and instrumental activities of daily living. *Gerontologist, 9*(3), 179–186.

Lichtenstein, M. J., Bess, F. H., & Logan, S. A. (1988). Validation of screening tools for identifying hearing-impaired elderly in primary care. *Journal of the American Medical Association, 259*(19), 2875–2878.

Lin, K., Lipsitz, R., Miller, T., & Janakiraman, S. (2008). Benefits and harms of prostate-specific antigen screening for prostate cancer: an evidence update for the U.S. Preventive Services Task Force. *Annals of Internal Medicine, 149*(3), 192–199.

Lund, B. C., Carnahan, R. M., Egge, J. A., Chrischilles, E. A., & Kaboli, P. J. (2010). Inappropriate prescribing predicts adverse drug events in older adults. *Annals of Pharmacotherapy, 44*(6), 957–963.

Morse, J. (2006). The safety of safety research: the case of patient fall research. *Canadian Journal of Nursing Research, 38*(2), 73–88.

Nelson, H. D., Helfand, M., Woolf, S. H., & Allan, J. D. (2002). Screening for postmenopausal osteoporosis: a review of the evidence for the U.S. Preventive Services Task Force. *Annals of Internal Medicine, 137*(6), 529–541.

Nelson, H. D., Tyne, K., Naik, A., Bougatsos, C., Chan, B. K., & Humphrey, H. (2009). Screening for breast cancer: an update for the U.S. Preventive Services Task Force. *Annals of Internal Medicine, 15*(10), 727–737.

Puchalski, C., & Romer, A. L. (2000). Taking a spiritual history allows clinicians to understand patients more fully. *Journal of Palliative Care, 3*(1), 129–137.

Rao, S. S. (2005). Prevention of falls in older patients. *American Family Physician, 72*(1), 81–88.

Rowe, J. W., & Kahn, R. L. (1998). Successful aging. *Aging: Clinical and Experimental Research, 10*(2), 142–144.

Rubenstein, L. Z. (2004). Comprehensive geriatric assessment: from miracle to reality. *Journal of Gerontology: Medical Sciences, 59A*(5), 473–477.

Saliba, D., Orlando, M., Wenger, N. S., Hays, R. D., & Rubenstein, L. Z. (2000). Identifying a short functional disability screen for older persons. *Journal of Gerontology: Medical Sciences, 55A*(12), M750–M756.

Scanlan, B. C. (2005). The value of comprehensive geriatric assessment. *Care Management Journals, 6*(1), 2–8.

Stewart, A., & Ware, J. E. (1992). The SF-36 Health Survey. Retrieved from www.sf-36.org/

Tinetti, M. E. (1986). Performance oriented assessment of mobility problems in elderly patients. *Journal of the American Geriatrics Society, 34*(2), 119–126.

Wei, L. A., Fearing, M. A., Sternberg, E. J., & Inouye, S. K. (2008). The Confusion Assessment Method: a systematic review of current usage. *Journal of the American Geriatrics Society, 56*(5), 823–830.

Williams, M. E. (2008). *Geriatric physical diagnosis: a guide to observation and assessment.* Jefferson, NC: McFarland & Company.

Wong, C. L., Holroyd-Leduc, J., Simel, D. L., & Straus, S. E. (2010). Does this patient have delirium? *Journal of the American Medical Association, 304*(7), 779–786.

Zecevic, A. A., Salmoni, A. W., Speechley, M., & Vandervoort, A. A. (2006). Defining a fall and reasons for falling: comparisons among the views of seniors, health care providers, and the research literature. *The Gerontologist, 46*(3), 367–376.

chapter 5

Symptoms and Syndromes

Kathleen Fletcher

ASSESSMENT

Assessment of a symptom-based problem or a geriatric syndrome in the older adult poses challenges to the health-care provider. Heterogeneity increases with age, so there are a greater number of possibilities to consider in formulating a diagnosis and the differential diagnosis can be quite broad. Working up a geriatric patient with a single symptom or cluster of symptoms using typical symptom analysis and clinical decision-making tools can be done, but it is often complicated by the fact that patients may ignore symptoms initially because they do not interfere with functional activities or because they attribute the symptoms to the aging process. Conversely, patients may fear loss of independence related to a subtle decline in functional abilities and deliberately choose to conceal this until it becomes apparent to others. Acuity of symptoms may be blunted because of changes in the efficiency of certain physiological mechanisms. New symptoms often appear in one organ system as an offshoot of preexisting disease in another organ system. Multiple symptoms may be present because of comorbidities. These factors can result in a delayed or atypical presentation. In many cases, the first hint of illness may be a change in cognitive function or mental status. In the case of the patient with an underlying dementia, the refusal to eat or drink or a change in the patient's behavior may signal an acute illness. The term *geriatric syndrome* refers to conditions that often have multiple underlying factors that may involve multiple organ systems; some of the most common are delirium, falls, dizziness, and incontinence. The literature reflects that shared risk factors across geriatric syndromes include older age, cognitive impairment, functional impairment, and impaired mobility. For each presenting symptom, the following descriptors should be used to guide the diagnosis:

- Mode of onset of the symptom (events coinciding with onset, similar past episodes, gradual or sudden, total duration)
- Location of the symptom
- Character of the symptom
- Radiation of the symptom
- Precipitating or aggravating factors
- Relieving or ameliorating factors
- Past treatment or evaluation (when, where, who; studies done and results)
- Course of the symptom
- Effect of the symptom on normal daily activities

If the symptom or the patient's demeanor indicates a problem in function or cognition, assess these areas. Perform a thorough medication history, including the use of over-the-counter (OTC) preparations, vitamins, herbal and homeopathic remedies, and any other dietary supplements, and consider their use in formulating diagnostic possibilities. Pharmacotherapeutic or other treatment modalities can complicate or even cause illness in older patients.

BOWEL INCONTINENCE

Description: Fecal or bowel incontinence (FI), involuntary loss of liquid or solid stool that is a social or hygienic problem, can be episodic and self-limiting or a chronic problem in the older adult. This socially and emotionally devastating situation interferes with quality of life and self-esteem.

Etiology: Overflow incontinence resulting from fecal impaction is a common cause of FI. Gastrointestinal (GI) dysfunction/disease with excessive stool volume and rapid gut transit, as well as loose stools from laxative abuse and dietary factors, can contribute. Rectal sphincter dysfunction related to sphincter damage and/or pudendal neuropathy affecting sphincters, puborectalis muscle, and rectal sensation may be seen with traumatic childbirth, anal surgery, rectal prolapse, and prolonged straining. Neuropathies associated with diabetes, vitamin B_{12} deficiency, and hypothyroidism can also result in pudendal nerve dysfunction and impaired sphincter contraction, thus leading to FI. Reservoir incontinence due to diminished colonic/rectal capacity is a less common type of FI. Reservoir incontinence involves a loss of compliance of the rectal wall leading to urgency, frequency, and leakage of stool. It is associated with colectomy, inflammatory bowel disease, chronic rectal ischemia, and prostate/cervical radiation. Central nervous system diseases that disturb neural pathways for continence include stroke, dementia, multiple sclerosis, and spinal cord trauma. Functional FI occurs when the physiological mechanisms to control evacuation are intact in a dependent elder but there are environmental barriers to bathroom facilities and/or inadequate assistance to help with toileting.

Occurrence: Prevalence in community-dwelling elders is 10% to 15% and more than 40% of nursing home residents. A substantial number of elders experience urinary incontinence along with FI.

Age: FI is found more frequently in older adults than in the general population.

Gender: FI occurs equally in men and women.

Ethnicity: Not significant.

Contributing factors: Diarrhea from GI disease (colitis, irritable bowel syndrome [IBS]), infectious causes such as *Clostridium difficile*, or medication side effects can contribute to acute, short-term bowel incontinence. Constipation from inadequate dietary fiber, insufficient fluid intake, or the effects of certain medications increases the risk for fecal impaction. Altered cognition related to delirium, dementia, or depression contributes to the inability to respond appropriately to the urge to defecate. Impaired mobility from acute musculoskeletal conditions, obesity, chronic degenerative changes, or neurological deficits affects toileting ability.

Signs and symptoms: Patients may not readily volunteer information about incontinence; asking directly about bowel habits and continence may elicit the problem. Determine the duration, frequency, severity, and character of the incontinence (gas, liquid, solid). Inquire if there is sensation of rectal fullness, awareness of passing stool or gas, and warning symptoms of cramping or urgency. Associated symptoms of abdominal pain and bloating, anorexia, diarrhea or constipation, nausea and/or vomiting, rectal bleeding, and urinary incontinence should be ascertained. Review prescription and OTC medications carefully; drugs increasing the risk of constipation and fecal impaction include narcotics, calcium channel blockers, antipsychotics, some antidepressants, diuretics, and iron. Magnesium-containing antacids, sorbitol sweeteners, proton pump inhibitors, selective serotonin reuptake inhibitors (SSRIs), cholinesterase inhibitors, stool softeners, and laxative overuse can contribute to loose stool and FI. Past medical history may be positive for diabetes, neurological and psychiatric diseases, GI disorders, cancers with radiation, and any condition limiting mobility. Surgical history may include hemorrhoidectomy, anal fissure repair, fistulectomy, anal dilation, or colon resection. Diet review may reveal low fiber and fluid intake and foods that may worsen FI such as caffeine, alcohol, chocolate, greasy or spicy foods, dairy products, and various raw fruits and vegetables. Physical examination includes checking weight for significant loss. The abdomen is examined for distention, hyperactive or absent bowel sounds, pain, masses, and bladder distention. The perineum is inspected for gaping of anus, an indication of severe sphincteric dysfunction, hemorrhoids, dermatitis, surgical scars, fissures, and fistulas. The clinician should check the "anal wink" (the reflex contraction of the anal sphincter when the skin around the anus is stroked bilaterally) to test sensation and pudendal nerve function. Asking the patient to bear down will reveal rectal prolapse. The digital rectal examination is performed to detect hemorrhoids or masses and evaluate baseline and squeeze sphincter tone, as well as the amount and character of stool. Neurological examination includes assessment of gait, general mobility, motor strength, and sensory testing.

Diagnostic tests: Tests are determined by the history and physical examination findings. With diarrhea, when an infectious or food-borne cause is suspected, stool tests guided by the clinical presentation are indicated. Exclusion of fecal impaction, particularly in nursing home patients, is essential. Plain abdominal radiograph may show a high impaction when no hardened stool is felt in the rectal vault. If organic bowel disease is suspected (inflammatory disease, ischemic colitis, neoplasm), stools for occult blood, flexible sigmoidoscopy, or colonoscopy is indicated. Anorectal manometry tests rectal sensation and compliance through the use of an intrarectal balloon and measures pressure, tone, and reflex contraction of the internal sphincter. It provides comprehensive information about anorectal function and is reasonable in the ambulatory and/or healthy elder who has failed conservative interventions. Other tests that may be considered include electromyography, anal ultrasound, and magnetic resonance imaging (MRI).

Differential diagnosis: Includes fecal impaction, gastroenteritis, food-borne illness, ruptured diverticulum, inflammatory bowel disease, ischemic colitis, IBS, anal fistula, diabetic neuropathy, rectal prolapse, upper motor neuron lesions secondary to cerebrovascular accident, multiple sclerosis, spinal cord compression, degenerative processes, dementia, depression with self-care deficits, and functional impairment.

Treatment: Fecal impaction requires disimpaction (manually, with enemas, and/or osmotic/stimulant laxatives) and establishment of a preventive bowel regimen (see section on constipation). With loose or liquid stools, a supplement of soluble dietary fiber may be beneficial; the ideal amount and type have yet to be determined, and response varies greatly. Increasing fiber gradually over a period of several days can help reduce symptoms of abdominal bloating and discomfort that may be associated with increased fiber intake. In the setting of fecal reservoir incontinence, avoidance of dietary fiber may be indicated. Habit training may be effective for elders with dementia and involves frequent and regular toileting, usually after a meal to take advantage of the gastrocolic reflex. Once infection is ruled out, fecal impaction is excluded, and no clear cause is determined for FI with diarrhea, antidiarrheal medications such as loperamide (drug of choice) and diphenoxylate may be considered (use caution in the setting of inflammatory bowel disease). For rectosphincter dysfunction, biofeedback with sphincter-strengthening exercises is an option for motivated, cognitively intact elders who have some degree of rectal sensation. Sacral nerve stimulation is also a promising, safe, minimally invasive treatment of FI related to rectosphincter dysfunction. Surgical sphincter repair may be considered when incontinence is severe, unresponsive to conservative interventions, and clearly related to anatomical defects, with best outcomes seen with repair of defined defects in the external sphincter.

Follow-up: Follow-up is indicated by cause. Ongoing monitoring is needed in all cases.

Sequelae: Complications of FI include perineal dermatitis, nonhealing wounds, recurrent urinary tract infections, anxiety, social isolation, and depression. FI, along with urinary incontinence, is a leading cause of institutionalization of elders.

Prevention/prophylaxis: Manage constipation. Optimize treatment of underlying medical conditions, such as diabetes and GI disturbances. Adjust diet and laxative use to address loose stools. Consider physical therapy/occupational therapy (PT/OT) intervention to address mobility and toileting ability. Reinforce a regular toileting program for the cognitively impaired and physically frail.

Referral: Urgent spinal imaging/neurosurgical consultation for new-onset fecal/urinary incontinence with lower extremity weakness and paresthesia to rule out spinal cord compression. Additional evaluation with "alarm" symptoms: change in bowel habits, rectal bleeding, weight loss to rule out GI malignancy.

Education: Provide clear information on normal bowel function, FI cause, and rationale for any diagnostic tests, preventive strategies, and treatments. Instruct in appropriate dilution and need for adequate fluid with fiber supplements. Direct to appropriate resources for incontinence pads and briefs as needed.

CLINICAL RECOMMENDATION	EVIDENCE RATING	REFERENCE
With loose or liquid stools, a supplement of soluble dietary fiber may be beneficial.	A	Bliss et al. (2001) Bliss & Norton (2010) Croswell, Bliss, & Savic (2010) Tjandra et al. (2007)
Habit training may be effective for elders with dementia and involves frequent and regular toileting.	C	Hagglund (2010)
Antidiarrheal medications, such as loperamide (drug of choice) and diphenoxylate, may be considered.	B	Cheetham, Brazzelli, Norton, & Glazener (2003) Scarlett (2004) Tjandra et al. (2007)
Provide biofeedback with sphincter-strengthening exercises.	B	Bartlett, Sloots, Nowack, & Ho (2011) Norton, Cody, & Hosker (2006) Tjandra et al. (2007)
Stimulate the sacral nerve.	A	Michelson et al. (2010) Ratto et al. (2010) Tjandra et al. (2007)

A = consistent, good-quality, patient-oriented evidence; B = inconsistent or limited-quality, patient-oriented evidence; C = consensus, disease-oriented evidence, usual practice, expert opinion, or case series. For information about the SORT evidence rating system, go to www.aafp.org/afpsort.xml.

CHEST PAIN

Description: Acute, nontraumatic chest discomfort, perceived as pain or as a sensation of tightness, pressure, or squeezing in the chest, is associated with actual or potential tissue damage.

Etiology: The many different pathophysiologies of chest pain (CP) may be attributed to segmental overlap of neurons of cardiopulmonary and noncardiopulmonary origin. CP may originate from organs within or outside of the thorax; cardiac, pulmonary, esophageal, large vessel, gastric, pancreas, biliary, and musculoskeletal pathology may be implicated. Life-threatening causes include acute coronary syndrome (ACS; includes acute myocardial infarction [MI] and unstable angina), thoracic aortic dissection, spontaneous pneumothorax, and pulmonary embolism.

Occurrence: CP is one of the most common causes of emergency department visits, with more than 5 million people evaluated yearly.

Age: The probability for serious conditions increases with age due to increasing prevalence of coronary artery disease (CAD), hypertension, lung cancer, cardiac arrhythmias, diabetes, and conditions associated with recent immobilization.

Gender: Atypical presentation of ACS is more common in females.

Ethnicity: African Americans report less typical anginal features than Caucasians. Hispanic women with MI report more prodromal chest pain/discomfort than African Americans and Caucasians.

Contributing factors: Esophageal disease not only can mimic but also coexists with MI in 50% of elders with CAD. A recent heavy, fatty meal can exacerbate reflux esophagitis. Panic disorder with a prevalence of 0.1% to 1.0% may manifest with hyperventilation, which has been linked to coronary artery and esophageal spasm. Medications, illicit drugs (cocaine), and prescriptions such as sildenafil (Viagra), which may cause hypotension, and sumatriptan (Imitrex) through coronary vasoconstriction, can trigger CP. Cancer, recent orthopedic surgery, and immobility may result in deep vein thrombosis, a risk factor for pulmonary emboli.

Signs and symptoms: Pain of ACS may be retrosternal or poorly localized; may radiate to arms, back, neck, or jaw; may occur at rest; may last longer than 20 minutes; and is unrelieved with nitroglycerin. It may occur with nausea, vomiting, diaphoresis, dyspnea, weakness, fatigue, lightheadedness, and/or anxiety. It may be precipitated by stress, exercise, or illness. Stable angina is substernal or precordial pressing, constricting, or heaviness precipitated by exertion and relieved with nitroglycerin. Elderly or diabetic patients with altered pain perception or altered ability to localize the discomfort commonly have atypical presentations. An absence of chest pain with ACS in elderly persons is common. Dyspnea, not chest pain, is the most common presenting symptom of acute myocardial infarction in patients over 85 years old.

Thoracic aortic dissection has abrupt onset and severe, retrosternal tearing pain that usually radiates to the back and both arms. Pulmonary embolism may present with acute dyspnea, cough, deep pleuritic chest pain that may not be severe, and hemoptysis. Tension pneumothorax is associated with acute unilateral pleuritic chest pain and dyspnea. Esophageal spasm/gastroesophageal reflux disease (GERD) may mimic myocardial ischemia, may be associated with eating, improves with upright position or antacids, and is accompanied by cough, hoarseness, and dysphagia. Acute pancreatitis may present with knifelike epigastric or lower chest pain radiating to the left shoulder associated with vomiting and relieved by leaning forward. Musculoskeletal pain is usually persistent and is aggravated by movement, cough, or deep respirations. Herpes zoster is described as sharp pain or paresthesia in the midthorax unilaterally. Pain may precede rash by several days. History may be positive for CAD with or without angina or risk factors thereof, including hypertension, diabetes, and hypercholesterolemia. Anemia may predispose to ischemia. Atrial fibrillation is associated with pulmonary emboli, as is recent orthopedic surgery, recent immobilization, deep vein thrombosis, and cancers. GI disorders, degenerative joint disease, and anxiety disorders, as well as smoking and alcohol abuse, can be clues to diagnosis. Signs of serious conditions include acute confusion or anxiousness, pallor/cyanosis, diaphoresis, tachycardia, bradycardia, tachypnea, and hypotension. A new S4 murmur or signs of heart failure (jugular venous distention, wet crackles, S3 murmur, extremity edema) suggest myocardial ischemia. Asymmetrical blood pressures, absent or asymmetrical extremity pulses, and aortic bruit may be present with aortic dissection. Tracheal deviation, unilateral diminished or absent breath sounds, and palpable subcutaneous crepitus may reveal pneumothorax. Rapid, irregularly irregular apical pulse suggests atrial fibrillation whereas unilateral lower extremity swelling and tenderness suggests DVT. Fever suggests an infectious cause. Localized abdominal tenderness with guarding and rebound points to GI origins. Costochondritis pain is worse with chest movement, sneezing, or cough and is not associated with fever, shortness of breath, tachycardia, or other cardiopulmonary symptoms. Diffuse tenderness is usually seen over one or more costochondral joints. Vesicular rash in a unilateral thoracic dermatome suggests zoster.

Diagnostic tests: If myocardial ischemia is suspected, immediate 12-lead electrocardiogram (ECG) is essential and may show ST-segment depression or elevation, T-wave inversion, new left bundle branch block (LBBB), or new Q waves. However, ECG may not change for hours or sometimes not at all. Elevations in cardiac markers (serum creatine kinase MB (CK-MB) and troponins I and T) 4 to 24 hours after the onset of pain indicate myocardial cell damage.

Additional tests include chest x-ray, which may reveal pulmonary edema, pneumothorax, pleural effusion, pneumonia, or lung mass. D-dimer and spiral computed tomography (CT) or ventilation/perfusion (V/Q) scan may confirm pulmonary emboli. Lower extremity Doppler ultrasound diagnoses DVT. Additional testing is guided by the clinical situation, history, and physical findings. Elderly patients with ACS are less likely to have typical ECG findings (i.e., ST-segment elevation). Unstable angina/non-ST elevation MI shows T-wave inversion, absent Q waves, and evolving ST-segment changes.

Differential diagnosis: Includes previously discussed emergent conditions, stable angina, pericarditis, pneumonia, pleurisy, lung/chest malignancy, esophageal spasm, esophagitis, GERD, cholecystitis, pancreatitis, peptic ulcer disease, costochondritis, herpes zoster infection, and psychogenic causes.

Treatment: If there is high suspicion of emergent conditions, such as ACS or aortic dissection, immediate transport to the emergency department by emergency medical services (EMS) is recommended. For institutionalized elders, conservative management of ACS in the facility may be reasonable. Immediate intervention for suspected ACS is supplemental oxygen, 160 to 325 mg chewed aspirin (if no allergy), and sublingual nitroglycerin when blood pressure is greater than 90 mm Hg systolic and heart rate is greater than 50 beats per minute. Supplemental oxygen to maintain oxygen saturation above 90% is indicated with other suspected emergent conditions. Treatment of stable angina includes aspirin, beta blockers, angiotensin-converting enzyme (ACE) inhibitors, nitrates, and statins. Long-acting calcium channel blockers may be used for symptom reduction if beta blockers are ineffective or contraindicated. Although only moderately successful, treatment options for esophageal spasm include calcium channel blockers, tricyclic antidepressants (exercise caution with use in the elderly), nitrates, botulinum toxin, and dilation. Proton pump inhibitors, H_2 blockers, and/or antacids are the mainstay for GERD. Weight loss is advised for the overweight patient. Costochondritis may respond to local cool or warm packs, rest, or topical or oral analgesics. Zoster requires oral antiviral medications and appropriate pain management. Reassurance, cognitive-behavioral therapy, and/or antidepressants may be indicated for psychogenic causes.

Follow-up: Guided by diagnosis and response to treatment.

Sequelae: A 20% to 60% rate of unrecognized MI in the elderly with inappropriate hospital discharge and delayed treatment results in poor outcomes and increased mortality.

Prevention/prophylaxis: Optimize treatment of diabetes, hypertension, CAD, and atrial fibrillation. Encourage daily exercise and smoking cessation. For reflux symptoms, recommend controlling weight, elevating head of bed on blocks, staying upright after meals, and avoiding caffeine, chocolate, spicy foods, peppermint, cigarettes, and alcohol. Encourage the patient to get the Pneumovax and Zostavax vaccinations.

Referral: Suspected life-threatening conditions or unstable status may be referred to the emergency department depending on the patient's and family's wishes. Physician consultation is indicated with uncontrolled pain, uncertain diagnosis, and poor response to treatment.

Education: Teach patients and families to immediately seek medical care with acute new-onset CP or when a change in chronic CP is experienced. Carefully explain causes of pain, appropriate testing and treatment, prevention strategies, and indications for follow-up.

CLINICAL RECOMMENDATION	EVIDENCE RATING	REFERENCE
If there is a high suspicion of an emergent condition, immediate transport to emergency department.	B	American College of Cardiology and American Heart Association (2007) van Schagen & Dibble (2011)
Immediate interventions for suspected ACS: supplemental oxygen, 160–325 mg aspirin, sublingual nitroglycerin.	B	American College of Cardiology and American Heart Association (2007) van Schagen & Dibble (2011)
All patients with coronary artery disease (CAD) should be taking the following medications unless contraindicated:		Rodney (2013)
• aspirin	A	
• lipid lowering agent if low-density lipoprotein (LDL) is above target	A	
• beta blocker for patients with a history of myocardial infarction (MI)	A	
• beta blocker for patients without a history of MI	B	

Continued

CLINICAL RECOMMENDATION	EVIDENCE RATING	REFERENCE
For patients with CAD and diabetes mellitus (DM)/left ventricular systolic dysfunction, add: Angiotensin-converting enzyme (ACE) inhibitor unless contraindicated.	A	
Immediate-acting nitroglycerine (sublingual/spray) provides relief of anginal symptoms.	B	Rodney (2013)
Treatment of esophageal spasm: long-acting calcium channel blockers.	B	Thompson (2009)
Treatment of esophageal spasm: calcium channel blockers, tricyclic antidepressants, nitrates, botulinum toxin, dilation.	C	Thompson (2009)
Treatment of GERD: proton pump inhibitors, H2-blocker, antacids.	A	American American Gastroenterological Association Institute (2009) Heidelbaugh (2009)
Treatment for GERD: controlling weight, elevating the head of the bed on blocks, staying upright after meals, avoiding specific foods and alcohol, smoking cessation.	C	American Gastroenterological Association Institute (2009) Heidelbaugh (2009)
Treatment for costochondritis: NSAIDs for pain.	C	Tudiviver (2011)
Treatment for herpes zoster: antivirals.	A	Hutchinson & Miller (2010)
Treatment of psychogenic causes: cognitive-behavioral therapy.	A	Huttunen & Pirkola (2010)

A = consistent, good-quality, patient-oriented evidence; B = inconsistent or limited-quality, patient-oriented evidence; C = consensus, disease-oriented evidence, usual practice, expert opinion, or case series. For information about the SORT evidence rating system, go to www.aafp.org/afpsort.xml.

CONSTIPATION

Description: Constipation is subjectively defined as decreased frequency, decreased volume, or straining at stool. In true clinical constipation, a large amount of stool is objectively found by the digital examination, or fecal loading is revealed by x-ray examination.

Etiology: Colonic motility depends on the integrity of the nervous system impulses and circular smooth muscle tone and motor complexes stimulated by increasing intraluminal pressure generated by bulk. Any pathophysiological process that interferes with this process can cause constipation. It is thought that changes in colonic motility are not age related but are influenced instead by extrinsic factors such as insufficient fluid, fiber, and exercise.

Occurrence: The constipation rate in the adult population has been estimated at 15%. Over $800 million are spent on OTC laxatives in the United States alone.

Age: Constipation is a frequent complaint of elderly persons, with self-reported constipation in 26% of women and 16% of men older than age 65, and in the subset of individuals older than age 85, it is 34% and 26%, respectively.

Ethnicity: Not significant.

Gender: At all ages, constipation is reported more frequently in women than in men. Elderly women are 2 to 3 times more likely to report constipation than their male counterparts.

Contributing factors: The functional factors described earlier contribute to constipation if they are not the primary etiology. Medications that may contribute to constipation include calcium channel blockers, calcium supplements, narcotics, iron supplements, aluminum-containing antacids, anti-Parkinson's drugs, NSAIDs, and any drug that has anticholinergic side effects. Certain types of laxatives also may be constipating, such as stimulant laxatives, which may cause cathartic colon and laxative dependency, and bulk laxatives taken with insufficient fluids. Neurological disorders, such as Parkinson's disease, stroke, spinal cord disorders, dementia, depression, metabolic factors, and nursing home placement, are also factors that increase the risk for constipation.

Signs and symptoms: Patients may not actively complain about constipation because they may not think it is important or are embarrassed to talk about it. Patients may describe constipation as an inability to pass or difficulty in passing stool, hard or dry stool, a feeling of abdominal or rectal fullness, and less than normal frequency or less than normal amount of passing stool. Ask the patient to describe specifically the frequency, character, and amount of stool. Determine the patient's fluid and fiber intake and exercise level. Conduct a thorough medication review to determine use of constipating drugs and laxatives. For cognitively impaired or communication-impaired individuals who are unable to self-report bowel frequency or elimination of discomfort, encourage the caregiver to maintain a record of the frequency and character of bowel elimination. The physical examination of the constipated patient should focus on a general assessment for signs of dehydration, such as inadequate skin turgor or dry mucous membranes. Perform an abdominal examination to check for distention and visible peristalsis. Auscultate bowel sounds, and check the patient for abdominal masses. Do a rectal examination, assessing for fissures and external hemorrhoids

and checking for anal stricture and sensation. Do a digital examination to assess for the presence of rectal masses and stool. The absence of stool found on examination does not exclude the possibility of constipation or fecal impaction. Key alarm features include weight loss, hematochezia, positive stool testing for occult blood, iron deficiency anemia, abdominal distention, nausea and vomiting, and sudden change in bowel habits.

Diagnostic tests: All individuals should have a fecal occult blood test at the initial visit of a complaint of constipation. Additional diagnostic tests should be done if they can inform contributing causes or alter the treatment. Laboratory tests might include complete blood count, glucose, thyroid-stimulating hormone, electrolytes, blood urea nitrogen (BUN), and creatinine. An abdominal radiograph may help to determine the extent and distribution of feces. Sigmoidoscopy or barium enema or both may be indicated in patients with a recent onset of constipation when a lesion is suspected. Checking colonic transit times may be indicated in patients who have a normal number of bowel movements but still complain of constipation. Colonic motility testing may be useful in identifying patterns of colonic activity. A colonoscopy should be done if the patient presents with alarm symptoms, anemia, or positive fecal occult blood.

Differential diagnosis: The differential diagnosis involved in evaluating a patient with a complaint of constipation involves first determining what the patient perception is of normal bowel frequency. The clinician then evaluates the etiology and contributing causes.

Treatment: After the specific etiology is established and factors contributing to constipation are identified, the appropriate pharmacological and nonpharmacological interventions are initiated. Nonpharmacological measures to treat constipation include encouraging fluids (1500 to 2000 mL/day minimum), increasing fiber intake (approximately 20 to 35 g/day), and prescribing exercise (20 to 30 minutes of walking daily when appropriate). Recent studies have demonstrated the efficacy of prunes and prune juice as compared to other fiber sources. Modify existing medication therapies if they are contributing to the constipation. If nonpharmacological measures are unsuccessful, the use of an osmotic laxative such as polyethylene glycol (PEG) or a chloride-channel activator such as lubiprostone may be appropriate. The clinician might also consider fiber or bulk agents such as psyllium or lactulose. Start bulk laxatives slowly, increasing the dose as the patient tolerates. Avoid bulk-forming laxatives in patients who cannot take adequate fluids and patients with swallowing difficulties. If these agents are unsuccessful, a suitable stimulant laxative such as senna, cascara, or bisacodyl might be added. Avoid long-term use of stimulant laxatives in older adults because these can cause malabsorption, electrolyte imbalance, dehydration, and cathartic colon. Mineral oil is always avoided in older adults, owing to the risk of aspiration and the depletion of fat-soluble vitamins. Newer agents such as guanylate cyclase (GC) activators, serotonergic enterokinetics, motilin agonists, or opioid receptor antagonists might be appropriate in some cases. Enemas and suppositories are used frequently in the geriatric population, but the evidence on their efficacy is limited. Rectal laxatives are often used as rescue therapy, but they have the potential for adverse effects. Enemas work through lavage and can cause fluid and electrolyte imbalance and can increase the risk of bowel perforation, particularly if the patient is not manually disimpacted first. Fecal softeners (docusate sodium) do not act as laxatives and are not useful in constipation, although they may reduce the strain associated with bowel elimination.

Follow-up: Chronically constipated individuals often need to have combined nonpharmacological with periodic pharmacological intervention. When laxatives are prescribed, these individuals need regular monitoring for the side effects and the responses to treatment.

Sequelae: Constipation, although uncomfortable, is rarely life threatening. When associated with pain, distention, or vomiting, constipation may be a sign of a life-threatening mesenteric infarction or a partial or complete bowel obstruction. Straining in elderly persons may have serious effects on the cerebral, coronary, and peripheral arterial circulation. If stool is not eliminated from the colon and the patient becomes dehydrated, stool may harden, resulting in fecal impaction. Hardened stool may back up farther into the colon and become difficult to remove with either cathartics or enemas. Some individuals have needed surgical intervention to remove hard stool that is obstructing the bowel. Delirium can also result from severe constipation.

Prevention/prophylaxis: Adequate dietary fluid and fiber and regular exercise habits help to promote colonic mobility. Bowel elimination patterns should be monitored regularly in individuals who are unable to report bowel habits or bowel discomfort.

Referral: Hospitalization may be necessary in some cases of severe constipation and/or impaction, anorexia, dehydration, or nausea or vomiting. Patients with recent-onset constipation associated with bleeding, anemia, or family history of colon cancer; patients with chronic constipation with anemia, abdominal pain, and weight loss; and patients with recent-onset fecal incontinence should be referred to a gastroenterologist. Referral to a specialist also should be considered when there is a failure to alleviate constipation despite escalating attempts.

Education: In addition to giving instruction in the dietary measures appropriate in preventing constipation, encourage older patients to maintain regular bowel habits and respond to the urge to defecate rather than suppress it. Patient education regarding diet and exercise is challenging when patients have cognitive impairments, mood disorders, uncontrolled pain, or significant muscle weakness. Patients should be taught to take advantage of the gastrocolic reflex, which is strongest about 30 minutes after meal consumption. All individuals should avoid the use of laxatives and OTC medications known to have constipating side effects.

CLINICAL RECOMMENDATION	EVIDENCE RATING	REFERENCE
Ask the patient about a feeling of incomplete evacuation, obstruction, digital manipulation, infrequent bowel movements, and abdominal bloating.	B	Hofford (2011)
Consider laboratory testing: CBC, electrolytes, BUN, creatinine, calcium, glucose, and thyroid-stimulating hormone if symptoms persist despite conservative treatment.	B	American College of Gastroenterology Task Force (2005)

CLINICAL RECOMMENDATION	EVIDENCE RATING	REFERENCE
Patients with red flags for malignancy or complicated disease should have a colonoscopy.	A	Hofford (2011)
The initial management of symptomatic constipation is typically dietary modification (high fiber, exercise, and fluid supplementation).	B	Hofford (2011)
Polyethelene glycol (PEG) and lubiprostone are effective for the management of chronic constipation.	A	Hofford (2011)

A = consistent, good-quality, patient-oriented evidence; B = inconsistent or limited-quality, patient-oriented evidence; C = consensus, disease-oriented evidence, usual practice, expert opinion, or case series. For information about the SORT evidence rating system, go to www.aafp.org/afpsort.xml.

COUGH

Description: Cough is the forceful expelling of air from the lungs involving the use of accessory muscles of the chest and constriction of the glottis.

Etiology: Cough is the voluntary or involuntary mechanism used to eject aspirants or noxious substances, including fluids, solid, dust, and gases from the body's upper and lower airways. Cough is also the body's mechanism to remove mucus from the upper or lower respiratory tracts.

Involuntary cough is regulated by the vagal afferent nerve, but higher central nervous system cortical modulation can inhibit cough or allow for voluntary cough.

Occurrence: Cough is one of the most common complaints for seeking medical attention. It is divided into three categories based on duration: acute, lasting less than 3 weeks; subacute, lasting between 3 and 8 weeks; and chronic, lasting more than 8 weeks.

Age: Occurs at any age.

Gender: No gender-specific differences.

Ethnicity: No direct ties to ethnicity have been documented.

Contributing factors: Smoking, as well as second-hand smoke, is the primary cause of chronic cough. Cigarette smoking is the most significant preventable cause of disease, and lung cancer is the number one cause of cancer deaths of both men and women in the United States. Cough from chronic obstructive pulmonary disease (COPD) worsens in intensity and duration if the patient continues to smoke. Bronchogenic cancers are often associated with cough, but metastatic cancers to the lungs seldom result in cough until late in the course of the disease.

Trauma that can contribute to cough includes assault, motor vehicle accidents, or falls leading to contusion of the lungs.

Environment, home, and work can be responsible for exposure to multiple different types of infectious agents such as common cold, tuberculosis (TB), or *Bordetella pertussis*. In addition, work environment can cause exposure to chemicals and dust.

Medications can contribute to cough. Angiotensin-converting enzyme (ACE) inhibitors cause cough as a side effect in 20% of users.

Signs and symptoms: A thorough history of the disease, the patient's risk factors, and the work and home environments is essential in narrowing the cause of cough. Risk factors for cough include smoking, stroke, immigrant status, use of ACE inhibitors, HIV–positive status, and heart disease. The cough may be productive or nonproductive, and the sputum may be a variety of colors or tinged with blood. Identify the onset, including if it is episodic or continuous or occurs only certain times of the day; the duration and character of the cough; and if it is associated with other symptoms, including fever, tachycardia, dyspnea, weight loss, or pain. The physical examination begins with vital signs that should include temperature, heart rate, respirations, and oxygen saturation. Next is a thorough examination of the nose and orophyaryngeal mucosa. Tenderness to percussion of the facial and maxillary sinuses and swollen, mucus-covered, boggy turbinates indicate allergic rhinitis. A "cobblestone" appearance from chronic posterior pharynx and swollen eyelids are other indicators of an allergic origin. Loss of tooth enamel can indicate GERD. The chest must be assessed for adventitious breath sounds. Wheezes indicate bronchitis or asthma caused by mucus in or constriction of the airways. Rhonchi or crackles are suspicions for pneumonia or infiltrates. Diminished or absent lung sounds by auscultation and dullness to percussion are highly suggestive of pneumonia's consolidation. Rhonchi or crackles with cardiomegaly on x-ray or ECG indicate congestive heart failure and may not be accompanied by edema.

Diagnostic tests: No specific tests are indicated when the patient has a cough. The selection and extent of testing depends on the findings of the history and physical examination, duration (acute, subacute, or chronic), previous evaluations, and whether services are available.

Acute cough associated with upper respiratory infection does not require further diagnostic evaluation. Acute cough with physical findings of life-threatening illness should be appropriately evaluated for the diagnosis of concern. A chest radiograph is appropriate for physical findings consistent with pneumonia (fever, heart rate above 100, respiratory rate greater than 24 breaths/min, chest examination with findings of local consolidation). Viral cultures, serologic assays, and sputum analysis should not be routinely performed in the diagnosis of acute bronchitis.

Subacute cough that has lasted more than 2 weeks without an apparent cause and is associated with post-tussive vomiting, inspiratory whooping, and paroxysms of coughing should have a nasopharyngeal aspirate or polymer swab of the nasopharynx for culture to confirm the presence of *B. pertussis*, whooping cough. Bacterial isolation is the only certain way to confirm the diagnosis. The testing for TB should occur when there is an increased risk of the population becoming infected, such as in nursing homes or prisons, in a patient with a recent visit to a country with high prevalence of TB, or in an immunocompromised patient. Tuberculin skin test may not be reliable if the patient is unable to mount a response. Sputum smears and cultures for acid-fast bacilli and chest radiograph provide more diagnostic benefit.

Chronic cough diagnostic testing in nonsmokers is guided by the elimination through treatment of the most common disorders: upper airway cough syndrome (UACS), previously known as postnasal drip syndrome secondary to rhinosinus diseases; GERD; and asthma. Medical history is crucial to determining progression of diagnostic tests for chronic cough. A chest radiograph is appropriate though most often negative. An abnormal study would guide further diagnostics; a mass suggestive of lung cancer could be followed up with high-resolution CT scan, bronchoscopy, and biopsy; congestive heart failure would lead to cardiovascular evaluation; evidence of infection such as TB would direct microbiologic diagnostics. UACS evaluation includes sinus imaging, either plain sinus films or sinus CT scan. Scans or films taken during the episode of a common cold are not diagnostic of bacterial sinus infection. Evaluation for asthma-induced chronic cough is bronchoprovocation challenge. GERD evaluation includes a barium swallow and 24-hour esophageal pH monitoring test.

Differential diagnosis: The most important first step is determining if the acute cough is potentially related to a life-threatening condition such as pneumonia, congestive heart failure, or pulmonary embolism. Most acute coughs are related to a respiratory tract condition such as common cold, flu, acute bronchitis, acute exacerbation of COPD, viral syndrome, or exposure to environmental irritant.

Subacute cough is usually a cough that lingers on from a respiratory tract infection, a postinfectious cough. Consider UACS, transient bronchial hyperresponsiveness, asthma, acute exacerbation of chronic bronchitis, and pertussis. If it appears to be a noninfectious cough, it should be managed and further evaluated as a chronic cough. Chronic cough most commonly is UACS, asthma, and GERD. Other potential causes may include nonasthmatic eosinophilic bronchitis (NAEB), COPD, drug-induced cough, fungal infection, and mediastinal masses. Diagnosis of unexplained cough or idiopathic cough requires an exhaustive evaluation by a specialist for uncommon causes before it is used. A nocturnal cough associated with shortness of breath suggests heart failure and without shortness of breath is more indicative of an allergy.

Treatment: Most often the source of the cough is isolated to the respiratory system and the condition is not life threatening. The following treatments are recommended:

Common cold, postnasal drip, and throat clearing: Treat with first-generation antihistamine/decongestant preparation to decrease and hasten the resolution of the cough. Naproxen, an NSAID, may also be used to decrease cough. It is thought to work by inhibiting the inflammatory process.

Acute bronchitis: This diagnosis is applicable in persons without signs or symptoms of acute exacerbation of COPD, acute asthma, common cold, or pneumonia. In the older adult a high suspicion of pneumonia should be considered until proven otherwise. Most acute bronchitis is viral and self-limiting; antibiotics do not shorten the course of the disease and should not be used. Albuterol is not recommended unless there is an asthma component. Expectorants such as guaifenesin may be used. Dextromethorphan or codeine may be used for cough suppression for severe coughing though research has only been done in chronic bronchitis. A cool mist humidifier in the bedroom may be helpful.

Bacterial pneumonia: Community-acquired pneumonia (CAP) is treated differently than health-care–associated pneumonia. It is of particular concern in elderly patients and those who are immunocompromised because their symptoms may be less intense. Pneumonia most often is caused by *Staphylococcus*, *Klebsiella*, or *Pseudomonas* in the otherwise healthy individual. If pneumonia is suspected, broad-spectrum antibiotic therapy should be initiated empirically. Patients with any respiratory distress and elderly patients with significantly elevated white blood cell (WBC) counts may need to be hospitalized.

Chronic bronchitis: Stable patients with a sudden change of symptoms, increase in cough, shortness of breath, purulent sputum, and increase in sputum production are to be considered as having an acute exacerbation. Treatment includes a combination bronchodilator, beta-agonists, and ipratropium as an inhaler or as a nebulizer, antibiotics, and oral steroids. Dextromethorphan or codeine may be used for cough suppression. Diagnosis and chronic management of COPD is addressed elsewhere in this text.

TB: Antituberculosis drugs should be begun with a positive tuberculin skin test and the patient referred to a health department.

Drug reaction: ACE inhibitor should be stopped and only restarted if there is compelling need for the category of drug.

Postinfectious cough: A treatment trial of inhaled ipratropium for a cough that is adversely affecting quality of life may be used. If ipratropium alone is not successful, use of inhaled corticosteroids can be considered. Antibiotics are not recommended. Severe symptoms may require use of an oral steroid for a short period while other causes of cough are being considered.

Chronic cough treatment: Treatment of UACS, asthma, and GERD in a stepwise, systematic approach is most likely to provide a high rate of success. Since UACS is the most common cause of chronic cough, a trial of first-generation antihistamine and decongestant should be tried. Cough should improve in 1 to 2 weeks; if the response is positive, the medication should continue because it may take several weeks for marked improvement. A partial response indicates more than one cause of the cough, and evaluation and treatment for asthma or GERD is reasonable.

Follow-up: The tenacity of follow-up depends on the severity of the illness and the impact on the patient's life. For pneumonia or bronchitis with minimal dyspnea, a call to check on the patient is appropriate. Rising temperature or increasing difficulty breathing requires immediate attention or emergency department evaluation. Patients with resolving pneumonia should be evaluated in 2 to 3 weeks; a repeat chest x-ray may be taken. Chronic cough may take multiple follow-up visits, evaluation, and treatment trials.

Referral: A referral to a specialist can be initiated anytime during the evaluation and treatment of a cough. Some results such as lesions suspicious for cancer on radiography require referral to a specialist immediately. A cough specialist, allergist, or pulmonologist referral is appropriate for a chronic cough that is persistent. Other specialists who may be helpful are a GI specialist for evaluation of GERD, an infectious disease specialist for infections and immunocompromised patients, and a cardiologist for heart conditions.

Prevention/prophylaxis: Preventive measures include smoking avoidance or cessation intervention, evaluation of the work and home environment, and humidification of the sleeping area with a cool mist humidifier. Patients should be provided vaccinations following Centers for Disease Control and Prevention guidelines, including annual flu shots, Pneumovax, and Tdap.

Education: Recommend smoking cessation classes and allergen avoidance training.

DIAGNOSIS	CLINICAL RECOMMENDATION	EVIDENCE RATING	REFERENCE
Common cold, postnasal drip, and throat clearing	First-generation antihistamine/decongestant preparation, naproxen.	B	Pratter (2006a, 2006b)
Acute bronchitis without signs or symptoms of pneumonia, COPD exacerbation, acute asthma, or common cold	Most acute bronchitis is viral and self-limiting; antibiotics do not shorten the course of the disease and should not be used.	B	Braman (2006a)
Bacterial pneumonia—community acquired	Broad-spectrum antibiotic therapy should be initiated empirically; elderly patients with significantly elevated WBC counts or patients with respiratory distress may need to be hospitalized.	B	File (2009)
Chronic bronchitis—sudden change in symptoms	Combination bronchodilator, beta agonists, and ipratropium as an inhaler or as a nebulizer, antibiotics, and oral steroids. Dextromethorphan or codeine may be used for cough suppression.	A	Irwin et al. (2006)
Drug reaction	ACE inhibitor should be stopped.	A	Dicpinigaitis (2006)
Postinfectious cough with other conditions ruled out	Treatment trial of inhaled ipratropium for cough if affecting quality of life; can consider inhaled corticosteroids or use 30–40 mg of prednisone for limited period of time for severe paroxysms. Cough suppression for failure of other treatments. Antibiotics are not recommended.	B	Braman (2006b)
Upper airway cough syndrome (UACS)	First-generation antihistamine and decongestant.	C	Pratter et al. (2006)

A = consistent, good-quality, patient-oriented evidence; B = inconsistent or limited-quality, patient-oriented evidence; C = consensus, disease-oriented evidence, usual practice, expert opinion, or case series. For information about the SORT evidence rating system, go to www.aafp.org/afpsort.xml.

DEHYDRATION

Description: Dehydration, or fluid volume depletion caused by too little fluid intake, too much fluid lost, or both, is a common condition in older patients. Fluid balance, intake equals output, is essential to health.

Etiology: Total body water decreases with age. The total body water of an adult age 61 to 74 is approximately 43% for women and 51% for men compared with 80% for children. Even small decreases in fluid intake can cause dehydration quickly in an older adult. The ability of the kidneys to concentrate urine declines with age, so that even when deprived of water, urination is not significantly reduced. Also, thirst decreases as a person ages, which is an important self-regulation against dehydration.

Dehydration can be defined as a fluid and electrolyte disturbance arising from either a water depletion or a sodium depletion in which there is accompanying water loss. It can be classified into three different types based on the possible causes (Table 5-1): isotonic, hypotonic, and hypertonic.

Occurrence: Dehydration has been reported to be the most common fluid and electrolyte imbalance in older adults. The prevalence is increasing, with hospitalizations for dehydration increasing by 40% from 1990 to 2000.

Age: Older people are particularly susceptible to dehydration because of age-related changes noted above, with individuals older than 85 at the highest risk.

Gender: Not significant.

Ethnicity: African Americans have a greater likelihood of dehydration than Caucasians (Stookey, Pieper, & Cohen, 2003).

TABLE 5-1	Types of Dehydration
TYPE OF DEHYDRATION	**DESCRIPTION**
Isotonic	A balanced loss of both sodium and water causes extracellular fluid loss that increased blood viscosity. Common causes: vomiting, diarrhea, osmotic effects of glucose.
Hypertonic	Excessive water loss results in raised sodium levels and shifts from the intracellular space to extracellular space. Common causes: renal tubular disease, osmotic diuresis, resistance to vasopressin.
Hypotonic	Excessive sodium loss results in extracellular fluid loss. Common causes: overuse of diuretics, chronic salt wasting.

Contributing factors: Decreased mobility and the presence of chronic diseases such as diabetes, cancer, and cardiovascular and renal disease make older adults more sensitive to fluid and electrolyte imbalance. Other risk factors for dehydration in the elderly include the following: dependency for eating or drinking, mouth pain, poorly fitted dentures, and difficulty swallowing. Vomiting, diarrhea, hemorrhage, and increased metabolic states that result in excess loss of fluids (fever, infection, excess sweating, excess urination) are also contributing factors. The use of certain medications, such as diuretics, anticholinergics, psychotropics, or laxatives, also may increase the risk. Dehydration is the most frequent secondary condition resulting from debilitating issues such as fever, confusion, pain, or pneumonia. Cognitive impairment (delirium, dementia, depression) has been associated with dehydration in older adults.

Signs and symptoms: A dry, furrowed tongue and mucous membranes, sunken eyes, confusion, concentrated or dark urine, and upper body muscle weakness may indicate dehydration. Clinical signs may not appear, however, until dehydration is far advanced. In addition, the usual signs of constipation, disorientation, dry mucous membranes, orthostatic hypotension, and weight loss may be caused by other factors. If one or more of these are present or are a change from baseline, dehydration may be the cause. Assessment of skin turgor at the sternum is not a reliable indicator of dehydration in the elderly. Signs and symptoms of hypovolemic shock include altered mental status, hypotension, tachycardia, cold clammy skin, and rapid deep respirations. The most reliable sign of general dehydration is dry tongue with longitudinal furrows.

Diagnostic test: Serum markers provide the most reliable indicators of dehydration and these include serum sodium, increased serum osmolality, and BUN-creatinine ratio. The serum albumin may be higher than normal when the patient is dehydrated.

Differential diagnosis: When dehydration is identified, it is important to identify the cause and contributing factors and address these. Weight gain and edema from congestive heart failure can conceal a patient's dehydrated status.

Treatment: Individualize treatment, depending on the type of dehydration. The route of administration (oral or IV or subcutaneous) is determined by what is safe and effective. The recommended daily intake of fluids for sedentary individuals should be ≥1600 mL/24 hours to ensure adequate hydration, and this is adjusted for climate and physical activity. Regular presentation of fluids to bedridden individuals can maintain adequate hydration status. Provide continuous verbal cues to encourage drinking fluids. Fluids given with medication can be an important source of fluids, so fluids should be encouraged at this time. Determine the patient's personal preferences of fluid.

Follow-up: See patient as indicated by cause and response to treatment.

Sequelae: Dehydration has severe consequences for the elderly and leads to constipation, falls, medication toxicity, and infection. Inadequate fluid intake can have serious medical consequences such as renal failure, hyperthermia, bowel obstructions, delirium, cardiovascular symptoms, and death.

Prevention/prophylaxis: Educate patients, families, and caregivers that to prevent dehydration one needs to ensure adequate fluid intake. All liquids are not the same in maintaining fluid balance. Water is the best and should be at least half of the daily intake of fluid.

Add milk, fruit and vegetable juices, and nonsalty soups for variety. Decrease coffee, tea, alcohol, colas, and liquid diet supplements because they may cause dehydration. The use of a 24-hour fluid balance chart can help determine if the patient is at risk or is dehydrated.

Referral: Refer as indicated by source of symptom. Hospitalization is indicated when the patient has severe signs and symptoms such as dizziness, altered mental status, or lethargy; is hemodynamically unstable; or cannot tolerate oral fluids.

Education: Explain causes of symptoms and measures taken to determine cause and treatment. Aim for 1600 mL of oral liquids per day unless contraindicated by certain medical conditions such as congestive heart failure. Allow adequate time for eating at mealtimes. Meals can provide two-thirds of daily fluids. Offer fluids regularly during the day. Encourage consumption of fluids with medications. Staff education is critical; staff should report any significant weight loss, change in fluid consumption, or other relevant symptoms such as dry mucous membranes.

CLINICAL RECOMMENDATION	EVIDENCE RATING	REFERENCE
The recommended daily intake of fluids should not be <1600 mL/24 hours to ensure adequate hydration.	A	Hodgkinson, Evans, & Wood (2003) Theerthakaria & Madlon-Kay (2011)
Hypodermoclysis is as effective as IV rehydration of older adults with mild-to-moderate dehydration.	A	Rochon et al. (1997) Thomas et al. (2008)
Verbal prompts have been shown to increase fluid intake in nursing home residents.	A	Simmons, Alessi, & Schnelle (2001)

A = consistent, good-quality, patient-oriented evidence; B = inconsistent or limited-quality, patient-oriented evidence; C = consensus, disease-oriented evidence, usual practice, expert opinion, or case series. For information about the SORT evidence rating system, go to www.aafp.org/afpsort.xml.

DELIRIUM

Description: Delirium presents as a disturbance of consciousness (decreased awareness of the environment) with a reduced ability to focus, sustain, or shift attention.

Cognitive change (poor memory, disorientation, speech disturbance) and perceptual disturbance are distinct from a preexisting, established, or evolving dementia.

The onset of the disturbance is rapid (hours to days) and typically fluctuates over the course of the day. Delirium frequently represents a sudden and significant decline from a previous level of functioning, and there is usually evidence from the history, physical examination, or laboratory tests of a direct physiological etiology of a general medical condition, substance intoxication or withdrawal, use of a medication, toxin exposure, or a combination of these factors. The *Diagnostic and Statistical Manual of Mental Disorders, Fourth Edition, Text Revision* (DSM-IV-TR) differentiates delirium by etiology:

1. Delirium due to a general medical condition
2. Substance-induced delirium
3. Delirium due to multiple etiologies
4. Delirium not otherwise specified

Etiology: Causes of delirium are numerous and in elderly hospitalized patients there are often multiple etiologies, including metabolic, infection, cardiac, neurological, pulmonary, sensory impairments, medications, and toxins. Regardless of cause, a consistent finding is significant reduction in regional cerebral perfusion during periods of delirium in comparison with blood flow patterns after recovery. A possible neurological common pathway may involve acetylcholine and dopamine, and the disruption in the sleep-wake cycle in delirium indicates melatonin as a possible factor.

Occurrence: Prevalence in the general population is 0.4% in adults age 18 years and older and rises with age to 1.1% in those age 55 and older. In the hospitalized medically ill the prevalence of delirium ranges from 10% to 30%. The prevalence of delirium in long-term care residents age 75 and older may be as high as 60% at any given time. In the hospitalized elderly, approximately 10% to 15% exhibit delirium on admission, and 10% to 40% may develop delirium during their hospital stay. Prevalence varies depending on the underlying condition(s), procedures and surgeries performed, and other medical interventions provided.

It is not uncommon for hospitalized cancer patients (25%) and hospitalized AIDS patients (30% to 40%) to develop delirium. Approximately half of postoperative patients develop delirium, and the majority of those with terminal illness (up to 80%) develop delirium as they approach death. Symptoms of subclinical delirium, such as restlessness, anxiety, irritability, distractibility, or sleep disturbance, may be manifested in the days before the onset of overt delirium and may progress to full-blown delirium over the course of a few days. The duration of delirium can range from less than 1 week to more than 2 months but typically resolves within 10 to 12 days.

Age: Any medically ill patient can develop delirium, but the elderly may be more prone due to preexisting conditions, aging processes, and greater vulnerability to acute opportunistic disease processes.

Ethnicity: No difference in vulnerability.

Gender: Males tend to have a higher incidence rate, and the male gender appears to be an independent risk factor for delirium.

Contributing factors: Changes in brain function, multiple general medical problems, polypharmacy, reduced hepatic metabolism of medications, multisensory declines, and brain disorders such as dementia make the elderly particularly vulnerable to delirium. A careful medical evaluation that includes attention to level of oxygenation, possible occult infection (e.g., urinary tract infection), and the role of medications is essential. Although many medications can be a causative factor, those with anticholinergic effects are frequently responsible.

Signs and symptoms: The clinical presentation may include difficulty sustaining and shifting attention; extreme distractibility; disorganized thinking; rambling, irrelevant, pressured, and incoherent speech; and impaired reasoning ability and goal-directed behavior. Patients with delirium also demonstrate disorientation to time and place, impairment of recent memory, misperceptions about the environment (including illusions and hallucinations), emotional instability, and psychomotor activity that fluctuates between agitation, purposeless movements, and a vegetative state. Disorientation to other persons occurs commonly, but disorientation to self is rare. Dysarthria is a frequent speech and language disturbance, and dysnomia (impaired ability to name objects), dysgraphia (impaired ability to write), or aphasia may be observed. Commonly associated features of delirium include disturbances in the sleep-wake cycle such as daytime sleepiness, nighttime agitation, and disturbances in sleep continuity. Complete reversal of the sleep-wake cycle or fragmentation of the circadian sleep-wake pattern can occur. Emotional disturbances may include anxiety, fear, depression, irritability, anger, euphoria, and apathy. Affective lability (rapid and unpredictable shifts from one emotional state to another) may occur. Possible autonomic signs associated with delirium include tachycardia, sweating, flushed face, dilated pupils, and elevated blood pressure.

Diagnostic and screening tests: Laboratory work will assist in identifying potential causative factors, and rating scales that measure cognition and establish diagnostic data, such as Folstein's Mini Mental State Examination (MMSE), the Confusion Assessment Method (CAM), the Delirium Rating Scale—Revised, or the Delirium Observation Screening Scale, assist in tracking progress and return to baseline functioning. However, because of fluctuating levels of consciousness and cognition, it may be difficult to assess mental status and cognitive function. When possible, obtain information from the medical record, medical staff, and others, especially family members. Culture and ethnicity should be taken into consideration when evaluating an individual's mental status and capacity. Some patients may not be familiar with information used in cognitive rating scales (general knowledge, geographical information, memory, and orientation/location), and many scales adjust for these factors, as well as educational level, in the interpretation of scores.

Differential diagnosis: The most common differential diagnostic challenge is whether the patient has a dementia versus delirium, has delirium alone, or has a delirium superimposed on a preexisting dementia. Although there are common cognitive disturbances in delirium and dementia, a primary difference is the patient with dementia is usually alert whereas the patient with delirium manifests overt disturbance of consciousness or arousal. The rapid onset and course of cognitive impairments and reversibility of symptoms are helpful in distinguishing between delirium and dementia. The severity of delirium symptoms typically fluctuates over the course of a day, whereas dementia symptoms generally do not fluctuate. Information from medical records, caregivers, and family members may help determination of whether dementia was present before the onset of delirium. Depression is another differential diagnosis because patients often manifest cognitive and psychomotor symptoms common to dementia and delirium.

Treatment: Appropriate treatment for delirium involves discovering the causes, many of which are reversible, and preventing complications through prompt treatment of specific, identified disorders. A thorough, comprehensive assessment; evaluation of medications, interactions, and contraindications; and ordering laboratory work will assist in ruling out/in the many etiologies of delirium. While assessing for probable etiology and definitive treatment, management should focus on ensuring safety from behavioral disturbances by combining environmental therapy, behavioral therapy, and pharmacotherapy.

Nonpharmacological interventions: A therapeutic environment would include frequent reassurance and reality orientation, clear communication, caregiver consistency, decreased stimuli (noise reduction, adequate lighting, do not rush the patient), decreased stress, and decreased anxiety through frequent reassurance. Providing a structured daily routine, maintaining comfort (eyeglasses, hearing aids, personal belongings), and reestablishing the sleep-wake cycle by controlling nighttime noise and unnecessary disruptions can help. Ensuring adequate daily fluid intake and that elimination needs are met; providing for physical activity, ambulation, and range of motion; and avoiding chemical or physical restraints are helpful. Medication should be used as a last resort.

Pharmacotherapy: Data support the use of first-generation (e.g., haloperidol) and second-generation (e.g., olanzapine, risperidone, ziprasidone, and quetiapine) antipsychotic medications to control behavioral symptoms of delirium and prevent injury to self or others. Cholinesterase inhibitors (e.g., donazepil and rivastigmine) also have shown success in managing delirium, but usually for reversing drug-induced delirium. The avoidance of benzodiazepines except for specific indications (e.g., alcohol or γ-hydroxybutyric acid [GHA] withdrawal delirium, delirium related to seizures) continues to be a recommendation.

Patients in critical care settings, who are receiving high doses of parenteral lorazepam, should be monitored closely for toxicity (e.g., renal dysfunction, hyperosmolar metabolic acidosis). It is important to periodically reassess the patient's mental status and other psychiatric symptoms and behaviors such as depression, suicidal ideation or behavior, hallucinations, delusions, aggression, agitation, anxiety, disinhibition, affective lability, cognitive deficits, and sleep disturbances because these symptoms can fluctuate rapidly. Regular monitoring and serial assessments of mental status and symptoms will allow for the adjustment of treatment strategies and may indicate the effectiveness of interventions and new or worsening medical conditions.

Follow-up: Close follow-up for treatment efficacy, appropriate laboratory and diagnostic studies to monitor resolution of the underlying cause, and monitoring of mental status and cognitive functioning are essential to ensure full recovery.

Sequelae: During overt periods of delirium, there is risk of injury to self or others due to confusion, altered perception, and impaired insight and judgment. Fear is often a precipitant to injury in patients with delirium and may result in their attacking others, falling out of bed, or pulling on IV lines, oxygen tubing, tracheotomy or GI tubes, urinary catheters, or other medical equipment. Although the majority of patients recover fully, delirium may progress to stupor, coma, seizures, or death. Full recovery is less likely in the elderly, and persistent cognitive deficits are common. Such deficits may be due to preexisting dementia that was not clearly established. The elderly have a significantly increased risk of developing complications, such as pneumonia and decubitus ulcers, which may result in longer hospital stays. In postoperative patients, delirium may limit recovery and contribute to poorer long-term outcomes. Increased risk for postoperative complications, longer postoperative recuperation periods, longer hospital stays, and long-term disability are associated with delirium. Delirious patients with alcohol or sedative-hypnotic withdrawal, cocaine intoxication, head trauma, hypoglycemia, strokes, or extensive burns are at increased risk for seizures. Delirium in the medically ill is associated with an increased mortality rate, and patients who develop delirium during a hospitalization also have a very high rate of death during the months following discharge.

Prevention/prophylaxis: Preventive measures to lessen the likelihood of delirium include elimination or minimization of risk factors. These measures include judicious use of high-risk medications (Beers List); timely management and good control of acute and chronic medical disease processes; correction of sensory deficits (eyeglasses, magnifying glasses, adequate lighting, hearing aids, cerumen removal); promotion of normal sleep patterns through good sleep hygiene measures; provision of adequate nutrition and hydration with oral/parenteral supplementation as necessary; prompt attention to elimination needs; participation in activities that maintain and stimulate cognitive and physical functioning; and provision of general supportive measures (environmental modifications, reality orientation, control of external stimuli). For hospitalized elders and long-term care residents, encourage frequent visits by family members to provide familiarity, reality orientation, reassurance, and comfort.

Referral: Patients with delirium should be hospitalized so that diagnostic testing, identification of underlying causes, and management can occur in a rapid, coordinated manner during concurrent treatment of acute symptoms to ensure patient safety and comfort. Care of the patient with delirium should be coordinated by the primary care provider and managed jointly with internal medicine, psychiatry, neurology, and other specialty physicians to ensure appropriate comprehensive evaluation and care.

Education: Patients and families should be educated about the etiology of delirium and the expected course of illness while providing reassurance that delirium is usually temporary and that the symptoms are part of a medical condition. Additional resources can be found at the following Web sites:

- National Library of Medicine: www.nlm.nih.gov/MEDLINEPLUS/ency/article/000740.htm
- National Cancer Institute: www.cancer.gov/cancertopics/pdq/supportivecare/delirium/Patient
- The Mayo Clinic: www.mayoclinic.com/health/delirium/DS01064

CLINICAL RECOMMENDATION	EVIDENCE RATING	REFERENCE
Delirium is associated with increased mortality, functional decline, and new nursing home placement.	A	Inouye et al. (1998)
The incidence of delirium superimposed on dementia is 22%–89%.	A	Fick, Agostini, & Inouye (2002)
The CAM tool for assessing delirium has sensitivity, specificity, and high interrater reliability.	A	Laurila, Pitkala, Strandberg, & Tilvis (2002)

A = consistent, good-quality, patient-oriented evidence; B = inconsistent or limited-quality, patient-oriented evidence; C = consensus, disease-oriented evidence, usual practice, expert opinion, or case series. For information about the SORT evidence rating system, go to www.aafp.org/afpsort.xml.

DIARRHEA

Description: Diarrhea is defined by the passage of three or more loose or watery stools or increased stool weight of >200 g in a day. Acute diarrhea is described as lasting less than 4 weeks and chronic diarrhea as lasting longer than 4 weeks. See Table 5-2 for types of diarrhea.

Etiology: Diarrhea occurs when food and liquids pass too quickly through the body and are excreted through the colon as loose or watery stool. *Clostridium difficile* infection as a cause of diarrhea should be suspected in the assessment of patients with watery diarrhea during or shortly after antibiotic therapy. Diarrhea may also be a symptom of a disease requiring surgical intervention in order to correct. Diarrhea in the older patient is often acute and self-limited.

Occurrence: The prevalence rate is approximately 5%.

Age: Occurs at any age, but the mortality rate is increased in infants and the frail elderly.

Ethnicity: No direct ties to ethnicity have been documented.

Gender: No gender-specific differences.

Contributing factors: The following can be contributing factors in the development of diarrhea: recent travel, family history of inflammatory/bowel disorders, recent antibiotic usage, exposures to either contacts or foods, whether or not the individual is immunocompromised such as with HIV, recent hospitalization, age of more than 65 years, extended stay in hospital or nursing home, recent chemotherapy, recent GI surgery including postpyloric tube feeding, and medications. The list of medications includes diuretics, beta blockers, NSAIDs, antibiotics, quinidine, chemotherapy, colchicine, laxatives, digitalis, theophylline, prostaglandins, cholinergic agents, and phenolphthalein.

Signs and symptoms: The history should include symptom assessment parameters, including onset, frequency, amount, and character of the stool (including the presence of blood, mucus, or atypical color) and any associated symptoms such as abdominal pain, cramping, fever, or bloating. The patient's baseline bowel pattern, usual dietary intake, food intolerance history, exposure to others with illness, and any recent dining out need to be identified. A thorough medication review including any OTC herbal remedies or laxatives needs to be conducted. A dietary history 2 days before onset of symptoms would be helpful, with particular attention to the ingestion of meat, dairy products, and seafood. The associated symptoms of fever, abdominal pain and distention, vomiting, myalgias, and headache with abrupt onset suggest acute diarrhea etiologies. On the other hand, fatigue, muscle weakness, weight loss, alternating diarrhea and constipation, incomplete evacuation, abdominal pain, and protracted or recurring symptoms suggest chronic diarrhea etiologies.

Physical examination should include vital signs, weight, and assessing for the presence of postural hypotension. Assess the skin for turgor and the condition of the tongue and mucous membranes. Check for evidence of jaundice, rashes, or lesions. Examine the thyroid for lesions. Perform a thorough examination of the abdomen for distention, rigidity, tenderness, bowel sounds, masses, hepatomegaly, or splenomegaly. Perform a rectal examination, including Hemoccult testing to assess for bleeding, hemorrhoids, polyps, fissures, fistulas, or evidence of malignancy. Include a general inspection for arthritis or lymphadenopathy. Stool should be examined for mucus and for the presence of blood.

TABLE 5-2 Types of Diarrhea		
TYPE OF DIARRHEA	**DESCRIPTION**	**CAUSES**
Watery	Secretor	Infection, toxins, drugs, endocrine disorders, motility disorders, ileal disorders, neuroendocrine tumors
	Osmotic	Use of osmotic laxatives, carbohydrate malabsorption (lactose, sorbital, mannitol, and fructose)
Inflammatory	Bloody or pus containing	Crohn's disease, ulcerative colitis, diverticulitis, *C. difficile*, TB, viral infections, parasitic infections, radiation colitis, microscopic colitis
Fatty	Malabsorption	Short bowel syndrome, celiac disease, postsurgical resection of bowel, mesenteric ischemia
	Maldigestion	Bile acid insufficiency, pancreatic disease

Diagnostic tests: Complete blood count (CBC), electrolytes, and renal function will help identify an infectious process and any electrolyte imbalance and the presence of dehydration. Abdominal x-rays are helpful to identify the presence of obstruction or ischemia. A barium enema can reveal malignancies, polyps, or abnormalities of the mucosal lining. Colonoscopy or sigmoidoscopy may be useful when symptoms are persistent and unexplained. If you suspect laxative abuse, you may order a stool laxative screen. You may send in stool samples to test for occult blood, *C. difficile*, salmonella, *Escherichia coli*, lactoferrin, salmonella, campylobacter, leukocytes, ova, and parasites. If the stool tests positive for leukocytes, the sample should be cultured to identify any bacterial etiology.

Differential diagnosis: Distinguish first between acute diarrhea and chronic diarrhea. In acute diarrhea, consider inflammatory bowel disease, fecal impaction, irritable bowel syndrome, diverticulitis, antibiotic-associated pseudomembranous colitis, bowel ischemia, drug side effects, food poisoning, and virus or bacteria exposure. In chronic diarrhea consider ulcerative colitis, Crohn's disease, microscopic colitis, celiac disease, IBS and bile acid malabsorption, occult neoplasm, postradiation enterocolitis, and functional problems. A fecal specimen should be obtained for anyone in cases of severe, bloody, inflammatory, or persistent diarrhea or if an outbreak is suspected.

Treatment: In many cases of diarrhea, replacing lost fluid and electrolytes is the only treatment needed, but treatment is dependent on the cause. Frail elderly persons are at increased risk for dehydration and multisystem failure from diarrhea. If diarrhea is severe, refer the patient for emergent evaluation and treatment. In the hospital, the elderly patient should be treated aggressively with IV fluid therapy with close monitoring of the patient's cardiopulmonary status, renal status, and electrolytes. In cases of acute-onset diarrhea in which a viral cause is likely, provide symptomatic treatment to maintain hydration and electrolyte balance.

Follow-up: Schedule follow-up visits as indicated by the cause of the diarrhea. In the case of acute diarrhea, reevaluate the patient after 3 days of following the initial treatment plan. If diarrhea persists, diagnostic studies may be indicated and the patient's hydration status reevaluated.

Referral: Refer to the hospital for consideration of an inpatient stay if IV fluids and/or electrolyte replacements are needed or if diarrhea persists. The patient may need to be evaluated by a nephrologist or an infectious disease specialist depending on the causative agent of the patient's diarrhea. Complications may include dehydration, malnutrition, peritonitis, sepsis, shock, anemia, or electrolyte imbalances, which can be life threatening (such as with hypokalemia).

Prevention/prophylaxis: Prevention depends on the cause. Oral replacement of fluids is first and foremost, but in severe cases IV replacement may be warranted.

Careful cooking and storage of food is important to avoid spoilage. Check expiration dates on dairy and meat products before using. Clean cutting boards and utensils. Educate about cross-contamination when cooking, such as with raw meats, to prevent exposure to pathogens. For individuals who are traveling to a foreign country, begin appropriate prophylactic treatment (WHO, 2012). Caution travelers about avoiding undercooked foods, raw foods, buffet food and unpasteurized dairy products, tap water, and ice. Carbonated drinks, bottled water, and boiled water are considered safe for drinking and to use for oral hygiene.

Prevention of transmission of diarrhea in hospitals and long-term care facilities is extremely important. Frequent hand washing by patients and health-care providers is the key to preventing transmission of infectious diarrhea. Avoidance of long-term laxative use and prudent use of antimicrobial agents are also important in preventing diarrhea.

Education: Explain to the patient, family, and caregivers the cause of symptoms, diagnostic and treatment measures, follow-up, and preventive strategies. Emphasize the need for early intervention to prevent dehydration.

CLINICAL RECOMMENDATIONS	EVIDENCE RATING	REFERENCE
Classify diarrhea into three categories (watery, bloody, or fatty) based on the history, physical examination, and testing.	C	Shiu (2012)

Continued

CLINICAL RECOMMENDATIONS	EVIDENCE RATING	REFERENCE
Specific therapy depends on the underlying cause.	C	Shiu (2012)
Teach patients the signs and symptoms of dehydration.	C	Shiu (2012)
Metronidazole 500 mg PO 3 times a day for 10–14 days is the initial and most cost-effective treatment for *C. difficile* diarrhea.	A	Ibrahim & Yeldia (2011)

A = consistent, good-quality, patient-oriented evidence; B = inconsistent or limited-quality, patient-oriented evidence; C = consensus, disease-oriented evidence, usual practice, expert opinion, or case series. For information about the SORT evidence rating system, go to www.aafp.org/afpsort.xml.

DIZZINESS

Description: *Dizziness* is an imprecise term commonly used to describe various subjective symptoms. Dizziness is described as a disturbance in a person's sense of relationship to space, exemplified by a sensation of unsteadiness and a feeling of movement occurring within the head. The practitioner must understand the patient's personal meaning of dizziness to classify the symptom and determine its cause. The most frequently used categories of dizziness are vertigo, unsteadiness, lightheadedness, and disequilibrium.

Etiology: Dizziness may result from neurological, cardiovascular, or psychiatric causes; medications; sensory deficits; peripheral or central vestibular disorders; or mixed pathologies. Benign paroxysmal positional vertigo (BPPV) is a very common cause of vertigo in the elderly. It is a disorder arising from the inner ear and is often described as a spinning sensation.

Occurrence: Dizziness is a common symptom reported by older adults at a primary care visit.

Age: Dizziness is a common complaint in individuals over 60 years old, occurring in an estimated 30% of this age group and increasing to >50% in individuals over age 85. Presbystasis is age-related disequilibrium that cannot be attributed to any pathology and is characterized by a gradual onset of difficulty walking. People greater than age 70 who have a neurological deficit or who lack vertigo should be investigated for the cause of their dizziness, looking at medications, the cardiac system, and neurological systems thoroughly.

Ethnicity: Not significant.

Gender: Dizziness occurs more frequently in women.

Contributing factors: Factors contributing to dizziness in older adults include use of medications, particularly antihypertensives, anticonvulsants, psychotropic drugs, and ototoxic drugs. Changes in body systems with age can affect coordination and equilibrium and cause delays in recovery of balance. Altered sensitivity of the baroreceptors over time increases the vulnerability to presyncope, and the sensory and motor pathways are diminished with aging.

Signs and symptoms: The patient's description of the symptom should help determine the type of dizziness experienced. What does the patient mean by the word *dizzy*? The parameters of symptom assessment include the onset and trigger for the symptom, relieving or aggravating factors, symptom pattern, and associated symptoms. A careful medication review needs to be completed.

Vertigo: Patients describe episodic, short, sporadic episodes in which the environment or they are spinning; an illusion of movement, continuous or positional; or the sensation of being pushed. Associated symptoms include nausea, vomiting, unsteadiness, hearing loss, visual disturbances, and tinnitus.

Presyncope: Patients have the sensation one feels when about to faint. Associated symptoms include perspiration, pallor, palpitations, and syncope. The patient may be orthostatic or an arrhythmia may be present.

Disequilibrium: Patients describe a sense of imbalance. It may be a sensation localized to the body and relieved by bracing oneself, sitting, or lying down.

Associated symptoms are numbness, poor coordination, and general weakness. Gait difficulty, hearing loss, or speech impairment may also be noted.

Lightheadedness: Patients may describe this as feeling woozy. Often it is associated with anxiety or depression; autonomic signs may also be present.

Physical examination: The physical examination should be comprehensive and include the following components:

General: Observe how the patient moves around in the physician's office. Does he or she hold onto the furniture or walls? Check vital signs, especially postural blood pressure. A drop in systolic blood pressure of ≥ 20 mm Hg or diastolic of 10 mm Hg without normalization after 2 minutes is significant. It is important to determine whether the test of abruptly going from a lying to a sitting or standing position reproduces the patient's sensation. Check for an irregular heart rate and presence of fever.

Head, eyes, ears, nose, and throat examination: Test for extraocular movement, watching for nystagmus, and check corneal reflexes. Rotatory nystagmus suggests a peripheral cause of dizziness; vertical nystagmus suggests a central lesion. Check the patient's static monocular or binocular visual acuity and dynamic visual acuity (decrease in visual acuity with head movement). Perform a funduscopic examination, looking for papilledema. Inspect the ears for accumulation of fluid, bulging tympanic membrane, inflamed tympanic membrane, presence of cerumen impaction, or pus accumulation and discharge. Perform Weber's and Rinne's hearing tests if gross hearing is diminished. Acute hearing loss is associated with Ménière's disease, acoustic neuroma, and vestibular neuronitis.

Cardiovascular examination: Assessment should include central and peripheral function. Auscultate for heart sounds and arrythmia and check the carotid artery for bruit.

Neurological examination: Assessment includes cerebellar testing. If the patient points past the examiner's finger, suspect a vestibular lesion. Intentional tremor or abnormal alternating movements suggest cerebellar dysfunction (point-to-point). Perform sensory testing, position sense, and Romberg's test. Patients with cerebellar disease have difficulty standing with their feet together. Patients with decreased position sense are able to compensate with eyes open but sway with eyes closed. Perform gait assessment (such as the Get Up and Go Test); patients with cerebellar disease perform this maneuver poorly. Check deep tendon reflexes. Lower extremity weakness should be evaluated because this represents a fall risk. The inclusion of psychological tests (mental status, depression, anxiety) is appropriate if a psychogenic cause is suspected.

Special diagnostic and screening tests: Have the patient breathe 20 to 30 times/minute for 2 to 3 minutes (forced hyperventilation). This normally causes dizziness and finger and perioral numbness. Determine whether these are the same sensations the patient has been feeling; if so, the dizziness may be related to anxiety.

Have the patient march in place for 30 seconds with the eyes closed and arms extended in front. Be careful not to orient the patient with any sounds (e.g., your voice or a ticking clock). Patients with absent or reduced vestibular function (from prior vestibular damage) rotate more than 30° to 45° while marching.

For the Hallpike maneuver, assist the patient quickly to lay down on the examination table with the head hanging over the back of the table at about a 30° angle and the face turned 45° to the right. While holding the patient's head in place for 1 minute, observe the patient for nystagmus and ask whether this reproduces the dizziness (vertigo) symptoms. Bring the patient back to a sitting position and observe for 1 minute. Repeat the test with the head turned 45° to the left. If vertigo is reproduced, the test should be repeated two or three times on the side that caused the most severe symptoms to determine if the nystagmus and symptoms begin to disappear. Patients with benign postural vertigo experience severe vertigo 5 to 15 seconds after the head is turned and nystagmus is induced. Position change must be completed in 2 seconds, the signs typically fade in less than 1 minute, and repeated testing causes the symptoms to disappear. This test procedure may be modified if the patient is frail or has neck or back problems.

Diagnostic tests: There are no routine tests to evaluate the complaint of dizziness. If indicated by history, selected testing might be done: CBC for anemia, serum glucose for hypoglycemia, ECG or Holter monitoring for arrhythmia, audiometery if hearing loss is present, or vestibular function tests (such as videonystagmography or electronystagmography). Neuroimaging (CT or MRI) may be ordered if neurological symptoms are present.

Differential diagnosis: Differentiate between vertigo (a sensation of movement), lightheadedness (a sensation of being about to faint), and syncope (an actual loss of consciousness). If dizziness has a predictable pattern associated with it (e.g., mid to late morning, mid to late afternoon, 2 to 4 hours after eating), suspect hypoglycemia.

Treatment: Patients are treated according to the cause of the dizziness. Physical therapy may be the primary therapy mode or it may supplement other management approaches.

Depending on the cause, this might include balance retraining or vestibular rehabilitation. Patients with benign positional vertigo can perform therapeutic exercises, such as the Epley maneuver, which loosens particles out of the posterior semicircular canal and back into the utricle. If the cause of lightheadedness is medication side effects or volume deficiencies, adjustments are indicated. Support stockings may help to reduce pooling in the lower extremities. Management of cardiovascular, cerebrovascular, or psychogenic conditions is appropriate. Medications for dizziness (e.g., meclizine), although they are commonly prescribed, have not been rigorously tested and can worsen the symptoms of dizziness and have anticholinergic side effects, which is particularly problematic in the elderly.

Follow-up: Patients should return for follow-up visits if symptoms worsen, change from one type of dizziness to another, or do not resolve within 2 weeks.

Sequelae: Sequelae depend on the underlying cause of the dizziness. Older adults with dizziness are at high risk for both falling (and injury potential) and the fear of falling (and self-induced immobility). Almost 60% of dizzy older primary care patients experience moderate or severe impact on everyday life due to dizziness.

Prevention/prophylaxis: Teach older adults to move extremities before rising from positions held for any length of time to compensate for age-related changes in vascularity. Try to determine if dizziness is from medication side effects before adding additional medications to combat the dizziness.

Referral: If the etiology remains unclear, refer the patient to a specialist. Consider neurology, cardiology, eyes/nose/throat, or psychiatry as appropriate if the symptom persists and is disabling or a new abnormality is detected.

Education: Explain the underlying cause, rationale for treatment, and importance of exercises. Teach the patient the exercises and ask him or her to demonstrate. Explain that this condition may return intermittently for several years. Encourage the use of assistive devices for safety until the condition resolves. Placement of handrails in the bathroom and halls may assist with safe ambulation. If the condition worsens (e.g., the patient develops a fever, increased dizziness, or tinnitus), advise the patient to seek medical attention.

CLINICAL RECOMMENDATIONS	EVIDENCE RATING	REFERENCE
Balance disorders and dizziness are the second- and third-leading causes, respectively, of falls in older adults.	A	Rubenstein & Josephson (2006)
Performing a medication history and review is important for adjusting medications to prevent/resolve medication-related dizziness.	A	Shoair, Nyandge, & Slattum, (2011)
No routine tests are indicated in the diagnosis of dizziness, but check glucose levels in diabetics and monitor cardiac rhythm in those >45 years old.	C	Labuguen (2009)
Vestibular rehabilitation is a safe, effective management for unilateral peripheral vestibular dysfunction.	B	Hillier & McDonnel (2011)

A = consistent, good-quality, patient-oriented evidence; B = inconsistent or limited-quality, patient-oriented evidence; C = consensus, disease-oriented evidence, usual practice, expert opinion, or case series. For information about the SORT evidence rating system, go to www.aafp.org/afpsort.xml.

DYSPHAGIA

Description: Dysphagia is a swallowing disorder involving the inability to get the food from the mouth to the stomach. The problem is commonly divided into oropharyngeal (the inability to initiate the act of swallowing) and esophageal (the sensation of impeded transit through the esophagus).

Etiology: The causes of dysphagia are multiple and diverse. Aging does not cause clinical dysphagia; however, some normal changes of aging, such as changes in nerve and sensory function, pharyngeal swallow, loss of esophageal sphincter tone, and oral cavity changes (impaired masticatory function, reduced salivary flow, xerostoma), can contribute to or aggravate any swallowing problems. Oropharyngeal dysphagia is usually related to neuromuscular impairments of the tongue, pharynx, and upper esophageal sphincter. Stroke is the most common cause of oropharyngeal dysphagia in the elderly, but others include central nervous system disorders such as extrapyramidal syndromes, tumors, and Alzheimer's disease; myogenic disorders such as myasthenia gravis or myopathies; or structural disorders such as Zenker diverticulum, cricopharyngeal stenosis, or tumors. Esophageal dysphagia is usually a result of a motor disorder (e.g., muscular dystrophy, myasthenia gravis, scleroderma), a motility or neurological disorder (e.g., achalasia, multiple sclerosis, or amyotrophic lateral sclerosis), or an obstruction from either an intrinsic (carcinoma, stricture, web, diverticula) or an extrinsic (mediastinal tumors, vascular anomalies) source. Achalasia is characterized by slow progressive dysphagia for liquids and solids with weight loss, and its etiology is unknown. Esophagitis is another etiology, usually secondary to GERD, herpes virus, or a retained pill (primary offenders include NSAIDs, quinidine, potassium, ferrous sulfate, tetracycline, and alendronate). Drugs with dopamine antagonist action such as phenothiazines and metoclopramide can cause dystonia and dsykinesia leading to dysphagia.

Xerostoma (dry mouth) is common, occurring in 16% of elderly men and 25% of elderly women and adversely affects swallowing by impairing initiation and transport of food/fluid.

Occurrence: Swallowing disorders occur in about 20% of individuals over 50 years old and 60% to 80% of nursing home patients.

Age: Dysphagia occurs predominantly in older adults, because the causes for this problem primarily affect the elderly. Symptomatic dysphagia occurs in 16% of individuals over 87 years old.

Ethnicity: Not significant.

Gender: Dysphagia occurs equally in males and females, although this varies based on the etiology of the disorder.

Contributing factors: Factors that contribute to dysphagia include changes in swallowing with aging, such as decreased facial muscle and masticatory strength, delay in pharyngeal swallow, delay in emptying of the esophagus, and decreased lower esophageal sphincter relaxation. Medications with anticholinergic side effects (e.g., antidepressants, opiates, sedatives, antipsychotics, antispasmodics, antihistamines, and some antihypertensives) may produce slowing or disruptions of the oral phase of swallowing and affect salivation. Other drugs can increase the likelihood of reflux (e.g., calcium channel blockers, β-adrenergic agents, aspirin, theophylline, nitrates, vitamin C, and NSAIDs), particularly if the patient has inadequate fluid intake. Inadequate fluid intake with medication or meals may contribute to dysphagia.

Signs and symptoms: Symptoms typically associated with oropharyngeal dysphagia include difficulty initiating swallowing, food sticking in the throat, nasal regurgitation, and coughing during the swallow. The onset of symptoms may assist in the differential diagnosis because sudden onset may suggest a cerebrovascular event whereas insidious onset is more characteristic of a myopathy, multiple sclerosis, or amyotrophic lateral sclerosis. Voice changes (wet vocal quality) may be associated with swallowing incompetence. Patients with esophageal dysphagia most commonly present with a complaint that food is stuck in the chest (sternum or suprasternal area) and may report choking or a feeling of pressure sensation. Reflux symptoms may be present. If total obstruction occurs, salivation increases, and vomiting may result. Weight loss and aspiration pneumonia may occur.

Weight gain may be a sign of dysphagia if the patient consumes significant amounts of processed foods such as milkshakes that have a higher calorie count.

Careful history helps to distinguish the type of dysphagia. It is important for the clinician to distinguish between difficulty swallowing solids, liquids, or both. In general, patients with obstructions (strictures, webs) complain of solid rather than liquid dysphagia.

The time of the presentation of signs and symptoms is important because a rapid onset may indicate infection, irritation, or a food impaction, whereas a more insidious onset suggests a motor disorder. Physical examination consists of checking the oral cavity in conjunction with a neuromuscular examination. The mouth should be assessed for signs of irritation, ill-fitting dentures, and any pharyngeal masses. The head and neck should be examined, checking for lymph node or thyroid enlargement. Dentures may block palatal mechanoreceptors, which can lead to poor bolus control, oral transit delays, and longer feeding times.

Neurological evaluation must be comprehensive and include a mental status evaluation, cranial nerve examination, and muscle weakness. A bedside swallow assessment to determine aspiration risk is often inadequate and misleading, so additional diagnostics may be in order.

Diagnostic tests: Videofluoroscopy (modified barium swallow) is important to assess aspiration risk and guide therapy. Other tests that may be indicated based on the history and physical examination include testing the stool for occult blood and a CBC with indices if associated esophagitis is suspected. Ambulatory 24-hour pH testing of intraesophageal pH and pressures has been found to be useful when evaluating for GERD. If malnutrition is suspected, a serum albumin level is appropriate. Laboratory screening may be helpful to exclude metabolic, systematic, myogenic disease. MRI or CT is used if a cerebrovascular event is suspected. Fiberoptic endoscopic evaluation is an option when the patient cannot be transported to the radiology department for the modified barium swallow. Additional swallowing studies include radiography, and manometry may be indicated to identify specific abnormalities.

Differential diagnosis: It is important to differentiate whether the patient has a feeding problem (inability to present food to the mouth) or a swallowing problem (inability to get food from the mouth to the stomach) or both. Cognitive impairments frequently are associated with feeding problems. Determination of specific motor, neurological, or obstructive cause needs to be accomplished. For the patient complaining of burning associated with swallowing, reflux esophagitis, esophageal infection, and tablet-induced esophagitis need to be explored.

Treatment: Treatment always targets the specific cause, compensates for mechanical problems, and eliminates or minimizes aspiration risk. Therapeutic strategies include diet modification and swallowing posture or techniques. Management of dysphagia after a stroke is directed toward increasing the sensory awareness of food and improving bolus movement by the chin-tuck and double-swallow technique. A percutaneous endoscopic gastrostomy or nasogastric tube may be used to feed stroke patients at high risk for aspiration, but there is no guarantee it will prevent aspiration. A nutritionist works to ensure appropriate consistency and nutritional content. Stable patients can be treated as outpatients. Hospitalization may be required when dysphagia is associated with total or near-total obstruction of the esophageal lumen. Esophageal dilation (pneumatic or bougie), surgical intervention for an esophageal stent, or laser therapy for late cancer also may be part of the treatment plan, depending on the etiology of the dysphagia. Patients with esophageal spasms can be given calcium channel blockers, and those with associated esophagitis may receive antacids or H_2 blockers, or, in cases of severe esophagitis, a proton pump inhibitor.

Follow-up: Patient monitoring depends on the specific etiology of the dysphagia.

Sequelae: Complications from dysphagia depend on its cause. The most common complications are malnutrition, aspiration, pneumonia, and death. Of stroke patients with dysphagia, 45% to 68% die within 6 months, largely due to dysphagia related to nutritional and pulmonary complications.

Prevention/prophylaxis: People with dysphagia should remain upright with the head midline and slightly flexed when eating or drinking. Extremely hot or cold foods may worsen symptoms of dysphagia. Aspiration precautions include modifying food and fluid consistencies, giving verbal and physical prompts, and allowing additional time for feeding to encourage double swallows and small amounts taken per mouthful.

Referral: A gastroenterologist should be consulted for the endoscopy and for possible hospitalization of patients with severe dysphagia. Other referrals may include a speech therapist, radiologist, and dentist.

Education: Patients and caregivers should be encouraged to provide foods and fluids at appropriate consistency. All foods, especially meat products, should be chewed thoroughly. Patients also should be informed that it is important to swallow all medications with plenty of fluid while in an upright position.

CLINICAL RECOMMENDATIONS	EVIDENCE RATING	REFERENCE
Patients with cough and their caregivers should be questioned regarding swallowing problems and if positive further evaluation for dysphagia is indicated.	C	Smith, Hammond, & Goldstein (2006)
Patients with dysphagia should undergo videofluoroscopic swallow evaluation or fiberoptic-endoscopic evaluation of swallowing to identify appropriate treatment.	C	Smith et al. (2006)
Patients with a decrease in the level of consciousness are at high risk for aspiration and should not be fed until the level of consciousness has improved.	C	Smith et al. (2006)

A = consistent, good-quality, patient-oriented evidence; B = inconsistent or limited-quality, patient-oriented evidence; C = consensus, disease-oriented evidence, usual practice, expert opinion, or case series. For information about the SORT evidence rating system, go to www.aafp.org/afpsort.xml.

FALLS

Description: Although it may appear intuitive, there are many definitions as to what constitutes a fall. Some include the event that results from a seizure, syncope; some include the "breaking of a fall" when the care provider lowers the patient to the floor; and sometimes the terms *slip, trip, near fall,* and *fall* are used interchangeably. Clarity in the definition is essential when we question the patient or caregiver about history of falls, to ensure consistency in reporting of falls within an institutional setting, and for fall research purposes. A *fall* is defined here as an unplanned descent to the floor (or an extension of the floor) with or without injury to the patient.

Etiology: A fall is often a result of multiple, complex, and interrelated etiologies that involve both intrinsic and extrinsic factors. Studies have reflected some of the most influential factors are a history of falls, weakness, gait and balance disorders, functional impairments, cognitive impairments, vision and hearing impairments, and the use of multiple drugs and psychotropic drugs.

Occurrence: Falls are a common and serious cause of morbidity and mortality in older adults. Falls, especially those without injury, are underreported. Each year an estimated one-third of older adults fall, and approximately 10% of these falls result in an injury. Long-term care residents have about twice the rate of

falling as the elderly living in the community. Falls account for about 2% of adverse events during hospitalization, and the elderly are twice as likely to experience this event as younger hospitalized patients.

Age: The risk of falling increases with advancing age, with 50% of individuals over 80 years old experiencing a fall.

Ethnicity: No known difference.

Gender: Males and females are equally likely to fall, but women report more fall-related injuries.

Contributing factors: The risk of a fall increases as the number of fall risk factors increases (about 27% for those with no or one risk factor and 78% for those with four or more risk factors). Environmental factors contribute to falls, including slippery floors, uneven surfaces, inadequate lighting, improper footwear, trips over pets or toys, and so on.

Signs and symptoms: All older adults should be assessed for falling by asking how often they have fallen in the past year, if an injury was sustained, and if they sought medical attention. It may also be valuable to ask all older adults about near falls, trips, or slips to further determine risk. Those who have a prior fall history or gait and balance disorder should be further evaluated and targeted for a multidimensional fall risk assessment. The patient with a prior fall history should be asked about the use of walking aides, the environmental conditions, and the circumstances surrounding the fall in order to identify risk factors that are the target for effective interventions. The medication history should be detailed and complete. If the primary reason for the assessment is a recent fall, the patient should be evaluated for injury (fracture, bleed, skin tear). Additional physical examination should focus on neurological (cognitive, proprioception), musculoskeletal (range of motion and strength, gait and balance), and cardiac factors (including postural blood pressure) and continence. If the fall occurred in an accessible setting, an environmental assessment should be done. Standardized fall risk assessment tools are more reliable than individual judgment of fall risk, though they vary in sensitivity and specificity. None has been found to be useful among various populations and across settings. Balance and stability tests such as the Timed Get Up and Go Test and the Tinetti Balance and Gait Assessment have proven helpful.

Diagnostic tests: There are none specific to identify fall risk or injury risk. The x-ray, CT, or MRI used selectively may identify an injury. Blood work may be done selectively to identify the cause or contributing factor to a fall.

Differential diagnosis: The differential would focus on both the cause and contributing factors to the fall and whether syncope, seizure, stroke, vertebrobasilar insufficiency, or alcohol-related events constitute a fall by definition.

Treatment: The treatment would address any injury, as well as the underlying cause and contributing factors to the fall.

Follow-up: Because the highest risk factor for a fall is a previous fall, all patients should be monitored closely. A "postfall huddle" of the interprofessional team is helpful to identify what happened, why it happened, and what interventions could be put into place to prevent a future fall.

Sequelae: Although most falls do not result in injury, some result in minor injuries, major injuries, or even death. Injuries after a fall might result in a premature placement in a long-term care facility. After a fall many patients experience a fear of falling and subsequently decline in function. If an individual is not discovered quickly and cannot access help after a fall, it may result in dehydration, a pressure ulcer, or rhabdomyolysis.

Prevention/prophylaxis: Exercise has been the most widely studied single intervention for fall prevention with a focus on strength, balance, and endurance. Vitamin D treatment effectively reduces the risk of falls in older adults, though the optimum dose is not clear. Evidence is contradictory on multifactorial interventions in the prevention of falls, though it is still better than usual care. Cost-effectiveness of single interventions shows that management of psychotropic medications and tai chi exercises cost the most whereas the best value is in home modification and vitamin D supplements.

Referral: Individuals with major injuries after a fall warrant hospitalization. Based on the assessment of fall risk factors and physical examination findings, additional specialty experts will be needed. Referral for physical therapy, occupational therapy, and a home safety assessment is often appropriate.

Education: Patients and their families need to be instructed in how to manage both the intrinsic and extrinsic risk factors for falls and how to take the necessary safety precautions to prevent a future fall. They need to be encouraged to report all falls or near falls to the health-care provider so that interventions may be put in place in a timely way.

CLINICAL RECOMMENDATIONS	EVIDENCE RATING	REFERENCE
Balance, strength, and endurance training for fall prevention is effective.	A	Tinetti & Kumer (2010)
Vitamin D treatment effectively reduces the risk of falls in older adults.	A	Kalyani et al. (2010)
The most effective strategy for reducing the rate of falls is intervening in multiple fall risk factors.	A	Chang et al. (2004) Gillespie, Gillespie, & Robertson (2004) Tinetti & Kumer (2010)

CLINICAL RECOMMENDATIONS	EVIDENCE RATING	REFERENCE
All older persons should be asked about falls. Patients at risk for falling or who have fallen warrant a detailed fall-related assessment.	B	Kristopaitis & Homan (2009)
Medications should be reviewed and appropriately modified with particular attention to psychotropic medications and polypharmacy.	B	Gillespie et al. (2007)

A = consistent, good-quality, patient-oriented evidence; B = inconsistent or limited-quality, patient-oriented evidence; C = consensus, disease-oriented evidence, usual practice, expert opinion, or case series. For information about the SORT evidence rating system, go to www.aafp.org/afpsort.xml.

FATIGUE

Description: Fatigue is a subjective state often described as a feeling of tiredness, weariness, or exhaustion that is unrelieved or only partially relieved by rest and often results in a decreased capacity for physical or mental work. Occasional fatigue is common, but pathological fatigue impairs mental and physical capacity. Chronic fatigue syndrome occurs when fatigue lasts longer than 6 months and is not relieved with rest.

Etiology: Physiological fatigue occurs normally with inadequate rest, excess exertion, or insufficient diet. Fatigue that interrupts the patient's activities of daily life (ADLs) may have a physical or psychological cause and be either acute or chronic. Fatigue is commonly linked to sleep disorders, depression, heart disease, Parkinson's disease, anemia, and fibromyalgia and is often a reported symptom in patients with cancer. Fatigue in older adults may be an early indicator of the aging process. Medications commonly associated with fatigue include psychotropics, muscle relaxants, opioids, antihistamines, antihypertensives, and antibiotics, although often the symptom persists for a short period of time.

Occurrence: Fatigue occurs in about 20% of the U.S. population. Underreporting and underrecognition make the actual prevalence unknown.

Age: Fatigue is common among the elderly. Among elders living in assisted living facilities, more than 50% report mild fatigue and 7% report severe fatigue.

Ethnicity: Not significant.

Gender: Fatigue is more common in women than in men.

Contributing factors: Poor dietary habits, overexertion, alcohol abuse, smoking, stress, chronic illness, drug interactions, misuse of drugs, and sleep apnea may contribute to fatigue. In the elderly it is compounded by a decrease in muscle strength, loss of muscle neurons, a decrease in hormone levels, and lack of exercise.

Signs and symptoms: Obtain a complete medical history and perform a physical examination because fatigue may indicate various psychological or physiological illnesses. Conduct a complete symptom assessment, including the onset, duration, severity, and precipitating, aggravating, and relieving factors. Identify other indicators or associated symptoms of fatigue, which may include decreased energy expenditure, decreased endurance, sleep disturbance, attention deficits, somatic complaints (aching body, tired eyes), and weakness. Carefully review the adequacy of the diet, any medication side effects, and potential causes or contributing factors. Identify the impact fatigue is having on the person's ADLs and quality of life and current stressors. The quality and quantity of sleep should always be evaluated. A complete physical examination is indicated. Distinguish between generalized fatigue and actual weakness by testing for muscle strength and presence of localized tenderness. A mental status examination should be included to screen for dementia.

Diagnostic tests: The benefit of testing is limited when fatigue is the only symptom. Diagnostic tests on all patients with persistent unresolved fatigue should include CBC with differential, erythrocyte sedimentation rate (ESR), and/or C-reactive protein because these are low cost and offer significant screening capacity. Other tests that may be appropriate include liver function tests, electrolytes, thyroid function, urinalysis and additional renal tests as indicated, and pulmonary function tests. An ECG may reveal cardiac arrhythmias, enlargement of the heart, myocardial infarction, or abnormalities in the conduction system.

Masked hyperthyroidism may present with a chief complaint of fatigue.

Differential diagnosis: Fatigue can be related to many psychological and physiological etiologies. Psychiatric disorders including depression and generalized anxiety disorder account for 70% of cases of fatigue. An underlying cause is determined in only 10% of all cases. Fatigue that cannot be relieved by rest or sleep is often a sign of disease.

Treatment: Treatment depends on the etiology identified in the comprehensive workup. Symptom management includes regular exercise, attention-restoring activities, psychosocial techniques, energy conservation measures, and good sleep hygiene. Pharmacological management is directed at the cause of the fatigue.

Psychostimulants may be considered for opioid-related somnolence, cognitive impairment, and depression.

Follow-up: Follow-up depends on the findings. Monitor the patient periodically as indicated by diagnosis or symptoms, symptom persistence, and disability associated with the symptom. The symptom may be a subclinical one.

Sequelae: The potential for complications relates to the cause of fatigue and the impact the symptom has on the person's function.

Prevention/prophylaxis: Optimal health maintenance, including maintaining a healthy diet and regular exercise and good sleep hygiene, may prevent or enable early recognition of signs and symptoms of systemic or psychological illness.

Referral: Referral to a specialist may be indicated based on the results of the workup.

Education: If the fatigue has a physiological cause, teaching should be related to the findings; psychological counseling, changes in the environment, behavior modification, and stress reduction may be needed. The goal of fatigue management is to provide the patient with self-help tools to eliminate or alleviate fatigue.

CLINICAL RECOMMENDATIONS	EVIDENCE RATING	REFERENCE
A thorough history and physical examination are crucial in determining the differential diagnosis and identifying the causative agent.	C	Bono & Sheflin (2011)
Graded aerobic exercise has been shown to improve symptoms and physical function in patients with fatigue.	A	Larun et al. (2009)
Cognitive-behavioral therapy is an effective treatment for adult outpatients with chronic fatigue syndrome.	A	Whiting et al. (2001)

A = consistent, good-quality, patient-oriented evidence; B = inconsistent or limited-quality, patient-oriented evidence; C = consensus, disease-oriented evidence, usual practice, expert opinion, or case series. For information about the SORT evidence rating system, go to www.aafp.org/afpsort.xml.

HEADACHE

Description: Headache refers to multiple problems in which the primary symptom is pain in the head, neck, or face. Headache is one of the most commonly encountered problems in primary care of older adults. Although the incidence of headache decreases with age, the problem interferes with optimal functioning and quality of life. Most causes of headache are benign, but some are life threatening. Multiple types of headaches exist. Tension headaches are the most common and are due to mostly extracranial causes, such as muscle tension. Migraine headaches decrease with age, although more than half of elderly patients who have an existing diagnosis of migraine continue to have active disease past age 65.

Occurrence: Headache is one of the 10 most common symptoms seen in primary care. In any year, 5% of all people in the United States seek medical care for headaches. Current estimates are that 90% of all people have headaches, with 45 million individuals reporting recurring headache.

Age: Headache is a common complaint in the elderly. The incidence of headache decreases with age; patients aged 65 to 74 have a 1-year headache prevalence of 56.7%, and patients aged 85 to 96 have a 1-year prevalence rate of 26.1%.

Ethnicity: Giant cell arteritis is more common in Caucasian populations. Ethnicity does not appear to be related to other headache types.

Gender: Women are affected more often than men; 76% of women and 57% of men report one headache per month. Migraine headaches are more common in women than in men, tending to begin in early adulthood. Cluster headaches are more common in men than in women, with a mean age of onset at 30 years. Giant cell arteritis is more commonly seen in women.

Contributing factors: Depending on the type of headache, multiple factors can contribute. Poor posture, cervical osteoarthritis, ill-fitting dentures, tooth pain, and jaw disorders can contribute to tension headaches. Depression, anxiety, sleep disorders, and general pain syndromes can also contribute to most headache types. Medication side effects, particularly with estrogen, calcium channel blockers, nitrates, anti-Parkinson's drugs, indomethacin, and theophylline, can contribute to headaches. Alcohol can trigger or worsen headaches. Migraine can be triggered by dietary factors such as aged or smoked cheese, chocolate, caffeine, and monosodium glutamate, as well as changes in sleep pattern, weather changes, and smoking. Genetics may play a role in migraine, cluster headache, and giant cell arteritis.

Signs and symptoms: Diagnosis of headache is frequently made on the basis of history because the physical examination is often normal. Headaches are characterized by manifestations including onset, location, duration, frequency, severity, character, triggering or aggravating factors, and alleviating factors. Associated symptoms are elicited and might include nausea and vomiting, eye tearing, nasal congestion, teeth grinding, and neck pain. For recurrent headaches, having the patient keep a headache diary is helpful in identifying patterns and identifying the impact the symptom has on function. Input from family and caregivers on the impact of the headaches on daily life is helpful.

Past history should be explored for a history of migraine or head trauma, and family history should be explored for migraine, cluster headache, or giant cell arteritis. Medications should be reviewed thoroughly. Alcohol and smoking consumption should be examined, because they frequently intensify headaches.

The physical examination should include observation of general appearance, including facies, and evaluation of mental status. Any sudden change in mental status or mood should be evaluated swiftly. Assess vital signs for extremes in blood pressure, which suggest a neurological event. Examine the head and palpate for tenderness, signs of trauma, pain over the temporal artery, and strength of the temporal arterial pulse. Test the cranial nerves. Perform a funduscopic examination to assess for papilledema, hemorrhages, exudates, and venous pulsations. Check for pupillary size and look at the cornea for haziness. Check extraocular movements and position of the eyelids. Evaluate gross and fine motor and sensory functions, including gait, balance, and tactile sense. Test deep tendon reflexes for presence and symmetry; measure muscle strength for grading and equality.

Conduct an examination of the head and neck for lymphadenopathy, thyroid enlargement, carotid bruits, trigger points, meningeal irritation, or limitation in normal range of motion. Check the temporomandibular joint for alignment, mobility, and clicking. Examine the ears, nose, throat, and teeth for contributing problems. Evaluate the patient for postural alignment problems, muscle spasms, or trigger points in the back or shoulders.

Differential diagnosis: Symptoms of headaches of various types and etiologies can mimic each other. Potentially serious causes include temporal arteritis, stroke, brain lesions, infectious disease, and hemorrhage. Severe or persistent pain, sudden-onset headaches that worsen over time, and early-morning head pain suggest an organic etiology.

Migraines are often unilateral, throbbing in quality, and associated with nausea and vomiting, photophobia, phonophobia, and visual disturbances. A prodrome may exist for several days before the onset of the headache and consists of fatigue, dizziness, aching muscles, stiff neck, change in mood and behavior, neurological changes, and loss of appetite. An aura is often present just before the onset of the headache and most commonly includes some type of visual phenomena. The headache onset is gradual, but the headache may linger for many days, is aggravated by exertion, and may only be relieved by vomiting or sleep. Most patients will experience a postdromal period following the headache that includes fatigue, lethargy, and depression. Migraine syndromes generally start in young adulthood but then persist throughout life. The characteristics of the migraine and accompanying symptoms have not been found to significantly differ in patients over 60 years old.

Tension headaches are bilateral and pressing in quality, are not aggravated by exertion, and last minutes to days. Often they are accompanied by muscular pain and stiffness. Generally, these are not accompanied by other symptoms such as nausea, vomiting, or visual changes. Daily activities are not disrupted by tension headaches. A variant of the tension headache is the chronic daily headache, with prevalence between 3.9% and 4.4% in individuals over 65 years old. The most common reason for the daily headache is overuse of analgesic medications. Daily headaches can present with migraine-like or tension-type characteristics. The treatment is generally to wean the patient from the analgesics and substitute more nonpharmacological approaches to treating the pain.

The cluster headache is characterized by severe unilateral orbital, periorbital, or temporal pain. The attacks are relatively short (15 to 90 minutes) but can recur up to 8 times in 1 day. The pain is worse in the supine position, which makes the patient very restless, and the patient often wants to pace or rock back and forth during an attack. There have been reports of patients committing suicide during an attack, due to the intensity of the pain. Autonomic symptoms are also associated with the pain and present as ipsilateral ptosis, miosis, lacrimation, rhinorrhea, and nasal congestion.

Some headaches may suggest a much more life-threatening situation. These are the headaches associated with hemorrhage, vasculitis, stroke, infectious disease, and acute angle-closure glaucoma. The most common acute cerebral bleed is a subarachnoid hemorrhage, which has its highest incidence in women greater than 70 years old, with a history including smoking, excessive alcohol ingestion, and hypertension. This individual generally presents with a "thunderclap" or the "worst headache of my life." The pain may be associated with other symptoms, such as confusion, vomiting, and seizures. This individual should be transported to the emergency department for a CT scan and of possibly surgery. More commonly, an elderly patient may present with a chronic subdural hematoma, which is defined as one that is more than 20 days old. The peak incidence is in ages 60 to 80 and up to 80% of the cases are in men. Most often a chronic subdural hematoma is associated with a fall or other type of minor trauma. Typically, they present with a headache and a change in mental status. The headache is described as mild and generalized all over the head. Although the individual does not appear to be in great distress, he or she should be transferred immediately, preferably to a location where neurosurgical consultation is possible.

Giant cell arteritis occurs predominantly in middle-aged and elderly individuals, with an average age of onset of 70 years. Women are affected more frequently than men. It generally presents with a temporal headache, along with some visual symptoms such as amaurosis, diplopia, and visual loss. Muscle pain and tension may also occur. Headache may also warn of an impending stroke but only in about 25% of all ischemic strokes. The incidence in hemorrhagic strokes is 40% to 60%. Infectious diseases, such as encephalitis and meningitis, may also present with a headache. Generally, both include other symptoms such as fever, altered mental status, and nuchal rigidity. The mortality rate for meningitis in patients older than 65 years is as high as 50% to 70%. When infectious disease is suspected, the patient should be immediately transferred.

Acute angle-closure glaucoma is an emergency more frequently seen in women. The first symptom generally experienced is the sudden onset of severe unilateral head pain. Normally, this is associated with nausea, vomiting, and blurred vision. On examination, the pupil is midposition and the cornea appears hazy. This presentation is considered a serious emergency, and the patient should be seen immediately by an ophthalmologist, because the main treatment is decreasing intraocular pressure.

Diagnostic tests: Individualize diagnostic tests according to the suspected cause of the symptom. Neuroimaging sometimes is indicated for emergency evaluation of suspected vascular, neoplastic, or infectious disease. Generally, MRI is preferred to CT scan. MRI is considered if the headache is of sudden onset, severe, worsening, unresponsive to treatment, and associated with neurological or constitutional symptoms. Blood tests are generally not helpful, unless anemia, infection, or electrolyte imbalance is suspected. ESR or C-reactive protein may be indicated if an inflammatory condition, such as giant cell arteritis, is under consideration. An elevated ESR warrants referral of the patient for temporal artery biopsy to confirm diagnosis. If thyroid abnormalities are a possibility, perform thyroid function studies. A lumbar puncture should be done for cerebrospinal fluid analysis if a diagnosis of subarachnoid hemorrhage or infection is being considered, although about 30% of lumbar punctures result in a low cerebrospinal fluid headache. Sinus or cervical spine x-rays may be indicated.

Treatment: Treatment of headache depends on its cause. Analgesics such as acetaminophen, aspirin, and NSAIDs in appropriate doses may be used cautiously. Caution is advised when using opioids in the treatment of headaches, because these have been known to cause rebound headaches and can lead to overuse of medications, which causes headaches. Nonpharmacological treatment, including biofeedback, imagery, progressive relaxation techniques, and other stress management strategies, should be tried initially for tension headaches. Additional treatments that may be effective include acupuncture, acupressure, transcutaneous electrical nerve stimulation, massage, intermittent use of a cervical collar, heat or cold application, and resting in a darkened room.

For frequent headaches, including daily, migraine, and cluster, prophylactic therapy may be instituted to prevent development of and decrease the impact of symptoms. Medication is taken daily for a trial period (usually 1 to 2 months) to evaluate the effect on headache frequency and strength. All categories of drugs should be started at low doses and incrementally increased to therapeutic dosing. Although beta blockers (propranolol [Inderal LA], 80 mg orally daily; atenolol [Tenormin], 50 to 100 mg orally daily; or nadolol [Corgard], 40 mg orally daily) have been used

prophylactically for migraine and cluster headaches, they are contraindicated in patients with a history of bronchospastic disease, asthma, diabetes, or congestive heart failure. ACE inhibitors (lisinopril) and angiotensin II receptor blockers have also been found to be effective for prophylaxis. However, the beta blockers continue to be the most effective.

Calcium channel blockers (verapamil, 240 mg orally daily in divided doses, or nifedipine, 30 to 180 mg orally daily) also have been used prophylactically to prevent migraines. Contraindications include congestive heart failure, heart block, hypotension, sick sinus syndrome, and atrial fibrillation. Antidepressants have been found to be effective for prophylaxis. Low doses of tricyclic antidepressants (amitriptyline [Elavil], 25 to 50 mg orally daily, or desipramine [Norpramin], 50 mg orally daily) have been used for prevention, although these agents may be contraindicated because of adverse effects on the cardiovascular system or anticholinergic effects. More recently, the serotonin/norepinephrine reuptake inhibitor (SNRI) venlafaxine (37.5 mg once a day, dosage range from 75 to 150 mg once a day) has been effective. However, SNRIs can be started at very low doses and titrated until effective.

Anticonvulsants have been found to be among the most effective agents for prophylaxis. Valproic acid (250 to 500 mg in daily divided doses), topiramate (100 to 200 mg in divided doses), and gabapentin (900 to 2400 mg/day) have been used successfully, particularly for migraine management. Each anticonvulsant can increase fatigue, and baseline liver and kidney function studies should be obtained before initiation. Topamax can cause kidney stones, so it is important that the patient increase fluids while taking the medication.

For abortive treatment of migraine or cluster headache, if nonprescription analgesics such as aspirin and acetaminophen are ineffective, the triptans are generally used. These drugs are categorized as selective serotonin agonists (e.g., sumatriptan) and have been used with some success in adults; however, there are general contraindications in patients with coronary artery disease or peripheral vascular disease, limiting their use in older patients. General guidelines now suggest that the first dose of the drug should be given under medical supervision for patients with risk factors but no known coronary heart disease. This group includes postmenopausal women and patients with controlled vascular risk factors such as diabetes mellitus, hypercholesterolemia, and hypertension. Various forms of the triptans are available in oral, injectable, and nasal forms. In cluster headaches, the same drugs may work in some cases, and if not contraindicated, prednisone, 40 to 60 mg orally daily for 1 week, then tapered off for another week, also may be prescribed. Intranasal lidocaine 4% topical solution, 1 mL in the nostril corresponding to the location of the headache, also has been effective in relieving migraine or cluster headaches. Ergotamine and dihydroergotamine (DHE 45) are effective in migraine treatment but are contraindicated for the elderly due to their effects on peripheral and central circulation. Botulinum toxin has been studied for the treatment of migraine and tension headaches; however, there is currently no evidence of efficacy.

For giant cell arteritis and cluster headaches, patients may take prednisone, 40 to 60 mg daily for several weeks, then tapered gradually to 10 to 20 mg daily and continued for 18 months. Long-term steroid therapy of this nature has important implications related to immune system function, GI bleeding, and bone deterioration. Additional medications for symptomatic care, such as antiemetics, should be used as needed.

Follow-up: Monitoring depends on cause and treatment strategies. Patients should be monitored for effectiveness of treatment. To ensure adjustment to the prophylactic regimen, patients and their caregivers should be seen frequently.

Sequelae: Sequelae depend on cause. Missed diagnosis of acute, life-threatening symptoms can prove fatal.

Most common causes have recurrence or chronicity, which affects quality of life. Potential for side effects from medications and medication overuse must be considered.

Prevention/prophylaxis: Preventive measures include avoidance of triggers, early intervention with medication as soon as symptoms present, and stress reduction techniques as appropriate. Use of alcohol, tobacco, and caffeine, in specific types of headache, should be monitored.

Referral: Refer patients to collaborating physician or neurologist when headaches associated with hemorrhage, vasculitis, stroke, infectious disease, or acute angle-closure glaucoma is suspected. Any abnormal MRI or CT scan results should be referred to a neurologist. Symptoms to warrant rapid referral to a facility with neurological and neurosurgical services include the following:

▓ Headache associated with any neurological changes
▓ Sudden change in mental status
▓ Headache associated with a fall or other unusual event
▓ New-onset migraine headache
▓ Patient complaint of the "worst headache" ever experienced

Education: Teach patients how to live with a chronic or recurrent problem, to avoid triggers, to reduce stress, and to promote self-care. If medications are prescribed, ensure that the patient understands proper use and safety considerations.

CLINICAL RECOMMENDATIONS	EVIDENCE RATING	REFERENCE
Nonpharmacological treatments for headache that might be effective include acupuncture, acupressure, transcutaneous electrical nerve stimulation, massage, intermittent use of a cervical collar, heat or cold application, and resting in a darkened room.	B	Diener et al. (2006) Linde et al. (2005)
Angiotensin-converting enzyme (ACE) inhibitors and angiotensin II receptor blockers (ARBs) have been found to be effective for prophylaxis of migraine; however, the beta blockers continue to be most effective.	A	Lim (2013)

CLINICAL RECOMMENDATIONS	EVIDENCE RATING	REFERENCE
Caution is advised when using opioids in the treatment of headaches, because these have been known to cause rebound headaches.	C	Lim (2013)
Image all patients with focal neurological deficits.	B	Detsky et al. (2006)

A = consistent, good-quality, patient-oriented evidence; B = inconsistent or limited-quality, patient-oriented evidence; C = consensus, disease-oriented evidence, usual practice, expert opinion, or case series. For information about the SORT evidence rating system, go to www.aafp.org/afpsort.xml.

HEMATURIA

Description: Hematuria is present when there are red blood cells in the urine. It can be classified as having either gross or microscopic blood in the urine. Gross hematuria is suspected when the urine appears either red or brown in color to the naked eye. Microscopic hematuria is identified usually by a urine sample being sent to the laboratory or when the urine is tested with a dipstick. The American Urological Association (AUA) defines clinically significant microscopic hematuria as three or more RBCs per high-power field on three or more samples of urine.

Etiology: Hematuria may result from glomerular or nonglomerular causes. Microscopic hematuria is a common finding on routine urinalysis of adults, and the etiologies range from life threatening to incidental causes. The most typical clinical situation for finding hematuria is during the evaluation of a patient suspected of having a urinary tract infection. The pathophysiology depends on the anatomical site from which blood loss occurred.

Occurrence: In patients older than 50 years of age the prevalence is estimated at 13%. The prevalence of asymptomatic microscopic hematuria ranges from 19% to 21%.

Age: Incidence increases with age. The younger the patient, the less likely it is that the etiology will be identified.

Ethnicity: Not significant.

Gender: Slightly higher incidence in females.

Contributing factors: The following are all contributing factors related to the development of a malignancy: age of more than 40 years, history of smoking, occupational exposures such as to chemicals or dyes (painters, printers, chemical plant workers), persistent gross hematuria, history of chronic cystitis, history of pelvic irradiation, any exposures to cytotoxic agents such as cyclophosphamide, ifosfamide, plus any history of analgesic abuse. Other contributing factors may be infection, kidney stone, trauma, anatomical defects such as rectocele, and anticoagulation therapy. A noticeable risk of malignancy is present in older patients (over 40 years old) even with transient hematuria.

Signs and symptoms: Obtaining the history is important in the assessment of hematuria. Ask about a history of vigorous exercise, recent prostate examination, vigorous exercise, and medications (analgesics, antibiotics, anticoagulants, NSAIDs). Gross hematuria would be recognizable by the red or brownish color of the urine, but there may not be any signs or symptoms related to microscopic hematuria. A patient may report urinary frequency or dysuria, which may indicate a urinary tract infection. Any complaints of flank pain, fever, chills, nausea or vomiting, or abdominal pain may represent kidney disease or a stone. An elevated creatinine may be indicative of renal disease. The physical examination would focus on abdominal and/or flank pain. Because the history and physical often fail to diagnose the etiology of hematuria, all patients need to be evaluated with diagnostic tests for glomerular disease.

Diagnostic tests: A urinalysis should be obtained and then repeated after a few days to confirm hematuria. If the patient is on anticoagulation therapy, a prothrombin time (PT), international normalized ratio (INR), and CBC may need to be obtained. Also, note if the patient is taking any other medications that would affect platelet function or decrease clotting abilities. If an infection is present, treat the infection and wait 6 weeks to repeat the urinalysis. If hematuria is persistent, obtain a comprehensive metabolic panel to correct any metabolic disarray. If the creatinine is elevated, kidney disease is likely contributing to the hematuria. A noncontrasted CT urography or IV pyelogram is indicated if there is suspicion for a stone, renal mass, or pelvicalyceal and ureteric transitional cell carcinomas. Cystoscopy is indicated in patients older than 40 years of age or patients younger than 40 if no other reason for hematuria is present. Cystoscopy is also used to diagnose bladder or prostatic cancers as well. Urine cytology is useful to identify the presence of any transitional or neoplastic cells (Up to Date, 2012). Urine dipstick evaluation may be misleading because it lacks the ability to distinguish red blood cells from myoglobin or hemoglobin.

Differential diagnosis: May include infection, glomerular disease, kidney stone, bladder cancer, trauma, anatomical defects, or too much anticoagulation therapy resulting in hematuria.

Treatment: Treatment is directed at the cause. If a stone is present, initial treatment may be hydration and narcotics or lithotripsy if the stone is too large to pass. Treating any urinary tract infection with the appropriate antibiotics may be all that is needed. Correcting metabolic disarray may also clear up the hematuria. If the patient is on anticoagulation therapy, medication adjustment may resolve the problem. If a glomerular source is ruled out, radiological imaging may be indicated to assess further for the cause of hematuria.

Follow-up: A repeat urinalysis should be obtained 6 weeks after initial treatment for any infection to make sure that the hematuria has cleared.

Referral to a nephrologist may be needed if hematuria persists. For those with idiopathic microscopic hematuria, a repeat at 6 months is appropriate.

Sequelae: Hematuria may be a sign of a malignancy and should not be ignored even if it occurs transiently. Hematuria may mean renal disease, especially when proteinuria is present. When in doubt, refer to a nephrologist for a second opinion. A diagnosis of a kidney stone does not rule out the coexistence of a malignancy.

Prevention/prophylaxis: The U.S. Preventive Services Task Force does not endorse routine screening for hematuria due to lack of effectiveness.

Referral: Have patient see his or her primary care provider initially to obtain preliminary testing to verify presence of hematuria. Refer to a nephrologist for proteinuria, red cell casts, and elevated serum creatinine levels. Patients with hematuria persisting after treatment for a urinary tract infection need to be evaluated as well. Of patients referred for evaluation of hematuria or specialty care, 2% to 13% have a urological malignancy—a risk highest among older men.

Education: Counsel patients and family members to seek medical advice about gross hematuria, plus signs and symptoms to report such as urinary frequency, dysuria, flank pain, and abdominal pain. Educate patients and families about side effects of OTC medications and prescribed medications. Educate the patient about the effects of anticoagulation therapy and to call immediately if the patient notices any hematuria, because this may mean the patient's drug levels are too high.

CLINICAL RECOMMENDATIONS	EVIDENCE RATING	REFERENCE
Although screening asymptomatic patients is not generally recommended, microscopic hematuria is still diagnosed incidentally by urine dipstick.	B	McDonald, Swagerty, & Wetzel (2006) USPSTF (2004)
The AUA recommends patients >40 years old and those who are younger but have risk factors for bladder cancer obtain cystoscopy to complete the evaluation for microscopic hematuria.	C	Grossfield et al. (2001)

CLINICAL RECOMMENDATIONS	EVIDENCE RATING	REFERENCE
Urinary dipsticks are useful in the detection of asymptomatic microscopic hematuria, although they cannot determine the source of the bleed.	B	Kaplan, Caloagu, & Slawson (2011)

A = consistent, good-quality, patient-oriented evidence; B = inconsistent or limited-quality, patient-oriented evidence; C = consensus, disease-oriented evidence, usual practice, expert opinion, or case series. For information about the SORT evidence rating system, go to www.aafp.org/afpsort.xml.

HEMOPTYSIS

Description: Coughing or spitting blood from the respiratory tract can either be described as blood-streaked or frank bleeding such as coughing up more than 100 to 600 mL in 24 hours, which is indicative of massive hemoptysis.

Etiology: There are many causes of hemoptysis. Hemoptysis refers to bleeding from the lower respiratory tract but it can also originate from the upper respiratory tract and the upper GI tract, which may mimic hemoptysis. There are multiple potential causes for hemoptysis, including, but not limited to, airway disease and trauma, pulmonary infections or inflammation, lung neoplasms, cardiac disease, cocaine use, and medication use (anticoagulant, antithrombotic, NSAIDs). The lungs receive blood from the pulmonary and bronchial arterial systems, and the low-pressure pulmonary system produces small-volume hemoptysis whereas the high-pressure bronchial system produces profuse bleeding. Infection causes mucosal inflammation that can lead to blood vessel rupture, and neoplasms cause mucosal invasion, which erodes the blood vessels. In the primary care setting the most common causes of hemoptysis are acute and chronic bronchitis, pneumonia, TB, and lung cancer.

Occurrence: The most common culprit of hemoptysis is airway disease. There is a strong seasonal trend with a peak incidence in the spring and a decreased incidence in late summer.

Age: May occur at any age.

Ethnicity: No direct ties to ethnicity have been documented, but immigrants and persons living in poverty are at higher risk for TB and other pulmonary infections.

Gender: No gender-specific factors.

Contributing factors: Smoking history of active or passive exposure, alcohol use, cocaine use, and any history of trauma, environmental exposures, hypertension, comorbidities, or medications such as aspirin, NSAIDs, or anticoagulants can either be causative or contributing factors. The following risk factors are associated with an increased risk of finding a malignancy with bronchoscopy: male sex, older than 40, greater than 40-pack-per-year smoking history, and duration of hemoptysis longer than a week.

Signs and symptoms: The quantity and characteristics of the blood and the length of time the symptoms have been occurring are the first questions to ask when assessing the patient. Also, has it increased in severity? Is the cough worse at night? What other associated symptoms are present? Hemoptysis of more than 100 mL in under 24 hours is potentially life threatening and requires treatment in an emergency department. Any sudden onset of hemoptysis with or without any other associated symptoms can be caused by a pulmonary embolism and needs emergent treatment. A comprehensive history of the disease, the patient's known risk factors, and the work and home environment are all helpful in narrowing the cause of the hemoptysis. Ask about signs and symptoms of infection (fever, cough, sputum production), malignancy (cachexia, weight loss, smoking history), trauma or foreign body, and immune deficiency, and complete a medication review.

Risk factors such as smoking, cocaine use, long-term alcohol abuse, stroke, older age, emigrant status, HIV positive status, and any heart disease are important to assess in trying to find the cause of bleeding. Use of tobacco with long-standing or increasingly severe hoarseness may indicate cancer of the mouth or throat. A history of persistent "heartburn" may be a clue to possible esophageal erosion as the source of bleeding. Chronic cough, dyspnea, and/or sputum production may suggest pulmonary disease.

Vital signs should include oxygen saturation. The physical examination should begin with a thorough examination of the nose and oropharyngeal mucosa. The lymph nodes in the neck and chest should be palpated to assess for infection, lymphoma, or other malignancies.

The chest must be assessed for abnormal sounds. Diminished or absent lung sounds by auscultation and dullness to percussion are highly suggestive of pneumonia. Rhonchi or crackles with cardiomegaly on x-ray or ECG indicate congestive heart failure (CHF). A prominent first heart sound, early diastolic snap, and rumbling diastolic murmur are signs of mitral valve stenosis. A patient's abdomen distended owing to ascites is likely to be accompanied by esophageal varices. The amount of blood loss usually is overestimated by patients and physicians, but an attempt to determine the volume and rate of blood loss should be made.

Diagnostic tests: The test of choice is the chest x-ray or chest CT. Diagnostic workup may also include the following laboratory tests: CBC, coagulation studies, comprehensive metabolic panel, arterial blood gas, sputum culture and smear, purified protein derivative, INR, d-dimer, ESR, CT angiogram, or bronchoscopy. A flexible bronchoscopy is useful even if the radiological studies are normal to rule out the possibility of an early neoplasm.

Differential diagnosis: Determine first if the blood is coming from the respiratory tract (hemoptysis) or from the GI tract (hematemesis). Patients with hematemesis typically have nausea and vomiting and a history of gastric or liver disease. The sputum more likely will be coffee ground in texture and a brown/black color. In hemoptysis the sputum is bright red or pink and a frothy liquid or clotted, and the patient has a history of lung disease. If the lung is determined to be the etiology, consider the possibility of infection, inflammation, malignancies, trauma, autoimmune disease, cardiovascular disease, and coagulopathy disorders, among others.

Treatment: The goals of management include bleeding cessation, aspiration prevention, and treatment of underlying cause. If the source of the bleeding has been reasonably isolated to the respiratory system and the condition is not life threatening, and if an infectious or inflammatory etiology is diagnosed, the following might be considered.

Acute bronchitis: Acute bronchitis is predominantly viral, and antibiotics do not shorten the course of the disease. If the patient smokes, he or she should be counseled to quit or to cut back significantly. Bronchodilators help open the airways; expectorants such as guaifenesin used to mobilize secretions are about as effective as drinking two additional glasses of water per day. Cough suppressants should be avoided except to help the patient sleep. A cool mist humidifier in the bedroom is useful in loosening secretions.

Chronic bronchitis: Chronic bronchitis needs a combination bronchodilator as an inhaler or as a nebulizer. Because chronic bronchitis is usually a result of smoking, the patient should be counseled to stop. Antibiotics or oral steroids should be reserved for acute exacerbations heralded by increasing shortness of breath, change in the color of the sputum to dark yellow or green, or fever.

Bacterial pneumonia: Pneumonia is most often caused by *Staphylococcus*, *Klebsiella*, or *Pseudomonas* in the otherwise healthy individual. If pneumonia is suspected, broad-spectrum antibiotic therapy should be initiated empirically. Immunocompromised patients, patients with any respiratory distress, and elderly patients with significantly low or elevated WBC counts may need to be hospitalized.

Fungal infection: A fungal infection should be suspected if the pneumonia does not respond to conventional antibiotic therapy. Appropriate antifungal therapy may be initiated, and the patient should be referred to a pulmonologist.

Tuberculosis: Antituberculosis drugs should be begun with a positive Mantoux test and/or a positive chest x-ray and the patient referred to the health department for reporting purposes.

Follow-up: The tenacity of follow-up depends on the severity of the illness. For pneumonia or bronchitis with minimal dyspnea, a call to check on the patient is appropriate. Worsening temperature, bleeding, or difficulty breathing requires immediate attention or emergency department evaluation. Patients with resolving pneumonia should be evaluated in 2 to 3 weeks.

Mild hemoptysis recurring sporadically over a few years is common in smokers who have chronic bronchitis punctuated with superimposed acute bronchitis.

Sequelae: Death can occur if the etiology is not identified quickly and treated, particularly if it causes cardiovascular collapse or acute respiratory insufficiency. The mortality rate depends on the etiology, and in patients with a malignancy and massive hemoptysis (more than 1000 mL/24 hours) the rate is 80%. Chronic lung disease may also result.

Prevention/prophylaxis: Counseling patients and their families about the benefits of smoking cessation and to decrease alcohol intake are worthwhile. Discussions to promote a healthy lifestyle are important, stressing activity and weight loss.

Referral: Massive hemoptysis requires treatment in the intensive care unit and pulmonary and cardiovascular surgeon consultation. If hemoptysis persists or increases, the patient may need to be referred to a pulmonologist for either bronchoscopy or laryngoscopy. Radiological imaging such as CT scan may be needed to rule out neoplasm followed by a referral to a surgeon or an oncologist.

Education: Discuss risk factors associated with pulmonary embolism such as immobility or hormonal replacement therapies. Provide patient education related to smoking cessation and cessation of street drugs and/or alcohol abuse.

CLINICAL RECOMMENDATIONS	EVIDENCE RATING	REFERENCE
The initial test of choice is a chest x-ray. A high-resolution CT is appropriate for patients with parenchymal disease identified by the x-ray.	C	McGuiness et al. (1994) Tasker & Flower (1999)
Patients with a mass on chest x-ray and those at risk for cancer should have a flexible bronchoscopy.	B	Colice (1997) O'Neil & Lazarus (1991)
Massive hemoptysis is a respiratory emergency. CT angiography (CTA) can play a crucial role in assessing the cause and origin of hemoptysis and directing the interventional radiologist before treatment.	C	Noe, Jaffe, & Molan (2011)
After careful assessment initially, closely follow smokers >40 years who have unexplained hemoptysis.	C	Bidwell & Pachner (2005)

A = consistent, good-quality, patient-oriented evidence; B = inconsistent or limited-quality, patient-oriented evidence; C = consensus, disease-oriented evidence, usual practice, expert opinion, or case series. For information about the SORT evidence rating system, go to www.aafp.org/afpsort.xml.

INVOLUNTARY WEIGHT LOSS

Description: Involuntary weight loss occurs when the number of calories available is less than the patient's daily needs. Recent, marked weight loss is a more ominous sign than gradual loss over many months or years; the rapidity of weight loss is an important clue. Recent loss is usually defined as a substantial loss of 10 or more lb occurring over the past 3 to 6 months. The Centers for Medicare and Medicaid Services defines involuntary weight loss that must be clinically investigated as 5% in 1 month, 7.5% in 3 months, or 10% in 6 months.

Etiology: Involuntary weight loss can be classified in three ways: inadequate nutrient intake, excessive energy expenditure that occurs in catabolism, and a combination of inadequate intake and excessive energy expenditure. Organic causes of inadequate nutrient intake include alcoholism, mechanical causes such as poor dentition, and dysphagia. Psychogenic causes of unexplainable weight loss include depression, anxiety, and dementia. Patients who have hyperthyroidism, diabetes mellitus, pheochromocytoma, malignancy, or fever lose weight because of excessive energy expenditure. For patients with neoplasms, infection, liver disease, renal disease, endocrine disorder, and GI disease, weight loss results both from anorexia and the excessive energy expended.

Occurrence: The occurrence of involuntary weight loss completely depends on the etiology and underlying disease (e.g., 71% of patients with COPD commonly lose weight). A high incidence of involuntary weight loss occurs with metastatic disease, alcoholism, dementia, depression, and AIDS. There is no universally accepted definition of clinically significant weight loss in the elderly, but most studies define it as a 5% or more reduction in body weight in 6 to 12 months. Weight loss is common in the elderly population, and it is not unusual for an older person to lose 5% of his or her body weight over 3 years. From 30% to 50% of long-term care residents have below-average body weight with low serum albumin levels, and there are many documented studies to validate that weight loss is associated with poor health outcomes.

Age: Age as an isolated factor has no documented significance; however, age-related changes (e.g., smell, taste) and chronic diseases common in the elderly predispose this age group to weight loss. About one-half of Americans over 65 years old have lost all their teeth. This tooth loss and teeth in poor repair may affect significantly the ability to eat a nutritious diet in adequate amounts.

Ethnicity: Not significant.

Gender: No documented significance; however, gender data are affected if the specific underlying disease causing the weight loss is more common in men or in women.

Contributing factors: Pulmonary and cardiac diseases, cancer, dementia, alcoholism, depression, medications, GI tract dysmotility, sensory changes, decreased functional status, hyperthyroidism, chronic infection, dentition, and smoking may cause or contribute to weight loss. In addition, family history of involuntary weight loss and history of exposure to hepatitis have been known to contribute to involuntary weight loss. Social factors such as lack of transportation and financial issues may have an influence on proper intake as well. Clinicians need to carefully review the patient's drug regimen for medications that contribute to weight loss, listed in Table 5-3.

Signs and symptoms: Patients may report depression, poor dentition, dysphagia, alcohol and drug use, persistent localized pain, sore tongue, paresthesia,

TABLE 5-3	Drugs That May Cause Weight Loss
DRUG	**EXAMPLES**
Psychiatric	Antidepressants, cholinesterase inhibitors, stimulants, drugs for Parkison's disease, lithium, phenothiazines, butyrophenones
Cardiovascular	Digoxin, amiodarone, procainamide, quinidine, spironolactone
Gastrointestinal	Cimetidine, interferon, diphenoxylate-atropine
Anti-infective	Metronidazole, griseofulvin, most antibiotics
Nutritional	Calcium carbonate, ferrous sulfate, potassium
Antirheumatic	Nonsteroidal anti-inflammatories, colchicine, penicillamine, aspirin
Pulmonary	Theophylline
Antineoplastic	
Malabsorptive agents	Laxatives, bile acid sequestrants, proton pump inhibitors, methotrexate, colchicine, neomycin
Metabolic agents	Stimulants, pseudoephedrine, thyroid replacement therapy (at incorrect doses)

anorexia, nausea, vomiting, change in stools, and diarrhea. Patients with accelerated metabolism may describe episodes of fatigue, fever, melena, heat intolerance, polydipsia, polyphagia, and polyuria. On physical examination, patients with significant weight loss appear pale and cachectic, with a malnourished appearance (hair loss, muscle wasting, and loss of subcutaneous fat, especially around the face). Look for evidence of loose skin, petechiae, cyanosis, clubbing of the fingers, and edema. There may be temporal wasting, icterus, dry mucous membranes, and flattened papillae of the tongue. The oral examination also should note denture fit; tooth and gum disease; and oral lesions such as ulcers, stomatitis, and candidiasis. Examination of the cardiorespiratory system may reveal loud or palpable murmurs and diminished breath sounds. Liver or spleen may be palpable. Check for masses in the abdomen, breasts, and rectum. Muscle wasting may be apparent on the extremities, and deep tendon reflexes may have a prolonged relaxation phase. Patients may have diminished position and vibratory sense. Check women for ovarian masses, cervical lesions, and any obvious neoplasia. In men, examine the prostate gland for enlargement. An early focus of the assessment should be screening for a functional cause of weight loss (i.e., is the patient able to prepare and eat an appropriate diet; if functional limitations are present, is adequate help consistently available to assist with ADLs). Weight loss in the elderly can cause skeletal muscle loss, which in turns increases the risk for falls, functional impairment, protein malnutrition, immune system compromise, anemia, and decreased cognition, all of which increase morbidity and mortality.

Diagnostic tests: There are no published guidelines to guide assessment and management for elderly patients with unintentional weight loss, and clinical responses vary from no intervention or diagnostics because the weight loss is viewed as a normal part of the aging process to extensive investigations because it is believed to be the result of an underlying malignancy. Physical findings and history indicate most organic causes of weight loss and guide the choice of diagnostic tests. A nutritional or diet history and calorie counts add objective data to evaluate the amount and quality of food intake. A complete review of medications is always a good idea, looking for medication effects on appetite, taste, mouth dryness, nutrient absorption, or increased indigestion or reflux. Standard screening tests are shown in Table 5-4.

Additional tests such as serum glucose and/or hemoglobin A1c (HgbA1c), liver function tests, urea and electrolytes, C-reactive protein and ESR, chest x-ray, urinalysis, and fecal occult blood testing may be appropriate based on the history and physical examination findings.

For patients whose nutrition is being monitored closely, an increase in the prealbumin of 1 mg/day indicates a good response to nutritional supplementation. A response of less than 2 mg/wk signifies an inadequate response or an inadequate level of nutritional support.

In the absence of localized symptoms, routine cancer screening is indicated in certain patients. Consider a neoplastic origin when benign causes of weight loss appear unlikely. Evidence of blood loss anemia on the CBC or one positive fecal occult blood result is a reason to perform GI imaging. In general, imaging studies performed in the hope that they will show something are expensive, are as likely to yield false-positive results as true-positive results, and are overused for general screenings. These methods have a higher diagnostic yield if directed at a specific organ, system, or region of the body. With frail older persons, however, before this kind of invasive and expensive workup is begun,

TABLE 5-4	Standard Screening Tests
TEST	RESULTS INDICATING DISORDER
Albumin (has a half-life of about 21 days and reflects level about 3 weeks in past)	2.9–3.5 g/dL, mild nutritional deficiency
	2.1–3 g/dL, moderate nutritional deficiency
	<2.1 g/dL, severe nutritional deficiency
Prealbumin	10.7–16 g/dL, moderate deficiency
	<10.7 g/dL, severe deficiency
Serum cholesterol	≤160 mg/dL, consider protein-calorie malnutrition if signs/symptoms of poor nutrition present
CBC with differential	Low total lymphocyte count or an unexplained normocytic anemia may indicate malnutrition. A blood loss anemia should raise concern of malignancy
Thyroid-stimulating hormone	1.9–5.4 μIU/mL, normal reference range
	Decreased levels in hyperthyroidism, often associated with weight loss
	Increased levels in hypothyroidism, associated with weight change (usually gain, but loss also occurs in elderly)
Transferrin	150–200 mg/dL, mild depletion
	100–150 mg/dL, moderate depletion
	<200 mg/dL, severe visceral protein depletion
	Limited use in monitoring response to therapy, but better than albumin; not specific to nutritional issues

it is important to address the question of treatment options with the patient and family. There is no need to proceed further if surgery, radiation, or other treatment options are not feasible or if the patient or family is not interested. If the cause of weight loss is not clear from these results, watchful waiting is recommended; watch for further weight loss or specific symptoms, and reconsider a functional cause of weight loss. If no abnormalities are detected from the standard tests, history, and physical examination, an organic cause is unlikely (<5%). When the findings from the initial workup are negative, psychological problems, particularly depression and anxiety, are among the most common reasons for weight loss. For gradual weight loss, the workup can take 6 months. In elderly patients with multiple or nonspecific complaints (often including weight loss), a high index of suspicion for depression is warranted. An adequate trial of an antidepressant is almost always appropriate.

Differential diagnosis: For weight loss that occurs with increased food intake, consider diabetes, thyrotoxicosis, malabsorption, leukemia, lymphoma, and adrenal insufficiency. For weight loss that occurs with normal or decreased food intake, consider alcoholism; malignancy; infection; GI, hepatic, renal, dental, endocrine, respiratory, cardiac, or psychological causes; anorexia nervosa; malnutrition; or a functional origin. After investigation, the cause of weight loss remains unknown in 16% to 28% of patients. Table 5-5 lists the causes of weight loss in the elderly.

Treatment: Watchful waiting is recommended if no organic cause is determined immediately. Otherwise, treat or manage the identified underlying cause. It is common in clinical practice for clinicians to order megestrol

TABLE 5-5	Meals-on-Wheels Mnemonic for Causes of Weight Loss in the Elderly
MNEMONIC	**CAUSES OF WEIGHT LOSS**
M	Medications
E	Emotional
A	Alcoholism, anorexia tardive, abuse
L	Late-life paranoia
S	Swallowing problems (dysphagia)
O	Oral problems
N	No money (poverty)
	Nosocomial infections
W	Wandering and other dementia-related problems
H	Hyperthyroidism
	Hypercalcemia
	Hypoadrenalism
E	Enteric problems (malabsorption)
E	Eating problems
	Enteral problems
L	Low-salt, low-cholesterol diet
S	Shopping and meal preparation problems
	Stones

acetate, mirtazapine, and other pharmacological agents to stimulate appetite; however, evidence underlying their use is limited, particularly in the elderly, and none has gained approval from the Food and Drug Administration. Consultation with a dietitian experienced in weight loss in the elderly is important. Nutritional supplements and extra snacks between meals are often ordered.

Many nondrug interventions can increase caloric intake. These include smaller meals more often, encouraging the patient to eat favorite foods, and minimizing dietary restrictions. Patients with dementia tend to consume most of their daily energy at breakfast, so high-energy foods should be served at this meal, and varying dietary texture can be helpful. Eating with assistance and in the company of others increases calorie intake. For elders in the community, Meals on Wheels programs are beneficial. Oral nutritional supplements should be consumed between meals. Problems with dentition and oral health need to be addressed. Regular exercise, especially resistance training, stimulates appetite and also prevents sarcopenia. All patients with involuntary weight loss should be assessed by a dietitian and screened for depression and cognitive impairment.

Follow-up: If results of the standard tests listed earlier are negative, and the history and physical examination are negative, the recommended approach is to watch for further weight loss and to reconsider functional causes. Have the patient or caregiver keep a daily record of food intake, activity levels, and symptoms, and schedule a return visit in 2 to 4 weeks.

Sequelae: Malnutrition is the first complication to consider in involuntary weight loss. Long-term unexplained weight loss may indicate failure to thrive and the beginning of a downward spiral in health and function. Many patients in acute and long-term care have unrecognized protein-calorie malnutrition. Protein-calorie malnutrition is a common iatrogenic complication of hospitalization.

Prevention/prophylaxis: Discuss proper nutrition and the need for dental care, if appropriate. Address functional, financial, and social issues that may affect nutrition (i.e., address depression, arrange for socialization at mealtime if feasible, arrange Meals on Wheels).

Referral: Refer to a specialist for rapid or acute decline; for positive diagnostic test results indicating malignancy, thyrotoxicosis, or other acute organic illnesses requiring sophisticated diagnostic workup or management; or for a patient condition beyond your current scope of practice. Refer patients for assistance if social or functional issues may be contributing to weight loss. Refer to an appropriate specialist or perform additional assessments to confirm patient's denial of problems (e.g., nutritional, psychological, in-home, functional).

Education: Instruct patients about proper nutrition and hydration. Encourage exercise to improve strength or function and to stimulate appetite. Teach patients about medication side effects that may affect nutrition and about signs or symptoms of overmedication or undermedication.

Appetite Questionnaire to Predict Weight Loss in Older Persons—SNAQ (Simplified Nutrition Appetite Questionnaire)

1. My appetite is
   A. very poor
   B. poor
   C. average
   D. good
   E. very good

2. When I eat
   A. I feel full after eating only a few mouthfuls
   B. I feel full after eating about one-third of a meal
   C. I feel full after eating over more than one-half of a meal
   D. I feel full after eating most of a meal
   E. I hardly ever feel full

3. Food tastes
   A. very bad
   B. bad
   C. average
   D. good
   E. very good

4. Normally I eat
   A. less than one meal a day
   B. one meal a day
   C. two meals a day
   D. three meals a day
   E. more than 3 meals a day

Instructions: Complete the questionnaire by circling the correct answers and then tallying the results based on the following numerical scale: A = 1, B = 2, C = 3, D = 4, E = 5.

Scoring: If the mini-SNAQ total score is less than 14, there is a significant risk of weight loss.

Source: Dutch Malnutrition Steering Group. Fight malnutrition. Retrieved from www.fightmalnutrition.eu/malnutrition/screening-tools/snaq-tools-in-english

---

CLINICAL RECOMMENDATIONS	EVIDENCE RATING	REFERENCE
Screen for depression if indicated.	A	University of Texas at Austin School of Nursing, Family Nurse Practitioner Program (2006)
Ensure adequate oral health.	A	University of Texas at Austin School of Nursing, Family Nurse Practitioner Program (2006)
Oral nutritional supplementation is associated with weight gain and reduced fatality.	A	University of Texas at Austin School of Nursing, Family Nurse Practitioner Program (2006)
Take a multivitamin to keep up with the increased metabolism and restore deficiencies.	B	University of Texas at Austin School of Nursing, Family Nurse Practitioner Program (2006)

Continued

CLINICAL RECOMMENDATIONS	EVIDENCE RATING	REFERENCE
Minimize dietary restrictions.	B	University of Texas at Austin School of Nursing, Family Nurse Practitioner Program (2006)
Eat in the company of others.	B	University of Texas at Austin School of Nursing, Family Nurse Practitioner Program (2006)
Protein/calorie supplements should be given between meals.	A	University of Texas at Austin School of Nursing, Family Nurse Practitioner Program (2006)
Drugs should not be used as first-line intervention.	B	University of Texas at Austin School of Nursing, Family Nurse Practitioner Program (2006)

A = consistent, good-quality, patient-oriented evidence; B = inconsistent or limited-quality, patient-oriented evidence; C = consensus, disease-oriented evidence, usual practice, expert opinion, or case series. For information about the SORT evidence rating system, go to www.aafp.org/afpsort.xml.

JOINT PAIN

Description: Joint pain is discomfort, tenderness, or pain in one or more joints. Joint pain can arise from muscular, bone, or systemic disease. The knee is the most commonly affected joint in older adults.

Etiology: The description, location, onset, and associated symptoms are crucial to diagnosing the etiology of joint pain. Narrowing down or clarifying the etiology of the pain depends on the clinical presentation, complete history, and findings from physical examination and appropriate diagnostic testing. The pain can be mild (from strained muscles or ligaments that support the joint), chronic (lasting more than 6 months, from degenerative joint disease, arthritis, osteoarthritis), inflammatory (from joint effusion, rheumatoid arthritis [RA]), or severe and acute (from trauma or infection). Drug-induced arthralgia can occur with some medications, including anti-infectives, biologicals, lipid-lowering drugs, cardiac drugs, and hormones. Acute joint pain may also be a flare of a chronic condition or an initial symptom of a chronic condition. Acute joint pain often becomes a chronic pain. Systemic causes include lupus, sarcoidosis, Lyme disease, hemophilia, and Raynaud's and Paget's disease.

Occurrence: Joint pain is a common complaint and accounts for 315 million office visits yearly. The prevalence of chronic joint problems is about 33%.

Age: Joint pain is found more frequently in the elderly patient as a result of age-related muscle atrophy, demineralization of trabecular bone, atrophy of cortical bone, chronic disease, and loss of bone density. Arthritis (degenerative and inflammatory) is the most common cause of disability in individuals over 75 years old, and it affects more than 80% of individuals in this age group, with joint pain being the dominant symptom.

Ethnicity: No documentation is found specifically for joint pain; however, the prevalence of certain types of inflammatory joint disease and systemic disorders is higher in various ethnic groups.

Gender: Joint pain occurs more frequently in women than in men.

Contributing factors: Factors that may lead to joint pain include overuse or strain, previous injury or trauma to the joint, alterations in gait or balance, past surgery or joint replacement, known history of arthritis or joint disease, and postmenopausal women with no hormonal replacement therapy. Weight, physical stature, smoking, and family history should be assessed in reviewing the risk factors for osteoporosis. Other contributing factors include obesity, poor nutritional habits, low calcium intake, alcohol consumption, medications, and exercise habits.

Signs and symptoms: The history should identify how many joints are affected and include the onset of the pain (sudden, insidious); character of the pain (dull, sharp); and duration and location of the pain (including radiation). Inquire about any associated symptoms, any alleviating or aggravating factors, and timing (e.g., worse in morning, better late in the day). Symptoms associated with joint pain may include erythema, redness, warmth, general weakness, stiffness, decreased range of motion, and inflammation.

Discuss normal activity levels and the possibility of overuse or strain. Has there been any old or recent trauma to the joint? If there was an injury, did the patient hear any popping or clicking? Discuss the limitation in joint mobility, and note the presence of edema, redness, or fever. Review if there is any associated muscle fatigue, joint deformity, or inability to perform certain movements. Ominous signs that heighten the urgency of the workup include unremitting pain, fatigue, systemic symptoms (fever, chills, weight loss), significant disability, and change in function. Up to 40% of individuals with severe radiographic changes in the joints are symptom free.

The physical examination includes a complete assessment of the patient, paying specific attention to any joint pain complaints. Inspect and palpate each joint and assess the appropriate range of motion, noting any pain or limitations in movement. Special tests, such as the anterior drawer sign, may be appropriate. Note the patient's gait, balance, and posture. Inspect each joint, noting the musculature, any atrophy, contractures, nodules, asymmetry, or gross deformity. Note any erythema, inflammation, or soft tissue swelling on or near the joint. Note the joint(s) affected (RA usually involves the metacarpophalengeal joints and the wrist, whereas distal involvement of the interphalangeal suggests osteoarthritis). Palpate for any tenderness or effusions on or around the joint. Check for crepitus, clicking, or popping in or around the joint. Sensory testing may reveal neurological or vascular involvement. Extra-articular signs (rashes, tophi, conjunctivitis, mouth ulcers) provide additional information toward a differential diagnosis.

Diagnostic tests: Laboratory tests are useful only if the provider suspects a diagnosis. No tests are specifically indicated with a complaint of joint pain. Problem-specific complaints and physical examination findings dictate which tests are required. A CBC with differential may be needed to rule out infection and an ESR may help determine inflammation. Marked elevations in alkaline phosphatase level are seen in patients with bone disease (e.g., Paget's disease, metastatic bone disease). Hypercalcemia with marked alkaline phosphatase is seen in patients with hyperparathyroidism or bone carcinoma. Serum creatine kinase (CK) isoenzymes are elevated in persons with muscle trauma and progressive muscular disease. If indicated, obtain a complete electrolyte panel and urinalysis, checking blood urea nitrogen and creatinine, to assess renal function. Rheumatoid factor may be of use but it is negative in approximately 30% of all RA cases. X-rays of the joint can be useful to detect fracture, joint space destruction or narrowing, erosion, arthritic changes, and degeneration. Joint aspirations may be done to distinguish inflammatory, noninflammatory, and infectious conditions and may provide symptomatic relief. Further evaluation with CT scans or MRI may be necessary, although experience with the diagnostic value of these modalities is limited.

Differential diagnosis: The disease processes associated with joint pain are considered in the differential diagnosis. Morning stiffness points toward an inflammatory arthritis, whereas postexercise stiffness indicates a degenerative process. Some other conditions to rule out include gout, pseudogout, psoriatic arthritis, connective tissue disease, Reiter's disease, multiple myeloma, scleroderma, lupus, septic arthritis, polymyalgia rheumatica, cervical radiculopathy, and spinal stenosis.

Treatment: The goal in acute joint pain is to reduce swelling and pain. The mnemonic PRICE is helpful: *Protection* (brace/wrap), *Rest, Ice* (15 minutes several times a day), *Compression* (elastic wrap), and *Elevation* (elevate the joint above the heart level). Medical management of joint pain depends on the findings of the comprehensive assessment. The goal to decrease pain may include physical therapy, analgesic and anti-inflammatory medications, moist heat, intra-articular steroid injections, assistive devices, and surgery. Pharmacological agents include NSAIDs, which primarily have a role in treating inflammatory pain notwithstanding the GI and renal adverse effects. Cyclooxygenase type 2 inhibitors and opioids may be used when other agents fail. Acetaminophen continues to be the first-line drug in osteoarthritis in that it has a low cost, has low toxicity, and has high efficacy. Newer agents useful in inflammatory arthritis include disease-modifying antirheumatic drugs and biological response modifiers. Intra-articular injections can provide short-term relief. Nonpharmacological therapies are useful in both acute and chronic pain and include transcutaneous electrical nerve stimulation and acupuncture. Cryotherapy and application of heat can help with knee and back pain. Emergency intervention is required if you suspect a fracture, avascular necrosis, or sepsis. Capsaicin, an enzyme found in hot pepper, depletes substance P when applied to the painful area 3 times a day for several weeks. Side effects may include burning and erythema, and it should never be applied to open or irritated skin.

Follow-up: Monitoring of patients depends on findings. Patients with acute or severe joint pain may need emergency care and intervention. Monitor patients with chronic pain frequently until the clinical workup is completed. Management of chronic joint pain or disease requires routine visits to monitor medications and laboratory and diagnostic test results.

Sequelae: The condition and prognosis relate to the etiology of the joint pain.

Prevention/prophylaxis: Prevention methods depend on the etiology of the joint pain. When applicable, use weight reduction to decrease stress on the joint; physical therapy and exercise for strengthening; and moist heat, topical medications, and steroid injections to reduce pain and spasms. Explore alternative methods of pain control (acupuncture, yoga, medication, or massage therapy). Address fall prevention for patients using assistive devices (canes, crutches, or walkers). Instruct the patient concerning joint protection and preservation. Discuss proper nutrition, calcium supplements, and smoking cessation.

Referral: Refer patients to a specialist pending the results of the workup. Refer patients to the appropriate emergency service if you suspect sepsis, fracture, or avascular necrosis. Referral to physical or occupational therapy for exercises to reduce pain and improve strength and endurance is advised.

Education: Teach patients about the appropriate dose of medications and the potential side effects that need to be reported. Instruct patients about appropriate follow-up and referrals. Tell the patient to report any persisting or worsening joint pain and any systemic involvement. Instruct patients on the appropriate methods for pain control. Review the use of any adaptive equipment and the role the patient plays in avoiding disability and slowing progression of the disease. Low-impact exercise is important for obese patients.

CLINICAL RECOMMENDATIONS	EVIDENCE RATING	REFERENCE
Diagnose RA and refer promptly for early treatment.	B	Palmer (2011)
Intra-articular corticosteroid injections provide short-term benefit with few adverse effects in the treatment of knee osteoarthritis.	A	Arroll & Goodyear-Smith (2004) Bellamy, et al. (2006)
NSAIDs and acetaminophen improve pain in persons with knee osteoarthritis.	A	Deeks, Smith, & Bradley (2002) Geba et al. (2002)

A = consistent, good-quality, patient-oriented evidence; B = inconsistent or limited-quality, patient-oriented evidence; C = consensus, disease-oriented evidence, usual practice, expert opinion, or case series. For information about the SORT evidence rating system, go to www.aafp.org/afpsort.xml.

PERIPHERAL EDEMA

Description: Peripheral edema is an increase in the interstitial fluid volume and is not clinically apparent until the interstitial volume has increased by 2.5 to 3 L. Lymphedema, or lymphatic obstruction, occurs when a compromised lymphatic system causes localized fluid retention and tissue swelling. There are numerous etiologies for peripheral edema ranging from benign to life-threatening clinical conditions.

Etiology: Normally the distribution of water between the blood and interstitial tissues is maintained by equilibrium. Starling's concept—the osmotic pressure of the plasma proteins balances the hydrostatic pressure in the capillaries—helps in the understanding of fluid dynamics. Fluid flows from the vessels to the interstitial area in response to intravascular hydrostatic pressure and the colloid osmotic pressure of the interstitial fluid. In the opposite direction, fluid enters the blood because of the interstitial tissue tension and the oncotic pressure of the plasma proteins. Interstitial fluid also is returned to the blood as lymph. Under steady-state conditions, net fluid flux out of the capillary is balanced by lymph flow back into circulation. Alteration in any of these compartments (intravascular, extravascular, lymphatic) upsets the equilibrium, and leg edema occurs. Two basic steps occur in edema formation: sodium and water are retained, and capillary hemodynamics are altered.

Leg edema, common in elderly persons, often has diverse etiologies, and more than one disorder can be causing edema in the same patient. The most common cause in patients older than 50 years of age is insufficiency of the leg veins. In elderly patients with leg edema, the most common causes are venous insufficiency; congestive heart failure; drug-induced edema; and other conditions, including lymphedema (primary or inherited; secondary caused by damage to the lymphatic system), ovarian and prostate cancers, postphlebitic syndrome, nephrotic syndrome, and chronic anemia (Table 5-6).

TABLE 5-6	Common Causes of Peripheral Edema
Unilateral, acute	Deep venous thrombosis, ruptured Baker's cyst, compartment syndrome
Bilateral, acute	Allergic reaction, trauma, burns, bilateral deep venous thrombosis, acute worsening of renal failure or congestive heart failure (CHF)
Unilateral, chronic	Venous insufficiency, lymphedema, pelvic tumor, and reflex sympathetic dystrophy
Bilateral, chronic	Venous insufficiency, pulmonary hypertension, CHF, lymphedema, medications, renal disease, idiopathic, dependent edema, anemia

Source: Adapted from O'Brien, J. G., & Miles, T. P. (2013). Edema. *Essential Evidence Plus.* Retrieved from http://www.essentialevidenceplus.com.proxy.its.virginia.edu/content/eee/29

Occurrence: The frequency of occurrence completely depends on the underlying etiology and combined etiologies.

Age: Peripheral edema occurs frequently in older adults.

Ethnicity: Not significant.

Gender: No documented significance is found, but gender statistics vary according to the specific etiology (e.g., idiopathic edema is more common in women; heart failure edema is more common in men).

Contributing factors: Physiological age-related changes increase the vulnerability to fluid retention. The older adult has a smaller amount of total body water overall (80% of body weight for a newborn, 60% for a young adult, 50% for an older adult), and of this, two-thirds is intracellular and one-third is extracellular fluid. As more intracellular fluid is lost over time, extracellular fluid volume starts to comprise more body water. Risk factors for leg edema from age-related changes include a decrease in the following:

■ Serum albumin—less than 2 g/dL can cause edema
■ Glomerular filtration rate
■ Hepatic blood flow
■ Sodium-concentrating ability of the kidney
■ Myocardial contractility and cardiac output
■ Baroreceptor sensitivity

Additional contributing factors include dependent positioning of the lower extremities; excessive intake of sodium; hot weather; and use of medicines that contribute to sodium retention, particularly hormones, NSAIDs, and antihypertensives.

Signs and symptoms: The patient may complain of fullness, discomfort, aching pain, shoes that are too tight, wounds, gait disturbance, self-image issues, or weight gain. The history should elicit the seven dimensions of the signs and symptoms of edema, emphasizing location (unilateral or bilateral) and chronological evolution (acute or chronic progression). Associated symptoms need to be elicited, particularly shortness of breath or awakening at night with difficulty breathing. The presence or absence of pain is helpful in determining the differential diagnosis. Ask about aggravating and alleviating factors, including the effect of prolonged sitting or standing, and determine the effect of passive leg elevation. A history of cardiac, renal, liver, or peripheral vascular disease is important. Ask about changes in diet, salt intake, and alcohol use. Has the patient started any new medications or had dose changes? Has the patient been on a trip recently or had periods or prolonged standing or sitting? Has the patient's weight changed over the past 6 months?

The physical examination begins with weight. Assess skin changes, including pigmentation and thickening, lesions, discoloration, texture, temperature, and induration. Evaluate the venous and arterial circulation, checking pulses throughout, capillary refill, and dependent rubor. Varicose veins are usually readily apparent with the inspection of the legs while the patient stands.

Assess the extremity for local or diffuse tenderness and for pitting or nonpitting edema. Measure and compare the circumference bilaterally from a fixed reference point above the ankle to the area of maximal edema (e.g., patella, calf, midcalf). Assess any localized enlargement.

Pitting edema is measured by applying firm pressure with your thumb over the area of edema for 5 seconds and then releasing it and observing the amount of time it takes for the skin to return to normal as graded below:

1+: 30 seconds or less
2+: 30 to 60 seconds
3+: 60 to 90 seconds
4+: 90 to 120 seconds

The Kaposi-Stemmer sign suggests lymphedema and is the inability to tent the skin over the dorsum of the foot at the base of the second toe. Examine body systems indicated by the history (e.g., cardiac, renal, endocrine, pulmonary).

In unilateral edema, a 1-cm difference in size above the ankle or a 2-cm difference at the calf is significant and should lead to further investigation.

Diagnostic tests: Diagnostic tests depend on the probable etiology of leg edema. Cardiac causes may warrant a chest x-ray, ECG, or echocardiogram. Thyroid panel evaluates thyroid-stimulating hormone and free thyroxine. CBC with differential, serum protein albumin level, and electrolyte values should be obtained. Renal and liver panels usually are done as part of an automated chemistry test. Additional studies include ultrasound, venogram, venous Doppler studies, lymphoscintigraphy, or the more invasive lymphangiography. CT scans or ultrasound for pelvic masses and lymphoma may be indicated, as well as a CA-125. Urine studies quantify protein losses and urine electrolytes.

Differential diagnosis: Leg edema is an important clinical sign, and its causes are diverse. The differential diagnosis is facilitated in part by noting if edema is unilateral or bilateral and recognizing distinctions between lymphedema, lipedema, and venous stasis. A multisystem approach that excludes major organ system dysfunction is useful, especially cardiac, liver, and renal disease. An accurate diagnosis is important because the mainstay of treatment is reversing the underlying disorder if possible. Lipedema is a bilateral, symmetrical deposition of fat in the lower extremities that spares the feet (a distinguishing feature) and occurs exclusively in obese women.

Treatment: Always direct treatment at the cause of leg edema: diuretics for heart failure, a high-protein diet for hypoalbuminemia, ACE inhibitors for proteinuria, and thrombolytics for acute deep venous thrombosis. Any drugs known to cause edema should be discontinued or decreased in dosage.

Compression stockings: Compression stockings decrease the capillary filtration rate, thus decreasing edema. They are especially useful in patients with venous insufficiency. There is no evidence to indicate that high compression (30 to 40 mm Hg) is clinically more advantageous than medium compression (20 to 30 mm Hg), and patients are more compliant with medium compression. The stockings can be difficult to pull on, and a stocking donner can be helpful. Give the patient a prescription for two sets to allow for laundering. They need to be replaced every 6 months because the compression properties decrease with wear. Stockings that zip are available. Send the patient to the medical supply store where trained fitters will ensure the proper fit. Compression stockings are not recommended for patients with peripheral artery disease (PAD), and if suspected, an ankle-brachial index (ABI) can be ordered to screen for PAD.

Behavioral modifications include intermittent periods of recumbency, the avoidance of environmental heat, and sodium and water restriction as indicated. Exercise improves the muscle pump action and strengthens leg muscles.

Follow-up: Closely monitor patients for effectiveness of therapy and adverse events. Monitor the weight and limb circumference measurements using the same reference points because a patient's weight may increase 10% before pitting edema is clinically evident.

Sequelae: When administering diuretics, the healthcare professional must be alert to potential volume depletion. Elderly patients are very sensitive to diuretics, and their administration may result in falls, weakness, confusion secondary to sodium and other electrolyte abnormalities, urinary incontinence, gout attacks, volume depletion, and acute renal failure. Patients with edema as a result of deep venous insufficiency are prone to recurrent ulceration.

Prevention/prophylaxis: For patients with recurrent lymphangitis and cellulitis, prescribe intermittent long-term antibiotic prophylaxis. For patients with leg swelling secondary to deep venous thrombosis, thrombolytics may limit the tissue loss, pulmonary embolus, and more extensive thrombosis of the deep venous system.

Referral: Regardless of the cause of leg swelling, you can achieve the best fluid removal while the patient is hospitalized. It would be rare to hospitalize a patient for most causes of peripheral edema, thus treatment is almost always outpatient. Even deep venous thromboses are treated outpatient most of the time now with Lovenox or Arixtra and initiation of Coumadin. This is particularly true when the process is an acute one such as deep venous thrombophlebitis or cellulitis. When thrombolytic therapy is indicated, consult a vascular specialist.

Education: Patients need specific information related to the edema and the management of symptoms. Typically the patient with edema is instructed to avoid highly salted foods (follow a 2 to 3 g sodium diet). If compression stockings are recommended, emphasize the importance of proper sizing and application technique to avoid excessive pressure. Instruct patients to elevate their legs above heart level to decrease peripheral vascular pressure for 10 to 15 minutes 3 to 4 times a day. Periodic active muscle contraction exercises are important for individuals who must sit for long periods. Teach patients with peripheral vascular disorders to avoid excessive heat and to reduce weight if indicated. Special care of the skin, including proper shoes and prevention of trauma, is important.

CLINICAL RECOMMENDATIONS	EVIDENCE RATING	REFERENCE
When deep venous thrombosis is suspected, use the Wells Clinical Rule, D-dimer, and selective use of imaging to confirm the diagnosis.	A	O'Brien & Miles (2013)
Begin by evaluating whether edema is unilateral or bilateral, painful or nonpainful, and acute or chronic.	B	O'Brien & Miles (2013)
Brain natriuretic peptide (BNP) is helpful for distinguishing heart failure from other causes of leg edema.	B	O'Brien & Miles (2013)

A = consistent, good-quality, patient-oriented evidence; B = inconsistent or limited-quality, patient-oriented evidence; C = consensus, disease-oriented evidence, usual practice, expert opinion, or case series. For information about the SORT evidence rating system, go to www.aafp.org/afpsort.xml.

PRURITUS

Description: Pruritus is defined as an irritating or itching sensation on the surface of the skin. it may be localized or generalized. Pruritus may be acute (<6 weeks) or may be chronic (>6 weeks). Characteristic features include scratching and inflammation.

Etiology: The pathophysiology of pruritus remains unknown. Inflammation results from activation of the immune response. Immunoglobulin E (IgE) in the skin surface cells triggers an inflammatory response in which histamines and other neurostimulators are released. Repetitive rubbing and scratching exacerbate the inflammation. As the skin ages, integumentary and vascular changes lead to decreased skin moisture, decreased sweat, and sebum production, all of which contribute to dry skin. The decline in immune function with age produces increased incidence of autoimmune diseases that can cause pruritus. Pruritus can be caused by inflammatory skin disease, exogenous trigger factors (scabies, mites, toxins, allergens, and wind), endogenous trigger factors (medications and pH changes), or systemic disease (diabetes, iron deficiency anemia, chronic renal insufficiency, liver disease, tumors, HIV). Psychogenic pruritus (somatoform pruritus) is another common condition. Medications can induce pruritus, including antihypertensives (ACE inhibitors, calcium channel blockers), antibiotics, opioids, and psychotropics. Drug-induced pruritus may be localized or generalized and may start after the first dose of a drug or many weeks or months after being on the drug.

Occurrence: The prevalence of pruritus is unknown but it is the most common symptom seen in dermatology, and various skin and systemic diseases are associated with it.

Age: Pruritus is the most common skin complaint in individuals over 65 years old, and the incidence is about 20% in those over 85 years old. Analysis of hospital admission data indicates that 11.5% of the elderly had a primary diagnosis of pruritus and two-thirds of patients in skilled nursing facilities experience it. Xerosis is the most common cause in the elderly.

Gender: Pruritus is more prevalent in women than in men.

Contributing factors: Once a pattern for pruritus has been initiated, continued scratching causes a cascade of inflammatory mediators that provoke the itch sensation and repeat scratching. Additional factors that contribute to dryness include winter weather (low environmental humidity), daily use of cleansers, and bathing without replacement emollients. Sleep deprivation can cause an increase in the release of an inflammatory mediator and though it is often a result of pruritus, it can also contribute to it.

Signs and symptoms: A thorough history and physical examination should be done in all patients with pruritus. Focused questions should include the following:

- How did it start (sudden or gradual)?
- Characterize the sensation—is it prickling, crawling, burning, stinging?
- How severe is it?

- How frequently does it occur and for how long?
- Does anything make it worse or better?
- Where does it itch (local or systemic)?

Asking if and how it might interfere with activities or sleep is important. Asking patients what they think the cause might be might help. Find out about allergies and if there was an exposure to new creams or detergents. Ask about systemic-associated symptoms such as weight loss, fever, heat/cold intolerance (thyroid disease), nausea and vomiting (chronic renal failure), and polyuria/polydipsia (diabetes). Additional history of importance is past medical history, including previous skin conditions, skin care routine, and current medications. Some brief psychological screening may provide some insights into the potential cause. A complete physical examination is warranted, including examining all surfaces of the skin including the hair and nails. Assess texture, temperature, moisture, and turgor of the skin. Assess lesions and document using drawings or photos accurately recording the location, shape, and characteristics. Look for secondary lesions such as lichenification (the thickening of the skin from continued scratching). The general physical is focused on identifying potential systemic causes and contributors to pruritus and includes palpating lymph nodes and the thyroid gland.

Diagnostic tests: No specific tests are indicated for a complaint of pruritus though it might include a CBC, ESR, and/or C-reactive protein to determine infection/inflammation. Patch testing or photo testing may be needed to establish a diagnosis. If a systemic disease is suspected, an appropriate thyroid panel, liver function, anemia, renal values, and HIV testing may be done.

Differential diagnosis: The differential diagnosis is quite broad; there may be more than one cause, and frequently a cause is never determined.

Treatment: Treatment goals are always tailored and include alleviating the itch and maintaining skin integrity. Treatment is aimed at the cause. Xerosis, the most common cause, is treated with emollients that rehydrate the skin and reduce inflammation, and some may additionally include a mild anesthetic that helps decrease the sense of itching. Topical steroids can reduce inflammation and itching, though these are avoided for generalized itching or for prolonged periods because they cause skin thinning. An antihistamine topical cream may be used or a menthol cream, which has a cooling effect. Topical immunomodulators act on nerve fibers, and capsaicin topically has been found to be helpful with neuropathic origins such as postherpetic neuralgia. Local anesthetics can decrease transmission in sensory fibers. Systemic medications that have antipruritic properties include SSRIs, mirtazepine, and tricyclic antidepressants. The antidepressants may be helpful in psychogenic causes. Antihistamines, neuroleptics, and opioid agonists and antagonists can be helpful in some circumstances. Systemic steroids should only be used in acute, severe forms of pruritus. Nonpharmacological measures include removing any environmental allergens if identified, using an occlusive dressing in a localized area to reduce scratching, cool dressings, psychotherapy, and acupuncture work in some cases. Phototherapy has been used for decades to treat various pruritic dermatoses.

Sequelae: Secondary infection is a risk when the skin is broken. Neglecting the symptom can have a negative effect on the patient's quality of life, especially through sleep deprivation.

Prevention/prophylaxis: Bathing less often in warm (not hot) water, increasing the humidity, and using a soft towel to pat dry gently are advised. Apply emollients after bathing (and never in the tub due to fall risk), applying them gently to avoid overstimulating the nerve endings. Eating a healthy diet and drinking plenty of water are advised.

Follow-up: Monitor the patient frequently to evaluate the effectiveness of treatment and reinforce adherence and watch for secondary complications.

Referral: Refer to a dermatologist or an allergist for severe cases or when treatment is ineffective.

Education: In addition to bathing techniques and how and when to use moisturizers, educate the patient to keep fingernails short, wear light and loose clothing, avoid alkaline and alcohol-based cleansers, and maintain comfortable temperature and humidification.

CLINICAL RECOMMENDATIONS	EVIDENCE RATING	REFERENCE
Keep cool, use emollients, and take short, tepid showers. Avoid soaking and use moisturizing soaps as opposed to antibacterial soaps.	C	Trikha & Ebell (2011)
First-line treatment is an H1-receptor blocker.	B	Pham (2011)
Psychological interventions reduce the severity of eczema or the intensity of itching and scratching in patients with atopic dermatitis.	A	Chida et al. (2007)

A = consistent, good-quality, patient-oriented evidence; B = inconsistent or limited-quality, patient-oriented evidence; C = consensus, disease-oriented evidence, usual practice, expert opinion, or case series. For information about the SORT evidence rating system, go to www.aafp.org/afpsort.xml.

SYNCOPE

Description: Syncope is defined as a sudden and transient loss of consciousness and postural tone resulting from a reduction in oxygen to the brain.

Etiology: Etiologies for syncope range from trivial to lethal. In most instances, the loss of consciousness reflects a temporary decrease in cerebral blood flow that is usually secondary to a fall in the systemic arterial blood pressure influenced by metabolic regulation, chemical regulation, and autoregulation. Reflex-mediated and orthostatic causes are usually more benign, whereas cardiac and neurological causes are more dangerous. Studies show that the cause of syncope remains elusive in 30% of cases of patients admitted for syncope.

Occurrence: There is a 42% chance of a syncopal event during the life of a person living 70 years. The Framingham Heart Study showed that 3% of men and 3.5% of women had experienced at least one syncopal episode. Syncope accounts for about 1% to 3% of all emergency department visits and 6% of all hospital admissions.

Age: The lifetime incidence of syncope may be 25% in the elderly, and 80% of all emergency department admissions for syncope are individuals older than 65 years of age. Some forms of syncope (i.e., vasovagal, carotid sinus hypersensitivity) are more common in younger persons than in older persons; other forms of syncope (i.e., cardiac, orthostatic, micturition related) occur more often in older than in younger individuals.

Ethnicity: Not significant.

Gender: Among younger adults, women have nearly twice the rate of syncope as men; among elderly adults, men have the greater incidence. This likely reflects the most common etiologies in the different age groups.

Contributing factors: Cerebral blood flow has been reported to decline 25% with physiological aging, thought to be related to vascular stiffening. Hormonal regulation of extracellular volume may become impaired with age. Cardiac reflexes and baroreceptor sensitivity also may become impaired. The kidneys' ability to conserve sodium and water declines. Chronic diseases, such as heart disease, diabetes, renal insufficiency, hypertension, and chronic pulmonary disease, are predisposing conditions. Medications used to treat these chronic diseases, such as diuretics, beta blockers, vasodilators, nitrates, antiarrhythmics, and antihypertensives, also may be offenders. Alcohol is a contributing factor in vasovagal syncope. An emotional response can cause neurally mediated syncope in susceptible individuals in stressful circumstances. Dehydration and orthostatic hypotension may be factors. Situational syncope can occur when the Valsalva maneuver is produced (micturition, defecation, cough, lifting heavy objects, or after meals related to postprandial hypotension). Prolonged recumbency can contribute to micturition syncope. Men with prostate enlargement who awaken from a supine sleep and stand to urinate are at highest risk.

Signs and symptoms: Sudden collapse with loss of motor tone, with or without injury, is the most common presentation of syncope. Self-report and eyewitness accounts of transient loss of consciousness are often unreliable—even when the eyewitness is a health-care professional. The most important first step is determining if it is true syncope. Obtain the patient's description of symptoms preceding the event and of activities that may have precipitated the event. Cardiac-related syncope may be sudden and without warning. A brief prodrome of symptoms, such as nausea, pallor, or diaphoresis, may suggest a vasovagal episode or a seizure. Many elderly patients report presyncopal episodes along with true syncopal events. Determine if any focal neurological symptoms were present (i.e., diplopia, motor and sensory symptoms). Review significant past medical history, prior history of an event, all medications being used, and alcohol intake. Ask about family history for sudden cardiac event.

The physical examination should start with checking the patient for evidence of trauma, then focus the physical examination on the cardiovascular and neurological components. Check blood pressure in both arms and positionally. Determine the compensatory pulse rate. Check the carotids for bruits. Carotid sinus compression sometimes is used to provoke symptoms, but this should be done cautiously and selectively and is contraindicated in patients with a bruit or a history of stroke or myocardial infarction. Examine the heart, assessing for murmurs, signs of arrhythmia, vascular disease, and left ventricular dysfunction. Check oxygen saturation rates. Perform a thorough neurological examination, paying particular attention to focal abnormalities that may suggest neurological syncope. Generalized anxiety disorders can cause hyperventilation and trigger a vasodepressor reaction; this should be evaluated during the physical examination.

Diagnostic tests: The ECG is the most important diagnostic test with a focus on the rate and rhythm. Cardiac diagnostic studies may include echocardiogram (valuable in estimating ejection fraction and valvular heart disease), ambulatory ECG monitoring, and electrophysiological studies. A chest x-ray, which may reveal cardiomyopathy, is indicated in patients with new abnormal findings, patients with dyspnea, and patients without a recorded baseline. Electroencephalogram and CT scan of the head are reserved for patients with focal neurological abnormalities. Tilt-table testing is useful in patients with syncope of unknown etiology or patients with recurrent syncope. Vasovagal syncope may be induced with this procedure; this may be done with or without isoproterenol. Laboratory evaluation is generally of low yield but may include a CBC with differential if infection or anemia is suspected. Renal function studies and electrolytes also may be considered.

Differential diagnosis: Distinguish syncope from seizures, dizziness, drop attacks, orthostasis, postprandial hypotension, carotid sinus sensitivity, and arrhythmias. Atypical presentations include myocardial infarction and pulmonary embolism. Dizziness does not involve a loss of consciousness and is often characterized further as vertigo, lightheadedness, disequilibrium, or presyncope (sensation of impending loss of consciousness). Drop attacks are sudden drops without warning and may be due to transient basilar artery insufficiency at times precipitated by head movement or neck hyperextension. Metabolic disorders (hypoglycemia, hypoxemia) cause coma/somnolence rather than syncope. Orthostatic hypotension reflects a drop in blood pressure of 20 mm Hg systolic or 10 mm Hg diastolic after changing from a lying to a standing position. Consider the relationship to meals with a drop in blood pressure. Carotid sinus sensitivity and arrhythmias (atrioventricular block, sick sinus syndrome, and supraventricular arrhythmias) increase with age. Supraventricular arrhythmias rarely cause syncope, but ventricular tachyarrhythmias, especially those with decreased ejection fraction, are a major concern.

Treatment: When you identify the specific cause of syncope, you can initiate the appropriate treatment. Vasodepressor syncope is best addressed with volume expansion. Antiarrhythmic therapy is initiated, if indicated, and drug-induced or idiopathic orthostatic hypotension is treated appropriately. Cardiac pacing may be appropriate. Cardiac surgery is the treatment of choice for obstructive heart disease. Always correct underlying anemia and metabolic imbalance, and optimize cardiac and pulmonary status in the elderly patient. Address any age-related, disease-related, or disuse-related changes that impair the patient's compensation for hypotensive stressors, such as dehydration, deconditioning, and orthostatic hypotension. Nonpharmacological approaches to vasodepressor syncope include tilt-table training and lower extremity muscle tensing.

Follow-up: Unknown causes precipitate a high incidence of syncopal events, and in one-third of patients syncope is a recurring event. Because recurrences may reflect lack of effective therapy or a failure to diagnose correctly, close monitoring is indicated.

Sequelae: Syncope from cardiovascular causes tends to be more dangerous. Sudden death with syncope has been attributed to arrhythmia. Patients with syncope are at risk for fall-related injury (fracture, subdural hematoma) and reduced functional capacity.

Prevention/prophylaxis: Patients with vasovagal syncope are taught to avoid triggers and, if premonitory symptoms occur, to lie down immediately and elevate the feet higher than the chest. Adequate fluid intake is a precaution, and for selected individuals with vasovagal syncope, a higher salt intake may be advised. Support hose may help prevent reduction in central plasma volume. Patients are encouraged to avoid a sudden change in position. For syncope caused by atrial fibrillation, low-dose warfarin or aspirin therapy may be prescribed. Micturition syncope can be avoided by advising men to sit down to urinate.

Referral: Hospitalization is necessary for patients in whom you suspect an arrhythmia or myocardial infarction as the cause of the syncope and for patients who sustain significant injury during the syncopal event. Consultation may be appropriate with a cardiologist for managing cardiac syncope and with a neurologist for managing neurally mediated syncope.

Education: In addition to teaching preventive strategies and the avoidance of triggering events, teach individuals with recurrent syncope safety precautions related to driving or the use of dangerous machinery. It is prudent for the health-care professional to understand the driving laws relative to loss of consciousness/syncope in the state.

CLINICAL RECOMMENDATIONS	EVIDENCE RATING	REFERENCE
A 12-lead ECG in all patients coming to the emergency department for syncope should be done.	A	Huff et al. (2007)
Serious outcomes following syncope are unlikely if the following risk factors are absent: systolic blood pressure >90 mm Hg, shortness of breath, ECG with new changes or nonsinus rhythm, history of heart failure, hematocrit less than 30%.	B	Miller (2011)

A = consistent, good-quality, patient-oriented evidence; B = inconsistent or limited-quality, patient-oriented evidence; C = consensus, disease-oriented evidence, usual practice, expert opinion, or case series. For information about the SORT evidence rating system, go to www.aafp.org/afpsort.xml.

TREMOR

Description: Tremor is the most common form of involuntary movement and is characterized by rhythmic oscillation of a body part that can be classified according to the circumstances under which it occurs. Only a small fraction of persons with tremor seek medical attention. Tremors may result from physiological or pathological processes.

Etiology: Because of the vast number of causes of tremor, etiological classification is not helpful. Terms used to describe the clinical phenomenology of tremor include rest tremors and action tremors. *Rest tremor* occurs when muscle is not activated voluntarily, and the relevant body part is fully supported against gravity, whereas *action tremor* is present with voluntary contraction of muscle. Action tremors can be subclassified further into postural, kinetic, and isometric tremor. *Postural tremor* is present while voluntarily maintaining a position against gravity. *Kinetic tremor* may occur during any form of voluntary movement of the affected body part. *Isometric tremor* occurs with muscle contraction against a rigid stationary object. The most common tremor is enhanced physiological tremor followed by essential tremor and then parkinsonian tremor.

Occurrence: Tremor is the most common movement disorder encountered in clinical practice. Everyone has a low-amplitude physiological tremor that can be observed when the arms are extended. Present in all muscle groups, it persists throughout the waking state. Enhanced physiological tremor is a physiological tremor that comes and goes with anxiety, caffeine, and fatigue. Estimates suggest that 3 to 4 million people in the United States have the most common form of pathological tremor, essential tremor, and most do not seek help until later age because of slow progression. In 50% of cases, the disease is familial (autosomal dominant, meaning 50% of an affected individual's children have it). More than 70% of patients with Parkinson's disease have tremor as the presenting symptom. Less common are cerebellar tremor, psychogenic tremor, dystonic tremor, and tremor associated with Wilson's disease.

Age: Most studies report a significant age-associated increase in the prevalence of essential tremor. Essential tremor begins in young to middle-aged people and gradually intensifies with age. Most studies report a significant age-associated increase in the prevalence

of essential tremor. Tremors in older adults are more likely to be of the essential or parkinsonian type.

Ethnicity: Tremor is more prevalent in whites than in blacks and is of intermediate prevalence in Hispanics.

Gender: Tremor afflicts both genders equally, with perhaps slightly more frequency in men than in women.

Contributing factors: During times of stress, the amplitude of a physiological tremor increases. Fatigue, anxiety, hyperthyroidism, systemic illness, use of medications, drug withdrawal (especially from alcohol), use of methylxanthines, and excess caffeine intake can exaggerate tremor. Medications that can cause or exacerbate tremor include those that stimulate the sympathetic nervous system and psychoactive medications.

Signs and symptoms: The first step in the evaluation of tremor is to categorize based on activation conditions, distribution, and frequency. Determine the duration and age of onset of symptoms, exacerbating or alleviating factors, and any family history of tremor or other neurological disorders. Include any associated symptoms, such as bradykinesia or rigidity (suggesting Parkinson's disease) or ataxia and nystagmus (suggesting cerebellar disease). The patient's medication history, any exposure to toxins, and the presence of illness should be noted. In assessment of the impact of tremor on patients' lives, functional disability in performing ADLs and the patient's subjective assessment of his or her quality of life are useful. History is important, but the diagnosis is based on clinical physical examination findings. Tremor may occur in various body parts, such as the hands, head, facial structures (chin, tongue, lips, and ears), vocal cords, trunk, and legs. Of all tremors, 94% occur in the hands, either unilaterally or bilaterally.

On physical examination it is important to conduct a thorough tremor-focused neurological examination: muscle tone is checked throughout the body, cranial structures (including the mouth and jaw) are examined at rest and in action, and the tongue is observed during rest and protrusion. To distinguish properly between resting and action tremors, patients should be evaluated while supine and when seated with the arms fully supported. (If patients are in a position that does not provide complete support, certain muscles may be active against gravity, producing a tremor that may be classified improperly as a resting tremor.) Once rest tremor is ruled out the patient performs other maneuvers.

The upper extremities are examined in an outstretched position with the hands supine (palms up), hands sideways (semiprone), and then prone (palms down). Semiprone enhances essential tremor whereas supine inhibits it. In the wing position (i.e., with apposition of the index fingers close to each other but not touching) proximal tremor may be identified. Goal-directed activities are performed, such as finger-to-nose, heel-to-shin, and toe-to-finger movements. The patient is asked to recite a standard paragraph and enunciate a sustained vowel. Handwriting samples are obtained (e.g., script, numbers, Archimedes spirals). Gait is evaluated for shuffling and unsteadiness, and Romberg (station) and balance testing are conducted. Careful evaluation is performed for signs associated with tremor syndromes. Bradykinesia and postural abnormalities are evaluated by observing difficulty rising from a seated position, decreased arm swing, and masked facies. Patients with essential tremor typically have handwriting that is shaky and large, whereas the handwriting of patients with Parkinson's disease initially may be of normal size and progressively become smaller (micrographia). Archimedes spirals drawn by essential tremor patients tend to illustrate natural fluctuations in tremor magnitude.

Diagnostic tests: No specific tests are routinely ordered for tremors. Electromyography is used to subdivide tremors according to their rate and their relationship to posture of limbs and volitional movement. Tremor frequency usually is categorized as low frequency (<4 Hz), medium frequency (4 to 6 Hz), and high frequency (>6 Hz).

The diagnosis of tremor is primarily clinical; however, laboratory testing may be necessary to exclude certain conditions that may be associated with tremor, such as metabolic disturbances, including hyperthyroidism (e.g., through thyroid function tests) and Wilson's disease. Brain imaging may be indicated for select patients, particularly patients with tremor that is unilateral, of sudden onset, or associated with atypical clinical features. For difficult cases, single-photon emission computed tomography (SPECT) to visualize the integrity of dopaminergic pathways may be useful in diagnosing Parkinson's disease.

Differential diagnosis: The differential diagnosis, in general practice, is almost always between Parkinson's disease and essential tremor.

Physiological tremor: A normal phenomenon, physiological tremor occurs in all contracting muscle groups. Although seldom visible to the naked eye, physiological tremor often may be detected when the fingers are firmly outstretched with a piece of paper placed over the hands.

Enhanced physiological tremor (or an intensification of physiological tremor to detectable levels): Physiological tremor may be enhanced under conditions of stress, anxiety, fatigue, exercise, cold, hunger, stimulant use, alcohol withdrawal, or metabolic disturbances such as hypoglycemia or hyperthyroidism. Although the tremor is typically low in amplitude and high in frequency (8 to 12 Hz), it may be clinically indistinguishable from essential tremor.

Essential tremor (4 to 12 Hz): Essential tremor is a persistent postural and kinetic tremor that predominantly affects the hands and forearms. Classically, to show the tremor, the patient is asked to extend the arms in front of the body. The legs are affected less often. Although less frequently involved, the presence of tremor in the head and/or voice is a strong indication of essential tremor and is especially useful in differentiating the syndrome from Parkinson's disease. Head tremor, which is also postural, disappears when the head is supported. Listening to the patient speak or having the patient hold a musical note as long as possible may reveal a quivering intonation. A resting component is present only rarely and typically occurs in the most advanced cases.

Parkinsonian tremor syndromes (4 to 6 Hz): Parkinsonian tremor syndromes involve resting tremor that is often asymmetrical. Tremor may be observed when muscles are relaxed, such as when the hands are resting on the lap, and may affect hands, feet, mandible, and lips. Tremor disappears during sleep. Typical is an alternating tremor of the thumb against the index finger—*pill-rolling* tremor. Although rest tremor is a diagnostic criterion for Parkinson's disease, other forms of tremor also may be present.

Treatment: Tremor should be treated if it causes disability. First-line treatment for tremor is oral medication. Beta blockers, anticholinergic medication, and levodopa are useful modalities for resting tremor. Kinetic tremor may respond to beta blockers, primidone, anticholinergics, and alcohol. When there is a lack of response to medical treatment or when tremor results in severe disability, a patient may be considered for neurosurgery. Specific treatments for the most common causes are noted below:

Physiological tremor: Usually no treatment is required for physiological tremor. When exaggerated, however, it may interfere with activities requiring extreme precision. Identify and remove precipitating causes and contributing causes. If the precipitating cause cannot be removed, propranolol may be effective.

Essential tremor: Varying degrees of control in essential tremor have been obtained with the beta blocker propranolol and the anticonvulsant agent primidone. Either agent may be considered an appropriate first-line therapy for the symptomatic management of essential tremor. When appropriate, these agents may be administered in combination with benzodiazepines, such as lorazepam or clonazepam. If the medication is of no benefit at a dose that causes adverse effects, dose levels should be tapered down gradually and eventually discontinued. If a medication is documented to be beneficial, it may be continued at the regulated doses, and the next medication may be added to the drug regimen. If the response to a drug is adequate and the dose is well tolerated, you may continue to monitor tolerance and possibly increase the dose. Physical and psychological measures may be helpful in managing mild tremor. Physical measures may include the application of weights to affected limbs to decrease tremor amplitude. Some patients have experienced benefits with biofeedback, relaxation methods, and other behavioral techniques through alleviation of anxiety or stress that may exacerbate tremor. Alcohol consumption may lead to transient improvement for many with essential tremor. The potential risk of alcohol dependence and abuse among essential tremor patients who drink alcohol to control symptoms is controversial. Alcohol has no impact on the tremor of PD.

Parkinsonian tremor: The tremor of Parkinson's disease results from a loss of striatal dopamine, and this is the rationale for treatment with either the dopamine precursor levodopa or dopamine receptor agonists. Dopaminergic and anticholinergic agents are equally effective, but dopaminergic substances additionally improve other parkinsonian signs, and the potential side effects of anticholinergic medications make these drugs undesirable in the elderly. The combination of levodopa and carbidopa reduces levodopa-induced nausea; a typical starting dose is one tablet of Sinemet 25/100 three times daily.

Patients with severe tremors that are resistant to pharmacotherapy may benefit from ablative surgery and/or deep brain stimulation.

Follow-up: Patients should be evaluated for therapeutic effects and side effects within 1 week of starting treatment. Annual monitoring for weight loss, depression, and decline in functional status is necessary.

Sequelae: Functional disabilities may occur in ADLs, including compromised eating, drinking, and preparing food. Decreased caloric intake and weight loss may be observed. Ambulation, especially on stairs, may be hazardous. Withdrawal from social situations may occur, and depression is common.

Prevention/prophylaxis: Reduce factors that can exacerbate the tremor. Continue medication regimen.

Referral: A neurologist should be consulted for cerebellar tremors, mixed tremors, or parkinsonian tremor or when a focal neurological deficit is identified. An ophthalmologist should be consulted when Wilson's disease is suspected. A mental health provider or psychiatrist should be consulted when a hysterical tremor is suspected. Physical therapy or occupational therapy may be helpful in advanced or disabling cases.

Education: Some patients, particularly patients with severe, disabling tremor, may limit their contacts. Patients must be encouraged to learn as much as they can about their disease to help them cope better with the condition's progression. When a diagnosis has been established, the natural history of the condition should be explained to patients. It also may be appropriate to recommend counseling. Use of appropriate coping strategies may reduce stress substantially, preventing possible augmentation of tremor owing to anxiety. Referral to appropriate patient-support organizations is helpful for most patients.

CLINICAL RECOMMENDATIONS	EVIDENCE RATING	REFERENCE
The diagnosis of tremor is based on clinical information from the history and physical examination.	C	Deuschl et al. (1998)
Propranolol and primidone are first-line treatments for essential tremor.	A	Pham (2011)

CLINICAL RECOMMENDATIONS	EVIDENCE RATING	REFERENCE
Tremor amplitude worsens over time if not treated.	C	Pham (2011)

A = consistent, good-quality, patient-oriented evidence; B = inconsistent or limited-quality, patient-oriented evidence; C = consensus, disease-oriented evidence, usual practice, expert opinion, or case series. For information about the SORT evidence rating system, go to www.aafp.org/afpsort.xml.

URINARY INCONTINENCE

Description: Urinary incontinence (UI) is defined by Agency for Healthcare Research and Quality (AHRQ) as the unintentional loss of urine. Because this is not a life-threatening condition in the older adult population, it is often not addressed during the history or review of systems and can have a significant impact on quality of life, depending on the individual's perception of the problem. Acute UI is generally a result of illness or the effects of medications and is self-limiting when the cause is determined and addressed. Chronic UI includes stress, urge, overflow, and functional incontinence. Many older women manifest a combination of urge and stress symptoms resulting in mixed incontinence.

Stress incontinence occurs as a result of weak pelvic floor support and increased intra-abdominal pressure, causing the loss of urine with maneuvers such as coughing or laughing. This lack of anatomical support, weak pelvic floor muscles, and changes in coaptation and softness of the urethra are changes due to estrogen deficiency. These changes can result in inadequate urethral resistance to increased intra-abdominal pressure and the leakage of urine. Stress incontinence is common in women and often goes unreported.

Urge incontinence, also known as overactive bladder (OAB), is the loss of urine associated with urgency that is not necessarily related to the quantity of urine in the bladder. Detrusor muscle instability is the primary feature of OAB and is also associated with frequency and nocturia. When detrusor muscle pressures exceed urethral pressure, this will result in urine leakage and UI. Neurological injuries, infectious and inflammatory disorders, medications, chronic illness, and lifestyle issues can contribute to OAB.

Overflow incontinence is the involuntary loss of urine associated with overdistention and incomplete emptying of the bladder. This can be an acute event, such as with the use of anticholinergic medications, diuretics, trauma to the pelvis, or fecal impaction. Overflow incontinence is often associated with bladder outlet obstruction, such as benign prostatic hypertrophy in men and pelvic organ prolapse in women. Neurogenic bladder can also present as overflow UI. Symptoms can present as constant dribbling, frequency, hesitation when initiating urination, and nocturia.

Functional UI is associated with factors unrelated to urinary tract anatomy and physiology, such as cognitive impairment, immobility, and dexterity that is inadequate to meet toileting needs. Adequate assistance and environmental factors to meet continence needs, such as eliminating stairs, and providing grab bars and a raised toilet seat, can promote an individual's ability to maintain urinary continence.

Etiology: The causes and management of UI are multifactorial, depending on the type of incontinence and also the severity and impact on quality of life for the individual. Anatomical changes, factors related to the individual's medical history, lifestyle, and acute and chronic illnesses, in addition to medications, can result in incontinence that can be permanent or reversible. Cognitive as well as chronic mental illness, depression, and functional barriers to continence can also affect an individual's ability to maintain urinary continence.

Occurrence: Urinary incontinence is often unreported, with the prevalence of UI being more common in women and increasing with age. Approximately 32% of women over 80 years old report symptoms of UI. In the long-term care setting, this rate increases to 43% to 77% of the population and is the cause of approximately 1 in 10 nursing home admissions.

Age: Urinary incontinence affects all age groups, with the highest prevalence in older adults who are institutionalized, have cognitive impairment, and are physically frail with functional limitations. Despite popular belief, prompted voiding can be an effective intervention when used for individuals with cognitive impairment. Schnelle et al. (2010), in a randomized, controlled trial, found that subjects with cognitive impairment were the most responsive to prompted voiding as an intervention for UI. It is believed that the inability to self-initiate behavior, such as scheduled toileting or responding to the urge to void, is the primary cause of incontinence in this population, unlike other individuals whose incontinence is a result of other physical, medical, and environmental causes.

Ethnicity: Not significant with regard to incontinence in general; however, some data indicate a higher prevalence of stress incontinence among Caucasian women, whereas black women were found to be at higher risk for urge incontinence.

Gender: Urinary incontinence is twice as prevalent in women as in men and increases with age, with institutionalized older adults at the highest risk. Women are at higher risk for stress incontinence; however, overflow incontinence is more prevalent in men.

Contributing factors: The many contributing factors for UI include pelvic muscle weakness, multiparity, estrogen depletion, pelvic organ prolapse, diabetes, stroke, multiple sclerosis, Parkinson's disease, spinal cord injury, benign prostatic hypertrophy, urinary tract infection, fecal impaction, poor fluid intake, excessive fluid intake, smoking, cognitive impairment, depression, immobility or impaired mobility, environmental barriers, impaired dexterity, visual impairment, obesity, and high-impact physical activities. The side effects of many medications, such as anticholinergics, diuretics, antispasmodics, opiates, hypnotics, calcium channel blockers, ACE inhibitors, alcohol, and caffeine, also can contribute to urinary incontinence.

Signs and symptoms: Screening for UI can be evaluated as to whether symptoms are transient or persistent in nature. Functional assessment of the older adult should include questions regarding urinary incontinence and the degree to which this condition affects quality of life. Direct questions will yield a better evaluation of UI symptoms.

As part of the review of systems, asking about urine loss when sneezing, coughing, or laughing or during physical activity will evaluate the likelihood of stress incontinence. Frequent trips to the toilet, urgency with a small volume of urinary output, and discomfort with voiding may indicate urge incontinence. Additionally, men with a complaint of urgency, dribbling of urine, and hesitancy should be further assessed for overflow incontinence and appropriately diagnosed and treated for the cause of these symptoms. Restlessness and pacing in the older adult male with cognitive impairment may warrant observation of voiding patterns by caregivers to assess for bladder outlet obstruction symptoms. A thorough review of systems and functional assessment including screening for cognitive dysfunction and depression are also revealing to diagnose functional incontinence.

Questioning about the use of pads or other incontinence products further indicates that UI is problematic for the patient. The use of a bladder diary for a few days, indicating frequency, incontinent episodes, fluid intake, products used, and frequency of bowel movements, is also helpful in assessing the cause and impact of UI on the individual's lifestyle and function. The effect of these symptoms on ADLs, socialization, and relationships, including sexual activity, also needs further investigation to assess the need for treatment. Considering that approximately 10% of nursing home admissions are a result of UI, discussion with patients and caregivers before long-term care placement about symptoms of UI has the potential to prolong the individual's ability to be maintained at home for an extended period of time.

A history of the problem should include onset, duration, aggravating and relieving factors, associated symptoms, and current self-management. Obtain a thorough drug history, including use of prescribed and OTC medications, herbal and homeopathic remedies, caffeine, and alcohol. A surgical history, including gynecological, colorectal, urological, and neurosurgical procedures, should be explored. A history of any concurrent chronic diseases, such as diabetes mellitus, multiple sclerosis, stroke, spinal stenosis, parkinsonism, congestive heart failure, hypertension, or cancer with past radiation therapy, is essential to provide appropriate treatment for UI. Also of significance is if the patient has been hospitalized recently or had an indwelling catheter. It is also important to ask if there is any history of constipation to evaluate the risk for fecal impaction. Investigate nutritional status and fluid intake, as well as caffeine, citrus, and use of the artificial sweetener aspartame, because they can affect continence.

Recent changes in functional status are also helpful to reveal the cause of urinary incontinence. Questioning with regard to functional limitations and access to toileting may also be revealing, such as if climbing stairs is necessary to access the toilet, whether the bathroom is equipped with safety equipment, or if assistance of another person is available if needed to toilet. Consultation with other providers, such as a home health nurse or therapist who may be involved in the care of the patient, may also be enlightening to assess for environmental barriers to continence.

Physical examination should include functional assessment, with special attention to mobility and dexterity, especially the person's ability to remove necessary clothing in time to use the toilet. Vital signs should be completed, looking for the presence of an elevated temperature. Respiratory rate and the presence of dyspnea on exertion may affect continence due to limited stamina to complete necessary tasks for maintaining continence. Mental status, including cognition and evidence of depression, should be assessed. The abdomen should be examined for clues such as bladder distention, pelvic masses, inguinal lymphadenopathy, or tenderness in the suprapubic region. Bladder distention can be found in overflow incontinence secondary to obstruction. In women, malignancy, uterine fibroids, or organ prolapse in the pelvic region creates pressure on the bladder seen in urge, stress, or mixed incontinence. A vaginal examination may also reveal poor perineal hygiene, skin breakdown from urine soaking, or redness and thinning of tissue typical of atrophic changes. Prolapse of genitourinary structures or the rectum may be seen.

To assess for pelvic floor muscle strength and relaxation, instruct the patient to bear down as though having a bowel movement, then tighten or squeeze by pulling up with the pelvic floor muscles. In patients with pelvic floor relaxation, you can see the inability to contract or weak contractions, and feel a lack of muscle tone when testing during the vaginal examination. Have the patient cough and determine if leakage occurs. Urethral discharge in male patients should also be assessed. Positive neurological findings in the perineal area include hypersensation, hyposensation, or absence of the bulbocavernosus (anal wink) reflex. A rectal examination may uncover fecal impaction, rectal prolapse, hemorrhoids, masses, or, in men, prostatic enlargement. Whenever possible, the examiner should observe the patient voiding, having the patient void into a measurable receptacle. This should be followed by evaluation of a postvoid residual urine catheterization (PVR) or ultrasound of the bladder. Studies are inconclusive with respect to the amount of PVR that is significant, with values ranging from >50 mL to >200 mL.

Diagnostic tests: Initial evaluation for urinary incontinence should include a urinalysis to rule out infection and renal abnormalities. This is especially a consideration when UI is an acute event. The presence of nitrites and leukocyte esterase in the urinalysis is usually indicative of an infectious process. When a urinary tract infection is suspected, a culture and sensitivity should be ordered to ensure appropriate antimicrobial therapy. Hematuria may indicate a number of differential diagnoses, including infection, obstruction, or malignancy. Proteinuria is revealing for renal disease and is often associated with poorly controlled diabetes. When renal, metabolic, or obstructive causes of urinary tract dysfunction are suspected, a basic metabolic panel is recommended to evaluate elevated BUN, creatinine, and calculation of creatinine clearance to evaluate for renal disease. Measurement of postvoid residual urine by a bladder ultrasound or catheterization is revealing for evaluating urinary retention.

When symptoms and basic noninvasive evaluation do not clearly indicate the type of urinary tract dysfunction, and the individual indicates that urinary incontinence is problematic enough to warrant further treatment, urodynamic testing and referral to a urologist or urogynecologist is indicated. Urodynamic testing evaluates all stages of lower urinary tract function, including filling and storage, as well as bladder outlet abnormalities. Subjective reporting by the patient of sensation such as urgency can also be evaluated with respect to bladder wall compliance, detrusor overactivity, pressure, and flow measurements during testing. Cystoscopy is indicated for evaluation of hematuria to visualize the bladder wall when cancer is suspected, and also when stricture or prostate enlargement is suspected with symptoms of urinary retention.

Differential diagnosis: Urinary incontinence is a symptom, not a diagnosis. The two mnemonics *DRIP* and *DIAPERS* often are used to differentiate transient (acute) from persistent urinary incontinence:

Mnemonic: DRIP
- **D**elirium
- **R**estricted mobility
- **I**nfection
- **P**harmaceuticals, polyuria

Mnemonic: DIAPERS
- **D**elirium
- **I**nfection, impaction, inflammation
- **A**trophic vaginitis

- **P**sychological, pharmaceuticals, psychotropics
- **E**ndocrine problem
- **R**estricted mobility
- **S**tool impaction

Treatment: Management of UI will depend on the type of incontinence, the patient's preference with regard to his or her perception of how UI affects his or her lifestyle, and also the patient's physical condition to tolerate treatments, surgical procedures, and risk for adverse effects and complications as a result of medications and treatment regimens. For transient UI, treating, eliminating, or modifying the cause usually alleviates the symptom. Delirium or a mild elevation in temperature from the patient's baseline, rather than a fever, may be the first indication of a urinary tract infection in the older adult. Appropriate antimicrobial therapy will generally resolve the UI as a result of the infection.

Behavioral therapies and pelvic muscle exercises or Kegel exercises can be an effective treatment for stress incontinence and OAB, performed alone or in combination with biofeedback, to help strengthen periurethral muscles. Toileting programs, such as bladder training, scheduled toileting, and prompted voiding, can be effective interventions for controlling UI, even in patients with cognitive impairment. Nocturia can be a very annoying problem and cause significant issues where quality of life is concerned. Control of comorbidities and symptoms such as edema, in addition to limiting fluids before bedtime, can be helpful to improve sleep hygiene.

Pharmacological treatment for urge urinary incontinence with anticholinergic drugs is an effective treatment for OAB symptoms; however, they are not without side effects, especially constipation, blurred vision, and cognitive changes in older adults. These medications, such as tolterodine and oxybutynin, seem to be better tolerated in long-acting and transdermal forms. Drugs that are more selective for M3 receptors, such as darifenacin and solifenacin, and also trospium, which does not appear to cross the blood-brain barrier, appear to have a better side-effect profile and are better tolerated in the older adult population. In the STAR trial, with 70% of subjects over age 65, efficacy and tolerability of solifenacin was found to have better outcomes with regard to incontinence than long-acting tolterodine. Comorbidities such as narrow-angle glaucoma and potential interactions with other medications are always a concern in the geriatric population, and should be considered before prescribing a drug

regimen for UI. Topical estrogen therapy (one-quarter applicator nightly) for 2 weeks, then 3 times a week ongoing, can be an effective remedy for UI as a result of vaginal atrophy. Studies have also indicated that the antidepressant duloxetine can be an effective treatment for stress UI, with approximately a 50% reduction in incontinence episodes and improved quality of life; however, nausea as a significant adverse effect may reduce compliance with this treatment regimen.

For patients with overflow incontinence secondary to prostatic hypertrophy, 5-alpha-reductase inhibitors (finasteride, dutasteride) are effective to reduce prostate volume by preventing the conversion of testosterone to dihydrotestosterone. These drugs should not be handled by women of childbearing age, because they can be harmful to the development of a male fetus. Selective alpha-adrenergic antagonists such as tamsulosin relax smooth muscle to reduce urethral resistance and improve urine flow. Nonselective alpha-1 blockers such as doxazosin and terazosin are effective for UI and can also be used in patients who also require antihypertensive therapy. The provider should consider, however, the cardiovascular side effects due to their nonselectivity, because orthostatic hypotension is an adverse reaction that can have serious consequences, such as increased fall risk and injuries, in the older adult patient. Postprostatectomy incontinence can be treated long after surgery with behavioral therapy such as pelvic floor muscle training. Studies have found an average of 55% reduction in incontinence using these strategies.

Other treatments for UI include bulking agents such as collagen for stress incontinence, botulinum toxin, sacral nerve stimulation for urge incontinence, and surgical interventions for stress incontinence in women and for prostatic hypertrophy in men. Referral to urology or urogynecology for surgical intervention is appropriate if the patient is inclined to consider surgical intervention and is physically able to tolerate the procedure. Surgical management for pelvic organ prolapse to improve organ support, such as retropubic suspension, sling procedures, and vaginal mesh, are viable options; however, patient education with regard to the high failure rate (5% to 12%) should be discussed when considering these options. In July 2011, the Food and Drug Administration released an advisory and is reassessing regulation of vaginal mesh implants due to risks associated with the procedure. When surgical treatment for UI as a result of pelvic organ prolapse is contraindicated, a pessary is a viable option. In addition to incontinence pads and briefs, pessaries, when properly fitted within the vaginal vault to correct organ prolapse and reduce stress UI, can often be managed by the patient or cared for by a qualified nurse at regular intervals. Nonsurgical management of persistent urinary overflow incontinence includes clean intermittent catheterization. Although the Centers for Medicare and Medicaid Services now reimburses for a single-use sterile catheter, there is no evidence to support a reduction in urinary tract infections with the use of sterile versus clean urinary catheter.

Follow-up: Follow-up visits will depend on the acuity and severity of symptoms. Treatment of infection and symptoms related to urinary retention requires closer and more frequent follow-up until the problem is resolved due to complications that can result in renal problems. Initially, medication management should be monitored closely for adverse effects, especially with anticholinergic medications, because the side effects of these medications can result in significant complications for the geriatric patient, such as blurred vision, dizziness, and somnolence, that can contribute to fall risk. Long-acting medications appear to have less of a risk profile, but individual monitoring is necessary to ensure patient safety. Additionally, dementia exacerbation can occur with the use of anticholinergic medications, resulting in hallucinations, psychosis, or changes in behavior that can result in injury to the individual or others. Constipation, a common adverse effect of anticholinergics, can exacerbate UI by causing a fecal impaction. Polypharmacy issues also need to be monitored closely with any medication change, requiring close follow-up when starting a new drug regimen.

Sequelae: Possible complications include urinary tract infection, hydronephrosis (with overflow or obstruction), renal failure, adverse drug events, or failure of behavioral therapy. Skin breakdown is a significant complication with persistent UI. Urosepsis can occur with unrecognized urinary tract infections. Falls can occur due to UI as a result of environmental factors and as a result of side effects of medication management. Social isolation as a result of uncontrolled urinary incontinence can have a significant impact on quality of life and result in the need for institutionalization if the patient or caregiver is unable to manage symptoms.

Prevention/prophylaxis: Ways to help prevent incontinence include the following:

- Early identification of acute or transient UI
- Teaching patients and family members/caregivers that UI is not a normal part of the aging process, and that treatment options are available

- Referral to appropriate specialists for treatment options
- Regular rectal examination in men to detect and treat early prostatic hypertrophy
- Recognition of polypharmacy and adverse reactions when initiating new medications in the geriatric population

Referral: Referral to urogynecology for the female patient to explore treatment options is appropriate if behavioral interventions and medication management are unsuccessful or if the patient's symptoms are affecting her quality of life. It is also appropriate to refer to a specialty practice if the patient does not respond to the treatment plan or the diagnosis is uncertain. Refer men with overflow incontinence for urological evaluation urgently if postvoid residual urine volume is significant, to prevent renal complications, and for surgical intervention if indicated. Certified continence nurse specialists may be an appropriate referral for behavioral therapies, such as biofeedback or for electrical stimulation treatments to improve continence. Further workup and referral to urology would be indicated if abnormalities in the urinalysis do not resolve after treatment for infection, such as persistent hematuria or proteinuria, or if the patient has a past medical history that includes surgeries for genitourinary diagnoses, or a history of pelvic cancer with or without radiation therapy. Patients with neurogenic bladder as a result of injury or a chronic neurological condition should be followed by a neurologist in collaboration with the primary care provider.

Education: Teach patients, family, caregivers, and health-care providers, as well as the community, that UI is *not* a normal part of aging and it is a treatable medical problem. Behavioral therapy can be provided in the primary care setting, such as Kegel exercises, as well as self-catheterization techniques. Written instructions given to the patient with possible adverse drug effects when starting a new medication can preempt serious consequences of drug effects/complications. Teach patients, especially women and men with bladder outlet obstruction, the signs and symptoms of urinary tract infection, including delirium as an indication of acute illness, and that a fever may not be a good indication of infection in the older adult. Dietary issues such as adequate fluid intake, limiting bladder irritants such as caffeine and alcohol, and prevention of constipation to avoid fecal impaction can help avoid bladder symptoms and infections. The importance of good perineal hygiene, especially for women and patients who do self-catheterization, should be emphasized when appropriate. When incontinence cannot be completely avoided, attention to skin care and instruction in the use of skin barriers such as zinc oxide or dimethacone-based products should be taught to the patient or caregivers to prevent skin breakdown.

DIAGNOSIS	CLINICAL RECOMMENDATIONS	EVIDENCE RATING	REFERENCE
Urinary incontinence	Combination behavioral therapy and medication management.	A	Hay-Smith & Dulmoulin (2007) Wallace, Roe, Williams, & Palmer (2007)
Stress urinary incontinence	Alpha-adrenergic medications, serotonin-norepinephrine reuptake inhibitors.	B	Alhasso, Glazener, Pickard, & N'Dow (2007) Mariappan et al. (2007)
Stress urinary incontinence	Surgical procedures.	B	Bezerra, Bruschini, Cody, & Bezerra (2007)
Urge urinary incontinence	Anticholinergic medications (antimuscarinic agents).	A	Nabi et al. (2007) Zinner et al. (2011)
Overflow urinary incontinence	Treatment of underlying cause of bladder outlet obstruction, urinary catheterization.	C	Amin (2011)
Functional urinary incontinence	Scheduled toileting.	A	Wallace et al. (2007)
Mixed urinary incontinence	Anticholinergic medications (antimuscarinic agents).	A	Nabi et al. (2007)

A = consistent, good-quality, patient-oriented evidence; B = inconsistent or limited-quality, patient-oriented evidence; C = consensus, disease-oriented evidence, usual practice, expert opinion, or case series. For information about the SORT evidence rating system, go to www.aafp.org/afpsort.xml.

WANDERING

Description: Wandering is characterized as an excessive ambulatory behavior initiated by a cognitively impaired and disoriented individual possibly to fulfill a particular need (Carson, 2012; Thomas, 1995). This problem is usually seen in patients with dementia and those with developmental disabilities. People who wander are thought to have impaired visual-spatial problems, depressive symptoms, and anxiety. The activity can be purposeful or purposeless wandering. This behavior is seen often in the moderate or middle stage of Alzheimer's with restlessness and pacing activity. The behavior presents safety problems in the home and the institutional setting (Chung & Lai, 2010; Douglas, Letts, & Richardson, 2011; Rowe, 2008).

Etiology: Individuals at highest risk for wandering are those patients diagnosed with the various forms of dementia, including Alzheimer's disease, frontotemporal dementia, Lewy body disease, and multi-infarct dementia (Algase, Antonakos, Beattie, Beel-Bates, & Yao, 2009). The loss of judgment puts these individuals at risk in the home setting and the long-term care setting. In the hospital a patient with delirium can also wander away, becoming confused because of the change in surroundings, medications, and current disease complications, such as decrease in oxygen or cardiac function, that have compromised the patient's cognitive ability.

Occurrence: There are 5.3 million people with Alzheimer's disease, the most common form of dementia, and it is the seventh-leading cause of death. The number of Alzheimer's cases is expected to rise to 7.7 million by 2030 (a 50% increase in cases) and to about 11 million to 16 million by 2050, due to the rapid aging of the population. At least 60% of individuals with Alzheimer's disease will wander at some point and may become lost (Alzheimer's Association, 2007, 2010).

Gender: Women are diagnosed more often with Alzheimer's disease. Women generally live longer than men and therefore are more likely to live to the age when Alzheimer's is more common.

Ethnicity: Older African Americans and Hispanics are more likely than Caucasians to be diagnosed with Alzheimer's disease and some of the other dementias.

Signs and symptoms: The symptoms of early dementia include memory problems. As the dementia progresses, problems are observed in judgment, becoming disoriented, becoming confused easily, and behavioral problems, including wandering. There are different types of wanderers. Some wandering is purposeful (trying to get to a place or a job, which may be linked with a former occupation or place of residence); some individuals display restless wandering that lacks a goal; and some are focused on "getting out," hovering around exit doors. Some individuals demonstrate patterns of wandering at certain times of the day or night.

Diagnostic tests: A thorough physical examination, checking medication effects, and laboratory testing to evaluate the individual may help identify the problem causing the wandering. Checking for an acute problem such as infection can determine if this could be the cause. Upper respiratory infections and urinary tract infections in the elder can present as confusion that could include agitation and wandering. Hospitalized patients suffering from delirium can be monitored for its acute presentation of symptoms, which can be caused by changes in environment, medication, or treatments (Rowe, 2008). Testing for dementia might also be appropriate if symptoms of wandering develop, though these are not the earliest symptoms that generally present. Many individuals do not obtain this diagnosis until midstage when wandering is seen as a symptom.

Treatment: Key items in treatment, once the cause of the wandering symptom has been identified, is to correct the problem if possible with medication, develop a treatment plan, and, most important, provide a safe environment for the patient. This might involve medication to calm the individual or, if diagnosed with dementia, anticholinergic medications and an NMDA antagonist to lessen the behavioral symptoms that accompany these disease processes (News Briefs, 2009). The patient with wandering requires close supervision and an environment free of hazards.

Sequelae: The wandering patient is at risk for injury if left in an environment that has hazards. News articles across the country provide stories of how patients wandered out of their home or long-term care facility and were found dead later (Carr et al., 2010). Research shows that if the wanderer is not located within 24 hours, the chance of being found alive decreases significantly. Wandering accompanied by gait disturbances can lend itself to falls with fractures. Weight loss is another problem with the wandering behavior. With the extra expenditure of calories and difficulty in getting the individual to sit still long enough to eat, this can result in unwanted weight loss in an already compromised patient. Wandering takes its toll on the caregiver as well. The caregiver in the home is ill equipped to monitor the wandering individual around the clock, 7 days a week. The caregiver can easily become overwhelmed with this responsibility. Both lay and professional caregivers experience extreme stress when the patient elopes. Legal claims are also a consequence of wandering and elopement behaviors (Algase, Beattie, Antonakos, Beel-Bates, & Yao, 2010; Moore, Algase, Powell-Cope, Applegarth, & Beattie, 2009).

Prevention/prophylaxis: Prevention is similar whether at home or in a long-term care setting. Assessment of the patient is key to preventing accidents occurring because of wandering. Extra monitoring is required whether at home or in a facility. Use devices such as alarm bracelets and secured doors in facilities (Futrell, Melillo, & Remington, 2008; Lang et al., 2009). Secured doors and door alarms can help facility staff monitor the wandering residents. At home this becomes much more of a challenge. Project Lifesaver has receivers and transmitters provided by local law enforcement that are loaned or sold to caregivers to assist them in home monitoring. This system can track the wandering individual should he or she escape the caregiver's watchful eye. You can access www.projectlifesaver.org/site for information on sources in your community. The Safe Return Program, sponsored by the Alzheimer's Association and Medic Alert, is also very valuable. Silver alert programs now exist in many states to identify and find cognitively impaired older adults. Providing a calm, uncluttered environment can lessen the anxiety of the individual, resulting in less agitation and wandering behavior. Making environmental modifications such as camouflaging a door or moving the locks near the top or bottom of the door may be helpful. Speaking in simple language with a calm tone can lessen the anxiety of a patient with dementia. Checking the individual to see if he or she is hungry, thirsty, or constipated or has to empty his or her bladder can assist the individual who may lack the ability to communicate these needs. Redirecting the wandering individual into another, less harmful activity can be helpful. For caregivers in the home, home health agency professionals can assist in providing education that may assist them in identifying dangers in the home and helpful information on dealing successfully with the wandering individual. Respite care is also helpful for the caregiver to provide some much-needed time to rest from the burden of full-time caregiving duties.

Referral: The individual with wandering symptoms demonstrates a need for scheduled follow-up and evaluation by his or her primary care provider. The provider will need to work with caregivers to determine their level of ability to care for the individual in the home. Referrals to home health agencies and other community resources to provide education and support to the caregiver are needed to maintain a safe environment. At each visit, explore with caregivers their evaluation of their ability to provide care and patient behavioral and health status to decide if long-term care placement may be needed. Referral for respite care and support groups may be helpful for the caregiver.

Education: Education of facility staff and caregivers is essential to improving the level of care provided for the wandering individual. This education can assist them in understanding the current disease process and how to effectively deal with this individual to provide a safe environment and promote the patient's quality of life.

CLINICAL RECOMMENDATIONS	EVIDENCE RATING	REFERENCE
Location, light, sound, proximity to others, and ambience are associated with wandering and may serve to inform environmental design and care practices.	C	Algase et al. (2010)
Assess for factors associated with wandering such as a lack of activity, cognitive impairment, socially inappropriate behavior, resistance to care, and greater impairment in activities of daily living.	B	University of Iowa Gerontological Nursing Interventions Research Center (2008)
Decrease wandering during structured activities by using social interaction of staff or visitors or music.	B	Futrell, Melillo, & Remington (2008)
Use technological devices to locate and monitor wandering.	B	Futrell et al. (2008)

A = consistent, good-quality, patient-oriented evidence; B = inconsistent or limited-quality, patient-oriented evidence; C = consensus, disease-oriented evidence, usual practice, expert opinion, or case series. For information about the SORT evidence rating system, go to www.aafp.org/afpsort.xml.

CASE STUDY

J. B. is a 77-year-old man who is known to your practice. He is brought in today by his daughter who reports a new onset of confusion accompanied by urinary incontinence (first noticed bed was wet a few nights ago). When you see the patient today, he is oriented to place and person (knows you and your office) but not time and does not recall much about events of the past few days. He says that he is eating and drinking as usual (but daughter is shaking her head to the contrary). He denies any change in bowel function but is fearful of sleeping, because he might "wet the bed." Daughter states that he has been drinking a lot more water than usual and urinating more frequently. He denies any pain, other than arthritis. He was a regular attendee at the local senior center but has not been there for a week and seems to have forgotten about it.

Past medical history: Known coronary artery disease, hypertension, hyperlipidemia, impaired fasting glucose, osteoarthritis of knees.

Medications: Lisinopril 20 mg orally (PO) once daily in evening. Hydrochlorothiazide 12.5 mg PO once daily in morning. Metoprolol 50 mg PO once daily in morning. Simvastatin 20 mg PO once daily. OTC medications include Aleve, 2 tablets every 12 hours when needed for severe knee pain (infrequent use); topical "Icy Hot" for knee pain daily; glucosamine-chondroitin preparation daily for joint health; multivitamin "male over 50 years" daily.

Vital signs: blood pressure (BP) 130/84 mm Hg; heart rate (HR) 60 beats/min, regular; respiratory rate 16 breaths/min; temperature 99.2°F orally; body mass index (BMI) 38.

Physical findings are unremarkable.

Using the guide to characterizing a symptom located in this chapter, focus on the following questions:

1. What additional subjective data are you seeking?

2. What additional objective data will you be assessing for?

3. What national guidelines are appropriate to consider?

4. What tests will you order? How will you decide on prioritizing in this patient with multiple symptoms?

5. What are the differential diagnoses that you are considering? For each one, map out your clinical reasoning for and against it and make a tentative plan to confirm it or rule it out.

6. Will you be looking for a consultation?

REFERENCES

Assessment

Inouye, S. K., Studenski, S., Tinetti, M. E., & Kuchel, G. A. (2007). Geriatric syndromes: clinical, research, policy implications of a core geriatric concept. *Journal of the American Geriatrics Society, 55*(5), 780–791.

Wasson, J. A., Walsh, B. T., Labrecque, M. C., Sox, H. C., Pantell, R., & Wasson, E. S. (2009). *The common symptom guide* (6th ed.). New York City, NY: McGraw-Hill.

Bowel Incontinence

Bartlett, L. M., Sloots, K., Nowack, M., & Ho, Y. H. (2011). Biofeedback therapy for faecal incontinence: a rural and regional perspective. *Rural Remote Health, 11*(2), 1630. Epub 2011 Mar 2.

Bliss, D. Z., Jung, H., Savik, K., Lowry, A., & Jensen, L. (2001). Supplementation with dietary fiber improves fecal incontinence. *Nursing Research, 50*(4), 203–213.

Bliss, D. Z., & Norton, C. (2010). Conservative management of fecal incontinence. *American Journal of Nursing, 110*(9), 1–15.

Boyle, D. J., Murphy, J., Gooneratne, M. L., Grimmer, K., Allison, M. E., Chan, C. L., & Williams, N. S. (2011). Efficacy of sacral nerve stimulation for the treatment of fecal incontinence. *Diseases of the Colon & Rectum, 54*(10), 1271–1278.

Brown, S. R., & Nelson, R. L. (2007). Surgery for faecal incontinence in adults. *Cochrane Database of Systematic Reviews, 18*(2), CD001757.

Cheetham, M., Brazzelli, M., Norton, C., & Glazener, C. M. (2003). Drug treatment for faecal incontinence in adults. *Cochrane Database of Systematic Reviews* (3), CD002116.

Croswell, E., Bliss, D. Z., & Savic, K. (2010). Diet and eating pattern modifications used by community-living adults to manage their fecal incontinence. *Journal of Wound, Ostomy and Continence Nursing, 37*(6), 677–682.

Gladman, M. A., Scott, S. M., & Williams, N. S. (2005). Assessing the patient with fecal incontinence. In S. D. Wexner, A. P. Zbar, & M. Pescatori (Eds.), *Complex anorectal disorders* (pp. 547–594). Heidelberg, Germany: Springer.

Hagglund, D. (2010, Feb 19). A systematic literature review of incontinence care for persons with dementia: the research evidence. *Journal of Clinical Nursing* (3–4), 303–312.

Harari, D. (2010). Constipation and fecal incontinence in old age. In H. M. Fillit, K. Rockwood, & K. Woodhouse (Eds.), *Brocklehurst's textbook of geriatric medicine and gerontology* (7th ed., pp. 909–925). Philadelphia, PA: Saunders.

Landefeld, C. S., Bowers, B. J., Feld, A. D., Hartmann, K. E., Hoffman, E., Ingber, M. J., . . . Rao, S. S. (2009). Fecal incontinence in the elderly. *Gastroenterology Clinics of North America, 38*(3), 503–511.

Michelsen, H. B., Thompson-Fawcett, M., Lundby, L., Krogh, K., Laurberg, S., & Buntzen, S. (2010). Six years of experience with sacral nerve stimulation for fecal incontinence. *Diseases of the Colon & Rectum, 53*(4), 414–421.

Norton, C. C., Cody, J. D., & Hosker, G. (2006). Biofeedback and/or sphincter exercises for the treatment of faecal incontinence in adults. *Cochrane Database of Systematic Reviews,* Issue 3. Art. No.: CD002111. doi:10.1002/14651858.CD002111.pub2

Ratto, C., Litta, F., Parello, A., Donisi, L., & Doglietto, G. B. (2010). Sacral nerve stimulation is a valid approach in fecal incontinence due to sphincter lesions when compared to sphincter repair. *Diseases of the Colon & Rectum, 53*(3), 264–272.

Scarlett, Y. (2004). Medical management of fecal incontinence. *Gastroenterology, 126*(1 Suppl. 1), 555–563.

Schnelle, J. F., Leung, F. W., Rao, S. S., Beuscher, L., Keeler, E., Clift, J. W., & Simmons, S. (2010). A controlled trial of an intervention to improve urinary and fecal incontinence and constipation. *Journal of the American Geriatrics Society, 58*(8), 1504–1511.

Shamliyan, T., Wyman, J., Bliss, D. Z., Kane, R. L., & Wilt, T. J. (2007, Dec). Prevention of urinary and fecal incontinence in adults. *Evidence Report: Technology Assessment* (161), 1–379.

Stevens, T. K., Soffer, E. E., & Palmer, R. M. (2003). Fecal incontinence in elderly patients: common, treatable, yet often undiagnosed. *Cleveland Clinic Journal of Medicine, 70*(5), 441–448.

Tariq, S. H. (2006). Sphincter function. In M. S. J. Pathy, A. J. Sinclair, & J. E. Morley (Eds.), *Principles and practice of geriatric medicine* (4th ed., Vol. 1, pp. 395–406). Chichester, England: John Wiley & Sons Ltd.

Tjandra, J. J., Dykes, S. L., Kumar, R. R., Ellis, C. N., Gregorcyk, S. G., Hyman, N. H., & Buie, W. D. (2007). Standards Practice Task Force of the American Society of Colon and Rectal Surgeons. Practice parameters for the treatment of fecal incontinence. *Essential Evidence Plus.* Retrieved from www.essentialevidenceplus.com/content/guideline/12542

Trock, B. J. (2008). National Institutes of Health state-of-the science conference statement: prevention of fecal and urinary incontinence in adults. *Annals of Internal Medicine, 148*(6), 449–459.

Chest Pain

American College of Cardiology (ACC) and American Heart Association (AHA). (2007). ACC/AHA 2007 guidelines for the management of patients with unstable angina/non–ST-elevation myocardial infarction. *Journal of the American College of Cardiology, 50*(7), e1–e157.

American Gastroenterological Association Institute. (2009). American Gastroenterological Association medical position statement on the management of gastroesophageal reflux disease. *Essential Evidence Plus.* Retrieved from www.essentialevidenceplus.com/content/e1-5

Buttaro, T. M., Aznavorian, S., & Dick, K. (2006). *Clinical management of patients in subacute and long-term care settings.* St. Louis, MO: Mosby.

Gerardo, M. P. (2007). Coronary artery disease and angina pectoris. In T. J. Wachtel & M. D. Fretwell (Eds.), *Practical guide to the care of the geriatric patient* (3rd ed., pp. 306–313). Philadelphia, PA: Mosby.

Heidelbaugh, J. J. (2009). Gastroesophageal reflux disease. *Essential Evidence Plus.* Retrieved from www.essentialevidenceplus.com/content/eee192

Hung, C. L., Hou, C. J. Y., Yeh, H., & Chang, W. (2010). Atypical chest pain in the elderly: prevalence, possible mechanisms and prognosis. *International Journal of Gerontology, 4*(1), 1–8.

Hutchinson, A., & Miller, M. (2010). Herpes zoster (shingles). *Essential Evidence Plus.* Retrieved from www.essentialevidenceplus.com/content/eee0313

Huttunen, M., & Pirkola, S. (2010). A patient with psychosomatic symptoms. *Essential Evidence Plus.* Retrieved from http://essentialevidenceplus.com/content/ebm00709(035.007)

Jonsbu, E., Dammen, T., Morken, G., Lied, A., Vik-Mo, H., & Martinsen, E. W. (2009). Cardiac and psychiatric diagnoses among patients referred for chest pain and palpitations. *Scandinavian Cardiovascular Journal, 43*(4), 256–269.

Kristopaitis, K., & Homan, D. (2009). Falls in elderly patients. *Essential Evidence Plus.* Retrieved from www.essentialevidenceplus.com/content/eee/799

Lenfant, C. (2010). Chest pain of cardiac and noncardiac origin. *Metabolism, 59*(Suppl. 1), S41–S46.

Monreal, M., & Lopez-Jiminez, L. (2010). Pulmonary embolism in patients over 90 years of age. *Current Opinion in Pulmonary Medicine, 16*(5), 432–436.

Rodney, K. Z. (2013). Coronary heart disease. *Essential Evidence Plus.* Retrieved from http:www.essentialevidenceplus.com.proxy.its.virginia.edu/content/eee/9

Thompson, A. B. (2009). Esophageal spasm and treatment. Retrieved from *Medscape.* Retrieved from http://www.medisuite.ir/medscape/A174975-bussiness.html a11

Tudiviver, F. (2011). Costochondritis and Tietze syndrome. *Essential Evidence Plus.* Retrieved from www.essentialevidenceplus.com/content/eee0385

van Schagen, J. E., & Dibble, P. J. (2011). Angina (unstable). *Essential Evidence Plus.* Retrieved from www.essentialevidenceplus.com/content/eee0010

Constipation

Bouras, E. P., & Tangelos, E. G. (2009). Chronic constipation in the elderly. *Gastroenterology Clinics of North America, 38*(3), 463–480.

Brandt, L. J., Prather, C. M., Quigley, E. M., Schiller, L. R., Schoenfeld, P., & Talley, N. J. (2005). Systematic review on the management of chronic constipation in North America. *American Journal of Gastroenterology, 100*(Suppl. 1), S5–S21.

Fleming, V., & Wade, W. E. (2010). A review of laxative therapies for treatment of chronic constipation in older adults. *American Journal of Geriatric Pharmacotherapy, 8*(6), 514–550.

Gallegos-Orozco, J. F., Foxx-Orenstein, A. E., Sterler, S. M., & Stoa, J. M. (2012). Chronic constipation in the elderly. *American Journal of Gastroenterology, 107*(1), 18–25.

Harari, D. (2010). Constipation and fecal incontinence in old age. In H. M. Fillitt, K. Rockwood, & K. Woodhouse (Eds.), *Brocklehurst's textbook of geriatric medicine and gerontology* (7th ed., pp. 909–925). Philadelphia, PA: Saunders Elsevier.

Harris, L. A. (2005). Prevalence and ramifications of chronic constipation. *Managed Care Interface, 18*(8), 23–30.

Hatari, D. (2009). Constipation. In J. B. Halter, J. G. Ouslander, M. E. Tinetti, S. Studenski, K. P. High, & S. Asthana (Eds.), *Hazzard's geriatric medicine and gerontology* (6th ed., pp. 1103–1122). New York City, NY: McGraw-Hill.

Hofford, R. A. (2011). Constipation (adult). *Essential Evidence Plus.* Retrieved April 15, 2012, from www.essentialevidenceplus.com/content/eee/176

Mugie, S. M., Benninga, M. A., & DeLorenzo, C. (2010). Epidemiology of constipation in children and adults: a systematic review. *Best Practice & Research: Clinical Gastroenterology, 25*(1), 3–18.

Rao, S. S. (2007). Constipation: evaluation and treatment of colonic and anorectal motility disorders. *Gastroenterology Clinics of North America, 36*(3), 687–711.

Rao, S. S., & Go, J. T. (2010). Update on the management of constipation in the elderly: new treatment options. *Clinical Interventions in Aging, 5,* 163–171.

Stewart, W. F., Liberman, J. N., Sandler, R. S., Woods, M. S., Sternhagen, A., Chee, E., . . . Farup, C. E. (1999). Epidemiology of Constipation (EPOC) study in the United States: relation of clinical subtypes to sociodemographic features. *American Journal of Gastroenterology, 94*(12), 3530–3540.

Cough

Braman, S. S. (2006a, January). Chronic cough due to acute bronchitis: ACCP evidence-based clinical practice. *Chest, 129*(1), 95S–103S.

Braman, S. S. (2006b, January). Postinfectious cough: ACCP evidence-based clinical practice guidelines. *Chest, 129*(1), 138S–146S.

Dicpinigaitis, P. V. (2006, January). Angiotensin-converting enzyme inhibitor–induced cough: ACCP evidence-based clinical practice guidelines. *Chest, 129*(1), 169S–173S.

File, T. M. (2009). The science of selecting antimicrobials for community-acquired pneumonia (CAP). *Journal of Managed Care Pharmacy, 15*(2), S5–S11.

Irwin, R. S., Baumann, M. H., Bolser, D. C., Boulet, L. P., Braman, S. S., Brightling, C. E., . . . Tarlo, S. M.; American College of Chest Physicians (ACCP). (2006, January). Diagnosis and management of cough executive summary: ACCP evidence-based clinical practice guidelines. *Chest, 129*(1 Suppl.), 1S–23S.

Pratter, M. R. (2006a, January). Chronic upper airway cough syndrome secondary to rhinosinus diseases (previously referred to as postnasal drip syndrome): ACCP evidence-based clinical practice guidelines. *Chest, 129*(1), 63S–71S.

Pratter, M. R. (2006b, January). Cough and the common cold: ACCP evidence-based clinical practice guidelines. *Chest, 129*(1), 72S–74S.

Pratter, M. R., Brightling, C. E., Boulet, L. P., & Irwin, R. S. (2006, January). An empiric integrative approach to the management of cough: ACCP evidence-based clinical practice guidelines. *Chest, 129*(1), 222S–231S.

Rosen, M. J. (2006, January). Chronic cough due to tuberculosis and other infections: ACCP evidence-based clinical practice guidelines. *Chest, 129*(1), 197S–201S.

Dehydration

Ciccone, A., Allegra, J. R., Cochrane, D. G., Cody, R. P., & Roche, L. M. (1998). Age related differences in diagnoses within the elderly population. *American Journal of Emergency Medicine, 16*(1), 43–48.

Hodgkinson, B., Evans, D., & Wood, J. (2003). Maintaining oral hydration in older adults: a systematic review. *International Journal of Nursing Practice, 9*(3), S19–S28.

Holman, C., Roberts, S., & Nicol, M. (2005). Promoting adequate hydration in older people. *Nursing Older People, 17*(4), 31–32.

Jequier, E., & Constant, F. (2010). Water as an essential nutrient: the physiological basis of hydration. *European Journal of Clinical Nutrition, 64*(2), 115–123.

Lavizzo-Mourey, R., Johnson, J., & Stolley, P. (1988). Risk factors for dehydration among elderly nursing home residents. *Journal of the American Geriatrics Society, 36*(3), 213–218.

Mentes, J. (2000). Hydration management protocol. *Journal of Gerontological Nursing, 26*(10), 6–15.

Metheny, N. M. (2000). *Fluid and electrolyte balance: nursing considerations* (4th ed.). Philadelphia, PA: Lippincott.

Rochon, P. A., Gill, S. S., Litner, J., Fischbach, M., Goodison, A. J., & Gordon, M. (1997). A systematic review of the evidence for hypodermoclysis to treat dehydration in older people. *Journals of Gerontology Series A: Biological Sciences and Medical Sciences, 52*(3), 169–176.

Simmons, S. F., Alessi, C., & Schnelle, J. F. (2001). An intervention to increase fluid intake in nursing home residents: prompting and preference compliance. *Journal of the American Geriatrics Society, 49*(7), 926–933.

Stookey, J. D., Pieper, C. F., & Cohen, J. H. (2003). Is the prevalence of dehydration among community-dwelling older adults really low? Informing current debate over the fluid recommendation for adults aged 70+. *Public Health Nutrition, 8*(8), 1275–1285.

Theerthakaria, P., & Madlon-Kay, D. (2011). Dehydration: adult. *Essential Evidence Plus.* Retrieved January 19, 2013, from www.essentialevidenceplus.com.proxy.its.virginia.edu/content/eee/122

Thomas, D. R., Cote, T. R., Lawhorne, L., Levenson, S. A., Rubenstein, L. Z., Smith, D. A., . . . Morley, J. E. (2008). Understanding clinical dehydration and its treatment. *Journal of the American Medical Directors Association, 9*(5), 292–301.

Warren, J. L., Bacon, W. E., Harris, T., McBean, A. M., Foley, D. J., & Phillips, C. (1994). The burden and outcomes associated with dehydration among US elderly, 1991. *American Journal of Public Health, 84*(8), 1265–1269.

Xiao, H., Barber, J., & Campbell, E. (2004). Economic burden of dehydration among hospitalized elderly patients. *American Journal of Health-System Pharmacy, 61*(23), 2534-2540.

Delirium

American Psychiatric Association. (2000). *Diagnostic and statistical manual of mental disorders, 4th ed., rev., text revision.* Washington, DC: American Psychiatric Association.

American Psychiatric Association. (1999). Practice guidelines: treatment of patients with delirium. *Psychiatry Online.* DOI: 10.1176/appi.books.9780890423363.42494

Borja, B., Borja, C. S., & Gade, S. (2007). Psychiatric emergencies in the geriatric population. *Clinics in Geriatric Medicine, 23*(2), 391–400.

Cook, I. A. (2004). *Guideline watch: practice guideline for the treatment of patients with delirium.* Arlington, VA: American Psychiatric Association.

Fick, D. M., Agostini, J. V., & Inouye, S. K. (2001). Delirium superimposed on dementia: a systematic review. *Journal of the American Geriatrics Society, 50*(10), 1723–1732.

Flacker, J. M. (2010). Delirium. In F. J. Domino (Editor-in-Chief), *The 5-Minute Clinical Consult* (5th ed., pp. 352–353). Philadelphia, PA: Wolters Kluwers/Lippincott Williams & Wilkins.

Inouye, S. K., Rushing, J. R., Foreman, M. D., Palmer, R. N., & Pompei, P. (1998). Does delirium contribute to poor hospital outcomes? A three site epidemiological study. *Journal of General Internal Medicine, 13*(4), 234–242.

Laurila, J. V., Pitkala, K. H., Strandberg, T. E., & Tilvis, R. S. (2002). Confusion Assessment Method in the diagnosis of delirium among aged hospital patients: would it serve better in screening than as a diagnostic instrument? *International Journal of Geriatric Psychiatry, 17*(12), 1112–1119.

Tullman, D. F., Mion, L. C., Fletcher, K., & Foreman, M. D. (2008). Delirium: prevention, early recognition, and treatment. In E. Capezuti, D. Zwicker, M. Mezey, & T. Fulmer (Eds.), *Evidence-Based geriatric nursing protocols for best practice* (3rd ed., pp. 111–125). New York City, NY: Springer.

Diarrhea

Ibrahim, F., & Yeldia, P. (2011). *Clostridium difficile* infection. *Essential Evidence Plus.* Retrieved January 21, 2012, from www.essentialevidenceplus.com.proxy.its.virginia.edu/content/eee/220

Shiu, M. L. (2012). Chronic diarrhea. *Evidence Plus.* Retrieved April 19, 2012, from www.essentialevidenceplus.com

Tabloski, P. (2007). *Clinical handbook for gerontological nursing.* Upper Saddle River, NJ: Pearson Education.

World Health Organization. (2012). Retrieved April 19, 2012, from www.who.org

Dizziness

Barin, K., & Dodson, E. E. (2011). Dizziness in the elderly. *Otolaryngologic Clinics of North America, 44*(2), 437–454.

Belal, A., Jr., & Glorig, A. (1986). Dysequilibrium of ageing (presbyastasis). *Journal of Laryngology and Otology, 100*(9), 1037–1041.

Dros, J., Maarsingh, O. R., Beem, L., van der Horst, H. E., ter Riet, G., Schellevis, F. G., & van Weert, H. C. (2011). Impact of dizziness on everyday life in older primary care patients: a cross-sectional study. *Health and Quality of Life Outcomes, 9,* 44. doi:10.1186/1477-7525-9-44

Hanley, K., & O'Dowd, T. (2002). Symptoms of vertigo in general practice: a prospective study of diagnosis. *British Journal of General Practice, 52*(483), 809–812.

Hillier, S. L., & McDonnel, M. (2011). Vestibular rehabilitation for unilateral peripheral vestibular dysfunction. Retrieved from *Cochrane Database of Systematic Reviews.* doi: 10.1002/14651858. CD005397.pub3

Jönsson, R., Sixt, E., Landahl, S., & Rosenhall, U. (2004). Prevalence of dizziness and vertigo in an urban elderly population. *Journal of Vestibular Research, 14*(1), 47–52.

Kerber, K. (2010). Dizziness in older people. In S. D. Eggers & D. S. Zee (Eds.), *Vertigo and imbalance: clinical neurophysiology of the vestibular system* (pp. 491–501). Philadelphia, PA: Elsevier.

Labuguen, R. H. (2009). Dizziness. *Essential Evidence Plus.* Retrieved from www.essentialevidenceplus.com.proxy.its.virginia.edu/content/eee/430

Maarsingh, O., Dros, J., Schellevis, F. G., van Weert, H. C., Bindels, P. J., & Horst, H. E. (2010). Dizziness reported by elderly patients in family practice: prevalence, incidence, and clinical characteristics. *BMC Family Practice, 11,* 2. doi:10.1186/1471-2296-11-2

Neuhauser, H. (2007). Epidemiology of vertigo. *Current Opinion in Neurology, 20*(1), 40–46.

Rubenstein, L., & Josephson, K. (2006). Falls and their prevention in elderly people: what does the evidence show? *Medical Clinics of North America, 90*(5), 807–824.

Shoair, O. A., Nyandge, A. N., & Slattum, P. (2011). Medication-related dizziness in the older adult. *Otolaryngologic Clinics of North America, 44*(2), 455–471.

Sloane, P. D., Coeytaux, R. R., Beck, R. S, & Dallara, J. (2001). Dizziness: state of the science. *Annals of Internal Medicine, 134*(9), 823–832.

Stevens, K. N., Lang, I. A., Guralnik, J. M., & Melzer, D. (2008). Epidemiology of balance and dizziness in a national population: findings from the English Longitudinal Study of Aging. *Age and Ageing, 37*(3), 300–305.

Tinetti, M., Williams, C., & Gill, T. (2000). Dizziness among older adults: a possible geriatric syndrome. *Annals of Internal Medicine, 132*(5), 337–344.

Wetmore, S. J., Eibling, D. E., Goebel, J. A., Gottshall, K. R., Hoffer, M. E., Magnusson, M., & Raz, Y. (2011). Challenges and opportunities in managing the dizzy older adult. *Otolaryngology Head and Neck Surgery, 144*(5), 651–656.

Dysphagia

Achem, S. R., & DeVault, K. R (2005). Dysphagia in aging. *Journal of Clinical Gastroenterology, 39*(5), 357–371.

Barer, D. H. (1990). The natural history and functional consequence of dysphagia after hemispheric stroke. *Journal of Neurology, Neurosurgery & Psychiatry, 52*(2), 236.

Bloem, B., Lagaay, A., van Beek, W., Haan, J., Roos, R. A., & Wintzen, A. R. (1990). Prevalence of subjective dysphagia in community residents aged over 87. *British Medical Journal, 300*(6726), 721.

Cook, I. J. (2009). Oropharyngeal dysphagia. *Gastroenterology Clinics of North America, 38*(3), 411–431.

Groher, M. E. (1986). The prevalence of swallowing disorders in two teaching hospitals. *Dysphagia, 1*(1), 3.

Heeneman, H., & Brown, D. (1986). Senescent changes in and about the oral cavity and pharynx. *Journal of Otolaryngology, 15*(4), 214.

Rhodus, N. L., Moller, K., Colby, S., & Bereuter, J. (1995). Dysphagia in patients with three different etiologies of salivary gland dysfunction. *Ear, Nose & Throat Journal, 74*(1), 39–42.

Schmidt, J., Holas, M., Halvorson, K., & Reding, M. (1994). Video-fluoroscopic evidence of aspiration predicts pneumonia and death but not dehydration following stroke. *Dysphagia, 9*(1), 7–11.

Smith Hammond, C. A., & Goldstein, L. B. (2006). Cough and aspiration of food and liquids due to oral-pharyngeal dysphagia: AACP evidence based clinical practice guidelines. *Chest, 129*(1 Suppl.), 154S–168S.

Steele, C. M., Greenwood, C., Ens, I., Robertson, C., & Seidman-Carlson, R. (1997). Mealtime difficulties in a home for the aged: not just dysphagia. *Dysphagia, 12*(1), 43–50, discussion 51.

Tibbin, L., & Gustaffson, B. (1991). Dysphagia and its consequences in the elderly. *Dysphagia, 6*(4), 200–202.

White, G. N., O'Rourke, F., Ong, B. S., Cordato, D. J., & Chan, D. K. (2008). Dysphagia: causes, assessment, treatment, and management. *Geriatrics, 63*(5), 15–20.

Falls

American Geriatrics Society/British Geriatric Society. (2010). Clinical practice guideline: prevention of falls in older persons. Retrieved January 21, 2013, from www.americangeriatrics.org/health_care_professionals/clinical_practice/clinical_guidelines_recommendations/prevention_of_falls_summary_of_recommendations

Bertera, E. M., & Bertera, R. (2008). Fear of falling and activity avoidance in a national sample of older adults in the United States. *Health and Social Work, 33*(1), 54–62.

Blake, A. J., Morgan, K., Bendall, M. J., Dallosso, H., Ebrahim, S. B., Arie, T. H., . . . Bassey, E. J. (1988). Falls by elderly people at home: prevalence and associated factors. *Age and Ageing, 17*(6), 365–472.

Centers for Disease Control and Prevention. (2008, March 7). Self-reported falls and fall-related injuries among persons aged ≥65 years—United States, 2006. *MMWR Weekly, 57*(9), 225–229.

Chang, J. T., Morton, S. C., Rubenstein, L. Z., Mojica, W. A., Maglione, M., Suttorp, M. J., ... Shekelle, P. G. (2004). Interventions for the prevention of falls in older adults: Systematic review and meta-analysis of randomized clinical trials. *British Medical Journal, 328*(7441), 680.

Deandrea, S., Lucentefortte, E., Brave, F., Foschi, R., La Vecchia, C., & Negir, E. (2010). Risk factors for falls in community dwelling older adults: systematic review and meta-analysis. *Epidemiology, 21*(5), 658–668.

Evans, D., Hodgkinson, G., Lambert, L., & Wood, J. (2001). Falls risk factors in the hospital setting: a systematic review. *International Journal of Nursing Practice, 7*(1), 38–45.

Frick, K. D., Kung, J. Y., Parrish, J. M., & Narrett, M. J. (2010). Evaluating the cost effectiveness of fall prevention programs that reduce fall-related hip fracture in older adults. *Journal of the American Geriatrics Society, 58*(1), 136–141.

Gillespie, L. D., Gillespie, J. H., Robertson, M. C., Lamb, S. E., Cummings, R. G., Rowe, B. H., & Gillespie, L. (2007). Interventions for preventing falls in elderly people. Cochrane Review. *Cochrane Library 2007,* Issue 1.

Gillespie, L. D., Gillespie, W. J., & Robertson, M. C. (2004). Intervention for preventing falls in elderly people. Retrieved from *Cochrane Database of Systemic Reviews*

Haines, T. P., Massey, B., Varghese, P., Flemming, J., & Gray, L. (2009). Inconsistency in classification and reporting of in-hospital falls. *Journal of the American Geriatrics Society, 57*(3), 517–523. doi:10.1111/j.1532-5415.2008.02142.x

Hartikainen, S., Lonnross, E., & Louhivuori, K. (2007). Medication as a risk factor for falls: critical systematic review. *Journal of Gerontology: Medical Sciences, 62A*(10), 1172–1181.

Kalyani, R. R., Stein, B., Valiyil, R., Manno, R., Maynard, J. W., & Crews, D. C. (2010). Vitamin D treatment for the prevention of falls in older adults: systematic review and meta-analysis. *Journal of the American Geriatrics Society, 58*(7), 1299–1310.

Kristopaitis, T., & Homan, D. (2009). Falls in elderly patients. *Essential Evidence Plus.* Retrieved January 21, 2013, from www.essentialevidenceplus.com.proxy.its.virginia.edu/content/eee/799

Leape, L. L., Brennan, T. A., Laird, N., Lawthers, A. G., Localio, A. R., Barnes, B. A., . . . Hiatt, H. (1991). The nature of adverse events in hospitalized patients. Results of the Harvard Medical Practice Study II. *New England Journal of Medicine, 324*(6), 377–384.

Lyons, S. S. (2005). Evidence based protocol: fall prevention in older adults. *Journal of Gerontological Nursing, 31*(11), 9–14.

O'Loughlin, J. L., Robitaille, Y., Boivin, J. F., & Suissa, S. (1993). Incidence of and risk factors for falls and injurious falls among the community-dwelling elderly. *American Journal of Epidemiology, 137*(3), 342–354.

Oliver, D., Daly, F., Martin, F. C., & McMurdo, M. E. T. (2004). Risk factors and risk assessment tools for falls in hospitalized in patients: a systematic review. *Age and Ageing, 33*(2), 122–130.

Rubenstein, L. Z. (1997). Preventing falls in the nursing home. *Journal of the American Medical Association, 278*(7), 595–596.

Rutledge, D. N., Donaldson, N. E., & Pravikoff, D. S. (1998). Fall risk assessment and prevention in healthcare facilities. *Online Journal of Clinical Innovations, 1*(9), 1–33.

Sari, A. B., Cracknell, A., & Sheldon, T. A. (2008). Incidence, preventability, and consequences of adverse events in older people: results of a retrospective case-note review. *Age and Ageing, 37*(3), 265–269.

Scott, V., Votava, K., Scanlan, A., & Close, J. (2007). Multifactorial and functional mobility assessment tools for fall risk among older adults in the community, home support, long term and acute care settings. *Age and Ageing, 36*(2), 130–139.

Thurman, D. J., Stevens, J. A., & Rao, J. K. (2008). Practice parameter: assessing patients in a neurology practice for risk of falls (an evidence-based review). *Neurology, 70*(6), 473–479.

Tinnetti, M. E. (2008). Multifactorial fall prevention strategies: time to retreat or advance. *Journal of the American Geriatrics Society, 56*(8), 1563–1565.

Tinneti, M. E., & Kumer, C. (2010). The patient who falls. *Journal of the American Medical Association, 303*(3), 258–266.

Tinetti, M. E., Speechley, M., & Ginter, S. (1998). Risk factors for falls among elderly persons living in the community. *New England Journal of Medicine, 19*(26), 1701–1707.

Zecevic, A. A., Salmoni, A. V., Speechley, M., & Vandervoot, A. A. (2006). Defining a fall and reasons for falling: comparisons among the views of seniors, health care professionals and the research literature. *Gerontologist, 43*(3), 367–376.

Fatigue

Avlund, K. (2010). Fatigue in older adults: an early indicator of the aging process? *Aging Clinical and Experimental Research, 22*(2), 100–115.

Bono, N., & Sheflin, K. M. (2011). Fatigue. *Essential Evidence Plus.* Retrieved January 21, 2013, from www.essentialevidenceplus.com.proxy.its.virginia.edu/content/eee/433

Borneman, T., Piper, B., Sun, V., Koczywas, M., Uman, G., & Ferrell, B. R. (2007). Implementing the fatigue guidelines at one NCCN member institution: process and outcomes. *Journal of the National Comprehensive Cancer Network, 5*(10), 1092–1101.

Darbinshire, L., Risdale, L., & Seed, P. T. (2003). Distinguishing patients with chronic fatigue from those with chronic fatigue syndrome: a diagnostic study in UK primary care. *British Journal of General Practice, 53*(491), 441–445.

Eldadah, B. A. (2010). Fatigue and fatigability in older adults. *American Academy of Physical Medicine and Rehabilitation, 2*(5), 406–413.

Larun, L., McGuire, H., Edmonds, M., Odgaard-Jensen J., & Price, J. R. (2009). Exercise therapy for chronic fatigue syndrome. *Cochrane Database of Systematic Reviews,* Issue 1.

Liao, S., & Ferrell, B. A. (2000). Fatigue in an older population. *Journal of the American Geriatrics Society, 48*(4), 426–430.

Poluri, A., Mores, J., Cook, D. B., Findley, T. W., & Cristian, A. (2005). Fatigue in the elderly population. *Physical Medicine and Rehabilitation Clinics of North America, 16*(1), 91–108.

Ricci, J. A., Chee, E., Lorandeau, A. L., & Berger, J. (2007). Fatigue in the U.S. workforce: prevalence and implications for lost productive work time. *Journal of Occupational and Environmental Medicine, 49*(1), 1–10.

Ridsdale, L., Evans, A., Jerrett, W., Mandalia, S., Osler, K., & Vora, H. (1993). Patients with fatigue in general practice: a prospective study. *British Medical Journal, 307*(6896), 103–106.

Rosenthal, T., Majeroni, B. A., Pretorius, R., & Malik, K. (2008). Fatigue: an overview. *American Family Physician, 78*(10), 1173–1179.

Whiting, P., Bagnall, A. M., Sowden, A. J., Cornell, J. E., Mulrow, C. D., & Ramirez, G. (2001). Interventions for the treatment and management of chronic fatigue syndrome: a systematic review. *Journal of the American Medical Association, 286*(11), 1360–1368.

Yu, D. S. F., Lee, D. T. F., & Man, N. W. (2009). Fatigue among older people: a review of the research literature. *International Journal of Nursing Studies, 47*(2), 216–228.

Headache

Benseñor, I. M., Lotufo, P. A., Goulart, A. C., Menezes, P. R., & Scazufca, M. (2008). The prevalence of headache among elderly in a low-income area of São Paulo, Brazil. *Cephalalgia, 28*(4), 329–333.

Camarda, R., & Monastero, R. (2003). Prevalence of primary headaches in Italian elderly: preliminary data from the Zabut Aging Project. *Neurological Science, 24*(Suppl. 2), S122–S123.

Dambro, M. (2002). *Griffith's 5-minute clinical consult: 2002.* Philadelphia, PA: Lippincott Williams & Wilkins.

Detsky, M. E., McDonald, D. R., Baerlocher, M. O., Tomlinson, G. A., McCrory, D. C., & Booth, C. M. (2006). Does this patient with headache have a migraine or need neuroimaging? *Journal of the American Medical Association, 296*(10), 1274–1283.

Diener, H.-C., Kronfeld, K., Boewing, G., Lungenhausen, M., Maier, C., Molsberger, A., . . . Meinert, R. (2006). Efficacy of acupuncture for the prophylaxis of migraine: a multicentre randomised controlled clinical trial. *Lancet Neurology, 5*(4), 310–316.

Evans, R. W. (2001). Diagnostic testing for headache. *Medical Clinics of North America, 85,* 865.

Evans, R. W. (2003). Headache case studies for the primary care physician. *Medical Clinics of North America, 87*(3), 589–607.

Iversen, H. K., Langemark, M., Andersson, P. G., Hansen, P. E., & Olesen, J. (1990). Clinical characteristics of migraine and episodic tension-type headache in relation to old and new diagnostic criteria. *Headache, 30*(8), 514–519.

Lim, C. (2013). Migraine headache. In F. Ferri, *Ferri's Clinical Advisor 2013* (1st ed.). Philadelphia, PA: Mosby/Elsevier.

Linde, K., Streng, A., Jürgens, S., Hoppe, A., Brinkhaus, B., Witt, C., . . . Melchart, D. (2005). Acupuncture for patients with migraine: a randomized controlled trial. *Journal of the American Medical Association, 293*(17), 2118–2125.

Liou, J., & Grudem, J. (2007, January). Teaching case: severe headaches in an elderly patient. *Headache*, pp. 153–155.

May, A. (2005). Cluster headache: pathogenesis, diagnosis, and management. *Lancet, 366*(9488), 843.

Mazzotta, G., Gallai, V., Alberti A., Billeci, A., Coppola, F., & Sarchielli, P. (2003) Characteristics of migraine in an outpatient population over 60 years of age. *Cephalalgia, 23*(10), 953–960.

Nadeau, M. T., & Parma, D. L. (2011). Headache: diagnosis. *Essential Evidence Plus*. Retrieved from http://www.essentialevidenceplus.com

Prencipe, M., Casini, A., Ferretti, C., Santini, M., Pezzella, F., Scaldaferri, N., & Culasso, F. (2001). Prevalence of headache in an elderly population: attack frequency, disability, and use of medication. *Journal of Neurology, Neurosurgery & Psychiatry, 70*(3), 377–381.

Purdy, R. A. (2001). Clinical evaluation of the patient presenting with headache. *Medical Clinics of North America, 85*(4), 847.

Rankin, L. M., & Bruhl, M. (2000). Migraine in older patients: a case report and management strategies. *Geriatrics, 55*(7), 70.

Seller, R. H. (2000). *Differential diagnosis of common complaints* (4th ed.). Philadelphia, PA: Saunders.

Silberstein, S. D., Lipton, R. B., & Dalessio, D. J. (Eds.). (2001). *Wolff's headache and other head pain* (7th ed.). New York City, NY: Oxford University Press.

Tanganelli, P. (2010). Secondary headaches in the elderly. *Neurological Science, 31*(Suppl. 1), S73–S76.

Tepper, S. J. (2008). A pivotal moment in 50 years of headache history: the First American Migraine Study. *Headache, 48*(5), 730–732.

Tonini, M. C., & Bussone, G. (2010). Headache in the elderly: primary forms. *Neurological Science, 31*(Suppl. 1), S67–S71.

Uthaikhup, S., Sterling, M., & Jull, G. (2009). Psychological, cognitive and quality of life features in the elderly with chronic headache. *Gerontology, 55*(6), 683–693.

Walker, R. A., & Wadman, M. C. (2007). Headache in the elderly. *Clinics in Geriatric Medicine, 23*(2), 291–305.

Wang, S. J., Liu, H. C., Fuh, J. L., Liu, C. Y., Lin, K. P., Chen, H. M., . . . Lin, K. N. (1997). Prevalence of headaches in a Chinese elderly population in Kinmen: age and gender effect and cross-cultural comparisons. *Neurology, 49*(1), 195–200.

Ward, T. N. (2004). Medication overuse headache. *Primary Care Clinics in Office Practice, 31*(2), 369–380.

Winer, P. (2003). Botulinum toxins in the treatment of migraine and tension-type headaches. *Physical Medicine and Rehabilitation Clinics of North America, 14*(4), 885–899.

Yoshikawa, T. T., Cobbs, E. L., & Brummel-Smith, K. (1998). *Ambulatory Geriatric Care* (2nd ed.). St. Louis, MO: Mosby.

Yoshikawa, T. T., & Norman, D. C. (1995). Treatment of infections of the central nervous system. *Medical Clinics of North America, 79*(3), 651–661.

Hematuria

Choyke, P. L. (2008). Radiologic evaluation of hematuria: guidelines from the American College of Radiology's appropriateness criteria. *American Family Physician, 78*(3), 347–352.

Grossfeld, G. D., Wolf, J. S., Litwin, M. S., Hricak, H., Shuler, C. L., Agerter, D. C., & Carroll, P. R. (2001). Asymptomatic microscopic hematuria in adults: summary of the AUA best practice

policy recommendations. *American Family Physician, 63*(6), 1145–1155.

Kaplan, M., Caloagu, M., & Slawson, D. (2011). Hematuria. *Essential Evidence Plus*. Retrieved January 21, 2013, from www.essentialevidenceplus.com.proxy.its.virginia.edu/content/eee/641

McDonald, M. M., Swagerty, D., & Wetzel, L. (2006). Assessment of microscopic hematuria in adults. *American Family Physician, 73*(10), 1748–1754.

Muraoka, N., Sakai, T., Kimura, H., Uematsu, H., Tanase, K., Yokoyama, O., & Itoh, H. (2008). Rare causes of hematuria associated with various vascular diseases involving the upper urinary tract. *RadioGraphics, 28*(3), 855–867.

Noble, M. J. (2004). Hematuria. In J. M. Potts (Ed.), *Essential urology: a guide to clinical practice* (1st ed., pp. 91–102). Totowa, NJ: Humana Press.

USPSTF. (2004, June 5). *Screening for bladder cancer in adults: recommendation statement*. Rockville, MD: AHRQ.

Wachtel, T. (2007). *Geriatric clinical advisor: instant diagnosis and treatment*. Providence, RI: Mosby.

Hemoptysis

Bidwell, J. L. (2011). Hemoptysis. *Essential Evidence Plus*. Retrieved from http://www.essentialevidenceplus.com

Bidwell, J. L., & Pachner, R. W. (2005). Hemoptysis: diagnosis and management. *American Family Physician, 72*(7), 1253–1260.

Brown, C. A., III. (2009). Hemoptysis. In J. A. Marx (Ed.), *Rosen's emergency medicine: concepts and clinical practice* (7th ed.). Philadelphia, PA: Mosby Elsevier.

Colice, G. L. (1997). Detecting lung cancer as a cause of hemoptysis in patients with a normal chest radiograph: bronchoscopy vs CT. *Chest, 111*(4), 877–884.

McGuinness, G., Beacher, J. R., Harkin, T. J., Garay, S. M., Rom, W. N., & Naidich, D. P. (1994). Hemoptysis: prospective high resolution CT/bronchoscopic correlation. *Chest, 105*(4), 1155–1162.

Noe, G. D., Jaffe, S. M., & Molan, M. P. (2011). CT and CT angiography in massive haemptysis with emphasis on pre-embolization assessment. *Clinical Radiology, 66*(9), 869–875.

O'Neil, K. M., & Lazarus, A. A. (1991). Hemoptysis: indications for bronchoscopy. *Archives of Internal Medicine, 151*(1), 171–174.

Tasker, A. D., & Flower, C. D. (1999). Imaging the airways. Hemoptysis, bronchiectasis, and small airways disease. *Clinics in Chest Medicine, 20*(4), 761–773.

Involuntary Weight Loss

Chapman, I. M. (2011). Weight loss in older persons. *Medical Clinics of North America, 95*(3), 579–593.

Fox, C. B., Treadway, A. K., Blaszczyk, A. T., & Sleeper, R. B. (2009). Megestrol acetate and mirtazapine for the treatment of unplanned weight loss in the elderly. *Pharmacotherapy, 29*(4), 383–397.

McMinn, J., Steel, C., & Bowman, A. (2011). Investigation and management of unintentional weight loss in older adults. *British Medical Journal, 342*, d1732.

Morley, J. E. (2007). Weight loss in older persons: new therapeutic approaches. *Current Pharmaceutical Design, 13*(35), 3637–3647.

University of Texas at Austin School of Nursing, Family Nurse Practitioner Program. (2006). Unintentional weight loss in the elderly. *Essential Evidence Plus*. Retrieved January 21, 2013, from www.essentialevidenceplus.com.proxy.its.virginia.edu/content/guideline/9435

Joint Pain

Arroll, B., & Goodyear-Smith, F. (2004). Corticosteroid injections for osteoarthritis of the knee: meta-analysis. *British Medical Journal, 328*, 869.

Bellamy, N., Campbell, J., Robinson, V., Gee, T., Bourne, R., & Wells, G. (2006). Intraarticular corticosteroid injections for osteoarthritis of the knee: meta-analysis. *Cochrane Database of Systematic Reviews* (2), CD005328.

Centers for Disease Control and Prevention. (2002). Morbidity and mortality weekly report: prevalence of self reported arthritis or chronic joint symptoms among adults—United States 2001. *Journal of the American Medical Association, 288*(24), 3103–3104.

Collyott, C. L., & Vasquez Brooks, M. (2008) Evaluation and management of joint pain. *Orthopedic Nursing, 27*(4), 246–250.

Deeks, J. J., Smith, L. A., & Bradley, M. D. (2002). Efficacy, tolerability, and upper gastrointestinal safety of celecoxib for treatment of osteoarthritis and rheumatoid arthritis: systematic review of randomised controlled trials. *British Medical Journal, 325*, 619.

Geba, G. P., Weaver, A. L., Polis, A. B., Dixon, M. E., Schnitzer, T. J., & Vioxx, Acetaminophen, Celecoxib Trial (VACT) Group. (2002). Efficacy of rofecoxib, celecoxib, and acetaminophen in osteoarthritis of the knee: a randomized trial. *Journal of the American Medical Association, 287*(1), 64–71.

Harrington, L., & Schneider, J. L. (2006). Atraumatic joint and limb pain in the elderly. *Emergency Medicine Clinics of North America, 24*(2), 389–412.

Kidd, B. (2006). Osteoarthritis and joint pain. *Pain, 123*(1–2), 6–9.

Lavelle, W., Lavelle, E. D., & Lavelle, L. (2007). Intra-articular injections. *Medical Clinics of North America, 91*(2), 242–250.

Palmer, T. (2011). Knee pain. *Essential Evidence Plus.* Retrieved January 21, 2013, from www.essentialevidenceplus.com.proxy. its.virginia.edu/content/eee/390

Palmer, T., & Toombs, J. (2004). Managing joint pain in primary care. *Journal of the American Board of Family Practice, 17*(Suppl.), S32–S42.

Quiceno, G. A., & Cush, J. J. (2007). Iatrogenic rheumatic syndromes in the elderly. *Rheumatic Disease Clinics of North America, 33*(1), 123–134.

Ringdahl, E., & Pandit, S. (2011). Treatment of knee osteoarthritis. *American Family Physician, 83*(11), 1287–1292.

Roberts, D. (2003). Alternative therapies for arthritis treatment. *Orthopedic Nursing, 22*(5), 335–342.

Uphold, C. R., & Graham, M. V. (2003). Joint pain. In C. R. Uphold & M. V. Graham (Eds.), *Clinical guidelines for family practice* (4th ed., pp. 812–815). Gainesville, FL: Barmarrae Books.

Peripheral Edema

Koo, L. W., Reedy, S., & Smith, J. K. (2010). Patient history key to diagnosing peripheral edema. *Nurse Practitioner, 35*(3):44–52.

O'Brien, J.G., & Miles, T.P. (2013). Edema. *Essential Evidence Plus.* Retrieved from: http://www.essentialevidenceplus.com.proxy.its. virginia.edu/content/eee/29

Schroth, B. E. (2005). Evaluation and management of peripheral edema. *Journal of the American Academy of Physician Assistants, 18*(11), 29–34.

Pruritus

Beauregard, S., & Gilchrest, B. A. (1987). A survey of skin problems and skin care regimens in the elderly. *Archives of Dermatology, 123*(12), 1638–1643.

Berger, T. G., & Steinhoff, M. (2011). Pruritus in elderly patients—eruptions of senescence. *Seminars in Cutaneous Medicine and Surgery, 30*(2), 113–117.

Chida, Y., Steptoe, A., Hirakawa, N., Sudo, N., & Kubo, C. (2007). The effects of psychological intervention on atopic dermatitis: a systematic review and meta-analysis. *International Archives of Allergy and Immunology, 144*(1), 1–9.

Cohen, K. R., Frank, J., Salbu, R. L., & Israel, I. (2012). Pruritus in the elderly: clinical approaches to the improvement of quality of life. *Pharmacy and Therapeutics, 37*(4), 227–239.

Cowell, F. (2009). Care and management of patients with pruritus. *Nursing Older People, 21*(7), 35–41.

Dalgard, F., Svensson, A., Holm, J., & Sundby, J. (2004). Self-reported skin morbidity in Oslo. Associations with sociodemographic factors among adults in a cross-sectional study. *British Journal of Dermatology, 151*(2), 452–457.

Hanifin, J. M., Cooper, K. D., Ho, V. C., Kang, S., Krafchik, B. R., Margolis, D. J., . . .Van Voorhees, A. S. (2004). Guidelines of care for atopic dermatitis, developed in accordance with the American Academy of Dermatology (AAD)/American Academy of Dermatology Association "Administrative Regulations for Evidence-Based Clinical Practice Guidelines." *Journal of the American Academy of Dermatology, 50*(3), 391–404.

Norman, R. A. (2003). Xerosis and pruritus in the elderly: recognition and management. *Dermatologic Therapy, 16*(3), 254–259.

Norman, R. A. (2006). Xerosis and pruritus in elderly patients, part 1. *Ostomy Wound Management, 52*(2), 12–14.

Norman, R. A. (2006). Xerosis and pruritus in elderly patients, part 2. *Ostomy Wound Management, 52*(3), 18–20.

Patel, T., & Yosipovitch, G. (2009). The management of chronic pruritus in the elderly. *Skin Therapy Letter, 15*(8), 5–9.

Reamy, B., & Bunt, C. (2011). A diagnostic approach to pruritus. *American Family Physician, 84*(2), 195–202.

Reich, A., Stander, S., & Szepietowski, M. D. (2011). Pruritus in the elderly. *Clinics in Dermatology, 29*(1), 15–23.

Stander, S., Weisshaar, E., Mettang, T., Szepietowski, J. C., Carstens, E., Ikoma, A., . . . Bernhard, J. D. (2007). Clinical classification of itch: a position paper of the International Forum for the Study of Itch. *Acta Dermato-Venereologica, 87*(4), 291–294.

Steinhoff, M., Cevikbas, F., Ikoma, A., & Berger, T. G. (2011). Pruritus: management algorithms and experimental therapies. *Seminars in Cutaneous Medicine and Surgery, 30*(2), 127–137.

Trikha, A., & Ebell, M. H. (2011). Pruritus. *Essential Evidence Plus.* Retrieved January 21, 2013, from www.essentialevidenceplus. com.proxy.its.virginia.edu/content/eee/761

Yalçin, B., Tamer, E., Toy, G. G., Oztas, P., Hayran, M., & Alli, N. (2006). The prevalence of skin diseases in the elderly: analysis of 4099 geriatric patients. *International Journal of Dermatology, 45*(6), 672–676.

Syncope

Alboni, P., Brignole, M., Menozzi, C., Raviele, A., Del Rosso, A., Dinelli, M., . . . Bottoni, N. (2001). Diagnostic value of history in patients with syncope with or without heart disease. *Journal of the American College of Cardiology, 37*(7), 1921–1928.

Ammirati, F., Colivicchi, F., & Santini, M. (2000). Diagnosing syncope in clinical practice: implementation of a simplified diagnostic algorithm in a multicentre prospective trial—the OESIL 2 study. *European Heart Journal, 21*(11), 935–940.

Ebell, M. H. (2006). Syncope: initial evaluation and prognosis. *American Family Physician, 74*(8), 1367–1370.

Hood, R. (2007). Syncope in the elderly. *Clinics in Geriatric Medicine, 23*(2), 351–361.

Huff, J. S., Decker, W. W., Quinn, J. V., Perron, A. D., Napoli, A. M., Peeters, S., . . . American College of Emergency Physicians. (2007). Clinical policy: critical issues in the evaluation and management of adult patients presenting to the ED with syncope. *Annals of Emergency Medicine, 49*(4), 431–444.

Miller, T. H. (2011). Syncope. *Essential Evidence Plus*. Retrieved from http://www.essentialevidenceplus.com

Ouyang, H., & Quinn, J. (2010). Diagnosis and evaluation of syncope in the emergency department. *Emergency Medicine Clinics of North America, 28*(3), 471–485.

Roussanov, O., Estacio, G., Capuno, M., Wilson, J., Kovesdy, C., & Jarmukli, N. (2007). New onset syncope in older adults: focus on age and etiology. *American Journal of Geriatric Cardiology, 16*(5), 287–294.

Sarasin, F. P., Louis-Simonet, M., Carballo, D., Slama, S., Rajeswaran, A., Metzger, J. T., . . . Junod, A. F. (2001). Prospective evaluation of patients with syncope: a population-based study. *American Journal of Medicine, 111*(3), 177–184.

Tremor

Crawford, P., & Simmerman, E. E. (2011). Differentiation and diagnosis of tremor. *American Family Physician, 83*(6), 697–702.

Deuschl, G., Bain, P., Brin, M., & Ad Hoc Scientific Committee. (1998). Consensus statement of the Movement Disorder Society on tremor. *Movement Disorders, 13*(Suppl. 3), 2–23.

Pham, C. (2011). Tremor: Essential or familial. *Essential Evidence Plus*. Retrieved January 21, 2013, from www.essentialevidenceplus.com.proxy.its.virginia.edu/content/eee/463

Velickovic, M., & Gracies, J. M. (2002). Movement disorders: keys to identifying and treating tremor. *Geriatrics, 57*(7), 32–36.

Urinary Incontinence

Agency for Health Care Policy and Research. (1996). Urinary incontinence in adults, clinical practice guideline update. Retrieved from www.ahcpr.gov/news/press/overview.htm

Alhasso, A., Glazener, C., Pickard, R., & N'Dow, J. (2007). Adrenergic drugs for urinary incontinence in adults (Cochrane Review). *Cochrane Library*, 1.

Amin, S. H. (2011). Urinary incontinence. *Essential Evidence Plus*. Retrieved from www.essentialevidenceplus.com/content/eee/652

Bezerra, C. A., Bruschini, H., Cody, D. J., & Bezerra, C. (2007). Traditional suburethral sling operations for urinary incontinence in women (Cochrane Review). *Cochrane Library*, 1.

Chapple, C. R., Martinez-Garcia, R., Selvaggi, L., Toozs-Hobson, P., Warnack, W., Drogendijk, T., . . . Bolodeoku, J. (2005). A comparison of the efficacy and tolerability of solifenacin succinate and extended release tolterodine at treating overactive bladder syndrome: results of the STAR trial. *European Urology, 48*(3), 464–470.

Doughty, D. B. (2006). *Urinary and fecal incontinence: current management concepts*. St. Louis, MO: Mosby.

DuBeau, C. E. (2012). Treatment of urinary incontinence. *UpTo Date*. Retrieved from www.uptodate.com/contents/treatment-of-urinary-incontinence?source=search_result&search=uinary+incontinence&selectedTitle=2%7E150

Goode, P. S., Burgio, K. L., Johnson, T. M., Clay, O. J., Roth, D. L., Markland, A. D., . . . Lloyd, L. K. (2011). Behavioral therapy with or without biofeedback and pelvic floor electrical stimulation for persistent postprostatectomy incontinence: a randomized controlled trial. *Journal of the American Medical Association, 305*(2), 151–159.

Hay-Smith, E. J. C., & Dulmoulin, C. (2007). Pelvic floor training versus no treatment, or inactive control treatments for urinary incontinence in women (Cochrane Review). *Cochrane Library*, 1.

Mai-Duc, C. (2011, July 13). FDA reevaluating vaginal mesh implants. *Los Angeles Times*. Retrieved from www.latimes.com/news/nationworld/nation/sc-dc-0714-fda-mesh-20110714,0,6030373.story

Mariappan, P., Alhasso, A., Ballantyne, Z., Grant, A., & N'Dow, J. (2007). Duloxetine, a serotonin and noradrenaline reuptake inhibitor (SNRI) for the treatment of stress urinary incontinence: a systematic review. *European Urology, 51*(1), 67–74.

Michel, M. C., & Barendrecht, M. M. (2008). Physiological and pathological regulation of the autonomic control of urinary bladder contractility. *Pharmacology & Therapeutics, 117*(3), 297–312.

Nabi, G., Cody, J. D., Ellis, G., Herbison, P., & Hay-Smith, J. (2007). Anticholinergic drugs versus placebo for overactive bladder syndrome in adults (Cochrane Review). *Cochrane Library*, 1.

Nygaard, I., Barber, M. D., Burgio, K. L., Kenton, K., Meikle, S., Schaffer, J., . . . Pelvic Floor Disorders Network. (2008). Prevalence of symptomatic pelvic floor disorders in U.S. women. *Journal of the American Medical Association, 300*(11), 1311–1316.

Offermans, M. P., Du Moulin, M. F., Hamers, J. P., Dassen, T., & Halfens, R. J. (2009). Prevalence of urinary incontinence and associated risk factors in nursing home residents: a systematic review. *Neurourology and Urodynamics, 28*(4), 288–294.

Resnick, N. M., Tadic, S. D., & Yalla, S. V. (2011). Geriatric incontinence and voiding dysfunction. In A. J. Wein (Ed.), *Campbell-Walsh urology* (Vol. 3). St. Louis, MO: Saunders.

Schnelle, J. F., Leung, F. W., Rao, S. S., Beuscher, L., Keeler, E., Clift, J. W., & Simmons, S. (2010). A controlled trial of an intervention to improve urinary and fecal incontinence and constipation. *Journal of the American Geriatrics Society, 58*(8), 1504–1511.

Sellers, D. J., & McKay, N. (2007). Developments in the pharmacotherapy of the overactive bladder. *Current Opinion in Urology, 17*(4), 223–230.

Thom, D. H., van den Eeden, S. K., Ragins, A. I., Wassel-Fyr, C., Vittinghof, E., & Subak, L. L. (2006). Differences in prevalence of urinary incontinence by race/ethnicity. *Journal of Urology, 175*(1), 259–264.

Trowbridge, E. R. (2010, October). *Managing complications of vaginal mesh kits for pelvic organ prolapse* [PowerPoint slides]. Presentation at A Day at Virginia Urology, Gynecology and Endocrine Disorders conference, Charlottesville, VA.

Wallace, S. A., Roe, B., Williams, K., & Palmer, M. (2007). Bladder training for urinary incontinence in adults (Cochrane Review). *Cochrane Library*, 1.

Zinner, N. R., Dmochowski, R. R., Staskin, D. R., Siami, P. F., Sand, P. K., & Oefelein, M. G. (2011). Once-daily trospium chloride 60 mg extended-release provides effective, long-term relief of overactive bladder syndrome symptoms. *Neurourology and Urodynamics, 30*(7), 1214–1219.

Wandering

Algase, D. L., Antonakos, C., Beattie, E. R. A., Beel-Bates, C. A., & Yao, L. (2009). Empirical derivation and validation of a wandering typology. *Journal of the American Geriatrics Society, 57*(11), 2037–2045.

Algase, D. L., Beattie, E. R. A., Antonakos, C., Beel-Bates, C. A., & Yao, L. (2010). Wandering and the physical environment. *American Journal of Alzheimer's Disease & Other Dementias, 25*(4), 340–346.

Alzheimer's Association. (2007). Wandering behavior: preparing for and preventing it. Retrieved from www.alz.org/living-withalsheimerswanderingbehaviors.asp

Alzheimer's Association. (2010). 2010 Alzheimer's disease facts and figures. *Alzheimer's & Dementia, 6*. Retrieved from http://www.alz.org/documents_custom/report_alzfactsfigures2010.pdf

Ata, T., Terada, S., Yokota, O., Ishihara, T., Fujisawa, Y., Sasaki, K., & Kuroda, S. (2010). Wandering and fecal smearing in people with dementia. *International Psychogeriatrics, 22*(3), 493–500. doi:10.1017/S1041610210000086

Carr, D., Muschert, G. W., Kinney, J., Robbins, E., Petonito, G., Manning, L., & Brown, J. S. (2010). Silver alerts and the problem of missing adults with dementia. *Gerontologist, 50*(2), 149–157. doi:10.1093/geront/gnp102

Carson, V. B. (2012). Wandering: a common challenging behavior. *Caring, 31*(1), 52–53.

Chung, J. C. C., & Lai, C. K. Y. (2010). Elopement among community dwelling older adults with dementia. *International Psychogeriatrics, 23*(1), 65–72.

Douglas, A., Letts, L., & Richardson, J. (2011). A systematic review of accidental injury from fire, wandering and medication self-administration errors for older adults with and without dementia. *Archives of Gerontology and Geriatrics, 52*(1), e1–e10.

Futrell, M., Melillo, K. D., & Remington, R. (2008, July). *Wandering.* Iowa City, IA: University of Iowa Gerontological Nursing Interventions Research Center, Research Translation Dissemination Core.

Lang, R., Rispoli, M., Machalicek, W., White, P. J., Kang, S., Pierce, N., . . . Lancioni, G. (2009). Treatment of elopement in individuals with developmental disabilities: a systematic review. *Research in Developmental Disabilities, 30*(4), 670–681.

Moore, D. H., Algase, D. L., Powell-Cope, G., Applegarth, S., & Beattie, E. R. (2009). A framework for managing wandering and preventing elopement. *American Journal of Alzheimer's Disease & Other Dementias, 24*(3), 208–219.

News Briefs. (2009). Cholinesterase inhibitors reduce aggression, wandering, and paranoia in Alzheimer's disease. *American Journal of Alzheimer's Disease & Other Dementias, 24*(2), 169–170.

Rowe, M. (2008). Wandering in hospitalized older adults: identifying risk is the first step in this approach to preventing wandering in patients with dementia. *American Journal of Nursing, 108*(10), 62–70.

Thomas, D. W. (1995). Wandering: a proposed definition. *Journal of Gerontological Nursing, 21*(9), 35–41.

University of Iowa Gerontological Nursing Interventions Research Center. (2008). Evidence-based practice guideline: wandering. *Essential Evidence Plus.* Retrieved January 21(9), 2013, from www.essentialevidenceplus.com.proxy.its.virginia.edu/content/guideline/12992

unit **III**

Treating Disorders

chapter 6

Skin and Lymphatic Disorders

Laurie Kennedy-Malone

ASSESSMENT

Proper assessment of an older adult's skin, hair, and nails reveals the patient's history of sun exposure, nutrition, socioeconomic status, and education as well as his or her surgical and medical history. The largest organ of the body, the skin, undergoes certain normal changes with age. The number of cells in the epidermis, such as Langerhans' cells, which are responsible for immune surveillance, begins to decline. Melanocytes also decrease, thereby reducing the skin's natural protection from the sun (Aasi & Choi, 2010; Williams, 2009).

Changes With Aging

As people age, the skin tends to be very thin, fragile, and often transparent (Gray-Vickrey, 2010). Skin renewal turnover time increases to approximately 87 days in elderly adults, compared with 20 days during youth. This fact becomes an important consideration in surgical and dermatological healing. The subcutaneous tissue that houses the eccrine, sebaceous, and apocrine glands thins, thereby providing less protection from heat exposure and less insulation, energy storage, and shock absorption. Secretions aiding temperature control, moisturization, and odor production are also reduced. The skin of older adults therefore tends to be very dry (xerosis). Fat is generally redistributed to the abdomen and thighs, leaving bony surfaces, such as the face, hands, and sacrum, exposed to potential injury, especially skin tears from shearing and friction forces and pressure ulcer development (Bates-Jensen, 2009). The skin's repair system becomes impaired,

with delayed cell regeneration and poor circulation (Aasi & Choi, 2010).

Common benign skins lesions in older adults include seborrheic keratoses, cherry angiomas, acrochorda (skin tags), and senile lentigo (Gray-Vickrey, 2010; Williams, 2009). Although the capillaries in older adults tend to be fragile, making the skin of older adults more susceptible to bruising, it is important to discern the cause of the ecchymosis, whether it is trauma-, pressure-, or medication-induced as in patients taking anticoagulants or corticosteroids (Gray-Vickrey, 2010). It is important to note, however, that "sudden appearance of seborrheic keratoses, telangiectasia or pigmented warty lesions (known as Leser-Trelat sign) may suggest internal malignancy" (Williams, 2009, p. 305).

All of these tissue changes represent a near-catastrophic scenario of aged skin poorly protected from the environment (especially the sun, heat, and cold) and slow to respond to immunological challenges, producing minimal or delayed urticaria and swelling.

Evaluation of Skin and Lymphatics

Assessment of the skins begins with the chief complaint and history, including the dermatological problem's onset, duration, and location, size of lesion, color, associated pain or itching, and lost or heightened sensation to touch.

- Investigate associated symptoms such as wheezing, loss of appetite, fever, malaise, headaches, and change in temperature perception.

■ Question current and chronic medication history; complete a focused nutritional assessment, and ask about relevant childhood diseases (especially asthma, atopic dermatitis, and chickenpox).

■ Ask about contact with chemicals, lifetime occupations, level of lifetime sun exposure, family history of skin cancer, contact with animals, change in environmental habits (plants, insects, water) or internal habits (e.g., change in soap or laundry detergents, use of any lotions or creams, recent travel, change in diet to include cooking products, exposure to new clothing items or metals such as nickel).

■ Ask whether the person has been treated for a similar condition in the past and if so, ask about the results.

■ Note whether the patient appears uncomfortable or pruritic.

■ Observe overall hygiene and grooming (Williams, 2009).

Proper equipment for inspection includes good overhead and tangential lighting, a magnifying glass, blades, and collection devices for biopsies and microscopic study. Gloves should be readily available. Inspect the skin for possible signs of neglect, abuse, or decreased function. Poorly healing wounds or chronic pressure ulcers may signal a problem not only with the patient but with the caregiver's ability to provide adequate care. Welts, lacerations, burns, and distinctive markings may indicate a need for intervention (Gray-Vickrey, 2010; Williams, 2009).

Inspect the hair and nails. The hair may be graying and thinner than in youth. Normally, nails start to form ridges after age 80. A recent (in the past year) change in quality of hair and nails is a significant finding. For example, the hair may have become dryer, duller, and thinner or the nails pitted or brittle and may be indicative of a systemic condition or nutritional deficiency (Gray-Vickrey, 2010).

Inspection of the skin for even color and overall quality and care is important. Lesions require close scrutiny, description, and classification. Description by type, shape, arrangement, and distribution is a widely accepted and usable format.

■ Type: Is the lesion a macule or papule? Is it eroded, excoriated, or hyperpigmented or hypopigmented?

■ Shape: Is the periphery of the lesions round, ulcerated, or linear?

■ Arrangement: Are multiple lesions grouped (serpiginous, zosteriform, arciform, iris, or bull's-eye pattern) with or without definable borders (LeBlond, Brown, & DeGowin, 2009)?

■ Distribution: Is the extent of the lesions isolated, regional, or generalized? Is the pattern symmetrical or over pressure sites, hairline, or sun-exposed areas? Is the distribution characteristic of scabies, seborrheic dermatitis, contact dermatitis, herpes zoster, or lupus?

The lesion may be classified as primary or secondary. Primary lesions (vesicles, tumors, burrows) arise from normal tissue. Secondary lesions (infections, crusts, and lichenification) arise from changes to the primary lesion (LeBlond et al., 2009). Palpate for moisture, temperature, mobility, and turgor. Testing skin turgor in older patients can be done by pinching the skin on the sternum or forehead. The skin should move easily and return back to place after release; a slower return of the skin may be indicative of dehydration. Lax skin may indicate weight loss, whereas fixed skin may be associated with sclerotic or scarred tissue. Lesions should also be palpated to check whether they are fluctuant, hard, or fixed. At the end of the examination, consider associated pathology, especially thyroid disorders, diabetes, autoimmune conditions, and anemia. Provide wellness instructions, including those concerning proper nutrition, moisturizing, and sun protection. Awareness of the high susceptibility of the elderly to hyperthermia and hypothermia secondary to reduced thermoregulation in the skin should be emphasized (Williams, 2009).

Guidelines for Prescribing Topical Medications

Lesions that concern you or the patient should be examined through biopsy. Lesions that warrant biopsy are those that have changed, bleed, or are painful. Treatment for skin lesions must take impaired absorption, duration, dosage, and delivery method (e.g., creams, powder, ointment, lotion) into consideration. Patients for whom treatment plans fail initially should be referred to a dermatologist.

When prescribing topical treatments, it can be a challenge to determine the quantity necessary to dispense. A guideline for determining the quantity was first described by Long and Finlay in 1991 with the introduction of the "fingertip unit." One fingertip unit (FTU) is the amount of ointment or cream dispensed from a tube with a 5-mm opening from the tip of the finger to the first crease. One FTU is equal to approximately 0.5 g.

Along with the concept of FTUs, the "Rule of Hand" was developed. This rule says that the body surface of the front and back of an adult hand requires 1 FTU for coverage. Each body part is described by its equivalent surface area in hands. Each arm is equal to 3 hands, the front torso is 7 hands, and so are the back and buttocks. Each leg is equal to 6 hands, and each foot is 2 hands. So, if you are treating lesions on one foot, a total of 2 FTUs will be required or 1 g per treatment. For treatments that are prescribed as twice a day (BID) for 2 weeks, a total of 28 g will be necessary. This guideline results in a more quantitative prescription than writing "dispense 1 week's supply."

BURNS

Signal symptoms: Erythema, blistering, serous exudates, eschar, pain, carbaceous sputum, paresthesia.

Description: Burn injury can be caused by multiple mechanisms. Flame and hot liquids are obvious sources of burn injury. Other causes of burn damage can occur from electricity from high power lines, household current, or lightning strike; radiation or sun exposure; and chemical corrosion. Patients may present with varying degrees and depth of tissue damage along with underlying trauma, thus requiring a very thorough physical examination. In addition to what is considered a true burn injury, many exfoliative and necrotizing skin disorders can present in a similar fashion and must be ruled out. Although these skin disorders are not true burns, they are increasingly treated in burn care facilities.

Etiology: Skin forms the largest organ in the body and is constantly in contact with a changing environment. It is composed of three layers: the epidermis, the dermis, and the subcutaneous tissue or hypodermis. The epidermis is the thin outermost layer of the skin. It contains keratinizing cells that migrate from the basal cell membrane and eventually shed over a 4-week period. At this level of the skin, melanocytes, which are responsible for skin color, are found. The dermis consists of a dense connective tissue that forms the bulk of the skin. This layer is vascular with its deeper layer containing hair follicles, associated muscle fibers, cutaneous glands, and nerve fibers. The subcutaneous layer or hypodermis is largely composed of adipose tissue, which provides padding and thermal regulation. Burn injury can affect all of these skin levels in addition to deeper structures such as muscle and bone. As one ages there are significant changes in the skin, which becomes thinner, thus providing a less effective barrier to external stimuli. With aging the dermis atrophies. There are fewer appendages and decreased vascularity. Thus the elderly are at particular risk for injury from burns. Thinner skin combined with decreased vascularity and diminished nerve function often results in a higher incidence of deeper burns. With advanced age there is a weakening immune system. All of these factors found in the elderly population, along with the burden of various comorbidities, lead to reepithelialization after burn injury, occurring slowly with delayed wound healing (Demling, Pereira, & Herndon, 2007).

Occurrence: In 2009 approximately 85% of all fire deaths were associated with fires in the home (Flynn, 2010). Each year more than 1200 individuals over the age of 65 die in fire-related deaths. Between ages 65 and 75, the mortality rate from burns is twice that of the national average. According to the American Burn Association (ABA), those between 75 and 85 years of age die at 3 times the national average from fire-related deaths. Although the leading cause of fire-related death in the home involves smoking at 37%, fires from heating, cooking, and candles follow closely. Fire-related injuries in those 65 years and older are most frequently related to home heating followed by smoking and cooking accidents (Flynn, 2010).

Age: Scald/contact burns are the main mechanism of injury in the very young whereas flame/fire predominates in the adult population. Age can be more predictive of burn survival than the total body surface area (TBSA) involved (ABA, 2011). It is the very young along with the elderly who are most likely to die in house fires (Flynn, 2010). This is particularly true with the addition of an inhalation injury. For those individuals 55 years and older, burns were the seventh leading cause of unintentional injury-related death in the United States (Centers for Disease Control and Prevention [CDC], 2007).

Gender: The vast majority of burn victims are male. Between 2001 and 2010, nearly 70% of all patients reported to the ABA's National Burn Registry were males.

Ethnicity: The ABA's National Burn Registry 2011 report outlines the following breakdown of reported ethnicity in burn injuries: 59.6% White, 18.9% Black, 14.9% Hispanic, 3.4% Other, 2.4% Asian, and 0.7% Native American. When analyzed by age group, it was found that minorities were overrepresented among those with burn injuries 5 years and younger. As the population ages into adulthood, this characteristic shifts and minorities were no longer found to predominate.

Contributing factors: Nearly 85% of all burn-related deaths were associated with house fires (Karter, 2010). Smoke and toxic fumes associated with house fires are larger contributors to death than the burn itself. Inhalation injury is particularly lethal when victims are more than 65 years of age. Among the major causes of house fires are smoking, faulty wiring, and home heating sources such as kerosene (Ahrens, 2011). In home fires related to smoking, the risk of death is further compounded by the use of home oxygen.

Human judgment plays a large role in activities that are related to fire death. The elderly have slow response times and may show impaired judgment due to comorbidities or medications. As sensory and physical abilities decline, there is increased risk. The ability to sense fire decreases and disabilities can impede escape. Many elderly individuals live alone or are dependent on an aging spouse for support. This isolation further increases the risk of injury and death from fire.

Signs and symptoms: Burn injuries involve a graduating zone of damage that occurs along a continuum. Sunburn represents the mildest thermal injury, and a deep full-thickness burn with an inhalation injury represents the severest thermal injury (Table 6-1). It is possible to observe burns with components of both mild and severe damage.

Diagnostic tests/tools: A complete physical examination and history is essential. Be aware when obtaining vital signs that oxygen saturation measured by pulse oximetry does not distinguish a hemoglobin molecule saturated with oxygen from one saturated with carbon monoxide, and this can result in misleading saturation levels. When an inhalation injury is suspected, obtain a carboxyhemoglobin (COHb) level. During this period, it will be necessary to map the percent of TBSA involved in the burn. For initial burn care, this percentage will be among your most valuable tools. Various methods are available for mapping. The simplest is to use the rule of nines (Fig. 6-1). For splatter, the examiner may use the patient's palm to estimate a 1% area. For large burns, it

TABLE 6-1	Classification of Burns
First-degree burn—epidermal burn	Nonblanching erythema, mild to moderately painful, usually nonedematous, not included when calculating TBSA, healing time 1 week
Second-degree burn—superficial, partial-thickness burn	Wet, pink wound bed with blistering, mild edema, very painful, healing time 10–14 days
Second-degree burn—moderate, partial-thickness burn	Red wound base with minimal exudates, edematous, moderately painful, healing time 2–4 weeks
Second-degree burn—deep, partial-thickness burn	Wound bed is dry, pale pink to white, rubbery in appearance, edematous, minimally painful, hair loss (damage at level of nerve endings and hair follicles), healing time 3–8 weeks
Third-degree burn—full-thickness burn	Wound bed dry, white or tan eschar, edematous, painless and insensate, will require excision and grafting to heal
Fourth-degree burn	Term more frequently used in Europe than in the United States; refers to burns involving underlying structures such as fat, fascia, muscle, or bone
Circumferential burn	Burn injury encompassing the entire circumference of a digit, extremity, or trunk; may constitute an emergency due to compartment syndrome with distal compromise noted by edema, loss of pulse, discoloration, pain, and paresthesia
Inhalation injury	Soot deposits in oropharynx, carbaceous sputum, singed nasal hair, facial edema, hoarseness, progressing airway edema, burns that occur in an enclosed environment, presence of carbon monoxide poisoning
	Carbon monoxide poisoning is characterized by headache, confusion, visual changes, nausea, vomiting, dizziness, disorientation and at higher levels, by tachycardia, tachypnea, seizures, and death.

Adapted from Bullocks, Hsu, Izaddoost, Hollier, & Stal (2008).

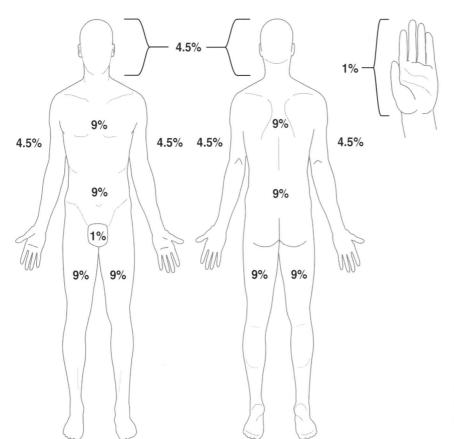

FIGURE 6-1. Estimated total body surface area using the rule of nines. *(Adapted from the Advanced Burn Life Support Manuel, ABA.)*

may be easiest to estimate the nonburn percentage and subtract from 100. An additional method for measuring the TBSA is to use a Lund and Browder chart (Table 6-2). This method allows for more detail by further breaking down the estimated areas by degree. Note that first-degree burns are not included when estimating TBSA.

Laboratory tests include a chemistry panel and complete blood count; in many institutions, these tests are included in a trauma panel. Additional testing may include toxicology for drug and/or ethanol ingestion. Pulmonary function should be assessed with chest x-ray, arterial blood gases, and COHb levels. Carbon monoxide has an affinity with hemoglobin 250 times greater than oxygen. While elevations in COHb levels >35% can result in death, the average levels in fire fatalities range between 25% and 85% (Peck, 2011). Chronic cigarette use results in elevated COHb levels between 4% and 6%.

Differential diagnosis:
- Erythema multiforme
- Stevens-Johnson syndrome
- Toxic epidermal necrolysis
- Erythema infectiosum
- Staphylococcal scald skin syndrome
- Necrotizing fasciitis
- Purpura fulminans
- Frostbite

Treatment: First, stop the burn. This should include removing and isolating the causative agent responsible for the injury while protecting the patient and your staff. If a scald has occurred, be certain that soaked clothing has been removed. If chemicals are suspected, irrigate the wounds with copious amounts of water (Lloyd, Rodgers, Michener, & Williams, 2012). Isolate clothing to be sure that others are not contaminated. In evaluating elderly burn patients, it is imperative to consider their physiological differences from younger adults, along with any associated comorbidities.

Assessment: Burn injury constitutes trauma, and as such the initial evaluation should always consist of a primary survey, including the ABCs: airway, breathing, and circulation. While undertaking this initial survey, take precautions to maintain cervical spine immobiliza-tion if indicated. After ensuring that these basics are completed, follow with a secondary survey, including a

TABLE 6-2	Lund and Browder Estimate of TBSA, Age vs. Area			
AREA	ADULT	SECOND-DEGREE BURN	THIRD-DEGREE BURN	TOTAL TBSA
Head	7			
Neck	2			
Anterior trunk	13			
Posterior trunk	13			
Right buttock	2.5			
Left buttock	2.5			
Genitalia	1			
Right upper arm	4			
Left upper arm	4			
Right lower arm	3			
Left lower arm	3			
Right hand	2.5			
Left hand	2.5			
Right thigh	9.5			
Left thigh	9.5			
Right lower leg	7			
Left lower leg	7			
Right foot	3.5			
Left foot	3.5			
Total				

Adapted from Bullocks, Hsu, Izaddoost, Hollier, & Stal (2008).

TABLE 6-3	American Burn Association Transfer Criteria

1. Partial-thickness burns greater than 10% of TBSA
2. Burns that involve the face, hands, feet, genitalia, perineum, or major joints
3. Third-degree burns in any age group
4. Electrical burns, including lightning injury
5. Chemical burns
6. Inhalation injury
7. Burn injury in patients with preexisting medical disorders that could complicate management, prolong recovery, or affect mortality
8. Any patient with burns and concomitant trauma in which the burn injury poses the greatest risk of mortality or morbidity; if trauma poses the greater immediate risk, the patient may be stabilized in a trauma center before transfer to a burn unit
9. Burned children in hospitals without qualified personnel or equipment for the care of children
10. Burn injury in patients who will require special social, emotional, and/or long-term rehabilitative intervention

Source: Guidelines for the operation of burn centers. (2007). *Journal of Burn Care & Research, 28*(1), 134–141.

head-to-toe assessment. This is the time to calculate the TBSA and to determine the category of burn injuries. Using the findings of these surveys and the ABA's criteria for transfer (Table 6-3), a decision must be made to transfer to a higher level of care or to continue management in the outpatient setting.

An important caveat is that any case of suspected elder abuse should be transferred via the emergency medical system to the appropriate emergency department to ensure proper follow-up and reporting. Suspicion of abuse should be triggered by any of the following:

■ Burn patterns that do not match the reported event
■ Straight or smooth transitions between the area burned and healthy skin resulting in a stocking- or glove-like appearance
■ A long delay between burn injury and request for treatment

Initial treatment: If it is determined that transfer to a higher level of care is appropriate, do not delay for wound débridement. Cover wounds with dry, clean sheets or towels. Maintain a warm environment to minimize the risk of hypothermia. Intravenous access should be obtained. During the first 24 hours, there is a shift of fluid and serum proteins from the vascular area to the interstitial spaces, resulting in edema, blisters, and weeping from open wounds. Fluid should be replaced based on the TBSA burned, age, and body weight. Lactated Ringer's solution is the preferred replacement agent, because it most closely resembles the body's normal physiological fluids (Ahrns, 2004). Various protocols exist for determining fluid replacement, with the Parkland and modified Brooke formulas being the most used (Kasten, Makley, & Kagan, 2011). In adults, the modified Brooke formula calls for fluid to be determined based on the following calculation: 2 mL/kg/TBSA burned. The Parkland formula uses a higher volume of 4 mL/kg/TBSA burned. Though each varies, the important caveat is to adjust delivery according to patient response. Urine output is closely followed to adjust fluids. Once the total required fluid dose is calculated, one-half is administered over the first 8 hours with the remainder given over the next 16 hours. An important consideration for outpatient management is the patient's ability to take in adequate fluids and nutrition.

Pain is best managed with small dosages of intravenous narcotics initially. This may be an important factor when considering the need for hospitalization. The elderly will require close monitoring of narcotics for both effectiveness and side effects. This monitoring may be difficult initially in an outpatient setting, especially in the case of elderly individuals with cognitive impairment, because they will require observation of nonverbal behavior and close monitoring of therapeutic response to analgesics (Titler et al., 2009). Adequate pain management is essential for successful wound care and physical therapy. All outpatients should be managed on oral analgesic agents.

Oxygen by nasal cannula would be appropriate for moderate-to-major burns and in any case where pulmonary distress is evident. In cases of suspected inhalation injury, 100% non-rebreather mask is indicated. Carbon monoxide has an affinity with hemoglobin that is 250 times higher than oxygen; however, it has a half-life of between 4 and 6 hours. Providing oxygen to a patient with suspected carbon monoxide exposure can rapidly decrease these levels in as little as 35 minutes. An excellent resource for practitioners interested in the emergency management of burn injuries is the Advanced Burn Life Support course developed and sponsored by the ABA (2007).

Wound management: After administration of appropriate pain medication, wounds should be initially doused with cool tap water to disperse any remaining heat in the tissue. The use of cold fluids is not advised, because this may cause further tissue damage as well as hypothermia. For routine wound care, tepid water is advised. Wounds should be cleaned with a mild soap and rinsed. Antibacterial soaps are not indicated. There are varying approaches to the management of blisters. One theory is that if left in place the blister provides a protective covering and will allow the wound to heal more quickly. Alternatively, plasmin inhibitors in the fluid of the blister may delay healing while the fluid itself can provide a medium for infection (Harford & Kealey, 2007). For small surface area burns, a good guide is to remove what tissue is loose during cleansing and allow intact blisters to remain. Gently wipe the wound in a circular manner, débriding any loose devitalized tissue and debris during this process. Wounds should be washed in this manner on a daily basis. Burns are not routinely managed with systemic antibiotic therapy. Topical agents are generally sufficient (Table 6-4).

When wrapping a burn wound, it is important to consider function. Digits should be wrapped individually in order to allow for gentle range of motion exercises. Extremities should be elevated while at

TABLE 6-4 Topical Agents and Dressings for Burn Wounds

NAME	USAGE	APPLICATION
Bacitracin	Prevention and treatment of infection in second-degree burns	Bacitracin ophthalmic without a dressing is preferred for facial wounds. Apply daily a thin layer of bacitracin to wound, then cover with a nonadherent dressing and sufficient gauze to absorb exudate.
Moisturizer/sun block	Apply to all healed burn wounds. Sunburn can be adequately managed with moisturizer.	Apply daily. Creams will adhere to closed wounds; if uncertain what areas are closed versus open, choose a good nonperfumed moisturizer.
Hydrocolloid dressings	Provide a moist protective covering for small-area, partial-thickness burns	Occlusive dressings may be left in place for 5 to 7 days for patients with low risk for complication.
Silver sulfadiazine 1%	Prevention and treatment of infection in second- and third-degree burns with eschar burden	Do not apply to face, cover burn area with a layer approximately 1/16 inch thick, wrap with sufficient gauze to absorb exudates, change daily, and discontinue use when necrotic tissue has sloughed because agent impedes epithelialization.
Xeroform	3% bismuth tribro-mophenate in a petrolatum blend on fine mesh gauze; bacteriostatic action for second-degree burns	May be used in cases of sulfa allergy, apply daily, cover with gauze wrapping sufficient to manage exudate.

rest, and Ace wraps or compression garments should be used to prevent edema.

Follow-up: It should be the goal to have all burn wounds closed within 1 month (Harford & Kealey, 2007). For wounds managed in the outpatient setting, evaluation should occur initially on a weekly basis (Lloyd et al., 2012). This will allow for evaluation for infection and appropriate wound care. At 2 weeks out from injury, small epithelial islands should be evident in the wound base, and a picture will begin to form as to whether or not the wound will heal spontaneously. A wound that has not begun to spontaneously close by 3 weeks will require surgical closure by means of grafting for an optimum outcome (Harford & Kealey, 2007).

Sequelae: Burn injuries can result in a host of sequelae as a consequence of physical, psychological, and financial trauma. While physical trauma is readily visible, associated financial trauma may be overlooked. Financial trauma can be associated with the possible loss of home or belongings, mounting health-care costs, and loss of gainful employment as a result of disability; it should not be left unaddressed.

Pain: Burn wounds are painful, and adequate medications must be available in order to allow for proper wound care, occupational therapy, and physical therapy. Initially and during hospitalization, burn wounds are managed with small, frequent doses of narcotic analgesia. As care progresses, patients can be transitioned onto an oral regimen of narcotics. It should be anticipated that for small burns the need for narcotics will be short lived as the wound heals. With deeper or larger burns, there may be benefit during the rehabilitative phase from adding pharmacological agents that act on neuropathic pain. Nonsteroidal anti-inflammatory agents may also be beneficial if platelet function is not a concern.

Pruritus: The process of healing triggers the mobilization of multiple agents, such as cytokines and histamine, into the wound bed. These agents, among others, can result in intense pruritus. However, although multiple causes for pruritus have been suggested, the exact causation remains unknown (Harford & Kealey, 2007). Individuals may cause significant disruption to their healing burns through the process of scratching. This can be particularly challenging in the elderly population, because antipruritic agents, such as diphenhydramine or hydroxyzine, can be sedating. Adequate analgesia in conjunction with these agents can be effective, but care must be taken to avoid oversedation. The use of moisturizers, including those that contain aloe vera, has proven helpful anecdotally. As the burn scar begins to mature, it is anticipated that pruritus will begin to diminish over a period of approximately 6 months.

Hypertrophy and contracture: In healing wounds, the production of collagen is increased. This can be even more exaggerated in infected wounds or in individuals prone to keloid formation. Wounds that remain open for 2 weeks or longer tend to be particularly prone to the development of hypertrophic scarring (Greenhalgh, 2007). Hypertrophy can lead to pain and loss of function through distortion of normal anatomy. The utilization of appropriate topical agents and dressings that act to facilitate a wound's timely closure will help prevent hypertrophy. In addition, the use of pressure garments over nearly closed or healed wounds will aid normal scar progression. Although the action is not completely understood, the use of silicone sheeting over areas of hypertrophy has been a successful adjunct to normal scar progression in some individuals. Management of scar bands that compromise function should include an evaluation for surgical release. The phenomenon of web creep occurs when hypertrophic scars begin to compromise the web spaces of the fingers and toes. Contractures and underlying tendon damage may result in impairments such as Boutonniere deformities. The resulting loss of function can be restored through surgical intervention. Healed scars at least 6 months out from injury that remain hyperemic and hypertrophic may benefit from resurfacing with a pulsed dye laser alternated with a fractional carbon dioxide laser to diminish inflammation and soften scars. Bands and contractures can develop many years after injury, and scars should be monitored for progression.

Infection: Burn wounds are frequently colonized with bacteria from the local environment, which can be managed with topical antibiotics. Systemic antibiotics are not routinely administered; however, they may play a role in the healing process if topical agents are not sufficient. Infected wounds remain inflamed. Inflamed wounds do not heal well and result in a host of other issues such as pruritus, hypertrophic scar formation, pain, and sepsis.

Burn wound care utilizes clean rather than sterile technique. Patients and families should be taught proper cleaning techniques, including frequent hand washing and management of supplies within their environment. Wounds should be examined daily during care for redness, swelling, purulent drainage, or odor. This should be reported promptly to the health-care provider, and the addition of systemic antibiotics should be considered.

Psychosocial trauma: Referral to social services or counseling services may be beneficial in helping individuals and families deal with the psychosocial impact of burn trauma (Blakeney, Rosenberg, Rosenberg, & Fauerbach, 2007). Consider the possibility of post-traumatic stress disorder when evaluating individuals, especially in their rehabilitative phase (Thomas, Meyer, & Blakeney, 2007).

Prevention/prophylaxis: In order for a burn injury to occur, there must be a coming together of multiple factors (Fig. 6-2). These factors include the host, the environment, and the vector. For example, an elderly patient falls asleep while smoking; his sheets ignite; and he is burned in a resulting house fire. It is the relationship between the man, his environment, and a potentially hazardous agent, his cigarette, that results in injury. The nurse practitioner can affect each of these components and possibly prevent the initial burn injury from occurring. By using three dimensions of prevention—primary, secondary, and tertiary—the nurse practitioner, by virtue of education, clinical expertise, and anticipatory guidance, plays a vital role in burn prevention (Grant, 2004).

Primary prevention constitutes product design, regulation, and legislation. This also includes educational programs designed to educate the public on safety. The individual smoking in bed would hopefully benefit from smoking cessation programs in his community. Regulation and product design in this scenario would affect the combustibility of clothing, linen, and housing materials exposed to the smoldering cigarette. During an annual physical examination, the nurse practitioner should include education on sound living habits and home safety. Included in this discussion should be a review of home fire safety protocols, including the proper use of smoke alarms, removal of hazards such as frayed electrical cords, visual aids for those with impaired sight, and the appropriate temperature setting for home hot water heaters. This is also an excellent opportunity to discuss the advantages of smoking cessation.

Secondary prevention includes actions that would serve to limit the extent of damage done such as cooling wounds initially and, for our client in the house fire, the initial application of 100% oxygen to decrease carbon monoxide levels rapidly, mitigating the effects of an inhalation injury. Occupational therapists provide compression garments and ensure proper splitting technique to maintain function. Physical therapists assist with mobilization though stretching and exercise programs. The injury has occurred, but these actions may limit the scope of damage done. Tertiary prevention addresses recovery and rehabilitation. Individuals continue to work with therapists to maximize function. Management of healed burn scars with moisturizers and sunscreen can prevent further skin damage. Through tertiary prevention the individual optimizes his or her level of functioning and minimizes disability resultant from the burn injury. Psychological counseling can help an individual or family work through post-traumatic stress. Social services can affect an individual's ability to regain control and return to the community.

The nurse practitioner can be instrumental in developing and/or referring clients to community-based programs that promote home safety for the elderly (Grant, 2004). Excellent educational programs are available through agencies such as the National Fire Protection Association, the Centers for

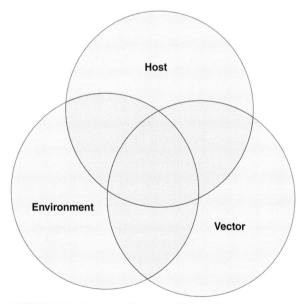

FIGURE 6-2. Required elements of burn injury.

Disease Control and Prevention, the ABA, and all verified burn centers.

Referral: Burns often require complex care and the involvement of multiple disciplines. In the elderly population, even a small burn may require fluid resuscitation that could complicate care due to pre-existing comorbidities and concomitant medications. The absence of support systems or the suspicion of elder abuse should prompt considerations for hospitalization and possible referral to a specialized burn care facility. The ABA has developed a list of criteria that should signal the need for referral to a burn center (see Table 6-3). A burn center verified by the ABA can provide services to a burn patient through all phases of the patient's care (Guidelines for the operation of burn centers, 2007).

For rehabilitation concerns related to nerve compression, development of scar bands, or contractures, it would be advantageous to make a referral to a plastic and reconstructive surgeon. Reconstruction after burn injury should also include evaluation of mature scars that have remained hyperemic and hypertrophic for possible photoablation with laser therapy. Occupational therapy and physical therapy are crucial in preserving and maintaining form and function for burn victims (Lloyd et al., 2012). Referral for these services should be made early in the care of the burn patient. A referral for social services or in-home assistance may be indicated to promote safe return to a living environment. Last, do not forego discussing the needs for emotional and spiritual support with clients and their families. Along with individual therapy, there are also many excellent community resources for support. Contact your nearest burn center for referral information. An excellent resource for support is the Phoenix Society, whose Web site can be accessed at www.phoenix-society.org.

Education: Education is an ongoing component of patient care. The treatment of burn wounds is systematic and manageable in an outpatient setting for those individuals with minor burn injuries and adequate support systems. The nurse practitioner should identify early on who will be providing wound care. This individual, or the patient if able, should demonstrate the ability to perform wound care before leaving the clinic or hospital setting. Patients should be provided with appropriate written instructions in clear language for wound care, indicators for infection or tissue compromise, and contact information should questions arise. In addition to wound care, there should be written instructions on medication, including dosing and possible side effects.

Patients should be instructed to minimize exposure to ultraviolet (UV) light. This should include the use of protective clothing and sunscreen. They should continue to utilize compression garments in the rehabilitative phase to minimize swelling and scar formation.

CLINICAL RECOMMENDATION	EVIDENCE RATING	REFERENCE
Education regarding fire safety and prevention is the most effective intervention to prevent loss of life and injury due to home fires and should be promoted at every visit.	A	American Burn Association Prevention Campaign (2010) Centers for Disease Control and Prevention (2010) National Fire Protection Association (2011)
Initial pain management for burn injuries with low-dose narcotics sufficient to allow for wound care and therapy. Adjunct therapy with NSAIDs and neuropathic pain modulators as indicated.	A	ABA (2007) Meyer, Patterson, Jaco, Woodson, & Thomas (2007)
Topical antibiotic use for burn wounds with avoidance of prophylactic systemic antibiotics.	A	Bessey (2007) Harford & Kealey (2007) Greenhalgh (2007)

Continued

CLINICAL RECOMMENDATION	EVIDENCE RATING	REFERENCE
Systematic daily care of burn wounds using clean technique, with goal of 1 month for wound closure.	A	Bessey (2007) Greenhalgh (2007) Harford & Kealey (2007)
Pressure garments and silicone sheeting to prevent swelling, decrease pruritus, and minimize hypertrophic scar formation.	B	Harford & Kealey (2007)
Evaluation for posttraumatic stress disorder and other psychiatric disorders associated with burn injury.	A	Blakeney et al. (2007) Thomas et al. (2007)

A = consistent, good-quality, patient-oriented evidence; B = inconsistent or limited-quality, patient-oriented evidence; C = consensus, disease-oriented evidence, usual practice, expert opinion, or case series. For information about the SORT evidence rating system, go to www.aafp.org/afpsort.xml.

CELLULITIS

Signal symptoms: Erythema, blisters, local tenderness, erysipelas.

Description: Cellulitis is a deep infection of the skin; it is most commonly caused by group A streptococci, *Staphylococcus aureus*, *Erysipelothrix rhusiopathiae*, *Vibrio vulnificus*, *Haemophilus influenzae*, or occasionally a gram-negative organism (Spellburg et al., 2009). Cellulitis also can be caused by specific pathogens from human or animal bites. Patients generally present with localized erythema, swelling, and tenderness to the affected area. Systemic symptoms may occur from the infection (Campbell, Burton-MacLeod, & Howlett, 2009; Petrou, 2011).

Etiology: Although cellulitis usually occurs when an organism enters the skin through an open area, it also can occur in intact but edematous skin. Cellulitis involves the dermis and subcutaneous tissue. A clear site of entry may not be evident in patients with obesity, edema, or lipedema.

Occurrence: Although the actual occurrence of cellulitis is unknown, approximately 600,000 patients are admitted each year with suspected cellulitis (Thorsteindottir, Tleyjeh, & Baddour, 2005).

Age: Cellulitis can occur at any age. Facial cellulitis is most common in people 50 years and older.

Gender: Cellulitis occurs equally among men and women.

Ethnicity: No known predominant ethnic group is associated with cellulitis incidence.

Contributing factors: Cellulitis can occur in patients who have arterial or venous insufficiency, diabetes mellitus, lacerations, lower extremity edema, lymphedema, human or animal bites (cat bites), tinea infections, recurring cellulitis, burns, trauma, stasis ulceration, ischemia, toe web maceration, and puncture wounds (Nazarko, 2008a; Tyrer & Thornalley, 2008). It also is associated with certain surgical procedures (such as mastectomies or any other surgery that involves the dissection of lymph nodes) and environmental and occupational hazards such as occupations that involve regularly handling poultry, fish, or meat. Intravenous drug use is another factor contributing to the development of cellulitis. Acute and chronic sinusitis can lead to periorbital or orbital cellulitis. Patients with a history of coronary artery bypass graft surgery with removal of the saphenous vein are susceptible to cellulitis. Consider cellulitis in patients who are on immunosuppressive medications or prescribed long-term use of corticosteroids (Price, 2009).

Signs and symptoms: Patients may complain of localized pain, fever, chills, rigors, malaise, anorexia, nausea, or headache, and, in severe cases, patients may have tachycardia, hypotension, and delirium (Nazarko, 2008b). Cellulitis most often appears on the lower extremities after a skin aberration, such as dermatitis, ulceration, trauma, or tinea pedis. Cellulitis can develop on the arms and the face as well. Scars from previous cardiovascular surgery are common sites for recurrent cellulitis (Price, 2009). Examine for skin temperature, note any breaks in the skin and ulcerations, and determine presence of pulses and sensation. Local erythema with edema and tenderness elicited by palpation are presenting signs of cellulitis. The skin can appear to look stretched, later taking on the appearance of an orange peel when the surface is infiltrated (Price, 2009). Depending on the organism of origin, large hemorrhagic bullae may be present. Because lymphangitis and regional lymphadenopathy also may occur with cellulitis, the clinician should examine for red streaks extending proximally to the infected area. If gas gangrene (anaerobic cellulitis) is suspected, the skin should be inspected for crepitus and foul-smelling exudates, and the surrounding area should be palpated for muscle tenderness. A positive Homans' sign (pain in the calf on dorsiflexion of the ankle of affected limb) or palpable venous cord may suggest deep vein thrombosis (DVT). A compete assessment of peripheral pulses is also warranted if DVT is suspected. If the cellulitis is located near a joint, carefully examine the area to note any articular swelling indicating possible septic arthritis. If systemic infection is suspected, assess for lymphadenopathy (Price, 2009; Schalock & Sober, 2009). A cardiac examination is warranted to assess for a heart murmur.

Diagnostic tests: Unless pus has formed in the wound, a tissue culture is usually not necessary. In cases of extensive infection or suspected systemic toxicity, blood cultures and a complete blood count (CBC) with differential should be obtained to determine the severity of illness and to identify the organism, including methicillin-resistant *Staphylococcus aureus* (MRSA). Leukocytosis is present in patients with anaerobic cellulitis, and the Gram's stain smear shows gram-positive encapsulated bacilli. C-reactive protein will be elevated in patients with severe cellulitis. In patients with rhabdomyolysis, creatine kinase will be elevated. Patients with diabetes mellitus should have a radiograph of the area to rule out the presence of osteomyelitis. Skin biopsies may be necessary to rule out the presence of fungal, viral, parasitic, or mycobacterial etiologies (Petrou, 2011).

Differential diagnosis:

- Lipodermatosclerosis (tender red plaque on the medial lower legs in patients with venous stasis or varicosities)
- Acute severe contact dermatitis (edema is superficial, itching is more prevalent)
- Acute gout (synovial fluid aspiration contains monosodium urate crystals)
- Necrotizing fasciitis (determined by magnetic resonance imaging [MRI] or computed tomography [CT]; patient presents with diffuse swelling or an arm or leg with associated bullae with clear or serosanguineous fluid)
- Thrombophlebitis (lower extremity Doppler ultrasound)
- Pseudogout (synovial fluid aspiration contains calcium pyrophosphate crystal deposition)
- Osteomyelitis (determined by radiographs, MRI, CT)
- Pyromyositis (determined by radiographs, MRI, CT)
- Early herpes zoster
- Atypical drug eruptions
- Erysipelas (superficial cellulitis found on the face originating as a bright reddened area)
- Venous or varicose eczema (absence of malaise, fever, and limited progression of erythemic area) (Nazarko, 2008a; Petrou, 2011; Price, 2009)

Treatment: Patients with an open wound initially should be asked when their last tetanus toxoid booster was given; if the most recent booster was ≥10 years ago, 0.5 mL of tetanus toxoid should be administered immediately. If the wound is grossly contaminated and the patient's last tetanus booster was 5 to 10 years ago, the practitioner should consider giving another booster at this time. An older adult who has not had primary immunization requires tetanus toxoid and tetanus immune globulin.

Patients with mild cellulitis may be given oral antibiotics. In a mild case of cellulitis found to be gram-negative bacilli in origin, antibiotics are not necessary unless the patient is at high risk (see under Referral). The drugs of choice include dicloxacillin, 125 to 500 mg 4 times daily; clindamycin, 300 mg 4 times daily; and a first-generation cephalosporin such as cephalexin, 250 to 500 mg 4 times daily. For streptococcal cellulitis, penicillin is the drug of choice. Oxacillin is also effective for streptococcus and staphylococcus. Cellulitis resulting from an anaerobe should be treated with a fluoroquinolone plus clindamycin or metronidazole. Oral therapy should be prescribed for 7 to 10 days, and extended medication may be needed. Treatment of MRSA should be guided by culture results. Patients with underlying tinea should be treated with topical antifungal medications as well as antibiotics (Schalock & Sober, 2009). Evaluation of patient's pain is needed. The use of NSAIDs or acetaminophen is recommended to reduce inflammation and pain (Price, 2009).

Consider the patient's renal function before prescribing any medication. Tell the patient to elevate the affected area, keep the area as clean as possible, and avoid any trauma to the area. Moist warm soaks can be applied to the affected area. Patients may require analgesics in appropriate dosages for pain. Patients with edema should take measures to control the edema by elevating the extremity. The use of compression bandaging has been recommended for patients with cellulitis of the lower extremity (Dutton, Paulik, & Jones, 2009). Blood glucose levels need to be monitored carefully if the patient has diabetes. Patients with complications (see under Referral) should be hospitalized for monitoring and to receive IV antibiotics.

Follow-up: Outpatients should be requested to contact their health-care providers within 1 week if no improvement with antibiotic use is noted or within 48 hours if fever or inflammation continues. On their return visit, patients should be examined for evidence of thrombophlebitis or recurrence of the cellulitis (Schalock & Sober, 2009).

Sequelae: In patients with cellulitis of the lower extremities, thrombophlebitis is a potential complication.

Additional problems arising from cellulitis include bacteremia, bullae, lymphangitis, and necrosis of the affected area, especially in patients with recurrent cellulitis (Petrou, 2011).

Prevention/prophylaxis: Preventive measures for cellulitis include reduction of chronic edema in patients with peripheral vascular disease, control of blood glucose in patients with diabetes, and meticulous hand washing. Wheelchair-bound patients should have protective measures to avoid trauma to their extremities (Nazarko, 2008b).

Referral: Patients should be hospitalized if they have high fever, diabetes, alcoholism, HIV, anaerobic cellulitis, necrotizing fasciitis, or cellulitis of the orbit or face or if they are experiencing extreme pain. Consultation with an infectious disease specialist may be necessary. Order a surgical consultation for patients who require incision and drainage of abscesses and débridement of necrotic tissue. Home IV treatment may be indicated to shorten hospital stay.

Education: Patients with cellulitis must be informed that completion of the antibiotic regimen is mandatory. Patients should not attempt to scratch the affected area but should keep the site meticulously clean to avoid superinfection. Advise patients with lower extremity involvement to maintain bed rest with bathroom privileges and to elevate the limb. Apprise them of the signs and symptoms of thrombophlebitis (Carter, Kilburn, & Featherstone, 2007).

CLINICAL RECOMMENDATION	EVIDENCE RATING	REFERENCES
The use of an institution-based clinical practice guideline recommending single gram-positive agent (vancomycin) in treating cellulitis in hospitalized patients reduced the duration of time exposed to antibiotic treatment and the use of broad-spectrum agents.	A	Jenkins et al. (2011)
The use of cycloidal vibration in combination with antibiotic therapy reduced hospital admission for community-based patients with cellulitis.	A	Tyrer & Thornalley (2008)
Obesity was found to be a significant factor in the development of lower extremity cellulitis.	B	McNamara et al. (2007) Thorsteinsdottir et al. (2005)

CLINICAL RECOMMENDATION	EVIDENCE RATING	REFERENCES
The use of antibiotics and compression bandages is recommended for patients with lower extremity cellulitis.	C	Dutton et al. (2009)

A = consistent, good-quality, patient-oriented evidence; B = inconsistent or limited-quality, patient-oriented evidence; C = consensus, disease-oriented evidence, usual practice, expert opinion, or case series. For information about the SORT evidence rating system, go to www.aafp.org/afpsort.xml.

CORNS AND CALLUSES

Signal symptoms: Hyperkeratotic overgrowths.

Description: Corns and calluses are aggregations of hyperkeratotic skin on the foot. A hyperkeratotic nodule that forms on the inner (web surface) between toes is known as a soft corn (clavus). Soft corns are commonly located on the fourth web space and at the medial side of the second proximal interphalangeal joint. A soft corn occurs when an extreme amount of moisture from perspiration is absorbed between the toes, resulting eventually in a deteriorated appearance of the skin. Hard corns or heloma duram are hypertrophic skin changes often found on the dorsolateral aspect of the fifth toe and over the metatarsal heads on the plantar aspect of the foot (Helfand, 2009; Schalock, & Sober, 2009). The hard corn is a dry, horny mass of keratosis with a hard central core. Calluses (tylomata) are diffuse hyperkeratotic lesions generally found on the sole of the foot under the metatarsal head. There are two types of calluses, namely, the discrete-nucleated and the diffuse shearing (Freeman, 2002). The discrete-nucleated callus has a central keratin plug; when palpated, tenderness is elicited. A diffuse shearing callus is spread over a wider area, is directly related to a shearing activity of the foot, and does not have a central plug. People with bunions often develop a callus over the bunion because of the friction of the bunion against the shoe.

Etiology: Increased rubbing of, pressure on, or friction to the dermis layer of skin on the foot causes corns and calluses. Hyperkeratosis is the body's protective response when the skin has been exposed to friction and rubbing (Freeman, 2002). Often the skin surrounding the corn will macerate, causing tenderness, and may become infected. The most common cause is poorly fitting shoes. Individuals with foot deformities or gait disturbances, or both, are also at high risk for developing calluses, especially over bony prominences (Helfand, 2009; Schalock & Sober, 2009).

Occurrence: Both corns and calluses are common in older adults. Studies report the prevalence of corns to affect 9% to 62% of the population and calluses approximately 20% to 50% of older adults (Stolt, Suhonen, Voutilainen, & Leino-Kilpi, 2010).

Age: Individuals more than 65 years old most commonly develop corns and calluses (Bennett, 2006).

Gender: More common in women secondary to restrictive footwear.

Ethnicity: The prevalence of corns and calluses was found to be higher in African Americans as compared to Caucasians and Hispanics (Dunn et al., 2004).

Contributing factors: Gait disturbance or imbalance secondary to weakness, arthritis, and normal aging changes of the foot; foot deformities such as hammer-toe deformity and bunions, bony prominences, irregularities of footwear; and use of improper footwear. High levels of ambulatory activity also can contribute to the formation of corns and calluses.

Signs and symptoms: Usually corns and calluses are asymptomatic. Thick calluses may cause a burning sensation in the foot. Depending on the location of the corn or callus, tight-fitting shoes may cause severe pain.

Diagnostic tests: Radiograph of the foot can be ordered to rule out abnormal bone structure.

Differential diagnosis:
- Plantar ulcers and plantar warts (verrucae)
- Tinea pedis (differentiate from soft corns) (Freeman, 2002).

Treatment: Mechanical paring of the corn, callus, or both is recommended. Improper footwear should be avoided. Use of accommodative padding, such as a metatarsal pad, helps to relieve pressure by changing the alignment of the toes. Silicone toe sleeves, polymer gel, cushions, and padding with foam or lamb's wool are available over the counter. Patients with soft corns are advised to soak the foot in a solution of potassium permanganate and then carefully apply absorbent lamb's wool to the macerated skin (Helfand, 2009; Landorf et al., 2011; Schalock & Sober, 2009).

Follow-up: Periodic physical examination of the foot is needed to assess the status of the healing.

Sequelae: Without correcting the causative agent of the corns and calluses, the cycle will continue, contributing to continued pain and nonhealing of the skin.

Prevention/prophylaxis: Relief of the pressure on the affected area can prevent development of corns and calluses. Shoes should be wide enough at the toe to allow the toes to extend straight ahead. Encourage women to avoid wearing shoes with high heels (Bennett, 2006).

Referral: Refer patients with complicated management to a podiatrist or orthopedic surgeon if relief is not experienced. Diabetic patients with corns and calluses should be receiving their foot care from a podiatrist (Schalock & Sober, 2009).

Education: Teach patients the importance of avoiding improper footwear. To prevent injury to the toes, 0.5 inch of extra space should be allowed in the toe box. Products that contain salicylic acid "should be avoided because they may damage surrounding normal tissues, especially in neuropathic and immunocompromised patients" (Bennett, 2006; Freeman, 2002, p. 2279).

CLINICAL RECOMMENDATION	EVIDENCE RATING	REFERENCES
Scalpel débridement of painful calluses is of small benefit to patients with painful plantar calluses.	A	Landorf et al. (2011)
Acrylic or wool fiber is absorbent, suggesting that patients with feet that perspire would benefit from socks made of these materials.	C	Bennett (2006)
Over-the-counter products that contain salicylic acid should not be used in patients with neuropathic foot conditions or in those patients who are immunocompromised. Damage can occur simultaneously to the surrounding unaffected tissue.	C	Freeman (2002)
The use of therapeutic padding, including foam pads, lamb's wool, and silicone sleeves, has been found to be beneficial in alleviating painful symptoms of corns and calluses.	C	Freeman (2002)

A = consistent, good-quality, patient-oriented evidence; B = inconsistent or limited-quality, patient-oriented evidence; C = consensus, disease-oriented evidence, usual practice, expert opinion, or case series. For information about the SORT evidence rating system, go to www.aafp.org/afpsort.xml.

HERPES ZOSTER

Signal symptoms: Cutaneous eruption of a dermatome distribution, burning or tingling skin sensation.

Description: Herpes zoster is an acute vesicular eruption caused by a virus histologically identical to the varicella (chickenpox) virus. Herpes zoster is human (alpha) herpes virus 3 (varicella-zoster virus [VZV]), a member of the herpes virus group.

Etiology: Recurrent VZV infection causes herpes zoster. The patient has initial contact with VZV in the form of chickenpox. The DNA virus resides within the neurons. During reactivation, the virus spreads across the sensory ganglion to other neurons, which causes a cutaneous eruption of a dermatome distribution (Fashner & Bell, 2011). Older adults have a decrease in cell-mediated immunity, which contributes to the risk of developing herpes zoster and postherpetic neuralgia (Barakzai & Fraser, 2008).

If herpes zoster affects bilateral dermatomes, it is considered to be disseminated herpes zoster (Sandy, 2005). Although chickenpox is one of the most readily communicable diseases, herpes zoster has a much lower rate of transmission. Nonimmune persons are considered contagious 8 to 21 days after exposure to VZV. Mode of transmission is coming into contact with the vesicle fluid. Patients with herpes zoster may be sources of infection for 1 week after the appearance of vesicle lesions. Nonimmune individuals can transmit the infection and should avoid contact with patients with herpes zoster (Fashner & Bell, 2011).

Occurrence: Herpes zoster occurs worldwide, more commonly in older adults. An estimated one-half of the population is affected by age 85 (Sampathkumar, Drage, & Martin, 2009). Approximately 1 million cases occur in the United States each year (Centers for Disease Control and Prevention, 2011). It is estimated that 3.2 cases of herpes zoster occur in every 1000 persons (Insinga, Itzler, Pellissier, Saddler, & Nikas, 2005).

Age: This infection is most common in adults over 55 years old. The incidence of herpes zoster increases with age (Dworkin et al., 2009).

Gender: Women are diagnosed with 60% of the cases of herpes zoster (Insinga et al., 2005).

Ethnicity: African Americans are one-fourth as likely as whites to develop herpes zoster.

Contributing factors: Individuals are more likely to develop herpes zoster if they are more than 55 years old, have diabetes mellitus, have had an organ transplant, are immunosuppressed (e.g., HIV-infected patients), have certain malignancies, are receiving long-term corticosteroids, are receiving chemotherapy, or are taking radiation treatments. Physiological or psychological stressors can precipitate the development of herpes zoster (Fashner & Bell, 2011; Johnson, Wasner, Saddier, & Baron, 2008).

Signs and symptoms: Patients usually experience hyperesthesia with a burning or tingling pain at the site 4 to 5 days before the eruption appears. Pain in a dermatomal pattern may precede the appearance of the vesicles by weeks, however. Patients often experience a sense of anxiety, malaise, headache, fever, and flu-like symptoms with the onset of herpes zoster. Patients may report sleep disturbances, decreased appetite, and depression. There may be a sense of dysesthesias and paresthesias along the dermatome (Ferri, 2007). Some patients complain of intense itching in the involved area (Dworkin et al., 2009). There may be reported pain around the eye if ophthalmic herpes zoster later develops. The eruption is maculopapular for a few hours and then becomes characterized as grouped vesicles on an erythematous base over one dermatome (usually). The vesicles are clear at first and then become cloudy within 3 to 5 days. T5 and T6 are the most common vertebral dermatomes involved, followed by cervical and sacral dermatomes. As vesicles age, they become pustular, then crust over after 3 to 4 days, finally healing in 2 to 4 weeks. Lesions may appear in irregular crops and are typically unilateral. Scarring and change in pigmentation may occur following the healing of the crusted vesicles. The most common distributions are on the trunk or face in elderly persons. Regional lymph nodes may or may not be swollen and tender (Fashner & Bell, 2011). The pain can last 6 to 12 months after disappearance of the rash (postherpetic neuralgia [PHN]). Ocular complications occur in about one-half of patients with involvement of the ophthalmic division of the trigeminal nerve; these complications may include keratitis, anterior uveitis, and corneal ulceration. Herpes zoster ophthalmicus occurs in 5% to 10% of patients with herpes zoster; permanent loss of vision or cranial nerve palsies can occur (Dworkin et al., 2009). Vesicles on the tip of the nose, known as Hutchinson's sign, have been found to be a precursor to corneal involvement in herpes zoster (Sampathkumar et al., 2009). Cutaneous or visceral dissemination, the appearance of numerous varicella-like lesions in extradermatomal sites, may cause pneumonitis, encephalitis, meningitis, myelitis, and hepatitis (Fashner & Bell, 2011). The reactivation of VZV in the geniculate ganglion produces vesicles in the mucocutaneous distribution of the peripheral nerves. Known as Ramsey-Hunt syndrome, patients may experience vesicles in the pharynx and external auditory canal, tinnitus, vertigo, one-sided hearing loss, and often paralysis on one side of the face (Sampathkumar et al., 2009).

Diagnostic tests: Diagnosis usually is based on clinical appearance and distribution of the eruption and on a careful history of when the rash appeared. The direct immunofluorescence with fluorescein-tagged antibody (DFA) or polymerase chain reaction (PCR) (if available) is preferred over the old standard Tzanck smear. These tests have far greater sensitivity and specificity than the Tzanck smear and allow differentiation between herpes simplex virus (HSV) and VZV infections. The DFA and PCR are useful in complicated cases and epidemiological studies (Sampathkumar et al., 2009). PCR is an expensive test, however, and the results of the test generally are not known for at least a day (Dworkin et al., 2007).

Differential diagnosis: When the pain of pre-eruptive herpes occurs, the differential diagnosis depends on the dermatome involved:

- Migraine
- Myocardial infarction
- Acute abdomen
- Renal colic
- Pericarditis
- Pleuritis
- Pulmonary embolism

Once the rash or eruption appears:

- Contact allergic dermatitis (linear vesicles)
- Grouped vesicles (viral infection) (Fashner & Bell, 2011; Sampathkumar et al., 2009)

Treatment: Antiviral agents are recommended in the presence of significant pain, serious herpes zoster, or involvement near the eye. Postherpetic neuralgia is not reduced by antiviral therapy, but these agents may help with healing in the acute phase by reducing viral shredding (Cadogan, 2010). Give acyclovir, 800 mg 5 times a day for 7 to 10 days; famciclovir, 500 mg orally every 8 hours for 7 days; or valacyclovir, 1000 mg orally every 8 hours for 7 days (Fashner & Bell, 2011). These drugs must be given within 72 hours after onset of rash to be effective, and their use must be monitored in patients with reduced renal function (Tyring, Beutner, Tucker, Anderson, & Crooks, 2000). Patients should be encouraged to stay hydrated and to avoid scratching (Cadogan, 2010). Patients with disseminated disease and those who are immunocompromised may need IV antiviral medications (Cadogan, 2010). Topical agents are also effective in treating herpes zoster. The use of cool compresses with 1:20 Burow's solution, calamine lotion, and topical lidocaine (Xylocaine) is recommended for the soothing local effect.

Analgesics may be necessary for the initial prodromal pain associated with herpes zoster. Acetaminophen is recommended initially. Tramadol, NSAIDs, and opiates can be used as recommended for severe pain.

Gabapentin is recommended for the treatment of PHN. Initial dose is 300 mg on the first day and is titrated up gradually until pain relief is safely reached. The maximum does of gabapentin is 3600 mg/day. Pregabalin is also recommended for the treatment of postherpetic neuralgia and can be administered 50 mg 3 times a day or 75 mg twice a day. The dosage can be increased to 300 mg daily after 3 to 7 days as tolerated, followed by 150 mg every 3 to 7 days. The maximum recommended dose is 600 mg/day. Caution is advised when prescribing gabapentin and pregabalin to older adults given the side effects of dizziness and ataxia (Christo, Hobelmann, & Maine, 2007).

The secondary amine tricyclic antidepressants, nortriptyline 10 mg orally or desipramine 10 to 25 mg orally both given at bedtime, may be helpful, and it may be necessary to gradually increase the dosage until reduction of pain occurs; however, because of the anticholinergic side effects, caution is warranted (Ahmad & Goucke, 2002).

The use of opioids in the treatment of PHN alone or in combination with other therapies has also been studied; greater pain relief was experienced by patients when a combined regimen was prescribed over a single agent (Gilron et al., 2005). The 5% lidocaine patch has been shown to be effective in treating the pain of PHN; 1 to 3 patches are applied in a 24-hour period. For PHN pain, capsaicin (Zostrix cream) can be applied topically. The capsaicin 8% patch can be applied by a health-care professional to the most painful skin areas (Christo et al., 2007). In cases of severe pain, a transcutaneous electrical nerve stimulator unit may be tried (Christo et al., 2007).

Follow-up: Patients should be reexamined in 2 to 4 weeks to monitor progression of rash and as needed for follow-up of PHN.

Sequelae: Postherpetic neuralgia is the primary complication, occurring almost exclusively in people over 60 years old. From 30% to 50% of people over the age of 80 diagnosed with herpes zoster develop PHN (Watson, 2010). This pain persists at least 6 weeks after skin lesions. The pain, characterized as constant, severe, sharp, or burning, may develop into a long-standing, debilitating problem. Postherpetic neuralgia usually lasts 1 year or less. Some patients experience a postherpetic itching sensation rather than pain (Dworkin et al., 2009; Oaklander, 2008). Another consequence of herpes zoster is secondary bacterial infection leading to cellulitis, caused by staphylococcus group A or group A β-hemolytic streptococcus.

Prevention/prophylaxis: The vaccine for herpes zoster (Zostavax) is available and is recommended for patients age 60 and older. The immunization may be given without any serologic testing, history of varicella, or history of herpes zoster. Lower incidence of herpes zoster has been found in individuals who have received the herpes zoster vaccine (Hurley et al., 2010; Lu, Euler, Jumaan, & Harpaz, 2009; Oxman et al., 2005; Tseng et al., 2011). Practitioners are advised to review the listed contraindications before administering the herpes zoster vaccine. Caution, however, has been advised in prescribing Zostavax to patients over 80 (Fried, 2010). High-risk individuals, such as immunosuppressed patients and individuals who have not had chickenpox, should be kept from exposure to patients with herpes zoster. Positive results were found in adults and older adults who participated in tai chi as a means to boost cell-mediated immunity, suggesting that the effect of the vaccine can be enhanced with regular relaxation and meditation techniques (Irwin, Olmstead, & Oxman, 2007).

Second cases of herpes zoster are rare in immunocompetent patients given that one incidence of herpes zoster boosts immunity and prevents subsequent outbreak (Dworkin et al., 2009).

Referral: Because of probable ocular involvement, patients with lesions on the nose or in the eye area should be referred to an ophthalmologist. Patients with disseminated herpes zoster should be referred to a specialist. Refer patients with severe uncontrollable PHN to a neurologist (Christo et al., 2007).

Education: Emphasize to the patient the need to stay home and get plenty of rest. Teach patients proper infection control measures and proper disposal of dressings or items of clothing that contain vesicle fluid, especially if they have known contacts that are vulnerable for developing varicella. Patients should avoid contact with immunosuppressed individuals, pregnant women, and individuals who have not had chickenpox.

CLINICAL RECOMMENDATION	EVIDENCE RATING	REFERENCES
Antiviral therapy should be initiated within 72 hours of onset of the maculopapular lesions to increase the healing of the herpes zoster.	A	Tyring et al. (2000)
Regular participation in tai chi boosted the cell-mediating effects of the herpes zoster vaccine.	B	Irwin et al. (2007)
In the treatment of PHN, combined use of morphine and gabapentin provided patients greater pain relief over a prescribed single agent.	A	Gilron et al. (2005)
The herpes zoster vaccine (Zostavax), unless contraindicated, should be given to persons >60 years old to prevent an outbreak of herpes zoster and subsequent development of PHN.	B	Hurley et al. (2010) Lu et al. (2009) Oxman et al. (2005)
The use of the high-concentration capsaicin patch provided sustained relief from pain in patients with PHN.	B	Irving et al. (2010)
The lidoderm 5% patch provided relief to patients experiencing pain from PHN.	B	Binder et al. (2009)

A = consistent, good-quality, patient-oriented evidence; B = inconsistent or limited-quality, patient-oriented evidence; C = consensus, disease-oriented evidence, usual practice, expert opinion, or case series. For information about the SORT evidence rating system, go to www.aafp.org/afpsort.xml.

PRESSURE ULCERS

Signal symptoms: Nonblanching erythema (darkly pigmented skin may not have visible blanching; its color may differ from the surrounding area), shallow or deep painful lesions, dry or exudating lesions, wound base colors vary from pink/red to yellow/white with slough (nonviable tissue) and those covered with black/brown eschar. Pressure ulcers may be firmer, softer, cooler, or warmer as compared to adjacent tissue (National Pressure Ulcer Advisory Panel [NPUAP] & European Pressure Ulcer Advisory Panel [EPUAP], 2009).

Description: A pressure ulcer is defined as localized injury to the skin and/or underlying tissue usually over a bony prominence as a result of pressure or pressure in combination with shear (NPUAP/EPUAP, 2009). Friction is assumed in the presence of shear, because friction generates shear. A number of contributing or confounding factors are also associated with pressure ulcers; the significance of these factors is yet to be elucidated. Common terms for pressure ulcer include bedsore, decubitus ulcer, pressure sore, and pressure ulcer. There are six pressure ulcer stages:

Stage I: Intact skin with nonblanchable redness of a localized area usually over a bony prominence. Darkly pigmented skin may not have visible blanching; its color may differ from the surrounding area. The area may be painful, firm, soft, warmer, or cooler as compared to adjacent tissue. Stage I may be difficult to detect in individuals with dark skin tones. May indicate "at risk" persons (a heralding sign of risk).

Stage II: Partial-thickness loss of dermis presenting as a shallow open ulcer with a red/pink wound bed, without slough. May also present as an intact or open/ruptured serum-filled blister. Presents as a shiny or dry shallow ulcer without slough or bruising (bruising indicates suspected deep tissue injury). This stage should not be used to describe skin tears, tape burns, moisture-associated dermatitis, maceration, or excoriation.

Stage III: Full-thickness tissue loss. Subcutaneous fat may be visible but bone, tendon, and muscles are not exposed. Slough may be present but does not obscure the depth of tissue loss. May include undermining and tunneling. The depth of a stage III pressure ulcer varies by anatomical location. The bridge of the nose, ear, occiput, and malleolus do not have subcutaneous tissue, and stage III ulcers can be shallow. In contrast, areas of significant adiposity can develop extremely deep stage III pressure ulcers. Bone/tendon is not visible or directly palpable.

Stage IV: Full-thickness tissue loss with exposed bone, tendon, or muscle. Slough or eschar may be present on some parts of the wound bed. Often includes undermining and tunneling. The depth of a stage IV pressure ulcer varies by anatomical location. The bridge of the nose, ear, occiput, and malleolus do not have subcutaneous tissue, and these ulcers can be shallow. Stage IV ulcers can extend into muscle and/or supporting structures (e.g., fascia, tendon, or joint capsule), making osteomyelitis possible. Exposed bone/tendons are visible or directly palpable.

Unstageable: Full-thickness tissue loss in which the base of the ulcer is covered by slough (yellow, tan, gray, green, or brown) and/or eschar (tan, brown, or black) in the wound bed. Until enough slough and/or eschar is removed to expose the base of the wound, the true depth, and therefore stage, cannot be determined. Stable (dry, adherent, intact without erythema or fluctuance) eschar on the heels serves as the body's natural (biological) cover and should not be removed.

Suspected deep tissue injury: Purple or maroon localized area of discolored intact skin or blood-filled blister due to damage of underlying soft tissue from pressure and/or shear. The area may be preceded by tissue that is painful, firm, mushy, boggy, warmer, or cooler as compared to adjacent tissue. Deep tissue injury may be difficult to detect in individuals with dark skin tones. Evolution may include a thin blister over a dark wound bed. The wound may further evolve and become covered by thin eschar. Evolution may be rapid, exposing additional layers of tissue even with optimal treatment.

Etiology: The exact mechanism of pressure ulcer development is poorly understood. Kottner, Balzer, Dassen, and Heinze (2009) describe four causation theories: ischemia caused by occlusion of the capillaries leading to vascular insufficiency, tissue anoxia, and cell death; reperfusion injury (i.e., cellular injury resulting from the reperfusion of blood to previously ischemic tissue); impairment of lymphatic function leading to a buildup of metabolic waste products; and mechanical deformation of tissue cells. The type of tissue involved is also important, with epidermis and dermis being more resilient to the effects of pressure than muscle (Kottner et al., 2009). Also, the type of force or combination of forces (i.e., pressure, shear, friction) exerted on the tissue is important. Pressure and shearing forces mainly affect deeper tissue layers, with friction affecting primarily superficial layers (Kottner et al., 2009). That said, pressure is believed to be a major causative factor in pressure ulcer formation. Several factors play a role, however, in determining whether pressure is sufficient to create an ulcer. The pathological effect of excessive pressure on soft tissue can be attributed to intensity of pressure, duration of pressure, and tissue tolerance (the ability of skin and its supporting structures to endure pressure without adverse sequelae).

Injury occurs to the skin and underlying tissues. Ischemia and hypoxia result as the pressure is applied to the area. Waste products accumulate as the ischemia continues, which produces toxins that cause further tissue breakdown.

Occurrence: Definitive information on the occurrence of pressure ulcers is limited. Studies to date have been encumbered by methodological issues such as variability in describing the lesions and in differentiating pressure ulcers from lesions of other etiologies (Salcido & Popescu, 2011). The incidence in hospitalized patients ranges from 2.7% to 29% and the prevalence in hospitalized patients ranges from 3.5% to 69%. Patients in critical care units have an increased risk of pressure ulcers, as evidenced by a 33% incidence and 41% prevalence. Elderly patients admitted to acute care hospitals for nonelective orthopedic procedures, such as hip replacement and treatment of long bone fractures, are at even greater risk, with a 66% incidence.

In the nursing home environment, the prevalence of pressure ulcers is in the range of 2.6% to 24%. The incidence has been as high as 25% in residents admitted from an acute care hospital. Patients with preexisting pressure ulcers demonstrate a 26% incidence of additional pressure ulcer formation over a 6-month period. The incidence in chronic care hospitals is reported to be 10.8%, whereas 33% of those admitted to a chronic care hospital have pressure ulcers. Long-term follow-up demonstrates that most ulcers healed within a year. Persons with spinal cord injury and associated comorbidity are also at increased risk. The incidence of pressure ulcers in this population is in the range of 25% to 66%.

Age: It is believed that comorbid conditions are associated with pressure ulcers, and age is considered a comorbid state. Prevalence of pressure ulcers in the elderly population is 11.6% to 27.5%, with the increased risk being assigned to those of advancing age. The incidence in skilled care and nursing home facilities is approximately 25%. Patients admitted to a hospital geriatric unit have similarly high prevalence rates: of patients under 70 years of age, only 6% have pressure ulcers; of patients over 70 years of age, the prevalence almost doubles to 11.6%.

Gender: Pressure ulcers occur equally in men and in women.

Ethnicity: Cited more recently in the literature and mentioned in the NPUAP 2007 Staging Document is that there may be some difficulty in detecting Stage I pressure ulcers in persons with darker skin pigmentation.

Contributing factors: The main contributing factors to pressure ulcer development are pressure, shear, friction, and malnutrition. Moisture (specifically incontinence) is cited as a related condition, because it alters the resiliency of the epidermis to external forces. An emerging concept is that of moisture-associated skin damage to assist the clinician in the differential diagnosis of pressure ulcers from those partial- or full-thickness tissue injuries that are not resultant from pressure (Gray et al., 2011).

Signs and symptoms: A detailed history of the ulcer should be obtained from the patient or caregiver, including chronic illness, hygiene, nutritional status, immobility, presence of prolonged moisture, ability to perform activities of daily living, psychological impact of ulcer, and sources of available support. Ask the patient if he or she has pain over bony prominences.

Clinical presentation can vary from nonblanching erythema to ecchymosis to frank necrosis. Nonblanching erythema results from damage to blood vessels and extravasation of blood into the tissue. Its presence suggests that tissue damage is imminent or has already occurred. The color of the skin can be an intense bright red to a dark purple; pressure-induced nonblanching erythema is often misdiagnosed as a hematoma or ecchymosis. When deep tissue damage is also present, the area is often either indurated or boggy when palpated. Note the ulcer size, depth, presence of exudate, epithelialization, granulation tissue, and findings such as necrotic tissue, sinus tracts, undermining, tunneling, and purulent drainage or other signs of infection.

Diagnostic tests: General laboratory tests for the patients with a pressure ulcer include wound culture and sensitivity. Particularly look for any of the following:

- Signs of local infection (erythema, edema, change in exudate to include purulent or foul-smelling drainage, pain, crepitus)

■ Signs of systemic infection (fever, leukocytosis); bone involvement (due to risk of osteomyelitis)

■ Presence of chronicity to determine if there is a causative organism

Evaluation of nutritional status should include total protein, albumin, and prealbumin; in patients with a pressure ulcer, often these clinical indicators are decreased because of inadequate nutritional stores present for tissue repair. A CBC may reveal increased red cell distribution, decreased lymphocyte count (malnutrition), and elevated leukocyte count (osteomyelitis). The erythrocyte sedimentation rate will be increased. X-rays of the appropriate area often reveal bony rarefaction (decreased density), periosteal elevation, and new bone formation.

Differential diagnosis:
■ Skin cancers
■ Fungal or yeast infections
■ Lower extremity wounds (venous, arterial, mixed etiology, and neuropathic etiology in origin)

Treatment: Effective pressure ulcer treatment with topical dressings requires consideration of numerous factors. Consider use of the following mnemonic (I DIP A MOP):

■ **I**nfection (eliminate, reduce bioburden)
■ **D**ébride necrotic tissue (consider: surgical/conservative, sharp, mechanical, enzymatic, biological, autolytic)
■ **I**nsulate the wound
■ **P**rotect periwound tissue
■ **A**bsorb excess exudate
■ **M**aintain a constant moisture level
■ **O**bliterate dead space
■ **P**revent further injury

Pharmacological management: Most moisture-retentive dressings are available without a prescription. Some antimicrobials (e.g., silver sulfadiazine) and some enzymatic débriding agents (e.g., collagenase) are prescriptive.

Follow-up: Practitioners need to objectively evaluate the patient's progress toward healing at least weekly using standardized methods of assessment (e.g., wound dimensions, amount of exudate, patient comfort, etc.). Immediate intervention is indicated if wound deterioration is observed sooner. If the wound deteriorates, is it in accordance with a decline in the patient's overall condition? It is important to communicate this decline as an expected result to patient, caregivers, and staff.

The patient's general health and nutritional intake, the stability of the comorbid conditions, the need for psychological support, and the patient's comfort level should be monitored. Signs and symptoms of complications need to be reported and recorded accurately.

Sequelae: Complications include, but are not limited to, cellulitis, bacteremia, osteomyelitis, and sepsis (secondary to pressure ulcers).

Prevention/prophylaxis: Conduct a valid and reliable risk assessment tool (e.g., Braden, Norton) at the first encounter and at regular intervals thereafter for patients at risk. Specific interventions are to be directed at the first encounter and at regular intervals following initial appraisal of skin and should be targeted toward improving subscale scores in any areas in which the patient's score falls below normal. Enlist the support of an interdisciplinary care team (e.g., nurse, physician, physical therapist, caregiver, dietitian, pharmacist) to ensure all goals of care are addressed adequately. Consider therapeutic support surfaces for bed and/or chair when decreased mobility is a risk factor.

Referral: Consider referral to a wound care specialist (wound, ostomy, and continence [WOC] nurse, plastic surgeon, infectious disease practitioner, dermatologist) if wounds fail to progress in spite of evidence-based interventions consistent with the overall plan of care.

Education: Practitioners should provide patients and their caregivers with information that highlights the applicable contributing factors to the development of pressure ulcer formation.

■ Review available and appropriate treatment modalities for each identified stage of wound progression as well as expected outcomes and anticipated time frames for healing.
■ Discuss reportable signs and symptoms of infection and complications.
■ Discuss advances in technology and dispel myths that may exist regarding wound care.
■ Identify informative Web-based resources, and explain that information available via electronic means and/or from well-meaning individuals may not be evidence based.
■ Discuss hand hygiene and disposal of soiled dressings.
■ Review the importance of positioning, sources of dietary protein, and the amount to be consumed during the wound repair process.

CLINICAL RECOMMENDATION	EVIDENCE RATING	REFERENCES
Identify persons at risk for pressure ulcer development by conducting a valid and reliable risk assessment tool (e.g., Braden, Norton) at the recommended intervals (often on admission, daily, weekly, or monthly—depending on care setting— and with any change in patient condition).	C	NPUAP & EPUAP (2009)
Screen and assess nutritional status for each individual with a pressure ulcer at admission and with each condition change and/or when progress toward pressure ulcer closure is not observed.	C	NPUAP & EPUAP (2009)
Assess all individuals for pain related to a pressure ulcer or its treatment.	B	NPUAP & EPUAP (2009)
Provide a support surface that is properly matched to the individual's needs for pressure redistribution, shear reduction, and microclimate control.	C	NPUAP & EPUAP (2009)
Relieve pressure under the heel(s) by placing legs on a pillow to "float the heels" off the bed or by using pressure redistribution devices with heel suspension.	B	NPUAP & EPUAP (2009)

A = consistent, good-quality, patient-oriented evidence; B = inconsistent or limited-quality, patient-oriented evidence; C = consensus, disease-oriented evidence, usual practice, expert opinion, or case series. For information about the SORT evidence rating system, go to www.aafp.org/afpsort.xml.

PSORIASIS

Signal symptoms: Erythematous patches, papules, and plaques with silvery scales that may be pruritic. Rare form with pustules.

Description: Psoriasis is a disease of abnormal keratin synthesis. Inflammation in the lesions results in hyperproliferation with a shortening of the cell cycle that results in 28 times the normal production of epidermal cells (Habif, 2010; Wolff, Johnson, & Fitzpatrick, 2009). This results in the development of papules with a fine scale that coalesce and form distinctive, well-demarcated, round to oval plaques with a silvery scale. If the scale is removed traumatically, the presence of bleeding points, Auspitz sign, is noted. When the lesion is present in intertriginous

areas, the moist environment macerates the scale, so the lesion appears as a smooth plaque. Less common forms of psoriasis include the guttate or acute eruptive psoriasis, which presents with small papules that are generalized over the trunk and extremities. Pustular in contrast to papular types include pustular psoriasis of the palms and soles or generalized pustular psoriasis (Zumbusch's psoriasis), which is an acute systemic illness that may be fatal. Ninety percent of those with psoriasis have involvement of either the fingernails or toenails (Habif, 2010; Menter et al., 2008; Wolff et al., 2009).

Psoriasis can affect the joints also, causing a seronegative spondyloarthropathy, psoriatic arthritis.

Other autoimmune diseases, such as inflammatory bowel disease, also may be present (Menter et al., 2008).

John Updike is credited with first describing the "heartbreak of psoriasis." The phrase was used in advertisement in the 1960s, but it is a genuine concern because psoriasis may have a more profound effect on the emotional health of patients than on the physical health. The prevalence of depression in patients with psoriasis may be as high as 60% (Menter et al., 2008; Wolff et al., 2009).

Etiology: Recent understanding of the pathogenesis includes the probability of psoriasis being an immune-mediated disorder. This is supported by the responsiveness of psoriasis to treatment with immunosuppressive drugs. Although there appears to be a genetic link to psoriasis, it is a polygenic trait with an 8% incidence when one parent has psoriasis, and it increases to a 41% rate if both parents have been affected. About one in three patients with psoriasis has a family history of the disease. In addition to the genetics, environmental factors are often the trigger: skin trauma (Koebner phenomenon), streptococcal or viral infection, and stress, medications, smoking, and alcohol consumption (Habif, 2010; Menter et al., 2008; Wolff et al., 2009).

Occurrence: Psoriasis affects about 2% of the population of the United States, or about 7.5 million Americans. About 10% of those also have psoriatic arthritis (National Psoriasis Foundation, 2012). Chronic stable plaque psoriasis is the most common type, affecting 80% to 90% of those with psoriasis. Guttate psoriasis most often occurs in younger adults and represents about 2% of patients with psoriasis (Menter et al., 2008).

Age: The peak incidence of psoriasis occurs at 22.5 years of age although it can occur even in childhood and may have a later onset at age 55 or over. Women tend to have earlier onset, and earlier onset is associated with more severity of the disease. Psoriatic arthritis occurs most often in those between the ages of 30 and 50 (National Psoriasis Foundation, 2012; Wolff et al., 2009).

Gender: There is an equal incidence of the disease in males and in females.

Ethnicity: Prevalence is highest among Scandinavians, with low incidence in West Africans, Japanese, and Inuits. There is a very low incidence among North and South American Indians. African Americans also have a low incidence of 1.3% compared with 2.5% of Caucasians.

Contributing factors: Classic links to the development of psoriasis include drugs, physical trauma (Koebner's phenomenon), infection, and stress. A streptococcal or viral infection often precedes the onset of guttate psoriasis by 2 weeks. Drugs that may precipitate or exacerbate psoriasis include lithium, beta blockers, antimalarial agents, and systemic steroids. Several lifestyle factors or behaviors have been associated with a higher rate of psoriasis. Smoking was reported by 37% of those with psoriasis, and 78% of those reported smoking before they were diagnosed. This compares to a rate of smoking of only 13% in the general population. Psoriasis is more prevalent in those who abuse alcohol and may increase the severity of the disease. Multiple studies have noted a relationship between obesity and the development of psoriasis (Menter et al., 2008).

Signs and symptoms: Patients may present with a papular rash that is getting worse, with shiny scales on the lesions. They may complain of pruritus. In guttate psoriasis, the lesions are distinct small papules with thin scales over the trunk and extremities. Chronic plaque psoriasis may involve a few plaques or may have many plaques scattered over the entire body. If the patient presents with a sudden onset of lesions, it is important to elicit a history of possible upper respiratory infection 2 to 3 weeks before the onset of the lesions.

Physical examination will reveal well-demarcated erythematous lesions with silvery scales. The scales may be thin or very thick. They are not easily removed, and if forcefully removed there may be points of bleeding, the Auspitz sign. The lesions of plaque psoriasis are generally symmetrical in distribution and may be located on the scalp, trunk, and buttocks, often affecting the extensor surface of the extremities. When the lesions form in the skinfolds, the moisture affects the development of scale, and the surface may be shiny. This inverse pattern psoriasis may be difficult to distinguish from *Candida* or tinea. The distinct demarcated border is helpful in differentiation. Nails also may be affected with the presence of pitting, onycholysis, subungual hyperkeratosis, red-brown coloring (oil drop sign), and nail plate dystrophy.

Diagnostic tests: The distinct presentation of the lesions of psoriasis makes a clinical diagnosis possible. When fungal infections are a possibility, KOH tests are the gold standard for that diagnosis. Biopsies to confirm the diagnosis of psoriasis are rare, but when they are necessary, it is essential to take the sample from an intact lesion that has not been scratched and is not bleeding. If biopsy is required, a referral to a dermatologist will ensure accurate testing.

Laboratory testing, including blood chemistry profile, liver function tests, serum uric acid, a CBC with differential, antinuclear antibody titer, or rheumatoid factor, is directed at the inflammatory process and to rule out the possibility of infection. If the patient is presenting with guttate-type psoriasis, a throat culture to screen for streptococcus should be considered.

Differential diagnosis:

Plaque psoriasis:
- Seborrheic dermatitis
- Nummular eczema
- Tinea corporis
- Lichen planus
- Pityriasis rubra pilaris
- Mycosis fungoides
- Atopic dermatitis

Guttate psoriasis:
- Secondary syphilis
- Pityriasis rosea
- Maculopapular drug eruption

Inverse psoriasis:
- Candidiasis
- Tinea

Psoriatic nails:
- Tinea unguium
- Onychomycosis caused by yeast or molds

Treatment: The staging of psoriasis helps to determine the choice of treatment. The National Psoriasis Foundation (2012) defines severity as follows:

- Mild, affecting 3% of the body
- Moderate, affecting 3% to 10% of the body
- Severe, affecting more than 10% of the body

The hand is representative of about 1% of the body. The emotional impact of psoriasis is also considered in determining the severity and may increase the ranking even with less severe involvement. Eighty percent of patients have mild-to-moderate disease.

In addition to severity, the age of the patient and the type of psoriasis needs to be considered. To ensure the appropriate choice of treatment, referral to a dermatologist should be initiated. Dermatologists are the experts who treat and manage the multiple nuances of this disease. However, primary care providers need to be knowledgeable regarding the treatment options, because the treatments have implications for ongoing primary follow-up.

Topical treatments: The first line of treatment and recommended for mild-to-moderate psoriasis. For most patients in that category, the topical treatments are safe and effective. The treatments are also used as adjunctive therapy for patients with more extensive disease who are receiving phototherapy or systemic therapy. When making a choice of topical treatments, the patient's goals are important to consider. The vehicle for the medication should be chosen to match those goals and the severity of the disease. Problems with topical treatments include the time needed for application, the need for prolonged treatment, and incomplete clearance of lesions. All of these factors influence the patient's likelihood of adherence to therapy. Patients may be on concurrent topical therapy with the use of more than one topical agent. Agents include corticosteroids, vitamin D analogues, retinoids, calcineurin inhibitors, salicylic acid, anthralin, coal tar, and nonmedicated topical moisturizers (Table 6-5) (Menter et al., 2009).

TABLE 6-5 Topical Treatment for Psoriasis		
TOPICAL TREATMENT	**MECHANISM OF ACTION**	**SIDE EFFECTS/PRECAUTIONS**
Corticosteroids	Anti-inflammatory, antiproliferative, immunosuppressive, vasoconstrictive	Skin atrophy, telangiectasia, striae distensai, acne, folliculitis, and purpura
		May exacerbate some superficial skin conditions: rosacea, tinea
		Rebound of psoriasis
		With high potency, possible systemic side effects
Vitamin D analogues	Binds to vitamin D receptors	Burning, pruritus, edema, peeling, dryness, erythema may improve with continued treatment
Calcipotriene topical	Inhibition of keratinocyte proliferation and enhancement of differentiation	Rarely systemic effects of hypercalcemia and parathyroid suppression
		Apply after UVA therapy

Continued

TABLE 6-5 Topical Treatment for Psoriasis—cont'd		
TOPICAL TREATMENT	**MECHANISM OF ACTION**	**SIDE EFFECTS/PRECAUTIONS**
Retinoids Tazarotene topical	Normalizes abnormal keratinocyte differentiation, diminishes hyperproliferation Decreases inflammation	Local irritation, may be reduced with lower concentrations; combine with moisturizers or topical steroids
Calcineurin inhibitors Pimecrolimus topical	Block the synthesis of inflammatory cytokines	Burning and itching reduced with continued therapy Cautious use with light therapy Not FDA approved for psoriasis
Salicylic acid	Keratolytic; reduce keratinocyte-to-keratinocyte binding Reduce pH stratum corneum	Risk of systemic toxicity; do not use with oral salicylates Use after UVA therapy
Anthralin	Prevent T lymph activation Normalize keratinocyte differentiation	Skin irritation and staining

Phototherapy: Requires treatment by a dermatologist. Narrow-band ultraviolet B (UVB) is often used in combination with topical therapies and offers the possibility of home therapy. A more aggressive treatment is chemophototherapy with psolarens (an oral medication) and long-wavelength UV light (PUVA). The treatment inhibits mitosis by stopping DNA replication. It increases the risk of squamous cell carcinoma and possibly melanoma. It also induces photoaging. Although it has more risk than UVB, it is more effective (Menter et al., 2008).

Systemic therapy: Reserved for those patients with severe disease and requires management by a dermatologist with expertise in treatment of psoriasis. Methotrexate is very effective but has the potential for hepatotoxicity and should be avoided in renal impairment (this will eliminate many older adults). Drug interactions are common. Biologicals include T-cell and tumor necrosis factor (TNF) inhibitors. Baseline laboratory data are essential and need to be repeated frequently to monitor for toxicities. Live vaccines must be avoided in patients being treated with biologicals. All of the TNF inhibitors carry the increased risk of infection, especially upper respiratory infection. Coordinating the care of older adults on systemic therapy with the dermatologist is essential to adequate management (Menter et al., 2008).

Follow-up: Follow-up should be on a case-by-case basis. A key to follow-up is coordination with the dermatologist, who, in other than the mildest cases,

should be managing the disease process. It is important to consider the "heartbreak of psoriasis." The incidence of depression and suicidal ideation is higher in psoriasis and may not be directly related to the severity of the disease. All patients should be screened for depression. Patients with psoriasis have a higher incidence of arthritis, heart disease, diabetes, cancer, and hypertension, and all of these are increased in older adults as well (Habif, 2010).

Sequelae: Psoriasis is a chronic disease with exacerbations and remissions. In a small percentage of those with psoriasis, more serious types, such as psoriatic erythroderma or generalized acute pustular psoriasis, may occur. These diseases have much higher morbidity and may even result in death. Five percent of those with psoriasis will develop psoriatic arthritis.

Prevention/prophylaxis: Triggers should be avoided: smoking, excess alcohol use, and skin trauma. Keeping the skin dry but well hydrated may decrease pruritus and the urge to scratch. Drugs known to exacerbate psoriasis should be avoided. Stress management, adequate rest, and a well-balanced diet to achieve ideal body weight are all important.

Referral: Except in the mildest cases of psoriasis, the patient should be comanaged with a dermatologist.

Education: In addition to ways to avoid triggers that can cause exacerbations, patients need to understand the treatment options and partner with providers to make choices that increase adherence. Teaching needs to include information regarding medication side effects and special considerations such as the importance of not getting live vaccines if currently being treated with biologicals. In the current healthcare environment, retail clinics and pharmacies are offering vaccines, so patients need to be especially conscious of the recommendations related to their treatments and the guidelines regarding vaccines. The emotional toll of this disease needs to be acknowledged, offering patients connection to support groups. Patients also need to be informed of reputable Internet sources on psoriasis.

CLINICAL RECOMMENDATION	EVIDENCE RATING	REFERENCES
Psoriasis is associated with depression and suicidal ideation. In one study of 217 patients with psoriasis, almost 10% indicated a wish to be dead, with 7.2% of patients with severe psoriasis indicating active suicidal ideation. This compares to a rate of 2.4%–3.3% in the general medical patient population. The recommendation to screen patients with psoriasis for depression and suicidal ideation is supported.	A	Gupta & Gupta (1998)
Early studies of topical calcineurin inhibitors, tacrolimus and pimecrolimus, did not show efficacy, but when used under occlusion, they were efficacious. The conclusion that they lacked the ability to penetrate thick plaque was supported by their successful use in the treatment of thin lesions on the face and in intertriginous areas. Although not FDA approved for treatment of psoriasis, two double-blind studies strongly support their effectiveness in treating psoriasis on the face or intertriginous areas, without the skin atrophy common with chronic steroid treatment.	A	Gribetz et al. (2004) Lebwohl et al. (2004)
Vitamin D analogue calcitriol, used in topical treatment of plaque psoriasis, was found to have slower onset of action but a longer disease-free period than betamethasone diproprionate. The risks of toxicity are minimal compared to topical steroids.	A	Camarasa, Ortonne, & Dubertret (2003)
Tumor necrosis factor (TNF) inhibitors are an effective treatment for severe psoriasis and psoriatic arthritis. Side effects may discourage their use. However, for treatment of psoriasis, TNF inhibitors are only approved as monotherapy while they are often combined with methotrexate in the treatment of rheumatoid arthritis and inflammatory bowel disease. The risks associated with the combination therapy may overestimate the risk when using TNF inhibitors alone.	C	Menter et al. (2008)

A = consistent, good-quality, patient-oriented evidence; B = inconsistent or limited-quality, patient-oriented evidence; C = consensus, disease-oriented evidence, usual practice, expert opinion, or case series. For information about the SORT evidence rating system, go to www.aafp.org/afpsort.xml.

SKIN CANCER

Signal symptoms: Telangiectasia, abnormal symmetry of lesion, crusting, and bleeding.

Description: Neoplasms of the skin are the most common type of cancers in humans. Three main types of skin cancer are basal cell carcinoma (BCC), which arises from the basal keratinocyte layer of the epidermis; squamous cell carcinoma (SCC), which originates in the squamous cells of the epithelium; and malignant melanoma (MM), which is a tumor arising in a pigmented area. Melanoma causes abnormal proliferation of specialized cells that produce melanin in the skin, eyes, and hair.

Etiology: The major risk factor for the development of skin cancers is exposure to ultraviolet radiation (UVR). Patients who have or had an occupation requiring them to spend extensive time outdoors are susceptible to the development of skin cancer. There is a high recurrence rate for BCC.

Occurrence: Each year, more than 1 million new cases of skin cancer are diagnosed in the United States. Annual diagnosis of skin cancer exceeds the incidence of breast, prostate, lung, and colon cancer combined (Heckman, Egleston, Wilson, & Ingersoll, 2008). BCC, the most common type of skin cancer, accounts for 65% to 80% of these cases. SCC constitutes 10% to 25% of all skin cancers. BCC and SCC are referred to as *nonmelanoma skin cancer* (NMSC). MM accounts for the remainder of skin cancers (Centers for Disease Control and Prevention, 2009). Seventy-five percent of skin cancer deaths, however, can be attributed to MM (Lin, Eder, & Weinmann, 2011). Melanoma, though deadly in the later stages of development, has an excellent prognosis if treated early (Rubin, 2010b).

Age: The incidence of all types of skin cancers increases with age, owing to sun exposure over an extended period.

Gender: Currently, more men than women develop BCC, but the number of women with BCC is increasing (Kiiski et al., 2010). SCC presents 3 times more frequently in men than in women (Nolen, Beebe, King, Bryn, & Limaye, 2011). MM is equally prevalent in men and in women. It poses significant mortality risk for both men and women (Jensen & Moriarty, 2008).

Ethnicity: All skin cancers are more prevalent in fair-skinned persons, blue-eyed persons (especially people with blonde, red, or light brown hair) and people of Celtic ancestry. In the United States, residents of states where year-round sunshine is abundant are at a high risk, especially those people who spend an extended time period outside. The highest incidence of BCC in the world occurs in Australia (Kiiski et al., 2010; Nolen et al., 2011). SCC is more common than BCC in African Americans.

Contributing factors: Certain patient phenotype characteristics are associated with risk for developing skin cancer: albinism, hair and eye color, tendency to burn, and skin freckling (Lin et al., 2011). Male sex and European descent are risk factors for developing BCC (Kiiski et al., 2010). Besides sun exposure as a contributing factor, skin cancer may occur as a result of tanning bed use, late sequelae to burns, scars, chronic ulcers, or radiodermatitis. Patients who report severe sunburns in childhood are at risk for developing skin cancer. Patients who have had ionizing radiation, whether as a treatment for a condition such as acne or accidental exposure, are at risk for developing BCC and SCC. Inorganic arsenic, pitch, tar, and radium exposure also have been linked to the development of skin cancer. Patients who have had a renal transplant and immunosuppression are also at risk for developing skin cancer and cancer of the lips (Nolan et al., 2011). Presence of multiple and atypical nevi is a known contributing factor (Rubin, 2010b). Human papillomavirus and xeroderma pigmentosum may play a role in the development of SCC. Certain genetic predispositions can contribute to the development of skin cancer, and there is a familial tendency to develop melanoma. For patients diagnosed with familial atypical mole and melanoma syndrome or dysplastic nevus syndrome, the lifetime risk of developing melanoma reaches close to 100% (Rubin, 2009).

Signs and symptoms: Patients need to be questioned about concerns of any new or changing lesions. Is the lesion painful? Does it itch or bleed? Has it healed and then reappeared? Ask about past history of any diagnosed skin cancers or any of the precursor lesions (described in greater detail below) or previously excised or treated lesions. Question patients about any family history of skin cancers. Patients need to be questioned regarding their history of sun exposure, severe sunburn, burns, scars, ulcers, radiation dermatitis, frequent use of tanning beds, prior occupation, and family history of skin cancer. The presentation of the skin cancer depends on the type of tumor.

There are three specific types of basal cell carcinoma: nodular, morpheaform, and superficial. Nodular BCC generally presents first as a dome-shaped, white-to-pink papule or nodule having a raised pearly border with prominent telangiectasia. BCC tumors can also have a brown to glossy black appearance (Gloster & Neal, 2006). Patients may describe this lesion as a pimple that did not heal. As the nodule enlarges, scaling, crusting, or central ulceration may become noticeable. It is important to note that the ulcerated areas can heal over with new scar tissue; however, the tumor grows deeper and the cycle of ulceration and healing begins again (Habif, 2004). Superficial BCC often appears on the trunk and extremities. Characteristic of the superficial BCC is the presence of a well-circumscribed translucent or bright pink to red patch of skin surrounded often by telangiectasia. This type of BCC resembles other chronic skin conditions such as psoriasis, eczema, discoid lupus erythematous, and Bowen's disease. The least common type of BCC is the sclerosing or morpheaform tumor. Found on the head and neck and occasionally the trunk of the body, the lesion appears to be a hypopigmented tumor that eventually is surrounded by irregular telangiectasia with atrophic scarlike appearance (Nolen et al., 2011).

Squamous cell carcinoma often originates at the site of chronic inflammation or old scars. Actinic keratoses, which appear as round or irregular-shaped erythematosus or tan plaques with a scaly or rough surface, are a precursor to SCC. Other precursor lesions of SCC include cutaneous horn, leukoplakia, and keratoacanthoma (although it has been suggested that these lesions are malignant given the rapid growth rate of a new lesion) (Nolan et al., 2011). Signs of malignancy of SCC include elevation, ulceration, or inflammation of the lesion; the original lesion also may have enlarged in size. In later stages of SCC, the surface may appear crusted, and a horn of keratin forms. SCC appears on sun-exposed as well as on non–sun-exposed areas of the body. These tumors may be tender to touch owing to their rapid growth and inflammatory process. Examine the scalp, ears, lower lip, and dorsa of the hands for SCC.

For patients with suspected melanoma, the mnemonic ABCDE guides the clinician in determining if the clinical characteristics of a suspicious lesion warrant close surveillance and/or biopsy for histological evaluation:

- Asymmetry
- Border irregularity
- Color variation
- Diameter >6 mm
- Elevation of a previously flat lesion, evolving and enlarging (Halpern, Marghoob, & Sober, 2009; Rubin, 2010b).

It is important to note, however, than only one-third of melanoma cases follow the classic ABCDE pattern of development, and many forms of melanoma mimic benign lesions (Rubin, 2009).

Major signs: Change in size, change in shape, change in color. If one or more major signs exist, refer for expeditious biopsy.

Minor signs: Inflammation, crusting or bleeding, sensory change, diameter of ≥7 mm. If three or four minor signs exist with a major sign, consider referral.

Patients may be concerned about a new, pigmented lesion or a change in an already existing one. Patients may report associated itching, burning, or pain in a mole. Superficial spreading melanoma is a flat to slightly raised pigmented lesion with irregular borders, commonly found on the backs of men and the lower legs of women. Lentigo maligna melanoma, an irregularly pigmented macula with notched borders, occurs on sun-exposed areas, especially on the faces of older adults. Nodular melanoma, brown or black papules usually located on the trunk, head, and neck, is characterized by rapid growth. Acral lentiginous melanomas, a rare melanoma subtype, is found proportionally higher in people of color. Acral lentiginous melanoma occurs on the palms, soles, fingers, and toes; a pigmented streak of the cuticle is diagnostic (Hutchinson's sign) (Bradford, Goldstein, McMaster, & Tucker, 2009; Bristow, de Berker, Acland, Turner, & Bowling, 2010). Clinical evaluation for skin cancer also includes a total body skin examination and palpation of regional lymph nodes, liver, and spleen (Rubin, 2010a).

Diagnostic tests: Skin cancer is diagnosed through biopsy. Biopsy of the suspected lesion is necessary to confirm the diagnosis via histological examination of the tissue; an adequate tissue sample should be excised, and an elliptical excision generally is necessary for larger lesions. Excisional biopsy is recommended for any pigmented lesion (Nolen et al., 2011).

Differential diagnosis:
- Actinic keratoses
- Seborrheic keratoses
- Keratoacanthoma
- Atypical nevi
- Blue nevus
- Dermatofibroma
- Venous lakes
- Pyogenic granulomas
- Intradermal nevus
- Sebaceous hyperplasia
- Molluscum contagiosum

- Psoriasis
- Eczema
- Discoid lupus erythematous
- Bowen's disease (Nolen et al., 2011).

Treatment: Several factors need to be considered before skin cancer therapy begins: the patient's age and general health, whether or not the patient is immunocompromised, size and location of the tumor, the pathology of the tumor, and the cosmetic concerns of the patient. BCC may be treated by excisional surgery, electrodessication and curettage, cryotherapy, ionizing radiation, and Mohs' micrographic surgery (MMS). A chemotherapeutic agent such as 5-fluorouracil, interferon, and retinoids are topical agents for superficial or small BCCs and early diagnosed SCC. SCC may be treated in the same manner as BCC; however, because of its more truculent growth pattern, wider excision and MMS are the preferred methods of treatment. Recurrent BCC and SCC should be treated with surgical excision (Nolan et al., 2011).

Treatment of MM is surgical. An excisional margin surrounding the tumor is made, depending on the thickness of the tumor. Chemotherapy and radiation are used for palliative measures in the treatment of metastatic disease.

A number of different treatment options are available for the management of actinic keratosis (AK), including field-directed treatments such as the retinoid difluormethylornithine (DFMO), a topical agent that inhibits polyamine synthesis. Some studies show that it reduces actinic keratosis numbers (Heckman et al., 2008). The use of 5-fluorouracil has been shown to reduce lesion count in patients with AK (Askew, Mickan, Soyer, & Wilkinson, 2009).

Topical imiquimod is an immune response modifier that is approved for AK and BCC (Watkins, 2010). Imiquimod 3.75% recently received Food and Drug Administration (FDA) approval for AK treatment of the entire face and balding scalp. It is prescribed in a pulse-type treatment regimen. Cryotherapy, which is a lesion-directed therapy, is a commonly used treatment for AK. It is relatively easy to use and is effective. Liquid nitrogen or compressed nitrous oxide that is applied to lesions destroys atypical cells and normal cells through irreversible intracellular ice formation. Other treatments can include electrodessication and curettage or photodynamic therapy. Combination therapies include both field-directed and lesion-directed therapy (Huang & Clark, 2011).

Follow-up: Follow-up for a patient with diagnosed skin carcinoma is essential, because the recurrence rate of skin cancer is high; 50% of persons with BCC and SCC have a reappearance of a cancerous lesion within 5 years. A person who is susceptible to skin cancer may develop another cancerous lesion at any time. Precancerous lesions should be examined regularly every 3 to 12 months using a head-to-toe skin examination, including a careful inspection of the previous site of a lesion. In patients with SCC, palpation of regional lymph nodes is suggested. During subsequent visits of patients with malignant melanoma, a thorough review of systems is imperative to elicit clinical signs and symptoms of metastasis.

Sequelae: BCC rarely metastasizes; however, if it is not treated early, the carcinoma may invade the surrounding tissue and bone. Advanced SCC lesions of the lips, pinna, and genitalia often metastasize. Recurrent NMSC has a higher rate of recurrence and eventually may lead to the development of metastatic disease (Kiiski et al., 2010; Nolan et al., 2011). The larger the NMSC in size, the higher the rate of recurrence. The anatomical location of the NMSC also influences the recurrence rate; lesions on the face, ears, vertex, and scalp are known as high-risk cancer areas. Five-year prognosis for MM is determined by the Breslow thickness of the tumor. Tumors <0.76 mm are associated with a 98% 5-year survival rate; tumors 0.76 to 1.49 mm, with an 87% to 94% 5-year survival rate; and tumors 1.50 to 3.99 mm, with a 66% to 83% 5-year survival rate. Patients with tumors >4.0 mm have a <50% 5-year survival (Rubin, 2010b).

Prevention/prophylaxis: Because the incidences of all skin cancers increase with age, it is important to discuss sun care protective behaviors with all older adults (Lin et al., 2011). The CDC recommends easy options for sun protection. Because UVR exposure increases the risk for skin cancer with all skin types, individuals need to seek shade when UVR is strongest, during the hours of 10:00 a.m. to 4:00 p.m., and avoid burning. According to the Skin Cancer Foundation, sunscreen should be a sun protective factor (SPF) of at least 30 or higher, broad spectrum, and water resistant for extended outdoor activity. Tanning itself and tanning beds or booths should be avoided (CDC, 2009). Areas of the body for sunscreen application include head, neck and ears, exposed areas of the front of torso, back of torso, each arm, dorsum of hand and shoulder, each upper and lower leg, and each foot. One teaspoon of sunscreen should be applied separately to the upper leg and one teaspoon applied to the lower leg. It is necessary to reapply sunscreen after toweling off from swimming or exercise and after heavy sweating. Wide-brim hats that shade the face, head, ears, and neck, long-sleeved shirts, and long pants are recommended. Sunglasses that are wrap-around type should be worn and can be purchased to block up to 100% of UVR (CDC, 2009). Patients need to be routinely asked about their ability to conduct skin self-examinations. Recommending partner participation can enhance one's thoroughness in examining hard-to-reach areas of the body (Robinson, Turrisi, & Stapleton, 2007). Providing individuals with printed directions on how to position mirrors to examine the body, the use of good lighting, and suggesting magnifying lenses for those with impaired eyesight can help ensure a thorough examination has been carried out by the patient. Taking the time to given patients adequate instructions in skin self-examination has been found to be a successful strategy in ensuring older adults routinely conduct or seek assistance in regular skin examinations and the use of sunscreen (Glanz, Schoenfeld, & Steffen, 2010; Janda et al., 2011). High-risk patients can be provided body maps to record areas of suspicious lesions to bring with them at the time of clinical examinations. These patients should be questioned if they are regularly being followed by a dermatology practice. If not, primary care providers are well positioned to begin triaging (to include referring patients to a dermatologist) patients who present with suspicious skin lesions (Goulart et al., 2011).

The yearly physical examination should include assessment of the head, scalp, and skin and an accurate recording of descriptions of any suspicious lesions. Patients should be fully undressed, including undergarments, to complete an accurate physical (Rubin, 2010b). If a patient has a new, unusual, or changed lesion or mole, evaluation with dermoscopy makes characterization more efficient than with the naked eye alone. A tutorial that discusses dermoscopy principles and effective use of the dermatoscope can be found at www.genomel.org/dermoscopy/toolkit.html (Genomel Production, 2009). A dermatologist should evaluate all precancerous lesions. Lesions that have variegated colors, irregular elevations, or irregular borders should be examined by biopsy. Immunosuppressed organ recipients are at high risk for developing skin cancer at rates faster than the general patient population; they should be scheduled for regular skin examinations.

Referral: When a suspicious lesion is found, referral to a dermatologist for evaluation and possibly biopsy is necessary. Whole-body photographs and epiluminescence microscopy may be used to follow patients with suspicious lesions. Oncology referral is needed for metastatic SCC and MM.

Education: Advise older patients that skin cancers are a common occurrence as one ages, especially for patients at risk. Older adults should perform a monthly self-evaluation of the skin; suggest the use of mirrors to examine lesions on the back. Any suspicious open lesion that does not heal in a reasonable time needs to be examined by a primary care provider. Patients also need to report any slow-growing, flesh-colored or pigmented lesion, noting if the lesion has irregular borders, changes in color, ulceration, bleeding, or horn formation. Sun exposure, especially during the hours of 10:00 a.m. to 4:00 p.m., should be avoided. Year-round broad-spectrum sunscreen that blocks ultraviolet A and ultraviolet B light is recommended. Vulnerable areas, such as the head and neck, should be covered with protective clothing. Showing patients actual pictures of early melanoma coupled with teaching them the mnemonic ABCDE has been shown to help patients to identify suspicious cancerous lesions (Girardi et al., 2006).

CLINICAL RECOMMENDATION	EVIDENCE RATING	REFERENCES
The use of photographs of early melanomas for teaching patients to recognize abnormal lesions was far superior than using just the ABCDE method of recognition alone.	B	Girardi et al. (2006)
Even patients with a confirmed melanoma do not regularly practice total skin self-examination. Patients need to involve a partner in the routine screening.	B	Loescher, Harris, Lim, & Su (2006)

Continued

CLINICAL RECOMMENDATION	EVIDENCE RATING	REFERENCES
Participation in an educational intervention did improve self-care practices, including increased use of sun-screen and sunglasses.	B	Glanz et al. (2010)
Application of 5-fluorouracil treatment for actinic keratosis has been shown to effectively reduce AK lesions over the duration of treatment.	B	Askew et al. (2009)

A = consistent, good-quality, patient-oriented evidence; B = inconsistent or limited-quality, patient-oriented evidence; C = consensus, disease-oriented evidence, usual practice, expert opinion, or case series. For information about the SORT evidence rating system, go to www.aafp.org/afpsort.xml.

SUPERFICIAL FUNGAL INFECTIONS

Signal symptoms:

Dermatophyte infection (tinea): Erythema, scale, raised border, clearing center, may present with vesicles if inflammatory.

Candidiais (moniliasis): Pustules, red, denuded, glistening surface with a scaling border and satellite pustules. In the oral cavity and vagina, the scale and inflammatory cells form the classic "cottage cheese curds."

Tinea versicolor (pityriasis versicolor): Hypopigmented macules and patches or scaly red or shades of brown macules or patches may be slightly pruritic.

Description: Superficial fungal infections include the dermatophytes, candidiasis, and tinea (pityriasis) versicolor. Dermatophyte infections are referred to clinically as tinea followed by the region of the body that is infected: tinea capitis (the head), tinea barbae (the beard area), tinea facea (the face except for the beard area), tinea manuum (the hand), tinea corporis (the body), tinea cruris (the groin), tinea pedis (the foot), and when there is nail involvement, tinea unguium or onychomycosis. Lay terms for the dermatophytes include ringworm, jock itch, and athlete's foot.

Candidiasis may be termed monilia, yeast, or thrush and generally presents in intertriginous areas or on mucous membranes.

Tinea (pityriasis) versicolor is a chronic scaling change in color that affects the areas of the body with increased sebaceous activity. It is not caused by a dermatophyte and therefore is not a true tinea.

Etiology:

Dermatophytes: The dermatophytes are a group of fungi that infect the dead keratin of the stratum corneum, the hair, and nails. They are responsible for most of the fungal infections of the skin, hair, and nails. In one study almost 78% of superficial fungal infections were attributed to dermatophytes (Das, Goyal, & Bhattacharya, 2007). Patients who are chronically infected may have a genetic predisposition to dermatophyte infection. One way to classify dermatophytes is by the origin of the infection: anthropophilic, transmission from person to person by fomites or direct contact; zoophilic, transmission from animal to person by fomites or direct contact; or geophilic, from the soil. The latter two sources result in a more rapid and more severe inflammatory response. Another classification is based on the tissue primarily involved: epidermomycosis when the epidermis is infected, trichomycosis when it involves the hair or hair shaft, and onychomycosis when the nail is affected. The dermatophytes within the stratum corneum disrupt the horny layer, lead to scaling, and create an inflammatory response. Three fungal species are primarily responsible for the infection: *Trichophyton, Epidermophyton,* and *Microsporum. T. rubrum* is the most common cause of skin and nail infection (Havlickova, Czaika, & Friedrich, 2008; Wolff, Johnson, & Fitzpatrick, 2009).

Cutaneous candidiasis: Candida albicans is an oval, yeastlike fungus that lives in the normal flora of the mouth and gastrointestinal tract. It reproduces through budding, the development of pseudohyphae and true hyphae. Conditions that compromise the immune system or alter the normal body flora contribute to the development of candida infections. The yeast infects the outer layer of the skin with the primary lesion a pustule that dissects under the outer skin layer and peels it away. The result is a glistening surface with a scaling advancing border and often the presence of satellite lesions. Candida grows best in warm, moist environments, and often the lesions end as they meet the area of dry skin.

Tinea (pityriasis) versicolor: Tinea or pityriasis versicolor is caused by organisms in the *Malassezias* species formerly known as *Pityrosporum,* is not a dermatophyte, and is not a true tinea (Panackal, Halpern, & Watson, 2009; Wolff et al., 2009). The organisms are lipophilic yeasts that reside in the keratin and hair follicles, areas with increased sebaceous activity (Habif, 2010; Wolff et al., 2009). It is not known to be contagious but is an overgrowth of a normal flora.

Occurrence: Immunosuppressed patients are at higher risk for fungal infections of all kinds and are more likely to have infections that do not resolve. Older adults are at higher risk for many fungal infections because of the decline in the immune system with aging as well as the increased incidence in comorbidities and the use of multiple medications. Functional compromise can lead to a decline in personal hygiene, which also increases the risk factors for fungal infection.

The feet and nails are the most common areas of the body affected by dermatophytes in the older adult. Tinea unguium (onychomycosis) increases in incidence with advancing age. When the dermatophytes are inaccurately diagnosed and treated with topical steroids, a phenomenon called tinea incognito may occur. The rash initially disappears, but when treatment with steroids is discontinued, the rash returns with much more extensive involvement and may appear without scale. It is not responsive to subsequent topical steroid treatment, and a thorough history is necessary to make the proper diagnosis of tinea.

Candida rarely causes infection in fingernails or toenails; the incidence has been noted to be 29.2% and 1.7%, respectively. In one study, initial cultures identified candida as the infectious agent, but repeat cultures in one-quarter of the cases found that the infection was due to dermatophytes (Loo, 2007). However, intertriginous *Candida* is most common in the very young and in those over 65 years old.

The prevalence of tinea (pityriasis) versicolor in the U.S. population is estimated to be between 2% and 8% (Panackal et al., 2009). Many of those afflicted with the disease do not seek treatment, so the exact incidence is unknown. Tinea (pityriasis) versicolor is less common in those over 65 years old.

Age: Tinea of the scalp and face (tinea capitis and tinea facialis) are primarily diseases of children. Tinea of the body, trunk, and extremities (tinea corporis) can occur at any age. The initial presentation of athlete's foot (tinea pedis) is most common in adults aged 20 to 50, and the initial presentation of tinea unguium (onychomycosis) commonly occurs in those aged 45 to 54. Adults older than 45 accounted for 71.6% of all ambulatory visits for tinea unguium made from 1995 to 2004 (Panackal et al., 2009). Tinea unguium can affect any age, but the incidence increases with aging and is most common in the oldest old. Approximately 50% of those over 70 years old are affected (Wolff et al., 2009).

Candida of the skin and nails occurs more often in older adults because of the decline in immune response with aging as well as a decline in hygiene among many older adults (Hedderwick & Kauffman, 1997).

Tinea (pityriasis) versicolor is more common when sebaceous glands are most active during puberty and in young adults ages 15 to 24. It is rare in older adults (Wolff et al., 2009).

Gender: Tinea barbae is an infection that only occurs in males and is more common in rural areas. Males also more often experience tinea cruris and tinea pedis and are more likely to have nails infected with dermatophytes than females; in one study the ratio of males to females was almost 2:1 (Das et al., 2007; Panackal et al., 2009). Gender differences have not been found in cases of *Candida* or tinea (pityriasis) versicolor.

Ethnicity: Although blacks are less likely than other races to be diagnosed with dermatophytosis, black children are at highest risk for tinea capitis. This is attributed to genetic and cultural factors as well as socioeconomic status (Panackal et al., 2009). Ethnic differences have not been seen with either *Candida* or tinea (pityriasis) versicolor.

Contributing factors: Fungal infections are more common in warmer climates. Excessive sweating increases risk. Any of the diseases that compromise the immune system, atopy, and topical and systemic steroids increase risk. Age also increases the risk, particularly of onychomycosis. Tinea manuum is rare in individuals who do not also have tinea pedis. A common presentation is two feet–one hand syndrome, which is believed to be a result of the patient touching or scratching the infected feet. Tinea pedis occurs more frequently in those who wear occlusive footwear that promotes warmth and sweating, the perfect environment for fungal growth. Socioeconomic status also appears to contribute to the incidence of dermatophyte infections; in a study of worldwide trends, tinea pedis was more prevalent in developed countries, whereas tinea capitis was more prevalent in poorer countries (Havlickova et al., 2008).

Cutaneous candidiasis is more common in adults with diseases that compromise the immune system, medications that cause immune decline, adults treated with broad-spectrum antibiotics, and poor hygiene that results in moist areas in intertriginous areas (Habif, 2010; Hedderwick & Kauffman, 1997; Loo, 2007). Other contributing factors include hot humid weather, tight underwear, poor hygiene, and inflammatory diseases occurring in skinfolds.

Like other fungal infections, tinea (pityriasis) versicolor is more common in an environment of heat and humidity. It grows best where sebaceous activity is highest and may be more common in those with oily skin. Immune-compromised individuals and those on steroids are also more susceptible (Habif, 2010; Wolff et al., 2009).

Signs and symptoms: Dry scaling is a hallmark of each of the superficial fungal infections.

Tinea capitis presents as hair loss (alopecia). Grey patch tinea capitis often is circular in shape with the presence of many broken-off hairs and the scalp assumes a dull grey color due to the arthrospores that are formed by the fungi. Black dot tinea capitis occurs when hairs break off near the surface and give the appearance of dots. The dots may be scattered over the scalp and not form a classic round patch. A kerion is an inflammatory mass on the scalp that is painful and may include pustules and result in cervical or occipital adenopathy.

Tinea of the face and body presents as the classic ringworm pattern with a clearing center and a raised, scaling leading edge. Tinea cruris presents as an erythematous pruritic rash that begins in the groin and spreads onto the thighs. It is usually unilateral and rarely involves the scrotum. The lack of scrotum involvement can help to differentiate from *Candida* of the groin where scrotum involvement is common (Habif, 2010).

Tinea pedis, athlete's foot, is a common dermatophyte infection and presents with many different signs and symptoms. Habif (2010) notes that although it may present in the classic ringworm

pattern, involvement between the toes or on the soles of the feet is more common. Three primary types are interdigital, moccasin type, and vesicular.

- Interdigital results in erythema and scaling present between the fourth and fifth toes, although any interdigital space can be affected. Secondary infection with bacteria is more common in the macerated toe space.
- Moccasin-type tinea pedis affects the entire sole of the foot, and the chronic silvery white scale may also occur on the palms of the hands, where it is referred to as painter's palm. The creases of the palms and the soles of the feet are thickened and the creases are white in color, hence the appearance of paint that was not fully washed away. Because of the mild nature of this infection and its subtle presentation, it may be present for years before the patient seeks treatment.
- Vesicular-type tinea pedis may appear on the sole or the top of the foot and may represent a secondary bacterial infection in someone with chronic interdigital tinea pedis. It can also occur as an id reaction to the fungal infection, in which case the blisters may even involve remote sites.

Toenails are most often infected with dermatophytes, and there are three classic presentations:

- Distal and lateral subungual onychomycosis (DLSO), which presents with onycholysis (the pulling away of the nail plate from the nail bed), hyperkeratosis, and yellow-brown discoloration.
- Superficial white onycomycosis (SWO), in which the dermatophyte invades the surface of the nail, and the dorsal nail plate is chalky white.
- Proximal subungual onychomycosis (PSO) appears as a chalky white color at the base of the nail.

Not every toenail with abnormal appearance is infected with fungus. Studies using the gold standard for diagnosis found that only 46% of abnormal appearing nails were infected (Garcia-Doval et al., 2010; Gupta, 2000). This is an important consideration in the diagnosis of tinea unguium or onychomycosis.

Cutaneous candidiasis occurs in large skinfolds, intertrigo, and interdigital areas as well as in nails. Habif (2010) describes two presentations of candida: (1) Pustules form, become macerated in the skinfold, and develop papules with a fringe of moist scale at the border and intact pustules outside the intertriginous area. (2) Red, moist, and shiny lesions form that lack the pustules, because they macerate as soon as they form. Small intact pustules appear outside the border, and these satellite lesions are helpful in making the diagnosis.

Tinea (pityriasis) versicolor appears as macular, well-demarcated lesions that are light brown on untanned skin and white on tanned skin. The lesions vary in size and may become confluent and cover large areas of the body. They are finely scaled and sometimes pruritic. The trunk is the most common area of the body affected, but the lesions can spread to the upper arms, neck, and face.

Diagnostic tests: History of the concern is critical in diagnosis, because in most superficial fungal infections, diagnosis is primarily presumptive, based on clinical presentation. The fungal lesions evolve and for the most part are asymptomatic, so they may be found coincidentally by the provider on physical examination or presented by the patient when self-treatments have failed. Taking the history along with inspection is recommended. Asking the patient to identify what part of the lesion looks like the initial presentation allows for identification of the primary lesion and can sort out confusing signs of lesions that are secondary and that may mask the primary disease.

For fungal skin involvement, the gold standard of diagnosis is direct microscopic examination of a potassium hydroxide wet mount preparation (Habif, 2010). Scale is obtained using a surgical blade and placed on a slide. Although fungal infection in the hair or nails may need to be cultured, most tinea does not require culture, because treatments are effective against any of the specific species. Culture may also be needed for definitive diagnosis of lesions on the foot. Because nail involvement will require prolonged oral treatment to eradicate the infective agent, clinical diagnoses should be confirmed by laboratory testing. Approximately 90% of nail infections are due to dermatophytes; 8% are caused by a mold, *Scopulariopsis;* and 2% are due to a yeast, *Candida,* that may not respond to treatments useful in treating dermatophytes (Habif, 2010; Loo, 2007). Garcia-Doval et al. (2010) present a clinical diagnostic rule for tinea unguium. In their study, they found that if the patient with suspected onychomycosis had greater than 25% of the sole of the foot with plantar desquamation and the presence of interdigital tinea pedis, the positive predictive value of the rule was 81%, which is higher than that of laboratory tests.

Differential diagnosis:

Scalp lesions:
- Seborrheic dermatitis
- Psoriasis
- Atopic dermatitis
- Alopecia areata
- Bacterial folliculitis
- Neoplasia needs to be considered with presence of a kerion

Lesions on the trunk:
- Allergic contact dermatitis
- Atopic dermatitis
- Nummular eczema
- Psoriasis
- Pityriasis rosea
- Tinea (pityriasis) versicolor

Lesions in the groin:
- Intertrigo
- Psoriasis
- Seborrheic dermatitis
- Erythrasma

Lesions on the feet:
Between the toes:

- Bacterial infections: erythrasma, impetigo, *Pseudomonas*
- *Candida* intertrigo

Moccasin type:

- Allergic contact dermatitis
- Atopic dermatitis
- Dyshidrotic eczema
- Psoriasis

Vesicular:

- Allergic contact dermatitis
- Dyshidrotic eczema
- Bacterial infection
- Bullous disease

Nail involvement:
DLSO:

- Psoriatic nails
- Onychogryphosis (thickening and hardening)
- Onychauxis (overgrowth or thickening)

SWO:

- Trauma
- Contact or irritant dermatitis

Tinea pityriasis versicolor:
- Vitiligo
- Pityriasis alba

- Seborrheic dermatitis
- Secondary syphilis
- Pityriasis rosea (Habif, 2010; Wolff et al., 2009)

Treatment: In older adults, response to treatment may be decreased due to slower cell turnover and comorbid conditions, particularly diabetes and peripheral vascular disease. Tables 6-6 and 6-7 offer topical and systemic treatment options, respectively. For topical agents, the treatment is twice a day for 2 to 4 weeks and should be continued for 1 week after the lesions clear. Application should extend beyond the leading edge of the lesion. Within a class of medication, the options are comparable and should be selected based on cost and the preferred base (lotion, cream, ointment). Topical treatments are not useful for tinea capitis, and failure is common in tinea manum and tinea unguium.

TABLE 6-7 Systemic Treatment for Superficial Fungal Infections

DRUG CLASS	PREPARATION	USE
Allylamines	Terbinafine	Tinea corporis, cruris, capitis, pedis
		Onychomycosis
Azoles	Itraconazole	Dermatophyte infections
	Fluconazole	Tinea (pityriasis) versicolor
		Onychomycosis
Mitotic Inhibitor	Griseofulvin	Tinea corporis, cruris, capitis, pedis
		Tinea (pityriasis) versicolor

TABLE 6-6 Topical Treatment for Superficial Fungal Infections

DRUG CLASS	PREPARATION	USE
Azoles	Clotrimazole	Dermatophytes of the trunk or extremities
	Miconazole	Cutaneous candidiasis
	Ketoconazole	Tinea (pityriasis) versicolor
	Econazole	
	Oxiconizole	
	Sulconizole	
Allylamines	Naftifine	Dermatophytes of the trunk or extremities
	Terbinafine	Tinea (pityriasis) versicolor
	Butenafine	
Naphthionates	Tolnaftate	Dermatophytes of the trunk or extremities
Pyridone	Ciclopirox	Dermatophytes of the trunk or extremities
		Candidiasis
		Tinea (pityriasis) versicolor
		Onychomycosis SWO
Polyene	Nystatin	Candidiasis

Newer agents are more likely to cure tinea pedis than the older generation of antifungals, including clotrimazole, which is fungistatic, whereas terbinafine is fungicidal. Terbinafine cannot be used more than 4 weeks. Econazole and ciclopirox also have antibacterial properties and may be the drugs of choice if bacterial involvement is suspected.

When tinea pedis is vesicular, the use of aluminum acetate solution is a helpful drying agent and facilitates the penetration of the topical antifungal treatment. In hyperkeratotic, moccasin-type tinea, keratolytic agents, such as ammonium lactate lotion or topical urea, can reduce the hyperkeratosis and allow for improved penetration. Applying a plastic occlusive dressing over the keratolytic agents enhances their effectiveness. For tinea pedis it is important to assess the condition of the nails and treat any reservoir that may be present.

Topical treatments are rarely useful in the treatment of tinea unguium, except for SWO. In the United States, the only topical treatment approved by the FDA is ciclopirox topical (Penlac Nail Lacquer). An intriguing alternative was presented by Derby, Rohal, Jackson, Beutler, and Olsen (2011). In a small study of the effectiveness of the lay treatment of onychomycosis with Vicks VapoRub applied topically once a day for 48 weeks, 83% of the participants reported satisfactory results, with 27.8% experiencing a complete clinical and mycological cure. This rate is comparable to the 34% noted in studies of ciclopirox 8% topical with the advantage of a much lower cost (Loo, 2007).

An alternative treatment of tinea (pityriasis) versicolor is selenium sulfide 2.5% lotion or shampoo applied for 10 to 15 minutes followed by showering off for 2 weeks. Weekly application for several additional months may prevent recurrence. The skin color alterations may take 1 to 2 months to resolve completely.

Research supports a variety of dosing options for all of the oral treatments from daily to once-a-month pulse therapy (Baran, Hay, & Garduno, 2008; Loo, 2007). The duration of therapy depends on the site of involvement as well as the response. Although oral terbinafine is least toxic of the antifungals, all of the agents have the potential of serious side effects. Before recommending any oral treatment, consultation is recommended.

Mechanical treatments of nails infected with fungus offer another option for resolution of the infection. Total nail removal is an option but can have unintended consequences.

Follow-up: Follow-up of the patient with superficial fungal infections needs to be addressed on a case-by-case basis. A follow-up in 4 weeks is a reasonable option, especially for those patients on oral therapy, where hepatitis may appear after 4 weeks of treatment (Baran et al., 2008). For oral therapy, a baseline CBC and liver function tests are recommended with retesting every 4 to 6 weeks (Habif, 2010). Infection of the toenails requires 6 weeks or longer to judge results, and in tinea (pityriasis) versicolor 1 to 2 months are required before the lesions resolve. Patient education regarding expected outcomes and possible side effects can help in the assessment of when or even whether follow-up is necessary.

Sequelae: The superficial fungal infections for the most part do not present a serious health threat to older adults. Their lack of symptoms is one reason they are often chronic before they are addressed. The risk of superinfection with bacteria and resulting severe consequences is greatest in those with diabetes, peripheral vascular disease, or immune compromise. The Candida species may have systemic consequences and are often painful; treatment and prevention are key. The side effects of the treatments may be more concerning than the disease, and these risks are important to weigh in decision making. Serious consequences include hepatic toxicity, CyP-450 interactions, neutropenia, and agranulocytosis.

Prevention/prophylaxis: All fungus grows best in warm humid environments. The key to prevention of all types is to keep the skin cool and dry. Avoiding occlusive footwear, wearing absorbent materials, and practicing good hygiene offer the best primary prevention. Tinea pedis, tinea manuum, and onychomycosis are difficult to completely eradicate; recurrence is common, and the diseases may become chronic in nature. The interdependence of these infections requires the complete resolution of all three in order to prevent recurrence. Tinea (pityriasis) versicolor is the result of the conversion of the normal *Malassezia* skin flora to a mycelial form that is pathological and causes the scaly lesions. Older age actually decreases the risk of this disease, because sebaceous activity declines with age. Prophylactic therapy with topical or oral antifungals has been effective in preventing recurrence. The *Candida* species are part of the normal flora in the mouth, gut, and vaginal tract. The key to prevention of recurrence is keeping the skinfolds dry. Use of a hairdryer to thoroughly dry the area after bathing, the use of aluminum acetate solution (Burow's), and the application of antifungal or absorbent powder have all been shown to prevent recurrence (Habif, 2010; Wolff et al., 2009).

Referral: When definitive diagnosis is needed for suspected fungal infections of the skin, hair, or nails, referral is often necessary so that direct visualization of a wet mount preparation can be performed. When the hair or nails are affected, systemic treatment is usually required. A culture is necessary to rule out the other diseases that can mimic fungal infection and to determine the causative organism.

Education: Patient education should center on the cause of the infection and the risk of reinfection/recurrence. Prevention requires avoidance of situations that cause occlusive, warm, moist environments. This can be accomplished by wearing absorbent materials, loose clothing, and open-toe shoes in the summer, and wearing protective footwear in showers and around pools. Patients can be reassured that tinea (pityriasis) versicolor is the result of a change in the normal body flora and not contagious and that coloration changes will resolve with treatment. Prophylactic antifungal therapy may be required, especially for tinea pedis, tinea manuum, or onychomycosis.

CLINICAL RECOMMENDATION	EVIDENCE RATING	REFERENCES
A rule for the clinical diagnosis of onychomycosis was developed. Data supported that the rule was at least as accurate as laboratory tests. When dermatologists considered onychomycosis was the most likely diagnosis and plantar desquamation affected >25% of the sole of the foot, treatment could be started without further confirmation. The rule needs to be validated with primary care practitioners.	B	Garcia-Doval et al. (2010)
The use of débridement as an adjunct to oral antifungal therapy is usually not necessary. This was demonstrated in two studies comparing oral therapy alone to oral therapy and chemical avulsion.	A	Gupta (2000)
Oral Ketoconazole is not a recommended treatment for dermatophyte infections. Newer antifungals are more effective, and it is the most toxic antifungal with the risk of hepatitis and drug interactions.	A	Baran et al. (2008) Gupta (2000) Habif (2010)
A small study of topical Vicks VapoRub applied to nails affected with fungus confirmed by microscopy and culture was found to be as effective as topical ciclopirox 8%, the only FDA-approved treatment for onychomycosis. Participants were followed for 48 weeks, and the outcome measure was clinical and mycological cure. Patient satisfaction was also measured. The cost of treatment is less than one-fourth that of the prescription treatment.	B	Derby et al. (2011)
White socks are not useful in the prevention of tinea pedis. The color of the socks does not make a difference; the fabric does. Cotton socks are preferable to synthetics.	C	Gupta (2000) Habif (2010)

A = consistent, good-quality, patient-oriented evidence; B = inconsistent or limited-quality, patient-oriented evidence; C = consensus, disease-oriented evidence, usual practice, expert opinion, or case series. For information about the SORT evidence rating system, go to www.aafp.org/afpsort.xml.

CASE STUDY

Mrs. Jones is a 70-year-old woman you are admitting to the skilled nursing facility after a total hip replacement. When you obtain her past medical history, she reports a problem with a chronic rash under her breasts and in her supra-gluteal fold. She has tried a number of topical antifungal treatments without success. She has never seen a dermatologist. While she finds the rash a nuisance and experiences an occasional increase in itchiness, it is something she can live with. Her primary care provider diagnosed the rash as Candida and encouraged her to keep the area clean and dry and to use antifungals. Recently, her 42-year-old daughter was diagnosed with psoriasis and asked about a family history of

CASE STUDY—cont'd

the disease. Mrs. Jones was unaware of anyone in her or her husband's family with that diagnosis.

On physical examination, you note a shiny, erythematous lesion with symmetrical distribution under both breasts. It is well demarcated without drainage and without the presence of any satellite lesions. Examination of the gluteal fold reveals a similar well-demarcated, shiny, erythematous lesion without drainage. On close inspection of the rest of the body around the umbilicus, you note an erythematous patch with silvery scale. You ask Mrs. Jones about the lesion, and she states that it has been there for years. The lesion is worse in the winter, but she attributes this to the closures on her skirts and pants causing irritation. She reports some improvement when applying over-the-counter hydrocortisone cream, although when she stops

using the cream, the lesion returns. For this case, the answers and rationale for your decision making need to be provided.

1. What clues in Mrs. Jones' history can help you determine her diagnosis?

2. What signs on physical examination are most helpful to defend or refute the differential?

3. How would you classify the severity of Mrs. Jones' disease? Be specific in your explanation.

4. What would be the treatment(s) of choice in her case?

5. What are some important points to include in patient education?

6. What would require a referral to a dermatologist?

REFERENCES

Assessment

Aasi, S. Z., & Choi, J. (2010). Dermatological diseases and disorders. In J. T. Pacala & G. S. Sullivan (Eds.), *The geriatrics review syllabus: a core curriculum in geriatrics* (7th ed.). New York City, NY: American Geriatrics Society.

Bates-Jensen, B. (2009). Pressure ulcers. In J. Halter, J. Ouslander, M. Tinetti, S. Studenski, K. High, S. Asthana, & W. Hazzard (Eds.), *Principles of geriatric medicine and gerontology* (6th ed.). New York City, NY: McGraw-Hill Medical.

Gray-Vickrey, P. (2010, March). Gathering "pearls" of knowledge for assessing older adults. *Nursing 2010*, pp. 34–42.

LeBlond, R. F., Brown, D. D., & DeGowin, R. L. (2009). *DeGowin's diagnostic examination* (9th ed.). New York City, NY: McGraw-Hill Medical.

Long, C., & Finlay, A. (1991). The fingertip unit—a new practical measure. *Clinical and Experimental Dermatology, 16*, pp. 444–447.

Williams, M. (2009). *Geriatric physical diagnosis*. Jefferson, NC: McFarland & Co.

Burns

Ahrens, M. (2011). *Home structure fires* (F. A. a. R. Division, Trans.). Quincy, MA: National Fire Protection Association.

Ahrns, K. S. (2004). Trends in burn resuscitation: shifting the focus from fluids to adequate endpoint monitoring, edema control, and adjuvant therapies. *Critical Care Nursing Clinics of North America, 16*(1), 75–98.

American Burn Association. (2007). Advanced burn life support course: provider's manual. Retrieved from http://ameriburn.org/ABLSProviderManual_20101018.pdf

American Burn Association. (n.d.). Fire and burn safety for older adults: educator's guide. Community Fire and Burn Prevention Programs. Retrieved August 26, 2011, from www.ameriburn.org/Preven/BurnSafetyOlderAdultsEducator'sGuide.pdf

American Burn Association. (2011). National burn repository, 2011 report. Retrieved October 15, 2011, from www.ameriburn.org/2011NBRAnnualReport.pdf?PHPSESSID=bb8aca1889fcfe96c3329571eece45c3

Bessey, P. Q. (2007). Wound care. In D. N. Herndon (Ed.), *Total burn care* (3rd ed., pp. 127–135). Philadelphia, PA: Saunders Elsevier.

Blakeney, P. E., Rosenberg, L., Rosenberg, M., & Fauerbach, J. A. (2007). Psychosocial recovery and reintegration of patients with burn injuries. In D. N. Herndon (Ed.), *Total burn care* (3rd ed., pp. 829–843). Philadelphia, PA: Saunders Elsevier.

Bullocks, J. M., Hsu, P. W., Izaddoost, S. A., Hollier, L. H., & Stal, S. (2008). Burns and frostbite. In *Plastic surgery emergencies: principles and techniques* (pp. 29–53). New York City, NY: Thieme.

Centers for Disease Control and Prevention. (2007). 10 Leading causes of injury deaths by age group highlighting unintentional injury deaths, United States—2007. Available from CDC Web-based Injury Statistics Query and Reporting System (WISQARS). Retrieved July 30, 2011, from www.cdc.gov/injury/wisqars/pdf/Unintentional_2007-a.pdf

Demling, R. H., Pereira, C. T., & Herndon, D. N. (2007). Care of geriatric patients. In D. N. Herndon (Ed.), *Total burn care* (3rd ed., pp. 496–499). Philadelphia, PA: Saunders Elsevier.

Flynn, J. D. (2010). Characteristics of home fire victims. (Fire, Analysis and Research Division.) Quincy National Fire Protection Association. Retrieved August 26, 2011, from www.nfpa.org/assets/files/pdf/os.homevictims.pdf

Grant, E. J. (2004). Burn prevention. *Critical Care Nursing Clinics of North America, 16*(1), 127–138.

Greenhalgh, D. (2007). Wound healing. In D. N. Herndon (Ed.), *Total burn care* (3rd ed., pp. 578–595). Philadelphia, PA: Saunders Elsevier.

Guidelines for the operation of burn centers. (2007). *Journal of Burn Care & Research, 28*(1), 134–141.

Harford, C. E., & Kealey, G. P. (2007). Care of outpatient burns. In D. N. Herndon (Ed.), *Total burn care* (3rd ed., pp. 67–80). Philadelphia, PA: Saunders Elsevier.

Karter, M. J. (2010). *Fire loss in the United States during 2009* (F. A. a. R. Division, Trans.). Quincy, MA: National Fire Protection Association.

Kasten, K. R., Makley, A. T., & Kagan, R. J. (2011). Update on the critical care management of severe burns. *Journal of Intensive Care Medicine, 26*(4), 223–236.

Lloyd, E. C., Rodgers, B. C., Michener, M., & Williams, M. S. (2012). Outpatient burns: prevention and care. *American Family Physician, 85*(1), 25–32.

Meyer, W. J., Patterson, D. R., Jaco, M., Woodson, L., & Thomas, C. (2007). Management of pain and other discomforts in burned patients. In D. N. Herndon (Ed.), *Total burn care* (3rd ed., pp. 797–818). Philadelphia, PA: Saunders Elsevier.

Peck, M. D. (2011). Structure fires, smoke production, and smoke alarms. *Journal of Burn Care & Research, 32*(5), 511–518.

Thomas, C. R., Meyer, W. J., & Blakeney, P. E. (2007). Psychiatric disorders associated with burn injury. In D. N. Herndon (Ed.), *Total burn care* (3rd ed., pp. 819–828). Philadelphia, PA: Saunders Elsevier.

Titler, M. G., Herr, K., Xie, X., Brooks, J. M., Schilling, M. L., & Marsh, J. L. (2009). Summative index: acute pain management in older adults. *Applied Nursing Research, 22*(4), 264–273.

Cellulitis

Campbell, S. G., Burton-MacLeod, R., & Howlett, T. (2009). A cellulitis guideline at a community hospital—we can reduce costs by standardizing care. *Journal of Emergency Primary Health Care, 7*(1), Article 990329.

Carter, K., Kilburn, S., & Featherstone, P. (2007). Cellulitis and treatment: a qualitative study of experiences. *British Journal of Nursing, 16*(6), S22–S28.

Dutton, M., Paulik, O., & Jones, P. (2009). A new concept for managing lower limb cellulitis. *Australian Nursing Journal, 16*(10), 40–41.

Jenkins, T. C., Knepper, B. C., Sabel, A. L., Sarcone, E. E., Long, J. A., Haukoos, J. S., . . . Burman, W. J. (2011). Decreased antibiotic utilization after implementation of a guideline for inpatient cellulitis and cutaneous abscess. *Archives of Internal Medicine, 171*(12), 1072–1079.

McNamara, D. R., Tleyjeh, I. M., Berbari, E. F., Lahr, B. D., Martinez, J. W., Mirzoyev, S. A., & Baddour, L. M. (2007). Incidence of lower-extremity cellulitis: a population-based study in Olmsted County, Minnesota. *Mayo Clinic Proceedings, 82*(7), 817–821.

Nazarko, L. (2008a). Infection control: cellulitis. *Nursing & Residential Care, 10*(4), 175–179.

Nazarko, L. (2008b). Providing outpatient antibiotic therapy for cellulitis in primary care. *British Journal of Community Nursing, 13*(11), 520–524.

Petrou, I. (2011, April). Cellulitis conundrum. *Modern Medicine,* pp. 35–36. Retrieved from www.modernmedicine.com/modern medicine/article/articleDetail.jsp?id=714667

Price, N. (2009). Management of cellulitis after insect bites. *Emergency Nurse, 17*(7), 24–27.

Schalock, P., & Sober, A. (2009). Approach to bacterial skin infections. In A. H. Goroll & A. G. Mulley (Eds.), *Primary care medicine* (6th ed.). Philadelphia, PA: Lippincott Williams & Wilkins.

Spellburg, B., Talbot, G., Boucher, H. W., Bradley, J., Gilbert, D., Scheld, W., . . . Bartlett, J. G. (2009). Antimicrobial agents for complicated skin and skin-structure infections: justification of noninferiority margins in the absence of placebo-controlled trials. *Clinical Infectious Diseases, 49*(3), 383–391. doi:10.1086/600296

Thorsteinsdottir, B., Tleyjeh, I. M., & Baddour, L. M. (2005). Abdominal wall cellulitis in the morbidly obese. *Scandinavian Journal of Infectious Diseases, 37*(8), 605–608. doi:10.1080/00365540510037957

Tyrer, A., & Thornalley, C. (2008). Cycloidal vibration for the treatment of cellulitis in a community setting. *British Journal of Nursing, 17*(20), S34–S37.

Corns and Calluses

Bennett, P. C. (2006). Foot care: prevention of problems for optimal health. *Home Healthcare Nurse, 24*(5), 325–329.

Dunn, J. E., Link, C. L., Felson, D. T., Crincoli, M. G., Keysor, J. J., & McKinlay, J. B. (2004). Prevalence of foot and ankle conditions in a multiethnic community sample of older adults. *American Journal of Epidemiology, 159*(5), 491–498.

Freeman, D. B. (2002). Corns and calluses resulting from mechanical hyperkeratosis. *American Family Physician, 65*(11), 2277–2280.

Helfand, A. (2009). Considerations in managing the older patient with foot problems. In J. Halter, J. Ouslander, M. Tinetti, S. Studenski, S. High, S. Asthana, & W. Hazzard (Eds.), *Principles of geriatric medicine and gerontology* (6th ed.). New York City, NY: McGraw-Hill Medical.

Landorf, K. B., Morrow, A., Spink, M. J., Nash, C. L., Novak, A., Bird, A. R., . . . Menz, H. B. (2011). Effectiveness of scalpel debridement for painful plantar calluses in older patients: a randomized trial. *Journal of Foot and Ankle Research, 4*(Suppl. 1), O23. Retrieved from www.jfootankleres.com/content/4/S1/O23

Schalock, P., & Sober, A. (2009). Management of corns and calluses. In A. H. Goroll & A. G. Mulley (Eds.), *Primary care medicine* (6th ed.). Philadelphia, PA: Lippincott Williams & Wilkins.

Stolt, M., Suhonen, R., Voutilainen, P., & Leino-Kilpi, H. (2010). Foot health in older people and the nurses' role in foot health care—a review of literature. *Scandinavian Journal of Caring Sciences, 24*(1), 194–201. doi:10.1111/j.1471-6712.2009.00700.x

Herpes Zoster

Ahmad, M., & Goucke, C. R. (2002). Management strategies for the treatment of neuropathic pain in the elderly. *Drugs & Aging, 19*(12), 929–945.

Barakzai, M. D., & Fraser, D. (2008). Assessment of infection in older adults. *Journal of Gerontological Nursing, 34*(1), 7–12.

Binder, A., Bruxelle, J., Rogers, P., Hans, G., Bosl, I., & Baron, R. (2009). Topical 5% lidocaine (lignocaine) medicated treatment for post-herpetic neuralgia: results of a double-blind, placebo-controlled, multinational efficacy and safety trial. *Clinical Drug Investigation, 29*(6), 393–408.

Cadogan, M. P. (2010). Herpes zoster in older adults. *Journal of Gerontological Nursing, 36*(3), 10–14. doi:10.3928/00989134-20100218-01

Centers for Disease Control and Prevention. (2011, January 10). About shingles (herpes zoster). Retrieved from: http://www.cdc.gov/vaccines/vpd-vac/shingles/dis-faqs.htm

Christo, P. J., Hobelemann, G., & Maine, D. N. (2007). Post-herpetic neuralgia in older adults: evidence-based approaches to clinical management. *Drugs & Aging, 24*(1), 1–19.

Dworkin, R. H., Johnson, R. W., Breuer, J., Gnann, J. W., Levin, M. J., Backonja, M., . . . Whitley, R. J. (2009). Recommendations for the management of herpes zoster. *Clinical Infectious Diseases, 44*(Suppl. 1), S1–S26.

Fashner, J., & Bell, A. (2011). Herpes zoster and postherpetic neuralgia: prevention and management. *American Family Physician, 83*(12), 1432–1437.

Ferri, F. F. (2007). *Ferri's Clinical Advisor 2008: Instant Diagnosis and Treatment.* St. Louis, MO: Mosby.

Fried, R. (2010). Zoster vaccine in older adults. *Journal of the American Geriatrics Society, 58*(9), 1799–1800. doi:10.111/j.1532-5415.2010.03023.x

Gilron, I., Bailey, J. M., Tu, D., Holden, R. R., Weaver, D. F., & Houlden, R. L. (2005). Morphine, gabapentin, or their combination for neuropathic pain. *New England Journal of Medicine, 352*(13), 1324–1334.

Hurley, L. P., Lindley, M. C., Harpaz, R., Stokley, S., Daley, M. F., Crane, L. A., . . . Kempe, A. (2010). Barriers to the use of herpes zoster vaccine. *Annals of Internal Medicine, 152*(9), 555–560.

Insinga, R. P., Itzler, R. F., Pellissier, J. M., Saddler, P., & Nikas, A. A. (2005). The incidence of herpes zoster in a United States administrative database. *Journal of General Internal Medicine, 20*(8), 748–753.

Irving, G. A., Backonja, M. N., Dunteman, E., Blonsky, E. R., Vanhove, G. F., Lu, S. P., & Tobias, J. (2011). A multicenter, randomized, double-blind, controlled study of NGX-4010, a high concentration capsaicin patch for the treatment of postherpetic neuralgia. *Pain Medicine, 12*(1), 99–109. doi: 10.1111/j.1526-4637.2010.01004.x

Irwin, M. R., Olmstead, R., & Oxman, M. N. (2007). Augmenting immune responses to varicella zoster virus in older adults: a randomized, controlled trial of tai chi. *Journal of the American Geriatrics Society, 55*(4), 511–517. doi:10.1111/j.1532-5415.2007.01109

Johnson, R., Wasner, G., Saddier, P., & Baron, R. (2008). Herpes zoster and postherpetic neuralgia: optimizing management in the elderly patient. *Drugs & Aging, 25*(12), 991–1006.

Lu, P. J., Euler, G. L., Jumaan, A. O., & Harpaz, R. (2009). Herpes zoster vaccination among adults aged 60 years or older in the United States, 2007: uptake of the first new vaccine to target seniors. *Vaccine, 27*(6), 882–887.

Oaklander, A. L. (2008). Mechanism of pain and itch caused by herpes zoster (shingles). *Journal of Pain, 9*(1 Suppl. 1), S10–S18.

Oxman, M. N., Levin, M. J., Johnson, G. R., Schmader, K. E., Straus, S. E., Gelb, L. D., . . . Shingles Prevention Study Group. (2005). A vaccine to prevent herpes zoster and postherpetic neuralgia in older adults. *New England Journal of Medicine, 352*(22), 2271–2284.

Sampathkumar, P., Drage, L. A., & Martin, D. P. (2009). Herpes zoster (shingles) and postherpetic neuralgia. *Mayo Clinic Proceedings, 84*(3), 274–280.

Sandy, M. C. (2005). Herpes zoster: medical and nursing management. *Clinical Journal of Oncology Nursing, 9*(4), 443–446.

Tseng, H., Smith, N., Harpaz, R., Bialek, S., Sy, L. S., & Jacobsen, S. J. (2011). Herpes zoster vaccine in older adults and the risk of subsequent herpes zoster disease. *Journal of the American Medical Association, 305*(2), 160–166. doi:10.1001/jama.2010.1983

Tyring, S. K., Beutner, K. R., Tucker, B. A., Anderson, W. C., & Crooks, R. J. (2000). Antiviral therapy for herpes zoster: randomized, controlled clinical trial of valacyclovir and famciclovir therapy in immunocompetent patients 50 years and older. *Archives of Family Medicine, 9*(9), 863–869.

Watson, P. (2010). Postherpetic neuralgia (updated). *Clinical Evidence.* Retrieved January 2, 2012, from http://clinicalevidence.bmj.com/ceweb/conditions/ind/0905/0905

Pressure Ulcers

Gray, M., Black, J. M., Baharestani, M. M., Bliss, D. Z., Colwell, J. C., Goldberg, M., . . . Ratliff, C. R. (2011). Moisture-associated skin damage: overview and pathophysiology. *Journal of Wound, Ostomy and Continence Nursing, 38*(3), 1–9.

Kottner, J., Balzer, K., Dassen, T., & Heinze, S. (2009). Pressure ulcers: a critical review of definitions and classifications. *Ostomy and Wound Management, 55*(9), 22–29.

National Pressure Ulcer Advisory Panel & European Pressure Ulcer Advisory Panel. (2009). *Prevention and treatment of pressure ulcers: clinical practice guideline.* Washington, DC: National Pressure Ulcer Advisory Panel.

Salcido, R., & Popescu, A. (2011, November 11). Pressure ulcers and wound care. Retrieved from http://emedicine.medscape.com/article/319284-overview

Psoriasis

Camarasa, J. M., Ortonne, J. P., & Dubertret, L. (2003). Calcitriol shows greater persistence of treatment effect than betamethasone dipropionate in topical psoriasis therapy. *Journal of Dermatological Treatment, 14*(1), 8–13.

Habif, T. P. (2010). *Clinical dermatology* (5th ed.). London, England: Mosby.

Gribetz, C., Ling, M., Lebwohl, M., Pariser, D., Draelos, Z., Gottlieb, A. B., . . . Menter, A. (2004). Pimecrolimus cream 1% in the treatment of intertriginous psoriasis: a double-blind, randomized study. *Journal of the American Academy of Dermatology, 51*(5), 731–738.

Gupta, M. A. & Gupta, A. K. (1998). Depression and suicidal ideation in dermatology patients with acne, alopecia areata, atopic dermatitis and psoriasis. *British Journal of Dermatology, 139*(5), 846–850.

Lebwohl, M., Christophers, E., Langley, R., Ortonne, J. P., Roberts, J., & Griffiths, C. (2003). An international, randomized, double-blind, placebo-controlled phase 3 trial of intramuscular alefacept in patients with chronic plaque psoriasis. *Archives of Dermatology, 139*(6), 719–727.

Menter, A., Gottlieb, A., Feldman, S. R., Van Voorhees, A. S., Leonardi, C. L., Gordon, K. B., & Bhushan, R. (2008). Guidelines of care for the management of psoriasis and psoriatic arthritis: Section 1. Overview of psoriasis and guidelines of care for the treatment of psoriasis with biologics [Consensus Development Conference Practice Guideline]. *Journal of the American Academy of Dermatology, 58*(5), 826–850. doi:10.1016/j.jaad.2008.02.039

Menter, A., Korman, N. J., Elmets, C. A., Feldman, S. R., Gelfand, J. M., Gordon, K. B., & Bhushan, R. (2009). Guidelines of care for the management of psoriasis and psoriatic arthritis. Section 3. Guidelines of care for the management and treatment of psoriasis with topical therapies [Practice Guideline]. *Journal of the American Academy of Dermatology, 60*(4), 643–659. doi:10.1016/j.jaad.2008.12.032

National Psoriasis Foundation. (2012). About psoriasis: statistics. Retrieved from www.psoriasis.org/learn_statistics

Wolff, K., Johnson, R. A., & Fitzpatrick, T. B. (2009). *Fitzpatrick's color atlas and synopsis of clinical dermatology* (6th ed.). New York City, NY: McGraw-Hill Medical.

Skin Cancer

Askew, D. A., Mickan, S. M., Soyer, H. P., & Wilkinson, D. (2009). Effectiveness of 5-fluorouracil treatment for actinic keratosis: a systematic review of randomized controlled trials. *International Journal of Dermatology, 48*(5), 453–463.

Bradford, P. T., Goldstein, A. M., McMaster, M. L., & Tucker, M. A. (2009). Acral lentiginous melanoma: incidence and survival patterns in the United States: 1986–2005. *Archives of Dermatology, 145*(4), 427–434.

Bristow, I. R., de Berker, D. A., Acland, K. M., Turner, R. J., & Bowling, J. (2010). Clinical guidelines for recognition of melanoma of the foot and nail unit. *Journal of Foot and Ankle Research, 3,* 25. Retrieved from www.jfootankleres.com/content/3/1/25

Centers for Disease Control and Prevention. (2009, March). *Skin cancer prevention and education initiatives* [White paper]. Retrieved from National Center for Chronic Disease Prevention and Health Promotion, www.cdc.gov/cancer/skin/basic_info/prevention.htm

Genomel Production. (2009). [Dermoscopy Tutorial]. *New Knowledge Directorate.* Retrieved from www.genomel.org/dermoscopy/toolkit.html

Girardi, S., Gaudy, C., Gouvernet, J., Teston, J., Richard, M. A., & Grob, J. J. (2006). Superiority of a cognitive education with photographs over ABCD criteria in the education of the general population to the early detection of melanoma: a randomized study. *International Journal of Cancer, 118*(9), 2276–2280.

Glanz, K., Schoenfeld, E., & Steffen, A. (2010). A randomized trial of tailored skin cancer prevention messages for adults: Project SCAPE. *American Journal of Public Health, 100*(4), 735–741.

Gloster, H. M., Jr., & Neal, K. (2006). Skin cancer in skin of color. *Journal of the American Academy of Dermatology, 55*(5), 741–760.

Goulart, J. M., Quigley, E. A., Dusza, S., Jewell, S. T., Alexander, G., Asagari, M. M., . . . Halpern, A. C. (2011). Skin cancer education for primary care physicians: a systematic review of published evaluated interventions. *Journal of General Internal Medicine, 26*(9), 1027–1036. doi: 10.1007/s11606-011-1692-y

Habif, T. P. (2004). *Clinical dermatology: a color guide to diagnosis and therapy* (4th ed.). New York City, NY: Mosby.

Halpern, A., Marghoob, A., & Sober, A. (2009). Clinical characteristics of melanoma. In C. Balch, A. Houghton, A. Sober, S. Soong, M. Atkins, & J. Thompson (Eds.), *Cutaneous melanoma* (5th ed., p. 162). St. Louis, MO: Quality Medical Publishing.

Heckman, C. J., Egleston, B. L., Wilson, D. B., & Ingersoll, K. S. (2008). A preliminary investigation of the predictors of tanning dependence. *American Journal of Health Behavior, 32*(5), 451–464.

Huang, W., & Clark, A. (2011). Understanding the therapies and adverse events helps in selecting the most appropriate option for each AK patient. *Advance for NPs & PAs.* Retrieved from http://nurse-practitioners-and-physician-assistants.advanceweb.com/Editorial/Content/PrintFriendly.aspx?CC=233268

Janda, M., Neale, R. E., Youl, P., Whiteman, D. C., Gordon, L., & Baade, P. D. (2011). Impact of a video-based intervention to improve the prevalence of skin self-examination in men 50 years or older. *Archives of Dermatology, 147*(7), 799–806. doi:10.1001/archdermatol.2011.48

Jensen, J., & Moriarty, C. (2008). Psychosocial factors associated with skin self-exam performance. *Journal of American College Health, 56*(6), 701–705.

Kiiski, V., de Vries, E., Flohil, S. C., Bijl, M. J., Hofman, A., Stricker, B. H. C., & Nijsten, T. (2010). Risk factors for single and multiple basal cell carcinomas. *Archives of Dermatology, 146*(8), 848–855.

Lin, J. S., Eder, M., & Weinmann, S. (2011). Behavioral counseling to prevent skin cancer: a systematic review for the U.S. Preventive Services Task Force. *Annals of Internal Medicine, 154*(3), 190–201.

Loescher, L. J., Harris, R. B., Lim, K. H., & Su, Y. (2006). Thorough skin self-examination in patients with melanoma. *Oncology Nursing Forum, 33*(3), 633–637.

Nolen, M. E., Beebe, V. R., King, J. M., Bryn, N., & Limaye, K. M. (2011). Nonmelanoma skin cancer: Part 1. *Journal of the Dermatology Nurses' Association, 3*(5), 260–279. doi:10.1097/JDN.06013e31822F1f77

Robinson, J. K., Turrisi, R., & Stapleton, J. (2007). Efficacy of a partner assistance intervention designed to increase skin self-examination performance. *Archives of Dermatology, 143*(1), 37–41.

Rubin, K. (2010a). Dysplastic nevi and the risk of melanoma. *Journal of the Dermatology Nurses' Association, 1*(4), 228–235.

Rubin, K. (2010b). Melanoma staging: a review of the revised American Joint Committee on Cancer Guidelines. *Journal of the Dermatology Nurses' Association, 1*(4), 254–259.

Watkins, J. (2010). Dermatology and the community nurse: actinic (solar) keratosis. *British Journal of Community Nursing, 15*(1), 6–11.

Superficial Fungal Infections

Baran, R., Hay, R. J., & Garduno, J. I. (2008). Review of antifungal therapy and the severity index for assessing onychomycosis: Part I [Review]. *Journal of Dermatological Treatment, 19*(2), 72–81. doi:10.1080/09546630701243418

Das, S., Goyal, R., & Bhattacharya, S. N. (2007). Laboratory-based epidemiological study of superficial fungal infections. *Journal of Dermatology, 34*(4), 248–253. doi:10.1111/j.1346-8138.2007.00262.x

Derby, R., Rohal, P., Jackson, C., Beutler, A., & Olsen, C. (2011). Novel treatment of onychomycosis using over-the-counter mentholated ointment: a clinical case series. [Research Support, Non-U.S. Government.] *Journal of the American Board of Family Medicine, 24*(1), 69–74. doi:10.3122/jabfm.2011.01.100124

Garcia-Doval, I., Cabo, F., Monteagudo, B., Alvarez, J., Ginarte, M., Rodriguez-Alvarez, M. X., . . . Gomez-Centeno, P. (2010). Clinical diagnosis of toenail onychomycosis is possible in some patients: cross-sectional diagnostic study and development of a diagnostic rule. [Research Support, Non-U.S. Government.] *British Journal of Dermatology, 163*(4), 743–751.doi: 10.1111/j.1365-2133.2010.09930.x

Gupta, A. K. (2000). Onychomycosis in the elderly [Review]. *Drugs & Aging, 16*(6), 397–407.

Habif, T. P. (2010). *Clinical dermatology* (5th ed.). London, England: Mosby.

Havlickova, B., Czaika, V. A., & Friedrich, M. (2008). Epidemiological trends in skin mycoses worldwide [Review]. *Mycoses, 51*(Suppl. 4), 2–15. doi:10.1111/j.1439-0507.2008.01606.x

Hedderwick, S., & Kauffman, C. A. (1997). Opportunistic fungal infections: superficial and systemic candidiasis [Review]. *Geriatrics, 52*(10), 50–54, 59.

Loo, D. S. (2007). Onychomycosis in the elderly: drug treatment options [Review]. *Drugs & Aging, 24*(4), 293–302.

Panackal, A. A., Halpern, E. F., & Watson, A. J. (2009). Cutaneous fungal infections in the United States: analysis of the National Ambulatory Medical Care Survey (NAMCS) and National Hospital Ambulatory Medical Care Survey (NHAMCS), 1995–2004. [Research Support, U.S. Government, P. H. S.] *International Journal of Dermatology, 48*(7), 704–712. doi:10.1111/j.1365-4632.2009.04025.x

Wolff, K., Johnson, R. A., & Fitzpatrick, T. B. (2009). *Fitzpatrick's color atlas and synopsis of clinical dermatology* (6th ed.). New York City, NY: McGraw-Hill Medical.

chapter 7

Head, Neck, and Face Disorders

Lori Martin-Plank

ASSESSMENT

A systematic and thorough examination of the head and neck begins with the inspection of the face, head, and scalp. Assess the shape, size, and symmetry of the patient's features. Examine the shape of the skull, palpating the bones of the head for any anatomical irregularities, masses, or areas of tenderness. Inspect the hair for distribution, quantity, and any balding patterns, noting any uniform alopecia, nits, or seborrhea. The scalp should be carefully inspected for any skin lesions on sun-exposed areas, noting pigment changes, tenderness, scales, or lumps. Assess for scars or bruising patterns. Note the symmetry of the patient's features, facial expressions, the presence of involuntary tics or tremors, periorbital edema, or facial drooping; palpate over the temples for any abnormality or tenderness in the temporal arteries. The presence of pain and nodules on palpation is not a normal finding even in very old individuals. Cranial nerve VII (facial nerve) should also be assessed at this time, noting any facial asymmetry, weakness, drooping of the lower eyelid, and unilateral paralysis (Bickley & Szilagyi, 2009; LeBlond, Brown, & DeGowin, 2009).

Eyes

Begin the inspection of the eyes by noting the position and symmetry of the surrounding skin and tissue as well as the presence and position of the eyebrows and eyelashes. Screen visual acuity before proceeding with any other examination of the eye. Using a Snellen chart from 20 feet or a handheld chart approximately 12 inches from the patient, assess visual acuity in each eye separately, then together; if the patient wears corrective lenses, he or she should have them on for this test. Note the condition of the skin around the eyes, check the sclera, and note the color of the conjunctiva. Assess the presence of exophthalmos, xanthelasma, pinguecula, ptosis, edema, and skin lesions. The lids should be carefully examined for the presence of hordeolum, chalazion, ectropion, and entropion, which is most common among elderly persons. Examine the cornea for any scarring, presence of pterygium, corneal arcus, and opacities. Note that basal and squamous cell carcinomas are common around the eye. Palpate for any tenderness over the lacrimal gland and assess the patency of the lacrimal duct. Examine the extraocular motions of the eye (cranial nerves III, IV, and VI). Check the visual fields (cranial nerve II), corneal reflexes (cranial nerve V), and pupillary reactions (cranial nerves II and III), with direct and consensual reactions. Carefully perform a funduscopic examination; most elderly patients need dilation for accurate assessment of the fundus. If you see the fundus, note the narrow, pale appearance of the arterioles common in elderly persons. Be careful to note any abnormalities in blinking (Parkinson's disease), dull or blank staring (hypothyroidism), residual facial paralysis (Bell's palsy or cerebrovascular accident), and skin changes. Decreased elasticity and turgor is a normal aging pattern; the skin around the eyes becomes thin and wrinkles appear. This is a normal change in older adults and makes skin turgor a poor determinant of hydration status (Bickley & Szilagyi, 2009; LeBlond et al., 2009).

159

Sinuses

Inspect and palpate over the frontal and maxillary sinus areas. Note any gross tenderness or inflammation in the sinus area or around the eyes.

Nose

Inspect the external nose for any asymmetry, inflammation, gross septal deviation, or deformities. If applicable, assess the function of the olfactory nerve (cranial nerve I) by having the patient identify a familiar-smelling item with the eyes closed. The olfactory sense greatly diminishes as a normal part of aging. Assess for patency of each nostril. Examine the internal nose, noting any discharge, bleeding, or edema. Check the status of the turbinates and position of the septum using a large otoscope speculum. The color and consistency of the inferior and middle turbinates as well as the presence of any polyps should be noted (Bickley & Szilagyi, 2009).

Ears

Carefully examine the external ears, noting their position and symmetry on the head, as well as any abnormal lesions, deformities, and the presence of tophi, keloids, or cysts. Estimate auditory acuity (cranial nerve VIII) by using the whisper test, testing each ear separately. Use the Weber and Rinne tests to assess for any conductive or sensorineural hearing loss. Palpate the tragus for any tenderness as well as for any preauricular or postauricular adenopathy. When examining the middle ear, note any inflammation, discharge, erythema, or cerumen in the canal. If visible, inspect the tympanic membranes and surrounding landmarks for abnormalities. Note any foreign bodies, dull membranes, alterations in the cone of light reflex, and presence of fluid or scarring. Be careful to inspect the posterior ear and helix for any skin lesions or carcinomas (LeBlond et al., 2009).

Oral Cavity

Perform a complete assessment of the lips, mouth, oral mucosa, and pharynx, noting the color, moisture, and presence of any abnormal lesions on and around the lips. Assess for any herpes simplex I, chancres, angular stomatitis, mucous retention cysts, angioedema, and fissures. Check oral mucosa for color, nodules, ulcers, or white patches (Bickley & Szilagyi, 2009). If the patient has dentures, these should be removed to do a complete oral examination. Examine the fit of the dentures and assess the consistency of the gums under the dentures. If natural teeth are present, note any loose or broken teeth as well as caries. Because periodontal disease is the primary cause of tooth loss in the adult, do a careful oral and gum examination. Examine the gums for bleeding, discoloration, swelling, and retractions. Note the attrition of the teeth (exposed dentin) and enamel loss from years of chewing. Note the condition of the hard palate and the presence of torus palatinus, thrush, or other lesions. Assess the gag reflex and rise of the palate (cranial nerves IX and X). Carefully examine the tongue for symmetry, enlargement (hypothyroidism), growths, protrusions, or abnormal movements (cranial nerve XII) and the dorsum for any papillary atrophy. A swollen, red, painful tongue may indicate vitamin B or riboflavin deficiency. Note any inflammation or obstruction in the parotid (Stensen) or submaxillary (Warton) ducts. Thoroughly examine the area underneath the tongue, the floor of the mouth, and the tonsils, soft palate, uvula, and posterior pharynx, noting any lesions, inflammation, or exudate and the color. Examine the strength and movement of the temporal and masseter muscles (cranial nerve V) as well as any crepitus in the mandible junction. Complete assessment should also include evaluation of the voice (cranial nerve X) and speech (cranial nerves V, VII, X, and XII).

Neck

Inspect the neck for symmetry, masses, scars, tracheal position, and deviation. Look for the presence of thyroid inflammation or goiters. Carefully palpate for any lymphadenopathy, noting that loss of lean muscle makes it easier to feel nodes in the cervical region of elderly persons. Assess supraclavicular, tonsilar, superficial, deep, and posterior cervical chains and submaxillary, submental, occipital, preauricular, and postauricular nodes, noting any inflammation, tenderness, or change in size, position, or shape. Hard, fixed nodes imply malignancy; tender nodes are typical of inflammation (Bickley & Szilagyi, 2009). Gently palpate and auscultate the carotid arteries one side at a time for any nodularity or bruits. Note any jugular vein distention that occurs when the patient is seated. Check to see if the patient uses any neck muscles to breathe. Carefully inspect and palpate the thyroid gland, noting any inflammation or nodules (unilateral). Examination of the range of motion of the neck should include flexion, extension, rotation, and lateral bending. Check the strength of the trapezius and sternomastoid muscles (cranial nerve XI).

A complete and thorough detailed examination of the head and neck has the potential to allow the examiner to discover multiple variants from the normal. Develop a clear and concise pattern of examination to ensure appropriate evaluation of these areas. Keep in mind the normal variants of the older person and how these differ from pathological or abnormal findings.

ACUTE GLAUCOMA

Signal symptoms: Unilateral eye pain, visual blurring with halos around lights, conjunctival injection, and photophobia; nausea and vomiting may also occur.

Description: Acute glaucoma, also known as *angle-closure* or *narrow-angle glaucoma*, is an obstruction to the outflow of aqueous humor from the posterior to the anterior chamber through the trabecular meshwork, canal of Schlemm, and associated structures. It results in an elevation of intraocular pressure, damaging the optic nerve and causing loss of peripheral vision, eye pain, and redness. This type of glaucoma is uncommon but may occur as a primary disease or secondary to other conditions and constitutes an ophthalmic emergency (Horton, 2012). Associated presenting symptoms may complicate diagnosis or result in misdiagnosis. There is still some confusion about the variations within angle-closure glaucoma, but acute angle-closure glaucoma must meet the following criteria:

- Two of these symptoms must be present—nausea/vomiting, history of intermittent visual blurring with halos, and ocular pain.
- Three of these signs must be identified—conjunctival injection, intraocular pressure (IOP) greater than 21 mm Hg, occlusion with a shallower chamber, corneal epithelial edema, and nonreactive mid-dilated pupil (Aherne & Dronen, 2012).

Etiology: The precise pathophysiology of acute glaucoma is unknown. In the acute form, pupillary blockage limits the progress of the aqueous humor through the trabecular network. The peripheral iris, which blocks the trabecular meshwork, is displaced forward. In susceptible persons, this may be precipitated by emotional stress, sudden darkness (such as in a theater when the lights go out), or medications such as sympathomimetics and anticholinergics. A recent theory suggests that susceptible individuals have an imbalance in autonomic tone with an increase in sympathetic tone. The conditions listed above are heightened, and a thickening of the middle-peripheral iris results in angle closure (Cronemberger, Calixto, de-Andrade, & Mérula, 2010).

Occurrence: Uncommon; accounts for 10% of all glaucoma. This is more common in families with prior history.

Age: The predominant age range is 60 to 70 years old.

Gender: Occurs more often in women.

Ethnicity: Acute and primary angle-closure glaucoma are more common in Inuit and Asian populations.

Contributing factors: Contributing factors include an anatomically narrow anterior chamber angle, requiring identification with the use of a special examination technique called *gonioscopy*. This examination technique is beyond the scope of the primary care practitioner, but the condition can be evaluated during the comprehensive eye examination. Other risk factors include hyperopia; small cornea; shallow anterior chamber; Eskimo ancestry; female gender; family history of glaucoma (first-degree relatives have a 2% to 5% risk over a lifetime); and use of certain cold remedies, antidepressants, antipsychotics, and other drugs with anticholinergic properties (e.g., atropine, preoperative medications, imipramine, inhaled ipratropium bromide) (Weizer, 2012).

Signs and symptoms: The presentation is often dramatic, but the diagnosis can be missed because of the associated symptoms (Horton, 2012). The history reveals severe, unilateral eye pain, blurred vision, lacrimation, reports of seeing colored halos around lights, and a red eye. Headache, nausea, and vomiting frequently accompany eye pain, causing eye pain to be overlooked. Emotional stress also is common. Examination reveals circumcorneal, conjunctival injection, tearing, and a fixed semidilated pupil that is nonreactive to light; the cornea is steamy or cloudy. Visual acuity, if evaluated, shows a loss in the affected eye.

Diagnostic tests: Immediately refer patients for a complete ophthalmic examination, including gonioscopy and tonometry (American Academy of Ophthalmology, 2005).

Differential diagnosis:
- Conjunctivitis
- Hyphema

- Uveitis
- Corneal trauma or infection

Treatment: The patient with acute glaucoma needs an immediate consultation with and referral to an ophthalmologist; permanent visual loss occurs within 2 to 5 days if this condition is untreated. Surgical treatment includes peripheral iridectomy or laser iridotomy. Intraocular pressure must be lowered preoperatively, which may require the use of an osmotic diuretic intravenously or orally and miotic eye drops. As the primary health-care provider, you must communicate to the specialist any medical conditions that need monitoring with the use of these agents. Bilateral treatment is indicated, because patients are at risk for developing the same problem in the other eye (Tsai & Cheng, 2011).

Follow-up: The ophthalmologist treating the patient determines follow-up treatment. Periodic eye examinations are recommended by preventive guidelines.

Sequelae: If treated promptly, acute glaucoma is not associated with sequelae. If untreated, permanent visual loss occurs.

Prevention/prophylaxis: Knowing the risk factors for acute angle-closure glaucoma, the health-care provider should educate patients with those risk factors (see under Education). Periodic eye examinations are recommended for prevention.

Referral: Refer the patient immediately on presentation and evaluation of symptoms.

Education: Teach patients with known risk factors (see under Contributing Factors) the importance of regular eye examinations and reporting of symptoms.

CLINICAL RECOMMENDATION	EVIDENCE RATING	REFERENCES
Acute angle-closure glaucoma is an ocular emergency that requires immediate lowering of IOP with topical/oral/parenteral medications and occasionally laser peripheral iridotomy.	A	Tsai & Cheng (2011)
For acute angle-closure glaucoma, topical and systemic agents are usually necessary to adequately decrease the IOP, and laser iridotomy is the definitive surgical treatment.	A	American Academy of Ophthalmology (AAO) (2005)

A = consistent, good-quality, patient-oriented evidence; B = inconsistent or limited-quality, patient-oriented evidence; C = consensus, disease-oriented evidence, usual practice, expert opinion, or case series. For information about the SORT evidence rating system, go to www.aafp.org/afpsort.xml.

CATARACT

Signal symptoms: Diminished vision in one or both eyes, poor night vision, sensitivity to glare; because progression is gradual, changes may go unnoticed until visual loss is advanced.

Description: A cataract is an opacification of the lens that interferes with the passage of light through the lens, decreasing visual acuity. The location, size, and density of this opacity influence the degree of visual impairment (Giaconi, Sarraf, & Coleman, 2010). Nuclear sclerotic cataracts affect contrast sensitivity,

progress slowly, and tend to preserve functional reading vision while frequently causing nearsightedness. In contrast, posterior subcapsular cataracts progress more rapidly and interfere with reading vision. Glucocorticoid treatment and radiation tend to be associated with a posterior, subcapsular location (Horton, 2012).

Etiology: Most cataracts are related to the aging process. The gradual thickening or hardening in the lens is believed to be caused by oxidative damage to the lens protein.

Occurrence: The rate of visually significant cataracts in persons 50 to 59 years old is 6.8%. Of persons over 80 years old, 68.3% have cataracts (Gambert, 2012). Cataracts tend to be bilateral, although the rate of progression varies between the eyes.

Age: Although subtle changes in visual acuity related to cataract formation occur by age 50, people over 75 years old experience most visually significant cataracts.

Gender: Cataracts occur equally in men and women.

Ethnicity: No ethnic groups are significantly more prone to cataracts.

Contributing factors: Diabetes mellitus, hypertension, poor nutrition, cigarette smoking, high alcohol intake, trauma to the eye, long-term exposure to ultraviolet (UV) B radiation (sunlight), and a strong family history of cataracts are risk factors. Use of certain substances, including oral glucocorticoids, also contributes to cataracts. An association between cataracts and glaucoma and intraocular inflammation exists (Jacobs, 2012). There is some evidence that inhaled corticosteroids, particularly in high doses, also contribute to cataract formation (Weatherall et al., 2009).

Signs and symptoms: The patient with a cataract initially may present with an improvement in near vision, requiring a new prescription for corrective lenses; distance vision will worsen (Jacobs, 2012). Patients also may experience blurred vision or sensitivity to glare from bright light or from automobile headlights during night driving. Complaints of having difficulty reading and distinguishing contrast sensitivities and of seeing a yellow tint or washed-out colors are common. Some patients may not seek evaluation of their symptoms by a health-care provider owing to denial or fear of loss of independence (driver's license being revoked), whereas other patients seek prompt assessment in the hope of early intervention. A recent history of falls, accidents, or injury is suspicious. On physical examination, visual acuity test results are abnormal for one or both eyes (evaluate near and distance vision). Examine the eye using an opaque light for opacification of the lens. The cataract may be visible to the naked eye. The red reflex may be absent, or the cataract may appear as a black area.

Diagnostic tests: No diagnostic testing is required other than that for visual acuity and examination of the eye, unless other visual problems are suspected. Refer the patient to an ophthalmologist for complete evaluation after initial screening. Pupillary dilation and slit lamp examination will reveal white, gray, or brownish opacities if the cataract is developed. Dark areas on the red reflex in a dilated eye indicate small cataracts; the red reflex may not be visible if the cataract is large (Jacobs, 2012).

Differential diagnosis:
- Corneal scarring
- Retinal detachment
- Macular degeneration
- Chronic glaucoma
- Diabetic retinopathy

Treatment: Treatment is determined after full evaluation by the ophthalmologist. Ultimately, surgical intervention is required with extraction of the cataract and immediate implantation of a plastic intraocular lens, unless contraindicated by other disease conditions (American Academy of Ophthalmology [AAO] Cataract and Anterior Segment Panel, 2011). Patients with posterior capsular opacification may require neodymium:yttrium-aluminum-garnet (Nd:YAG) laser capsulotomy; this should not be performed at the same time as other cataract surgery. Collaboration with the ophthalmologist is indicated for patients with severe cardiac, respiratory, or neuromuscular conditions that may prevent the patient from lying still or supine as required during the surgery. Patients with diabetes and hypertension should be instructed in medication use preoperatively. Patients receiving anticoagulant therapy also should be managed collaboratively and individually. Patients on clopidogrel after cardiac stent are encouraged to delay surgery until the clopidogrel is no longer needed. There is no hard and fast rule for patients on aspirin or warfarin maintenance (Jacobs, 2012). Patients who are or have been on alpha receptor therapy, such as tamulosin for prostatic enlargement, may experience intraoperative floppy iris syndrome (IFIS); treatment of these patients may require special techniques during surgery to prevent this (AAO Cataract and Anterior Segment Panel, 2011; Handzel, Briesen, Rausch, & Kälble, 2012).

The degree of visual impairment and its influence on the patient's usual daily functioning determine the timing of the surgery (AAO Cataract and Anterior Segment Panel, 2011; Servat, Risco, Nakasato, & Bernardino, 2011). Initially a conservative treatment plan may include prescription of corrective lenses and periodic reevaluation by the ophthalmologist, coupled with a plan for environmental safety and optimization of the patient's functional abilities within his or her visual limitations. Preoperative medical clearance (history and physical) is required before surgery. The American Academy of Ophthalmology (AAO) and a recent Cochrane review (Keay, Lindsley, Tielsch, Katz, & Schein, 2009) determined that preoperative testing increases costs and does not improve outcomes of surgery. Surgery is performed in an outpatient or short procedure unit, with the patient returning home immediately after discharge.

Follow-up: Immediate postsurgical care includes eye protection and application of topical agents prescribed by the ophthalmologist. The patient may be cautioned to avoid straining, lifting, or bending. Postoperative follow-up is usually within 24 to 48 hours. The family or health-care team should heighten precautions for environmental safety to avoid injury. Intensive supervision of mentally compromised patients is required to prevent damage to the operative site. Future follow-up includes a reevaluation of visual acuity, prescription of corrective lenses as indicated, and monitoring of the unaffected eye for cataract development.

Sequelae: Possible sequelae to cataract surgery include faulty wound closure with aqueous humor leakage, blindness secondary to choroidal hemorrhage, endophthalmitis, toxic anterior segment syndrome (TASS), inflammation, retinal detachment, prolapse of the iris into the corneal wound, and secondary glaucoma (AAO Cataract and Anterior Segment Panel, 2011; Jacobs, 2012).

Prevention/prophylaxis: The patient should be protected from exposure to UV B radiation by wearing sunglasses designed for this and by wearing a hat with a wide brim.

Referral: After the initial visual screening, refer the patient to an ophthalmologist for complete examination and treatment, including postsurgery follow-up.

Education: Provide the patient with information on age-related visual changes and the importance of protecting the eyes from sunlight with UV-blocking sunglass lenses, maintaining a nutritionally balanced diet including green, leafy vegetables (Renzi, 2007), avoiding tobacco and high alcohol intake, and having periodic eye examinations every 2 years. Instruct the patient to seek prompt evaluation of any vision changes, and reassure the patient that with proper treatment cataracts do not result in permanent loss of visual acuity (Horton, 2012).

CLINICAL RECOMMENDATION	EVIDENCE RATING	REFERENCES
There is no evidence from randomized, controlled trials (RCTs) that supplementation with antioxidant vitamins (beta carotene, vitamin A, or vitamin E) prevents or slows the progression of age-related cataract.	A	Mathew, Ervin, Tao, & Davis (2012)
The decision to recommend cataract surgery should be based on consideration of the following factors: visual acuity, visual impairment, and the potential for functional benefits.	B	AAO Cataract and Anterior Segment Panel (2011)
Ophthalmologists and other physicians managing patients taking alpha antagonists should be aware of the risks of intraoperative floppy iris syndrome (IFIS).	B	AAO Cataract and Anterior Segment Panel (2011)
Extracapsular cataract surgery by phacoemulsification with intraocular lens (IOL) implantation provides safe and effective treatment for patients with cataract.	A	Packer (2011)

A = consistent, good-quality, patient-oriented evidence; B = inconsistent or limited-quality, patient-oriented evidence; C = consensus, disease-oriented evidence, usual practice, expert opinion, or case series. For information about the SORT evidence rating system, go to www.aafp.org/afpsort.xml.

CHRONIC GLAUCOMA (PRIMARY OPEN-ANGLE GLAUCOMA)

Signal symptoms: None initially; tunnel vision, night blindness, halos around lights.

Description: Chronic open-angle or primary open-angle glaucoma is an insidious optic neuropathy characterized by increased IOP severe enough to damage the optic nerve. Progressive over time with a gradual visual field loss, chronic glaucoma is called the *silent blinder*, because it often goes unnoticed until the later stages. Variants occur in which IOP does not increase, but the optic nerve still becomes damaged; this is termed *normal tension glaucoma* (Koby, 2012) and is common in Asian populations (Jacobs, 2012a, 2012b). Conversely, some patients have increased IOP but show no optic nerve changes or visual defects; these are referred to as glaucoma suspects (Bell, 2012) or those with ocular hypertension (Quigley, 2011). Secondary glaucomas are the result of prior or concurrent ocular disease or trauma; they may have open angles caused by steroid-induced pressure increases.

Etiology: The etiology of chronic glaucoma is unknown, but the disease is associated with increased intraocular pressure, optic nerve degeneration, and visual field loss. Current theories include vascular dysfunction resulting in optic nerve ischemia, immune-mediated damage to the nerve, oxidative stress, or excitotoxicity from too much retinal glutamate (Bell, 2012; Jacobs, 2012a, 2012b). Because IOP is the one factor that can be measured, most reevaluation and treatment decisions are influenced by this measurement (Heijl et al., 2002).

Occurrence: Prevalence of chronic glaucoma increases in persons over 40 years old, approaching 15% by age 75; 80% of cases are the open-angle type. Primary open-angle glaucoma causes 15% to 20% of all blindness in the United States and is the primary cause of blindness in African Americans (Bell, 2012; Varma, Lee, Goldberg, & Kotak, 2011).

Age: The incidence increases in persons over 40 years old, with another increase in incidence in persons between ages 60 and 75. Onset is earlier in African Americans.

Gender: Chronic glaucoma occurs equally in men and in women.

Ethnicity: African Americans, Afro-Caribbeans, and Hispanics are at a higher risk than the general population

for developing chronic glaucoma (AAO Glaucoma Panel, 2010a).

Contributing factors: Risk factors include old age, a positive family history, African American ancestry or Latino/Hispanic ethnicity, type 2 diabetes mellitus, hypertension, myopia, low ocular perfusion, thinner central cornea, and genetic mutations (AAO Glaucoma Panel, 2010a). There is some association with migraine headache, but further research is needed to confirm this. Risk factors for secondary open-angle glaucoma include long-term use of topical or oral corticosteroids. It is important to note if the patient had prior LASIK surgery, because this can alter corneal thickness. Cataract surgery can also lower IOP, so this history is essential (AAO Glaucoma Panel, 2010b).

Signs and symptoms: The disease is asymptomatic in the early stages; by the time symptoms develop, significant neural damage has occurred. Eye health specialists frequently discover chronic open-angle glaucoma during routine eye examinations. Patients may present with a complaint of blurred vision, a request for new corrective lenses, or occasionally a report that they see a halo around lights (Jacobs, 2012a; Quigley, 2011).

On routine vision screening, visual acuity may be normal or unchanged from previous screening; visual fields may be decreased, however. The skilled examiner may detect changes in the cup-to-disc ratio on funduscopic examination—a cup with a diameter of more than 50% of the vertical disc diameter is highly suspect for glaucoma (Jacobs, 2012a, 2012b). Because it is difficult to perform a funduscopic examination on older patients without the benefit of a mydriatic agent, referral for specialized ophthalmological examination is essential. The ophthalmological examination may reveal increased IOP or signs of optic nerve damage without increased pressure.

Diagnostic tests: Visual acuity should be measured and compared with prior measurements; pupillary assessment should be included. A dilated funduscopic examination and slit lamp examination of the anterior segment is conducted, assessing cup-to-disc ratio, asymmetry between discs, or other abnormalities. Applanation tonometry with the Goldmann applanation criterion standard should be measured to determine IOP. IOP has a circadian rhythm and is highest in the morning. Time of day, method, and measurements in both eyes are noted and compared with any prior measurements. If glaucoma is suspected, pachymetry should be used to measure central corneal thickness. If corneal thickness is outside of an established normal range, an adjustment in the IOP number is made based on this, raising or lowering the number. Because a thin central cornea is a risk factor, those with thicker central corneas but increased IOP have a correction factor calculated into the adjusted IOP (AAO Chronic Glaucoma, 2012; Bell, 2012).

Automated visual field testing is done to rule out any visual field deficits (visual field assessment by confrontation is of no value) (Jacobs, 2012a). Gonioscopy is done to rule out other causes of IOP increase, including angle-closure glaucoma. Various imaging modalities, including fundus photography, optical coherence tomography, and scanning laser polarimetry, are used to preserve a permanent visual picture of the optic disc and are to be repeated later for comparison or evidence of disease progression (Koby, 2012). At this time, imaging is still an evolving tool and its full contribution as a diagnostic entity is yet to be realized (AAO Glaucoma Panel, 2010a, 2010b).

Differential diagnosis:
- Cerebral neoplasia
- Other optic neuropathies

- Vascular occlusive disease
- Trauma

Treatment: Chronic open-angle glaucoma cannot be cured; the goal of treatment is to halt progression of the disease and preserve existing vision as follows:

- IOP control within an identified range
- Stable visual fields
- No further progression of optic nerve damage

Mainstay treatment modalities include the following:

- Topical eye drops that reduce aqueous production or encourage outflow
- Laser trabeculoplasty
- Trabeculectomy or filtering surgery

Medical treatment with eye drops is usually first-line therapy unless there are contraindications. Consultation between primary care provider and ophthalmologist may be indicated for patient safety and accurate identification of comorbidities and current medications (Table 7-1).

If topical ophthalmic agents do not effectively lower IOP, systemic carbonic anhydrase inhibitors are added. These also may be used before surgery to lower the IOP. If medical therapy is unsuccessful, selective laser trabeculoplasty or filtration surgery

TABLE 7-1 Glaucoma Drugs				
DRUG CLASS	**ACTION**	**EXAMPLES**	**SIDE EFFECTS**	**CONTRAINDICATIONS**
Prostaglandin analog	Lower IOP 25%–30% by increasing trabecular or uveoscleral outflow Once-daily dosing	Lantanoprost Travoprost Bimatoprost Tafluprost	Iris color change, uveitis, eyelash growth, conjunctival injection	History of herpes keratitis, macular edema
Beta blockers	Decrease aqueous production; lower IOP 20%–25%	Betaxalol Carteolol Levobunolol Metipranolol (OptiPranolol) Timolol gel	Fatigue, bronchospasm, hypotension, bradycardia, corneal toxicity, depression, impotence	Congestive heart failure (cardiology consult) Nonselective are contraindicated in asthma, chronic obstructive pulmonary disease Hypotension, >first-degree heart block
Adrenergic agonists	Decrease aqueous production, enhance aqueous outflow; lower IOP 20%–25%	Apraclonidine Brimonidine Dipivefrin Epinephrine	Conjunctival injection, fatigue, headache	Use of monoamine oxidase inhibitors

TABLE 7-1	Glaucoma Drugs—cont'd			
DRUG CLASS	**ACTION**	**EXAMPLES**	**SIDE EFFECTS**	**CONTRAINDICATIONS**
Parasympathomimetic agents	Increase trabecular outflow; lower IOP 20%–25%	Pilocarpine Carbachol	Corneal toxicity Increased myopia Cataract Decreased vision	Other types of malignant glaucoma
Carbonic anhydrase inhibitors (primarily oral route)	Decrease aqueous production; lower IOP 15%–20%	*Topical:* Dorzolamide Brinzolamide *Oral:* Acetazolamide Acetazolamide sustained release Dichlorphenamide Methazolamide	*Topical:* Corneal edema, metallic taste, conjunctivitis *Oral:* Stevens-Johnson syndrome Metallic taste Renal calculi Aplastic anemia Thrombocytopenia	Sulfa allergy Sickle cell disease Renal calculi Thrombocytopenia

(trabeculectomy), to improve aqueous outflow, is indicated. The laser treatment is considered for elderly patients who cannot tolerate surgery, although the outcome is not as desirable as with surgery. In either case, medication still may be required after surgery (AAO Glaucoma Panel, 2010a; Jacobs, 2012b).

The Food and Drug Administration (FDA) has approved the use of a miniscule device called the Glaukos iStent® Trabecular Micro-Bypass Stent for patients with glaucoma and cataract. At the conclusion of cataract surgery, this stent is inserted into the canal of Schlemm, allowing the aqueous humor to bypass trabecular obstruction and drain directly from the anterior chamber into Schlemm's canal, lowering IOP (AAO Podcast, 2012; Nichamin, 2009).

Follow-up: Monitor patients for compliance with the treatment regimen. If eye drops are used, ensure that the patient can instill these, or teach a family member or neighbor to do it. Monitor medications for adverse effects; the range and frequency of side effects to glaucoma medications are significant. Ensure that patients have regular ophthalmological follow-up visits. If visual loss is severe, evaluate the environment for safety and risk of falls or injury. If the patient is still a licensed motor vehicle operator, driver's license retesting may be indicated in the interest of public safety.

Sequelae: If initial presentation is monocular, the other eye may become affected. Changes in the patient's overall health may have implications for the treatment plan.

Prevention/prophylaxis: The U.S. Preventive Services Task Force (USPSTF) found insufficient evidence to recommend screening for glaucoma (USPSTF, 2005). A more recent Cochrane Review concurred with insufficient evidence for screening (Hatt, Wormald, Burr, & Wormald, 2009). Primary care providers need to be aware of risk factors and discuss these with patients who have not been diagnosed but are at risk. Patients who are glaucoma suspects or have actual primary open-angle glaucoma must be reminded of the need for eye examinations, continued monitoring, and adherence to the prescribed regimen. African Americans should have periodic eye examinations every 3 to 5 years, beginning at age 40. Anyone with a family history of glaucoma should have an annual eye examination, beginning at age 40. Patients with hypertension or diabetes should have regular eye examinations, as recommended by their health-care provider. All patients over 65 years old should have annual eye examinations (AAO Glaucoma Panel, 2010a, 2010b). Recently, Li, Ervin, Scherer, Jampel, and Dickersin (2009) identified areas for research related to the Preferred Practice Patterns of the AAO and the need to measure outcomes of interventions.

Referral: Refer patients initially for ophthalmological examination and diagnosis. Collaborate on the management plan if the patient has significant medical conditions that affect treatment options, particularly pharmacological choices. Refer patients for periodic follow-up eye examinations or for treatment of complications if they arise.

Education: Educate the patient about the chronic and progressive nature of the disease, the need to follow the treatment regimen as prescribed, and the need for regular follow-up eye examinations and reporting of symptoms if any. Reassure the patient that, although the disease is not curable, it can be managed. Educate patients with known risk factors about the need for eye examinations despite the absence of symptoms. Asymptomatic patients may question the need for regular treatment; explain that treatment is preventing disease progression, which is why there are no symptoms. The frequency or complexity of the medication regimen may influence compliance; reinforce the role of medication in controlling IOP and preventing visual loss.

CLINICAL RECOMMENDATION	EVIDENCE RATING	REFERENCES
Prostaglandin analogs are the most effective drugs at lowering IOP and can be considered as initial medical therapy unless other considerations, such as cost, side effects, intolerance, or patient refusal, preclude this.	A	AAO Glaucoma Panel (2010b)
IOP is measured in each eye, preferably by Goldmann applanation tonometry, before gonioscopy or dilation of the pupil.	A	AAO Glaucoma Panel (2010a, 2012b)
Measurement of central corneal thickness (CCT) aids the interpretation of IOP readings and helps to stratify patient risk for ocular damage.	B	AAO Glaucoma Panel (2010a, 2012b)
The IOP can be lowered by medical treatment, laser therapy, or incisional glaucoma surgery (alone or in combination). The choice of initial therapy depends on numerous considerations, and discussion of treatment with the patient should include the relative risks and benefits of the three options.	B	AAO Glaucoma Panel (2010a)

A = consistent, good-quality, patient-oriented evidence; B = inconsistent or limited-quality, patient-oriented evidence; C = consensus, disease-oriented evidence, usual practice, expert opinion, or case series. For information about the SORT evidence rating system, go to www.aafp.org/afpsort.xml.

EPISTAXIS

Signal symptom: Bleeding from the nose.

Etiology: Epistaxis results from a spontaneous rupture of a blood vessel in the nose, usually in the anterior septum in Kiesselbach's plexus (Nguyen, 2012). The bleeding may be secondary to local infections, systemic infections, drying of the nasal mucous membrane, trauma, arteriosclerosis, hypertension, or bleeding disorders. Trauma is usually the primary mechanism of disruption of the nasal mucosa. Posterior epistaxis can result in nausea and respiratory compromise. In older adults, nasal and paranasal tumors may be involved (Mäkitie, 2010).

Occurrence: Most people have at least one episode of minor, nonrecurring epistaxis. Because self-treatment is often effective and the episode is not reported, statistical data are scarce. Several sources indicate a lifetime incidence of 60% with more than 10% requiring medical intervention (Nguyen, 2012). The incidence of epistaxis is higher in winter when heating causes drying and cracking of nasal mucosa. Epistaxis is rare without trauma in patients with hypertension or hemophilia but is characteristic of von Willebrand's disease (Ruhl, 2011).

Age: Epistaxis occurs most frequently in children and in elderly persons.

Gender: Epistaxis occurs more frequently in males than in females (Cusik & Clenney, 2005; Nguyen, 2012).

Ethnicity: No ethnic groups are significantly more prone to epistaxis.

Contributing factors: Local trauma to the anterior portions of the nose (digital, as in picking the nose, and blunt, as in nasal fractures) is usually the cause of epistaxis. Foreign bodies, intranasal polyps or neoplasms, irritants (smoking), intranasal steroids, local infections such as rhinitis and sinusitis, systemic medications such as anticoagulants, antiplatelets, NSAIDs, and aspirin may contribute secondarily to the occurrence of epistaxis. Septal deviation or perforation is also a contributing factor. Systemic problems including hypertension and bleeding disorders, such as aplastic anemia, leukemia, thrombocytopenia, liver disease, and hereditary coagulopathies, may also contribute to the occurrence of epistaxis (Blomgren, 2011; Cusik & Clenney, 2005; Nguyen, 2012).

Signs and symptoms: Usually no signs or symptoms are associated with epistaxis other than the awareness of blood dripping down the posterior nasopharynx as well as external bleeding.

Diagnostic tests: No laboratory studies are indicated for minor and nonrecurring epistaxis. For more substantial or recurrent epistaxis, a complete blood count including platelet count, bleeding time, prothrombin time, and partial thromboplastin time may be useful. In a patient who is on warfarin therapy, an international normalized ratio (INR) should be drawn if epistaxis occurs (Konkle, 2012). If bleeding is severe and the need for blood replacement is anticipated, type and crossmatch should also be done.

Differential diagnosis:
- Trauma
- Inflammation due to rhinitis or infection
- Vascular disorders
- Clotting disorders and blood dyscrasias
- Intranasal foreign bodies
- Hereditary telangiectasia
- Tumors

Treatment: Most episodes of epistaxis are mild and self-limited, resolving spontaneously. Epistaxis may be controlled by pinching the nasal alae together for 5 to 10 minutes, keeping the patient in an erect sitting position with head tilted forward to prevent blood from going down the posterior nasopharynx. A nasal vasoconstrictor, such as oxymetazolone 0.05% or phenylephrine, may be placed in the vestibule of the nose and pressed against the bleeding site to promote vasoconstriction. An ice pack can be applied over the nose for additional therapy. The mucous membrane can be anesthetized with 4% lidocaine topically, and a silver nitrate stick can be applied to the site of bleeding once it is located. Other devices include nasal tampons such as Merocel or balloons for packing. The user must be skilled in handling these devices properly. Older patients must be assessed for any breathing problems as well as for heavy bleeding. Comorbidities may necessitate admission or referral to an ears, nose, and throat (ENT) specialist for management (Bamimore & Silverberg, 2012). If packing is needed, adequate pain management must be prescribed also.

Follow-up: For recurrent episodes, follow-up visits are recommended as needed. If medications have been implicated as likely causes, follow-up by a home health nurse for medication management education may be helpful.

Sequelae: Anemia can be a complication of excessive or frequent bouts of epistaxis. Infection can result from nasal packing as well as from septal perforation.

Prevention/prophylaxis: Discourage patients from picking, constant rubbing, and excessively forceful blowing of the nose and advise them to increase the humidity in the home, especially in winter months. Some patients may be prescribed bacitracin or petrolatum topical to instill twice weekly in the area of Kiesselbach's plexus (Nguyen, 2012).

Referral: Consultation with an ENT specialist is indicated for the following conditions:

- Bleeding that is not controlled after 15 minutes of compression
- Evidence of massive bleeding

- Recurrent bleeding within the first hour
- Second episode of epistaxis within 1 week
- Uncontrolled bleeding from the posterior nasopharynx

The consulting physician may initiate interventions such as the insertion of Merocel nasal tampons or an intranasal balloon to control bleeding. Intractable epistaxis may require transantral arterial ligation or embolization (Bamimore & Silverberg, 2012).

Education: Discourage picking of the nose and advise patients to increase the humidity in the home, especially in winter months, by means of a humidifier. Petrolatum may be rubbed over the nasal septum twice daily to decrease dryness of mucosa. Teach the patient how to manage simple epistaxis at home, and instruct him or her to seek medical attention for excessive (bleeding for more than 1 hour) or recurrent epistaxis. Use of nasal saline spray for humidification is encouraged. Prolonged hot showers and hot, spicy foods should be avoided. Instruct the patient to avoid nose blowing and to open the mouth when sneezing (Nguyen, 2012).

CLINICAL RECOMMENDATION	EVIDENCE RATING	REFERENCES
Simple measures are helpful in stopping most nosebleeds: nose blowing to clear clots, pinching the nose for 15 minutes, and topical decongestants.	C	Ruhl (2011)
Cauterizing visible bleeding vessels with silver nitrate (AgNO$_3$) or electrocautery are equally effective.	B	Ruhl (2011)
Patients with resistant or posterior bleeds are likely to need posterior packing, surgery, or embolization.	C	Ruhl (2011)
Routine coagulation tests for epistaxis are not useful unless the patient is taking an anticoagulant.	B	Ruhl (2011)

A = consistent, good-quality, patient-oriented evidence; B = inconsistent or limited-quality, patient-oriented evidence; C = consensus, disease-oriented evidence, usual practice, expert opinion, or case series. For information about the SORT evidence rating system, go to www.aafp.org/afpsort.xml.

HEARING LOSS

Signal symptoms: Can hear but not understand, especially in a group; turning up radio or television louder to hear (noted by family or neighbors); inability to hear in one ear; tinnitus; feeling like people are "mumbling." Because presbycusis is gradual and insidious, hearing loss may go unnoticed until it has progressed significantly.

Description: Hearing loss is the decreased ability or complete inability to hear. The loss may involve the external, middle, or inner ear and can be unilateral or bilateral.

Etiology:

Sensorineural: A lesion in the organ of Corti or in the central pathways, including the eighth nerve and auditory cortex, causes sensorineural hearing loss. Presbycusis, noise-induced hearing loss, and ototoxic drug-related hearing loss all are sensorineural. Because there is no cure for this, amplification is usually required (Yueh & Shekelle, 2007).

Conductive: Conductive hearing loss is caused by a lesion involving the outer and middle ear to the level of the oval window. Various structural abnormalities, cerumen impaction, perforation of the tympanic membrane, middle ear fluid, damage to the ossicles from trauma or infection, otosclerosis, tympanosclerosis, cholesteatoma, middle ear tumors, temporal bone fractures, injuries related to trauma, and congenital problems are some of the causes.

Mixed: Mixed hearing loss includes sensorineural and conductive components.

Retrocochlear: Retrocochlear hearing loss is caused by a lesion between the cochlea and the brain such as an acoustic neuroma or a meningioma.

Occurrence: From 20% to 40% in adults over 50 years old and more than 80% for those over 80 years old; it is the most common sensory deficit in older adults (Lin, Thorpe, Gordon-Salant, & Ferucci, 2011).

Age: Sensorineural hearing loss increases with age.

Ethnicity: No ethnic groups are significantly more prone to hearing loss.

Gender: Presbycusis is more severe in men than in women; this is attributed to environmental causes.

Contributing factors: Exposure to loud noises; heredity; ototoxic drugs, such as aminoglycoside antibiotics, salicylates, loop diuretics, cisplatin, and quinine; eustachian tube obstruction; chronic middle ear infections; and chronic cerumen impaction are contributing factors. Most cases of sudden unilateral hearing loss in elderly persons are due to thrombotic or embolic obstruction of the internal auditory artery.

Signs and symptoms: The patient may complain that people mumble. There may be difficulty hearing associated with pain, pressure, discomfort, vertigo, or loss of balance. Associated symptoms may include tinnitus, dizziness, blockage, popping, pressure, crackling, trouble hearing distant sounds, or stiffness. A history of noise exposure, prior ear problems, or familial hearing problems is significant.

Otoscopic examination and inspection of the external auditory canal and middle ear may reveal redness, foreign objects, discharge, scaling, lesions, fluid, or cerumen impaction. Expect to see minimal cerumen, a pink color, and hairs in the outer one-third of the ear. The tympanic membrane should have no perforations and should be a translucent pearly gray; changes in the tympanic membrane may be consistent with conductive hearing loss.

Diagnostic tests: Awareness on the part of primary care providers to ask about or screen for hearing loss in older adults is a critical first step to diagnosis (Bentur, Valinsky, Lemberger, Ben Moshe, & Heymann,

2012). The self-administered Hearing Handicap in the Elderly (HHIE-S) is a 10-question instrument that can be given to patients in the waiting room or administered in the long-term care setting (Bushman, Belza, & Christianson, 2012; Chou, Dana, Bougatsos, Fleming, & Beil, 2011; Yueh & Shekelle, 2007). Alternatively, asking a single question,—"Do you have a hearing problem now?"—can be effective in uncovering a problem. Use of a portable pure-tone audiometer in the primary care office is also a quick screening test, and a medical assistant or office nurse can be instructed in how to administer the test and record results. Anyone with a hearing threshold of 40 dB or greater should be referred to audiology for evaluation. If there is a history of trauma or sudden hearing loss, urgent consultation with an otolaryngologist is warranted, and a computed tomography (CT) may be ordered. The Weber and Rinne are not good screening tests for hearing loss, but they can help to identify if the loss is sensorineural or conductive (Pacala & Yueh, 2012).

Differential diagnosis:
- Ménière's disease
- Acoustic neuroma (unilateral, with tinnitus)
- Cholesteatoma (unilateral)
- Embolic or thrombotic phenomenon, associated with hypertension (sudden onset, unilateral)
- Meningioma (unilateral)
- Trauma (history of ear trauma, unilateral)
- Otitis media with effusion (retracted tympanic membrane, fluid behind tympanic membrane)
- Acute otitis media (unilateral, ear pain; bulging, immobile tympanic membrane)
- Central auditory processing disorder (seen in dementia)

Treatment: Treat the cause or refer the patient as appropriate. Encouragement, follow-up, and support are important for the patient with hearing loss.

Cerumen impaction: Treat the patient with cerumenolytic agents, manual removal, or irrigation followed by manual removal as needed (Roland et al., 2008). If cerumen impaction is a chronic problem, instruct the patient on instillation of an over-the-counter (OTC) agent to soften cerumen.

Acute otitis media: Antibiotic treatment; an analgesic, such as acetaminophen or an NSAID, may be indicated for pain initially.

In the presence of *tympanic perforation, ossicle damage, tumor, tympanosclerosis, otosclerosis, sudden hearing loss,* or *temporal bone injury,* refer the patient to a specialist (Weber, 2012b, 2012d).

Presbycusis: Educate and support the patient so that no further damage occurs. Have the patient reduce noise exposure and avoid ototoxic medications. Refer to an audiologist for hearing aid evaluation. Refer the patient for lip-reading instruction when appropriate, and instruct the family to speak clearly. Consult a hearing rehabilitation company about the availability of special audio equipment. Patients with profound hearing loss should also be evaluated for suitability for cochlear implant (Blevins, 2012; Raman et al., 2011).

Follow-up: See patients as indicated by the cause of the symptom.

Sequelae: Possible complications depend on the cause of the symptom but may include permanent hearing loss. The patient may need a hearing aid or assistive listening device. Middle ear problems may progress to chronic ear problems such as perforations and cholesteatoma. Social isolation and depression may result from inability to communicate.

Prevention/prophylaxis: Advise the patient to use protective devices to guard against occupational or recreational hearing loss, to equalize ear pressure when diving, to chew gum or use decongestants in airplanes, to avoid flying or diving if upper respiratory infection is present, and to avoid ototoxic medications. Teach the patient proper techniques for cerumen removal and avoidance of Q-tips–type ear swabs or other foreign bodies in the ear. Hearing screening tests are recommended for persons over 65 years old and persons who report hearing difficulty. The USPSTF recently revised its recommendation and does not recommend periodic screening for hearing loss in asymptomatic adults (USPSTF, 2012). The American Speech-Language-Hearing Association recommends screening every 3 years for adults more than 50 years of age (American Speech-Language-Hearing Association, 1997). Residents of long-term care facilities should be screened for hearing loss on admission and as needed thereafter (Adams-Wendling, Pimple, Adams, & Titler, 2008).

Referral: Refer to or consult with appropriate specialist as indicated by cause of symptom. All patients with unexplained hearing loss should have an otoscopic and audiometric evaluation.

Education: Explain cause of symptoms, measures taken to determine the cause, and symptomatic treatment if any. Advise the patient when to seek medical care. Teach the importance of using hearing aids, if indicated, because this can make a significant difference in the patient's quality of life. Older patients with multiple comorbidities may require the services of a multidisciplinary team to learn how to use a hearing aid effectively (Pacala & Yueh, 2012). Advise the patient to contact rehabilitation centers to learn lip-reading skills or sign language if a hearing aid is not indicated. Hearing rehabilitation services can also assess the need for assistive devices such as flashing smoke detector alarms, an amplified telephone, or an amplified television device. Provide support, and help the patient resist the temptation to withdraw socially. Caution the patient to avoid solicitation by hearing aid salespeople, particularly if they are offering a device without proper testing of the patient or a device that is very inexpensive. For patients in a long-term care setting, education of staff is essential to enhance communication and improve quality of life (Adams-Wendling et al., 2008; Harkin & Kelleher, 2011).

CLINICAL RECOMMENDATION	EVIDENCE RATING	REFERENCES
The USPSTF concludes that the current evidence is insufficient to assess the balance of benefits and harms of screening for hearing loss in asymptomatic adults ≥ 50 years. This recommendation applies to asymptomatic adults ≥ 50 years. It does not apply to persons seeking evaluation for perceived hearing problems or for cognitive or affective symptoms that may be related to hearing loss. These persons should be assessed for objective hearing impairment and treated when indicated.	B	USPSTF (2012)
Sudden hearing loss warrants urgent evaluation and treatment by a specialist.	C	Gross (2011a)

CLINICAL RECOMMENDATION	EVIDENCE RATING	REFERENCES
Patients who report hearing loss should be referred for full audiometry.	C	Gross (2011a)
Order imaging and/or ears, nose, and throat referral if vertigo, sudden onset, neurological symptoms, unilateral loss, or primarily low-frequency loss.	C	Gross (2011a, 2011b)
Patients with presbycusis may benefit from amplification or assistive listening devices.	C	Gross (2011b)

A = consistent, good-quality, patient-oriented evidence; B = inconsistent or limited-quality, patient-oriented evidence; C = consensus, disease-oriented evidence, usual practice, expert opinion, or case series. For information about the SORT evidence rating system, go to www.aafp.org/afpsort.xml.

HORDEOLUM AND CHALAZION

Signal symptoms: Increased lacrimation with lump on eyelid.

Description: A hordeolum (stye) is an acute, purulent area of inflammation in the meibomian gland or gland of Zeis, commonly referred to as a "stye." The hordeolum typically contains *Staphylococcus aureus* bacteria; it can occur internally (underside of the eyelid) or externally at the lid margin (Ghosh & Ghosh, 2012). A chalazion is a mass on the eyelid caused by an inflammation of a meibomian (oil-secreting) gland of the upper or lower eyelid. Meibomian glands lubricate the lid margins. The chalazion is more chronic in nature, painless, and lipogranulomatous without erythema. It can interfere with vision at times and develops a rubbery consistency (Papier, Tuttle, & Mahar, 2007).

Etiology: Blockage in a duct leading to the eyelid surface from the meibomian gland or obstruction of the gland of Zeis results in inflammation or infection (usually from *Staphylococcus*)—hordeolum. If the blockage becomes chronic, progressing to the formation of a hard granulomatous mass, it is called a chalazion.

Occurrence: Common.

Age: Hordeolum and chalazion can occur at any age.

Gender: Hordeolum and chalazion occur equally in men and in women.

Ethnicity: No ethnic groups are significantly more prone to hordeolum or chalazion.

Contributing factors: Previously unresolved blepharitis, poor hygiene, immunosuppression, and skin conditions, such as acne rosacea or seborrheic dermatitis, all are contributing factors to development of hordeolum or chalazion (Bron, 2012).

Signs and symptoms: A hordeolum is painful and erythematous; it may present initially as a grossly swollen and tender eyelid, then localize (Bessette, 2012). A chalazion is a slow-developing painless hard mass, with inflammation of the meibomian gland and possible involvement of the surrounding tissue. Physical examination with inversion of the eyelid reveals a red elevated mass that may become large and press against the cornea.

Diagnostic tests: None unless recurrent, then biopsy of lesion to rule out malignancy.

Differential diagnosis:
- Foreign body
- Contact dermatitis
- Rosacea
- Atopic dermatitis
- Blepharitis
- Orbital cellulitis
- Sebaceous gland carcinoma (Papier et al., 2007)

Treatment: Warm compresses are applied to the affected eyelid for 10 minutes, 4 times daily, to facilitate opening and drainage. Allow purulent lesions to drain without squeezing them. Massage of the eyelid after warm compresses may help to soften secretions. In cases of secondary infection, antibiotic eye drops or ointment may be used; combination antibiotic and steroid should be used only by an ophthalmologist. If the hordeolum progresses to preseptal cellulitis, prescribe a systemic antibiotic such as cephalexin or dicloxacillin. Treatment of chalazion includes warm compresses for 15 minutes 4 times a day. Incision and drainage by an ophthalmologist may be needed if there is no resolution after 2 months. A large nondraining hordeolum or chalazion may require emergency treatment if cellulitis occurs (Bessette, 2012).

Follow-up: See patient in 2 to 4 weeks to evaluate treatment (Ehrenhaus & Sturridge, 2012).

Sequelae: Complete resolution may take several weeks to months; frequent recurrence may indicate underlying malignancy.

Prevention/prophylaxis: Prevention strategies include advising the patient to perform proper lid hygiene (helps prevent recurrence) by gently scrubbing lids with diluted baby shampoo daily or directly applying baby shampoo with cotton-tipped applicator, then rinsing. Frequent hand washing is advised. Warm compresses should be initiated at the first sign of eyelid irritation or if chalazion starts to return; a clean cloth should be used for each warm compress to eye (Ehrenhaus & Sturridge, 2012).

Referral: Refer to or consult with an ophthalmologist if the patient has a visual change, eye pain, or impairment to the eye or if the chalazion does not heal spontaneously in 6 weeks, because surgical removal may be necessary.

Education: Explain the problem and treatment. Discuss prevention strategies.

CLINICAL RECOMMENDATION	EVIDENCE RATING	REFERENCES
Initial treatment includes warm compresses 4 times daily and topical erythromycin ointment for hordeolum.	C	Wolter (2011)
Lesions refractory to treatment should be referred for incision and drainage (both hordeolum and chalazion).	C	Wolter (2011)
Intralesional triamcinolone is an effective alternative to incision and drainage of chalazion.	C	Ben Simon et al. (2005)
Sebaceous carcinoma should be suspected in patients who are middle-aged and older with persistent chalazia.	C	Wolter (2011)

A = consistent, good-quality, patient-oriented evidence; B = inconsistent or limited-quality, patient-oriented evidence; C = consensus, disease-oriented evidence, usual practice, expert opinion, or case series. For information about the SORT evidence rating system, go to www.aafp.org/afpsort.xml.

AGE-RELATED MACULAR DEGENERATION

Signal symptoms:

Dry, atrophic: Insidious loss of central vision, blurred or fuzzy vision (late), straight lines appear wavy.

Wet, exudative or neovascular: Dramatic, accelerated central vision loss in a period of weeks to a couple of months.

Description: Age-related macular degeneration (ARMD) is a disorder affecting the macula in the middle of the retina. The macula comprises millions of photoreceptor cells containing visual pigments for central vision; these are nourished by the retinal pigment epithelium (RPE), part of a complex basement membrane that becomes sclerotic with age. There are two types of ARMD, wet and dry. Dry ARMD is most common, accounting for 90% of cases. Onset of visual loss is gradual and may not be noticed if only one eye is affected. The cause is unknown, but there is disintegration of the retinal pigment epithelium and light-sensing cells (Klingler & Bakri, 2012). A small percentage of dry ARMD progresses to wet ARMD (Arroyo, 2012). Wet ARMD occurs in 10% of cases but accounts for 90% of all ARMD blindness. Neovascularization of the choroid area with leakage of new blood vessels and fluid into the retinal pigment epithelium causes scarring and damage to the macula (Moutray & Chakravarthy, 2011).

Etiology: Unknown; for wet ARMD, it is hypothesized that an angiogenic, hypoxia-related factor is responsible for neovascularization of retina and iris. This factor is called vascular endothelial growth factor (VEGF) (Klingler & Bakri, 2012; Moutray & Chakravarthy, 2011).

Occurrence: Common; macular degeneration is the leading cause of legal blindness in adults over 55 years old. Risk rises with age; occurrence is 30% in adults over 75 years old. According to the National Eye Institute, more than 2 million people ages 50 years and older have advanced ARMD, the stage leading to significant vision impairment.

Gender: Most sources report equal distribution between male and female, but some identify women as having increased risk (Prall, Ciulla, Criswell, & Harris, 2012).

Ethnicity: Caucasians are more likely to experience visual loss from AMD than are African Americans.

Contributing factors: Risk factors for ARMD include family history, smoking, exposure to sunlight, and nutritional deficits. Genetic factors and obesity are also risk factors; recent research points to polymorphisms in the complement pathway, some of which are inflammatory and others of which are protective (AAO Retina Panel, 2008; Moutray & Chakravarthy, 2011; Prall et al., 2012). History of ARMD in one eye is a risk factor for developing it in the other eye; 10% have binocular ARMD within 1 year (Koby, 2012).

Signs and symptoms: In dry ARMD, there are no symptoms initially, particularly if it is monocular. Later, patients may note a decrease in visual acuity or blurred vision that improves in bright light. In wet ARMD, straight lines appear wavy, and there may be a hole in central vision. White-yellow drusen spots are seen on funduscopic examination; Amsler grid test reveals wavy lines or missing lines in central vision. Funduscopic examination reveals choroidal neovascular membranes (CNVMs); subretinal fluid, hemorrhage, and subretinal lipid deposits may also be present (Arroyo, 2012a; Prall et al., 2012).

Diagnostic tests: All patients should have a comprehensive eye examination by an ophthalmologist, including visual acuity with best correction, funduscopic examination, Amsler grid, fluorescein angiography, and fundus photos, including optical coherence tomography (OCT) (AAO Retina Panel, 2008; Koby, 2012).

Differential diagnosis:
- Unexplained loss of visual acuity
- Diabetic retinopathy
- Ocular histoplasmosis
- Trauma with scar
- Hypertension

Treatment: There is no treatment for dry ARMD at present. The Age-Related Eye Disease Study (AREDS) found that patients at high risk of advanced ARMD lowered their risk by 25% when treated with high doses of vitamin C, vitamin E, beta carotene, zinc oxide, and cupric oxide; use of beta carotene is associated with an increased risk of lung cancer in smokers. There was no benefit to this therapy seen in patients without ARMD or with early ARMD, and subsequent analysis has called results of the AREDS into question (Evans & Lawrenson, 2012). The AREDS II evaluating the effect of lutein and omega-3 fish oil on macular degeneration is currently under analysis (www.areds2.org). Low-vision enhancement aids are available to help patients with dry ARMD.

Several new treatment options for wet or exudative ARMD are currently being used, with more in development (Arroyo, 2012b; Moutray & Chakravarthy, 2011; Prall et al., 2012). First-line therapy includes monoclonal antibodies that have anti-VEGF abilities. These drugs are injected directly into the vitreous area of the eye. They bind with the angiogenic VEGF or receptor and interrupt the neovascularization. They are not able to repair the basic defect or attack the source of VEGF, so they must be used repeatedly to suppress the angiogenic process (Arroyo, 2012b; Klingler & Bakri, 2012). Ranibizumab and bevacizumab are two humanized monoclonal antibodies that are used to treat wet ARMD successfully, although they are not successful in all patients with wet ARMD (AAO Retina Panel, 2008; Arroyo, 2012b; Moutray & Chakravarthy, 2011; Prall et al., 2012). They are injected intravitreally at monthly intervals; current focus is on determining optimal spacing and length of treatment for best results. Local side effects include eye pain, uveitis, and endophthalmitis. There are also potential systemic cardiovascular and thrombotic effects from these drugs, although they have proved minimal (Moutray & Chakravarthy, 2011). Pegaptanib, an earlier anti-VEGF drug, was not shown to be as effective in treatment and is no longer recommended in the United Kingdom (National Institute for Health and Care Excellence [NICE], 2008/2012); nor is it used much in the United States. Aflibercept is a newer agent that improves visual outcomes with less frequent injections; preliminary studies show it to be as effective as ranibizumab, with better outcomes in visual acuity and less frequent dosing or maintenance; further studies are in progress (Arroyo, 2012b; Prall et al., 2012). Laser photocoagulation therapy is no longer first-line treatment since the advent of anti-VEGF therapies. Photodynamic therapy is now being studied as a possible combination therapy with anti-VEGF treatment (Arroyo, 2012b). Research into retinal cell transplantation and submacular surgery has yielded disappointing results; likewise, use of statins for ARMD has not shown positive results (Arroyo, 2012b; Prall et al., 2012). Research is currently underway to find safe, effective treatments for both dry and wet ARMD.

Follow-up: All patients with ARMD should be seen periodically by an ophthalmologist for reevaluation of disease progression and, where applicable, further treatment. Patients may be given an Amsler grid to use weekly or monthly to check for visual changes. A recent study suggesting sustained increases in IOP after repeated anti-VEGF injections in all patients, not just those with known glaucoma, is concerning, and further research is needed. IOP should be monitored in patients receiving anti-VEGF therapy (Hoang et al., 2012).

Sequelae: Loss of central vision limits functional capacity and ability to read. Most ARMD patients cannot drive. Environmental safety also is compromised; falls and hip fractures can occur in patients with ARMD. Patients using high-dose vitamin and mineral therapy may have yellowing of skin; smokers are at increased risk of lung cancer from beta carotene.

Prevention/prophylaxis: There is no specific prevention. The USPSTF has determined that there is not enough evidence to support visual screening of older adults for ARMD (USPSTF, 2009). Annual eye examinations in persons over 65 years old can facilitate early detection and, in the case of wet AMD, early intervention to limit visual loss. Smokers should be encouraged to quit.

Referral: All patients over 65 years old should be referred to an ophthalmologist for an annual eye examination. Patients under 65 years old with visual symptoms also should be referred. Patients with ARMD should be referred to the local chapter of the Blind Association for services, vision enhancement devices, and support groups.

Education: Teach patients the importance of seeking evaluation for visual symptoms as soon as they occur. Explain disease process and community support services. Educate family about need for environmental safety. Caution patients to avoid unproven remedies.

CLINICAL RECOMMENDATION	EVIDENCE RATING	REFERENCES
Anti-VEGF injections are first-line agents to treat wet ARMD.	A	Federici (2011)
Patients with early ARMD or a family history of ARMD should be encouraged to have regular dilated eye examinations for the early detection of intermediate-stage ARMD.	A	AAO Retina Panel (2008)
Dry ARMD cannot be treated.	C	Federici (2011)

A = consistent, good-quality, patient-oriented evidence; B = inconsistent or limited-quality, patient-oriented evidence; C = consensus, disease-oriented evidence, usual practice, expert opinion, or case series. For information about the SORT evidence rating system, go to www.aafp.org/afpsort.xml.

ORAL CANCER

Signal symptoms: Nonhealing sore in the mouth or lip, unexplained lymph node swelling in head/neck area.

Description: Oral cancer is a malignant tumor of the oral squamous epithelium. The most common sites are the floor of the mouth, tongue, oropharynx, and lips. The rare tumors of the upper gingiva and hard palate are usually salivary gland adenocarcinomas (Goldstein & Goldstein, 2012; Kademani, 2007).

Etiology: Oral cancers are associated with chronic irritation of the squamous epithelial lining of the oral cavity. Tobacco (cigarette, pipe, cigar) smoking, use of smokeless tobacco, and heavy alcohol use are risk factors. In younger patients, human papillomavirus (HPV) has been implicated as a primary factor in oral cancer (Contessa, Lloyd, & Decker, 2011).

Occurrence: The National Cancer Institute Surveillance Epidemiology and End Results (SEER) estimates that in 2013, 41,380 people in the United States will be diagnosed with cancer of the oral cavity and pharynx, and 7890 men and women will die of this disease; this does not include cancer of the tongue. In recent years, the incidence of lip cancer has declined, whereas the number of tongue cancers has increased.

Age: The median age at diagnosis for cancer of the tongue from 2005 to 2009 in the United States was 61 years of age; the median age for death from this cancer was 66 years old. The median age at diagnosis for cancer of the oral cavity and pharynx was 62 years between 2005 and 2009, with 67 years being the median age of death (SEER stat fact sheets, 2012).

Gender: Previously, men were 3 to 4 times more likely to have oral cancer, but the gap is narrowing.

Ethnicity: The incidence of oral cancer is declining among white men but is increasing among African American men and all women. Worldwide, Southeast Asians have the highest rates of oral cancer.

Contributing factors: Tobacco use and heavy alcohol consumption, alone or synergistically, are strongly related to the development of oral cancer. Pipe smoking and sun exposure have been implicated in lip cancer. Leukoplakia and erythroplasia are often precursors to oral cancer. Relationships between oral cancer and Epstein-Barr virus, HPV, herpes simplex virus, and immunodeficiency states also have been found (Stenson, 2011). No strong association exists between irritation from dentures or teeth and oral cancers. In Asian populations, several genetic polymorphisms, combined with environmental carcinogens, have been implicated in the development of oral cancer (Chu et al., 2012; Zhang et al., 2011). Chewing Betel leaves and areca nuts in conjunction with smoking is common in India and accounts for 40% of all malignancies in that country (Kademani, 2007).

Signs and symptoms: Nonhealing, ulcerative lesions on the lip, tongue, or oral mucosa usually are noted first. Leukoplakia, a white patch on the mucosa that cannot be rubbed off, is the most common precancerous lesion. Erythroplasia, a nonpainful, red, velvety lesion, typically on the floor of the mouth, can be carcinoma in situ. Patients may complain that dental appliances are not fitting properly and that they have difficulty chewing (Poon & Stenson, 2012). Oral pain and bleeding lesions are usually late signs of malignancy. Occasionally patients may complain of numbness in the skin around the chin when the lesion involves a nerve. Enlarged submandibular or submental lymph nodes may be found in advanced disease. Unexplained weight loss may be a late symptom.

Diagnostic tests: Depending on location and potential extent of oral cancer and the possibility of second primary site or distant metastases, various diagnostic strategies will be employed by the specialist seeing the patient. Magnetic resonance imaging (MRI), CT, positron emission tomography (PET), or PET/CT will show extent of infiltration, regional lymph node spread, second primary tumors, or distant metastases. These studies are recommended before biopsy, because biopsy will distort the anatomy and may give false results on subsequent imaging studies.

Biopsy of the lesion after 2 weeks of nonhealing is recommended. In early diagnosis, a panendoscopy with selective focus (e.g., larynx, esophagus, bronchus), depending on symptoms, may be sufficient for diagnosis (Contessa et al., 2011; Poon & Stenson, 2012). If syphilis is suspected, a rapid plasma reagin (RPR) or Venereal Disease Research Laboratory (VDRL) test should be drawn.

Differential diagnosis:

- Oral candidiasis (white patches are scraped off and bleed underneath)
- Melanotic macule (rare)
- Oral lichen planus (lacy white lesions on buccal mucosa)
- Oral hairy leukoplakia
- Peutz-Jeghers syndrome (multiple lentigines of oral mucosa, associated intestinal polyposis)
- Xerostomia
- Gingivitis
- Secondary syphilitic lesion (split papules at the angle of the mouth, positive RPR or VDRL) (Gonsalves, Chi, & Neville, 2007b; Gonsalves, Wrightson, & Henry, 2008)

Treatment: The cancer is staged by oncology specialists using the American Joint Committee on Cancer (AJCC) staging system and the Union for International Cancer Control (UICC) system. Surgical excision and radiation therapy depend on the size and location of the tumor and on the presence or absence of metastases. Early-stage lesions are smaller than 4 cm. Various options for surgery in early-stage oral cancer are available, including laser and robotic minimally invasive types (Gross, Lee, Okuno, & Rao, 2012). In some cases, radiation may be the primary treatment modality. Chemotherapy is currently not a first-line therapy in early-stage oral cancers but may be used in conjunction with adjuvant therapy in more advanced cases. For patients with locoregionally advanced oral cancer, initial multidisciplinary approach includes the surgeon, radiation oncologist, and medical oncologist (Wu, Lee, Gross, & Okuno, 2011). In all patients, abstinence from tobacco and alcohol is emphasized.

Follow-up: Lifetime surveillance is recommended; second primary cancers occur in 10% to 30% of cases. During the first year, the patient should be seen frequently for focused oral examinations and to assess for recurrence of symptoms, in addition to yearly complete physical examinations. Thereafter, follow-up visits should occur as scheduled by the surgeon or oncologist. The 5-year overall survival rate by stage is approximately 80% for localized disease, 50% for regional disease, and 15% for metastatic disease (Contessa et al., 2011).

Sequelae: Complications of oral cancer include disfigurement and xerostomia from surgery and radiation treatments, malnutrition resulting from difficulty chewing, infection, second primary cancers, or metastases to the lungs, regional lymph nodes, or adjacent organs. Patients with dentures may need to abstain from wearing them for 1 year when radiation is performed.

Prevention/prophylaxis: Smoking cessation, treatment for alcoholism, adequate nutrition, and yearly oral examinations can help prevent oral cancer. Edentulous patients should remove dentures for oral examination. Wearing a hat with a brim or using lip gloss with sunscreen can prevent sun exposure of lips. The USPSTF (2004), Cochrane Database of Systematic Reviews (Brocklehurst et al., 2010), and American Dental Association Council on Scientific Affairs Expert Panel (Rethman et al., 2010) all agree that there is insufficient evidence to justify screening for oral cancer in the general population. A recent Cochrane Review found good evidence that dentists were effective in counseling patients to quit tobacco when seen for an annual examination (Carr & Ebbert, 2012).

Referral: Refer the patient to an oncologist; initial consultation with a dentist who specializes in oral cancer detection may also be indicated. Also refer the patient or his or her family to the National Cancer Institute Helpline (1-800-4-CANCER) for information about resources and support and to a local support group if available. If nutrition is a problem, refer to a nutritionist who works with cancer patients.

Education: Teach patients about the risk factors for developing oral cancer, including smoking, chewing tobacco, alcohol abuse, and poor nutrition. Discuss strategies to help the patient deal with these issues. Advise patients to report any nonhealing oral lesion within 2 weeks of onset.

CLINICAL RECOMMENDATION	EVIDENCE RATING	REFERENCES
Curative treatment for oropharyngeal cancer typically consists of surgery, radiation therapy, or radiation therapy in combination with chemotherapy.	C	National Comprehensive Cancer Network Guidelines (2012)

CLINICAL RECOMMENDATION	EVIDENCE RATING	REFERENCES
Risk factors for oropharyngeal cancer include tobacco and alcohol use as well as human papillomavirus (HPV) infection.	B	Contessa et al. (2011)
Patients presenting with metastatic disease may benefit from systemic chemotherapy, local radiation to palliate symptoms, or both.	B	Contessa et al. (2011)

A = consistent, good-quality, patient-oriented evidence; B = inconsistent or limited-quality, patient-oriented evidence; C = consensus, disease-oriented evidence, usual practice, expert opinion, or case series. For information about the SORT evidence rating system, go to www.aafp.org/afpsort.xml.

RETINOPATHY

Signal symptoms: Blurred vision, painless visual loss, poor night vision, poor color vision, floaters.

Description: Retinopathy, a disease of the retina, includes hypertensive; diabetic; and, less commonly in older adults, sickle cell; polycythemia vera; and infectious causes such as toxoplasmosis or cytomegalovirus in HIV.

Etiology: The pathology of the retinopathy relates to the underlying cause. Systemic causes common to older adults include hypertension (arteriosclerotic retinopathy), diabetes (diabetic retinopathy), and ARMD (see earlier). Hypertensive or arteriosclerotic retinopathy is related to the severity of the hypertension. Diabetic retinopathy is a highly specific vascular complication of type 1 and type 2 diabetes. It is related directly to the duration of diabetes, the patient's age at onset, and glycemic control. Diabetic retinopathy is either proliferative or nonproliferative. Nonproliferative retinopathy is most common in type 2 diabetics and is characterized by dilation of veins, microaneurysms, retinal edema and hemorrhages, and hard exudates. Proliferative retinopathy is common in type 1 diabetics and includes neovascularization, vitreous hemorrhage, and retinal detachment; secondary glaucoma also can occur because of blockage of outflow channels by new vessels. Diabetic retinopathy often coexists with hypertensive retinopathy.

Occurrence: Diabetic retinopathy is the leading cause of new blindness in people 20 to 74 years old. Type 1 diabetics usually have some retinopathy present within 5 years of diagnosis; it is found in 21% of type 2 diabetics at the time of diagnosis. Diabetic retinopathy develops earlier in older patients, but proliferative retinopathy is less common. Proliferative retinopathy is more common with insulin use. According to the National Eye Institute, diabetic retinopathy affects 4.4 million people ages 40 years and older. Hypertensive retinopathy is seen with poorly controlled hypertension (AAO, 2011).

Age: Elderly patients are more likely to have hypertensive or diabetic retinopathy because of the increase in chronic disease with age; approximately one-half of all diabetes cases occur in persons over 55 years old.

Gender: Men develop diabetic retinopathy sooner than women.

Ethnicity: Diabetes is more common in Native Americans, Asian Americans, African Americans, Hispanic Americans, and Pacific Islanders than in whites. Hypertension is also more prevalent among African Americans.

Contributing factors: Contributing factors in diabetic retinopathy include age at onset, type of diabetes, duration of disease, poor glycemic control (persistent elevated hemoglobin A1c), dyslipidemia, nephropathy, smoking, and stage at which retinopathy is detected (early detection of nonproliferative is preferred) (Fraser & D'Amico, 2011a, 2011b). Several experts (AAO Retina Panel, 2008; Fraser & D'Amico, 2011b; Rosenblatt & Benson, 2008) state that duration of disease is the best predictive factor for retinopathy.

Causes of other types of retinopathy include poorly controlled hypertension and ARMD. Multiple sclerosis, sarcoidosis, and coagulopathies are also associated with proliferative retinopathy (Bearelly, Mathura, & Jampol, 2008).

Signs and symptoms: The presenting symptom may be the insidious painless onset of decreased visual acuity. Patients may report blurred vision, poor night vision, poor color vision, or "floaters and flashers." The ophthalmoscopic examination may be the first point of detection in an asymptomatic patient. All patients with known diabetes or hypertension should have regular comprehensive eye examinations, including a funduscopic examination. The funduscopic changes seen in patients with hypertension include arteriolar narrowing, arteriovenous nicking, changes in arteriolar light reflex, and tortuosity of vessels. Classic nonproliferative changes in patients with diabetes are microaneurysms and hard and soft exudate. Clinical findings in patients with proliferative retinopathy are cotton-wool spots, deep hemorrhages, and neovascularization.

Diagnostic tests: Dilated funduscopic examination and comprehensive eye examination, fundus photos, ocular coherence tomography (OCT), and fluorescein angiography are used to diagnose diabetic retinopathy (AAO Retina Panel, 2008; Koby & Ferri, 2013). Hypertensive retinopathy is a clinical diagnosis based on physical examination findings during slit-lamp examination. Hypertensive retinopathy presents as disc edema and can be classified by ophthalmology using the Keith-Wagener-Barker classification or the Scheie classification (Rogers, 2008). Hypertensive retinopathy is often associated with a systemic disease such as left ventricular heart failure, pulmonary edema, stroke, or myocardial infarction (Rogers, 2008). Although not specific for the diagnosis of retinopathy, regular monitoring of hypertension and blood glucose is essential in disease management and prevention of complications.

Differential diagnosis:
- Retinal detachment
- Cytomegalovirus retinitis (usually associated with HIV)
- Toxoplasmosis (associated with latent infection)
- Retinal vasculitis
- Retinal vein occlusion
- Hyperviscosity syndromes

Treatment: Prevention and early detection are fundamental to preserving vision. Annual ophthalmological examinations are required. For patients with diabetes, the goal is to optimize glucose control, particularly if proliferative changes have not occurred (Fraser & D'Amico, 2011b; McCulloch, 2011). Patients with hypertension or hypertension and diabetes should be treated to control blood pressure (goal is 130/80 mm Hg for diabetics, 140/90 mm Hg for nondiabetics). Blood pressure reduction should be slow and deliberate to minimize end-organ damage; treatment of the underlying pathology is essential. The parameters and goal of treatment in patients with hypertension and diabetes should be clear and concise.

For diabetic patients with nonproliferative retinopathy, macular edema is responsible for most vision loss. If macular edema is clinically significant, treatment with focal photocoagulation should be instituted (Fraser & D'Amico, 2011b; Rosenblatt & Benson, 2008). Intravitreal steroid injection or anti-VEGF injection is also used. For diabetics with severe nonproliferative disease, panretinal laser photocoagulation can lower the risk of progression to proliferative diabetic retinopathy (Fraser & D'Amico, 2011a, 2011b; Rosenblatt & Benson, 2008). For diabetic patients with vitreous hemorrhage and advanced neovascularization, vitrectomy can be of significant benefit (Fraser & D'Amico, 2011b; Rosenblatt & Benson, 2008).

Follow-up: Follow-up depends on the findings. A retinal specialist should follow up with patients with retinopathy. The primary care provider is responsible for regular disease management. The staging of retinopathy and the treatment plan require specialty follow-up.

Sequelae: Not all retinopathy is progressive. The condition and its outcome are related to the cause of the retinopathy and the degree of successful disease management. For hypertensive retinopathy, arteriovenous nicking and arteriolar narrowing are irreversible (Rogers, 2008).

Prevention/prophylaxis: Elderly patients should have an annual ophthalmological examination. During routine office visits, perform a funduscopic examination on the eyes of diabetics and hypertensives. Promptly refer the patient to a retinal specialist at the earliest report of vision change or abnormal examination findings. Patients with diabetes and hypertension should be aware of the goals of treatment and the need to control blood pressure and blood glucose. Home monitoring of blood glucose and blood pressure may be advised.

Referral: A retinal specialist should see all patients with retinopathy. All patients with diabetes and hypertension need to see an ophthalmologist annually. Communication between specialist and primary care provider is essential for optimal patient treatment.

Education: Patients should report any alteration in vision. Patients should know how the goals of blood pressure and blood glucose control relate to prevention of complications. Finally, patients should understand the importance of follow-up care. The goals of treatment should be a partnership between patient and health-care provider.

CLINICAL RECOMMENDATION	EVIDENCE RATING	REFERENCES
Refer patients with macular edema, severe nonproliferative retinopathy, or any degree of proliferative retinopathy to an ophthalmologist immediately for treatment.	A	Laufgraben & Meattey (2011)
Optimal glycemic control reduces the risk and progression of retinopathy.	B	Diabetes Control and Complications Trial (DCCT) Research Group (1993)
Optimal blood pressure control reduces the risk and progression of retinopathy.	A	Adler et al. (2000)
Laser photocoagulation reduces the risk of vision loss in patients with proliferative retinopathy, clinically significant macular edema, and some cases of severe nonproliferative retinopathy.	A	ACCORD Study Group & ACCORD Eye Study Group (2010)
Aspirin therapy does not prevent the progression of retinopathy, nor is it contraindicated for prevention of cardiovascular disease in the presence of retinopathy, because it does not increase the risk of retinal hemorrhage.	A	ACCORD Study Group & ACCORD Eye Study Group (2010)

A = consistent, good-quality, patient-oriented evidence; B = inconsistent or limited-quality, patient-oriented evidence; C = consensus, disease-oriented evidence, usual practice, expert opinion, or case series. For information about the SORT evidence rating system, go to www.aafp.org/afpsort.xml.

RHINITIS

Signal symptoms: Sneezing, postnasal drip, nasal congestion and itching, and rhinorrhea; may be accompanied by eye tearing or throat irritation.

Description: Rhinitis is an inflammation of the nasal mucosa.

Etiology: Rhinitis may be either allergic or nonallergic. Allergic rhinitis results as a response of the nasal mucosa to airborne allergens in atopic genetically prone individuals. This response is mediated by the production of immunoglobulin E (IgE). IgE antibodies produced in response to the initial and subsequent exposure to allergens bind to the nasal mucosa. With repeated exposure, immediate type 1 hypersensitivity reactions may occur (Simoens & Laekeman, 2009). Antigen-specific T cells are activated through the lymphatic system in response to the antigen. The activated antigen-specific T cells activate B cells, and IgE is created in lymphoid tissue and at local tissue sites (Adelman, Casale, & Corren, 2002; Novak, 2009). The newly created antigen-specific IgE is released by plasma cells and binds to high-affinity IgE receptors located on the basophils and mast cells. This leads to the sensitization of the cells in the tissues of the nose, lung, or skin (Adelman et al., 2002; Cirillo, Pistorio, Tosca, & Ciprandi, 2009). IgE also binds with the antigen protein, beginning degranulation of the mast cells and basophils. These actions start the allergic cascade. Mediators are released as a result of the degranulation and include histamine, proteoglycans, enzymes, leukotrienes, cytokines, and many others. The chain in the release of mediators is responsible for the immediate and late phase responses of the cells. Histamine may be fully released within 30 minutes of degranulation, whereas cytokines may be released over many hours (Adelman et al., 2002; Derendorf & Meltzer, 2008).

Allergic rhinitis may be seasonal, caused by pollens from trees, grass, or weeds pollinating in the spring or fall. Pollen from flowers is rarely allergenic, because the pollen is heavier and is carried by bees from plant to plant (Asthma Task Force, 2009). Perennial allergic rhinitis is often related to environmental exposure to pollutants, animal dander, dust, and indoor and outdoor molds. Irritants, such as cigarette smoke, and pollution and odors, such as perfumes and diesel, may cause rhinitis but are not IgE mediated.

The subtypes of nonallergic rhinitis include vasomotor, atrophic nonallergic, rhinitis medicamentosa, drug-induced, hormonal, gustatory, or infectious. Nonallergic rhinitis is defined as episodic or persistent perennial rhinitis symptoms that are not mediated by the production and interaction of IgE. Vasomotor rhinitis, caused by an idiopathic hyperactive nasal mucosa, produces symptoms similar to those of allergic rhinitis. One theory of vasomotor rhinitis proposed that a neurogenic dysfunction causes vascular and glandular hyperactivity of the nasal mucosa. Environmental conditions, including temperature changes, inhaled irritants, and odors, are implicated. Atrophic nonallergic rhinitis is probably due to degeneration and atrophy of nasal membranes and bony structures. Rhinitis medicamentosa is frequently due to the overuse of topical OTC nasal decongestants. Drug-induced rhinitis may occur with use of angiotensin-converting enzyme inhibitors, methyldopa, beta blockers, amitriptyline, chlorpromazine, aspirin, nonsteroidal anti-inflammatory drugs, and estrogens. Hormonal rhinitis may occur in patients with hypothyroidism or those who are pregnant. Gustatory rhinitis can occur after food or alcohol ingestion and is thought to be mediated vagally. Infectious rhinitis is most commonly caused by acute viral syndrome. Chronic infectious rhinitis results from a secondary bacterial infection.

Occurrence: Allergic rhinitis occurs in 9% to 21% of the population, or more than 20 million people in the United States. Nonallergic rhinitis occurs in 20% to 60% of the population.

Age: Allergic rhinitis is most common between ages 10 and 39, declining after age 40. Vasomotor rhinitis is a condition of adulthood and is more common in the elderly. Atrophic rhinitis is associated with aging.

Gender: Men and women ages 40 and older have roughly the same incidence of rhinitis.

Ethnicity: No prevalence for rhinitis exists among ethnic groups.

Contributing factors: Most important, allergic rhinitis usually is associated with a strong family history of atopic disorders, including asthma, atopic eczema, urticaria, food allergy, stinging-insect-venom allergy, and anaphylaxis. Exposure to airborne allergens in the environment, such as animal dander, dust mites, molds, or seasonal pollens, triggers allergic rhinitis. A variety of factors are thought to contribute to nonallergic rhinitis, including anatomical abnormalities, infections, medications (especially in the elderly), immunodeficiency, tumors of the nasopharynx and paranasal sinuses, Wegener's granulomatosis, pregnancy, hypothyroid disease, and leakage of cerebrospinal fluid. Vasomotor rhinitis can be triggered by strong odors or fumes, temperature or barometric pressure changes, and psychological factors. Age-related changes in the geriatric population should be considered, because physiological changes in this age-group as well as medication side effects and drug–drug interactions may contribute to the development of symptoms (Wallace et al., 2008).

Signs and symptoms: Patients with seasonal allergic rhinitis report rhinorrhea, sneezing, obstructed nasal passages, and pruritic eyes, nose, and oropharynx during the spring and fall. Patients with perennial allergic rhinitis have similar symptoms associated with exposure to environmental allergens typically in their homes. Physical examination may reveal a pale, boggy nasal mucosa, injected conjunctiva, enlarged turbinates, dark discoloration or bags under the eyes, and mouth breathing; absence of pale, boggy nasal mucosa does not rule out allergic rhinitis.

Postnasal discharge and congestion are common complaints in vasomotor rhinitis; symptoms associated with allergic rhinitis may coexist. Individuals with atrophic rhinitis report a bad taste along with congestion and thick postnasal discharge. In nonallergic rhinitis, pink-to-red, dry nasal mucosa is found on examination.

Review of symptoms: Questions to ask patients with symptoms of rhinitis include the following: Does the patient associate the symptoms with a season, place, time of day, or activity? Is there a family history of allergic diseases? Do symptoms seem to occur during times of stress or during weather or temperature changes? Does the patient use intranasal drugs such as cocaine? Symptoms of infection, such as fever, purulent nasal discharge, and tenderness over the sinuses, should be ruled out on history and physical examination.

Although the patient history is key in establishing the diagnosis, the physical examination will assist in ruling out other differential diagnoses. A full head, eyes, ears, nose, and throat (HEENT) and respiratory examination should be performed. The examination should always include a careful HEENT examination, looking for allergic symptoms of the nose and eyes, including sclera erythema and injection, allergic shiners from venous engorgement, swollen pink nasal turbinates, and tonsillary enlargement.

Diagnostic tests: Specialized allergy skin prick testing may be performed. Scratch testing involves scratching the surface of the skin with a single stylus for each allergen. This form of allergy testing is safer, more rapid, and less uncomfortable to patients than intradermal testing (Krau & McInnis, 2010). Depending on the practice, providers may begin with scratch testing and proceed to intradermal testing if the results are negative (Sporik, Henderson, & Hourihane, 2008). Radiographic sinus films or CT scan may be made if infection is suspected. Patients with chronic rhinitis may be referred for evaluation of obstructive sleep apnea in the presence of sleep-disordered breathing (Wallace et al., 2008).

Differential diagnosis:
- Viral or bacterial upper respiratory infection
- Acute or chronic sinusitis
- Otitis media
- Nasal polyps
- Deviated nasal septum
- Hypothyroid disease
- Tumor
- Foreign body in the nose

Treatment:

Allergic rhinitis: Pharmacological therapy is directed at control of the specific patient symptoms. Avoid first-generation antihistamines, such as diphenhydramine, because of safety issues related to sedating effects. The lowest possible dose of these medications should be used in elderly persons to avoid excessive sedation. Because of their anticholinergic effects, these drugs may worsen certain conditions that are common in the elderly patient such as benign prostatic hypertrophy, bladder neck obstruction, and narrow-angle glaucoma.

Second-generation antihistamines are relatively free of central nervous system (CNS) and anticholinergic side effects and effectively relieve allergic rhinitis symptoms.

- Loratadine (Claritin), 10 mg once daily (10 mg every other day in hepatic or renal insufficiency with glomerular filtration rate less than 30 mL/min)
- Cetirizine (Zyrtec), 10 mg once daily (5 mg once daily with hepatic or renal insufficiency)
- Levocetirizine 5 mg once daily
- Fexofenadine (Allegra), 180 mg once daily, 60 mg twice daily (60 mg once daily with decreased renal function)

These antihistamines should not be prescribed for patients taking antifungal medications, macrolide antibiotics, tricyclic antidepressants, or class Ia antiarrhythmics, because their interaction with these drugs may cause life-threatening cardiac dysrhythmias. They are also contraindicated for patients with a history of congestive heart failure, coronary artery disease, or liver disease.

Pseudoephedrine is best used intermittently for only short periods, because it has many CNS side effects. Decongestants are contraindicated in elderly patients with poorly controlled hypertension, coronary artery disease, and a history of cerebrovascular accident. These medications are recommended to decrease severe nasal congestion and enhance the penetration of topical therapies. Decongestant medications decrease nasal mucosa swelling but have little effect on the other symptoms of rhinitis.

Topical corticosteroid nasal sprays are the most effective treatment in most types of rhinitis when used regularly (Wallace et al., 2008). These sprays are available in once- and twice-a-day doses and in aqueous or aerosol preparations to suit patient preferences. Topical nasal preparations are helpful in avoiding systemic side effects but may cause local irritation and dryness of the nasal mucosa.

Topical antihistamine: azelastine (Astelin) nasal spray, 2 sprays each nostril twice daily

Intranasal corticosteroids:

- Fluticasone furoate (Veramyst), 2 sprays each nostril once daily
- Budesonide (Rhinocort), 2 sprays each nostril twice daily
- Flunisolide (Nasarel, Nasalide), 2 sprays each nostril twice daily
- Fluticasone propionate (Flonase), 2 sprays each nostril once daily or 1 spray each nostril twice daily
- Mometasone furoate (Nasonex), 2 sprays each nostril once daily
- Triamcinolone acetonide (Nasacort), 2 sprays each nostril once daily

Nonallergic rhinitis:

- Avoid known irritants.
- Nasal corticosteroids (see earlier) for nonallergic rhinitis with eosinophilia syndrome (NARES).
- Nasal corticosteroids and elimination of topical decongestant sprays in rhinitis medicamentosa.
- Ipratropium bromide (Atrovent) nasal spray 0.03%, 0.06%, 2 sprays each nostril 2 to 4 times daily, is an anticholinergic for local control of rhinorrhea.
- Pseudoephedrine, 30 to 60 mg orally every 4 hours, a decongestant, decreases nasal mucosa swelling but has little effect on other rhinitis symptoms; it is best used briefly and intermittently because of CNS side effects. It is contraindicated in elderly patients with poorly controlled hypertension, coronary artery disease, and a history of cerebrovascular accident. Oral corticosteroids are recommended only for severe nasal obstruction, such as that caused by rebound rhinitis or nasal polyps, and require individualized dosing.

Follow-up: Have the patient return in 3 to 4 weeks to review his or her response to medications and the avoidance procedures discussed as well as to assess his or her understanding of the management plan and prevention.

Sequelae: Epistaxis, acute and chronic sinusitis, and the development of nasal polyps are complications of rhinitis.

Prevention/prophylaxis: Teach patients with allergic rhinitis to avoid irritants and to try to control environmental risk factors. Discuss the need to take antihistamines or to use nasal sprays before exposure to irritants, to prevent symptoms.

Referral: When symptoms persist or worsen, refer the patient to an otolaryngologist or allergist (Wallace et al., 2008). In patients with chronic rhinitis or sinusitis, the otolaryngologist may prescribe a short-term course of antibiotics along with oral prednisone. Sinus surgery may be indicated in order to correct obstruction, a major component of recurrent sinusitis. An allergist may skin prick test patients in order to determine their sensitivities and place the patient on allergy immunotherapy. Controlling the production of clear mucus will help to control the other, more significant component of recurrent sinusitis.

Education: Discuss specific environmental control with the patient. Avoid the use of OTC nasal sprays for more than 3 consecutive days. Teach the patient about the potential sedating side effects of first-generation antihistamine medications and the need to use their medications on a routine basis. Waiting until symptoms have progressed may result in the lack of efficacy of either the oral antihistamine and/or the topical nasal steroid.

For control of seasonal pollen from trees and grass in the spring and weeds in the summer and fall, it is essential that patients keep their windows closed and air conditioning on during periods of high pollen counts, especially from 5 a.m. to 10 a.m. Pollen easily enters the screens of windows and deposits on furniture and bedding. Therefore, bed linens should be changed weekly and washed in hot water. High-efficiency particulate air (HEPA) filters can be used in bedrooms and living areas. Patients should also be encouraged to shower and change their clothes when coming in from the outside. Clothes should be dried in an automatic dryer, not outdoors. Outdoor mold exposure can be decreased by avoiding areas of decaying plants, rotting leaves, and other debris. Wearing a mask when working outside can also be of benefit (National Institute of Environmental Health Sciences, n.d.).

Patients with animal dander sensitivity can be more difficult to treat if the family chooses to keep the pet. Pets must be kept out of the patient's room at all times, and a HEPA filter should be run in the bedroom. Because animal dander is sticky, bed clothes should be clean before entering the bedroom. Washing the hands and face after pet exposure is also advised (National Institute of Environmental Health Sciences, n.d.).

CLINICAL RECOMMENDATION	EVIDENCE RATING	REFERENCES
Topical corticosteroid nasal sprays are the most effective treatment in most types of rhinitis when used regularly.	A	Wallace et al. (2008)
Patients with chronic rhinitis may be referred for evaluation of obstructive sleep apnea in the presence of sleep-disordered breathing.	A	Wallace et al. (2008)
Patients with animal dander sensitivity can be more difficult to treat if the family chooses to keep the pet. Pets must be kept out of the patient's room at all times, and a HEPA filter should be run in the bedroom. Because animal dander is sticky, bed clothes should be clean before entering the bedroom. Washing the hands and face after pet exposure is also advised.	A	National Institute of Environmental Health Sciences (n.d.)
Outdoor mold exposure can be decreased by avoiding areas of decaying plants, rotting leaves, and other debris. Wearing a mask when working outside can also be of benefit.	A	National Institute of Environmental Health Sciences (n.d.)
Specialized allergy skin prick testing may be performed. Scratch testing involves scratching the surface of the skin with a single stylus for each allergen. This form of allergy testing is safer, more rapid, and less uncomfortable to patients than intradermal testing but is not as sensitive as intradermal testing.	B	Krau & McInnis (2010)
Depending on the practice, providers may begin with scratch testing and proceed to intradermal testing if the results are negative.	B	Sporik et al. (2008)

A = consistent, good-quality, patient-oriented evidence; B = inconsistent or limited-quality, patient-oriented evidence; C = consensus, disease-oriented evidence, usual practice, expert opinion, or case series. For information about the SORT evidence rating system, go to www.aafp.org/afpsort.xml.

CASE STUDY

A 76-year-old woman presents today with complaints of running nose, clearing of throat, and occasional nasal congestion, especially on waking in the morning. She has recently moved into an independent living center after living in her home for 40 years. She states that, although she has had these symptoms before, generally the symptoms appeared in the spring, and she associated the running nose with pollination. Because it is winter, she could not identify the trigger of her symptoms.

Chief Complaint: Persistent running nose for 3-week duration, associated clearing of throat, and nasal congestion on awakening in the morning.

Objective: Blood pressure (BP) 130/84, temperature 98.6, pulse 78, respiratory rate 20.

1. How will you use this information to prepare for today's visit?

2. What additional subjective data are you seeking, to include history of any allergies?

3. What additional objective data will you be assessing for?

4. What are the differential diagnoses that you are considering?

5. What laboratory tests will help you rule out some of the differential diagnoses?

6. What is your treatment, and what specific information about the prescription will you give to this patient?

7. What are the potential complications from the treatment ordered?

8. What additional specific laboratory tests will you consider ordering?

9. What additional patient teaching may be needed?

10. What type of specialist will you be consulting for this patient?

REFERENCES

Assessment of the Head, Neck, and Face

Bickley, L. S., & Szilagyi, P. S. (2009). *Bates' guide to physical examination and history taking* (10th ed.). Philadelphia, PA: Wolters Kluwer Health/Lippincott Williams & Wilkins.

LeBlond, R. F., Brown, D. D., & DeGowin, R. L. (2009). *DeGowin's diagnostic examination* (9th ed.). New York City, NY: McGraw-Hill Medical.

Acute Glaucoma

Aherne, A., & Dronen, S. C. (2012). Acute angle-closure glaucoma. *Medscape*. Retrieved from http://emedicine.medscape.com/article/798811

Cronemberger, S., Calixto, N., deAndrade, A. O., & Mérula, R. V. (2010). New considerations on papillary block mechanism. *Arquivos Brasileiros de Oftalmologia, 73*(1), 9–15.

Horton, J. C. (2012). Disorders of the eye. In D. L. Longo, A. S. Fauci, D. L. Kasper, S. L. Hauser, J. L. Jameson, & J. Loscalzo (Eds.), *Harrison's principles of internal medicine* (18th ed., pp. 230–235). New York City, NY: McGraw-Hill Medical.

Preferred Practice Patterns Committee. (2005). *Comprehensive adult medical eye evaluation*. San Francisco, CA: American Academy of Ophthalmology, 1–15.

Tsai, H. C., & Cheng, J. H. (2011). Glaucoma. *Essential Evidence Plus*. Retrieved from http://www.essentialevidenceplus.com

Weizer, J. S. (2012). Angle-closure glaucoma. *UpToDate*. Retrieved from http://www.uptodate.com

Cataracts

American Academy of Ophthalmology Cataract and Anterior Segment Panel Preferred Practice® Guidelines. (2011). *Cataract in the adult eye*. San Francisco, CA: American Academy of Ophthalmology. Retrieved from www.aao.org/ppp

Gambert, S. R. (2012). Keeping an eye on healthy vision. *Clinical Geriatrics, 20*(2). Retrieved from www.clinicalgeriatrics.com/articles/Keeping-Eye-Healthy-Vision

Giaconi, J. A., Sarraf, D., & Coleman, A. I. (2010). Visual impairment. In J. T. Pacala & G. W. Sullivan (Eds.), *Geriatrics review syllabus: A core curriculum in geriatric medicine* (7th ed., pp. 187–196). New York City, NY: American Geriatrics Society.

Handzel, D. L., Briesen, S., Rausch, S., & Kälble, T. (2012). Cataract surgery in patients taking alpha-1 antagonists: know the risks, avoid the complications. *Deutsches Ärzteblatt International, 109*(21), 379–384.

Horton, J. C. (2012). Disorders of the eye. In D. L. Longo, A. S. Fauci, D. L. Kasper, S. L. Hauser, J. L. Jameson, & J. Loscalzo (Eds.), *Harrison's principles of internal medicine* (18th ed., pp. 224–241). New York City, NY: McGraw-Hill Medical.

Jacobs, D. S. (2012). Cataract in adults. *UpToDate*. Retrieved from http://www.uptodate.com

Keay, L., Lindsley, K., Tielsch, J., Katz, J., & Schein, O. (2009). Routine preoperative medical testing for cataract surgery. *Cochrane Database of Systematic Reviews* (2):CD007293.

Mathew, M. C., Ervin, A.-M., Tao, J., & Davis, R. M. (2012). Antioxidant vitamin supplementation for preventing and slowing the progression of age-related cataract. *Cochrane Database of Systematic Reviews*, Issue 6. Art. No. CD004567.

Packer, M. (2011). Cataract. *Essential Evidence Plus*. Retrieved from http://www.essentialevidence.com

Renzi, L. M. (2007). Lutein and age related ocular disorders in the older adult: a review. *Journal of Nutrition for the Elderly, 26*(3–4), 139–157.

Servat, J. J., Risco, M., Nakasato, Y. R., & Bernardino, C. R. (2011). Visual impairment in the elderly: impact on functional ability and quality of life. *Clinical Geriatrics, 19*(7), 49–56.

Weatherall, M., Clay, J., James, K., Perrin, K., Shirtcliffe, P., & Beasley, R. (2009). Dose-response relationship of inhaled corticosteroids and cataracts: a systematic review and meta-analysis. *Respirology, 14*(7), 983–990.

Chronic Glaucoma

AAO Podcast. (2012). i-Stent. Retrieved July 20, 2012, from www.aao.org/one

American Academy of Ophthalmology Glaucoma Panel. Preferred Practice Pattern® Guidelines. (2010a). *Primary open-angle glaucoma.* San Francisco, CA: American Academy of Ophthalmology. Retrieved from www.aao.org/ppp

American Academy of Ophthalmology Glaucoma Panel. Preferred Practice Pattern® Guidelines. (2010b). *Primary open-angle glaucoma suspect.* San Francisco, CA: American Academy of Ophthalmology. Retrieved from www.aao.org/ppp

Bell, J. A. (2012). Primary open-angle glaucoma. *Medscape.* Retrieved from http://emedicine.medscape.com/article/1206147

Hatt, S. R., Wormald, R., Burr, J., & Wormald, R. (2009). Screening for prevention of optic nerve damage due to chronic open angle glaucoma (Cochrane Review). In *The Cochrane Library 2009,* Issue 2. Chichester, UK: John Wiley & Sons, Ltd.

Heijl, A., Leske, M. C., Bengtsson, B., Hyman, L., Bengtsson, B., Hussein, M., & Early Manifest Glaucoma Trial Group. (2002). Reduction of intraocular pressure and glaucoma progression: results from the Early Manifest Glaucoma Trial. *Archives of Ophthalmology, 120*(10), 1268–1279.

Jacobs, D. S. (2012a). Open-angle glaucoma: epidemiology, clinical presentation, and diagnosis. *UpToDate.* Retrived from http://www.uptodate.com

Jacobs, D. S. (2012b). Open-angle glaucoma: treatment. *UpToDate.* Retrieved from: http://www.uptodate.com

Koby, M. (2012). Glaucoma, open-angle. In F. Ferri (Ed.), *Ferri's clinical advisor 2013* (1st ed.). St. Louis, MO: Mosby/Elsevier.

Li, T., Ervin, A. M., Scherer, R., Jampel, H., & Dickersin, K. (2010). Setting priorities for comparative effectiveness research: a case study using primary open-angle glaucoma. *Ophthalmology, 117*(10), 1937–1945. doi:10.1016/j.ophtha.2010.07.004

Nichamin, L. D. (2009). Glaukos iStent® Trabecular Micro-Bypass. *Middle East African Journal of Ophthalmology, 16*(3), 138–140. doi:10.4103/0974-9233.56227

Quigley, H. A. (2011). Glaucoma. *Lancet, 377*(9774), 1367–1377.

U.S. Preventive Services Task Force. (2005). Screening for glaucoma: recommendation statement. *Annals of Family Medicine, 3*(2), 171–172.

Varma, R., Lee, P. P., Goldberg, I., & Kotak, S. (2011). An assessment of the health and economic burdens of glaucoma. *American Journal of Ophthalmology, 152*(4), 515–522.

Epistaxis

Bamimore, O., & Silverberg, M. A. (2012). Management of acute epistaxis. *Medscape.* Retrieved from http://emedicine.medscape.com/article/764719-overview

Blomgren, K. (2011). EBM guidelines: epistaxis. Article ID: ebm00866 (038.046) © Duodecim Medical Publications Ltd. Retrieved from http://www.essentialevidenceplus.com

Cusik, C. J., & Clenney, T. (2005). Management of epistaxis. *American Family Physician, 71,* 305–312.

Konkle, B. (2012). Bleeding and thrombosis. In D. L. Longo, A. S. Fauci, D. L. Kasper, S. L. Hauser, J. L. Jameson, & J. Loscalzo (Eds.), *Harrison's principles of internal medicine* (18th ed., pp. 457–463). New York City, NY: McGraw-Hill Medical.

Mäkitie, A. (2010). EBM: Tumours of the nasal and paranasal cavities. Article ID: ebm00874 (038.062) © Duodecim Medical Publications Ltd. Retrieved from http://www.essentialevidenceplus.com

Nguyen, Q. A. (2012). Epistaxis. *Medscape.* Retrieved from http://emedicine.medscape.com/article/863220-overview

Ruhl, T. S. (2011). Epistaxis and nosebleeds. *Essential Evidence Plus.* Retrieved from http://www.essentialevidenceplus.com

Hearing Loss

Adams-Wendling, L., Pimple, C., Adams, S., & Titler, M. G. (2008). Evidence-based guideline: nursing management of hearing impairment in nursing facility residents. *Journal of Gerontological Nursing, 34*(11), 9–17. doi:10.3928/00989134-20081101-09

American Speech-Language-Hearing Association. (1997). Guidelines for audiologic screening. Rockville, MD: American Speech-Language-Hearing Association. Retrieved from www.asha.org/docs/html/GL1997-00199.html

Bentur, N., Valinsky, L., Lemberger, J., Ben Moshe, Y., & Heymann, A. D. (2012). Primary care intervention programme to improve early detection of hearing loss in the elderly. *Journal of Laryngology & Otology, 126*(6), 574–579.

Blevins, N. H. (2012). Presbycusis. *UpToDate.* Retrieved from http://www.uptodate.com

Bushman, L.A., Belza, B., & Christianson, P. (2012). Older adult hearing loss and screening in primary care. *Journal for Nurse Practitioners, 8*(7), 509–514.

Chou, R., Dana, T., Bougatsos, C., Fleming, C., & Beil, T. (2011). Screening adults aged 50 years or older for hearing loss: a review of the evidence for the U.S. Preventive Services Task Force. *Annals of Internal Medicine, 154*(5), 347–355.

Gross, S. R. (2011a). Hearing loss in adults: diagnostic approach. *Essential Evidence 2011.* John Wiley & Sons, Inc. Retrieved from http://www.essentialevidenceplus.com

Gross, S.R. (2011b). Presbycusis. *Essential Evidence 2011.* John Wiley & Sons, Inc. Retrieved from http://www.essentialevidenceplus.com

Harkin, H., & Kelleher, C. (2011). Caring for older adults with hearing loss. *Nursing Older People, 23*(9), 22–28.

Lin, F. R., Thorpe, R., Gordon-Salant, S., & Ferrucci, L. (2011). Hearing loss prevalence and risk factors among older adults in the United States. *Journals of Gerontology Series A: Biological Sciences and Medical Sciences, 66*(5), 582–590. doi:10.1093/gerona/glr002

Pacala, J. T., & Yueh, B. (2012). Hearing deficits in the older patient. "I didn't notice anything." *Journal of the American Medical Association, 307*(11), 1185–1194.

Raman, G., Lee, J., Chung, M., Gaylor, J. M., Sen, S., Rao, M., & Lau, J. (2011). Effectiveness of cochlear implants in adults with sensorineural hearing loss. Tufts Evidence-based Practice Center; Technology Project Report. Project ID: AUDT0510.

Roland, P. S., Smith, T. L., Schwartz, S. R., Rosenfeld, R. M., Ballachanda, B., Earll, J. M., . . . Wetmore, S. (2008). Clinical practice guideline: cerumen impaction. *Otolaryngology—Head and Neck Surgery, 139*(3 Suppl. 2), S1–S21.

U.S. Preventive Services Task Force. (2012). *Screening for hearing loss in older adults: U.S. Preventive Services Task Force Recommendation Statement.* AHRQ Publication No. 11-05153-EF-2, Retrieved from http://www.uspreventiveservicestaskforce.org/uspstf11/adulthearing/adulthearrs.htm

Weber, P. C. (2012a). Etiology of hearing loss in adults. *UpToDate.* Retrieved from http://www.uptodate.com

Weber, P. C. (2012b). Evaluation of hearing loss in adults. *UpToDate.* Retrieved from http://www.uptodate.com

Weber, P. C. (2012c). Hearing amplification in adults. *UpToDate.* Retrieved from http://www.uptodate.com

Weber, P. C. (2012d). Sudden sensorineural hearing loss. *UpToDate*. Retrieved from http://www.uptodate.com

Yueh, B., & Shekelle, P. (2007). Quality indicators for the care of hearing loss in vulnerable elders. *Journal of the American Geriatrics Society, 55* (Suppl. 2), S335–S339.

Hordeolum and Chalazion

Ben Simon, G. J., Huang, L., Nakra, T., Schwarcz, R. M., McCann, J. D., & Goldberg, R. A. (2005). Intralesional triamcinolone acetonide injection for primary and recurrent chalazia: is it really effective? *Ophthalmology, 112*(5), 913–917.

Bessette, M. J. (2012). Hordeolum and stye in emergency medicine. *Medscape*. Retrieved from http://emedicine.medscape.com/article/798940-overview

Bron, A. (2012). Ocular rosacea. *UpToDate*. Retrieved from http://www.uptodate.com

Ehrenhaus, M. P., & Sturridge, K. A. (2012). Hordeolum. *Medscape*. Retrieved from http://emedicine.medscape.com/article/1213080-overview

Ghosh, C., & Ghosh, T. (2012). Eyelid lesions. *UpToDate*. Retrieved from http://www.uptodate.com

Papier, A., Tuttle, D. J., & Mahar, T. J. (2007). Differential diagnosis of the swollen red eyelid. *American Family Physician, 76*(12), 1815–1824.

Wolter, B. R. (2011). Hordeolum and chalazion. *Essential Evidence Plus*. © 2011 John Wiley & Sons, Inc. Retrieved from http://www.essentialevidenceplus.com

Age-related Macular Degeneration

American Academy of Ophthalmology Retina Panel. Preferred Practice Pattern® Guidelines. (2008). Age related macular degeneration. San Francisco, CA: American Academy of Ophthalmology. Retrieved from www.aao.org/ppp

Arroyo, J. G. (2012a). Age-related macular degeneration: epidemiology, etiology, and diagnosis. *UpToDate*. Retrieved from http://www.uptodate.com

Arroyo, J. G. (2012b). Age-related macular degeneration: treatment and prevention. *UpToDate*. Retrieved from http://www.uptodate.com

Evans, J. R., & Lawrenson, J. G. (2012). Antioxidant vitamin and mineral supplements for preventing age-related macular degeneration. *Cochrane Database of Systematic Reviews*, Issue 6. Art. No.: CD000253.

Federici, T. J. (2011) Macular degeneration. *Essential Evidence Plus*. © 2011 John Wiley & Sons, Inc. Retrieved from http://www.essentialevidenceplus.com

Hoang, Q. V., Mendonca, L. S., Della Torre, K. E., Jung, J. J., Tsuang, A. J., & Freund, K. B. (2012). Effect on intraocular pressure in patients receiving unilateral intravitreal anti-vascular endothelial growth factor injections. *Ophthalmology, 119*(2), 321–326.

Klingler, K. N., & Bakri, S. J. (2012). Age-related macular degeneration: a primer for the primary care provider. *Medscape*. Retrieved from www.medscape.com/viewarticle/765123

Koby, M. (2012). Macular degeneration. In F. Ferri (Ed.), *Ferri's clinical advisor 2013* (1st ed.). St. Louis, MO: Mosby/Elsevier.

Moutray, T., & Chakravarthy, U. (2011). Age-related macular degeneration. *Therapeutic Advances in Chronic Disease, 2*(5), 325–331.

National Institute for Health and Care Excellence (NICE). (2008/2012). NICE technology appraisal guidance TA155. Ranibizumab and pegaptanib for the treatment of age-related macular degeneration. Retrieved from www.nice.org.uk/TA155 and http://publications.nice.org.uk/ranibizumab-and-pegaptanib-for-the-treatment-of-age-related-macular-degeneration-ta155

Prall, R., Ciulla, T., Criswell, M. H., & Harris, A. (2012). Exudative age-related macular degeneration. *Medscape Ophthalmology*. Retrieved from http://emedicine.medscape.com/article/1226030

U.S. Preventive Services Task Force. (2009). Screening for impaired visual acuity in older adults: U.S. Preventive Services Task Force recommendation statement. *Annals of Internal Medicine, 151*(1), 37–43.

Oral Cancer

Brocklehurst, P., Kujan, O., Glenny, A. M., Oliver, R., Sloan, P., Ogden, G., & Shepherd, S. (2010). Screening programmes for the early detection and prevention of oral cancer. *Cochrane Database of Systematic Reviews* (11):CD004150.

Carr, A. B., & Ebbert, J. (2012). Interventions for tobacco cessation in the dental setting. *Cochrane Database of Systematic Reviews*, Issue 6. Art. No.: CD005084. doi:10.1002/14651858.CD005084.pub3

Chu, Y. H., Tzeng, S. L., Lin, C. W., Chien, M. H., Chen, M. K., & Yang, S. F. (2012). Impacts of microRNA gene polymorphisms on the susceptibility of environmental factors leading to carcinogenesis in oral cancer. *PLoS One, 7*(6), e39777. Epub June 28, 2012.

Contessa, J.N., Lloyd, S., & Decker, R. (2011). Oropharyngeal cancer. *Essential Evidence Plus*. Retrieved from http://www.essentialevidenceplus.com

Goldstein, B. G., & Goldstein, A. O. (2012). Oral lesions. *UpToDate*. Retrieved from http://www.uptodate.com

Gonsalves, W. C., Chi, A. C., & Neville, B. W. (2007a). Common oral lesions: Part I. Superficial mucosal lesions. *American Family Physician, 75*(4), 501–506.

Gonsalves, W. C., Chi, A. C., & Neville, B. W. (2007b). Common oral lesions: Part II. Masses and neoplasia. *American Family Physician, 75*(4), 509–512.

Gonsalves, W. C., Wrightson, A. S., & Henry, R. G. (2008). Common oral conditions in older persons. *American Family Physician, 78*(7), 845–852.

Gross, N. D., Lee, N. Y., Okuno, S., & Rao, S. S. (2012). Treatment of early (stage I and II) head and neck cancer: the oral cavity. *UpToDate*. Retrieved from http://www.uptodate.com

Kademani, D. (2007). Oral cancer. *Mayo Clinic Proceedings, 82*(7), 878–887.

National Comprehensive Cancer Network (NCCN) Guidelines. (2012). Version 1.2012: Cancer of the oral cavity. Retrieved from www.nccn.org

Poon, C. S., & Stenson, K. M. (2012). Overview of the diagnosis and staging of head and neck cancer. *UpToDate*. Retrieved from http://www.uptodate.com

Rethman, M. P., Carpenter, W., Cohen, E. E., Epstein, J., Evans, C. A., Flaitz, C. M., . . . American Dental Association Council on Scientific Affairs Expert Panel on Screening for Oral Squamous Cell Carcinomas. (2010). Evidence-based clinical recommendations regarding screening for oral squamous cell carcinomas. *Journal of the American Dental Association, 141*(5), 509–520.

SEER stat fact sheets: Oral cavity and pharynx. (2012). Bethesda, MD: National Cancer Institute. Retrieved July 8, 2012, from http://seer.cancer.gov/statfacts/html/oralcav.html

Stenson, K. M. (2011). Epidemiology and risk factors for head and neck cancer. *UpToDate*. Retrieved from http://uptodate.com

U.S. Preventive Services Task Force. (2004). Screening for oral cancer: best evidence update. Retrieved from www.uspreventiveservicestaskforce.org/3rduspstf/oralcan/oralcanup.htm

Wu, A., Lee, N. Y., Gross, N. D., & Okuno, S. (2011). Treatment of locoregionally advanced (stage III and IV) head and neck cancer: the oral cavity. *UpToDate.* Retrieved from http://www.uptodate.com

Zhang, Z. J., Hao, K., Shi, R., Zhao, G., Jiang, G. X., Song, Y., . . . Ma, J. (2011). Glutathione S-transferase M1 (GSTM1) and glutathione S-transferase T1 (GSTT1) null polymorphisms, smoking, and their interaction in oral cancer: a HuGE review and meta-analysis. *American Journal of Epidemiology, 173*(8), 847–857.

Retinopathy

ACCORD Study Group & ACCORD Eye Study Group. (2010). Effects of medical therapies on retinopathy progression in type 2 diabetes. *New England Journal of Medicine, 363*(3), 233–244.

Adler, A. I. , Stratton, I. M., Neil, H. A. W., Yudkin, J. S., Matthews, D. R., Cull, C. A., . . . Holman, R. R. (2000). Association of systolic blood pressure with macrovascular and microvascular complications of type 2 diabetes (UKPDS 36): prospective observational study. *British Medical Journal, 321*(7258), 412–419.

American Academy of Ophthalmology. (2011). Eye health statistics at a glance. Updated April 2011. Retrieved from www.aao.org/newsroom/upload/Eye-Health-Statistics-April-2011.pdf

American Academy of Ophthalmology Retina Panel. Preferred Practice Pattern® Guidelines. (2008). *Diabetic retinopathy.* San Francisco, CA: American Academy of Ophthalmology. Retrieved from www.aao.org/ppp

Bearelly, S., Mathura, J. R., & Jampol, L. M. (2008). Proliferative retinopathies. In M. Yanoff & J. S. Duker (Eds.), *Ophthalmology* (3rd ed., pp. 640–645). St. Louis, MO: Mosby/Elsevier.

Diabetes Control and Complications Trial (DCCT) Research Group. (1993). The effect of intensive treatment of diabetes on the development and progression of long-term complications in insulin-dependent diabetes mellitus. *New England Journal of Medicine, 329*(14), 977–986.

Fraser, C. E., & D'Amico, D. J. (2011a). Classification and clinical features of diabetic retinopathy. *UpToDate.* Retrieved from http://www.uptodate.com

Fraser, C. E., & D'Amico, D. J. (2011b). Prevention and treatment of diabetic retinopathy. *UpToDate.* Retrieved from http://www.uptodate.com

Koby, M., & Ferri, F. F. (2013). Diabetic retinopathy. In F. F. Ferri (Ed.), *Ferri's Clinical Advisor 2013.* (1st ed.). St. Louis, MO: Mosby/Elsevier.

Laufgraben, M. J., & Meattey, H. (2011). Diabetic retinopathy. In *Essential Evidence Plus.* Retrieved from http://www.essentialevidenceplus.com

McCulloch, D. K. (2011). Pathogenesis of diabetic retinopathy. *UpToDate.* Retrieved from http://www.uptodate.com

Rogers, A. H. (2008). Hypertensive retinopathy. In M. Yanoff & J. S. Duker (Eds.), *Ophthalmology* (3rd ed., pp. 584–588). St. Louis, MO: Mosby/Elsevier.

Rosenblatt, B. J., & Benson, W. E. (2008). Diabetic retinopathy. In M. Yanoff & J. S. Duker (Eds.), *Ophthalmology* (3rd ed., pp. 613–621). St. Louis, MO: Mosby/Elsevier.

Rhinitis

Adelman, D. C., Casale, T. B., & Corren, J. (2002). *Manual of allergy and immunology.* Philadelphia, PA: Lippincott Williams & Wilkins.

Asthma Task Force at the Children's Hospital, Denver. (2009). Environmental control and asthma. *CRS—Pediatric Advisor,* 1.

Cirillo, I., Pistorio, A., Tosca, M., & Ciprandi, G. (2009). Impact of allergic rhinitis on asthma; effects on bronchial hyperreactivity. *Allergy, 64*(3), 439–444.

Derendorf, H., & Meltzer, E. O. (2008). Molecular and clinical pharmacology of intranasal corticosteroids: clinical and therapeutic implications. *Allergy, 63*(10),1292–1300.

Krau, S. D., & McInnis, L. A. (2010). Allergy skin testing: what nurses need to know. *Critical Care Nursing Clinics of North America, 22*(1), 75–82.

National Institute of Environmental Health Sciences. (n.d.). Allergens and irritants: mold. Retrieved December 1, 2010, from www.niehs.nih.gov/health/topics/conditions/asthma/mold.cfm

Novak, N. (2009). New insights into the mechanism and management of allergic diseases: atopic dermatitis. *Allergy, 64*(2), 265–275.

Simoens, S., & Laekeman, G. (2009). Pharmacotherapy of allergic rhinitis: a pharmaco-economic approach. *Allergy, 64*(1), 85–95.

Sporik, R., Henderson, J., & Hourihane, J. B. (2008). Clinical immunology review series: an approach to the patient with allergy in childhood. *Journal of Translational Immunology, 155*(3), 378–386.

Wallace, D. V., Dykewicz, M. S., Bernstein, D. I., Blessing-Moore, J., Cox, L., Khan, D. A., . . . American Academy of Allergy, Asthma and Immunology. (2008). The diagnosis and management of rhinitis: an updated practice parameter. *Journal of Allergy and Clinical Immunology, 122*(2 Suppl.), S1–S84. Retrieved October 2, 2011, from www.guideline.gov/content.aspx?id=12999&search=rhinitis

chapter 8

Chest Disorders

Lori Martin-Plank

ASSESSMENT OF THE CARDIOVASCULAR SYSTEM

Key symptoms for cardiovascular assessment include dizziness, syncope, orthopnea, angina, edema, and claudication (Kane, Ouslander, Abrass, & Resnick, 2008). Differentiating normal from abnormal cardiac function in an older adult can be a challenge because one in two older persons has cardiac disease. More specifically, almost one-half of all individuals older than age 60 have severe coronary artery narrowing with a respective increase in myocardial demand. Of these, less than 50% have clinical signs and symptoms of this process. Cardiovascular disease is the most prominent cause of disability in this age group and the leading cause of death, accounting for about one-half of all deaths among elderly persons.

ASSESSMENT OF RISK FACTORS FOR CORONARY ARTERY DISEASE

Although some risk factors for coronary artery disease (CAD) can be remedied, others cannot. The two most important risk factors for atherosclerosis that cannot be remedied are advanced age and male gender. The major remediable risk factors are high blood pressure (BP), cholesterol levels, and smoking.

Since the 1970s, the mortality rate from CAD has shown a pronounced decline in the United States. Most of this decline can be attributed to changes in lifestyle.

The decline in cardiovascular disease has occurred in older as well as younger age groups, suggesting that the effects of risk factor modification persist well into later life.

Blood Pressure

The systolic blood pressure (SBP) rises with age; the diastolic blood pressure (DBP) remains the same or drops a bit. Established hypertension is a risk factor for cardiovascular disease in the geriatric age group, with systolic elevations posing a greater risk than diastolic elevations. Overall, the risk for both genders of experiencing a cardiovascular event or death is 2 to 3 times higher in those with significant hypertension than in those who are normotensive.

Isolated systolic hypertension (ISH) is defined as a SBP greater than 160 mm Hg and a diastolic BP of less than 90 mm Hg. Aggressive treatment of ISH has demonstrated a significant reduction in stroke, myocardial infarction, and sudden cardiac death.

Cholesterol

Serum cholesterol levels rise with age, up to age 60; thereafter, these levels begin to drop. The risk of the effects of an elevated cholesterol level persists from middle age to extreme old age. Aggressive efforts are often indicated to lower low-density lipoprotein (LDL) levels and raise high-density lipoprotein (HDL) levels for cardiac protection. Controversy exists about the role of statins in primary prevention of low-risk older adults (Greenland et al., 2010; Taylor et al., 2011).

Smoking

Smoking is an independent significant risk factor for atherosclerosis and coronary heart disease (Rubenfire & Jackson, 2012). Smoking cessation is strongly advised as both primary prevention (Greenland et al., 2010) and secondary prevention for those with known CAD or peripheral vascular disease (American Heart Association [AHA]/American College of Cardiology [ACC], 2006).

Additional proven or postulated risk factors for cardiovascular disease in the elderly include obesity, lack of exercise, left ventricular hypertrophy, and impaired glucose tolerance. Elderly individuals are most likely to have a combination of risk factors, which has a cumulative effect of increasing the risk of CAD. Control of hypertension is clearly the most potentially remediable risk factor. Evidence is compelling for discontinuation of cigarette smoking at any age. More information is needed regarding the effectiveness and feasibility of lowering cholesterol levels, weight reduction, improved exercise plans, and strict control of blood glucose levels, with respect to the incidence of coronary heart disease (CHD), particularly in those of most advanced age.

Cardiac risk assessment tools, including the Global Framingham Risk Assessment, are available at www.nhlbi.nih.gov/health/prof/other/index.htm#tools. Assessment for metabolic syndrome and obesity, including body mass index (BMI), and waist circumference also enhances risk assessment.

Physiological Changes

The size of the heart remains essentially unchanged, although some increase in left ventricular wall thickness has been demonstrated even in older individuals who do not have cardiovascular disease. Left ventricular hypertrophy is usually due to increased cardiac demand, most likely caused by an increase in peripheral resistance. Peripherally, the vessels become atherosclerotic and arteriosclerotic, and the SBP increases with age. Structural and physiological changes in the aging cardiovascular system cause decreased capacity to endure stresses, decline in physical activity performance, and limited functional reserve capacity (Lakatta & Levy, 2003). Fat deposits accumulate around the sinoatrial (SA) node. The number of pacemaker cells usually has decreased by age 75. Baroreceptors become less sensitive with age, and the response to changes in BP often is blunted.

These physiological changes have little functional impact on the aging heart at rest, but with exercise or stress, they render the aging heart less capable of increasing and sustaining an increase in cardiac output. The maximal heart rate declines approximately 30% between ages 20 and 80. Cardiac dilation and increased stroke volume compensate somewhat for the diminished heart rate during exercise (Laketta & Levy, 2003).

Symptom Assessment

Using the Onset, Location, Duration, Characteristics, Aggravating factors, Relieving factors, Timing (OLDCART) or Precipitating/Palliating factors, Quality, Radiation, Severity, Timing (PQRST), ask the patient about chest pain, shortness of breath, dizziness, palpitations, or edema. Establish the patient's usual baseline activities of daily living (ADLs) and activity level and ask how symptoms are affecting this. Some older adults experience palpitations as "feeling nervous," so include that in your questioning. Chest pain may be presented as heartburn or indigestion, particularly if the patient also has gastroesophageal reflux disease (GERD). Shortness of breath may be felt as anxiety but is a more common presentation of an acute coronary event than chest pain. Atypical presentation for myocardial infarction includes vague symptoms such as nausea, decreased ADL status, and fatigue without chest pain (Ham, Sloane, Warshaw, Bernard, & Flaherty, 2006).

CLINICAL EXAMINATION FEATURES

In the actual physical assessment of the older adult, the apical impulse is difficult to locate as the chest wall undergoes changes due to the intercostal muscles weakening, resulting in an increased anteroposterior diameter (Bickley & Szilagyi, 2009).

Auscultation in the geriatric patient frequently reveals changes in normal heart sounds, extra heart sounds, bruits, and murmurs. The S_1 is more easily heard, and splits of the first heart sound are more easily detected because of an ejection sound that occurs when the aortic valve cusp tissue fails to fold into the vessel wall during ejection. A change in the loudness of S_1, accompanied by a slow heart rate, may indicate heart block. The S_2 split on inspiration is narrower or absent because of decreased compliance of the pulmonary vasculature. An opening snap occurs when the mitral or tricuspid valve produces minor vibrations of increased intensity caused by more rapid cusp movement or a resistance to inflow caused by cusp fusion

(Bickley & Szilagyi, 2009). An audible opening snap is the best physical sign of mitral stenosis, but it becomes less obvious in the older adult whose valves are rigid and calcified.

Ventricular filling sounds, best heard with the stethoscope bell, are caused by the halting of the ventricle after ventricular filling. The physiological S_3, heard most clearly at the apex, disappears by the fourth decade as the ventricle stiffens and filling becomes less rapid. An S_3 in an individual more than 50 years old is usually pathological and reflects an increased filling rate, indicating heart failure or mitral regurgitation (Bickley & Szilagyi, 2009). Early diastolic filling is reduced in healthy elderly persons, resulting in an end-diastolic volume maintained by an increase in atrial contribution to left ventricular filling. This condition may cause an S_4, which in the absence of other findings, is considered normal in elderly persons.

The carotid arteries should be assessed routinely for the presence of bruit. Asymptomatic carotid bruit is a risk factor for stroke (Bickley & Szilagyi, 2009). Studies demonstrate that a vessel is occluded more than 50% by the time a bruit can be heard. In elderly persons, assess the top level of the internal jugular pulsation when evaluating jugular venous pressure. Do not use the external jugular veins, because they may be sclerosed and appear to be falsely distended or may yield a falsely low pressure reading.

Prolonged extra heart sounds (murmurs), particularly systolic ones, are quite common in elderly individuals. Systolic murmurs, which often indicate aortic valve disease, occur in more than 50% of individuals over age 70. The soft systolic ejection murmur is due to the dilation and the decrease in compliance of the aorta caused by stiffening of the aortic cusps without obstruction (aortic sclerosis). Loud murmurs, which usually indicate aortic stenosis, are often accompanied by a slow rising carotid pulse and left ventricular hypertrophy. An apical pansystolic or late systolic murmur also occurs frequently in older persons, resulting from floppy valves that become regurgitant over time. The two most common causes of mitral regurgitation are papillary muscle dysfunction (usually due to myocardial infarction) and mitral annular calcification. Diastolic murmurs, which are always pathological in elderly persons, may be caused by heart block, aortic regurgitation, or mitral stenosis (Lakatta & Levy, 2003).

In the older adult, additional features of cardiac disease may be seen on physical examination of systems other than the heart. The eye examination may reveal the thick corneal arcus seen with lipid abnormalities or the funduscopic findings of atherosclerosis. The skin may demonstrate xanthomas or cholesterol nodules and changes in skin temperature, indicating a metabolic or peripheral vascular disease causing or contributing to cardiac disease. The presence of edema must be determined. The following lists the clinical cardiac examination features in the geriatric patient:

- Structural wall changes are common.
- S_1 is more easily heard.
- S_2 split is narrower.
- S_4 is common.
- Systolic murmurs are common.
- Bruits (carotid, abdominal) are common.

ASSESSMENT OF THE RESPIRATORY SYSTEM

Key symptoms warranting evaluation include increasing dyspnea and persistent cough (Kane et al., 2008). In order to assess the respiratory system accurately in the older adult, the nurse practitioner (NP) must be familiar with changes in tissue and in the musculoskeletal and respiratory systems that are caused by aging.

The aging process is characterized by a loss of elasticity and flexibility in collagen and elastin tissue components; this impedes the normal expiratory recoil of the lung. The concurrent decrease in body water composition dries mucous membranes and interferes with the protective functions of the upper airway in expelling foreign material. Loss of elastin also affects the alveoli and the basement membrane of the capillary wall, where gas exchange occurs. A thickening occurs in both areas, limiting the amount of diffusion (Bickley & Szilagyi, 2009). Musculoskeletal changes, including calcification of costal cartilage and weakening of inspiratory muscles, result in a relaxation of the skeletal contours and an increased anteroposterior diameter, causing a barrel chest, although not as pronounced as that found in patients with chronic obstructive pulmonary disease (COPD). An exaggeration of the thoracic curvature may also occur, with some tracheal displacement. Expiratory muscles must work harder because expiration is no longer a passive act, resulting in use of accessory muscles. The residual capacity of the lungs is increased and inspiratory reserve capacity lessened. Air tends to fill the apices and not the bases. Because of decreased muscular strength, the cough reflex is not as forceful or as effective. All of these changes occur gradually and are hardly noticeable unless a physiological challenge or stress arises. Even in such an event, exertional dyspnea may be the only observed change in the healthy older adult. Healthy lifestyle behaviors also serve to mitigate these age-related changes.

Healthy older adults or those with stable, chronic problems are unlikely to seek care unless there is a change in functional capabilities related to breathing, such as decreased exercise tolerance, shortness of breath with exertion, or easy fatigability. In frail elderly persons, an increase in respirations, sweating, or anorexia may be the only indication of a respiratory problem. History questions should address the symptom(s) using the OLDCART or PQRST symptom analysis format. Is there a prior history of the problem(s) or of any respiratory problem(s)? Does the patient use tobacco, or has he or she used it in the past? Is there a history of occupational exposures or lung problems? Has the possibility of tuberculosis been eliminated? Is the patient a silent aspirator? Any changes in medications, including the use of over-the-counter (OTC), herbal, and homeopathic remedies, should be addressed. Is there a cough, sputum production, or hemoptysis? Is the patient wheezing? If there is pain, have cardiac or musculoskeletal causes been ruled out? If there is dyspnea, is it related to activity, or does it occur at rest or when lying down? How many pillows are used? Specific questions about changes in endurance, stair-climbing, or ADLs are necessary to quantify the extent of the problem. Does the problem interfere with eating? Has there been a 10-lb weight loss or gain in the past 6 months? Has the patient received the influenza vaccine and pneumococcal vaccine? Is HIV a consideration?

Physical assessment of the respiratory system begins with general observation of the patient: rate and ease of respirations at rest, conversational ability (limited by breathing problems), use of accessory muscles, posture, color, pursed lips, circumoral or nailbed cyanosis, and capillary refill. The chest and upper back should be exposed for full inspection and examination. Are both sides symmetrical, with equal respiratory effort and diaphragmatic movement? Is there any evidence of kyphosis, lordosis, or scoliosis? Rapid respiratory rates are common with pneumonia, fever, or COPD.

Palpation of the posterior chest to confirm equal chest expansion is done by placing the thumbs on the chest wall near the vertebrae at T9 and T10 and spreading the hands. A small fold of skin should be between the thumbs. When the patient takes a deep breath per your instruction, the thumbs should move apart symmetrically. If pneumonia or consolidation is suspected, palpating for tactile fremitus may be helpful. Using the ball of the hand (metacarpophalageal area of the palm) or the ulnar side of the hand, feel the vibrations in a side-to-side pattern while the patient says "ninety-nine." The vibrations should feel the same on either side and should be stronger in the upper areas. Increased fremitus occurs with marked consolidation, such as lobar pneumonia. Percussion of the posterior chest for resonance and symmetry is the next step, again using a side-to-side approach. Dullness is indicative of increased density as found with pneumonia, tumor growth, or pleural effusion. Hyperresonance is found with air trapping in emphysema or with pneumothorax. Auscultation of posterior breath sounds for symmetry, presence or absence of adventitious sounds, and air movement is done with the patient seated and the arms resting on the knees to retract the scapulae. The patient is instructed to take a deep breath through the mouth, with the mouth open, inhaling and exhaling. Decreased breath sounds are common with emphysema, pleurisy, or pleural effusion. Wheezing is commonly heard with asthma or acute bronchitis, although it may also be part of the background of chronic bronchitis or COPD. Crackles are heard with congestive heart failure (CHF), pulmonary edema, or pneumonia; basilar crackles that clear with coughing or deep breathing are not pathological. Older patients become lightheaded with deep breathing and may need this part of the examination to be spaced out over time. If pneumonia is suspected, vocal fremitus techniques such as bronchophony, egophony, or whispered pectoriloquy may be indicated. Examination of the anterior chest follows the same sequence. The right middle lobe is auscultated anterolaterally.

ASTHMA

Signal symptoms: Wheezing, shortness of breath, cough (especially at night), chest tightness.

Etiology: The Global Initiative for Asthma (GINA) describes an operational definition of asthma as a chronic inflammatory disorder of the airways in which many cells and cellular elements play a role. The chronic inflammation is associated with airway hyperresponsiveness that leads to recurrent episodes of wheezing, breathlessness, chest tightness, and coughing, particularly at night or early in the morning. These episodes are usually associated with widespread, but variable, airflow obstruction within the lung that is often reversible either spontaneously or with treatment (Global Strategy for Asthma Management and Prevention, 2011 update).

Both GINA and the National Asthma Education and Prevention Program Expert Panel Report–3 (NAEPP-EPR-3) (2007) cite a lack of agreement on definition and etiology due to the complexity and variation in manifestation of asthma as well as the lack of identification of the phenotype qualities of asthmatics. Characteristics that are agreed on are inflammation, airway hyperresponsiveness, airway obstruction, and clinical symptoms (NAEPP-EPR-3, 2007).

Occurrence: In the United States, asthma is more prevalent in African Americans—the age-adjusted rate for those over 18 years of age is 10.5%; the rate for Caucasians is 7.8%; and the rate for Hispanics/Latinos is 6.9% (U.S. Department of Health and Human Services, Centers for Disease Control and Prevention, National Center for Health Statistics, 2012). Estimates for occurrence of asthma worldwide is 300 million individuals (Global Strategy for Asthma Management and Prevention, 2011 update).

Age: The age-adjusted rate for adults 65 to 74 years old is 8.7%; for age 75 and older it is 7.4% (U.S. Department of Health and Human Services, Centers for Disease Control and Prevention, National Center for Health Statistics, 2012).

Gender: In adult asthma there are more females with the disease than males (Litonjua & Weiss, 2012). The age-adjusted rate for females over 18 years old is 10.3%; for males it is 5.8% (U.S. Department of Health and Human Services, Centers for Disease Control and Prevention, National Center for Health Statistics, 2012).

Contributing factors: Exposure to allergens, respiratory infections, family history/genetic predisposition, atopy, occupational irritants, tobacco smoke (smoking and second-hand smoke exposure) (Eisner et al., 2008), living in an urban area, and obesity; rhinitis is a specific factor in older adults (Boulet, 2008; Global Strategy for Asthma Management and Prevention, 2011 update; Litonjua & Weiss, 2012). Research into genetic phenotypes is ongoing (Fanta & Fletcher, 2012; Ferri, 2012).

Signs and symptoms: Wheezing, recurrent wheezing, cough (especially occurring at night), recurrent chest tightness, and recurrent breathing difficulty (NAEPP-EPR-3, 2007). Symptoms may occur in conjunction with a respiratory infection, weather changes, contact with environmental allergens, strong emotional reactions, animal fur, mold, exercise, or other triggers. Drugs, including aspirin, NSAIDs, and beta blockers, can also exacerbate symptoms. Older adults are less likely to sense dyspnea related to airway obstruction, even in the presence of cough, chest tightness, or wheezing (Enright & Barr, 2012; Gillman & Douglass, 2012; Mathur, 2010). Other symptoms may include rhinorrhea with postnasal drip.

Diagnostic tests: Spirometry or pulmonary function testing, particularly forced expiratory volume in 1 second (FEV_1), FEV_6, forced vital capacity (FVC), and FEV_1/FVC ratio before and after bronchodilator challenge, showing an improvement of 12% and 200 mL, indicates reversible airway obstruction; this is helpful in differentiating asthma from COPD, particularly in an older adult with a prior smoking history. A history of atopy or allergen testing may establish an allergic component. In a patient with dyspnea, measurement of brain natriuretic peptide, also known as B-type natriuretic peptide (BNP), and a chest x-ray may be needed to eliminate other conditions. If spirometry is near normal, bronchoprovocation such as a methacholine challenge test may help to differentiate other conditions with a similar presentation (Irvin, 2011; NAEPP-EPR-3, 2007). Older adults tend to have increased hyperresponsiveness to bronchoprovocation even when adjusting for the baseline amount of airway obstruction, atopy, or smoking status (Mathur, 2010). Enright and Barr (2012) suggest that in response to a low provocative challenge (PC-20), a PC-20 threshold for hyperresponsiveness should be decreased to less than 4 mg/mL in lieu of the standard less than 8 mg/mL. The American Thoracic Society (ATS) has endorsed the use of FENO, the fractional nitrous oxide measurement in exhaled breath, as a biomarker for eosinophilic inflammation and a complementary tool to assess airway disease, including asthma (Dweik et al., 2011). At the present time, use and utility of this test are still evolving.

Differential diagnosis:
- COPD
- CHF
- Pneumonia
- Upper respiratory infection (URI)
- Pulmonary embolism
- Anxiety disorder
- Vocal cord dysfunction (VCD)
- Cough secondary to drugs
- GERD
- Allergic bronchopulmonary aspergillosis (ABPA)

Treatment: The NAEPP-EPR-3 (2007) has identified four components of asthma management:

- Assessment and monitoring measures, including patient history, physical examination, and objective testing such as spirometry to diagnose asthma and determine severity and initial and ongoing level of control
- Patient, family, and professional education for partnership in asthma management
- Control of comorbidities and environmental factors affecting asthma
- Pharmacotherapy

Treatment in older adults may need to be individualized based on comorbidities. Recommendations from the NAEPP-EPR-2 (1997) relevant to older adults that are incorporated into current asthma guidelines include the following:

- Review of patient technique in using inhaler medications/devices is essential; functional, visual, or cognitive impairments may require more intense and prolonged instruction for safe and efficacious use.
- A comprehensive medical history is essential to safely integrate asthma medications without aggravating preexisting medical conditions such as osteoporosis, glaucoma, or cardiac problems. Conversely, medications such as beta blockers or aspirin prescribed for a preexisting condition may need to be reevaluated if they are exacerbating the asthma.
- COPD may coexist with asthma; a trial of systemic corticosteroids will establish reversibility and benefit.

Assessment and monitoring: Initial assessment of severity is optimized when the patient has not been started on long-term controller therapy. Asthma is classified as intermittent or persistent; persistent is further classified as mild, moderate, or severe based on certain parameters (NAEPP-EPR-3, 2007). See Figure 8-1.

Once the severity is established, treatment goals at all levels aim to control asthma and evaluate responsiveness to the plan of care (Fig. 8-2), using a stepwise approach to management (Fig. 8-3).

Asthma is a chronic health problem, just as hypertension and diabetes are. Regular chronic maintenance visits are required for optimal management. Depending on level of control, patients should be seen every 1 to 6 months for reevaluation. An interval symptom history is highly important in ongoing monitoring of control and adjustment of stepped treatment. An increase in symptoms indicating that asthma is not well controlled necessitates stepped up management and more frequent monitoring. A printable asthma action plan including information on controlling environmental triggers is available at www.nhlbi.nih.gov/health/public/lung/asthma/asthma_actplan.pdf. All patients who are able to read and comprehend should have an asthma action plan that is updated whenever changes in treatment are made (Rance, 2011; Yawn, 2011). The plan may need to be adapted to older adults who cannot or will not perform peak flow monitoring. A small ($n = 300$) randomized clinical trial compared two groups of older adults with moderate to severe asthma who received identical instructions in symptom management, with one group receiving additional instruction on use of peak flow meter use. Over a 2-year period, there was no additional benefit seen in the peak flow group in terms of health-care utilization, lung function, or quality of life (Buist, Vollmer, Wilson, Frazier, & Hayward, 2006).

Pharmacotherapy for asthma follows the guidelines in the NAEPP-EPR-3 (2007) outlined in Figure 8-3.

For intermittent asthma, a short-acting beta agonist (SABA) such as albuterol used as required for symptoms is the only treatment. Levalbuterol is an alternative with fewer side effects than albuterol. Patients are instructed to contact their primary care provider if symptoms increase, necessitating more frequent use of the SABA, or if their use of the medication does not alleviate symptoms.

For persistent asthma, initiate stepwise therapy with the goal of well-controlled asthma. For patients with mild persistent asthma by severity classification, Step 2 therapy with a low-dose inhaled corticosteroid (ICS) such as fluticasone should be initiated. The patient should be followed up in 2 to 6 weeks to evaluate level of control and modify treatment as indicated.

Patients with moderate persistent asthma should be started on Step 3 therapy with either a medium-dose ICS or a combined low-dose ICS and long-acting beta agonist (LABA) such as fluticasone/salmeterol, budesonide/formoterol, or momentasone/formoterol. Follow up at 2 to 6 weeks for evaluation of response and adjustments to therapy.

Patients with severe persistent asthma should be started on Step 4 treatment with a medium-dose ICS and LABA combination and reassessed at 2 to 6 weeks for response and level of control.

Assessing severity and initiating treatment for patients who are not currently taking long-term control medications

Components of Severity		Classification of Asthma Severity ≥12 years of age			
			Persistent		
		Intermittent	Mild	Moderate	Severe
Impairment Normal FEV₁/FVC: 8–19 yr 85% 20–39 yr 80% 40–59 yr 75% 60–80 yr 70%	Symptoms	≤2 days/week	>2 days/week but not daily	Daily	Throughout the day
	Nighttime awakenings	≤2x/month	3–4x/month	1x/week but not nightly	Often 7x/week
	Short-acting beta₂-agonist use for symptom control (not prevention of EIB)	≤2 days/week	>2 days/week but not daily, and not more than 1x on any day	Daily	Several times per day
	Interference with normal activity	None	Minor limitation	Some limitation	Extremely limited
	Lung function	• Normal FEV₁ between exacerbations • FEV₁ >80% predicted • FEV₁/FVC normal	• FEV₁ >80% predicted • FEV₁/FVC normal	• FEV₁ >60% but <80% predicted • FEV₁/FVC reduced 5%	• FEV₁ <60% predicted • FEV₁/FVC reduced 5%
Risk	Exacerbations requiring oral systemic corticosteroids	0–1/year	≥2/year ──────────────────────────▶		
		Consider severity and interval since last exacerbation. Frequency and severity may fluctuate over time for patients in any severity category. Relative annual risk of exacerbations may be related to FEV₁.			
Recommended Step for Initiating Treatment		Step 1	Step 2	Step 3 and consider short course of oral systemic corticosteroids	Step 4 or 5
		In 2–6 weeks, evaluate level of asthma control that is achieved and adjust therapy accordingly.			

Key: FEV₁ forced expiratory volume in 1 second; FVC, forced vital capacity; ICU, intensive care unit

FIGURE 8-1. Classifying asthma severity and initiating treatment in youths ≥12 years of age and adults. FEV₁, forced expiratory volume in 1 second; FVC, forced vital capacity. *(National Asthma Education and Prevention Program. [2007, August]. Third Expert Panel on the Diagnosis and Management of Asthma. Expert Panel Report 3: Guidelines for the diagnosis and management of asthma. Section 4: Stepwise approach for managing asthma in youths ≥12 years of age and adults. Bethesda, MD: National Heart, Lung, and Blood Institute. Available from www.ncbi.nlm.nih.gov/books/NBK7222)*

For Steps 2 through 4 alternative treatments include a leukotriene modifier antagonist (LTRA) such as montelukast, either alone (Step 2) or in combination with an ICS (Steps 3 through 4). A recent Cochrane review (Chauhan & Ducharme, 2012) found that LTRAs were safe but not as effective as monotherapy ICS for asthma. Research continues into the role of leukotrienes in asthma (Hallstrand & Henderson, 2010). Theophylline is also listed as an alternative treatment in Steps 2 through 4; Enright and Barr (2012) discourage the use of this medication in older adults due to toxicity and adverse effects. Other considerations in older adults with comorbidities include individualizing therapy—for example, for a patient with heart disease, increasing the dose of ICS and avoiding a LABA is prudent; for a patient with glaucoma or osteopenia, adding a LABA or LTRA instead of increasing the dose of ICS is preferable (Enright & Barr, 2012; Peters, McCallister, & Pascual,

Components of Control		Classification of Asthma Control ≥12 years of age		
		Well Controlled	Not Well Controlled	Very Poorly Controlled
Impairment	Symptoms	≤2 days/week	>2 days/week	Throughout the day
	Nighttime awakenings	≤2x/month	1–3x/week	≥4x/week
	Interference with normal activity	None	Some limitation	Extremely limited
	Short-acting beta$_2$-agonist use for symptom control (not prevention of EIB)	≤2 days/week	>2 days/week	Several times per day
	FEV$_1$ or peak flow	>80% predicted/ personal best	60%–80% predicted/ personal best	<60% predicted/ personal best
	Validated questionnaires ATAQ ACQ ACT	 0 ≤0.75* ≥20	 1–2 ≥1.5 16–19	 3–4 N/A ≤15
Risk	Exacerbations requiring oral systemic corticosteroids	0–1/year	≥2/year	
		Consider severity and interval since last exacerbation.		
	Progressive loss of lung function	Evaluation requires long-term follow-up care		
	Treatment-related adverse effects	Medication side effects can vary in intensity from none to very troublesome and worrisome. The level of intensity does not correlate to specific levels of control but should be considered in the overall assesment of risk.		
Recommended Action for Treatment		• Maintain current step. • Regular follow-ups every 1–6 months to maintain control. • Consider step down if well controlled for at least 3 months.	• Step up 1 step and • Reevaluate in 2–6 weeks. • For side effects, consider alternative treatment options.	• Consider short course of oral systemic corticosteroids • Step up 1–2 steps, and • Reevaluate in 2 weeks. • For side effects, consider alternative treatment options.

*ACQ values of 0.76–1.4 are indeterminate regarding well-controlled asthma.
Key: EIB, exercise-induced bronchospasm; ICU, intensive care unit

FIGURE 8-2. Assessing asthma control and adjusting therapy in youths ≥12 years of age and adults. EIB, exercise-induced bronchospasm. *(National Asthma Education and Prevention Program. [2007, August]. Third Expert Panel on the Diagnosis and Management of Asthma. Expert Panel Report 3: Guidelines for the diagnosis and management of asthma. Section 4: Stepwise approach for managing asthma in youths ≥12 years of age and adults. Bethesda, MD: National Heart, Lung, and Blood Institute. Available from www.ncbi.nlm.nih.gov/books/NBK7222)*

2012). In short, guidelines are not meant to be absolute and do not preclude the use of clinical judgment.

For patients with severe persistent asthma, initiate therapy at Step 5, with a high-dose ICS/LABA and possible addition of omalizumab for patients with an allergic component. Studies have demonstrated that omalizumab, a humanized monoclonal antibody, is safe and effective for difficult-to-control asthma in older adults who meet allergic criteria (Korn et al.,

2010; Maykut, Kianifard, & Geba, 2008; Pelaia et al., 2011; Thomson & Chaudhuri, 2012). Practitioners must be prepared to treat anaphylaxis in the unlikely event that it occurs.

Step 6 is reserved for patients who are not well controlled at Step 5. Therapy includes high-dose ICS and LABA and oral corticosteroid. Omalizumab should also be considered for those with an allergic component. Close follow-up of these patients is essential to avoid

Intermittent Asthma	Persistent Asthma: Daily Medication
	Consult with asthma specialist if step 4 care or higher is required. Consider consultation at step 3.

Step 1

Preferred:
SABA PRN

Step 2

Preferred:
Low-dose
ICS

Alternative:
Cromolyn,
LTRA,
nedocromil, or
theophylline

Step 3

Preferred:
Low-dose
ICS + LABA
OR
Medium-dose
ICS

Alternative:
Low-dose ICS
+ either LTRA,
theophylline,
or zileuton

Step 4

Preferred:
Medium-dose
ICS + LABA

Alternative:
Medium-dose
ICS + either
LTRA,
theophylline,
or zileuton

Step 5

Preferred:
High-dose
ICS + LABA
AND
Consider
omalizumab
for patients who
have allergies

Step 6

Preferred:
High-dose
ICS + LABA +
oral
corticosteroid
AND
Consider
omalizumab
for patients who
have allergies

Step up if
needed

(first, check
adherence,
environmental
control, and
comorbid
conditions)

*Assess
control*

Step down if
possible

(and asthma is
well controlled
at least
3 months)

Each step: Patient education, environmental control, and management of comorbidities.
Steps 2–4: Consider subcutaneous allergen immunotherapy for patients who have asthma.

Quick-Relief Medications for All Patients
• SABA as needed for symptoms. Intensity of treatment depends on severity of symptoms: up to 3 treatments at 20-minute intervals as needed.
• Use of SABA >2 days a week for symptom relief (not prevention of EIB) generally indicates inadequate control and the need to step up treatments.

Alphabetical order is used when more than one treatment option is listed within either preferred or alternative therapy.
EIB, exercise-induced bronchospasm; ICS, inhaled corticosteroid; LABA, long-acting inhaled beta$_2$-agonist; LTRA, leukotriene receptor antagonist; SABA, inhaled short-acting beta$_2$-agonist

FIGURE 8-3. Stepwise approach for managing asthma in youths ≥12 years of age and adults. EIB, exercise-induced bronchospasm; ICS, inhaled corticosteroid; LABA, long-acting inhaled beta-2 agonist; LTRA, leukotriene receptor antagonist; SABA, inhaled short-acting beta-2 agonist. *(National Asthma Education and Prevention Program. [2007, August]. Third Expert Panel on the Diagnosis and Management of Asthma. Expert Panel Report 3: Guidelines for the diagnosis and management of asthma. Section 4: Stepwise approach for managing asthma in youths ≥12 years of age and adults. Bethesda, MD: National Heart, Lung, and Blood Institute. Available from www.ncbi.nlm.nih.gov/books/NBK7222)*

further morbidity and even mortality due to asthma. Oral corticosteroid therapy should be limited to short "bursts" to avoid drug-related events.

Asthma exacerbations in older adults frequently result in emergency department visits or hospital admissions. Aggressive treatment with SABAs and systemic (IV or oral) glucocorticoids is the standard of care along with frequent spirometric assessment (Fanta, 2011; Humphrey, 2009). Patients who do not respond well within 4 to 6 hours should be

hospitalized (Fanta, 2012). Despite this, follow-up studies have shown that less than 50% of the patients have filled their prescription for either oral corticosteroid or ICS 1 week after discharge (Krishnan et al., 2004).

Stepping down therapy is a gradual process compared to stepping up treatment. If a patient has been stable and well controlled for 3 months or more, consider stepping the patient down to the next lower level of treatment.

Follow-up: Regular monitoring at 1- to 6-month intervals is recommended, depending on the level of control and severity. After initial diagnosis until the patient is stable and when making stepwise changes, follow up at intervals of 2 to 6 weeks (Ferri, 2012; NAEPP-EPR-3, 2007). If step-down is anticipated, monitoring every 3 months is advised.

Sequelae: Asthma in older adults is associated with increased bronchial hyperresponsiveness and a more rapid decline in lung function than in older adults without asthma (Mathur, 2010). Older adults also have increased treatment-related adverse events. Comorbidities such as COPD, cardiovascular disease, osteoporosis, glaucoma, diabetes mellitus, and other health problems complicate management and may limit treatment options. Older adults have the highest rate of asthma-associated mortality.

Prevention/prophylaxis: There is no known strategy to prevent asthma. Patients with asthma should be given influenza vaccine annually. Immunization with the pneumococcal pneumonia vaccine is also advised if the patient has not already been immunized. Partnership with the patient/family in education to recognize triggers, identify changes in status, and seek prompt medical assistance to avoid complications is key to success. Avoidance of environmental factors is also essential.

Referral: According to the NAEPP-EPR-3 (2007) report, consultation with an asthma specialist is advised at Step 4, with a suggestion to consider a consultation at Step 3. Older adults who have multiple comorbidities, have been treated in the emergency department, or have been hospitalized due to an asthma exacerbation within the past year should also be managed in collaboration with an asthma specialist. Patients who require ongoing oral corticosteroids or more than two courses of oral corticosteroids in a year should be referred to an asthma specialist. Patients having any complications that affect asthma or those who require further testing should be also referred (Fanta, 2012; Humphrey,

2009; NAEPP-EPR-2, 1997); patients with characteristics of both asthma and COPD fall into this category (Zeki, Schivo, Chan, Albertson, & Louie, 2011). Patients/families may also be referred to a community-based asthma education program, although many of these initiatives are more focused on childhood asthma. Referral to case management through local Area Agency on Aging services can be helpful if the patient has unmet care needs or financial problems with obtaining medications.

Education: Patient/family education is an important component of asthma management in older adults. In addition to educating patients on the disease and the need for frequent monitoring and immediate reporting of increased symptoms, a written asthma action plan should be initiated, detailing how to identify and deal with environmental triggers, medications (including dosage and frequency), and when to seek emergent care. Instruction in use and care of inhalers and spacers, if used, is also important. If the patient is on an ICS, instruct on the need for daily use and oral hygiene to prevent a fungal infection. Clarification of the action and role of quick relief inhaler versus daily controller therapy is essential for medication adherence. The role of patient as partner in asthma management should be emphasized (Rance, 2011).

A recent survey (patient self-report) of asthma control in adults and children in 64 primary care practices nationwide revealed that factors predictive of uncontrolled asthma in adults were less education, a BMI of more than $30 \, kg/m^2$, insurance status, history of gastroesophageal symptoms, and current tobacco use (Stanford et al., 2010). Gearing education to the health literacy level of the patient is critical to gaining patient understanding and partnership. Patients who are still smoking should receive brief motivational counseling at each visit and referral to a Quitline or community-based smoking cessation program when ready to quit. Referral to the local Area Agency on Aging for assistance with insurance issues may also be beneficial.

CLINICAL RECOMMENDATION	EVIDENCE RATING	REFERENCE
The hallmark of asthma is partial reversibility of airflow obstruction on spirometry following beta-2 agonist administration.	B	Kraft & DeSimone (2011)

Continued

CLINICAL RECOMMENDATION	EVIDENCE RATING	REFERENCE
Short-acting beta-2 agonists (SABAs) are indicated only as needed rather than on a scheduled basis for all levels of asthma severity.	A	Kraft & DeSimone (2011)
Inhaled corticosteroids (ICSs) are the preferred controller medication for all but mild intermittent asthma.	A	Kraft & DeSimone (2011)
Long-acting beta agonists are the preferred add-on agent due to lack of control, but they should never be used as monotherapy without ICSs.	A	Kraft & DeSimone (2011)
It is important to educate patients on the proper technique for inhaled medications and triggers.	B	Kraft & DeSimone (2011)
Early treatment of asthma exacerbations is the best strategy for management and improved outcomes.	A	EPR-3 (2008) Humphrey (2011)
Initial treatment (of asthma exacerbation) should include oxygen for most patients, SABA for all patients, ipratropium bromide for severe exacerbations, and systemic corticosteroids for most patients.	A	EPR-3 (2008)
Response to initial treatment in the emergency department is a better predictor of need for hospitalization than severity of the attack on presentation.	C	Rowe et al. (2007)

A = consistent, good-quality, patient-oriented evidence; B = inconsistent or limited-quality, patient-oriented evidence; C = consensus, disease-oriented evidence, usual practice, expert opinion, or case series. For information about the SORT evidence rating system, go to www.aafp.org/afpsort.xml.

CARDIAC ARRHYTHMIAS

Signal symptom: No symptoms at times; feeling of heart "beating out of the chest."

Description: An arrhythmia is a disturbance of cardiac rhythm. Cardiac arrhythmias, which occur in either the presence or absence of underlying heart disease, may be life threatening or may be an incidental finding. Arrhythmias may be differentiated by type or mechanism.

Atrial fibrillation is the most common sustained rhythm disorder. Atrial fibrillation consists of numerous fibrillatory P waves that vary in shape, size, and timing. The ventricular response is often chaotic and rapid if the atrioventricular (AV) conduction is intact. Atrial fibrillation can be clinically classified as follows:

- Paroxysmal, less than 7 days and self-terminating
- Persistent, greater than 7 days and requires intervention to terminate
- Permanent, which is refractory to cardioversion or is determined to be the final rhythm (Knight, Sorrentino, Delaughter, & Shah, 2010)

Other prevalent forms of arrhythmias in a geriatric population are as follows:

Sick sinus syndrome: (1) Pathological bradyarrhythmia with an alternating supraventricular tachyarrhythmia (bradycardia-tachycardia syndrome). (2) Supraventricular tachyarrhythmia—three primary categories.

Arrhythmias primarily of atrial origin: Atrial premature beats, ectopic atrial rhythms, multifocal atrial tachycardia, atrial flutter, and atrial fibrillation.

Arrhythmias arising primarily within the AV node: AV nodal reentrant tachycardia, junctional premature beats, and nonparoxysmal junctional tachycardia.

Arrhythmias partially supraventricular in origin: Preexcitation syndromes.

Ventricular arrhythmias: Ventricular ectopic beats are the most common variety.

Etiology: Most arrhythmias are thought to be caused by abnormalities either in impulse formation (disordered automaticity) or in impulse conduction (allowing reentry), or by a combination of the two. Increased automaticity is an accentuation of the inherent ability of many cardiac tissues to generate an independent rhythm. Reentry consists of a wave of excitation repeatedly circulating around a fixed anatomical obstacle. Triggered arrhythmias are caused by altered cellular depolarization.

Occurrence: Studies show that asymptomatic older patients with no known structural heart disease have an incidence of up to 40% of sinus arrhythmia, supraventricular or ventricular premature beats, or supraventricular tachycardia.

Age: The prevalence of ventricular arrhythmia increases with age, occurring in 80% of healthy older adults ages 60 to 85. Atrial fibrillation is diagnosed in 4.8% of women and 6.2% of men over age 65 at baseline examination, and its prevalence is strongly associated with advanced age, particularly in women. Although no specific data are available, the incidence of junctional arrhythmias and tachycardias related to the accessory pathway may be lower in elderly individuals because of an age-related reduction in accessory pathway conduction.

Ethnicity: Not significant.

Gender: Arrhythmias occur slightly more often in men than in women. (See also Age.)

Contributing factors: Preexisting heart disease is a contributing factor to arrhythmias, with structural disease becoming more prevalent with age. The muscular response and contractility decreases as the patient ages. The patient experiences a reduction in cardiac function and contractility. This reduction is responsible for a decreased stroke volume and ejection fraction. The average elderly person does not experience adverse symptoms with normal everyday activities. However, stressors (whether they are physical, psychological, environmental, or social) can increase the risk of illness in the patient. These illnesses are taxing to the patient's system, and the increased energy demands place an increased demand on the cardiac system. The aging process can also have an adverse effect on the cardiac valves. The valves tend to become thick and stiff secondary to arteriosclerosis and atherosclerotic plaques. Fibrosis or calcification in the vicinity of the AV node causes conduction disturbances. Atrial arrhythmias may be caused by a mechanical obstruction to atrial emptying with subsequent left atrial dilation, myocardial ischemia, and increased sympathetic activity.

An age-related factor associated with tachyarrhythmias is increased left atrial size. This enlargement may contribute to the increase in supraventricular ectopy. Increases in ventricular ectopic beats may be related to left ventricular enlargement. The overload of ionized calcium in the older myocardium may contribute to ectopy. Age-related factors associated with bradyarrhythmias include an age-related decline in the number of pacemaker cells and the presence of fat deposits around the SA node. His bundle cells are replaced with fibrous tissue, and adipose tissue and amyloid are deposited; this is also associated with conduction disturbance.

Systemic diseases (i.e., thyrotoxicosis, infection, hypoxemia, hypercapnea) can cause circulatory disturbances that may provoke an arrhythmia. Drugs that can cause an arrhythmia include digitalis and other antiarrhythmics, aminophylline, and alcohol. Electrolyte disturbances, particularly hyperkalemia, hypokalemia, hypercalcemia, and hypocalcemia, can precipitate ectopic beats. Family history of sudden cardiac death may indicate a predisposing factor for rhythm disorder, such as hypertrophic obstructive cardiomyopathy, congenital prolonged QT syndrome, or the presence of an aberrant conduction pathway.

Signs and symptoms: The history, physical examination, and electrocardiogram (ECG) studies represent the cornerstone to evaluation of arrhythmias. Arrhythmias may cause symptoms due to a reduced blood flow or inadequate cardiac pump function. In the history, the patient may describe sensations that accompany abnormal cardiac rhythm such as pounding, racing, or skipped beats. Older adults are less likely to complain of palpitations and more likely to present with manifestations of heart failure or hypoperfusion (i.e., impaired mental function, dizziness, syncope). There appears to be a peak in syncopal episodes above age 65 in both men and women. The Framingham study showed an increased incidence of syncope after age 70 years, from 5.7 events per 1000 person-years in men ages 60 to 69, to 11.1 in men ages 70 to 79 (Moya et al., 2009). Along with the history of present illness, previous diagnosis and treatment for arrhythmia and cardiac disease should be elicited.

In the physical examination, concentrate on the cardiac and peripheral vascular systems. Check the pulses for 1 full minute to determine rate and regularity (Bickley & Szilagyi, 2009; Goolsby & Grubbs, 2011). Assess normal and extra heart sounds. S_1 intensity may provide information about the relation of atrial to ventricular contraction. The longer the PR interval, the softer the S_1. Note intermittent extra heart sounds (S_3 and S_4). The jugular vein must be assessed. In AV dissociation (when the atria and ventricles contract independently), giant A waves (cannon waves) may be observed. Provoking maneuvers should not be attempted by the advanced practice nurse but may be attempted by a cardiologist. These maneuvers include carotid massage (for atrial arrhythmias only), mild exercise, psychological stress, pharmacological stress, and electrical programmed stimulation (EPS).

Other indicators of hemodynamic response to an arrhythmia include level of consciousness and skin temperature and color. The history should guide the remainder of the episodic examination because it is also helpful in identifying the contributing factors that may precipitate or aggravate an arrhythmia.

Diagnostic tests:

TEST	RESULTS INDICATING DISORDER
Rhythm strip	Rhythm disturbance may be present, or if transient, it may be absent
12-lead ECG	Acute myocardial infarction or ischemia, prolonged QT intervals, and pre-excitation may be identified as precipitators of an arrhythmia
Ambulatory ECG monitoring	Quantifies arrhythmias with reference to symptoms
	Identifies patients at risk for sudden death by documenting ventricular arrhythmias and heart rate variability
Implantable loop recorder	In infrequent syncope this long-term device (14 months) may identify the precipitant
Echocardiogram	Identifies structural, functional, and hemodynamic abnormalities in the cardiovascular system
Cardiac electrophysiological study	Evaluates specific arrhythmias to distinguish these, determine location and characteristics, and guide therapy
Implantable cardioverter-defibrillator (ICD)	ICD firings may be due to recurrent arrhythmia
Electrolyte panel	Identify electrolyte disturbance (i.e., hypokalemia, hyperkalemia, hypomagnesemia, hypocalcemia) that may be causative or contributory

Diagnostic testing: Diagnostic testing includes a 12-lead ECG done with a rhythm strip, lasting at least 2 to 3 minutes. Include exercise testing for those with a clinical history suggesting exercise-induced arrhythmia. Ventricular arrhythmias can occur in individuals with or without cardiac disorders. The standard resting 12-lead ECG is indicated in all patients who are evaluated for ventricular arrhythmias (Zipes et al., 2006). An ambulatory 24-hour ECG (Holter monitoring) helps to quantify arrhythmias with reference to symptoms. Ambulatory ECG is indicated when there is a need to clarify the diagnosis by detecting arrhythmias, QT interval changes, T-wave alternans, or ST changes; to evaluate risk; or to judge therapy (Zipes et al., 2006). Event recorders are best suited for documenting less-frequent but more-prolonged bouts of arrhythmias. Patient-activated loop memory devices, which record the ECG before the symptomatic event, are most useful.

His bundle electrograms involve the insertion of a transvenous electrode catheter into the right ventricle, to record depolarizations and the intervals. This method is most useful for distinguishing AV block from an ectopic focus.

Echocardiography is recommended in patients with ventricular arrhythmias who are suspected of having structural heart disease (Zipes et al., 2006). An echocardiogram is used more commonly than magnetic resonance imaging (MRI) or cardiac computed tomography (CT) because it is inexpensive in comparison. The echocardiogram is a useful tool in assessing for valvular disorders, left ventricular function and wall motion, and the ejection fraction. The electrophysiological (EP) testing is performed using intracardiac recordings, electrical stimulation, and drugs to assess and document ventricular tachycardia, guide ablations, and evaluate loss of consciousness in patients with arrhythmias as the suspected cause. EP testing is recommended for diagnostic evaluation of patients with remote myocardial infarction with symptoms suggestive of ventricular tachyarrhythmias, including palpitations, presyncope, and syncope (Zipes et al., 2006). EP testing is recommended in patients with syncope of unknown cause with impaired left ventricular function or structural heart disease (Zipes et al., 2006).

In EPS, multipolar catheter electrodes are introduced into the venous or atrial circulation and advanced to various intracardiac positions to monitor the electrical activity or to induce an arrhythmia. EPS is most useful for determining sinus node dysfunction, AV block, intraventricular conduction disturbances, pre-excitation syndromes, supraventricular tachycardia, ventricular tachycardia, and unexplained syncope or palpitations. It is used also to monitor cardiac activity in survivors of sudden cardiac death.

Differential diagnosis: Clarify the diagnosis with precision. Note reversible and precipitating causes of an arrhythmia and coexisting diseases.

Treatment: The incidence of asymptomatic arrhythmias of questionable clinical significance is high. Arrhythmias are never treated in isolation; some are benign and some are lethal. Patients with hemodynamic compromise resulting from arrhythmia need to be hospitalized as soon as possible. Prehospital care for threatening hemodynamic instability secondary to tachyarrhythmia may include direct current cardioversion, and the nurse practitioner should be skilled in this intervention. After thorough investigation, the goals of arrhythmia treatment include the alleviation of bothersome symptoms, the prevention of complications from sustained arrhythmias, and the avoidance of sudden death associated with certain arrhythmias.

The risk of treatment is considerable. Aggressive therapeutic treatment is indicated when patients are symptomatic and the urgency of therapy depends on the associated hemodynamic disturbance.

A comprehensive treatment plan must address the three cornerstones of AF management: rate control, rhythm control, and prevention of thromboembolism. Goals of the therapy should be to obtain symptom control, stroke prevention, and a reduction in hospital recidivism (Knight et al., 2010).

Three major factors determine how well a patient tolerates an arrhythmia: heart rate, duration of the arrhythmia, and presence and severity of associated underlying heart disease. Arrhythmias often cannot be controlled unless underlying cardiac problems are discovered and treated. No antiarrhythmic "wonder drug" exists, and the bothersome and potentially dangerous side effects necessitate determination of clear indications and use of the utmost caution. Pharmaceutical agent selection is based on the electrophysiology of the rhythm disturbance, the mechanism of action, and the side effects of the drug. Dabigatran is useful as an alternative to warfarin for the prevention of stroke and systemic thromboembolism in patients with paroxysmal to permanent atrial fibrillation and risk factors for stroke or systemic embolization who do not have a prosthetic heart valve or hemodynamically significant valve disease, severe renal failure, or advanced liver disease (Wann et al., 2011). Conditions common in the elderly that can affect the choice, dosing, efficacy, and safety of antiarrhythmic therapy include decreased hepatic or renal function, decreased serum albumin levels, and electrolyte abnormalities.

The broad categories of arrhythmia treatment include medications, pacemakers, antitachycardia devices, implantable automatic cardioverter-defibrillators, catheter ablative procedure, and specific maneuvers. Defibrillation is the required intervention in ventricular fibrillation or pulseless ventricular tachycardia and is the most important determinant of survival in cardiac arrest. A 1-minute delay in defibrillation is associated with a reduction in odds of survival of up to 21% (Scottish Intercollegiate Guidelines Network, 2007). Vagal maneuvers (carotid massage or the Valsalva maneuver) may terminate or slow AV nodal reentry or AV reentry types. These maneuvers are associated with a high risk of emboli dislodgment. The carotid arteries should be assessed for bruit before administering massage.

Because of the high mortality rate associated with antiarrhythmic surgery, it is not recommended in elderly individuals. The specifics of treatment are not detailed in this text, because all assessment and management must be done in close collaboration with a physician; much of the treatment is initiated by the specialist in the hospital setting.

Follow-up: Because of their low therapeutic ratio, drug dosing and plasma concentrations of the antiarrhythmics are based on therapeutic monitoring. Side effects are significant and include the negative inotropic effect, which can precipitate heart failure or proarrhythmia in the presence of structural heart disease. Extracardiac side effects can also be significant, including anticholinergic effects, gastrointestinal effects, and neurological toxicity with some antiarrhythmic agents. Monitor patients after pacemaker insertion with regular follow-up appointments and ECG testing, specifically looking for pacemaker failure, infection, thromboembolism, perforation or dislodgment, and complicating arrhythmias.

Sequelae: Regardless of age, the nature and severity of underlying heart disease are of much greater prognostic significance than the arrhythmia alone. The following rhythm disturbances have been reported to carry a poor prognosis in patients with CAD: frequent ventricular premature contractions (VPCs) (greater than 10/min), multiform VPCs, ventricular couplets, R-on-T phenomenon, and ventricular tachycardia.

Syncope can occur secondary to asystole. Syncope is an intermittent symptom that may be caused by an underlying arrhythmia with or without cardiac disease. Treatment goals are prevention of symptom recurrence, improvement of quality of life, and prolongation of survival. Permanent cardiac pacing may relieve the symptoms but may not affect the survival rate. Syncope recurs in approximately 20% of the patients (Moya et al., 2009). Bradycardia can contribute to complete heart block and to the development of heart failure in patients with associated ventricular dysfunction. Tachycardia can precipitate angina and circulatory arrest in patients with CAD. Bradyarrhythmias or tachyarrhythmias can cause systemic embolism and stroke. Atrial fibrillation can result in heart failure and a low cardiac output state. The risk of stroke related to atrial fibrillation increases with age.

The Cardiac Arrhythmia Suppression Trial (CAST) demonstrated that patients treated for prognostically significant arrhythmias may have a higher mortality rate from sudden cardiac death if Class IC (flecainide and encainide) agents are used (Greenberg et al., 1995).

Prevention/prophylaxis: All patients with atrial fibrillation should be considered for long-term low-intensity warfarin therapy. Aspirin, though less effective in preventing stroke, is an alternative for some patients in whom warfarin is contraindicated. Electrolyte imbalances should be monitored and metabolic disturbances treated. Patients receiving digitalis should be monitored for toxicity.

Referral: All patients with treatable arrhythmias require collaborative management. Clinically significant ventricular arrhythmias or any symptomatic arrhythmia is managed by the specialist in the coronary care unit. A primary care physician may handle many atrial arrhythmias and low-grade ventricular arrhythmias; however, a specialist should be consulted for all clinically significant ventricular arrhythmias, arrhythmias resistant to routine therapy, or arrhythmias whose clinical significance is in doubt.

Education: Carefully instruct all patients receiving antiarrhythmics about the therapeutic effects, side effects, and potentially adverse effects of these medications. Because patients with pacemakers are vulnerable to external electrical fields, they should be instructed to recognize this potential and avoid exposure. Patients with pacemakers must also be aware of signs and symptoms of pacemaker failure.

CLINICAL RECOMMENDATION	EVIDENCE RATING	REFERENCE
Dabigatran is useful as an alternative to warfarin for the prevention of stroke and systemic thromboembolism in patients with paroxysmal to permanent atrial fibrillation and risk factors for stroke or systemic embolization who do not have a prosthetic heart valve or hemodynamically significant valve disease, severe renal failure, or advanced liver disease.	C	Wann et al. (2011)

CLINICAL RECOMMENDATION	EVIDENCE RATING	REFERENCE
A 1-minute delay in defibrillation is associated with a reduction in odds of survival of up to 21%.	C	Scottish Intercollegiate Guidelines Network (2007)
Permanent cardiac pacing may relieve the symptoms but may not affect the survival rate. Syncope recurs in approximately 20% of the patients.	C	Moya et al. (2009)
EP testing is recommended in patients with syncope of unknown cause with impaired left ventricular function or structural heart disease.	C	Zipes et al. (2006)
EP testing is recommended for diagnostic evaluation of patients with remote myocardial infarction with symptoms suggestive of ventricular tachyarrhythmias, including palpitations, presyncope, and syncope.	C	Zipes et al. (2006)
Echocardiography is recommended in patients with ventricular arrhythmias who are suspected of having structural heart disease.	C	Zipes et al. (2006)
Ambulatory ECG is indicated when there is a need to clarify the diagnosis by detecting arrhythmias, QT-interval changes, T-wave alternans, or ST changes, to evaluate risk.	C	Zipes et al. (2006)
The standard resting 12-lead ECG is indicated in all patients who are evaluated for ventricular arrhythmias.	C	Zipes et al. (2006)

A = consistent, good-quality, patient-oriented evidence; B = inconsistent or limited-quality, patient-oriented evidence; C = consensus, disease-oriented evidence, usual practice, expert opinion, or case series. For information about the SORT evidence rating system, go to www.aafp.org/afpsort.xml.

CHRONIC OBSTRUCTIVE PULMONARY DISEASE

Signal symptoms: Dyspnea, chronic cough with sputum production, decreased activity tolerance, wheezing.

Description: COPD (also called chronic obstructive lung disease [COLD]) encompasses a group of conditions distinguished by ongoing expiratory airflow limitation (Shapiro, Reilly, & Rennard, 2010). COPD is preventable and treatable and includes multisystemic manifestations that may influence disease severity (Remels, Gosker, van der Velden, Langen, & Schols, 2007). COPD is defined by the Global Initiative for Chronic Obstructive Lung Disease (GOLD, 2011) as persistent airflow limitation that is progressive and associated with heightened inflammatory responses of a chronic nature in the lung and airways in the presence of noxious gases or particulate. The pulmonary component includes an abnormal inflammatory response to noxious stimuli, principally tobacco, but also occupational and environmental pollutants. The hallmark of chronic bronchitis is a daily chronic cough with increased sputum production lasting for at least 3 consecutive months in at least 2 consecutive years, usually worse on awakening; this may or may not be associated with COPD (GOLD, 2011). Emphysema is characterized by obstruction to airflow caused by abnormal airspace enlargement distal to terminal bronchioles. Recent evidence indicates that fibrosis occurs and the walls of the airspaces are destroyed, because inflammatory mediators, including polynuclear and mononuclear phagocytes, select T cells, and B cells, infiltrate the airways, resulting in chronic inflammation and remodeling. Air becomes trapped, hindering effective O_2 and CO_2 exchange. Although most patients with COPD have a combination of chronic bronchitis and emphysema, usually one predominates. Most authorities do not consider asthma as part of COPD, but it frequently coexists with COPD (Qaseem et al., 2011; Stephens & Yew, 2008; Yawn, 2009; Zeki, Schivo, Chan, Albertson, & Louie, 2011).

Etiology: Cigarette smoking is the primary etiological agent in COPD. Airway hyperreactivity and chronic inflammation are also factors. Currently studies are underway to identify phenotypes and gender variations. Alpha-1 antitrypsin deficiency is a known genetic determinant for one type of COPD (MacNee, 2008). Because COPD is a collection of heterogeneous conditions, precise etiological parameters are still evolving. Many patients with COPD are not smokers and have never smoked (Shapiro et al., 2010).

Occurrence: Those with a long history of cigarette smoking are at high risk for COPD. COPD affects more than 24 million people in the United States. It is the third leading cause of death in the United States (American Lung Association, n.d.) and the fourth leading cause of death in the world (GOLD, 2011).

Age: Highest incidence is in males over 40 years; older age groups have the greatest prevalence of both chronic bronchitis and emphysema (Cooper & Dransfield, 2008).

Ethnicity: Caucasians have the highest rate of COPD, followed by non-Hispanic blacks.

Gender: COPD is more common in men than in women. Women with COPD have fewer pack-years of smoking than men and progress to severe COPD more rapidly than men. Women die from COPD more frequently than men. Women tend to have more chronic bronchitis, whereas men have more emphysema (Martinez et al., 2007).

Contributing factors: Frequent exposure to tobacco smoke either by direct or second-hand smoke inhalation; industrial gases or fumes, dust particles, use of biomass fuels for heat and cooking, aerosol sprays, dander; frequent respiratory infections; and repeated allergic responses all contribute to the development of COPD (Buist et al, 2007; Ferri, 2012; GOLD, 2011; Radin & Cote, 2008; Wise & Tashkin, 2007).

Signs and symptoms: The patient may experience changes in appetite or activity tolerance. Symptoms may include chronic cough with copious sputum, wheezing, recurrent respiratory infections, fatigue, and mild exertional dyspnea progressing to difficulty breathing at rest. Signs may include neck vein distention during expiration in absence of heart failure, increased anteroposterior diameter of thorax, use of accessory muscles for respiration, prolonged expiration, hyperresonance on percussion, decreased heart and breath sounds, tachypnea, ruddy or cyanotic skin color, and clubbing of nail beds. Nocturnal and seasonal exacerbation of symptoms is common. Dyspnea is usually a late finding in older adults (Hall & Ahmed, 2007). Because the older COPD patient usually has several manifestations of COPD, symptoms often vary.

A careful history regarding onset and timing of symptoms, changes in activity and exercise patterns, smoking, and occupational background helps to establish the diagnosis. Physical examination will not reveal early stages of COPD but does help in establishing a baseline and uncovering comorbidities. Initially, the patient may present frequently with sinus or respiratory infections. As the disease progresses, changes in the respiratory pattern (such as prolonged expiration, pursed-lip breathing, and use of accessory muscles of respiration) can be seen. Weight loss is frequently seen in the later stages of emphysema when the patient becomes dyspneic while trying to eat. Right-sided heart failure and cor pulmonale seen in the later stages may present as jugular venous distention, hepatomegaly, or peripheral edema. The patient's color may appear ruddy or dusky, depending on oxygenation. In the early to middle stages, chest auscultation may reveal longer expirations, with wheezing on forced expiration. Later, as the chest hyperinflates, breath sounds become distant and percussion is hyperresonant. Wheezes can sometimes be heard (most frequently with chronic bronchitis); the presence of crackles suggests possible pulmonary edema or pneumonia. The chest takes on a barrel-like appearance. Hyperinflation restricts diaphragmatic movement. As the cardiovascular system attempts to compensate, tachycardia or a gallop rhythm commonly occurs (Table 8-1).

TABLE 8-1	Global Initiative for Chronic Obstructive Lung Disease: Post-Bronchodilator FEV$_1$ Classification of Severity of Airflow Limitation

Patient criteria: FEV$_1$/FVC <0.70	
FEV$_1$ ≥80% predicted	GOLD 1: Mild
50% ≤FEV$_1$ <80% predicted	GOLD 2: Moderate
30% ≤FEV$_1$ <50% predicted	GOLD 3: Severe
FEV$_1$ <30% predicted	GOLD 4: Very Severe

Adapted from *GOLD Pocket Guide to COPD Diagnosis, Management, and Prevention, A Guide for Health Care Professionals*, 2011.

Differential diagnosis: Carcinoma of the lung, asthma, interstitial lung disease, CHF, pneumonias, bronchiectasis, chronic rhinitis, chronic sinusitis, pulmonary embolism, obstructive sleep apnea.

Diagnostic tests: Spirometry is the gold standard for measuring airflow limitation. Airflow limitation that is not fully reversible is evident if postbronchodilator FEV$_1$/FVC is less than 0.70 and FEV$_1$ is less than 80% predicted (Pocket guide to COPD diagnosis, management, and prevention, 2011). The U.S. Preventive Services Task Force (USPSTF) recommends spirometry only in symptomatic patients, that is, those who present to their health-care provider with chronic cough, increased sputum production, wheezing, or dyspnea. In these individuals, spirometry would be indicated as a diagnostic test for COPD, asthma, and other pulmonary diseases (Qaseem et al., 2011). Although the Global Initiative for Chronic Obstructive Lung Disease (GOLD, 2011) guidelines are focused on spirometry results, FEV$_1$ decreases with age, with the average man experiencing a decrease of 14 to 30 mL/year in FVC and a decrease of 23 to 32 mL/year in FEV$_1$. Women have a decline of 14 to 24 mL/year (FVC) and 19 to 26 mL/year (FEV$_1$). This age-related change needs to be factored into interpretation of spirometry results. Pulmonary function test results alone are inadequate in characterizing COPD in the older adult (Celli et al., 2004; Cote & Celli, 2007; Nazir, Al-Hamed, & Erbland, 2007).

A complete blood count (CBC) helps to measure the degree of secondary polycythemia (advanced COPD with hypoxemia), detecting the presence of infection by an increased white blood cell (WBC) count, or if eosinophilia is present, considering an allergic or asthmatic component. Chest x-ray in those having advanced COPD with emphysema may reveal hyperinflation, bullae or blebs, and a flat hemidiaphragm. In chronic bronchitis, increased markings suggest dirty lungs, and cardiomegaly may be present. A chest x-ray may be indicated also when pneumonia is suspected, or to rule out other pulmonary problems. Unless you suspect hypoxemia or hypercapnia, evaluation of arterial blood gases (ABGs) is not necessary. Pulse oximetry, frequently used to determine oxygen saturation, is readily available, noninvasive, and a reliable guide to monitoring oxygen therapy. If cardiac involvement is severe, an ECG in advanced COPD may demonstrate evidence of right-axis deviation, sinus tachycardia, and pulmonary hypertension with the presence of ongoing S waves in the lateral precordial leads.

Several pulmonary experts recommend using the BODE scale to assess severity and possible mortality in COPD. The BODE scale consists of measurement of **B**ody mass index, airflow **O**bstruction as measured by spirometry, the patient's subjective report of **D**yspnea measured by the Medical Research Council questionnaire, and **E**xercise capacity measured by the 6-minute walk test; the higher the score, the more predictive of early mortality. Results can be used for advanced care planning or other interventions (Celli et al., 2004; Cote & Celli, 2007).

Treatment: Individualize treatment goals according to the stage of disease, comorbidities, and patient goals. Treatment is targeted toward improvement of health status and functional status, prevention of disease progression, avoidance of exacerbations or complications, prevention of treatment side effects, and management of exacerbations (GOLD, 2011). Optimal symptom management and quality of life are also included. The GOLD syllabus identifies four segments of a COPD management program: (1) risk factor reduction, (2) assessment and monitoring, (3) stable chronic management, and (4) management of exacerbations.

Risk factor reduction:

■ Smoking cessation is the most effective and cost-effective intervention and should be promoted at every visit (GOLD, 2011). Brief motivational counseling, use of office literature, and use of community resources are helpful. Nicotine replacement therapy can be considered as well as bupropion or varenicline; careful and individual evaluation is necessary because both of these medications now have black box warnings. Follow-up phone calls weekly for the first few weeks may help maintain the patient's motivation.

■ If environmental pollution is present, public health resources should be contacted for abatement. Patients should be instructed to monitor air quality and remain indoors if adverse external conditions prevail.

▪ Adequate hydration and nutrition are important.

▪ Vaccination for influenza and pneumonia should be mandatory unless contraindicated.

Assessment and monitoring of stable COPD:

▪ Establish partnership with the patient and family. Teach patients to recognize signs of instability and contact their primary care provider. Instruct in medication management and the importance of adherence. Explain self-management for chronic disease concept.

▪ Health coaches, home health nurse, or telephonic monitoring is associated with less frequency of exacerbations when compared to usual care. The deciding factor was patient initiation of contact when symptoms changed or a question arose.

▪ Pulmonary rehabilitation consisting of exercise training, muscle strengthening, nutritional counseling, energy conservation, ADLs, breathing modifications, medication education including use of inhaler devices, and oxygen use is beneficial particularly in moderate to severe COPD but benefits all COPD patients (GOLD, 2011).

▪ Supplemental oxygen therapy in patients with hypoxemic COPD improves survival (GOLD, 2011; Qaseem et al., 2011). Additional benefits include reductions in nocturnal hypoxemia and arrhythmias, reduction in polycythemia, dyspnea, increased exercise tolerance, and improved cognitive status. Criteria for oxygen therapy must be met, including $PaO_2 = 55$ mm Hg or $SaO_2 = 88\%$ with or without hypercapnia; $PaO_2 = 55$ to 60 mm Hg; or $SaO_2 = 89\%$ if there is evidence of pulmonary hypertension, polycythemia, or peripheral edema suggesting CHF.

▪ Assess patients periodically for depression and quality of life status as part of regular assessment and monitoring. Attention to the whole patient can facilitate self-management and self-care.

▪ Pharmacological management is a cornerstone of COPD treatment and is directed toward symptom management and prevention of complications. The GOLD (2011) guidelines offer a staged approach to pharmacological intervention. These guidelines can be used broadly to incorporate categories of pharmacological agents, but the emphasis on changes in FEV_1, which defines the stages, does not adjust for age-related decline in FEV_1. Treatment should be individualized in the older adult to optimize

symptom management, control comorbidities, and promote adherence.

▪ When dyspnea is unrelieved by medications and interferes with functioning and quality of life, consider evaluation for surgical options. Lung volume reduction therapy, lung resections, transplants, and laser bullectomy are available in selected circumstances.

▪ Clinician-patient communication should include a discussion of disease progression and patient choices for care, including high technology (intensive care unit [ICU], ventilator), subacute, long-term ventilator dependent, long-term care, home care, and surgical options.

▪ Advance directives and palliative care with hospice option should be discussed (GOLD, 2008). Emphasize partnership with the patient and the need to review options periodically. Palliative care focuses on symptom management and quality of life; communication and support for the emotional, psychosocial, and spiritual needs of patient and caregivers; and maintaining the highest level of physical functioning possible within the limitations of the disease. The palliative care team can include a social worker, pastoral counselor, nurse, physician, psychologist, dietitian, and physical or occupational therapist. When end-stage COPD is identified, the patient can be transitioned to hospice if desired (Johannes, 2007; Nazir et al., 2007).

Stable chronic management:

▪ Includes components of risk reduction and assessment and monitoring.

▪ Chronic management visits every 3 to 6 months as agreed on with patient and provider, including interval history, physical and functional assessment, spirometry if indicated, and reevaluation of patient goals.

Pharmacological management: No current drug therapy has been proven to influence the progressive decline in lung function of COPD (VA/DOD clinical practice guideline, 2007). Pharmacotherapy reduces symptoms, improves exercise tolerance and overall health status, and decreases frequency and severity of exacerbations (GOLD, 2011). The American College of Physicians (ACP), American College of Chest Physicians (ACCP), ATS, and European Respiratory Society (ERS) indicate that use of inhaled bronchodilators may be useful in stable COPD patients, having respiratory symptoms and FEV_1 from 60% to 80% predicted

(Qaseem et al., 2011); they recommend treatment with inhaled bronchodilators for COPD patients who are stable, have an FEV_1 of less than 60% predicted, and are symptomatic (Qaseem et al., 2011). Monotherapy with either LABAs or long-acting inhaled anticholinergics is recommended for COPD patients who are symptomatic and have an FEV_1 of less than 60% predicted; patient preference, adverse reactions, and cost are important determinants of specific drug monotherapy (Qaseem et al., 2011). Combination inhaled therapy with LABAs, ICSs, or long-acting inhaled anticholinergics may be used for stable COPD patients with symptoms and FEV_1 of less than 60% (Qaseem et al., 2011).

Bronchodilators are the foundation of symptomatic management (GOLD, 2010; Qaseem et al., 2007); beta agonists, anticholinergics/antimuscarinics, and methylxanthines are included in this category. Short-acting bronchodilators containing albuterol are prescribed for as-needed use. Other SABAs include pirbuterol acetate, terbutaline sulfate, and levalbuterol. The effects of beta agonists are antagonized by beta blockers. Beta agonists are sympathomimetic agents that cause transient tachycardia, nervousness, and elevation in BP. Use beta agonists cautiously with cardiovascular disease, and note that concurrent therapy with xanthines (e.g., theophylline) or other sympathomimetics (often found in OTC decongestants or cold remedies) will exaggerate side effects. A combination of albuterol and a short-acting anticholinergic, ipratropium, can be prescribed for regular use. Long-acting bronchodilators are more effective and convenient for regular use (Appleton et al., 2006; Barr, Bourbeau, & Camargo, 2009; GOLD, 2010). Formoterol is a LABA that comes as a dry powder with an inhaler device; salmeterol xinafoate (Serevent Diskus) is a LABA that comes in a preloaded disk. Instruct patients that LABAs are *NOT* for relief of acute symptoms. Tiotropium is a long-acting anticholinergic/antimuscarinic that comes as a dry powder tablet with a Handi-Haler device with once-daily dosing. Patient education on side effects and use of administration devices is key to success and avoidance of complications. Anticholinergics should be used cautiously in patients with narrow-angle glaucoma, prostatic hypertrophy, or bladder neck obstruction, and they are contraindicated in patients who are allergic to atropine. Because of the route of administration (inhalation), side effects are minimal. Studies have demonstrated that tiotropium is superior to placebo and ipratropium in reducing symptoms, improving quality of life, and reducing exacerbations and hospitalizations in patients with moderately severe COPD

(GOLD, 2011). The use of methylxanthines, such as theophylline and aminophylline, has decreased significantly. Dosage is individualized, with the timed-release forms being preferred. Significant side effects occur, including increased nervousness or agitation, increased heart rate, and gastrointestinal effects. Many drug interactions are associated with the methylxanthines, including H_2 blockers, fluoroquinolones, and macrolide antibiotics. Frequent drug level measurements are required to monitor for methylxanthine toxicity; subtherapeutic drug levels, especially in older patients, are not usually adjusted because of lack of monitoring. Doses should be reduced in the presence of hepatic or cardiac disease or a history of seizures. Theophylline is a nonspecific phosphodiesterase inhibitor. It increases intracellular cyclic adenosine monophosphate within airway smooth muscle. High doses are required for bronchodilator effects, contributing to toxicity. Roflumilast is a new oral, once-daily phosphodiesterase-4 inhibitor currently being used selectively to improve FEV_1 in patients with moderate to severe COPD who are being treated with tiotropium or salmeterol; it has also been shown to reduce exacerbations in severe COPD (Fabbri et al., 2009). Use is limited by cost and side effects, including depression, suicidal ideation, anxiety, impulsiveness, and insomnia. It should not be used with hepatic problems (www.frx.com/pi/Daliresp_pi.pdf).

ICSs are used in combination with LABAs for optimal symptom management in persistent symptoms. Monotherapy with ICS is not recommended (Pocket guide to COPD diagnosis, management, and prevention, 2011; Qaseem et al., 2011). Oral glucocorticoids are used for short-term treatment in a COPD exacerbation. Long-term monotherapy with oral corticosteroids is not recommended (Pocket guide to COPD diagnosis, management, and prevention, 2011).

Combination pharmacotherapy for COPD has demonstrated superior efficacy in symptom management and spacing of exacerbations. In some cases it has also reduced the complexity of dosage scheduling, which favors greater adherence. Currently available combinations include a LABA and an ICS, fluticasone/salmeterol, and budesonide/formoterol. Instruct the patient to rinse the mouth after using. Monitor closely for changes suggestive of pneumonia.

Management of exacerbations: Exacerbations of COPD are defined as acute diversions from the baseline dyspnea, cough, and sputum that are beyond usual daily variations (GOLD, 2011). It is part of the natural course of the disease but may require a change in medication to support the patient. Causes of acute exacerbations may be viral, bacterial, inflammatory, or unknown. In some cases exacerbations can be managed in the outpatient or long-term care setting but others require in-hospital care. In the usual scenario, increasing breathlessness sends the patient to the emergency department. The patient is evaluated to rule out heart failure, arrhythmias, myocardial infarction, or pulmonary embolism. Chest x-ray, pulse oximetry, ABGs, ECG, CBC, and metabolic profile are obtained. If heart failure is suspected, a BNP will be drawn; serial enzymes may be measured if acute myocardial infarction is high on the differential list. Once the diagnosis of COPD exacerbation is confirmed, patients are treated with IV or oral corticosteroids, bronchodilators, and oxygen. Criteria for antibiotic use include increased dyspnea, sputum volume and purulence, or need for mechanical ventilation (Pocket guide to COPD diagnosis, management, and prevention, 2011). Decisions about admission or discharge are individualized depending on the patient's physical and mental status, frequency of exacerbations, availability of home support system, severity of symptoms, and functional abilities. Close monitoring and prevention of exacerbations is a goal of COPD management. Exacerbations have a very negative effect on quality of life and can accelerate the decline in lung function. Frequent exacerbations are predictive of impending mortality. Treatment with an oral corticosteroid burst for 10 to 14 days has been shown to shorten hospital stay and reduce treatment failures. Use of steroids for longer than 2 weeks is associated with adverse effects and no further benefit (Pocket guide to COPD diagnosis, management, and prevention, 2011).

Follow-up: A newly diagnosed patient should be seen frequently until an optimal treatment plan is in place and disease education has been completed. For stable patients who are maintaining their usual ADLs, routine reassessment every 3 to 6 months is advisable, with instructions to the patient or caregiver to schedule an interim visit if there is a change in status, increased symptoms, or an infection. For stable patients with other significant comorbidities, visits every 3 months are advisable. A team model for chronic care has been very effective; if insurance and resources permit, this approach would be optimal for COPD management. Periodic reassessment of pulmonary function and assessment of patient report of breathing status can guide therapy. Patients who are

unstable or have had an acute exacerbation will need more frequent follow-up visits initially. Collaborative management with these patients is strongly advised; during the immediate postacute period, a pulmonary specialist should manage the patient.

Sequelae: COPD is a multisystem disease and can lead to infections, particularly respiratory (pneumonia, recurrent bronchitis, viral infections), cor pulmonale, pulmonary hypertension, malnutrition, acute or chronic respiratory failure, steroid-induced myopathy or Cushing's syndrome, bullous lung disease, polycythemia, and sleep-related hypoxemia. Depression is frequently associated with COPD (Remels et al., 2007; Shapiro et al., 2010).

Prevention/prophylaxis: COPD is almost 100% preventable by avoidance of smoking. All COPD patients should have annual influenza vaccines unless they are allergic to a component; the pneumococcal polysaccharide vaccine should also be given to all COPD patients at age 65 years. If they had the vaccine previously and they were under 65 years, they can be revaccinated once after a 5-year period has elapsed (Centers for Disease Control and Prevention [CDC], 2012).

Referral: Collaborative management is advised in all but stable, moderately ill patients. Refer patients to a pulmonary specialist during instability, for hospital and postacute care and for determination of the need for oxygen therapy. Refer patients to a surgeon if the option of surgery is deemed appropriate. Refer patients to physical therapy for reconditioning; occupational therapy may also be helpful in teaching breathing techniques and energy-conserving measures. Consult with a dietary health professional when eating is problematic. Postacute COPD patients dwelling in the community should be referred for home care. Also, refer all patients to community resources and support groups. Palliative care and hospice options have already been discussed.

Education: Teach the patient, family, and/or caregivers about the disease process and its management, the role of smoking in causing the disease, the possibility of reversibility in the early/moderate stage with smoking cessation, medications, oxygen therapy precautions, and the need to seek care early if infection develops, dyspnea increases, or a change in cognitive status occurs. Advise patients of the need for regular follow-up visits, even if no symptoms are present.

CLINICAL RECOMMENDATION	EVIDENCE RATING	REFERENCE
Smoking cessation is the most effective and cost-effective intervention and should be promoted at every visit.	A	GOLD (2011)
In patients with respiratory symptoms, particularly dyspnea, spirometry should be performed to diagnose airflow obstruction. Spirometry should not be used to screen for airflow obstruction in asymptomatic individuals.	B	Qaseem et al. (2011)
Pulmonary rehabilitation consisting of exercise training, muscle strengthening, nutritional counseling, energy conservation, ADLs, breathing modifications, medication education (including use of inhaler devices), and oxygen use is beneficial particularly in moderate-to-severe COPD.	A	GOLD (2011) Qaseem et al. (2011)
Supplemental oxygen therapy in patients with hypoxemic COPD improves survival.	A	GOLD (2011) Qaseem et al. (2011)
Bronchodilators are the foundation of symptomatic management; they are given on an as-needed basis for symptom management.	A	GOLD (2011)
ACP, ACCP, ATS, and ERS recommend that clinicians prescribe monotherapy using either long-acting inhaled anticholinergics or long-acting inhaled beta agonists for symptomatic patients with COPD and FEV_1 <60% predicted. Clinicians should base the choice of specific monotherapy on patient preference, cost, and adverse effect profile.	B	Qaseem et al. (2011)
Long-term monotherapy with oral corticosteroids is not recommended in COPD.	A	GOLD (2011)
Regular treatment with inhaled corticosteroids improves symptoms, lung function, and quality of life and reduces exacerbations in COPD patients with an FEV_1 <60% predicted.	A	GOLD (2011)
Education improves patient response to exacerbations.	B	GOLD (2011)
Prospective end-of-life discussions can lead to effective end-of-life decisions as a result of understanding advance directives.	B	GOLD (2011)

A = consistent, good-quality, patient-oriented evidence; B = inconsistent or limited-quality, patient-oriented evidence; C = consensus, disease-oriented evidence, usual practice, expert opinion, or case series. For information about the SORT evidence rating system, go to www.aafp.org/afpsort.xml.

HEART FAILURE

Signal symptoms: Dyspnea on exertion, orthopnea, paroxysmal nocturnal dyspnea, progressive activity intolerance, weakness.

Description: Heart failure is a clinical syndrome caused by the heart's inability to eject enough blood to maintain tissue perfusion. As a cardiac syndrome, heart failure is a secondary process that is associated with multisystem pathophysiology involving the cardiac muscle and wall function. The older term *congestive heart failure* does not represent symptom presentation in all heart failure patients; therefore it has been replaced with the preferred term, *heart failure.*

Etiology: CAD and hypertension are the most common causes of heart failure. Heart failure is also caused by valvular heart disease, dysrhythmias (e.g., atrial fibrillation), COPD, obstructive sleep apnea, fluid volume overload, and metabolic disorders such as diabetes, hypothyroidism, or hyperthyroidism. Heart failure with reduced left ventricular ejection fraction (LVEF), previously referred to as *systolic heart failure*, is due to a large thin left ventricular wall that has lost the elasticity required to effectively eject enough blood to maintain normal cardiac output (American Heart Association [AHA], 2010; Hunt et al., 2005). In contrast, heart failure with preserved LVEF, previously referred to as *diastolic heart failure*, is due to thick, stiff-walled ventricles and may occur with normal or near-normal LVEF (AHA, 2010; Hunt et al., 2005). Occurrences of heart failure with preserved LVEF and reduced LVEF are evenly distributed.

Occurrence: Both incidence and prevalence of heart failure increase with age. An estimated 5.8 million Americans older than age 20 have heart failure. Prevalence rates within the nursing home setting are estimated between 10% and 45% depending on the site and population studied. When compared to those 45 to 64 years old, the incidence of heart failure is 4 times higher in those over 65 and more than 6 times higher in those above 80 years of age (AHA, 2010). The 5-year mortality rate is higher in men (59%) than in women (45%) following onset of symptoms (AHA, 2010). Heart failure is the most common hospital discharge diagnosis in those over age 65. Hospital readmissions within the first 30 day are directly correlated with increased mortality (Bueno et al., 2010).

Gender: In the general population, heart failure is more common in men. In the nursing home setting, the prevalence is higher in women (Daamen, Schols, Jaarsma, & Hamers, 2010).

Ethnicity: African Americans have higher rates of heart failure hospitalizations.

Contributing factors: Nonmodifiable risk factors include gender and race. Advanced age is an independent risk factor for heart failure. Modifiable risk factors for heart failure are tobacco use, SBP of more than 140 mm Hg, fasting glucose of more than 125 mg/dL, elevated cholesterol, obesity, and physical inactivity. Use of NSAIDs, COX-2 inhibitors, glucocorticoids, and thiazolidinediones are common precipitating factors for heart failure in the geriatric population (American Medical Directors Association [AMDA], 2010; Feenstra, Eibert, Grobbe, & Stricker, 2002; Hunt et al., 2005).

Pathophysiology: Heart failure is caused by myocardial structural or functional damage. To maintain cardiac output, stroke volume, and vital organ perfusion, the sympathetic nervous system and renin-angiotensin-aldosterone system (RAAS) are activated to release neurohormones (Jackson, Gibbs, Davies, & Lip, 2000).

Angiotensin II, the end product of the RAAS and a potent vasoconstrictor, leads to increased systemic vascular resistance, enhances the release of catecholamines from noradrenergic nerve endings, and directly stimulates the adrenal cortex to increase secretion of aldosterone (Dunlap & Peterson, 2002). Vasopressin (antidiuretic hormone) and aldosterone secretion cause sodium and fluid retention with subsequent increase in blood volume. Increased systemic vascular resistance, decreased arterial pressure, increased venous pressure, increased blood volume, and decreased venous compliance further increase ventricular wall stress and myocardial oxygen demand (Jackson et al., 2000). Ultimately, these normal physiological responses become maladaptive and result in damage to the heart, cardiopulmonary, renal, and systemic vasculature and cause progression of heart failure (Dunlap & Peterson, 2002; Jackson et al., 2000).

Signs and symptoms: Geriatric residents with severe heart failure may be asymptomatic, whereas others with mild disease can suffer incapacitating symptoms (Jackson et al., 2000). The primary disease process that causes left ventricular heart failure leads to pulmonary venous congestion with subsequent right ventricular dysfunction and portal and systemic venous congestion.

Clinical symptoms of dyspnea on exertion or at rest, orthopnea, dry cough (worse in recumbent position), and/or paroxysmal nocturnal dyspnea due to increased pulmonary venous congestion are clues to possible left ventricular failure. Ankle swelling (not due to venous insufficiency or hypoalbuminemia) and abdominal symptoms (pain, distention, nausea) due to hepatic enlargement are symptoms suggestive of right ventricular failure or systemic venous congestion.

Signs that suggest heart failure include weight gain, tachycardia, S_3 or S_4 heart sound, laterally displaced point of maximum impulse (PMI), neck vein distention, rales in bilateral lower lobes that are not due to atelectasis, positive hepatojugular reflux, and ascites. Patients with dementia may present with alteration in mental status, restlessness, and/or decreased oxygenation without classic signs and symptoms of peripheral lower extremity edema, lung congestion, and dyspnea (Harrington, 2006).

Signs and Symptoms of Heart Failure

"A N-E-W L-E-A-F"
- **A:** Acute Agitation/Anxiety
- **N:** Nighttime shortness of breath or ↑ nighttime urination
- **E:** Edema in lower extremities
- **W:** Weight gain (2–4 lb/week)
- **L:** Lightheadedness
- **E:** Extreme shortness of breath lying down
- **A:** Abdominal symptoms (nausea, pain, decreased appetite, distention)
- **F:** Fatigue

© 2005 Candace Harrington, DNP, GNP-BC, ANP-BC. Permission to Reproduce with Acknowledgement.

Heart failure classification is based on risk, cardiac structural changes, symptom presentation, and functional impairment. The New York Heart Association (NYHA) classifies heart failure based on functional limitation (Hunt et al., 2005). This system is difficult to use with the elderly population, who may have functional decline related to comorbid conditions. In 2002, the American College of Cardiology/American Heart Association (ACC/AHA) introduced a new heart failure rating system based on risk factors, structural changes, and history of heart failure symptoms. The ACC/AHA system classifies heart failure in four stages as the syndrome progresses along the natural trajectory and is

used in conjunction with, not as a replacement for, the NYHA functional classification system.

Stages A and B refer to risk factors and present opportunities for primary and secondary prevention measures.

Stage A: Risk factors are present for heart failure without structural changes, history of signs or symptoms, or functional limitations.

Stage B: Risk factors and structural changes in the heart are present without signs or symptoms of heart failure.

Stage C: Risk factors, structural changes in the heart, and past or current signs or symptoms of heart failure are present. At this stage, the patient is diagnosed with heart failure that does not regress back to former stages.

Stage D: Heart failure is refractory despite maximum medical management. Patients are symptomatic at rest or with minimal exertion.

Diagnostic tests:

Two-dimensional echocardiography combined with Doppler flow studies: Two-dimensional echocardiogram is considered the most useful diagnostic tool for evaluation of ventricular ejection fraction and structural abnormalities. Two-dimensional echocardiograms are essential to accurate diagnosis and treatment plan development (Hunt et al., 2005; Kirkpatrick, Vannan, Narula, & Lang, 2007).

Electrocardiography: ECGs may indicate left atrial enlargement, left ventricular hypertrophy, arrhythmias, or ST-T wave changes associated with myocardial infarction or ischemia.

Cardiac angiography: Cardiac catheterization may benefit geriatric patients who are candidates for revascularization and may reveal hemodynamic abnormalities, the presence and severity of valvular heart disease, or CAD.

Chest x-ray: Chest x-ray may reveal cardiomegaly, increased pulmonary vascularities, interstitial edema, or pulmonary edema.

Brain natriuretic peptide (BNP) or N-terminal proBNP (NT-proBNP): BNP and NT-proBNP are helpful in narrowing differential diagnoses or establishing prognosis. BNP elevation occurs slowly; therefore, levels are not helpful in acute heart failure episodes. BNP levels of less than 100 pg/mL indicate that heart failure is unlikely. Levels between 100 and 500 pg/mL are indeterminate. Levels of more than 500 pg/mL may suggest heart failure, but they cannot be used as a stand-alone test, because levels are elevated in CAD, older patients, women, and other disease processes.

Blood chemistries and CBC: CBC, comprehensive metabolic profile (CMP), and thyroid-stimulating hormone (TSH) levels should be obtained initially and periodically to evaluate renal, liver, metabolic, and hemodynamic status.

Serial cardiac enzymes: Cardiac enzymes (CK-MB, troponin) may reveal myocardial ischemia or infarction. Cardiac enzymes require time-sensitive processing and therefore have limited value in the long-term care setting.

Differential diagnosis: Atypical symptom presentation in geriatric patients necessitates a thorough health history that includes evaluation of risk factors with correlation to physical examination findings and diagnostic test results.

Dyspnea on exertion, the most common heart failure symptom, may be caused by numerous disease processes, including asthma, COPD, anemia, renal failure, dysrhythmias, cardiomyopathies, valvular heart disease, pulmonary emboli, abdominal masses, deconditioning, and anxiety neurosis. Differentiation between heart failure with preserved LVEF or reduced LVEF is crucial and best determined by two-dimensional echocardiography (Hunt et al., 2005).

Treatment: Treatment options for heart failure are targeted at symptom management, treatment of the causative disease process(es), and the resulting multisystem pathophysiology (Zile & Brutsaert, 2002). Fragility, multiple comorbid disease processes, polypharmacy, age-related changes in pharmacokinetics and pharmacodynamics, and prevalence of geriatric syndromes require individualized treatment plans (Ahmed, 2003a, 2003b, 2003c; Rich, 2005).

Angiotensin-converting enzyme inhibitors: Unless contraindicated, angiotensin-converting enzyme (ACE) inhibitors are first-line agents in the treatment of asymptomatic heart failure with reduced LVEF or in patients with recent or remote history of myocardial infarction regardless of LVEF. Additionally, ACE inhibitors are recommended for all patients with Stage C heart failure unless contraindicated. ACE inhibitor contraindications include unilateral or bilateral renal artery stenosis, hypersensitivity to ACE inhibitors, angioedema, pregnancy, serum potassium more than 5.5 mEq/L that cannot be reduced, and hypotension in patients at risk for cardiogenic shock. ACE inhibitor therapy should be discontinued as a last resort in heart failure patients due to cardioprotective properties.

Obtain baseline serum potassium, serum creatinine, and blood urea nitrogen (BUN) before initiation and with dosage adjustments. Assess for fluid volume deficit, because this may precipitate hypotension. All ACE inhibitors should be started at low doses (captopril, 6.25 to 12.5 mg 3 times daily; enalapril, 2.5 mg twice daily; lisinopril, 2.5 to 5 mg once daily; fosinopril, 5 to 10 mg once daily). Ramipril and trandolapril have specific indications for treatment after myocardial infarction. Dosages should be gradually titrated over several weeks to achieve target doses (captopril, 50 mg 3 times daily; enalapril, 10 to 20 mg twice daily; lisinopril, 20 to 40 mg daily; fosinopril, 20 to 40 mg once daily; ramipril, 5 mg twice daily or 10 mg once daily; trandolapril, 4 mg once daily) based on renal function, potassium levels, and BP (more than 90 mm Hg). ACE inhibitor cough is a common side effect and is characterized as a dry nonproductive cough that starts as a tickling cough and is worse at night. ACE inhibitor cough is a classwide side effect and is not dose dependent. If intolerant to ACE inhibitors, angiotensin II receptor blockers (ARBs) are an appropriate alternative. Isosorbide dinitrate and hydralazine combination therapy is an appropriate alternative in patients who experience hypotension, hyperkalemia, angioedema, or renal insufficiency with ACE inhibitor or ARB therapy, and those who do not respond to treatment with ACE inhibitor and beta blocker. Geriatric patients may be sensitive to the vasodilatory effects of ACE inhibitors and may benefit from a test dosage with close monitoring of BP over 1 to 5 hours following dosage to evaluate tolerance and fall risk due to orthostatic hypotension.

Beta-adrenergic blockers: Carvedilol, metoprolol succinate, and bisoprolol are the only beta blockers indicated for treatment of heart failure and with evidence to support morbidity and mortality reductions in heart failure patients (Omnicare, 2010). Unless otherwise contraindicated (heart block, bradycardia, hypotension, severe respiratory disease), beta blockers are recommended for patients with recent or remote history of myocardial infarction regardless of LVEF. Use of carvedilol or metoprolol succinate has been shown to decrease morbidity and mortality in heart failure patients and is recommended in patients with Stage C heart failure and/or a history of myocardial infarction regardless of LVEF. Beta blockers are strongly associated with reduced risk of mortality and reduced rehospitalization during 30-, 60-, and 90- day follow-up periods (Fonarow, 2007; Omnicare, 2010). Carvedilol is the best option in those with advanced heart failure. Beta blockers should be used in combination with ACE inhibitors, if possible, for synergistic effect. Monitor geriatric patients closely for volume status, emotional side effects, and functional decline. Contraindications include bronchospastic lung disease (e.g., asthma), symptomatic bradycardia, or advanced heart block without a pacemaker. Beta blocker initiation should be started only in a euvolemic patient. Initial dosages should be low and titrated slowly based on response to treatment and tolerance. Carvedilol may have a greater hypotensive effect in the geriatric patient due to the vasodilatory effect of alpha-1 receptor blockade properties (Dulin, Haas, Abraham, & Krum, 2005). Metoprolol succinate may be better tolerated in those with lower baseline BP levels. Consider carvedilol or bisoprolol in patients who require crushed medications.

Diuretic therapy: Loop diuretics are used to reduce symptoms of peripheral or pulmonary congestion. No long-term blinded randomized clinical control trials evaluating the efficacy of loop or thiazide diuretics in heart failure patients have been done. Use of diuretics in the treatment of heart failure without ACE inhibitors, ARBs, or beta blockers activates the RAAS and may hasten progression of heart failure. Caution should be used when diuresing a patient in heart failure with preserved LVEF to avoid exacerbation of heart failure symptoms caused by overdiuresis. Most heart failure patients are resistant to the effects of hydrochlorothiazide; therefore, loop diuretics are preferred diuretics in heart failure treatment. When used in equipotent dosages, loop diuretics appear to have comparable diuretic effects (1 mg bumetanide = 40 mg furosemide = 10 to 20 mg torsemide). Furosemide should be initiated at 20 mg daily oral dosage in the elderly patient with mild symptoms. The usual maintenance dose is 40 mg daily, but dosage is titrated based on effect and tolerance. Bumetanide is 40 times more potent than furosemide and is less ototoxic, but it is associated with myalgias in some patients. Metolazone (2.5 to 5 mg daily), a thiazide-like agent, is a long-acting diuretic that is effective in increasing the effects of loop diuretics if given 30 minutes before the loop diuretic dosage. Combination therapy with metolazone requires close monitoring of potassium and magnesium levels. Torsemide may be advantageous, because absorption is unimpaired and the response is less variable than the other loop diuretics. Amiloride, triamterene, and ethacrynic acid should only be considered if there is life-threatening allergy to sulfa due to side effects and inability to protect against damaging neurohormonal activity. Spironolactone, an aldosterone receptor blocker, is an effective therapy in conjunction with ACE inhibitors or ARBs to more completely block the deleterious effects of the RAAS in patients with Stage C and D Class III–IV heart failure with reduced LVEF and in patients with LVEF of 40% or less who have adequate renal function without hyperkalemia. Additionally, providers should consider ability to monitor for renal dysfunction and hyperkalemia before initiation of therapy. Spironolactone is recommended at low dosages of 12.5 to 25 mg once daily and should not be initiated in men with serum creatinine of 2.5 or more; in women with serum creatinine of 2.0 or more; or potassium levels of more than 5.0.

Digoxin: Digoxin is recommended in the treatment of heart failure patients without bradycardia who have persistent symptoms despite optimal therapy with diuretics, ACE inhibitors, and beta blockers. In addition, digoxin is recommended to control ventricular response due to atrial fibrillation and men with heart failure with LVEF of less than 50% (Aronow, 2006a; Hunt et al., 2005). There is no evidence to support use of digoxin in men with heart failure with preserved LVEF. Mortality rate increases by 20% in women regardless of LVEF and increases 80% if the serum digoxin level is 1.2 ng/mL or higher (Aronow, 2006a; Hunt et al., 2005). To reduce morbidity and mortality, lower therapeutic range (0.5 to 0.8 ng/mL) is advised (Aronow, 2006a; Hunt et al., 2005). Evidence from several trials supports the use of digoxin to improve functional status and decrease heart failure hospitalization without improvement in mortality. Geriatric dosages should not exceed 0.125 mg daily (Aronow, 2006a; Beers, 1997; Hunt et al., 2005). In geriatric patients with renal dysfunction, every-other-day dosage scheduling may be appropriate.

There is general consensus that ACE inhibitors, beta blockers, diuretics, nitrates, and calcium channel blockers are helpful in treating heart failure with preserved LVEF. Concurrent treatment with beta blockers and non-dihydropyridine agents is contraindicated.

Implantable cardioverter-defibrillator (ICD) therapy will improve total mortality in certain patient populations who are at risk for sudden cardiac death; however, it will not improve quality of life or symptoms. ICDs must be deactivated with imminent death. Long-term infusions of positive inotropes may be harmful and are not recommended for patients with current or prior symptoms of heart failure with reduced LVEF. Calcium channel blockers are not indicated in routine treatment of heart failure in patients with current or past symptoms of heart failure with reduced LVEF and may exacerbate symptoms in this situation.

Follow-up: Ask the patient about the presence of symptoms of heart failure as noted previously. Determine and document the most strenuous activity that the patient can perform without significant symptoms. Ask general questions related to the patient's quality of life such as sleep patterns, sexual difficulties, symptoms of depression, and coping behaviors. Assess for caregiver overburden. Complete review of all medications, including nonprescription medications, is necessary. Laboratory work should be done as needed, including electrolytes, serum creatinine, BUN, and digoxin levels when indicated.

Sequelae: Complications of heart failure involve hepatic and renal end-organ disease. Fifty percent of heart failure sufferers die from sudden cardiac death.

Prevention/prophylaxis: Reducing cardiac risk factors in elderly persons affects coronary disease as strongly as it does in younger age groups. Encourage risk factor reduction using age-specific guidelines to facilitate changes in lifestyle. Patients with heart failure are at risk for a vascular event, although there is conflicting evidence regarding efficacy of prophylactic antithrombotic treatment (aspirin or warfarin) without other indications.

Referral: Warning signs for the need for hospitalization include weight gain that is resistant to diuresis, palpitations, persistent or recurrent dizziness, agitation or cognitive changes, inability to sleep because of paroxysmal nocturnal dyspnea, abdominal pain, and inability to walk.

Most patients with heart failure can be managed by the primary care provider. Referral to a cardiologist may be indicated when the diagnosis is unclear, if the patient remains symptomatic despite appropriate therapy, and in patients with significant cardiac disease. Hospice and palliative treatment should be considered when a patient has Stage D Class IV heart failure, has an ejection fraction of 20% or less, is unable to tolerate optimal therapy due to hypotension or renal failure, or has symptoms that are not controlled with maximized medical management.

Education: Education and use of support groups are important for patients with heart failure, because noncompliance is a major cause of morbidity and unnecessary hospital admissions. Instruct patients and their families about the natural progressive trajectory of heart failure, necessary medications, dietary restrictions, heart failure symptoms that necessitate contact with provider, and prognosis. Discussions regarding advance directives should begin early in the trajectory. Explain typical symptoms of worsening heart failure (orthopnea, paroxysmal dyspnea, leg edema, or exercise intolerance), and instruct patients to contact their health-care provider if these occur. Mild aerobic exercise increases functional capacity and improves the quality of life for heart failure patients but should be undertaken with provider supervision. Dietary sodium should be restricted to 2 or 3 g/day. Discourage alcohol use and tobacco use. Fluid restriction is not necessary unless there is hyponatremia, but patients with heart failure should avoid excessive fluid intake.

Advise patients to contact the health-care provider if weight increases more than 2 pounds in a day or 4 pounds in a week. Nurse practitioners should recommend that patients with heart failure receive vaccination against influenza and pneumococcal disease.

CLINICAL RECOMMENDATION	EVIDENCE RATING	REFERENCE
ACE inhibitors are recommended for all patients with Stage C heart failure unless contraindicated.	A	Hunt et al. (2005) Jackson et al. (2000) Muth, Gensichen, Beyer, Hutchinson, & Gerlach (2009) Pharmacy Benefits Management Strategic Healthcare Group & Medical Advisory Panel (2007)
Beta blockers should be used in combination with ACE inhibitors if possible for synergistic effect.	A	Hunt et al. (2005) Muth et al. (2009) Ruffolo & Feuerstein (1997)

CLINICAL RECOMMENDATION	EVIDENCE RATING	REFERENCE
Beta blocker initiation should be started only in a euvolemic patient. Initial dosages should be low and titrated slowly based on response to treatment and tolerance.	A	Gibbs, Davies, & Lip (2000) Hunt et al. (2005)
Beta blockers are recommended for patients with recent or remote history of myocardial infarction, regardless of LVEF.	A	Gibbs et al. (2000) Hunt et al. (2005)
Loop diuretics should be used to reduce symptoms of peripheral or pulmonary congestion, because most heart failure patients are resistant to the effects of hydrochlorothiazide.	C	American Medical Directors Association (AMDA) (2010) Hunt et al. (2005)
Avoid use of diuretics in the treatment of heart failure without ACE inhibitors, ARBs, or beta blockers (activates the renin-angiotensin-aldosterone system and may hasten progression of heart failure).	C	Domanski et al. (2003) Litaker & Chow (2003)
Spironolactone in conjunction with ACE inhibitors or ARBs to more completely block the deleterious effects of the renin-angiotensin-aldosterone system in patients with Stage C and D Class III–IV heart failure with reduced LVEF, LVEF ≤40%, and adequate renal function without hyperkalemia. Providers should consider ability to monitor for renal dysfunction and hyperkalemia before initiation of therapy.	A	Hunt et al. (2005) Parker, Miller, & DeBusk (2001) Zannad, Alla, Dousset, Perez, & Pitt (2000)
Digoxin is recommended in the treatment of heart failure with reduced LVEF to control ventricular response due to atrial fibrillation as an add-on agent and in those without bradycardia for control of heart failure symptoms resistant to ACE inhibitors, beta blockers, and diuretics unless contraindicated.	A	Aronow (2006a) Hunt et al. (2005)
Encourage risk factor reduction using age-specific guidelines to facilitate changes in lifestyle.	C	AMDA (2010) Hunt et al. (2005)
Mild aerobic exercise increases functional capacity and improves the quality of life for heart failure patients but should be undertaken with provider supervision.	C	AMDA (2010) Hunt et al. (2005)

Continued

CLINICAL RECOMMENDATION	EVIDENCE RATING	REFERENCE
Dietary sodium should be restricted to 2 or 3 g/day. Fluid restriction is not necessary unless there is hyponatremia or Stage D Class IV symptom management.	C	AMDA (2010) Hunt et al. (2005)
Discourage alcohol use and tobacco use.	C	AMDA (2010) Hunt et al. (2005)
Vaccination against influenza and pneumococcal disease is recommended unless contraindicated for heart failure patients.	A	CDC (1997) Hunt et al. (2005) Moberley, Holden, Tatham, & Andrews (2008)

A = consistent, good-quality, patient-oriented evidence; B = inconsistent or limited-quality, patient-oriented evidence; C = consensus, disease-oriented evidence, usual practice, expert opinion, or case series. For information about the SORT evidence rating system, go to www.aafp.org/afpsort.xml.

HYPERTENSION

Signal symptoms: No clear symptoms or warning signs.

Description: Hypertension is a chronic disease characterized by elevation of BP and is classified as either essential or secondary. There is no specific cause to explain essential hypertension, which accounts for approximately 90% to 95% of cases (Chobanian et al., 2003; Lakatta, 2007; Supiano, Hogikyan, Sidani, Galecki, & Krueger, 1999; Vasan et al., 2002). Although the pathophysiology of essential hypertension remains under constant research, mechanisms leading to essential hypertension can be linked to many risk factors that may include age, race/ethnicity, family history, being overweight or obese, leading a sedentary lifestyle, use of tobacco and tobacco products, high dietary intake of sodium, stress, and certain chronic conditions including high cholesterol, diabetes, and kidney disease. Secondary hypertension results from other underlying conditions such as kidney disease, adrenal tumor, or pheochromocytoma (Celermajer et al., 1994). Persistent hypertension, the leading cause of chronic renal failure, is one of the risk factors for strokes, myocardial infarction, heart failure, and aneurysm (Kithas & Supiano, 2010). Delays in the detection and treatment of hypertension are common and may result in the development of target organ damage and other conditions such as CHD, left ventricular hypertrophy, heart failure, transient ischemic attack, stroke, dementia, peripheral vascular disease, and retinopathy (Stokes, 2009).

Controlling hypertension in older adults is necessary to reduce the risk of cardiovascular disease, stroke, chronic kidney disease, atrial fibrillation, CHF, and cognitive impairment (Kithas & Supiano, 2010; Obisesan et al., 2008). A reduction in the SBP by 10 mm Hg and a reduction in the DBP by 5 mm Hg significantly decreases the incidence of myocardial infarction, stroke, CHF, and overall mortality in older adults. The estimated prevalence of hypertension in adults older than 65 years is 50% to 75%. For women over age 75, the value exceeds 75% (Chobanian et al., 2003). Overall, hypertension control in older adults is low, thus reflecting a need for more aggressive approaches to treatment and management (Kithas & Supiano, 2010).

Classification: The seventh report of the Joint National Committee (JNC 7) current classification of BP makes no adjustment for age. Through research findings, the JNC 7 guidelines indicate that cardiovascular risk increases with increasing BP. The risk starts to increase above a BP level of 115/75 mm Hg. The "pre-hypertension" category was added to the JNC 7 report and is defined as SBP 120 to 139 mm Hg or DBP 80 to 89 mm Hg. The JNC 7 classification of BP is illustrated in Table 8-2.

TABLE 8-2	JNC 7 Classification of Blood Pressure		
TYPE	SYSTOLIC (MM HG)		DIASTOLIC (MM HG)
Normal	<120	AND	<80
Pre-hypertension	120–139	OR	80–89
Stage 1 hypertension	140–159	OR	90–99
Stage 2 hypertension	>160	OR	>100

Source: Adapted from JNC 7: The Seventh Report of the Joint National Committee on Prevention, Detection, Evaluation and Treatment of High Blood Pressure.

Etiology: The etiology of hypertension is complex with several factors contributing to its development. In essential hypertension, it is difficult to identify a single causative factor regardless of age. It is most likely due to an array of physiological and lifestyle factors. Age-related pathophysiological changes include arterial stiffness, especially of the large arteries; decreased baroreceptor sensitivity; increased sympathetic nervous system activity; endothelial dysfunction; sodium sensitivity, particularly a decreased ability to excrete a sodium load; and decreased plasma renin activity and insulin resistance. Lifestyle factors include being sedentary, central adiposity, and a diet high in sodium and fat. In general, systolic hypertension with an increase in pulse pressure is the most common form of hypertension in the elderly and is associated with arterial stiffness (Chobanian et al., 2007). In addition, alterations in autonomic nervous system functioning, RAAS dysfunction, endothelial dysfunction of the blood vessels, and genetic influences may lead to the development of hypertension.

Occurrence: In older adults, hypertension is closely associated with increased sodium sensitivity, ISH, increase in arterial stiffness, increased incidence of endothelial dysfunction, and increased frequency of the "white coat effect" (Stokes, 2009). Lifestyle factors include being sedentary, central adiposity, and a diet high in sodium and fat (Chobanian et al., 2007).

Age: Disease typically appears between ages 30 and 50. From 50% to 75% of adults greater than 65 years have increased prevalence. For women over age 75, the value exceeds 75% (Chobanian et al., 2007).

Ethnicity: U.S.-born adults have higher levels of hypertension (30.8%) than foreign-born adults (24.9%). Non-Hispanic blacks have a higher risk for hypertension and hypertension-related complications (e.g.,

stroke, diabetes, and chronic kidney disease) than non-Hispanic whites and Mexican Americans (Keenan & Rosendorf, 2011).

Gender: In both men and women, the prevalence of hypertension increases with age. Women who are older than 55 are at a higher risk for developing hypertension. From 55 years and above, a higher percentage of women have a higher BP than men. Men who are older than 45 are at a higher risk of developing high BP. Men are at an increased risk for hypertension as compared to women until age 45.

Contributing factors: Certain medical conditions may contribute to the development of hypertension. Pre-hypertension (120 to 139 mm Hg/80 to 89 mm Hg) increases the risk of individuals developing chronic hypertension. Diabetes, due to hypoinsulinemia, contributes to the development of hypertension. Approximately 60% of individuals with diabetes also have hypertension. Individual behaviors can contribute to the development of hypertension. These include increased sodium intake, being overweight/obese, lack of physical activity, increased alcohol intake, and smoking. Heredity and genetics are also contributing factors to the development of hypertension.

Signs and symptoms: Hypertension is often asymptomatic. Individuals may report confusion, ear noise or buzzing, fatigue, headache, irregular heartbeat, epistaxis, and visual changes. Some individuals will have varying degrees of target organ disease, which may not appear until 10 to 20 years of disease progression:

- Cardiac system: CAD, left ventricular hypertrophy, left ventricular dysfunction, or cardiac failure
- Cerebrovascular system: transient ischemic attacks or stroke
- Peripheral vascular system: absence of one or more of the major pulses in extremities with or without intermittent claudication; aneurysm
- Renal system: microalbuminuria, proteinuria, and elevated serum creatinine levels
- Eyes: hemorrhages or exudates with or without papilledema

Signs of hypertension may be classified by actual BP measurements. A normal BP reading is SBP of less than 120 mm Hg and DBP of less than 80 mm Hg. Pre-hypertension is classified as SBP of 120 to 139 mm Hg or DBP of 80 to 89 mm Hg. Stage 1 hypertension is SBP of 140 to 159 mm Hg or DBP of 90 to 99 mm Hg. Stage 2 hypertension is SBP greater than or equal to 160 mm Hg or DBP greater than or equal to 100 mm Hg (Beevers, Lip, & O'Brien, 2001).

In older adults, signs and symptoms are associated with increased sodium sensitivity, ISH, increase in arterial stiffness, increased incidence of endothelial dysfunction, and increased frequency of the "white coat effect" (Stokes, 2009). Sodium sensitivity is the extent of the rise in arterial BP with an increase in sodium chloride intake (Weinberger, Miller, Luft, Grim, & Fineberg, 1986). A complex process is involved in factors mediating the relationship between sodium status and change in BP in older adults. The factors include an increased responsiveness of volume homeostasis to the level of salt intake, a salt-induced impairment of vascular nitric oxide (NO) production, and an increase in arterial stiffness (Bagrov & Lakatta, 2004). The systolic pressure is affected more than the diastolic pressure.

ISH is characterized by SBP greater than or equal to 140 mm Hg, DBP of less than 90 mm Hg, and a high pulse pressure (Stokes, 2009). ISH is characterized by decreased arterial compliance, usually expressed as an increase in arterial stiffness that may be attributed to the effect of age-related loss of distensibility in the major central arteries as elastic tissue is progressively replaced with collagen and increased arterial stiffness due to endothelial dysfunction. Although both factors most likely contribute, the loss of distensibility due to endothelial dysfunction is the cause more easily corrected using pharmacological agents (Stokes, 2009).

Endothelial dysfunction is caused by free oxygen radicals in the arterial wall and by the upstream effects of reduced distal vascular flow reserve (Kojda & Harrison, 1999). Accumulation of free oxygen radicals results from age-related cardiovascular risk factors that include atherosclerosis, diabetes mellitus, renal impairment, and hypertension (Kojda & Harrison, 1999). When there is endothelial dysfunction, NO-mediated vasodilation in the peripheral circulation is diminished (Stokes, 2009). The loss of vasodilator potential results in increased amplitude and early return of the reflective wave, causing high pulse pressure (O'Rourke, 2005). Tonometry reveals the typical characteristics of the pulse wave in groups of elderly patients with treatment-resistant ISH (Stokes, 2006; Stokes & Ryan, 1997).

The "white coat effect" occurs when the BP is increased temporarily through an autonomic neural reaction triggered by the actual process of measurement. This effect increases with age (Stokes, 2009). As the systolic component often rises more than the diastolic, the type of hypertension due to the white coat effect can be confirmed by finding a major discrepancy between automated BP values within the normal range and observed readings that are high (Stokes, 2009).

Differential diagnosis: It is important to correctly identify individuals who are truly hypertensive rather than pseudohypertensive, particularly in the elderly. Pseudohypertension occurs when the cuff pressure is inappropriately high as compared with the intra-arterial pressure because of excessive atheromatosis and/or medial hypertrophy in the arterial tree (Messeril, 1986). An elevated indirect (sphygmomanometer) BP determination associated with a lower direct (intra-arterial) BP determination occurs when arteries are stiff and noncompressible (Wright & Looney, 1997). This is a significant consideration for the health-care provider to avoid prescribing a treatment regimen to an older adult that lowers the intra-arterial pressure to hypotensive levels.

Diagnostic tests: Hypertension is diagnosed on the basis of a persistently high BP identified on three sphygmomanometer measurements at least 1 week apart (Clement et al., 2003). The initial evaluation of individuals with hypertension includes an assessment for the presence of other cardiovascular risk factors, target organ damage, concomitant diseases affecting prognosis and treatment, identifiable causes of hypertension, and contributing lifestyle factors. Physical examination should include an appropriate measurement of BP with verification in the contralateral arm; examination of the optic fundi; calculation of BMI; auscultation for carotid, abdominal, and femoral bruits; palpation of the thyroid gland; examination of the heart and lungs; examination of the abdomen for enlarged kidneys, masses, or abnormal aortic pulsation; palpation of the lower extremities for edema and pulses; and neurological assessment. Routine laboratory and diagnostic studies should be performed to evaluate cardiovascular risk and to rule out secondary causes.

Before initiating therapy, the following laboratory tests are recommended: ECG; urinalysis, blood glucose, and hematocrit; serum potassium; creatinine or the corresponding estimated glomerular filtration rate (GFR) and calcium; and a lipid profile, after a 7- to 12-hour fast that includes HDL cholesterol and LDL cholesterol and triglycerides. Optional tests include measurement of urinary albumin excretion or albumin/creatinine ratio (Chobanian et al., 2003).

Once hypertension is diagnosed, evaluation is focused on assessing the individual's lifestyle and identifying other risk factors, revealing identifiable causes of hypertension and assessing the presence or absence of target organ damage and cardiovascular disease (Chobanian et al., 2003).

Treatment: The treatment of hypertension is multi-faceted and involves lifestyle modification, pharmacological intervention, and consistent follow-up and monitoring. The goal of antihypertensive therapy is the reduction of cardiovascular and renal morbidity and mortality. The primary focus should be on achieving the SBP goal, especially for those ages 50 years and older, because most persons with hypertension will reach the DBP goal once the SBP goal is achieved. To decrease cardiovascular complication, treating SBP and DBP to targets that are less than 140/90 mm Hg is desirable. In patients with hypertension and diabetes or renal disease, the BP goal is less than 130/80 mm Hg.

Nonpharmacological interventions contribute to controlling hypertension through the promotion of healthy lifestyles (Chobanian et al., 2003). The adoption of healthy lifestyles by all persons is a critical part of preventing hypertension and management. The benefits of lifestyle modification include a reduction in BP, the enhancement of antihypertensive therapy, and decreased cardiovascular risk. A combination of two or more lifestyle modifications can achieve better results. Major lifestyle modifications to lower BP include weight reduction (Chobanian et al., 2003; Redón et al., 2008). Because body weight increases with age, hypertension is more prevalent in older, overweight adults. Body mass and waist circumference may have a direct impact on the development of hypertension (Redón et al., 2008). Although weight loss through dieting may vary among individuals, weight loss should be considered in any older adult with a BMI greater than 26 (Redón, et al., 2008); adoption of the Dietary Approaches to Stop Hypertension (DASH) eating plan (Appel et al., 2006); and dietary sodium reduction. A low-sodium diet of no more than 100 mEq/L (2.4 g sodium or 6 g sodium chloride) may be effective in older adults with mild ISH (Gates, Tanaka, Hiatt, & Seals, 2004; He, Markandu, & MacGregor, 2005). Adequate reduction of dietary sodium leads to an average decrease in SBP of 5 mm Hg and DBP of 4 mm Hg (He et al., 2005). Considerations for placing older adults on a low-sodium diet includes the individual's willingness to modify salt intake and a history of gout or diuretic-induced adverse events (Stokes, 2009) as well as physical activity (Brennan et al., 2005; Stewart et al., 2005; Whelton, Chin, Xin, & He, 2002). Regular aerobic exercise has been associated with modest BP reduction in hypertensive individuals in general

(Whelton et al., 2002). Regular aerobic exercise lowers the SBP an average of 5 mm Hg and the DBP an average of 4 mm Hg (Whelton et al., 2002). Overall, the research differs on the effect of aerobic exercise on reducing BP (Brennan et al., 2005; Ferrier, 2001). However, aerobic exercise, in general, increases plasma HDL cholesterol and lowers overall cardiovascular risk, especially in older hypertensive adults who have lipid disorders and diabetes mellitus (Stewart et al., 2005). Reduction of alcohol intake to a moderate level may help to reduce cardiovascular risk (Xin et al., 2001). Smoking cessation has also been found to reduce mortality and morbidity (Appel & Aldrich, 2003; Donzé, Ruffieux, & Cornuz, 2007; Fiore et al., 2008; Suskin, Sheth, Negassa, & Yusuf, 2001).

Pharmacological management involves several classes of antihypertensive agents used in the treatment of hypertension, including thiazide diuretics, ACE inhibitors, ARBs, calcium channel antagonists, beta-receptor antagonists, alpha-receptor antagonists, and aldosterone antagonists. Several factors contribute to age-related increases in BP and influence the selection of antihypertensive medications. These include increased arterial stiffness, decreased baroreceptor sensitivity, increased sympathetic nervous system activity, endothelial dysfunction, sodium sensitivity (primarily a decreased ability to excrete a sodium load), low plasma renin activity, insulin resistance, and the resulting effect on carbohydrate metabolism. A general approach to selecting antihypertensive therapy in older adults includes the use of agents based on the individual's comorbidities such as diabetes, CHF, and CHD. The SBP is the primary target of therapy (SBP 135 to 140 mm Hg); an SBP less than 130 mm Hg is the treatment goal for patients with type 2 diabetes (Chobanian et al., 2003; Kithas & Supiano, 2010). Typically, treatment involves the use of a low-dose diuretic in uncomplicated hypertension, starting at one-half the usual dose and increasing slowly (Chobanian et al., 2003). The focus is on the SBP, avoiding excessive lowering of the DBP. In patients with an SBP of more than 20 mm Hg above their target, two drugs may be initiated (Chobanian et al., 2003).

Current recommendations suggest combinations of a low-dose thiazide diuretic with an ACE inhibitor, an ARB, or a long-acting calcium channel antagonist (CCA) (Chobanian et al., 2003; London, Schmieder, Calvo, & Asmar, 2006; Somes, Pahor, Shorr, Cushman, & Applegate 1999). There is no universal agreement on the approach to choosing alternative agents or combination therapy. Decisions are made based on patient comorbidities and considering the advantages and disadvantages of a specific drug.

Thiazide diuretics: These are recommended as first-line therapy in most older adults with uncomplicated Stage 1 hypertension (Chobanian et al., 2003; Clement et al., 2003; London, Schmieder, Calvo, & Asmar, 2006; Somes et al., 1999). At low doses, they reduce mortality, stroke, and cardiovascular events and lower SBP. They also have fewer side effects of hypokalemia, hyperuricemia, hypomagnesemia, hypertriglyceridemia, and glucose intolerance when used at recommended doses. They are also low cost and can be taken as a once-daily dose. The thiazide diuretics can also be combined with other classes such as the ACE inhibitors, ARBs, and calcium channel antagonists (CCAs) (Chobanian et al., 2003; Clement et al., 2003; Somes et al., 1999). Some important considerations when prescribing thiazide diuretics include the need to carefully monitor the patient's potassium level to avoid arrhythmias, because higher doses have been shown to increase the incidence of sudden cardiac death as well as impairment of glucose tolerance. Also, the thiazides are often ineffective with serum creatinine levels greater than 2 mg/dL or creatinine clearance below 30 to 40 mL/min.

Angiotensin-converting enzyme inhibitors: These have been shown to be effective in lowering BP in older adults. They are well tolerated and are an acceptable first-line therapy or can be used in combination with a thiazide diuretic (Chobanian et al., 2003; Clement et al., 2003; Somes et al., 1999). They lack significant central nervous system or metabolic side effects and have demonstrated benefits in patients with diabetes and those with left ventricular systolic dysfunction. In several clinical conditions, this class is associated with preservation of renal function. General side effects include cough, angioedema, hyperkalemia (especially in the presence of renal insufficiency or in combination with NSAIDs or potassium-sparing diuretics), and acute renal failure in patients with bilateral renal artery stenosis.

Angiotensin receptor blockers: This class is generally not recommended as first-line therapy in uncomplicated hypertension, because there are no randomized controlled trials comparing ARBs with diuretics and their effects on treatment outcomes in older adults (Chobanian et al., 2003; Jamerson et al., 2008; Kithas & Supiano, 2010). They may be considered in patients with diabetes, CHF, or chronic kidney disease who do not tolerate ACE inhibitors. There is rarely angioedema, and they do not cause a cough.

Calcium channel antagonists: CCAs have shown effectiveness in reducing BP in older adults. In general, because of age-related pharmacokinetic changes such as decreased clearance and increased plasma levels, lower CCA dosages should be used in older adults (Chobanian et al., 2003; Jamerson et al., 2008; Kithas & Supiano, 2010). Long-acting formulations are preferred because short-acting CCAs lower SBP rapidly. Side effects include headache, lower extremity edema, gingival hyperplasia, worsening of gastroesophageal reflux symptoms due to relaxation of the lower esophageal sphincter, and constipation.

Beta-receptor antagonists: The drugs in this classification are less effective than low-dose thiazide diuretics with regard to improving BP and cardiovascular outcomes as initial therapy. They are more likely to be discontinued due to adverse side effects. JNC-7 designates these as second-line therapy, and they should not be considered as first-line therapy in uncomplicated hypertension in older adults (Clement et al., 2003; Cushman et al., 2002; Dahlöf, et al., 2005; Khan &McAlister, 2006; Kjelden et al., 2005; Lindholm, Carlbert, & Samuelson, 2005). They are indicated in the older adult with certain comorbidities such as CAD, in secondary prevention after myocardial infarction, and in some patients with systolic dysfunction.

Alpha-receptor antagonists: Although these drugs reduce peripheral vascular resistance and lower BP, the development of symptomatic postural hypotension limits their use in the older adult population (Chobanian et al., 2003). They may be considered as additional therapy, particularly in older hypertensive men with benign prostatic hypertrophy.

Aldosterone antagonists: These drugs may prove useful as first-line agents in older adults with uncomplicated hypertension (Brown et al., 2000; Oberleithner et al., 2007). Like thiazide diuretics, the aldosterone antagonists lower SBP. They also antagonize aldosterone's metabolic effects of increasing sodium resorption, altering renal hemodynamics, and increasing afterload and vascular stiffness.

Summary of recommendations includes the following:

▪ Without comorbidities, start low-dose diuretics and increase gradually as first-line treatment.
▪ For patients with diabetes mellitus, ACE inhibitors are considered first line. Use ARBs if there is a cough with the ACE inhibitors.
▪ In patients with systolic heart failure, use a multidrug approach of ACE inhibitors, diuretics

(thiazide or loop, depending on renal function), and aldosterone antagonists.

- In the presence of CAD, use beta-receptor antagonists (without sympathomimetic activity).
- Patients with renal insufficiency with proteinuria should be managed with ACE inhibitors, ARBs, and CCAs.

Follow-up: The frequency of office visits is based on the level of hypertension at presentation. For most patients, except for those with SBP greater than 180 mm Hg, visits should be scheduled 1 to 2 months for dosage adjustment. Decreasing BP levels rapidly through overtreatment should be avoided, because it could lead to decreased cerebral and coronary perfusion, resulting in postural or postprandial hypotension. Supine and standing BPs should be determined at each visit. Before increasing dosages, the individual's adherence to therapy should be thoroughly assessed. Medication lists should also be reviewed to identify interactions that may worsen BP control. If an individual's BP is still not at target, carefully increase the dose, add another agent, or switch to another class of medication. If target BP is not achieved on a three-drug regimen with documented compliance, the individual should be evaluated for resistant or secondary hypertension. After more than a year of stable BP control at target levels, a step-down in therapy may be considered, especially in individuals who have been successful in lifestyle modifications. All patients should be encouraged to continue lifestyle modifications (Viera, Kshirsagar, & Hinderliter, 2008).

Sequelae: Complications of hypertension include aortic dissection, blood vessel damage such as arteriosclerosis, CHF, myocardial infarction, peripheral artery disease, stroke, loss of vision, chronic kidney disease, and brain damage.

Prevention/prophylaxis: Lifestyle modification. Lifestyle is characterized by a collection of behaviors that makes sense to the individual. At least 80% of premature deaths from cardiovascular disease could be avoided by adopting lifestyle behaviors such as eating a healthy diet, taking regular physical activity, and avoiding tobacco smoke (World Health Organization, 2011). Adults over 18 should have their BP checked routinely. Lifestyle changes that may help to control BP include smoking cessation; limiting alcohol to no more than one drink a day for women and two for men; consumption of a diet that includes fruits, vegetables, and low-fat dairy products while reducing total and saturated fat intake (DASH diet); engaging in regular exercise for 30 minutes on most days; maintaining tight control of blood glucose if diabetic; weight reduction; and stress management.

Referral: Refer immediately if the individual has signs of accelerated (malignant) hypertension (BP greater than 180/110 mm Hg with signs of papilledema and/or retinal hemorrhage) or suspected pheochromocytoma. Possible signs include labile or postural hypotension, headache, palpitations, pallor, and diaphoresis. Consider referral if the individual has unusual signs and symptoms; the individual has signs or symptoms suggesting a secondary cause; the individual's management depends critically on the accurate estimation of his or her BP; or the individual has symptoms of postural hypotension or a fall in SBP when standing of 20 mm Hg or more (Chobanian et al., 2003).

Education: Teach the patient, family, and/or caregivers about the disease process and its management. Have individuals monitor BP routinely. Obtaining reliable home values is important. Patients should be educated in appropriate BP techniques. As with office measurements, the patient needs to be sitting quietly for 5 to 10 minutes with the back supported in a chair, feet flat on the floor, and arm supported at heart level (Chobanian et al., 2003).

CLINICAL RECOMMENDATION	EVIDENCE RATING	REFERENCE
Pharmacological Management		
SBP is a primary target of therapy (SBP 135–140 mm Hg)	B	Kithas & Supiano M. (2010)
SBP <130 mm Hg in type 2 diabetes is treatment goal.	A	U.S. Department of Health and Human Services, National Institutes of Health, National Heart, Lung and Blood Institute (2004)

Continued

CLINICAL RECOMMENDATION	EVIDENCE RATING	REFERENCE
Low-dose diuretic in uncomplicated stage I hypertension (no comorbidities); start with one-half the usual dose (<25 mg HCTZ) and increase slowly.	A	Cushman et al. (2002) London, Schmieder, Calvo, & Asmar (2006) Somes et al. (1999) U.S. Department of Health and Human Services, National Institutes of Health, National Heart, Lung and Blood Institute (2004)
In patients with SBP >20 mm Hg above target, initiate two drugs: combinations of a low-dose thiazide diuretic with an ACE inhibitor, ARB, or long-acting CCA.	A	Clement et al. (2003) Somes et al. (1999) U.S. Department of Health and Human Services, National Institutes of Health, National Heart, Lung and Blood Institute (2004)
ACE inhibitor used as alternative first-line treatment for diabetics and left ventricular dysfunction; ACE inhibitor may be combined with a thiazide-type diuretic	A	Clement et al. (2003) Somes et al. (1999) U.S. Department of Health and Human Services, National Institutes of Health, National Heart, Lung and Blood Institute (2004)
ARBs not recommended as first-line therapy in uncomplicated hypertension; consider as first-line therapy in patients with diabetes, CHF, or chronic kidney disease who do not tolerate ACE inhibitors (i.e., cough, angioedema). Currently no randomized trials comparing ARBs with diuretics and their effects on treatment outcomes in the elderly.	A B	Stokes (2009) U.S. Department of Health and Human Services, National Institutes of Health, National Heart, Lung and Blood Institute (2004) Kithas & Supiano (2010)
Long-acting CCAs should be used in lower doses in older adults. No role for short-acting CCAs in treating hypertension in older adults due to rapid lowering of SBP and side effects including headaches, lower extremity edema, gingival hyperplasia, worsening of gastroesophageal reflux symptoms due to sphincter relaxation, and constipation.	A B	Jamerson et al. (2008) U.S. Department of Health and Human Services, National Institutes of Health, National Heart, Lung and Blood Institute (2004) Kithas & Supiano (2010)

CLINICAL RECOMMENDATION	EVIDENCE RATING	REFERENCE
Avoid beta antagonists in older hypertensive patients without a specific indication such as CAD.	A	Clement et al. (2003) Cushman et al. (2002) Dahlöf et al. (2005) Khan & McAlister (2006) Kjelden et al. (2005) Lindholm, Carlbert, & Samuelson (2005) Psaty et al. (1997)
Limited use of alpha-receptor antagonists due to development of symptomatic postural hypotension in older adults.	A	Cushman et al. (2002) U.S. Department of Health and Human Services, National Institutes of Health, National Heart, Lung and Blood Institute (2004)
Aldosterone antagonists may be useful agents in the older adult when combined with other agents.	A	Brown et al. (2000) Oberleithner et al. (2007)
Nonpharmacological Management		
Weight reduction; maintain normal body weight (BMI) 18.5–24.9 kg/m^2.	A	Bramlage et al. (2004) Redón et al. (2008)
Restrict dietary sodium; reduce dietary sodium intake to no more than 100 mEq/L (2.4 g sodium or 6 g sodium chloride). Adopt DASH Eating Plan; consume a diet rich in fruits, vegetables, and low-fat dairy products with a reduced content of saturated and total fat.	A	He, Markando, & MacGregor (2005) Appel et al. (2006)
Physical activity; engage in regular aerobic physical activity such as brisk walking (at least 30 min/day, most days of the week).	A	Brennan (2005) Stewart et al. (2005) Whelton, Chin, Xin, & He (2002)
Moderate alcohol consumption; limit consumption to no more than 2 drinks/day (10 oz or 30 mL ethanol in most men and no more than 1 drink/day in women and lighter-weight persons).	A	Xi (2001)

Continued

CLINICAL RECOMMENDATION	EVIDENCE RATING	REFERENCE
Smoking cessation.	A	Appel & Aldrich (2003) Donzé, Ruffieux, & Cornuz (2007) Fiore et al. (2008) Suskin et al. (2001)

A = consistent, good-quality, patient-oriented evidence; B = inconsistent or limited-quality, patient-oriented evidence; C = consensus, disease-oriented evidence, usual practice, expert opinion, or case series. For information about the SORT evidence rating system, go to www.aafp.org/afpsort.xml.

ISCHEMIC HEART DISEASE

Signal symptoms: Chest pain, tightness, or discomfort.

Description: Ischemic heart disease (IHD) is an imbalance between the supply and demand for blood flow to the myocardium.

Etiology: The pathophysiology of myocardial ischemia in younger or older adults is related to an imbalance between myocardial demand and coronary perfusion. This imbalance precipitates ischemia, which frequently is manifested as angina but instead may present silently as an acute event (i.e., sudden death or myocardial infarction). The main cause is coronary atherosclerosis with plaque formation. Specific pathological mechanisms also may include spasms of the coronary arteries, changes in the normal arterial tone, thrombus formation, or arteritis. The amount of oxygen required by the myocardium (demand) is determined by the BP, heart rate, left ventricular size and thickness, and contractility state.

Occurrence: Although IHD is decreasing in incidence, it remains the leading cause of death for elderly men and women. One of every six deaths in the United States is caused by coronary heart disease (Roger et al., 2012).

Age: The prevalence increases dramatically with age. In the fourth to sixth decade, prevalence of IHD is equal in men and women (6%). During the sixth to seventh decade, this rate triples for men (22.8%) and doubles for women (13.9%). By the eighth decade, men are at a prevalence rate of 35.5% and women at 20.8% (Roger et al., 2012).

Ethnicity: Cardiovascular disease is the most frequent cause of death. Of all the cardiovascular diseases, 49.9% are due to CHD, which caused about one of every six deaths in the United States in 2008. CHD among whites is 6.4%, African Americans 6.3%, Hispanics 5.2%, Asians 4.9%, Native Americans 5.9%, and Pacific Islanders 19.7%. There are some differences among different ethnic groups.

Gender: The incidence of CHD is greater in men. In women, CHD increases steadily with age. Both men and women peak in their 80s. In the fourth to sixth decade, prevalence of CHD is equal between men and women at 6%. At the sixth to eighth decade, prevalence of CHD is 22.8% for men and 13.9% for women. At the eighth decade and beyond, men's prevalence is 35%, and for women it is 20.8% (Roger et al., 2012).

Contributing factors: Age-related changes in myocardial and circulatory pathophysiology include reduced left ventricular compliance, amyloid deposits, diastolic dysfunction, increased aortic impedance, and peripheral vascular resistance. Other factors predictive of risk for CHD include elevations in the SBP (33.5% of U.S. adults 20 years and older have hypertension), plasma glucose and diabetes (8% of adults have diabetes), BMI (67.3% of U.S. adults are overweight, and of this group 33.7% are obese), total serum cholesterol (15% prevalence among adults 20 years and older), inactivity (33% of adults report engaging in no aerobic leisure-time physical activity), and smoking (Americans 18 years and older: 21.2% men and 17.5% of women smoke) (Roger et al., 2012).

Signs and symptoms: Chest pain, or angina pectoris, is intermittent and caused by transient, reversible myocardial ischemia. Three variants are recognized:

- Stable angina is chest pain associated with particular levels of exertion. The descriptor of this pain is crushing or squeezing substernal heaviness that can radiate down the left arm or be referred to the jaw. Pain is usually relieved by rest or drugs such as nitroglycerin, which dilates the coronary artery and thus increases blood flow. Often patients show signs of autonomic dysfunction, including elevated heart rate, elevated BP, and diaphoresis.

■ Prinzmetal angina occurs at rest and is caused by a coronary artery spasm. This pain also responds to nitroglycerin and calcium channel blockers.

■ Unstable angina pain is characterized by increasingly frequent pain associated with less activity and/or rest (Mitchell, 2012).

The key symptom of IHD is chest pain, but other common symptoms include arm pain, lower jaw pain, shortness of breath, and diaphoresis. These symptoms are referred to as angina equivalents and can also include fatigue or breathlessness. Some patients may have no symptoms or atypical ones so that CAD may not be diagnosed until they experience a myocardial infarction.

The average person with prolonged rest angina does not seek medical care for approximately 2 hours after the symptoms start. Women wait longer than men. The reason commonly expressed is that patients expect that a heart attack would present dramatically with severe, crushing chest pain and that there would be no doubt what was occurring. Most commonly the symptom experienced was a gradual onset of discomfort involving midsternal chest pressure or tightness with other associated symptoms often increasing in intensity. The ambiguity of the expected symptoms and the actual experience resulted in uncertainty about the diagnosis, and most waited to see what would happen before seeking help. Many expressed that they were afraid of being embarrassed if symptoms turned out to be a false alarm, and they were reluctant to trouble others (Anderson et al., 2011). Chest discomfort may not always be the presenting symptom. As many as one-half of all myocardial infarctions may be clinically unrecognized. Patients without chest discomfort tend to be older women who have diabetes and prior heart failure. They delay longer before going to the hospital and are less likely to be diagnosed as having a myocardial infarction when admitted. They are also less likely to receive fibrinolysis or percutaneous coronary intervention (PCI), aspirin, beta blockers, or heparin. Patients with silent myocardial infarctions are over 2 times more likely to die during the hospitalization. Dyspnea without angina has more than twice the risk of death than for typical angina. Dyspnea is now seen as an independent predictor of cardiac and total mortality and as a risk factor for sudden cardiac death (Anderson et al., 2011).

The major objective of the physical examination is to identify possible precipitating causes for the anginal symptoms such as hypertension, thyrotoxicosis, or gastric bleed. This can guide the practitioner to identify the most likely diagnosis and treatment. In addition, the examination can identify possible comorbid conditions that could affect the therapeutic choices and risks involved. Vital signs, including BPs in both arms and a thorough cardiothoracic examination assessing for rales, gallops, or murmurs, may suggest CAD; back pain or unequal pulses may suggest aortic dissection; acute dyspnea, pleuritic chest pain, and differential breath sounds may suggest pneumothorax.

Diagnostic tests:

TEST	RESULTS INDICATING DISORDER
ECG	ST-segment depression or elevation or T-wave inversion in the absence of left ventricular hypertrophy supports the diagnosis of ischemia
	Q waves may be evidence of an old myocardial infarction
Exercise stress testing	Reproduces ischemic symptoms
	Defects in myocardial perfusion with exercise
	Cardiac risk identified in patients with a decrease in the blood pressure (BP), S_3, rales, or prolonged downsloping ST-segment depression after exercise
Myocardial perfusion imaging	Perfusion defects
	Left ventricular dysfunction
Echocardiogram	Assesses the severity of left ventricular dysfunction
Stress echocardiogram	Multiple reversible wall motion abnormalities
Cardiac catheterization	For patients who fail pharmacological therapy, have had a myocardial infarction, or have unstable angina, to determine the severity of disease

Differential diagnosis: IHD must be differentiated from other, superimposed diseases that may increase myocardial oxygen demand and decrease its supply (i.e., anemia, infection, hyperthyroidism, and arrhythmias).

Chest pain from IHD must be differentiated from pleuritic, costochondral, or pericardial pain. This type of pain also can mimic GERD, herpes zoster, and panic disorder (Uphold & Graham, 2003, p. 465).

Treatment: The immediate goal of treatment is to decrease oxygen consumption and increase the blood supply to the myocardium by reducing vascular tone, improving collateral flow, and preventing platelet plugs and thrombosis. The treatment regimens are similar for symptomatic and asymptomatic elderly persons.

Bedrest with continuous ECG monitoring for arrhythmias may provide a decrease in oxygen demands. Nitroglycerin, either sublingually or by spray, is followed by continuous IV administration for immediate relief of ischemia by decreasing preload and increasing dilation of the coronary arteries (Braunwald et al., 2000). Morphine is given IV to relieve symptoms or when acute pulmonary congestion or severe agitation is present. Supplemental oxygen may increase the oxygen supply. Aspirin is given to reduce platelet adhesion. If not tolerant to aspirin, clopidogrel is given (Braunwald et al., 2000). Beta blockers are given if there is ongoing chest pain. In patients with continuing or frequently recurring ischemic symptoms or when beta blockers are contraindicated (reversible airway disease), calcium channel blockers, such as verapamil or diltiazem, may be given in the absence of severe left ventricular dysfunction. ACE inhibitors may be started when hypertension persists in patients with left ventricular dysfunction or CHF or with a diagnosis of diabetes (Braunwald et al., 2000).

Acetylsalicylic acid (ASA), 75 to 325 mg, affords a protective benefit to individuals with angina. ASA is given after an acute myocardial infarction to reduce platelet aggregation. Daily doses of ASA are continued for at least 2 years after the myocardial infarction and indefinitely for many patients. The risk of gastric irritation and gastrointestinal bleeding exists even with low doses of ASA. For ASA-sensitive patients, clopidogrel might work to block platelet aggregation and reduce reoccurrence and progression. High-dose atorvastatin (80 mg) drugs may be added if myocardial infarction is suspected, because they may stabilize plaque (Lavie & Milani, 2010).

Invasive intervention therapy also includes IV thrombolytic therapy in patients with known or suspected acute myocardial infarction (see under Myocardial Infarction). Mechanical intervention with percutaneous transluminal coronary angioplasty (PTCA) is used to revascularize patients with acute or chronic manifestations of CAD. Patients with all forms of angina tolerate well and benefit from PTCA, particularly patients with comorbid factors that limit the appropriateness of a surgical procedure (i.e., coronary artery bypass graft [CABG] surgery). A high rate of restenosis occurs after PTCA. Other percutaneous interventions available include lasers, atherectomy devices, stents, and intra-aortic balloon counterpulsation.

The long-term goals for patients who have end-organ damage from IHD are to relieve symptoms and allow patients to resume their preferred lifestyle. CABG surgery is a revascularization procedure that is effective in alleviating ischemic symptoms. CABG surgery has an advantage over PTCA in that its results are more durable, and revascularization is more complete. The patient most likely to benefit maximally is one with the potential to return to an active lifestyle who can tolerate the 3 to 4 months of cardiac rehabilitation. Comorbid factors known to affect the outcome negatively include diabetes, cerebral and peripheral vascular disease, a history of recent myocardial infarction, systemic hypertension, renal insufficiency, pulmonary disease, and obesity. Elderly women have a considerably higher risk of death and complications from IHD than their male counterparts.

Follow-up: Patients with IHD must be monitored for the effectiveness of prescribed drugs and any potential adverse effect. Changes in features of symptoms and disease progression should be determined.

Sequelae: Silent ischemia has the same prognosis as symptomatic ischemia. Angina is associated with a twofold to threefold increase in the risk of death when ECG abnormalities are also present. ECG abnormalities compatible with ischemia are associated with mortality even in the absence of chest pain.

Complications from CAD include CHF, acute myocardial infarction and associated problems, arrhythmias, and sudden death.

Prevention/prophylaxis: Risk factor modification includes control of systolic hypertension, cholesterol levels, and elimination of smoking. A sedentary lifestyle predisposes an individual to CAD, particularly in the presence of other risk factors. Physical conditioning tends to lower the BP; individuals who are physically active have slightly higher plasma HDL levels than sedentary individuals. Other strategies to manage risk include weight control, stress reduction, and cholesterol management, if indicated. Low-dose aspirin therapy (325 mg every other day) may reduce the risk of myocardial infarction; however, its use is associated with adverse effects. Its risk and benefits must be examined individually in patients. Studies show potential benefits of ACE inhibitors and beta blockers after myocardial infarction in reducing risk of future coronary events.

Referral: Unstable patients with IHD require hospitalization because approximately 20% of these patients have myocardial infarction. Collaborate closely with the physician regarding patients who are refractory to treatment.

Education: Advise patients to report changes in the pattern or intensity of angina. All patients should be instructed to call emergency services when experiencing chest pain, because the differential diagnosis is difficult to determine without technological equipment. Each patient needs a plan for risk factor reduction and education related to this plan.

CLINICAL RECOMMENDATION	EVIDENCE RATING	REFERENCE
Unstable Angina/Non–ST-Elevation Myocardial Infarction		
ASA should be administered to UA/NSTEMI patients as soon as possible after hospital presentation and continued indefinitely in patients who tolerate.	A	Wright et al. (2011)
Unstable Angina/NSTEMI managed by Conservative Strategy		
Initiate anticoagulant therapy: • Enoxaparin or UFH or • Fondaparinux • Clopidogrel therapy	A B A	Anderson (2011)
Consider adding IV eptifibatide or tirofiban.	B	Anderson (2011)
If subsequent events: YES: angiography. NO: stress test.	B	Anderson (2011)
Continue ASA indefinitely.	A	Anderson (2011)
Continue clopidogrel for at least 1 month.	B	Anderson (2011)
Discontinue anticoagulant therapy.	A	Anderson (2011)
Unstable Angina/NSTEMI Managed by Invasive Strategy		
Initiate anticoagulant therapy: • Enoxaparin or UFH. • Bivalirudin or fondaparinux.	A	Anderson (2011)
Before angiography initiate: • One or • Both.	A	Anderson (2011)
Clopidogrel, IV GP IIb/IIa inhibitor	B	Anderson (2011)

Continued

CLINICAL RECOMMENDATION	EVIDENCE RATING	REFERENCE
Unstable Angina/NSTEMI Managed by CABG		
Continue ASA.	A	Anderson (2011)
Discontinue: • clopidogrel 5–7 days before CABG. • IV GP IIb/IIa 4 hours before CABG. • Enoxaparin 12–24 hours before CABG. • fondaparinux 24 hours before CABG. • Bivalirudin 3 hours before CABG.	B	Anderson (2011)
Continue UFH.	B	Anderson (2011)
Unstable Angina/NSTEMI Managed by PCI		
Continue ASA.	A	Anderson (2011)
Loading dose of clopidogrel is not started.	A	Anderson (2011)
IV GP IIb/IIa is not started.	A	Anderson (2011)
Discontinue anticoagulant after PCI for uncomplicated cases.	B	Anderson (2011)
IHD Long-Term Management		
Aspirin should be started at 75–182 mg per day and continued indefinitely in all patients unless contraindicated.	A	Fraker & Fihn (2007)
Use of warfarin in conjunction with aspirin and/or clopidogrel is associated with an increased risk of bleeding and should be monitored closely.	B	Fraker & Fihn (2007)
ACE inhibitors should be started and continued indefinitely in all patients with left ventricular ejection fraction ≤40% and in those with hypertension, diabetes, or chronic kidney disease unless contraindicated.	A	Fraker & Fihn (2007)
ARBs are recommended for patients who have hypertension, have indications for but are intolerant of ACE inhibitors, have heart failure, or have had myocardial infarction with left ventricular ejection fraction ≤40%.	A	Fraker & Fihn (2007)
ARBs may be considered in combination with ACE inhibitors for heart failure due to left ventricular systolic dysfunction.	B	Fraker & Fihn (2007)

CLINICAL RECOMMENDATION	EVIDENCE RATING	REFERENCE
Aldosterone blockade is recommended for use in post-myocardial infarction patients without significant renal dysfunction or hyperkalemia who are already receiving therapeutic doses of an ACE inhibitor and beta blocker, have a left ventricular ejection fraction ≤40%, and have either diabetes or heart failure.	A	Fraker & Fihn (2007)
It is beneficial to start and continue beta blocker therapy indefinitely in all patients who have had myocardial infarction, acute coronary syndrome, or left ventricular dysfunction with or without heart failure symptoms, unless contraindicated.	A	Fraker & Fihn (2007)
An annual influenza vaccination is recommended for patients with cardiovascular disease.	B	Fraker & Fihn (2007)
Chelation therapy is not recommended for the treatment of chronic angina or arteriosclerotic cardiovascular disease and may be harmful because of its potential to cause hypocalcemia.	C	Fraker & Fihn (2007)
Risk reduction:		
Smoking cessation and avoidance of exposure.	B	Fraker & Fihn (2007)
Blood pressure control according to JNC 7.	A	Fraker & Fihn (2007)
Lipid management: LDL cholesterol <100 mg/dL; reduction of LDL cholesterol <70 mg/dL or high-dose statin therapy is reasonable.	A	Fraker & Fihn (2007)
Where appropriate, exercise test to guide exercise prescription. Medically supervised cardiac rehabilitation for recent acute coronary syndrome or revascularization, heart failure.	B	Fraker & Fihn (2007)
BMI/waist circumference assessed regularly. Goal of weight loss therapy should be to gradually reduce body weight by approximately 10% from baseline.	B	Fraker & Fihn (2007)
Diabetes management: should include lifestyle and pharmacotherapy measures to achieve a near-normal HbA1c.	B	Fraker & Fihn (2007)

A = consistent, good-quality, patient-oriented evidence; B = inconsistent or limited-quality, patient-oriented evidence; C = consensus, disease-oriented evidence, usual practice, expert opinion, or case series. For information about the SORT evidence rating system, go to www.aafp.org/afpsort.xml.

LUNG CANCER

Signal symptoms: Cough, dyspnea, weight loss, anorexia, hemoptysis.

Description: Lung cancer is a malignant neoplasm originating in the parenchyma of the lung or airways (Midthun, 2012a, 2012b). Approximately 95% of all lung cancer is classified as non–small cell lung cancer (NSCLC) or small cell lung cancer (SCLC). NSCLC includes adenocarcinoma, squamous cell cancer, and large cell cancer (Carr, Finigan, & Kern, 2011).

Etiology: Research has shown conclusively that more than 85% of lung cancer cases are associated with tobacco smoking. Radon is the second leading cause of lung cancer (National Cancer Institute [NCI] Fact Sheet, 2012). The inhalation of other carcinogens, such as asbestos, arsenic, nickel, and chromium, usually through occupational exposure, accounts for most other cases of lung cancer; second-hand smoke is also a factor. Use of biomass fuel, coal, or wood increases risk of lung cancer (Hosgood et al., 2010). Patients with preexisting diseases that involve the lungs, such as COPD, prior lung cancers, sarcoidosis, and scleroderma, are at increased risk for developing lung cancer. Radiation exposure may cause lung cancer. Genetic predisposition to carcinoma of the lung continues to be studied (Midthun, 2012a, 2012b).

Occurrence: Lung cancer is the most common cause of cancer-associated deaths in the United States. It is the second most common cancer among men and women. Annually, more than 180,000 new cases are diagnosed. Lung cancer is responsible for 32% of cancer deaths in men and 25% of cancer deaths in women. The incidence in women is increasing rapidly.

Age: Lung cancer can occur at any age, but there is a dramatic increase in new diagnosis after age 40 years. Most recent statistics show 31.3% diagnosed between 65 and 74, 28.3% between 75 and 84, and 8.4% among those age 85 years and older (Howlader et al., 2012).

Ethnicity: African American men younger than 54 years old have a higher incidence than white men. No significant difference exists between African American and white women.

Gender: More men have lung cancer than do women, but the incidence rate for women is rising.

Contributing factors: The cumulative dose or pack-years for cigarette smoking is related directly to the risk of developing lung cancer. The more cigarettes smoked per day and the longer the individual has smoked, the higher the risk of developing lung cancer. The risk of lung cancer is 30 times higher in smokers than in non-smokers. Cigar and pipe smokers and passive smokers have double the risk. The risks of developing NSCLC steadily decline for people who quit smoking and approach that of a nonsmoker after 15 years of abstinence. Individuals who have smoked for more than 20 years probably always will have a slightly increased risk of developing the disease, even after 15 years as a nonsmoker. There is no change in risk of SCLC with smoking cessation; early age at beginning to smoke is a significant risk factor. Asbestos exposure alone increases the risk of developing pulmonary carcinoma, but when combined with smoking, the risk increases to 100 times that of a nonsmoker. Other inhaled agents implicated in the development of the disease are radon, arsenic, nickel, chromates, halo ethers, alkylating compounds, and polycyclic aromatic hydrocarbons. Radon is a risk factor; air pollution also is thought to contribute to the development of lung cancer. Sarcoidosis carries a threefold increased risk; scleroderma increases risk of bronchoalveolar cancer.

Signs and symptoms: Signs and symptoms of lung cancer are usually present only after the disease has progressed beyond the early stages. Routine screening for the disease with chest x-ray examination is not recommended because it is neither specific nor sensitive. A recent National Lung Screening trial randomized heavy smokers to either low-dose CT or chest x-ray annually for 3 years. Mortality rate in the group decreased by 20%, particularly in the low CT group (The National Lung Screening Trial Research Team, 2011; Midthun, 2012a, 2012b). Despite this clinical trial, there are many confounding elements from other trials that remain and the evidence is insufficient to recommend screening at this point, according to the American College of Chest Physicians (Silvestri & Jett, 2010). The National Comprehensive Cancer Network guidelines for non–small cell lung cancer (2011) has endorsed screening (see Prevention/Prophylaxis). Symptoms suggestive of lung cancer include a new or changing cough, hoarseness, hemoptysis, anorexia, cachexia, unexplained weight loss, dyspnea, hypoxia, wheezing, unresolving pneumonia, and chest wall pain (Collins, Haines, Perkel, & Enck, 2007; Midthun, 2012a, 2012b). Patients initially may present with symptoms related to extrathoracic disease, including tracheal obstruction, esophageal obstruction with dysphagia, laryngeal nerve paralysis, phrenic nerve paralysis with elevated hemidiaphragm, sympathetic nerve paralysis or Horner's syndrome, pleural effusion owing to lymphatic obstruction, Pancoast's syndrome involving the eighth cervical and first and second thoracic nerves, or superior vena cava syndrome from vascular obstruction (Spiro, Gould, & Colice, 2007).

Patients with pericardial and cardiac extension of tumor may have symptoms of arrhythmia, tamponade, or failure. The presenting illness in patients with lung cancer may be paraneoplastic syndromes, including hypercalcemia, hypophosphatemia, hyponatremia with syndrome of inappropriate antidiuretic hormone, and hypercoagulable states. Occasionally, skeletal-connective syndromes, clubbing, and osteoarthropathy are initial symptoms of lung cancer.

Diagnostic tests: After a history and physical examination suggestive of disease, the following tests are recommended (note that tissue biopsy results are required for diagnosis):

Noninvasive testing:

▨ Chest x-ray—this may show nonspecific abnormalities, hilar masses, atelectasis, pleural effusions or masses, and infiltrates.
▨ CT scan, preferably with contrast; CT can assist in defining the characteristics, size, and location of the primary tumor, lymphadenopathy if present, and any abnormalities of the liver and adrenal glands, if performed through the adrenals (Silvestri & Jett, 2010).
▨ Fluorodeoxyglucose positron emission tomography (FDG-PET) is a test that measures the metabolic uptake of glucose by cells; lung cancer cells have a higher cellular glucose uptake than normal cells. It is helpful in diagnosing metastatic disease (Carr et al., 2011).

Invasive testing:

▨ Sputum for cytology—this is positive in most centrally located tumors.
▨ Transthoracic needle aspiration is usually reserved for specific circumstances.
▨ Fiberoptic bronchoscopy with biopsies has a very high sensitivity rating for diagnosis.
▨ Bronchoscopy with CT-guided transbronchial needle aspiration has an important role in diagnosis and staging of lung cancer.
▨ Endoscopic ultrasound, endobronchial ultrasound, and mediastinoscopy also contribute to staging; mediastinoscopy is considered the gold standard for identifying mediastinal involvement (Silvestri & Jett, 2010).

If abnormalities suggest more extensive cancer, further testing will be conducted looking for extrathoracic, metastatic disease.

Staging:

▨ NSCLC staging was revised in 2009 and follows the tumor, node, metastasis (TNM) classification (Edge et al., 2009). Correct staging is essential at diagnosis to identify treatment options, prognosis, and potential for recurrence.
▨ SCLC staging follows the two-stage Veterans Administration Lung Study Group staging system of limited disease (LD) and extensive disease (ED). Limited disease is that confined to one hemithorax, the mediastinum, and the supraclavicular lymph nodes on the same side as the tumor. Extensive disease is any disease extending beyond this, including disease in the contralateral nodes or pleural effusion (Silvestri & Jett, 2010).

Differential diagnosis: Tuberculosis, infectious granuloma, pneumonia, empyema, bronchiectasis, abscess, sarcoidosis, pneumonitis, and asbestosis all can mimic lung cancer.

Treatment: Surgical resection, radiation therapy, and occasionally chemotherapy are indicated for NSCLC; staging of the disease, patient's functional status, and histology of the tumor determine the treatments. Recent advances in genotyping and targeting of altered signal mechanisms in lung cancer have allowed targeted treatment with monoclonal antibodies, anti–vascular endothelial growth factor (anti-VEGF) agents, and other modalities (Bonanno, Favaretto, Rugge, Taron, & Rosell, 2011; Cagle & Chirieac, 2012). Multimodal chemotherapy and radiation is the treatment of choice for SCLC-LD; cisplatin and etoposide are the preferred agents. Prophylactic cranial irradiation is done in select patients. In some patients with very limited disease, surgical resection may be done (Neal, Gubens, & Wakelee, 2011). Treatment of SCLC-ED is chemotherapy alone with cisplatin or carboplatin, up to six cycles, then watchful waiting. Use of PCI is controversial due to side effects. Treatment after relapse is dependent on response to initial chemotherapy; if there is a positive response, repeating the treatment is done. If nonresponsive to initial chemotherapy, "salvage chemotherapy" with a nonplatinum, single agent such as gemcitabine or a taxane is attempted (Neal et al., 2011). Clinical trials are now underway with other chemotherapy agents.

Treatment for older adults should be individualized. A comprehensive geriatric assessment is often conducted and used in determining treatment options; the

Karnofsky Performance Scale is also used by some specialists (www.hospicepatients.org/karnofsky.html).

Follow-up: Follow-up is individualized; generally patients should be seen for follow-up every 2 months after treatment for lung cancer. During years 2 to 5, follow-up should be every 3 months. Yearly examinations are advised thereafter.

Sequelae: Disability and death are the chief sequelae of lung cancer. The 5-year survival rate is 13% for NSCLC and is less than 10% for SCLC.

Prevention/prophylaxis: Prevention of lung cancer should focus on smoking cessation. Ask about and record the tobacco use status of every patient, advise patients who smoke to quit, and offer smoking cessation treatment at every office visit. Screening for lung cancer in asymptomatic patients is not advised. Screening in high-risk patients has not demonstrated any decrease in mortality; newer methodologies studying biomarkers have not been proven to date (Bach, Silvestri, Hanger, & Jett, 2007). The National Comprehensive Cancer Network (NCCN) has issued guidelines endorsing screening with low-dose helical CT in high-risk patients (NCCN, 2011). High risk includes those ages 50 to 74 years with a 30 pack-year smoking history and smoking cessation of less than 15 years or those ages 50 years and older with a 20 pack-year smoking history and one additional risk factor other than second-hand smoke (NCCN, 2011). The American College of Chest Physicians has written a comprehensive, evidence-based practice guideline addressing the failure of chemoprevention efforts such as vitamin therapy and the need for more studies on other agents (Gray et al., 2007).

Referral: On suspecting lung cancer, refer the patient to a pulmonary specialist. At a later stage, referral to palliative care or hospice may be indicated. Give patient information on the National Cancer Institute information line (1-800-4-CANCER). Referral to a mental health specialist is indicated in severe depression unresponsive to treatment.

Education: Many smoking cessation programs are available. Examples include the National Cancer Institute Tobacco Quitline, the American Academy of Family Physicians Stop Smoking Kit, various pamphlets from the American Cancer Society, and A Healthy Beginning Counseling Kit from the American Lung Association; the Web site www.smokefree.gov is another resource. The primary health-care provider can assess the smoker's motivation to quit and offer brief motivational interventions at each visit. Provide information about support groups and community programs available to help with smoking cessation.

Once the patient is diagnosed with lung cancer, education about type of cancer, treatment options, and prognosis is very important; this is typically done by the oncology team, but primary care providers can monitor for patient questions and communicate this to the specialty team.

CLINICAL RECOMMENDATION	EVIDENCE RATING	REFERENCE
For individuals with a smoking history >20 pack-years or a history of lung cancer, the use of beta carotene supplementation is not recommended for primary, secondary, or tertiary chemoprevention of lung cancer.	A	Gray et al. (2007)
For individuals who are at risk for lung cancer and patients with a history of lung cancer, the use of vitamin E, retinoids, N-acetylcysteine, and aspirin is not recommended for primary, secondary, or tertiary prevention of lung cancer.	A	Gray et al. (2007)
Surgery is the treatment of choice for patients with local or only locally advanced non–small cell carcinoma (Stage I through Stage IIIA).	B	Manser et al. (2009) National Comprehensive Care Network guidelines for non–small cell lung cancer (NCCN) (2009)

CLINICAL RECOMMENDATION	EVIDENCE RATING	REFERENCE
Treatment for unresectable non–small cell carcinoma may involve radiotherapy and chemotherapy.	C	NCCN (2009) Stewart (2009)
Chemotherapy, combined with radiotherapy in limited disease, is the mainstay of treatment for small cell carcinoma.	C	Pijls-Johannesma et al. (2009)
Both radiotherapy and chemotherapy are used in treatment of superior vena cava (SVC) syndrome because of non–small cell or small cell lung cancer.	B	Rowell, Gleeson, & Rowell (2008)
Suspect paraneoplastic syndromes in patients with cancer who have fatigue, weakness, myalgias, or electrolyte abnormalities that cannot be explained by their condition or treatment.	C	Giffi & Zimrin (2011)

A = consistent, good-quality, patient-oriented evidence; B = inconsistent or limited-quality, patient-oriented evidence; C = consensus, disease-oriented evidence, usual practice, expert opinion, or case series. For information about the SORT evidence rating system, go to www.aafp.org/afpsort.xml.

MYOCARDIAL INFARCTION

Signal symptoms: Typical symptom is prolonged chest pain (more than 20 minutes' duration); atypical symptoms include shortness of breath, neurological symptoms (confusion, weakness), and worsening of heart failure.

Description: Myocardial infarction (MI) is necrosis of heart tissue caused by lack of blood and oxygen supply to the heart. MIs can be classified as acute ST elevation MI (STEMI) or non–ST elevation MI (NSTEMI). The terms *Q-wave MI*, denoting transmural infarction or full thickness, and *non–Q-wave MI*, denoting nontransmural infarction, or partial thickness, were used previously; however, due to many anatomical inconsistencies noted, this terminology is used less frequently (Venkatesan, 2008).

Etiology: Atherosclerotic plaque formation has been noted in persons younger than 20 years of age. Gradually, this atherogenic plaque builds up inside the intimal linings of the coronary artery(ies), resulting in both hardening of the arterial walls and narrowing of the coronary vessels. This atherosclerotic plaque contains lipid (cholesterol)–rich content, covered by a fibrous cap, which can ulcerate or fissure. Rupture of this vulnerable plaque can result in thrombosis, which

partially or totally occludes the lumen of the affected artery(ies), either at the location where the thrombus formed or further downstream where a smaller artery could be blocked. The results are essentially the same—an abrupt decrease in coronary blood flow to the myocardium, termed *myocardial ischemia*. Prolonged myocardial ischemia can lead to tissue death and MI. Although there are other causes of MI due to reduced myocardial blood flow, including hypotension and prolonged coronary vasospasm, or severe hyperthyroidism (which can increase the heart's demand for oxygen), the most frequent cause of MI is due to atherosclerosis. Another factor that plays an important role in acute coronary syndrome (ACS) is platelet activation and aggregation (Davi & Patrono, 2007; Nathan, 2010). Damaged blood vessels result in exposed collagen fiber in the basement membrane. Platelets subsequently adhere to this collagen fiber and become activated. Upon activation, platelets then release chemicals including adenosine diphosphate (ADP) and thromboxane (a vasoconstrictor), which causes additional platelet aggregation. A platelet plug (or clot) is formed, which decreases blood flow to the blood vessel (Nathan, 2010).

Occurrence: When looking at all-cause mortality, coronary disease is the most frequent cause of death in the United States. In persons age 55 to 74 in the United States, coronary disease occurs more frequently in men, but by age 75, this gender gap narrows (Maroo, Lavie, & Milani, 2008). In persons older than age 65, coronary disease contributes to significant morbidities and mortality (Aronow, 2008). In persons age 65 years or older who present with MI, more than 60% have NSTEMI with associated in-hospital mortality, accounting for approximately 80% of all in-patient hospital deaths (Kyriakides, Kourouklis, & Kontaras, 2007; Tullman, Haugh, Dracup, & Bourguignon, 2007). In addition, persons older than 65 with MI are associated with higher postdischarge mortality, theoretically because of the higher incidence of diffuse coronary disease and existing poor myocardial perfusion. Data published by the CDC (2007) on coronary disease and MI found that males overall had a significantly higher myocardial rate than females (no specific age group identified); however, with successive age groupings, the prevalence of MIs significantly increased. When identifying level of education with MI and coronary disease, persons who had less than a high school diploma experienced almost twice the occurrences of these conditions when compared with those who had college education.

Age: Postmortem studies show that coronary atherosclerosis is widespread even among asymptomatic adults. Aging itself may be a risk factor for MI in both men and women (CDC, 2007; Khot et al., 2003).

Ethnicity: The incidences and occurrences of patients having MIs and CHD by race and ethnicity have been reported by the CDC (2007). Specific groups were identified at increased risk, including those persons who are multiracial, American Indians, and Alaskan natives, who have substantially higher prevalence of MI than non-Hispanic whites, whites, or blacks (CDC, 2007). Overall, in patients with NSTEMI, black patients (when compared to whites) were younger, with concomitant comorbidities including hypertension, renal insufficiency, diabetes, and heart failure (Kyriakides et al., 2007; Sonel et al., 2005).

Gender: Before menopause, due to estrogenic cardioprotective effect, women have a lower occurrence of MI than men. Coronary disease is much more prevalent in men than in women up to age 74, after which the occurrence increases steeply with age in both genders. On average, women develop heart disease 10 years later than men and suffer MIs and sudden death 20 years later than men. Thus, by age 75, postmenopausal women have an equal risk to men of coronary disease and MI.

Contributing factors: Risk factors for heart disease and MI in elderly individuals are essentially the same as in the younger population. Risk factors include hypertension, hyperlipidemia, diabetes, insulin resistance, physical inactivity and sedentary lifestyle, overweight or obesity, family history of heart disease, poor diet, sleep apnea, alcohol, and stress (www.nhlbi.nih.gov/health/health-topics/topics/hd). Cigarette smoking is associated with new coronary events for elderly men and women. The risks of MI drop rapidly after smoking cessation, and at 5 years, the risk for new coronary events is similar to that of a nonsmoker (Aronow, 2008). An emerging risk factor includes high levels of C-reactive protein (CRP). High-sensitivity CRP is a protein "marker" in blood associated with inflammation in the body. Elevated levels have been correlated with increased risk for CAD and MI, sudden death, stroke, and peripheral artery disease (Shishehbor, Bhatt, & Topol, 2003).

Aging alters the cardiovascular system in ways that reduce cardiac reserve and efficiency, thus compromising the ability to respond to stress or illness. The cardiovascular system becomes less compliant as diastolic filling of the ventricles declines and afterload increases secondary to increased stiffness in the ascending aorta. The result is moderate left ventricular hypertrophy, which creates a more precarious balance between myocardial oxygen supply and demand. Other changes in the elderly cardiovascular system include decreased responsiveness to beta-adrenergic stimulation, decreased baroreceptor sensitivity, and an increased dependence on a higher end-diastolic volume to maintain cardiac output (Aronow, 2008).

Signs and symptoms: With advancing age the presentation of acute MI will be less likely to include the classic symptoms of crushing substernal chest pain, nausea, vomiting, and diaphoresis. Rather, atypical symptoms such as a vague ache or discomfort may be present. Elderly persons may not recognize that throat, shoulder, arm, jaw, or abdominal pain may be referred cardiac pain or angina equivalent. Dyspnea is the second most common symptom of MI in both younger and older populations. For patients 85 and older, syncope, acute confusion, or stroke may be the only presenting symptom. Some elderly patients may present only with faintness, weakness, giddiness, or restlessness (Tullman et al., 2007).

On physical examination, the patient may be anxious and weak and may appear cyanotic. Arrhythmias may be noted on the ECG. The skin may be diaphoretic, cold, and clammy. Thrills, heaves, and an abnormal PMI may be palpated. Peripheral pulses may be irregular, slow, fast, or thready. Auscultation may reveal an S_3 or S_4, pericardial friction rub, murmurs, or crackles. The physical examination must focus on ruling out diagnoses other than MI.

Diagnostic tests: Along with a chest x-ray examination, CBC, clotting profile, electrolytes, and cardiac biomarkers including troponin, evaluation for acute MI includes serial 12-lead ECGs (O'Connor et al., 2010). Changes on the ECG indicative of STEMI include ST-segment elevation in leads facing the infarction. ST-segment depression is sometimes present. With the increased incidence of NSTEMI, the presence of a single normal ECG does not rule out MI, and therefore serial ECGs are necessary. However, ECG findings may be nondiagnostic or difficult to interpret in elderly people because of possible abnormalities such as left bundle branch block, left ventricular hypertrophy, and previously unrecognized MIs.

In older adults, the cardiac enzyme profile may be atypical. Creatine kinase (CK), an enzyme found in myocardial cells, is released into the bloodstream when cells are damaged approximately 6 to 8 hours after the onset of pain. Because the baseline CK in elderly patients may be significantly lower than normal, even those with MI may not develop CK levels high enough to be interpreted as abnormal, owing to decreased muscle mass. CK-MB, an isoenzyme of CK, is released upon the death of myocardial cells and not during ischemia. The presence of CK-MB is also found in skeletal muscle, which can result in false-positive results from noncardiac conditions such as renal failure, head or chest trauma, pulmonary embolus, acute and chronic muscular disorders, hypothyroidism, or hyperventilation. Therefore, CK-MB measurements do not provide additional information to the algorithms of STEMI and are not preferred over cardiac troponins (Saenger, 2010). Cardiac troponin T (cTnT) is a cardiac-specific marker for MI, with rises in concentration levels soon after chest symptoms begin (de Lemos et al., 2010). Although elevations may not occur for 6 to 12 hours after onset of symptoms, in approximately 80% of patients, use of cTnT alone can result in a definitive diagnosis of STEMI. Lactate dehydrogenase levels are occasionally useful in patients with delayed presentation because this enzyme remains elevated for several days. Other tests for MI may include echocardiography or stress thallium scans (Saenger, 2010).

Differential diagnosis: The pain from MI can be similar to that of acute pericarditis, pulmonary embolism, acute aortic dissection, or costochondritis. Many conditions can present as cardiac disease in the elderly, including cor pulmonale, pneumonia, esophageal spasm, GERD, hiatal hernia, gallbladder disease, osteoarthritis of the spine, inflammation at the chondrocostal junction, muscle injury, and panic disorder (McPhee & Papadakis, 2008).

Treatment: The American College of Cardiology and the American Heart Association have examined pharmacological and interventional treatments for acute MI and established guidelines for care. Nitrates, the cornerstone of therapy for ischemic pain, reduce preload and improve coronary perfusion. Chest pain should be treated with sublingual nitroglycerin, repeated 3 times, 5 minutes apart, unless the patient is hypotensive, has right ventricular infarction, or has aortic stenosis (Kushner et al., 2009). IV nitrates have been shown to limit infarct size and reduce pain, complications, and mortality. IV nitroglycerin is started at 5 mcg/min on an infusion pump and titrated to desired effect. Frequent monitoring is required because harmful effects can be seen if the SBP drops below 90 mm Hg. Morphine sulfate, 2 to 4 mg IV, repeated at 5- to 15-minute intervals, is also effective for pain relief and can be given with anxiolytics (O'Connor et al., 2010). Supplemental oxygen (2 to 6 L/min nasal cannula) should be given if oxygen saturation is less than 94% or arterial oxygen saturations are low.

Thrombolytics: Reperfusion in patients who present to hospitals with percutaneous coronary angioplasty and intervention (PCI) capability has become the standard of care (Morse, Todd, & Stouffer, 2009). In hospitals without PCI capability and where patients cannot be transferred to a hospital with PCI capability within 90 minutes, treatment with fibrinolytic (thrombolytic) therapy initiated within 30 minutes of presentation should be performed unless contraindicated (Lambert et al., 2010). The use of thrombolytics in STEMI patients has been shown to decrease mortality by up to 30% (Morse et al., 2009). Thrombolytic agents include tissue-type plasminogen (tPA) and streptokinase (SK). Indications for thrombolysis are based on the existence of chest pain and specific ECG changes. Studies show that this therapy is frequently omitted for elderly patients. Reasons for this include frequent delay in seeking medical care, atypical presentation of MI, and a higher prevalence of NSTEMIs. Fear of hemorrhage following use of thrombolytics must be weighed against the proven gains in survival for all age groups, especially for those presenting early with MI. A variety of studies suggest that SK may be as beneficial as tPA in treating the elderly MI patient. It is considerably less expensive (Morse et al., 2009).

Aspirin: Aspirin therapy in post-PCI STEMI patients without demonstrated aspirin resistance should be initiated at 162 to 325 mg daily and, depending of the type of stent implanted, continued for a minimum of 1 month to 1 year at the higher dosages, then continued indefinitely at the lower dosages. In patients at risk for increased bleeding after stent implantation, lower-dose aspirin is reasonable. Aspirin (non–enteric coated) should be given as soon as possible if there is no obvious contraindication.

Patients taking nonselective NSAIDs (excluding aspirin) and cyclooxygenase-2 inhibitors should have these agents discontinued at the time of presentation with STEMI and not readministered during the course of hospitalization due to increased risk of mortality, reinfarction, myocardial rupture, heart failure, shock, or hypertension (Kushner et al., 2009).

Thienopyridines: Concurrent use of dual antiplatelet therapy (aspirin and thienopyridines) in MI patients (STEMI or NSTEMI) following PCI with stent implantation is the gold standard for secondary prevention of subsequent cardiovascular events. Use of thienopyridines including clopidogrel or prasugrel is important to decrease the risk of death and stroke and to prevent reinfarction or in-stent thrombosis (Nathan, 2010; Spinler, 2010). Thienopyridines should be initiated as a loading dose early, either before or at the time or primary or nonprimary PCI, and continued for a minimum of 12 months after bare metal stent placement in patients who are not at high risk for bleeding (Kushner et al., 2009). In patients for whom nonemergent coronary artery bypass is planned, thienopyridine therapy should be discontinued for a minimum of 5 days for those patients receiving clopidogrel and 7 days for those patients receiving prasugrel (Kushner et al., 2009).

Parenteral anticoagulants are recommended in all patients with acute coronary syndrome or myocardial patients regardless of whether or not reperfusion therapy was received. Low-molecular-weight heparin (LMWH), unfractionated heparin, bivalrudin, enoxaparin, or fondaparinux is recommended in patients undergoing PCI (Kushner et al., 2009; Kyriakides et al., 2007). If coronary artery bypass grafting is planned, anticoagulants should be withheld for 5 to 7 days before the procedure due to risks of excessive bleeding.

For patients not receiving thrombolytics, low-dose subcutaneous heparin or LMWH is indicated for prophylaxis of deep venous thrombosis. Elderly patients with large anterior MIs and heart failure, as well as those with documented left ventricular thrombus, should receive full heparin anticoagulation.

Angiotensin-converting enzyme inhibitors: ACE inhibitors reduce mortality in post-MI patients. ACE inhibitors are recommended and should be continued indefinitely for every patient recovering from an STEMI and for those with MI with an LVEF less than 40% and no obvious contraindication(s) to their use. For patients with preserved LVEF with hypertension, chronic kidney diseases, or diabetes, ACE inhibitors are recommended unless contraindicated (Kushner et al., 2009; O'Connor et al., 2010).

Angiotensin receptor blockers: ARBs are recommended in those patients who are intolerant of ACE inhibitors, who have heart failure with LVEF of 40% or less, or those patients who have hypertension. A combination of ACE inhibitor and ARB can be used in patients with systolic dysfunction heart failure.

Aldosterone blockade is recommended for post-MI patients without severe renal dysfunction or hyperkalemia, with heart failure, with LVEF of 40% or less or with diabetes who are already on a therapeutic dose of ACE inhibitor and beta blockade (Aronow, 2008; Kushner et al., 2009).

Beta blockers, which have been shown to limit infarct size, decrease chest pain, improve prognosis, and reverse cardiovascular remodeling, are generally well tolerated in patients ages 65 to 75 (Crane, Oles, & Kennedy-Malone, 2006). Conditions that contraindicate the use of beta blockers in the elderly include bronchospastic lung disease, marked bradycardia, hypotension, depression, acute heart failure, and diabetes. Studies show that beta blockers are underused in the elderly; age alone should not determine their use. In acute MI, metoprolol or atenolol is given 2.5 to 5 mg IV every 5 minutes, for a total of 15 mg and 10 mg, respectively. Beta blockers should be initiated in the emergency department before PCI and within 24 hours in patients presenting with STEMI, MI, acute coronary syndrome, or left ventricular dysfunction with or without heart failure unless contraindicated. Contraindications to beta blocker therapy include heart failure, evidence for a low cardiac output state, or risk for cardiogenic shock (Kushner et al., 2009).

Statins and lipid-lowering therapy: A lipid profile that includes total cholesterol, LDL, HDL, and triglycerides should be performed and assessed on all acute coronary syndrome or MI patients within 24 hours of admission. Lipid-lowering therapy is recommended before discharge, with the LDL goal to be less than 100 mg/dL, preferably with further LDL reduction to less than 70 mg/dL (Kushner et al., 2009). Dietary therapy is recommended for all patients, including consumption of omega-3 fatty acids, weight management, and physical activity.

Calcium channel blockers have limited use in STEMI and NSTEMI patients. Hypotension-induced tachycardia has been associated with the use of short-acting calcium channel blockers. Long-acting calcium channel blockers should be used sparingly if needed, with additional precautions in those patients already taking digoxin or beta blockers (Kyriakides et al., 2007).

In terms of interventional management of elderly MI patients, guidelines by both the AHA and the ACC have established "door to needle" time of less than 30 minutes and "door to balloon" time within 90 minutes of initial presentation to the hospital for the best possible outcomes (Kushner et al., 2009). PTCA with PCI may be a valuable alternative in those for whom thrombolytics are contraindicated. CABG is preferred for patients with left main stenosis and those with moderately severe left ventricular depression. Emergency PTCA or CABG in elderly patients presenting with cardiogenic shock or heart failure is associated with high morbidity and mortality.

Glucose control: Hyperglycemia (defined as blood sugar greater than 180 mg/dL) in patients with STEMI have been associated with adverse outcomes, including increased morbidity and mortality, as well as prolonged hospitalizations (Kushner et al., 2009). Maintaining glucose control may decrease the inflammatory response and improve LVEF (Wiener, Wiener, & Larson, 2008).

Follow-up: Risk stratification for future cardiac events following stabilization from MI is necessary. Tests to evaluate for ischemia or myocardium at risk include low-level exercise test, nuclear perfusion scanning, and dobutamine echocardiography. Left ventricular function can be determined by echocardiography or radionuclide ventriculogram. Routine coronary angiography is not recommended for all MI patients but should be performed on patients with demonstrable ischemia. Patients at high risk for sudden death from arrhythmias should undergo EP evaluation.

Sequelae: Increasing age is associated with more complications after MI, including heart failure, arrhythmias, pulmonary edema, cardiogenic shock, cardiac rupture, and death.

Prevention/prophylaxis: Secondary prevention in the elderly MI patient includes use of aspirin, beta blockers, and ACE inhibitors unless there are absolute contraindications to these agents. Lipid-lowering therapy is also beneficial. Reduction of risk factors is necessary. Cardiac rehabilitation can be as beneficial in older MI patients as in younger ones. Emotional support remains important.

Referral: Suspicion of acute MI should prompt transfer of the patient to an environment equipped with cardiac monitoring and the ability to administer advanced cardiac life support. As hospitalization continues, consultation with a variety of disciplines, such as surgery, social work, and physical therapy, may be necessary.

Education: Individualized teaching following MI for each patient and family should be provided, using age-specific teaching methods. Teach the basic definitions of CAD, angina, and MI. Patients need information on the healing process following MI, when to return to work or resume normal daily activities, and when to resume sexual relations. Give an exercise prescription. Involve patients and families in a discussion of the psychological adjustment following MI. Encourage risk factor reduction. Health-care practitioners should work with patients to set goals and design plans. Give patients information on community resources, such as the AHA or support groups in their area. Smoking cessation should be strongly encouraged and pharmacological and nonpharmacological therapies discussed. Medication teaching and review are very important. Health-care providers should be aware of all medications prescribed for the patient and of any OTC medications, including vitamins, minerals, and supplements. Patients should bring in all of their medications at each visit. Teach patients about the desired effects and common side effects of their medications. Emphasize the importance of taking aspirin and anticoagulants as directed to prevent in-stent thrombosis. Review what to do if medication cannot be taken or obtained. Discuss the use of nitrates for any chest pain while avoiding the usage of nitrates in patients taking medications such as sildenafil, tadalifil, or vardenafil, due to sudden drops in BP, resulting in hypotension.

Teach elderly patients about altered pain perception that can occur with age and with diseases such as diabetes. Teach patients and their families about warning signs such as chest pain or pressure, shortness of breath, indigestion, choking, sweating, dizziness, palpitations, severe weakness, and loss of consciousness. Establish a clear plan for obtaining prompt medical attention.

CLINICAL RECOMMENDATION	EVIDENCE RATING	REFERENCE
The presence of elevated cardiac enzymes associated with clinical or ECG evidence of ischemia is diagnostic for myocardial infarction.	A	Thygesen, Alpert, & White (2007)
Treat all patients with oxygen, pain control medications, and antiplatelet therapy including aspirin and heparin (or enoxaparin).	A	O'Rourke & Hashimoto (2007)
Nitroglycerin may be given to relieve ischemic chest pain, except in patients with hypotension and right ventricular infarction.	A	O'Rourke & Hashimoto (2007)
Give thrombolysis within 30 minutes when percutaneous cardiac intervention (PCI) is not available or when >90 minutes of delay is expected in door to balloon time.	A	Thygesen et al. (2007)
Treat most patients with aspirin or clopidogrel, beta blockers, and statins (LDL target of 70–100 mg/dL) if no contraindications are noted.	A	O'Rourke & Hashimoto (2007)

A = consistent, good-quality, patient-oriented evidence; B = inconsistent or limited-quality, patient-oriented evidence; C = consensus, disease-oriented evidence, usual practice, expert opinion, or case series. For information about the SORT evidence rating system, go to www.aafp.org/afpsort.xml.

PNEUMONIA

Signal symptoms: Fever, chills, or hypothermia, new cough with or without sputum, chest discomfort or dyspnea, fatigue, headache; some older adults will not be symptomatic but may experience falls or confusion (Donowitz & Cox, 2007).

Description: Community-acquired pneumonia (CAP), an acute lower respiratory tract infection of the lung parenchyma, can be bacterial or viral. Bacterial pneumonia is the most common type in older adults (Marrie & Tuomanen, 2012).

CAP refers to pneumonia that begins outside of the hospital or is diagnosed within 48 hours of admission; the patient must not have resided in a long-term care facility for 14 days before symptom onset. Pneumonia also is classified as nosocomial or health-care acquired (acquired from a hospital or nursing home) (File, 2012).

Ventilator-associated pneumonia (VAP) is the most frequent ICU-acquired infection in mechanically ventilated patients (Chastre & Luyt, 2011). Placement of an endotracheal tube allows bacterial entry into the lower respiratory tract and increases the risk of VAP by 6-fold to 20-fold. Bacterial clearance by host defenses is hindered (Craven, Hudcova, & Lei, 2011).

Etiology: The most common cause of CAP is *S. pneumoniae*. Other common pathogens include *Staphylococcus aureus*, *H. influenzae*, and other gram-negative and anaerobic bacteria. In patients with COPD, *S. pneumoniae*, *H. influenzae*, *M. catarrhalis*, and *Legionella* predominate. Aspiration pneumonia is caused most often by anaerobes and *S. pneumoniae*. Nosocomial infections in older patients are caused by a variety of organisms, including *Enterobacteriaceae*, *Klebsiella pneumoniae*, *S. pneumoniae*, *S. aureus*, *H. influenzae*, *Pseudomonas aeruginosa*, *Escherichia coli*, anaerobes, *Legionella*, and *Chlamydia*. It is often the norm to have a mixture of organisms. Methicillin-resistant *S. aureus* (MRSA) is found in both VAP and CAP

(Donowitz, 2010). In addition to the above organisms, *Proteus, Acinetobacter* species, and *Stenotrophomonas maltophilia* are found in VAP (Craven et al., 2011).

Occurrence: CAP is not a reportable disease, so occurrence in the ambulatory population is difficult to ascertain. Incidence is 1 in 100 persons in the community; in the nursing home setting it is 8 in 1000 persons/year. In the United States, CAP is the leading cause of mortality from an infectious disease and the eighth leading cause of death. The rate of hospitalization for pneumonia is 15% to 20%. The mortality rate from CAP is less than 5% in the outpatient setting. In hospitalized patients the mortality rate is 10%, rising to 30% in ICU patients (Nair & Niederman, 2011). Incidence of VAP is 4%; crude mortality rate is 20% to 50%.

Age: Pneumonia is the most common cause of death from infectious disease in older patients. Elderly persons are at 5 to 10 times the risk of younger adults for dying of pneumonia.

Ethnicity: Not significant.

Gender: More men than women are diagnosed with pneumonia.

Contributing factors: Comorbidities, influenza, chronic pulmonary conditions, smoking, alcoholism, malnutrition, colonization of the oropharynx by gram-negative bacteria, institutional setting, decline in immune function, hospitalization, use of sedating medications, recent surgery or trauma, and diminished cough reflex may contribute to development of pneumonia (Chastre & Luyt, 2011; Donowitz, 2010). Swallowing problems from esophageal or neurological conditions or the presence of a feeding tube can lead to aspiration pneumonia (File, 2012). Risk factors for pneumonia-related death include age of more than 65 years, comorbid disease (e.g., diabetes, renal insufficiency, COPD, CHF), active malignancy, leukopenia, fever higher than 101°F, immunosuppressed state, pneumonia caused by *S. aureus* or gram-negative rods, aspiration, and airway obstruction (File, 2012; Nair & Niederman, 2011). Signs and symptoms associated with pneumonia-related mortality include dyspnea, chills, altered mental status, tachypnea, hypotension, hypothermia, and hyperthermia. Laboratory abnormalities associated with increased mortality are hyponatremia, hyperglycemia, abnormal liver function studies, hypoalbuminemia, azotemia, hypoxemia, and azotemia. Risk factors for drug-resistant *S. pneumoniae* (DRSP) include age of more than 65 years, alcoholism, antimicrobial therapy within the past 3 months,

exposure to children in daycare, multiple comorbidities, or immunocompromise (Nair & Niederman, 2011). Risk factors for VAP include the insertion of an endotrachial tube and device-related issues, immunocompromise, adult respiratory distress, COPD, patient positioning, medications, and personnel related (breach in technique) (Augustyn, 2007).

Signs and symptoms: Typical symptoms include fever, chills, cough, and rusty or thick sputum, with associated gastrointestinal upset or anorexia, malaise, and diaphoresis; pleuritic chest pain may also be present (Ferri, 2012). These characteristic symptoms are frequently absent, particularly in the frail elderly, leading to a lag time before diagnosis. In the older patient, mental status changes (i.e., confusion), new onset or increased frequency of falls, increased respiratory rate, hypotension, anorexia, a marked functional decline, and new onset of urinary incontinence are typical symptoms (Nair & Niederman, 2011). Caregivers or family members may report that the patient is not his or her usual self. Physical examination of the chest reveals crackles that do not clear with cough or deep breathing. Increased respiratory rate (more than 24 breaths/min) is typical. If the patient is not able to deep breathe adequately, crackles may be absent. Dullness to percussion, egophony, and bronchial breath sounds may be present. A fever of 100°F, with tachycardia, may be present. Signs of dehydration may occur. The patient may appear anxious, restless, or withdrawn. Concurrent symptoms of CHF may appear. Overall sensitivity of clinical diagnosis is 70% to 90%; specificity is between 40% and 70% (Nair & Niederman, 2011).

In VAP, signs and symptoms include a fever higher than 100.4°F; leukopenia less than 4000/mm^3 or a leukocyte count of more than 12,000/mm^3 *and* worsening oxygen requirements, or change in suctioning needs/onset of purulent secretions or Critical Pulmonary Infection Score (CPIS); calculator available at www.surgicalcriticalcare.net/Resources/CPIS.php (Craven et al., 2011).

Diagnostic tests: Chest x-ray is the gold standard for diagnosis, although radiological findings may lag behind clinical findings. Dehydration can make interpretation more difficult. The typical pattern for pneumococcal pneumonia is lobar consolidation; aspiration pneumonia most commonly involves the right upper lobe and viral pneumonias show diffuse infiltrates (Bartlett, 2012a, 2012b; Bruns et al., 2007; Ferri, 2012; Nair & Niederman, 2011).

Other diagnostic tests usually are reserved for candidates for hospital admission, following the Infectious

Disease Society of America/American Thoracic Society (IDSA/ATS) (Mandell et al., 2007), and relate to ICU admission. Sputum for Gram stain is recommended for all patients but is difficult to obtain in practice, particularly in an outpatient setting. For hospitalized patients, CBC and differential and CMP are standard. In ICU admissions, if *Legionella* is suspected, a urinary antigen assay test for *Legionella* serogroup 1 should be done; likewise, a urinary antigen test for pneumococcal disease is indicated (Sordé et al., 2011). Liver function testing, sputum for Gram stain, and culture and two pretreatment blood cultures should be obtained in ICU admissions. Selected patients may require tuberculosis, HIV, and other tests. In patients with comorbidities affecting oxygenation, pulse oximetry or ABGs are indicated to evaluate oxygen saturation and need for oxygen therapy.

Diagnostic testing for VAP includes chest x-ray or CT scan, endotrachial aspirate for Gram stain, and bacterial culture or bronchiolar lavage or protected specimen brush to obtain secretions (Chastre & Luyt, 2011; Craven et al., 2011). Diagnosis of VAP is divided into two stages. Early stage VAP, occurring within 48 hours of intubation, is usually not drug resistant; later stage VAP after 3 to 5 days of intubation is more complex and associated with DRSP or other difficult to treat organisms (Augustyn, 2007; Craven et al., 2011).

Differential diagnosis:
- Influenza or parainfluenza
- Adenoviruses
- Fungal agents
- Toxoplasma
- Tuberculosis
- Pulmonary embolism with infarction
- Vasculitis of the pulmonary bed
- Pneumothorax

Differential diagnosis for VAP includes ventilator-associated respiratory infection (VARI) and ventilator-associated tracheobronchitis (VAT) (Craven et al., 2011).

Treatment: A crucial element in treatment is determining the severity and deciding on the choice of setting (Yealey, 2011). For community-dwelling older patients, the presence of a responsible caregiver and a supportive home environment is necessary. Temporary measures to increase support and monitor status of response may be introduced by ordering home health services. If the patient fails to recover or deteriorates despite these interventions, hospitalization should be

contemplated. Infectious Diseases Society of America guidelines advocate the use of the PORT (Pneumonia Patient Outcome Research Team) Pneumonia Severity Index (PSI) prediction rule as a guideline for determining outpatient treatment versus hospitalization (this can be accessed at http://pda.ahrq.gov/clinic/psi/psicalc.asp).

Another tool with more clinical utility at point of care is the CURB-65 or CRB-65 Criteria, which eliminates the BUN measurement (Table 8-3).

Use of any prediction rule should be tempered by clinical judgment. Objective criteria for hospital admission include the following:

- Inability to take oral medications or fluids
- Acute mental status changes
- Severe acute metabolic, hematological, or electrolyte abnormalities
- Acute concomitant medical condition (e.g., malignancy, hepatic disease, renal insufficiency, cardiac disease)
- Hypoxemia on room air (PaO_2 <60 mm Hg)
- Multilobar involvement on chest x-ray
- Secondary suppurative infection (e.g., meningitis, endocarditis, empyema)
- Severe vital sign abnormality (SBP <90 mm Hg, pulse >125/min, respirations >30/min)

TABLE 8-3	CURB-65 Criteria for Evaluation of Pneumonia Severity and Treatment Site
CLINICAL FACTOR	**SCORING**
	0–1: Low risk; consider outpatient treatment
	2: Brief inpatient hospitalization or closely monitored outpatient treatment
	≥3: Hospitalize; severe pneumonia, consider ICU
Confusion (new disorientation)	1
BUN >19 ng/dL	1
Respiratory rate ≥30 breaths/min	1
BP: Systolic <90 mm Hg	1
OR	
Diastolic <60 mm Hg	1

Adapted from Dunphy, Winland-Brown, Porter, & Thomas. (2012). *Primary care: The art and science of advanced practice nursing* (3rd ed.). F.A. Davis.

The latest consensus guidelines from the IDSA/ATS for CAP include the following recommendations (Mandell et al., 2007):

- Outpatient treatment for previously healthy adults with no risk factors for DRSP should consist of a macrolide or doxycycline.
- For those with comorbidities, including diabetes mellitus, malignancies, alcoholism, chronic lung disease, cardiovascular disease, chronic liver or renal disease, immunosuppressive conditions or immunosuppressive drugs, or risk for DRSP such as antimicrobial use in the past 3 months, the following drug classes are advised: respiratory fluoroquinolone, beta-lactam, and a macrolide concurrently.
- For those in an area with more than 25% macrolide-resistant *S. pneumoniae*, consider alternatives such as respiratory fluoroquinolone; ceftriaxone, cefpodoxime, and cefuroxime (500 mg twice daily); doxycycline (level II evidence) is an alternative to the macrolide.
- For inpatient treatment outside the ICU, a respiratory fluoroquinolone or a beta-lactam and macrolide concurrently; cefotaxime, ceftriaxone, and ampicillin are preferred; ertapenem for selected patients; doxycycline (level III evidence) is an alternative to the macrolide.
- For severe CAP requiring ICU admission, treat with a beta-lactam antibiotic, plus azithromycin or a respiratory fluoroquinolone.
- Patients with risk factors for *Pseudomonas* should be treated with a beta-lactam antibiotic (piperacillin/tazobactam, imipenem/cilastatin, meropenem, doripenem, or cefepime), plus an aminoglycoside and azithromycin or an antipseudomonal fluoroquinolone (levofloxacin or ciprofloxacin).
- For risk factors for MRSA, treat with vancomycin or linezolid (Watkins & Lemonovich, 2011).
- Treatment should be instituted as soon as possible. Transition from IV to oral therapy should occur as soon as the patient is hemodynamically stable and shows clinical improvement, can ingest oral medications, and has no gastrointestinal tract problems. Duration of therapy is 5 to 7 days, provided the patient is afebrile for 48 to 72 hours.
- In addition to antimicrobial treatment measures, supportive and restorative measures are necessary for optimal recovery. Oxygen therapy is based on determinations of ABGs or pulse oximetry during the acute phase. Nutritional supplementation also may be indicated. Physical therapy measures for strengthening and ambulation may be initiated during the acute recovery period and continued during convalescence or replaced by restorative nursing measures.

Treatment for VAP is guided by ATS guidelines (Niederman, Craven, Bonten, & American Thoracic Society and Infectious Diseases Society of America, 2005). Once the potential for VAP is identified and specimens have been obtained, rapid empirical treatment with broad-spectrum antimicrobials is instituted. Knowledge of local resistance patterns, extent of MRSA, and other regional factors is essential. When the organism is identified from blood cultures or respiratory tract aspirates, therapy is changed to monotherapy with an antibiotic that is sensitive to the infection. Treatment is limited to short duration (most show good response within 7 to 8 days) to avoid colonization with antibiotic-resistant bacteria (Chastre & Luyt, 2011).

Follow-up: Follow-up depends on comorbidities and response to prescribed treatment regimen. Independent community-dwelling older adults or caregivers should be instructed to call if symptoms worsen, if no response occurs after 3 to 5 days of treatment, or if symptoms recur. A follow-up office visit after completion of treatment, to assess response and further interventions, is recommended. Patient teaching regarding self-care and increasing functional status can be given at this time, with further visits depending on individual status. Follow-up chest x-ray is usually not indicated; it is advised in smokers to rule out any other respiratory problems such as malignancy. The chest x-ray should be delayed for at least 6 weeks because radiological resolution of the pneumonia takes 6 to 12 weeks (Tang, Eurich, Minhas-Sandhu, Marrie, & Majumdar, 2011). Frail elderly persons in a long-term care facility need more frequent and prolonged monitoring after an acute episode of pneumonia.

Sequelae: The older patient with comorbidities is especially prone to complications, including severe deconditioning and decline in level of ADLs. If nutrition is poor, coexisting lung disease is present, or both, the patient may never return to baseline. Adult respiratory distress syndrome or multiple organ dysfunction syndrome also may occur, resulting in significant morbidity and mortality. Superinfections, recurrence, or opportunistic infections may occur in susceptible patients.

Prevention/prophylaxis: Older patients should have an annual influenza vaccine unless highly allergic. All health-care workers should have an annual influenza vaccine. The pneumococcal vaccine is administered once in patients 65 years and older. Patients who are hospitalized for pneumonia may be immunized before discharge. Antibiotics should be prescribed prudently. Teach patients with comorbidities to avoid contact with persons having known respiratory infections.

Prevention of VAP is facilitated by maintaining endotracheal tube cuff pressure above 20 cm H_2O (to avoid leakage of bacteria around the cuff into the lower respiratory tract), positioning patients semirecumbent, meticulous oral care with chlorhexidine, and promptly reintubating those who are failing extubation (Chastre & Luyt, 2011).

Referral: Refer patients with comorbidities to infectious disease, internal medicine, or pulmonary specialists for inpatient management and initial follow-up. Manage patients in long-term care facilities collaboratively until a return to baseline is achieved. Refer patients to a dietitian for nutritional guidance and to physical therapy for reconditioning, strengthening, and increasing level of ADLs. Refer patients to home care services (nursing, physical therapy, home health aide) as needed for in-home support.

Education: Provider education regarding appropriate prescribing of antibiotics is helpful in decreasing drug-resistant organisms. Teach groups of older adults (especially adults with comorbidities) about preventive measures. Educate patient and caregivers in management, including the importance of nutrition and hydration and deep breathing exercises. Smoking cessation education is critical in current smokers.

CLINICAL RECOMMENDATION	EVIDENCE RATING	REFERENCE
Consider pneumonia in patients with cough, dyspnea, or sputum production, especially if accompanied by fever, altered breath sounds, or rales.	C	Bartlett et al. (2000)
Perform a chest x-ray to confirm the diagnosis of pneumonia.	C	Detterline (2010)
Routine diagnostic tests are optional for outpatients, because most do well with empirical antibiotic treatment.	C	Fine et al. (1997)
Sputum gram stain and culture as well as legionella and pneumococcal antigen testing are recommended for inpatients, particularly those with severe pneumonia, in whom identification of an organism is more likely to prompt a change in the antibiotic agent.	C	Mandell et al. (2007)
The Pneumonia Severity Index and CURB-65 are validated prognostic models that may be used to help determine site of treatment in patients with CAP.	A	Mandell et al. (2007)
Administer antibiotic therapy as soon as possible after the diagnosis is made and before leaving the emergency department if the person is being admitted.	C	Mandell et al. (2007)
Treat previously healthy outpatients with a macrolide (azithromycin, clarithromycin, or erythromycin) or optionally doxycycline.	B	Mandell et al. (2007)
Treat inpatients with a respiratory fluoroquinolone (moxifloxacin, gemifloxacin, or levofloxacin).	A	Mandell et al. (2007)

CLINICAL RECOMMENDATION	EVIDENCE RATING	REFERENCE
VAP Evidence		
In the absence of medical contraindications, elevate the head of the bed at an angle of 30–45 degrees for a patient at high risk for aspiration (e.g., a person receiving mechanically assisted ventilation and/or who has an enteral tube in place).	A	Institute for Clinical Systems Improvement (ICSI) (2011)
Cuff pressure should be maintained at 20–25 cm H_2O. Minimal leak technique is discouraged.	B	American Thoracic Society (ATS) Documents (2004) ICSI (2011)
Effective infection control measures: staff education, compliance with alcohol-based hand disinfection, and isolation to reduce cross-infection with multidrug-resistant pathogens should be used routinely.	A	ATS Documents (2004)
Intensive insulin therapy is recommended to maintain serum glucose levels between 80 and 110 mg/dL in ICU patients to reduce nosocomial bloodstream infections, duration of mechanical ventilation, ICU stay, morbidity, and mortality.	A	ATS Documents (2004)

A = consistent, good-quality, patient-oriented evidence; B = inconsistent or limited-quality, patient-oriented evidence; C = consensus, disease-oriented evidence, usual practice, expert opinion, or case series. For information about the SORT evidence rating system, go to www.aafp.org/afpsort.xml.

PULMONARY EMBOLISM

Signal symptoms: dyspnea, acute onset, chest pain on inspiration, anxiety. Presentation is variable and symptoms are nonspecific; some pulmonary emboli are asymptomatic (Le Gal, Testuz, Righini, Bounameaux, & Perrier, 2005; Stein, Matta, Musani, & Diaczok, 2010).

Description: Pulmonary embolism is the occlusion of one or more pulmonary vessels by a traveling thrombus originating from a distant site. Although a blood clot is the most common embolism, fat, air, bone marrow, tumor cells, and foreign material also can occlude the pulmonary vasculature (Thompson & Hales, 2012). Pulmonary embolism is one component of venous thromboembolism (VTE), which also encompasses deep vein thrombosis (DVT).

Etiology: Pulmonary embolism usually is caused by a dislodged thrombus from one of the veins of the legs or pelvis (DVT); thrombi distal to the popliteal area are less likely to migrate and cause pulmonary embolism.

Occurrence: Between 600,000 and 700,000 cases are diagnosed each year, with up to 300,000 deaths annually; many pulmonary embolisms are diagnosed at autopsy (Stein, 2007). From 8% to 10% of pulmonary embolism victims die within the first hour (Ferri, 2012).

Age: The incidence of pulmonary embolism increases steadily with age (Ouellette, 2012).

Ethnicity: Pulmonary embolism is significantly more frequent in African Americans than Caucasians; Asians/Pacific Islanders and Native Americans have the lowest incidence (Schneider, Lilienfeld, & Im, 2006).

Gender: Men are affected more frequently than women (Ouellette, 2012; Schaffer & McKean, 2010).

Contributing factors: Risk factors for pulmonary embolism are indicated by Virchow's triad of stasis or prolonged immobility, hypercoagulation, and venous trauma (endothelial injury with inflammation of the vessel lining). Stasis may be occupational or medical (e.g., CHF, postsurgical paralysis, chronic illness or debilitation, tumor compression). Venous trauma damaging the deep veins of the legs; orthopedic procedures from arthroscopy to hip, knees, or pelvic repair; or trauma from falls, burns, or crush injuries may contribute to thrombus formation and lead to pulmonary embolism. Prolonged air travel is another risk factor. Hypercoagulation is associated with connective tissue diseases, malignant tumors, and stroke. Presence of a central venous catheter and insertion of a pacemaker are also risk factors. Autoimmune diseases including systemic lupus erythematosus, AIDS, rheumatoid arthritis, or inflammatory bowel disease are predisposing factors. Other risk factors include use of estrogen, advanced age, obesity, and malignancy. A past history of DVT or pulmonary embolism is associated with recurrence. Thrombophilias including factor V Leiden mutation, protein C or protein S deficiency, polycythemia vera, acquired protein C resistance without factor V Leiden, or antithrombin III deficiency also pose risks (Hunt & Bull, 2011; Jankowich & Ferri, 2012; Schaffer & McKean, 2010). Intravenous drug abuse, varicose veins, and heparin-associated thrombocytopenia (HIT) are additional risk factors.

Signs and symptoms: Signs and symptoms of pulmonary embolism tend to be nonspecific, so the diagnosis is frequently missed. In the Prospective Investigation of Pulmonary Embolism Diagnosis (PIOPED II) study, older patients presented with the same symptoms as younger ones (Stein et al., 2007). The problem may occur when these symptoms are attributed to aging or existing comorbidities. Dyspnea (acute onset), anxiety or apprehension, pleuritic chest pain, cough, tachypnea, and accentuation of the pulmonic component of S_2 are frequently present and may be accompanied by diaphoresis, syncope, tachycardia, S_3 or S_4 gallop, hypoxemia, or hemoptysis (Hunt & Bull, 2011). Physical examination usually reveals tachypnea. Auscultation of the lungs may be normal or may show localized wheezing, consolidation, or friction rub. Jugular venous distention and atrial arrhythmia may be present. Examination of the legs, especially of the iliofemoral and popliteal areas, may reveal signs of DVT; the arms, abdomen, and pelvic areas also should be examined for pain, erythema, or palpable vein cords. In the case of a massive pulmonary embolism, hypotension, circulatory instability, and cyanosis may be present.

Diagnostic tests: Clinical judgment in conjunction with clinical prediction scoring tools and diagnostic studies is recommended. The Wells Clinical Prediction Scoring Tool for Pulmonary Embolism (www.mdcalc.com/wells-criteria-for-pulmonary-embolism-pe) considers clinical symptoms, tachycardia, recent immobility or surgery, hemoptysis, malignancy, and prior DVT/pulmonary embolism. The Revised Geneva Score (Le Gal et al., 2006) uses similar criteria for scoring. Both instruments have been validated and are considered reliable in all age categories (Righini, Le Gal, Perrier, & Bounameaux, 2005). The Simplified Pulmonary Embolism Severity Index (PESI) (www.mdcalc.com/simplified-pesi-pulmonary-embolism-severity-index) is a prediction rule for 30-day mortality from symptomatic pulmonary embolism; this tool is used more selectively as appropriate.

The chest x-ray is used primarily to rule out other causes of symptoms such as pneumonia or CHF. ECG is also not valuable in diagnosing pulmonary embolism; signs of right ventricular strain, new-onset right bundle branch block, S1Q3T3 complex, tachycardia, or atrial fibrillation may be seen in acute pulmonary embolism (Hunt & Bull, 2011; Tapson, 2008). In a patient deemed to be at low or intermediate risk of pulmonary embolism, a negative enzyme-linked immunosorbent assay (ELISA) D-dimer test can rule out the possibility of pulmonary embolism; the D-dimer sensitivity is 95% regardless of age. The specificity of D-dimer tests decreases with increased age; inflammation, malignancies, and cardiopulmonary disease further limit the utility of the test. In hemodynamically stable older adults over 70 years with suspicion of pulmonary embolism, the D-dimer can be used in conjunction with venous compression ultrasonography for a reasonable noninvasive diagnosis of pulmonary embolism. D-dimer is not advised in hemodynamically unstable or hospitalized patients (Guyatt, Akl, & Crowther, 2010; Righini et al., 2005). Multidetector CT pulmonary angiography (CTPA) has largely replaced the pulmonary angiogram for diagnosis of pulmonary embolism. The CTPA is indicated in patients at high risk of pulmonary embolism for diagnosis (Bettman et al., 2012). In patients with a positive D-dimer but low clinical suspicion of pulmonary embolism, the multidetector CTPA is also the test of choice. The CTPA is equal to pulmonary angiography but not invasive and so has a lower rate of complications; interpretation of results is not affected by age. Limitations for using a CTPA include patients with renal dysfunction; in this case a ventilation/perfusion (V/Q) scan may be done. If there is a high suspicion of pulmonary embolism but a negative CTPA, a V/Q scan may be ordered also. To date, magnetic resonance angiography has not proven valuable in detecting pulmonary embolism. In patients with a massive pulmonary embolism, transesophageal echocardiography (TEE) should be done to assess right ventricular function. BNP or NT-proBNP have no role in diagnosis of pulmonary embolism, but they have been shown to forecast right ventricular dysfunction and mortality along with elevated troponin levels, so these should also be drawn in the case of a massive pulmonary embolism (Guyatt et al., 2010; Thompson & Hales, 2012).

Differential diagnosis:

- Pneumonia
- Myocardial infarction
- Pericarditis
- CHF
- Pleural effusion
- Panic attacks
- Hyperventilation syndrome
- Pneumothorax
- Esophageal rupture
- Gastritis
- Gastric or duodenal ulcer
- GERD
- Asthma
- Musculoskeletal pain
- Mediastinitis

Treatment: Anticoagulation is the cornerstone of treatment. Anticoagulation reduces the incidence of fatal pulmonary embolism by approximately 60% to 70% and should be initiated immediately in patients with high or moderate suspicion of pulmonary embolism who have no contraindications due to excessive bleeding or in those with low suspicion where a workup will not be completed within the first 24 hours (Guyatt, Akl, Crowther, Gutterman, & Schünemann, 2012; Tapson, 2012; Valentine & Hull, 2012).

In patients with a massive pulmonary embolism, IV therapy including dextran should be administered. Treatment should be individualized, and use of vasopressors may be required if hypotension does not respond to IV therapy, oxygenation, and other acute interventions. If anticoagulation is contraindicated, a vena cava filter may be placed. Options such as thrombolysis or embolectomy may also be considered in hemodynamically unstable patients (Guyatt et al., 2010).

In patients at low risk for bleeding, LMWH, subcutaneous fondaparinux, IV unfractionated heparin (UH), or subcutaneous UH can be used. LMWH or fondaparinux is preferred (Valentine & Hull, 2012). In patients with a creatinine clearance less than 30 mL/min, UH is the choice because of ease in monitoring via activated partial thromboplastin time (aPPT) testing. Use IV UH in patients with sustained hypotension from massive pulmonary embolism, those in whom thrombolysis is being contemplated, morbidly obese patients (questionable subcutaneous absorption), or those at high risk of bleeding (Valentine & Hull, 2012). Oral anticoagulation with warfarin (Coumadin) is initiated simultaneously with or shortly after heparin. Heparin therapy is continued for approximately 5 days after beginning the warfarin to ensure adequate anticoagulation. International normalized ratio (INR) is maintained in the therapeutic range of 2.0 to 3.0. Warfarin is used for long-term maintenance of 6 months or more, with measurements of the INR 3 times during the initial week of therapy, tapering to twice weekly for 2 weeks, then once weekly or every other week. Dosage is adjusted based on these results. Patients with genetic hypercoagulability or recurrent thrombus may be maintained on anticoagulants for life. Experts differ on optimal length of therapy and dosing adjustments in specific situations (Guyatt et al., 2012; Holbrook et al., 2012; Valentine & Hull, 2012). Absolute contraindications to anticoagulation include active internal bleeding, hemorrhagic stroke, or gastrointestinal bleeding (Guyatt, Akl, & Crowther, 2010). Risk of hemorrhage in the older patient is increased even when comorbid conditions are controlled for; older women are at a higher risk of hemorrhage than men.

Hemodynamically stable low-risk adults with a community-based support system can be managed successfully on home therapy (Guyatt, Akl, & Crowther, 2010).

Follow-up: Follow-up visits are on an individualized basis. Anticoagulation usually is continued for a minimum of 3 to 6 months after pulmonary embolism. Further therapy is based on risk factors for pulmonary embolism, potential for recurrence, and risks associated with anticoagulation. Close monitoring for control of anticoagulation is essential (Guyatt et al., 2012; Holbrook et al., 2012; Schaffer & McKean, 2010).

Sequelae: Unrecognized pulmonary embolism can be fatal; many are diagnosed at autopsy. Other complications include alveolar collapse, atelectasis, and pulmonary infarction. The condition tends to recur. Complications from anticoagulation include uncontrolled bleeding and hematoma.

Prevention/prophylaxis: Patients should avoid controllable risk factors for pulmonary embolism. Encourage frequent ambulation, use of antiembolic stockings or graded compression hose, safety precautions to avoid injury to lower extremities, evaluation of possible hypercoagulation pathology, and prophylactic anticoagulation after orthopedic and other surgery; intermittent pneumatic compression also is recommended, unless contraindicated. Prolonged sitting should be avoided. Consideration of prophylactic anticoagulation in any immobilized hospitalized patient, particularly ICU patients, is currently an area of controversy, with experts not agreeing (Guyatt et al., 2012). Detailed recommendations for prophylaxis in specific circumstances is available from Holbrook et al. (2012).

Referral: Refer patients to internal medicine or emergency medicine for emergent evaluation and initial treatment plan. When stable, patients can be managed on warfarin with INR testing in their usual place of residence (Spurzem & Geraci, 2010).

Education: Provider education about awareness of pulmonary embolism in differential for chest pain or dyspnea is needed. Teach the patient, family, or caregiver about risk factors and preventive measures, disease pathology, monitoring for signs of recurrence, and need for compliance with anticoagulation therapy. Instruct the patient to use a soft toothbrush and an electric razor and to report bleeding gums, hemoptysis, and any blood in stool or urine. Advise patients to avoid aspirin, to consult with their health-care provider before taking any OTC medications, and to take precautions to avoid bumping or bruising.

CLINICAL RECOMMENDATION	EVIDENCE RATING	REFERENCE
Prevention of VTE should be considered according to the patient's baseline risk.	A	Gurza (2011)
Diagnosis begins with estimating probability based on a validated clinical decision rule, then using a validated diagnostic algorithm integrating findings from D-dimer, ventilation/perfusion (V/Q) scan, lower extremity ultrasound, and spiral (helical) CT scanning with IV contrast (i.e., CT pulmonary angiography [CT-PA]).	A	Goldhaber & Bounameaux (2012) Gurza (2011) Qaseem et al. (2007)
In patients with acute pulmonary embolism, we recommend early initiation of vitamin K antagonist (VKA) (e.g., same day as parenteral therapy is started) over delayed initiation, and continuation of parenteral anticoagulation for a minimum of 5 days and until the INR is 2.0 or above for at least 24 hours.	B	Kearon et al. (2012)
In patients with acute pulmonary embolism, we recommend initial treatment with parenteral anticoagulation (LMWH, fondaparinux, IV UFH, or subcutaneous UFH) over no such initial treatment.	A	Kearon et al. (2012)

A = consistent, good-quality, patient-oriented evidence; B = inconsistent or limited-quality, patient-oriented evidence; C = consensus, disease-oriented evidence, usual practice, expert opinion, or case series. For information about the SORT evidence rating system, go to www.aafp.org/afpsort.xml.

PULMONARY TUBERCULOSIS

Signal symptoms: Initially asymptomatic, later productive, prolonged cough; fatigue; low-grade fever; night sweats; poor appetite; hemoptysis; weight loss. Fever and sweats are less common in older patients (Basgoz, 2010). Symptoms in older adults are often attributed to other comorbidities (Pratt, Winston, Kammerer, & Armstrong, 2011).

Description: Pulmonary tuberculosis is a chronic necrotizing infection caused by a slow-growing acid-fast bacillus (AFB), *Mycobacterium tuberculosis*. Tuberculosis is the most common cause of death related to infectious disease worldwide (World Health Organization [WHO], 2011). The primary site for most cases of tuberculosis is the lungs; extrapulmonary tuberculosis, which can affect any organ or tissue, is more common among individuals infected with HIV.

Etiology: The infection spreads by inhalation of airborne particles or droplets produced by persons with active pulmonary or laryngeal tuberculosis during coughing, sneezing, singing, and other expiratory efforts. The development of infection after exposure depends on the exposed person's ability to mount an effective immune response on the cellular level. In the initial 2 to 4 weeks before cellular immunity response occurs, direct pulmonary infection may develop, or lymphohematogenous circulation may lead to miliary, meningeal, or tuberculosis adenitis. When T cells recognize the specific antigen, they become sensitized, engaging the macrophages in destroying or containing the tubercle bacilli. This leads to healing, with no residual or calcified lymph nodes in the pulmonary or tracheobronchial areas (Herchline, 2012). This latent stage is typical of 90% to 95% of infected persons, leaving them at lifelong risk for reactivation. Tuberculin skin testing documents exposure at 2 to 10 weeks after exposure. The majority of tuberculosis cases in older adults are latent, also known as reactivation or recrudescent tuberculosis.

Occurrence: Tuberculosis occurs worldwide. According to the WHO, in 2010 there were between 8.5 and 9.2 million cases of tuberculosis worldwide, with an estimated 1.1 million deaths from tuberculosis in those without HIV co-infection. Deaths in HIV patients with tuberculosis accounted for an additional 0.35 million (WHO, 2011). In the United States, 10,521 new cases of tuberculosis were reported in 2011, the lowest rate of new cases since 1953 when tuberculosis became a reportable disease (CDC, 2012). Both worldwide and U.S. trends show a progressive decline in new infection, and the number of drug-resistant tuberculosis cases has remained stable (CDC, 2012; WHO, 2011).

Age: Children and adolescents are more likely to have primary disease; adults and elderly are more likely to have recrudescent disease (Pai & Menzies, 2012). Older adults have a higher burden of disease than younger adults; in 2008, the incidence rate for older adults was 6.4 per 100,000 compared to 5.0 per 100,000 for younger adults (Pratt et al., 2011).

Ethnicity: Persons born in geographical areas where tuberculosis is more prevalent, including Asia, Africa, and Latin America, are at higher risk. Non-Hispanic Asians currently have the highest rate of infection. In U.S.-born minorities, non-Hispanic blacks have the highest rate of infection (CDC, 2012).

Gender: Tuberculosis occurs in men more frequently than in women (WHO, 2011).

Contributing factors: Contributing factors include the following:

- HIV infection
- Substance abuse (especially IV drug use)
- Recent infection with *M. tuberculosis* (less than 2 years ago)
- Chest x-ray findings suspicious of previous tuberculosis with no treatment or ineffective treatment
- Diabetes mellitus
- Silicosis
- Cancer of the head and neck
- Hematological and reticuloendothelial diseases
- End-stage renal disease
- Intestinal bypass or gastrectomy
- Chronic malabsorption syndromes
- Low body weight (less than 10% ideal body weight)

Chronic corticosteroid therapy, transplant immunotherapy drugs, and tumor necrosis factor alpha–antagonist drugs can hasten the conversion of latent tuberculosis infection (LTBI) to active tuberculosis (Pratt et al., 2011).

Other factors associated with increased risk include homelessness, residence in a congregate setting (nursing home, boarding home, prison, mental health facility), low socioeconomic status, and health-care work in a high-risk area. The incidence of tuberculosis in nursing home residents is 2 to 4 times greater than that of noninstitutionalized older adults (Pratt et al., 2011).

Signs and symptoms: Typical presentation includes cough, hemoptysis, weight loss, anorexia, adenopathy, fever, night sweats, decreased activity level, and pleuritic pain. In the average population, the onset is gradual and may go undetected for some time. In the older patient, these findings are not usually present, or they are so subtle and intermingled with other chronic illness symptoms as to be undistinguishable. Weight loss, dyspnea, or anorexia may be the only symptoms (Basgoz, 2010). Typical simulations include pneumonia, bronchitis, or CHF with pleural effusion. Extrapulmonary tuberculosis may manifest with symptoms typical to the site involved (e.g., urinary incontinence or frequency and urgency for bladder tuberculosis).

Physical examination may be unrevealing; nonspecific signs such as fever or weight loss may be the only findings. In some persons, a positive tuberculin test reaction is the only manifestation. Many older adults will not have a positive tuberculin skin test due to a lower immune response (Pratt et al., 2011). Chest examination may show post-tussive apical rales. If pleural effusion is present, percussion in the area may be dull.

Diagnostic and screening tests: Current recommendations call for targeted testing of at-risk individuals. The standard Mantoux tuberculin skin test (TST) is an intradermal test to screen for exposure to tuberculosis or to detect an active case of tuberculosis, using 5 units of intermediate purified protein derivative (PPD). The test is technique specific; if administered too deeply, without producing the required bleb, it is invalid and must be repeated at another site. Interpretation of the result is also subject to error; the area of induration or hardness, not erythema, must be measured with a millimeter ruler 48 to 72 hours after the agent is administered. The results show the ability of the person tested to mount a delayed-type hypersensitivity response to prior infection. Appropriate measurement parameters for reactive and nonreactive results are as follows:

TEST	RESULTS INDICATING EXPOSURE	SELECTED POPULATION
PPD tuberculin skin test	5 mm	HIV-positive persons; recent contacts of tuberculosis case
		Persons with fibrotic changes on chest x-ray consistent with old healed tuberculosis
		Patients with organ transplants and other immunosuppressed patients
	10 mm	Recent arrivals from high-prevalence countries
		Injection drug users
		Residents and employees of high-risk congregate settings
		Mycobacteriology laboratory workers
		Persons with clinical conditions that place them at high risk
		Children <4 years old
		Children/adolescents exposed to high-risk adults
	15 mm	Persons with no known risk factors for tuberculosis

When reporting or recording results, specify reactive or nonreactive and the millimeter measurement for induration.

Many patients have an impaired delayed-type hypersensitivity response to the tuberculin testing; a negative reaction does not exclude disease. This absence of a response is known as anergy and is found in immunosuppressed individuals, including HIV-positive persons, persons on immunosuppressive drugs or corticosteroid therapy, persons with sarcoidosis, persons with Hodgkin's disease, and persons with recent vaccination with bacille Calmette-Guérin (BCG). Anergy testing is no longer recommended as part of a routine tuberculosis screening program for HIV-positive individuals. Two-step testing is recommended initially for adults who will be retested periodically, such as health-care workers and long-term congregate living residents. The TST is administered; if negative, a second TST is given 1 to 3 weeks later. If the second TST is positive, it probably represents a boosted response to a prior infection, so it is treated as infection and should be addressed accordingly. If the second TST is negative, the person is considered uninfected, and any subsequent positive TST indicates a new infection (www.cdc.gov/tb/publications/ LTBI/diagnosis.htm). See Mazurek et al. (2010) for extensive information on when to screen with TST versus interferon-gamma release assays (IGRAs), or both.

TEST	RESULTS INDICATING DISORDER
In vitro blood test; interferon-gamma release assay (IGRA) test using antigens specific to *Mycobacterium tuberculosis;* screens for latent as well as active tuberculosis. There are several tests available. The test is not affected by prior immunization with BCG vaccine and does not require an additional visit for reading results.	Positive result indicates probable infection; negative result indicates infection is unlikely. Indeterminate result is suggestive of immune system problem and frequently is accompanied by a negative TST.
Chest x-ray, posterior anterior view. *Note:* Abnormalities are suggestive of but not diagnostic for tuberculosis; this test may be used to rule out pulmonary tuberculosis in a person with a positive tuberculin test and no symptoms of disease. In select cases, other views, such as apical lordotic, may be indicated.	*Active disease:* Abnormalities seen in apical or posterior segments of upper lobe or superior segments of lower lobe. In HIV-positive or immunosuppressed persons, lesions may appear anywhere in lungs and may differ in size, shape, density, and cavitation. *Latent or old healed lesions:* Dense pulmonary nodules in hilar or upper lobes, with or without cavitation. Have "hard," sharply demarcated margins. Smaller, nodular or fibrotic lesions in upper lobes and a positive tuberculin test indicate latent infection and should be treated accordingly. Calcified granulomas usually do not progress to active tuberculosis.
CT scanning: If chest x-ray results are questionable, CT may give clarity.	Dense, homogeneous parenchymal consolidation in primary tuberculosis; patchy, nodular, masslike, or linear consolidation may also occur. In reactivation of LTBI, a tuberculoma may be seen; linear opacities or poorly defined nodules may be present. Patchy or focal heterogeneous consolidation in the posterior and apical segments of the upper lobes as well as superior segments in the lower lobes is typical (Jeong & Lee, 2008).
Technetium scanning.	Technectium CT for a solitary pulmonary nodule has good predictability for distinguishing tuberculosis from malignancy (Herchline, 2012).
Sputum for AFB.	Detection of AFB in stained smears is suggestive but not diagnostic; may be other mycobacteria. Negative smear does not rule out tuberculosis.
Sputum culture should be done on all specimens regardless of AFB result.	Positive culture for *M. tuberculosis* is diagnostic. Drug sensitivity testing should be done on all initial cultures.

Differential diagnosis: Pneumonia, lymphoma, fungal infections, CHF, pleural effusion, and lung cancer can mimic tuberculosis.

Treatment: Before treatment, obtain baseline values for liver function, bilirubin, CBC, BUN, creatinine, and serum uric acid; an HIV test should be administered also if status is unknown. if ethambutol (EMB) is used, baseline visual acuity should be measured. The goal of treatment is safety and efficacy in the shortest time period. For newly diagnosed, active tuberculosis, initial treatment consists of combined therapy using four first-line drugs: isoniazid (INH), rifampin (RIF), pyrazinamide (PZA), and EMB, until culture results are complete.

Follow-up cultures should be done, usually monthly until negative, to determine response to treatment. If culture is not negative after 3 months, suspect drug resistance or noncompliance and reevaluate. After culture is negative, obtain one further culture at treatment completion; for drug-resistant tuberculosis, different culture guidelines apply. Several treatment options are available. The most commonly used is presented here (for further information, consult with the CDC).

The basis for treatment is availability of two drugs to which the bacterium is susceptible. Prolonged treatment is needed. Compliance is key to successful control of disease.

Basic Tuberculosis Disease Treatment Regimens

PREFERRED REGIMEN	ALTERNATIVE REGIMEN	ALTERNATIVE REGIMEN
Initial Phase:	Initial Phase:	Initial Phase:
Daily INH, RIF, PZA, and EMB* for 56 doses (8 weeks)	Daily INH, RIF, PZA, and EMB* for 14 doses (2 weeks), then twice weekly for 12 doses (6 weeks)	Thrice-weekly INH, RIF, PZA, and EMB* for 24 doses (8 weeks)
Continuation Phase:	Continuation Phase:	Continuation Phase:
Daily INH and RIF for 126 doses (18 weeks)	Twice-weekly INH and RIF for 36 doses (18 weeks)	Thrice-weekly INH and RIF for 54 doses (18 weeks)
or		
Twice-weekly INH and RIF for 36 doses (18 weeks)		

*EMB can be discontinued if drug susceptibility studies demonstrate susceptibility to first-line drugs.
Note: HIV-positive individuals require specific modifications in therapy, and CDC guidelines should be consulted. Multidrug-resistant tuberculosis also requires different regimens; see CDC guidelines.
Source: www.cdc.gov/tb/topic/treatment/tbdisease.htm

Follow-up: Follow-up should be done by experienced tuberculosis expert health-care personnel. Follow-up chest x-ray examination may be done at therapy termination to evaluate response. Periodic liver enzymes are necessary, especially if the patient is taking INH, to monitor for effects on hepatotoxicity. For the frail elderly adult in a long-term care facility, more frequent monitoring for adverse effects of treatment, including anorexia, polyneuropathy, or development of medication-induced hepatitis, is warranted. Directly observed therapy (DOT) is the norm in these settings, so adherence is less of a concern. Refer community-dwelling elderly to the local or state health department for follow-up, monitoring of medication compliance and side effects, patient and family education, and testing of close contacts. Tuberculosis is a reportable disease. Refer HIV-positive patients or those with drug-resistant tuberculosis to an infectious disease expert. Refer to pulmonary specialist for bronchoscopy if indicated; refer to public health department charged with tuberculosis surveillance and control. Many agencies charged with monitoring and control have outreach services, such as home visits. Emphasize to patients that adherence is crucial to successful control. If no follow-up visitation is available through the monitoring agency, see the patient for monthly follow-up visits in the office.

Sequelae: Possible complications include development of drug-resistant organisms, particularly if a patient is nonadherent with the prescribed treatment. Secondary infection of cavitary lesions and development of treatment-associated hepatitis or polyneuropathy are possible. If treatment is ineffective, spread of disease to other close contacts can occur.

Prevention/prophylaxis: For older patients residing in long-term care facilities, TST testing before admission to the facility is required unless there is documented evidence of a positive test result in the past. Two-step testing (described earlier) is recommended initially. Annual retesting is recommended. Patients with a positive TST reaction need a chest x-ray to evaluate for active or latent disease. Staff members are required to have tuberculin skin testing at initial employment and annually.

When targeted testing reveals a positive tuberculin skin reaction but no evidence of active tuberculosis, it is referred to as *latent tuberculosis infection*. The person has been exposed to and infected with *M. tuberculosis* but does not have active disease and cannot infect others.

The decision to institute chemoprophylaxis is a clinical judgment, based on a comparison of individual factors with the risk of developing tuberculosis (see under Contributing Factors) versus the risk of INH toxicity. Chemoprophylaxis is with INH, 300 mg orally daily for 9 months by self-administration or INH twice weekly for 9 months by DOT. Older adults in congregate settings such as nursing homes and other health care facilities are considered priority for this treatment (CDC, 2012). For HIV-positive persons or close contacts of patients with drug-resistant tuberculosis, see CDC recommendations. Alternative regimens are available for healthy adults, including a 3-month regimen of rifapentine and INH (Sterling et al., 2011).

Referral: Patients may be referred to a government-associated community agency such as the health department or to an infectious disease or pulmonary specialist for initial evaluation and management recommendations. Refer patients with concurrent positive HIV status, confirmed AIDS, or drug-resistant tuberculosis to specialized treatment services or collaborate in management with specialists in this area (Kliiman & Altraja, 2009). Refer patients with severe anorexia or malnutrition to a dietitian.

Education: Teach patient, caregivers, close contacts, and paraprofessional providers about the nature of the disease, its mode of transmission, screening and control measures, and follow-up required. Teach the patient or caregiver about medications, drug actions and possible side effects, length of treatment, and need for adherence.

CLINICAL RECOMMENDATION	EVIDENCE RATING	REFERENCE
Screen only high-risk patients for tuberculosis.	C	Potter & Acevedo (2011)
If a screen for tuberculosis is positive, patient needs a chest x-ray, and if pulmonary tuberculosis is suspected, three induced sputums.	B	Potter & Acevedo (2011)
Active tuberculosis should be treated with a 2-month initiation phase with four drugs and a 4- to 7-month continuation phase.	A	Potter & Acevedo (2011)
Repeat sputum cultures at the end of the 2-month initiation phase. If the culture is positive, consider prolonging or changing treatment.	B	Potter & Acevedo (2011)
Screening for tuberculosis may be performed with the tuberculin skin test (TST).	C	Potter & Acevedo (2011)
The QuantiFeron-TB Gold test (QFT-G) can be used in place of TST, especially in patients who do not have known exposure to tuberculosis and have had the bacille Calmette-Guérin (BCG) vaccination.	C	Potter & Acevedo (2011)

A = consistent, good-quality, patient-oriented evidence; B = inconsistent or limited-quality, patient-oriented evidence; C = consensus, disease-oriented evidence, usual practice, expert opinion, or case series. For information about the SORT evidence rating system, go to www.aafp.org/afpsort.xml.

RESTRICTIVE LUNG DISEASE

Signal symptoms: Rapid, shallow respirations; dyspnea; decreased activity tolerance; easy fatigability; nonproductive, irritating cough provoked by deep breathing or exertion.

Description: Restrictive lung disease refers to a heterogeneous group of disorders that share a common abnormal ventilatory function. Restricted breathing is characterized by small tidal volume and rapid rate. The hallmark restrictive pattern is a decrease in lung volumes, principally total lung capacity and vital capacity (Kanaparthi, 2012).

Etiology: Restrictive lung diseases, which have a variety of etiologies, are divided into subgroups based on the location of the pathology:

Restrictive/parenchymal/interstitial/intrinsic: In addition to a decrease in total lung capacity and vital capacity, residual volume is decreased. Forced expiratory flow rates are maintained.

▪ Sarcoidosis
▪ Idiopathic pulmonary fibrosis
▪ Pneumoconiosis

■ Occupational lung disease
■ Drug/radiation-induced interstitial lung disease

Restrictive/extraparenchymal/extrinsic: Abnormalities can be predominantly in inspiration or in inspiration and expiration.

Neuromuscular:
■ Diaphragmatic weakness/paralysis
■ Myasthenia gravis (limitations may be inspiratory and expiratory)
■ Muscular dystrophies (limitations may be inspiratory and expiratory)
■ Cervical spine injuries (limitations may be inspiratory and expiratory)
■ Guillain-Barré syndrome (limitations may be inspiratory and expiratory)

Chest wall:
■ Kyphoscoliosis
■ Obesity
■ Ankylosing spondylitis (limitations may be inspiratory and expiratory)

Occurrence: The incidence of restrictive lung disease is undeterminable because several distinct entities are involved. Statistics are available for select causes of restrictive lung disease. Studies reference an overall prevalence of 3 to 6 cases per 100,000 persons for intrinsic lung diseases. Prevalence of idiopathic pulmonary fibrosis (IPF) is 27 to 29 cases per 100,000 persons; in adults over age 75 years, the prevalence increases to over 175 cases per 100,000 persons (Kanaparthi, 2012). Occupational lung diseases are common in farmers and in people who work with silica, asbestos, beryllium, organic solvents, or cotton. The prevalence of sarcoidosis in the United States is 10 to 40 cases per 100,000 persons.

Age: Occupationally induced disease and IPF are seen predominantly in the older population; other restrictive lung diseases may occur at any age.

Ethnicity: African Americans in the United States have a prevalence of sarcoidosis that is 10 to 17 times greater than whites.

Gender: The incidence is higher in men than women for occupational types of restrictive lung disease.

Contributing factors: Risk factors vary with etiology, including exposure to occupational dust, abnormalities in skeletal structure, genetics, and autoimmune disorders (King, 2012).

Signs and symptoms: Patients have a gradual onset of dyspnea, initially occurring only with exertion and progressing to dyspnea at rest. The breathing pattern is rapid and shallow. A nonproductive cough may be present (Behr, 2012). A careful, detailed history is essential, including prior systemic diseases, occupational or environmental exposures, family history, social history, and history of drug use (Alhamed & Cosgrove, 2011). Amiodarone, nitrofurantoin, hydralazine, gold, chemotherapeutic agents, and procainamide can cause drug-induced disease (Kanaparthi, 2012). Prior radiation can result in fibrosis. Use of tobacco also should be ascertained; it is common for patients to have a mixed pattern of obstructive and restrictive disease. Physical findings may reveal skeletal abnormalities, such as kyphoscoliosis, limiting lung expansion. The initial presentation of breathing problems often occurs after an acute respiratory viral infection.

Physical assessment of the lung initially may be unremarkable. In intrinsic disease, with progression of the disease, inspiratory crackles ("Velcro") typically are heard at the bases. Cyanosis and clubbing of fingers and toes may occur in IPF. In the end-stages, signs of right-sided heart failure, including cor pulmonale, appear (Behr, 2012; Kanaparthi, 2012; King, 2012).

Diagnostic tests: Because of the diverse nature of the conditions leading to restrictive lung disease, it is challenging to address diagnostic testing and results. Many results are specific to the causative condition. Routine testing including CBC, chemistry profile, and liver function tests is standard.

TEST	RESULTS INDICATING DISORDER
PFT	Normal FEV_1/FVC ratio but decreased FVC and FEV_1; decreased total lung capacity, residual volume, and functional residual capacity. Residual volume–to–total lung capacity ratio is normal to low. Most have a gas exchange problem with marked decrease in single breath diffusing lung capacity for carbon monoxide. Diagnosis of restriction and extent of restriction is based on total lung capacity (Kanaparthi, 2012).

Chest x-ray	Increased interstitial markings, especially in lower fields. Hilar and mediastinal lymphadenopathy in sarcoidosis, some lymphomas, and silicosis. Pleural effusion and thickening with collagen-vascular disease, lymphoma, and asbestosis. A scattered reticulonodular pattern and ground glass opacities are common (Behr, 2012).
High-resolution CT	In idiopathic pulmonary fibrosis, patchy, peripheral bibasilar reticular abnormalities in the subpleural area; with advanced disease, subpleural fibrosis and honeycomb pattern are present.

In the late stages, ABGs help to identify the degree of hypoxemia and carbon dioxide retention. In select cases, bronchoscopy and biopsy may be indicated (Gulati, 2011).

Differential diagnosis:

- Infectious or neoplastic diseases
- COPD
- CHF
- Wegener granulomatosis
- Goodpasture syndrome
- Bechet disease
- Sjögren syndrome
- Systemic sclerosis
- Pneumoconiosis
- Tuberous sclerosis
- Eosinophilic pneumonia

Treatment: Therapy depends on the cause of disease; specific diagnosis obtained from clinical evaluation, imaging, and lung biopsy; and the disease progression. Occupational exposures should be avoided. Therapy with corticosteroids, cytotoxic agents, and immunosuppressive agents has been the primary treatment for most interstitial diseases. Duration of treatment is still unknown, and objective data to support use of cytotoxics and immunosuppressants is lacking or low quality (Kanaparthi, 2012). Cytotoxic agents, including azathioprine (Imuran) and cyclophosphamide (Cytoxan), are given concurrently with prednisone or in place of it if the patient cannot tolerate high-dose prednisone therapy (Kanaparthi, 2012).

The ATS and other global organizations have recently issued an official statement on the evidence-based treatment of IPF (Raghu et al., 2011), citing the weakness of the evidence for current treatments including corticosteroids, cytotoxics, immunosuppressants, and other miscellaneous drugs and encouraging individual patient and specialist discussion before implementing any drug therapy. The ATS statement recommends against treatment of IPF with corticosteroids alone or in combination with cytotoxics or immunosuppressants (Raghu et al., 2011). Research indicates that IPF is related more to fibroblastic proliferation than inflammation (Cerri, Spagnolo, Luppi, & Richeldi, 2012). Lung transplantation is the only treatment to prolong survival in IPF (King, Pardo, & Selman, 2011); post-transplant the patient will be on immunosuppression for life (Whelan, 2012). Studies using stem cells are ongoing; prior studies with tumor necrosis factor inhibitors and other atypical drugs have proven unsuccessful (King et al., 2011).

In the end-stage of restrictive lung diseases, administer supplemental oxygen for supportive care; consider palliative care and hospice.

Follow-up: Follow-up visits are scheduled as indicated by symptoms and comorbidities. Periodic chest x-rays or pulmonary function tests (PFTs) may help to chart diseases course and to evaluate response to treatment.

Sequelae: Use of corticosteroids or immunosuppressives may result in increased risk of infection. Pulmonary hypertension and right-sided heart failure may occur. Restrictive lung diseases are chronic and there is no known cure.

Prevention/prophylaxis: Give patients pneumococcal pneumonia and influenza vaccine. Advise patients to avoid known exposures, tobacco use, and persons with acute, infectious upper respiratory illness.

Referrals: Initially refer patients to a pulmonary specialist for bronchoscopy and possible biopsy; thereafter, collaborative management is appropriate. If immunosuppressives are used, refer the patient for initial recommendations and periodic reevaluation.

Education: Teach the patient and family about chronic disease management, regular self-care habits, and early intervention in acute illness. Discuss prognosis and preferred choices for end-stage disease.

CLINICAL RECOMMENDATION	EVIDENCE RATING	REFERENCE
Interstitial lung disease diagnosis can be made with a chest x-ray, pulmonary function tests (PFTs) consistent with restrictive lung disease, and typical findings on high-resolution CT. Lung biopsy is necessary in atypical cases.	C	ATS (2002)
No treatment has been shown to have consistent benefit.	C	Reust (2011)
Corticosteroids, supplementary oxygen, and pulmonary rehabilitation may provide symptomatic relief.	C	Reust (2011)
Standard treatment regimens have included corticosteroids plus azathioprine or cyclophosphamide. However, a recent Cochrane review concluded that there is little good-quality information on the efficacy of noncorticosteroid agents for IPF.	C	Davies, Richeldi, Walters, & Davies (2007)
At present, there is no evidence for an effect of corticosteroid treatment in patients with IPF. On the other hand, other fibrotic lung diseases, such as nonspecific interstitial pneumonia (NSIP), are reported to show a better response to corticosteroids. Making a clear distinction between IPF and other entities grouped under the umbrella term *interstitial lung disease* is, therefore, essential, because this may have therapeutic and prognostic implications.	C	Richeldi, Spagnolo, Davies, et al. (2010)

A = consistent, good-quality, patient-oriented evidence; B = inconsistent or limited-quality, patient-oriented evidence; C = consensus, disease-oriented evidence, usual practice, expert opinion, or case series. For information about the SORT evidence rating system, go to www.aafp.org/afpsort.xml.

UPPER RESPIRATORY TRACT INFECTION

Signal symptoms: Nasal congestion, rhinorrhea/mucopurulent discharge, sore throat, cough, headache, malaise.

Description: Upper respiratory tract infection (URI), most frequently the common cold, usually is caused by a virus and results in inflammation of the nasal passages. Most URIs are self-limiting and accompanied only by minor somatic complaints. In addition to the common cold, acute laryngitis, acute rhinosinusitis, and acute pharyngitis are included as URIs (Meneghetti, 2012).

Etiology: URIs usually are caused by a virus such as rhinovirus; influenza A, B, and C viruses; parainfluenza viruses; respiratory syncytial viruses; coronaviruses; adenoviruses; and enteric cytopathogenic human orphan (ECHO) viruses (Lee & Treanor, 2010). New viruses, including the metapneumovirus and bocaviruses, have been recently identified (Sexton & McClain, 2011). The rhinovirus is the most common agent implicated in URI. The usual mode of transmission is hand-to-hand from contaminated nasal secretions. The incubation period is 1 to 3 days, with the usual URI lasting 6 to 10 days.

Occurrence: URIs are the most common cause of short-term disability in the United States; there are more than 62 million cases of the common cold annually. Acute URIs are the most frequent reason for seeking a health-care provider in the United States.

Age: URIs occur much more frequently in children than in adults.

Ethnicity: Noncontributory.

Gender: URIs occur equally in men and women.

Contributing factors: Risk factors for developing URIs include exposure to infected individuals and contact between nose or conjunctiva and contaminated fingers. Older persons with diabetes get more frequent URIs than the general population.

Signs and symptoms: The most common signs and symptoms include nasal obstruction and stuffiness, sneezing, and scratchy throat. Other signs and symptoms include cough, hoarseness, malaise, headache, and fever higher than 100°F (less than 1%). Physical examination may reveal mucopurulent nasal drainage, nasopharyngeal mucosal swelling, and lymphadenopathy.

Diagnostic tests: No diagnostic tests are indicated for the nonspecific URIs. Diagnosis is clinical based on symptoms. If symptoms persist for more than 10 days, a CBC may be ordered to rule out other causes. A throat culture or rapid strep test is used if streptococcal pharyngitis is suspected.

Differential diagnosis:

- Influenza
- Chronic rhinitis
- Sinusitis
- Epstein-Barr virus
- Mumps
- Pneumonia
- VCD
- Psittacosis

The use of medications such as nasal sprays (when use is continuous), antihypertensives, hormones, psychotropic drugs, aspirin, and NSAIDs can cause symptoms similar to those of URIs.

Treatment: URIs usually are managed on an outpatient basis. Patients with significant COPD or cardiac disease should be evaluated on an individual basis. URIs are treated with rest, increased fluid intake, and symptom relief measures such as humidified air (not recommended for asthma patients). OTC medications may be taken for pain, fever, congestion, or cough relief. A recent Cochrane review found some benefit to various OTC combination agents, including analgesics, antihistamines, and decongestants, in terms of limiting duration and symptoms when compared to no treatment (DeSutter, van Driel, Kumar, Lesslar, & Skrt, 2012). Antihistamine-decongestant combinations were most efficacious although more side effects occurred in those who used combination therapy. Controversy still remains about the use of antihistamines

for viral illness unless an allergic component has been identified (Lee & Treanor, 2010).

Topical nasal and oral decongestants are available, with topical decongestants preferred owing to fewer systemic side effects. The nasal decongestant of choice is oxymetazoline; use of nasal decongestants for more than 3 days may result in rebound vasocongestion and is not recommended. Nasal and oral decongestants are associated with elevated BP and should be used cautiously in older adults. A Cochrane review on the use of nasal saline irrigation for acute URIs found limited benefit for symptom alleviation (Kassel, King, & Spurling, 2010). Likewise, a Cochrane review of Echinacea products for prevention or treatment (limiting duration of symptoms) of URIs was confounded by the variability of Echinacea products on the market; there was some evidence that *Echinacea purpurea* administration limited duration of symptoms (Linde, Barrett, Wölkart, Bauer, & Melchart, 2006). *Antibiotics are not indicated* for viral URIs (Chow et al., 2012; Institute for Clinical Systems Improvement [ICSI], 2011; Khandelwal, Lathren, & Sloane, 2012; Spellberg et al., 2011). Guidelines are in agreement that consideration of bacterial illness should be deferred until the patient has had symptoms for 1 week or more that are worsening despite self-care measures. If a reevaluation at that time determines that a bacterial infection is likely, treatment with amoxicillin or amoxicillin clavulanate is instituted. Results of a large study in an ambulatory health network demonstrated a high volume of inappropriate antibiotic prescribing in URIs (Gill et al., 2006).

If streptococcal pharyngitis is indicated by a positive rapid strep test or a positive culture, initiate treatment with penicillin.

Follow-up: See the patient if symptoms last more than 6 to 10 days or if the patient develops fever associated with systemic symptoms, difficulty breathing, or purulent nasal drainage.

Sequelae: Possible complications include lower respiratory tract infection, sinusitis, and aggravation of asthma symptoms; in older individuals with comorbidities, URI may contribute to exacerbation of other symptoms (e.g., COPD, hyperglycemia, CHF) or may lead to pneumonia.

Prevention/prophylaxis: Advise the patient to perform frequent proper hand washing, avoid touching the face, and avoid contact with infected people. Pneumococcal and influenza vaccinations are recommended for all older adults.

Referral: Usually neither referral nor consultation is necessary if the patient has an uncomplicated URI.

Education:

Provider education: Diagnosis of nonspecific URI or acute rhinopharyngitis denotes an infection that is typically viral and in which sinus, pharyngeal, and lower airway symptoms may be present but not prominent (University of Michigan Health System, 2011).

Antibiotic treatment of adults with nonspecific URI does not improve illness resolution and is not recommended. There are no studies specifically testing the impact of antibiotic treatment on complications of acute URIs in adults. Life-threatening complications of URIs are rare.

Purulent nasal or pharyngeal secretions (commonly seen in patients with uncomplicated URIs) do not predict bacterial infection and do not benefit from antibiotic treatment.

Patient education: Explain the disease process, signs and symptoms, and treatment (including side effects of medications). Discuss prevention strategies, including hand washing, and when to contact a health-care provider. Educate patients and families about the dangers of antibiotic resistance owing to inappropriate prescribing.

CLINICAL RECOMMENDATION	EVIDENCE RATING	REFERENCE
The diagnosis of upper respiratory tract infection is based on clinical signs and symptoms. This is an acute infection that is typically viral in origin and in which sinus, pharyngeal, and lower airway symptoms are present but not prominent.	B	Wong (2009)
Purulent nasal discharge or sputum does not predict bacterial infection or benefit from antibiotics.	A	Wong (2009)
Antibiotics are ineffective for the treatment of the common cold in children and adults.	B	Wong (2009)
Antihistamine and decongestant combinations may help alleviate nasal symptoms in older children and adults. Newer-generation nonsedating antihistamines are ineffective.	B	Wong (2009)

A = consistent, good-quality, patient-oriented evidence; B = inconsistent or limited-quality, patient-oriented evidence; C = consensus, disease-oriented evidence, usual practice, expert opinion, or case series. For information about the SORT evidence rating system, go to www.aafp.org/afpsort.xml.

VALVULAR HEART DISEASE

Signal symptoms: Asymptomatic in early stages. Fatigue and exertional dyspnea.

Description: Valvular heart disease (VHD) is damage to a valve or valves of the heart, causing cardiac dysfunction. The most prevalent types of VHD in elderly persons are calcific and degenerative aortic valve disease.

Aortic stenosis: An abnormal narrowing of the aortic valve orifice.

Aortic regurgitation: Retrograde blood flow through an incompetent aortic valve into the left ventricle during ventricular diastole.

Mitral stenosis: An abnormal narrowing of the mitral valve orifice.

Mitral regurgitation: Retrograde blood flow during systole from the left ventricle into the left atrium through an incompetent mitral valve.

Mitral valve prolapse: Mitral regurgitation associated with a bulging of one or both mitral valve leaflets into the left atrium during ventricular systole.

Etiology: The most common causes of VHD in the elderly include age-related degenerative calcifications, myxomatous degeneration, papillary muscle dysfunction, infective endocarditis, and rheumatic disease. With valvular regurgitation, a portion of the ejected blood leaks back into the upstream cardiac chamber. Valvular stenosis usually results in elevated pressures in the chamber upstream from the stenosis.

Occurrence: Moderate valvular heart disease is found in an estimated one in eight people age 75 years and older. Occurrence of VHD varies according to the type of disease; only limited information is available.

Age: Present in 2% to 9% of persons over age 65, aortic stenosis is the most clinically significant cardiac valve lesion (Faggiano, 2006). Isolated aortic regurgitation is rarely seen and is usually accompanied by some degree of mitral valve involvement. Mitral regurgitation is more common than mitral stenosis in elderly individuals. Mitral valve disease, commonly caused by rheumatic heart disease, is usually acquired by younger patients; however, the effects may not be seen until they are in their forties or fifties. Mitral valve stenosis has a progressively slow course with latent symptoms over 20 to 40 years followed by rapid acceleration in later life.

Ethnicity: Not significant.

Gender: Mitral annular calcifications (a frequent cause of mitral regurgitation) affects women 2 to 3 times more frequently than it does men. Mitral valve prolapse is more common in elderly men than in elderly women.

Contributing factors: Age-related fibrotic thickening of valvular tissue or dilation and calcification of the valve annulus can contribute to and cause hemodynamic abnormalities. Valvular stenosis of rheumatic origin can progress gradually throughout adult life. Other factors that may contribute to or cause valvular disease include metastatic carcinoid tumors; drugs, including methysergide and ergotamine (used to treat migraines) and appetite-suppressing drugs fenfluramine and phentermine; rheumatoid arthritis (can produce nodules in the leaflets); systemic lupus (can cause small vegetations, thickening, and regurgitation in the leaflets); myocardial infarction (can cause the leaflets to tether); antiphospholipid syndrome; and radiation therapy.

Signs and symptoms:

Aortic stenosis: Many of these patients are asymptomatic. Prognosis is poor for patients who exhibit symptoms. The survival rate decreases to 2 to 3 years for the patients who exhibits symptoms (Yeo & Low, 2007). Angina is an early and more common symptom. Presyncope followed by effort syncope occurs in about one-third of the patients with symptoms. Exertional dyspnea indicates left ventricular dysfunction and CHF.

Physical findings include a prolonged, rough aortic systolic ejection murmur (ASEM) that radiates to the right coronary artery and is heard best at the upper right sternal boarder second intercostal space (Soriano, Fernandez, Cassel, & Leipzig, 2007). This murmur, which peaks in intensity in mid to late systole, may be associated with a thrill. S_1 is often soft, and the aortic component of S_2 is soft or absent. An S_4 is common. The pulse pressure is narrow; there is a slow rise in the carotid pulse and sustained brachial or apical beat.

Aortic regurgitation: Patients with chronic aortic regurgitation may be asymptomatic for many years. When the left ventricle can no longer manage the increased stroke volume, patients may experience signs of CHF (exertional dyspnea, fatigue, paroxysmal nocturnal dyspnea, orthopnea) or angina. Once the patient presents with symptoms of tachycardia and dyspnea, which are signs of pulmonary venous congestion, the patient will decompensate quickly.

Physical findings with chronic aortic regurgitation include wide pulse pressures and possibly bounding pulses. Systolic and diastolic thrills may be present on the precordium. S_1 is normal or soft. S_2 maybe physiologically split, but A_2 may be soft or not heard owing to a high-frequency, early diastolic blowing murmur heard best a the left sternal border. An atrial gallop and S_3 are often present. An apical rumble mid or late diastolic murmur, the Austin Flint murmur, may be heard.

Mitral stenosis: The symptoms of mitral stenosis, dyspnea on exertion and lethargy resulting from elevated left atrial and pulmonary venous pressures, and decreased cardiac output generally are associated with valve areas of less than 2.5 to 1.5 cm^2 (normal: 4 cm^2) (Halter et al., 2009). Later symptoms include those of right ventricular overload, such as neck vein distention, ascites, and edema.

The clinical findings include a loud S_1 and an apical diastolic rumble and presystolic accentuation. An opening snap, which occurs 0.04 to 0.10 second after the S_2, may also be present. Severity of mitral stenosis can be determined by the distance of the S_2 to the opening snap (Carabello, 2005). The opening snap maybe soft or not heard at all because the valves are stiff or calcified. In the early stages the murmur may be difficult to appreciate.

Mitral regurgitation: Mitral valve regurgitation may result from the surrounding structures that comprise the mitral apparatus or the valve leaflets. Some of the common causes of mitral regurgitation are rheumatic heart disease, mitral valve prolapse, and ischemic heart disease (Maganti, Rigolin, Sarano, & Bonow, 2010). Patients with mitral regurgitation may not become symptomatic for decades. The main complaints are fatigue and a gradual decrease in exercise tolerance, which occurs only when the ventricle begins to fail.

The clinical features vary, depending on the pathological cause; however, a pansystolic murmur at the apex that radiates to the axilla is nearly a constant feature. If the disease is severe, the apex beat is usually brisk, hyperdynamic, and displaced laterally. An S_3 and diastolic murmur may be present with left ventricular dysfunction (Maganti et al., 2010).

Mitral valve prolapse: Chest pain and palpitations are the most prominent symptoms in elderly and young patients, although most patients are asymptomatic. Other symptoms that may represent an arrhythmic etiology are dizziness, syncope, and early fatigue.

The clinical findings include a midsystolic click and a late systolic or holosystolic murmur characteristic of mitral regurgitation. In some patients, the murmur, click, or both are not appreciated until the patient stands or performs the Valsalva maneuver. An apical S_3–S_4 gallop usually is present at the time of heart failure.

Diagnostic tests: In aortic stenosis, the ECG is abnormal in most cases, demonstrating QRS or T-wave changes reflecting left ventricular hypertrophy. Chest x-ray examination usually reveals aortic dilation; rounded apex, rounded left ventricular border, and dense calcification are generally seen on lateral film. Chest films may show cardiac enlargement when CHF is advanced. Echocardiography demonstrates thickening and calcification of the aortic valve with decreased mobility of the leaflets. Doppler measurement of intracardiac blood velocity can help determine hemodynamic severity. Cardiac catheterization measurement of the systolic pressure gradient across the aortic valve is the definitive method for assessing aortic stenosis in patients being considered for surgery or when there is a discrepancy between the clinical findings and the diagnostic tests.

In aortic regurgitation, if the process is acute, the ECG findings may be normal. If chronic, a left ventricular hypertrophy and strain are seen. Cardiomegaly found on the chest x-ray examination is demonstrated with left ventricular enlargement. Echocardiography shows left ventricular muscle thickness and early diastolic fluttering of the anterior mitral valve leaflet. Color Doppler imaging can further determine the presence of aortic regurgitation; however, its severity is best determined by the more invasive cardiac catheterization with angiography.

In mitral stenosis, P waves may suggest left atrial enlargement, and (in the elderly) the ECG more commonly reveals atrial fibrillation. Chest x-ray examination nearly always reveals left atrial enlargement. Echocardiography with Doppler flow studies is diagnostic of thickening of the mitral leaflet, reduced motion, and parallel movement of anterior and posterior leaflets in diastole; the flow study also assesses the severity of the stenosis. Cardiac catheterization is sometimes performed in those with an uncertain degree of stenosis after noninvasive studies and in those being considered for surgery.

In mitral regurgitation, the ECG shows left atrial enlargement or atrial fibrillation, and the chest x-ray examination shows left ventricular dilation; in nonrheumatic forms of mitral regurgitation these are less distinctive. Echocardiography delineates overall ventricular function and Doppler studies show the jet and severity of the regurgitation. Transesophageal echocardiography is a more precise way of visualizing the regurgitant jet.

In mitral valve prolapse, the ECG may show left ventricular enlargement and atrial hypertrophy, and atrial fibrillation is a frequent finding in the elderly. The chest x-ray examination will display pulmonary congestion with moderate cardiac enlargement.

Differential diagnosis: The diagnosis of VHD in elderly persons is sometimes overlooked because the early symptoms are vague and nonspecific. Murmurs in older adults are common and frequently determined to be functional or insignificant. The barrel chest of an older individual may obscure a murmur; in fact, with an increased anteroposterior diameter, a left ventricular hypertrophy may not be detected.

Murmurs have been associated with conditions other than valvular disease (i.e., hypertension, anemia, thyroid disease), so this differential must be considered.

Patients with established valvular heart disease need to have a specific determination of the etiologies of valvular involvement.

Treatment:

Aortic stenosis: No medical therapies are available to delay the progression of aortic stenosis. The patient with asymptomatic aortic stenosis will need to be frequently monitored for the development of symptoms and progression of disease (Bonow et al., 2008; European Task Force, 2007). Symptoms of aortic stenosis (angina, heart failure, syncope) are associated with substantial valvular obstruction and a risk of sudden death; therefore, surgical management is necessary. Aortic valve replacement is associated with a higher mortality rate (9% to 12%) in elderly persons than in younger individuals. Factors associated with greater operative risk include emergency surgery, left ventricular dysfunction, right-sided heart failure, female gender, significant coronary disease, cachexia, additional valve replacement, renal insufficiency, or concomitant CABG. The proper selection of the type of valve is important in elderly patients. The bioprosthetic valves have fewer structural failures and are advantageous in that their use obviates the need for anticoagulation (which is associated with substantial morbidity and mortality in the elderly). The disadvantage of this valve type is that the tissue degrades and so 30% to 40% of the patients will require reoperation in 10 years. Mechanical valves are more durable and have better hemodynamic profiles, but these require lifelong anticoagulation therapy.

Aortic balloon valvuloplasty should be considered as an alternative method of treatment; however, because it is associated with rapid restenosis and significant residual outflow obstruction, it is reserved as a palliative procedure for the symptomatic patient who is not a surgical candidate or as a bridge to surgery.

Secondary to advanced age, 30% of the patients with symptomatic, severe aortic stenosis are not able to undergo surgery to replace the aortic valve. There has been a rapid growth in the use of a new procedure called transcatheter aortic valve implantation. This procedure involves implanting a biprosthetic valve within the diseased aortic valve through a catheter. So far, the studies have shown that a rate of death for any cause at 1 year is about 25% (Leon et al., 2010).

Aortic regurgitation: Acute aortic regurgitation warrants surgery if the symptoms are moderate or severe. Chronic aortic regurgitation requires medical treatment of the early signs of heart failure with ACE inhibitors, calcium channel blockers, digitalis, diuretics, and vasodilators (reduces wall stress and afterload). Surgical treatment (aortic valve reconstruction or replacement) is indicated before the ejection fraction decreases below 55%.

Mitral stenosis: Therapies for the symptomatic patient with mitral stenosis include medical therapy, percutaneous balloon mitral valvuloplasty, commissurotomy, and mitral valve replacement. Patients with symptoms of mild heart failure are managed with diuretics and salt restriction to decrease left atrial pressures. Because atrial fibrillation occurs in most patients with moderate-to-severe stenosis, anticoagulation and rate control (with digitalis, beta blockers, or calcium channel blockers) often are indicated (Halter et al., 2009). Because of the high risk associated with anticoagulation in elderly patients, however, a less aggressive approach to therapy may be taken. When the patient has severe symptoms of mitral stenosis, valve replacement is indicated.

Mitral regurgitation: Medical management of mitral regurgitation includes use of ACE inhibitors, digitalis, diuretics, and vasodilators to reduce the symptoms of heart failure and reduce the regurgitant volume. Mitral valve surgery is considered in asymptomatic and symptomatic patients with progressive disease before signs of irreversible left ventricular dysfunction are present. The mortality rate associated with mitral valve replacement could be as high as 14% in the elderly patient.

Mitral valve repair is associated with a lower operative mortality than mitral valve replacement and is preferred in that preservation of the existing valve architecture allows synchrony of left ventricular contraction. When mitral annular calcification is the cause, medical therapy is prudent because the operative risk is substantially higher in patients with this disease process. Acute mitral regurgitation from papillary muscle rupture or chordal rupture requires patient stabilization followed by surgery, which still carries a high mortality rate.

Mitral valve prolapse: Medical management with beta blockers may stabilize patients; anticoagulation to prevent emboli is warranted. Mitral valve surgery is needed in patients who have developed symptoms, atrial fibrillation, severe pulmonary hypertension, worsening left ventricular function, and left ventricular enlargement.

Follow-up: For patients treated medically for valvular disease, close follow-up to monitor the effectiveness of treatment, adverse effects of medication, and progressiveness of the disease process is indicated. Medication therapy, particularly the use of anticoagulation therapy, requires meticulous attention. Surgically treated patients are monitored for valve function, fluid balance, and anticoagulation. Periodic echocardiographic, electrocardiographic, and chest x-ray monitoring is indicated.

Sequelae: Valve replacement risks include thrombus formation, infection, or rupture at the attachment points to the valve ring. Infective endocarditis, which may occur with artificial valves, has a high risk of mortality and requires reoperation. There is a high prevalence of gallstones in patients with prosthetic valves, thought to be due to low-grade intravascular hemolysis.

In patients who are not surgical candidates, the symptoms of heart failure are progressive and disabling. Even in surgical patients, the symptoms of heart failure may recur or persist.

Prevention/prophylaxis: In patients with prosthetic valves, the risk of thromboembolism decreases with an individualized antithrombolytic regimen. The specific therapy is determined based on the comorbid state and the patient's overall status.

Consider prophylactic antibiotic therapy (endocarditis prophylaxis) before any surgical or dental procedures in all patients with valvular disease, especially patients with valve replacement, rheumatic heart disease, aortic regurgitation, or mitral valve prolapse with significant mitral regurgitation murmurs.

Referral: All patients with symptoms of progressive valvular disease must be managed collaboratively with the physician. Many require further collaboration with a cardiologist. The *Practice Guidelines for Cardiothoracic Surgery Concerning Valvular Heart Disease* include the indications for surgery. In general, these include symptoms that cannot be controlled with medical therapy or indications of a threat to survival (i.e., angina, dyspnea, effort syncope or progressive impairment of ventricular contractility, and infective endocarditis).

Education: Elderly persons constitute 40% to 60% of all cases of endocarditis. Instruct all at-risk patients in the importance of good dental care and antibiotic prophylaxis. Patients are taught to monitor and report febrile illness.

Teach all patients with valve disease requiring medication therapy to report lack of therapeutic effect or any adverse effects of the drugs. Teach patients to be aware of drug-food interactions (e.g., green leafy vegetables and anticoagulants). Teach patients to have prothrombin time/INR checked on a regular basis if they are taking anticoagulant medications. Teach the patient with disabling heart failure about energy-conserving measures. Patients with hemodynamically significant valvular heart disease may need to limit vigorous physical activity. Deterioration may be rapid and symptoms insidious, so patients are taught to report any change in condition.

CLINICAL RECOMMENDATION	EVIDENCE RATING	REFERENCE
In asymptomatic patients, hemodynamic measurements with cardiac catheterization are not recommended for the severity of aortic stenosis and assessment of left ventricular function.	C	Bonow et al. (2008)
Echocardiology is recommended in patients with aortic stenosis for the assessment of left ventricular function, size, and wall thickness.	B	Bonow et al. (2008)
Chronic therapy with vasodilators is indicated for patients with severe aortic regurgitation who have left ventricular dysfunction or symptoms when surgery is not recommended because of additional cardiac or noncardiac factors.	B	Bonow et al. (2008)
For patients with atrial fibrillation (permanent, persistent, or paroxysmal) and mitral stenosis, anticoagulation is indicated.	B	Bonow et al. (2008)

A = consistent, good-quality, patient-oriented evidence; B = inconsistent or limited-quality, patient-oriented evidence; C = consensus, disease-oriented evidence, usual practice, expert opinion, or case series. For information about the SORT evidence rating system, go to www.aafp.org/afpsort.xml.

CASE STUDY

You are assigned to see R. G., a 66-year-old man, known to the practice where you have your clinical experience. You go to review his chart, and it is in the inactive file; he has not been seen for more than 7 years. His last visit was for bronchitis, and he was prescribed albuterol metered-dose inhaler (MDI) as needed. He was given laboratory slips for a complete metabolic profile, ECG, and PFTs, but there are no results on the chart. A follow-up postcard was sent to him 2 months after the visit.

On review of his chart you note that he has never come for a comprehensive visit, only episodic problems. He was diagnosed with hypertension 10 years ago and was prescribed hydrochlorothiazide, 12.5 mg orally once daily; his last refill was 2 years ago. History is sketchy since he was seen mainly for sick visits. Here is what you can glean from the record:

Divorced; worked as a carpenter, also did handyman jobs

Last insurance through carpenters' union

Significant family history: father died from heart problem at age 42; mother died from lung cancer at age 60; younger brother has type 2 diabetes mellitus, heart disease

Smoker, 1½ packs/day since age 15 years

Occasional alcohol; during military service drank four six-packs of beer every weekend

Denies any drug use, uses OTC Advil for "aches and pains on the job"

Reported that he had a tetanus booster in the emergency department 8 years ago for a work-related injury

Last visit: BP 130/84, heart rate (HR) 76, respiratory rate (RR) 18, BMI 28

1. How will you use this information to prepare for today's visit?

Today's visit:

Chief Complaint: "I'm really feeling my age these days...there are times when I feel like I can't catch my breath. [Pause to breathe] I know I've put on a few pounds but I didn't think I'd feel so winded. This retirement is for the birds; I can't seem to get into the groove." [Pause to breathe]

Objective: BP 150/92, HR 110, RR 28, BMI 27

66-year-old Caucasian male, ruddy complexion, fingertips yellowed, prominent sternocleidomastoids, looks older than stated age

Diminished breath sounds, crackles at bases of lungs bilaterally

Heart sounds distant, possible S_4

Feet cyanotic when dependent, +2 edema bilaterally

2. What additional subjective data are you seeking?
3. What additional objective data will you be assessing for?
4. What national guidelines are appropriate to consider?
5. What tests will you order?
6. What are the differential diagnoses that you are considering?
7. What is your plan of care?
8. Are there any Healthy People 2020 objectives that you should consider?
9. What additional patient teaching may be needed?
10. Will you be looking for a consultation?

REFERENCES

Assessment of the Cardiac and Respiratory Systems
American Heart Association/American College of Cardiology. (2006). AHA/ACC guidelines for secondary prevention for patients with coronary and other atherosclerotic vascular disease: 2006 update., *Circulation, 113*(19), 2363–2372.

Bickley, L. S., & Szilagyi, P. G. (2009). *Bates' guide to physical examination and history taking* (10th ed.). Philadelphia, PA: Wolters Kluwer/Lippincott Williams & Wilkins.

Greenland, P., Alpert, J. S., Beller, G. A., Benjamin, E. J., Budoff, M. J., Fayad, Z. A., . . . Wenger, N. K. (2010). 2010 ACCF/AHA guideline for assessment of cardiovascular risk in asymptomatic adults: executive summary. A report of the American College of Cardiology Foundation/American Heart Association Task Force on Practice Guidelines. *Journal of the American College of Cardiology, 56*(25), 2182–2199. doi:10.1016/j.jacc.2010.09.002

Ham, R. J., Sloane, P. D., Warshaw, G. A., Bernard, M. A., & Flaherty, E. (Eds). (2006). *Primary care geriatrics: a case-based approach* (5th ed.). St. Louis, MO: Mosby.

Kane, R. L., Ouslander, J. G., Abrass, I. B., & Resnick, B. (2008). *Essentials of clinical geriatrics* (6th ed.). New York City, NY: McGraw-Hill.

Lakatta, E. G., & Levy, D. (2003). Arterial and cardiac aging: major shareholders in cardiovascular disease enterprises: Part II: the aging heart in health; links to heart disease. *Circulation, 107*(2), 346–354.

Rubenfire, M., & Jackson, E. (2012). Cardiovascular risk of smoking and benefits of smoking cessation. *UpToDate.* Retrieved from www.uptodate.com

Taylor, F., Ward, K., Moore, T. H. M., Burke, M., Davey Smith, G., Casas, J. P., & Ebrahim, S. (2011). Statins for the primary prevention of cardiovascular disease. Retrieved from *Cochrane Database of Systematic Reviews,* Issue 1. Art. No.: CD004816. doi:10.1002/14651858.CD004816.pub4

Asthma

Boulet, L. P. (2008). Asthma guidelines and outcomes. In N. F. Adkinson (Ed.), *Middleton's allergy: principles and practice* (7th ed.). Philadelphia, PA: Mosby.

Buist, A. S., Vollmer, W. M., Wilson, S. R., Frazier, E. A., & Hayward, A. D. (2006). A randomized clinical trial of peak flow versus symptom monitoring in older adults with asthma. *American Journal of Respiratory and Critical Care Medicine, 174*(10), 1077–1087.

Chauhan, B. F., & Ducharme, F. M. (2012). Anti-leukotriene agents compared to inhaled corticosteroids in the management of recurrent and/or chronic asthma in adults and children. *Cochrane Database of Systematic Reviews,* Issue 5. Art. No.: CD002314. doi:10.1002/14651858.CD002314.pub3

Dweik, R. A., Boggs, P. B., Erzurum, S. C., Irvin, C. G., Leigh, M. W., Lundberg, J. O., . . . Taylor, D. R. (on behalf of the American Thoracic Society Committee on Interpretation of Exhaled Nitric Oxide Levels (FENO) for Clinical Applications). (2011). An official ATS clinical practice guideline: interpretation of exhaled nitric oxide levels (FENO) for clinical applications. *American Journal of Respiratory and Critical Care Medicine, 184*(5), 602–615. doi:10.1164/rccm.912011ST

Eisner, M. D., Iribarren, C., Yelin, E. H., Sidney, S., Katz, P. P., Ackerson, L., . . . Blanc, P. D. (2008). Pulmonary function and the risk of functional limitation in COPD. *American Journal of Epidemiology, 167*(9), 1090–1101. doi:10.1093/aje/kwn025

Enright, P. L., and Barr, R. G. (2012). Diagnosis and management of asthma in older adults. *UpToDate.* Retrieved from http://www.uptodate.com

Fanta, C. H. (2011). Treatment of acute exacerbations of asthma in adults. *UpToDate.* Retrieved from http://www.uptodate.com

Fanta, C. H., & Fletcher, S. W. (2012). An overview of asthma management. *UpToDate.* Retrieved from http://www.uptodate.com

Ferri, F. F. (2012). Asthma. In F. F. Ferri (Ed.), *Ferri's Clinical Advisor 2013* (1st ed.). Philadelphia, PA: Mosby/Elsevier.

Gillman, A., & Douglass, J. A. (2012). Asthma in the elderly. *Asia Pacific Allergy, 2*(2), 101–108. doi:10.5415/apallergy.2012.2.2.101

Global Strategy for Asthma Management and Prevention. (2011 update). Retrieved from www.ginasthma.org/uploads/users/files/GINA_Report2011_May4.pdf

Hallstrand, T. S., and Henderson, W. R., Jr. (2010). An update on the role of leukotrienes in asthma. *Current Opinion in Allergy and Clinical Immunology, 10*(1), 60–66. doi:10.1097/ACI.0b013e32833489c3

Humphrey, D. A. (2009). Asthma, acute exacerbation. *Essential Evidence Plus.* Retrieved from http://www.essentialevidenceplus.com

Irvin, C. G. (2011). Bronchoprovocation testing. *UpToDate.* Retrieved from http://www.uptodate.com

Irvin, C. G. (2012). Use of pulmonary function testing in the diagnosis of asthma. *UpToDate.* Retrieved from http://www.uptodate.com

Korn, S., Schumann, C., Kropf, C., Stoiber, K., Thielen, A., Taube, C., & Buhl, R. (2010). Effectiveness of omalizumab in patients 50 years and older with severe persistent allergic asthma. *Annals of Allergy, Asthma & Immunology, 105*(4), 313–319.

Kraft, W. (2011). Asthma (chronic management). *Essential Evidence Plus.* Retrieved from http://www.essentialevidenceplus.com

Krishnan, J. A., Riekert, K. A., McCoy, J. V., Stewart, D. Y., Schmidt, S., Chanmugam, A., . . . Rand, C. S. (2004). Corticosteroid use after hospital discharge among high-risk adults with asthma. *American Journal of Respiratory and Critical Care Medicine, 170*(12), 1281–1285.

Litonjua, A. A., & Weiss, S. T. (2010). Natural history of asthma. *UpToDate.* Retrieved from http://www.essentialevidenceplus.com

Litonjua, A. A., & Weiss, S. T. (2012). Risk factors for asthma. *UpToDate.* Retrieved from http://www.uptodate.com

Mathur, S. K. (2010). Allergy and asthma in the elderly. *Seminars in respiratory and critical care medicine, 31*(5), 587–595. doi:10.1055/s-0030-1265899

Maykut, R. J., Kianifard, F., & Geba, G. P. (2008). Response of older patients with IgE-mediated asthma to omalizumab: a pooled analysis. *Journal of Asthma, 45*(3), 173–181.

National Asthma Education and Prevention Program. (2007). *Expert panel report III: guidelines for the diagnosis and management of asthma.* (NIH publication no. 08-4051.) Bethesda, MD: National Heart, Lung, and Blood Institute. Retrieved from www.nhlbi.nih.gov/guidelines/asthma/asthgdln.htm

National Asthma Education and Prevention Program, National Heart, Lung, and Blood Institute. (1997). *Expert panel report 2: guidelines for the diagnosis and management of asthma.* (NIH publication no. 97-4051.) Bethesda, MD: National Institutes of Health.

Pelaia, G., Gallelli, L., Renda, T., Romeo, P., Busceti, M. T., Grembiale, R. D., . . . Vatrella, A. (2011). Update on optimal use of omalizumab in management of asthma. *Journal of Asthma and Allergy, 4,* 49–59.

Peters, S., McCallister, J. W., & Pascual, R. (2012). Treatment of moderate persistent asthma in adolescents and adults. *UpToDate.* Retrieved from http://www.uptodate.com

Rance, K. S. (2011). Helping patients attain and maintain asthma control: reviewing the role of the nurse practitioner. *Journal of Multidisciplinary Healthcare, 4,* 299–309. doi:10.2147/JMDH.S22966

Rowe, B. H., Bretzlaff, J. A., Bourdon, C., Bota, G. W., Camargo, C. A., & Rowe, B. (2007). Magnesium sulfate for treating exacerbations of acute asthma in the emergency department (Cochrane Review). In *The Cochrane Library 2007,* Issue 1. Chichester, UK: John Wiley & Sons, Ltd.

Stanford, R. H., Gilsenan, A. W., Ziemiecki, R., Zhou, X., Lincourt, W. R., & Ortega, H. (2010). Predictors of uncontrolled asthma in adult and pediatric patients: analysis of the Asthma Control Characteristics and Prevalence Survey Studies (ACCESS). *Journal of Asthma, 47*(3), 257–62.

Thomson, N. C., & Chaudhuri, R. (2012). Omalizumab: clinical use for the management of asthma. *Clinical Medicine Insights: Circulatory, Respiratory and Pulmonary Medicine, 6,* 27–40. doi:10.4137/CCRPM.S7793

U.S. Department of Health and Human Services, Centers for Disease Control and Prevention, National Center for Health Statistics. (2012, January). Summary health statistics for U.S. adults: National Health Interview Survey, 2010. *Vital Health Statistics,*

Series 10, No. 252. Retrieved from www.cdc.gov/nchs/data/series/sr_10/sr10_252.pdf

Yawn, B. P. (2011). The role of the primary care physician in helping adolescent and adult patients improve asthma control. *Mayo Clinic Proceedings, 86*(9), 894–902. doi:10.4065/mcp.2011.0035

Zeki, A. A., Schivo, M., Chan, A., Albertson, T. E., & Louie, S. (2011). The asthma-COPD overlap syndrome: a common clinical problem in the elderly. *Journal of Allergy (Cairo), 2011,* 861926. doi:10.1155/2011/861926

Cardiac Arrhythmias

Bickley, L. S., & Szilagyi, P. G. (2009). *Bates' guide to physical examination and history taking* (10th ed.). Philadelphia, PA: Wolters Kluwer/Lippincott Williams & Wilkins.

Goolsby, M. J., & Grubbs, L. (2011). *Advanced assessment: interpreting findings and formulating differential diagnoses* (2nd ed.). Philadelphia, PA: F.A. Davis.

Greenberg, H. M., Dwyer, E. M., Hochman, J. S., Steinberg, J. S., Echt, D. S., & Peters, R. W. (1995). Interaction of ischaemia and encainide/flecainide treatment: a proposed mechanism for the increased mortality in CAST I. *British Heart Journal, 74*(6), 631–635.

Knight, B. P., Sorrentino, M., Delaughter, M. C., & Shah, D. P. (2010). Practical rate and rhythm management of atrial fibrillation. Adapted from the ACC/AHA/ESC 2006 guidelines for the management of patients with atrial fibrillation, *Heart Rhythm Society,* January 2010 update.

Moya, A., Sutton, R., Ammirati, F., Blanc, J., Brignole, M., Dahm, J., . . . Wieling, W. (2009). Guidelines for the diagnosis and management of syncope. Version 2009. *European Heart Journal, 30*(21), 2631–2671.

Scottish Intercollegiate Guidelines Network. (2007, February) *Cardiac arrhythmias in coronary heart disease. A national clinical guideline.* Edinburgh, Scotland: Scottish Intercollegiate Guidelines Network.

Wann, L. S., Curtis, A. B., Ellenboegen, K. A., Estes, N. A. M., 3rd, Ezekowitz, M. D., Jackman, W. M., . . . Tracy, C. M. (on behalf of the 2006 ACC/AHA/ESC Guidelines for Management of Patients with Atrial Fibrillation Writing Committee). (2011). ACCF/AHA/HRS focused update on the management of patients with atrial fibrillation (update on dabigatran): a report of the American College of Cardiology Foundation/American Heart Association Task Force on Practice Guidelines. *Heart Rhythm, 8*(3), e1–e8.

Zipes, D. P., Camm, A. J., Borggrefe, M., Buxton, A. E., Chaitman, B., Fromer, M., . . . Tracy, C. (2006). ACC/AHA/ESC 2006 guidelines for management of patients with ventricular arrhythmias and the prevention of sudden cardiac death—executive summary: a report of the American College of Cardiology/American Heart Association Task Force and the European Society of Cardiology Committee for Practice Guidelines (Writing Committee to Develop Guidelines for Management of Patients with Ventricular Arrhythmias and the Prevention of Sudden Cardiac Death). *Journal of the American College of Cardiology, 48*(5), 1064–1108.

Chronic Obstructive Pulmonary Disease

American Lung Association. (n.d.). November is COPD awareness month. Retrieved from www.lung.org/about-us/our-impact/top-stories/november-is-copd-awareness-1.html

Appleton, S., Jones, T., Poole, P., Lasserson, T. J., Adams, R., Smith, B., & Muhammed, J. (2006). Ipratropium bromide versus long-acting beta-2 agonists for stable chronic obstructive pulmonary disease. Retrieved from *Cochrane Database of Systematic Reviews.* doi: 10.1002/14651858.CD006101

Barr, R. G., Bourbeau, J., & Camargo, C. A. (Cochrane Airways Group). (2009). Tiotropium for stable chronic pulmonary disease. Retrieved from *Cochrane Database of Systematic Reviews.*

Buist, A. S., McBurnie, M. A., Vollmer, W. M., Gillespie, S., Burney, P., Mannino, D. M., . . . BOLD Collaborative Research Group. (2007). International variation in the prevalence of COPD (the BOLD Study): a population-based prevalence study. *Lancet, 370*(9589), 741–750.

Celli, B. R., Cote, C. G., Marin, J. M., Casanova, C., Montes de Oca, M., Mendez, R. A., . . . Cabral, H. J. (2004). The body-mass index, airflow obstruction, dyspnea, and exercise capacity index in chronic obstructive pulmonary disease. *New England Journal of Medicine, 350*(10), 1005–1012.

Centers for Disease Control and Prevention. (2012). Recommended adult immunization schedule—United States, 2012. *Morbidity and Mortality Weekly Report, 61*(04), 1–7. Retrieved from www.cdc.gov/mmwr/preview/mmwrhtml/mm6104a9.htm

Cooper, C. B., & Dransfield, M. (2008). Primary care of the patient with chronic obstructive pulmonary disease—Part 4: understanding the clinical manifestations of a progressive disease. *The American Journal of Medicine, 121*(7 Suppl.), S33–S45.

Cote, C. G., & Celli, B. R. (2007). Predictors of mortality in chronic obstructive pulmonary disease. *Clinics in Chest Medicine, 28*(3), 515–524.

Department of Veterans Affairs; Department of Defense. (2007). VA/DOD clinical practice guideline for management of outpatient chronic obstructive pulmonary disease. Retrieved from www.healthquality.va.gov/chronic_obstructive_pulmonary_disease_copd.asp

Evensen, A. E. (2010). Management of COPD exacerbations. *American Family Physician, 81*(5), 607–613.

Fabbri, L. M., Calverley, P., Izquierdo-Alonso, J. L., Bundschuh, D. S., Brose, M., Martinez, F. J., & Rabe, K. F. (2009). Roflumilast in moderate-to-severe chronic obstructive pulmonary disease treated with longacting bronchodilators: two randomised clinical trials. *Lancet, 374*(9691), 695–703. doi:10.1016/S0140-6736(09)61252-6

Ferri, F. F. (2012). COPD. In F. F. Ferri (Ed.), *Ferri's clinical advisor 2013* (1st ed.). Philadelphia, PA: Mosby/Elsevier.

Global Initiative for Chronic Obstructive Lung Disease (GOLD). (2008). Global Strategy for the diagnosis, management, and prevention of chronic obstructive pulmonary disease. Accessed July 25, 2009. Retrieved from http://www.goldcopd.org

Global Initiative for Chronic Obstructive Lung Disease (GOLD). (2010). Spirometry for health care providers. Retrieved from www.goldcopd.org/uploads/users/files/GOLD_Spirometry_2010.pdf

Global Initiative for Chronic Obstructive Lung Disease (GOLD). (2011). Global strategy for the diagnosis, management, and prevention of chronic obstructive pulmonary disease (revised 2011). Retrieved from www.goldcopd.org/uploads/users/files/GOLD_Report_2011_Feb21.pdf

GOLD Pocket guide for COPD diagnosis, management, and prevention. A guide for health care professionals (2011). Retrieved from www.goldcopd.org/uploads/users/files/GOLD_Pocket_May2512.pdf

Hall, W. J., & Ahmed, B. (2007). Pulmonary Disorders. In E. Duthie, P.R. Katz, & M. Malone (Eds.), *The Practice of Geriatrics* (4th ed.). Philadelphia, PA: Saunders/Elsevier.

Hopewell, P. C., & Kato-Maeda, M. (2010). Tuberculosis. In R. J. Mason (Ed.), *Murray and Nadel's textbook of respiratory medicine* (5th ed.). Philadelphia, PA: Saunders Elsevier.

Hurst, J. R., & Wedzicha, J. A. (2007). The biology of a chronic obstructive pulmonary disease exacerbation. *Clinics in Chest Medicine, 28*(3), 525–536. doi:10.1016/j.ccm.2007.05.003

Kilgore, D., & Najm, W. (2010). Common respiratory diseases. *Primary Care: Clinics in Office Practice, 37*(2), 297–324.

Lange, N. E., Mulholland, M., & Kreider, M. E. (2009). Spirometry: don't blow it! *Chest, 136*(2), 608–614.

Lee, F. E.-H., & Treanor, J. (2010). Viral infections. In R. J. Mason (Ed.), *Murray and Nadel's textbook of respiratory medicine* (5th ed.). Philadelphia, PA: Saunders Elsevier.

MacNee, W. (2008). Pathogenesis of chronic obstructive pulmonary disease. *Clinics in Chest Medicine, 28*, 479–513.

Martinez, F. J., Curtis, J. L., Sciurba, F., Mumford, J., Giardina, N. D., Weinmann, G., . . . Wise, R. (for the National Emphysema Treatment Trial Research Group). (2007). Sex differences in severe pulmonary emphysema. *American Journal of Respiratory Critical Care Medicine, 176*(3), 243–252.

Nazir, S. A., Al-Hamed, M. M., & Erbland, M. L. (2007). Chronic obstructive pulmonary disease in the older patient. *Clinics in Chest Medicine, 28*(4), 703–715. doi:10.1016/j.ccm.2007.07.003

Qaseem, A., Wilt, T. J., Weinberger, S. E., Hanania, N. A., Criner, G., van der Molen, T., . . . Shekelle, P. (for the American College of Physicians, the American College of Chest Physicians, the American Thoracic Society, and the European Respiratory Society). (2011). Diagnosis and management of stable chronic obstructive pulmonary disease: a clinical practice guideline update from the American College of Physicians, American College of Chest Physicians, American Thoracic Society, and European Respiratory Society. *Annals of Internal Medicine, 155*(3), 179–191.

Radin, A., & Cote, C. (2008). Primary care of the patient with Chronic Obstructive Pulmonary Disease—Part 1: frontline prevention and early diagnosis. *The American Journal of Medicine 121*(7 Suppl.), S3–S12.

Remels, A. H., Gosker, H. R., van der Velden, J., Langen, R. C., & Schols, A. M. (2007). Systemic inflammation and skeletal muscle dysfunction in chronic obstructive pulmonary disease: state of the art and novel insights in regulation of muscle plasticity. *Clinics in Chest Medicine, 28*(3), 537–552.

Ries, A. L., Bauldoff, G. S., Carlin, B. W., Casaburi, R., Emery, C. F., Mahler, D. A., . . . Herrerias, C. (2007). Pulmonary rehabilitation: Joint ACCP/AACVPR evidence-based clinical practice guidelines. *Chest, 131*(5), S4–S42.

Shapiro, S. D., Reilly, J. J., Jr., & Rennard, S. I. (2010). Chronic bronchitis and emphysema. In R. J. Mason (Ed.), *Murray and Nadel's textbook of respiratory medicine* (5th ed.). Philadelphia, PA: Saunders Elsevier.

Stephens, M. B., & Yew, K. S. (2008). Diagnosis of chronic obstructive pulmonary disease. *American Family Physician, 78*(1), 87–92.

Wise, R. A., & Tashkin, D. P. (2007). Preventing chronic obstructive pulmonary disease: what is known and what needs to be done to make a difference to the patient? *American Journal of Medicine, 120*(8A), S14–S22.

Yawn, B. P. (2009). Differential assessment of asthma versus chronic obstructive pulmonary disease. *Medscape Journal of Medicine, 11*(1), 20.

Yohannes, A. M. (2007). Palliative care provision for patients with chronic obstructive pulmonary disease. *Health and Quality of Life Outcomes, 5*, 17. doi:10.1186/1477-7525-5-17

Zeki, A. A., Schivo, M., Chan, A., Albertson, T. E., & Louie, S. (2011). The asthma-COPD overlap syndrome: a common clinical problem in the elderly. *Journal of Allergy (Cairo), 2011*, 861926. doi:10.1155/2011/861926

Heart Failure

Agency for Healthcare Research and Quality. (2005). Heart failure quality measures.

Ahmed, A. (2003a). American College of Cardiology/American Heart Association chronic heart failure evaluation and management guidelines: relevance to geriatric practice. *Journal of the American Geriatrics Society, 51*(1), 123–126.

Ahmed, A. (2003b). DEFEAT heart failure: clinical manifestations, diagnostic assessment, and etiology of geriatric heart failure [Electronic Version]. *Heart Failure Clinics, 3*(4), 389–402.

Ahmed, A. (2003c). Treatment of chronic heart failure in long-term care facilities: implications of recent heart failure guidelines recommendations. *Archives of Gerontology and Geriatrics, 37*(2), 131–137. doi:10.1016/S0167-4943(03)00027-X

Ahmed, A., Jones, L., & Hays, C. I. (2008). DEFEAT heart failure: assessment and management of heart failure in nursing homes made easy. *Journal of the American Medical Directors Association, 9*(6), 383–389.

American Heart Association. (2010). Heart disease and stroke statistics: 2010 update. Retrieved January 13, 2012, from lern.la.gov/index.php/download_file/view/128/227/

American Medical Directors Association. (2010). *Heart failure clinical practice guideline*. Columbus, MD: American Medical Directors Association.

Arling, M. L. (1998). Outcomes of ACE inhibitor use in nursing facility residents with congestive heart failure. *Annals of Long Term Care, 6*(8), 237–241.

Aronow, W. S. (2003). Mortality with nursing home patients with congestive heart failure. *Journal of the American Medical Directors Association, 4*(4), 201–202. doi:10.1097/01.JAM.0000073962.72130.D1

Aronow, W. S. (2006a). Appropriate use of digoxin in treating older nursing home patients with heart failure. *Journal of the American Medical Directors Association, 7*(9), 604–606.

Aronow, W. S. (2006b). Treatment of systolic and diastolic heart failure in the elderly. *Journal of the American Medical Directors Association, 7*(1), 29–36. doi:10.1016/j.jamda.2005.07.008

Barents, M., Hillege, H., de Boer, R., Koster, J., Muskiet, F., & de Jongste, M. (2008). BNP and NT-proBNP, predictors of 1-year mortality in nursing home residents. *Journal of the American Medical Directors Association, 9*(8), 580–585.

Beers, M. H. (1997). Explicit criteria for determining potentially inappropriate medication use by the elderly: an update. *Archives of Internal Medicine, 157*(14), 1531–1536.

Beier, M. T., Lawhorne, L. W., & Phillips, N. G. (1998). The utilization of echocardiography for community nursing facility residents with congestive heart failure. *Annals of Long Term Care, 6*(12), 376–381.

Bhalla, V., Willis, S., & Maisel, A. S. (2004). B-type natriuretic peptide: the level and the drug? Partners in the diagnosis and management of congestive heart failure. *Congestive Heart Failure, 10*(1 Suppl. 1), 3–27. doi:10.1111/j.1527-5299.2004.03310.x

Boxer, R. S., Dolansky, M. A., Frantz, M. A., Prosser, R., Hitch, J. A., & Pina, I. L. (2011). The bridge project: improving heart failure care in skilled nursing facilities. *Journal of the American Medical Directors Association, 13*(1), 83.e1–e7 doi:10.1016/j.jamda.2011.01.005

Bueno, H., Ross, J. S., Wang, Y., Vidan, M. T., Normand, S. T., & Curtis, J. P., . . . Krumholz, H. M. (2010). Trends in length of stay and short-term outcomes among Medicare patients hospitalized with heart failure: 1993–2006. *Journal of the American Medical Association, 303*(21), 2141–2147. doi:10.1001ama2010.748

Centers for Disease Control and Prevention. (1997). Prevention and control of influenza. Recommendations of the advisory committee on immunizations. *Morbidity and Mortality Weekly Report Recommendations and Reports, 46*(9), 1–25.

Cleland, J. G. F., Loh, H., & Windram, J. (2005). Are there clinically important differences between beta-blockers in heart failure? *Heart Failure Clinics, 1*(1), 57–66. doi:10.1016/j.hfc.2004.12.004

Clinical Pharmacology. (2009, November 25). Metoprolol succinate. Retrieved August 28, 2010, from www.clinicalpharmacology-ip.com/Forms/Monograph/monograph.aspx?cpnum=3978sec=monmech

Daamen, M. A., Schols, J. M., Jaarsma, T., & Hamers, J. P. (2010). Prevalence of heart failure in nursing homes: a systematic literature review. *Scandinavian Journal of Caring Sciences, 24*(1), 202–208. doi:10.1111/j.1471-6712.2009.00708.x

Domanski, M., Norman, J., Pitt, B., Haigney, M., Hanlon, S., & Peyster, E. (2003). Diuretic use, progressive heart failure, and death in patients in the Studies of Left Ventricular Dysfunction (SOLVD). *Journal of the American College of Cardiology, 42*(4), 705–708. doi:10.1016/S0735-1097(03)00765-4

Dulin, B. R., Haas, S. J., Abraham, W. T., & Krum, H. (2005). Do elderly systolic heart failure patients benefit from β-blockers to the same extent as the non-elderly? *American Journal of Cardiology, 95*(7), 896–898.

Dunlap, M. E., & Peterson, R. C. (2002). ACE inhibitors vs ARBs: is one class better for heart failure? *Cleveland Clinic Journal of Medicine, 69*(5), 433–438.

Feenstra, J. H., Eibert, R., Grobbee, D. E., & Stricker, B. H. (2002). Association of nonsteroidal anti-inflammatory drugs with first occurrence of heart failure and with relapsing heart failure: the Rotterdam Study. *Archives of Internal Medicine, 162*(3), 265–270. doi:10.1001/archinte.162.3.265

Fonarow, G. C. (2007). Performance measures for patients hospitalized with heart failure: are they predictive of clinical outcomes? *Congestive Heart Failure, 13*(6), 342–346. doi:10.1111/j.1527-5299.2007.07233.x

Forman, D. E., & Rich, M. W. (2003). Heart failure in the elderly. *Congestive Heart Failure, 9*(6), 311–323. doi:10.1111/j.1527-5299.2003.00798.x

Gambassi, G., Forman, D. E., Lapane, K. L., Mor, V., Sgadari, A., Lipsitz, L. A., & Bernabei, R. (2000). Management of heart failure among very old persons living in long-term care: has the voice of trials spread? The SAGE study group. *American Heart Journal, 139*(1 Pt. 1), 85–93.

Gibbs, C. R., Davies, M. K., & Lip, G. Y. (2000). ABC of heart failure. Management: Digoxin and other inotropes, β blockers, and antiarrhythmic and antithrombotic treatment. *BMJ, 320*(7233), 495–498.

Harrington, C. (2006). Assessing heart failure in long-term care facilities. In M. G. Titler (Series Ed.), *Series on evidence-based practice for older adults.* Iowa City, IA: University of Iowa Gerontological Nursing Interventions Research Center Research Translation and Dissemination Core.

Harrington, C. (2008). Assessing heart failure in long-term care facilities. *Journal of Gerontological Nursing, 34*(2), 9–14.

Hines, P. A., Yu, K., & Randall, M. (2010). Preventing heart failure readmissions: is your organization prepared? *Nursing Economics, 28*(2), 74–86.

Hobbs, F. D. (2000). Management of heart failure: evidence versus practice. Does current prescribing provide optimal treatment for heart failure patients? *British Journal of General Practice, 50*(1), 735–742.

Hunt, S. A., Abraham, W. T., Chin, M. H., Feldman, A. M., Francis, G. S., Ganiats, T. G., . . . Riegel, B. (2005). ACC/AHA 2005 guideline update for the diagnosis and management of chronic heart failure. *Circulation, 112*(2), 1825–1852. Retrieved July 16, 2011, from www.circulationaha.org. doi:10.1161/CIRCULATIONAHA.105167587

Hunt, S. A., Abraham, W. T., Chin, M. H., Feldman, A. M., Francis, G. S., Ganiats, T. G., . . . Yancy, C. W. (2009). 2009 focused update incorporated into the ACC/AHA 2005 guidelines for the diagnosis and management of heart failure in adults: a report of the American College of Cardiology Foundation/American Heart Association task force on practice guidelines developed in collaboration with the International Society for Heart and Lung Transplantation. *Journal of the American College of Cardiology, 53*(15), e1–e90. doi:10.1016/j.jacc.2008.11.013

Jackson, G., Gibbs, C. R., Davies, M. K., & Lip, G. Y. (2000). ABC of heart failure. *BMJ, 320*(7228), 167–170.

Kirkpatrick, J. N., Vannan, M. A., Narula, J., & Lang, R. M. (2007). Echocardiography in heart failure: application, utility, and new horizons. *Journal of the American College of Cardiology, 50*(5), 381–396. doi:10.1016/j.jacc.2007.03.048

Kleinpell, R., & Gawlinski, A. (2005). Assessing outcomes in advanced practice nursing practice: the use of quality indicators and evidence-based practice. *AACN Clinical Issues, 16*(1), 43–57.

Litaker, L. R., & Chou, J. Y. (2003). Patterns of pharmacologic treatment of congestive heart failure in elderly nursing home residents and related issues: a review of literature. *Clinical Therapeutics, 25*(7), 1918–1935.

Moberley, S., Holden, J., Tatham, D. P., & Andrews, R. M. (2008). Vaccines for preventing pneumococcal infection in adults. *Cochrane Database of Systematic Reviews.* Art. No.: CD000422. doi:10.1002/14651858.CD000422.pub2

Muth, C., Gensichen, J., Beyer, M., Hutchinson, A., & Gerlach, F. M. (2009). Systematic guideline review: method, rationale, and test on chronic heart failure. *BMC Health Services Research, 9*(74), 1–15.

Omnicare. (2010). *Geriatric pharmaceutical care guidelines.* Philadelphia, PA: Omnicare.

Oxberry, S. G., & Johnson, M. J. (2008). Review of the evidence for the management of dyspnoea in people with chronic heart failure. *Current Opinion in Supportive and Palliative Care, 2*(2), 84–88. doi:10.1097/SPC.0b013e3282ff122e

Parker, K. M., Miller, N. H., & DeBusk, R. F. (2001). Optimal use of spironolactone for treatment of heart failure. *Congestive Heart Failure, 7*(6), 315–318. doi:10.1111/j.1527-5299.2001.00270.x

Pharmacy Benefits Management Strategic Healthcare Group & Medical Advisory Panel. (2007). *The pharmacological management of chronic heart failure* (PBM-MAP Publication No. 00-0015). Retrieved March 24, 2010, from www.vaww.pbm.va.gov

Reddersen, L. A., Keen, C., Nasir, L., & Berry, D. (2008). Diastolic heart failure: state of the science on best treatment practices. *Journal of the American Academy of Nurse Practitioners, 20*(10), 506–514. doi:10.1111/j.1745-7599.2008.00352.x

Rich, M. W. (2005). Heart failure in the oldest patients: the impact of comorbid conditions. *American Journal of Geriatric Cardiology, 14*(3):134–141.

Ross, J. S., Chen, J., Lin, A., Bueno, H., Curtis, J. P., Keeman, P. S., . . . Krumholz, H. M. (2010). Recent national trends in readmission rates after heart failure hospitalization. *Circulation, 3*(1), 97–103. doi:10.1161.CIRCHEARTFAILURE.109.885210

Ruffolo, R. R., & Feuerstein, G. Z. (1997). Pharmacology of carvedilol: rationale for use in hypertension, coronary artery disease, and congestive heart failure [Abstract]. *Cardiovascular Drugs and Therapy, 11*(1), 247–256.

Ruths, S., Straand, J., Nygaard, H. A., & Hodneland, F. (2000). Drug treatment of heart failure—do nursing-home residents deserve better? *Scandinavian Journal of Primary Health Care, 18*(4), 226–231.

Shishehbor, M. H., & Litaker, D. (2007). Performance measures and outcomes for patients hospitalized with heart failure. *Journal of the American Medical Association, 297*(14), 1547; author reply 1548–1549. doi:10.1001/jama.297.14.1547-a

Silver, M. A., Maisel, A., Yancy, C. W., McCullough, P. A., Burnett, J. C., Francis, G. S., . . . Hollander, J. (2004). BNP consensus panel 2004: a clinical approach for the diagnostic, prognostic, screening, treatment monitoring, and therapeutic roles of natriuretic peptides in cardiovascular diseases. *Congestive Heart Failure, 10*(5 Suppl. 3), 1–30. doi:10.1111/j.1527-5299.2004.03271.x

Simonson, W., Han, L. F., & Davidson, H. E. (2011). Hypertension treatment and outcomes in U.S. nursing homes: results from the U.S. National Nursing Home Survey. *Journal of the American Medical Directors Association, 12*(1), 44–49. doi:10.1016/j.jamda. 2010.02.009

Zannad, F., Alla, F., Dousset, B., Perez, A., & Pitt, B. (2000). Limitation of excessive extracellular matrix turnover may contribute to survival benefit of spironolactone therapy in patients with congestive heart failure: insights from the Randomized Aldactone Evaluation Study (RALES). *Circulation, 102*(22), 2700–2706. doi:10.1161/01.CIR.102.22.2700

Zile, M. R., & Brutsaert, D. L. (2002). New concepts in diastolic dysfunction and diastolic heart failure: Part II: causal mechanisms and treatment. *Circulation, 105*(12), 1503–1508. doi:10.1161/hc1202.105290

Hypertension

Appel, D. W., & Aldrich, T. K. (2003). Smoking cessation in the elderly. *Clinics in Geriatric Medicine, 19*(1), 77–100.

Appel, L. J., Brands, M. W., Daniels, S. R., Karanja, N., Elmer, P. J., Sacks, F. M., & American Heart Association. (2006). Dietary approaches to prevent and treat hypertension: a scientific statement from the American Heart Association. *Hypertension, 47*(2), 296–308.

Bagrov, A. Y., & Lakatta, E. G. (2004). The dietary sodium-blood pressure plot "stiffens." *Hypertension, 44*(1), 22–24.

Beevers, G., Lip, G. Y. H., & O'Brien, E. (2001). ABC of hypertension. The pathophysiology of hypertension. *British Medical Journal, 322*(7291), 912–916.

Bihorac, A., Tezcan, H., Ozener, C., & Oktay, A. (2000). Association between salt sensitivity and target organ damage in essential hypertension. *American Journal of Hypertension, 13*(8), 864–872.

Borghi, C., Dormi, A., D'Addato, S., Gaddi, A., & Ambrosioni, E. (on behalf of the Brisighella Heart Study Working Party). (2004). Trends in blood pressure control and antihypertensive treatment in clinical practice: the Brisighella Heart Study. *Journal of Hypertension, 22*(9), 1707–1716.

Brennan, P., Pescatello, L. S., Bohannon, R. W., Marschke, L., Murphy, M., Coble, D., & Hasson, S. (2005). Time spent moving is related to systolic blood pressure among older women. *Preventive Cardiology, 8*(3), 160–164.

Brown, M. J., Palmer, C. R., Castaigne, A., de Leeuw, P. W., Mancia, G., Rosenthal, T., & Ruilope, L. M. (2000). Morbidity and mortality

in patients randomised to double-blind treatment with a long-acting calcium-channel blocker or diuretic in the International Nifedipine GITS study: intervention as a Goal in Hypertension Treatment (INSIGHT). *Lancet, 356*(9227), 366–372.

Celermajer, D. S., Sorensen, K. E., Spiegelhalter, D. J., Georgakopoulos, D., Robinson, J., & Deanfield, J. E. (1994). Aging is associated with endothelial dysfunction in healthy men years before the age-related decline in women. *Journal of American College of Cardiology, 24*(2), 471–476.

Chobanian, A. V., Bakris, G. L., Black, H. R., Cushman, W. C., Green, L. A., Izzo, J. L., Jr., . . . the National High Blood Pressure Education Program Coordinating Committee. (2003). The seventh report of the Joint National Committee on prevention, detection, evaluation, and treatment of high blood pressure: the JNC 7 report. *Journal of the American Medical Association, 289*(19), 2560–2572.

Clement, D. L., De Buyzere, M. L., De Bacquer, D. A., de Leeuw, P. W., Duprez, D. A., Fagard, R. H., . . . Office versus Ambulatory Pressure Study Investigators. (2003). Prognostic value of ambulatory blood-pressure recordings in patients with treated hypertension. *New England Journal of Medicine, 348*(24), 2407–2415.

Cushman, W. C., Ford, C. E., Cutler, J. A., Margolis, K. L., Davis, B. R., Grimm, R. H., . . . ALLHAT Collaborative Research Group. (2002). Success and predictors of blood pressure control in diverse North American settings: the antihypertensive and lipid-lowering treatment to prevent heart attack trial. *Journal of Clinical Hypertension, 4*(6), 393–404.

Dahlöf, B., Sever, P. S., Poulter, N. R., Wedel, H., Beevers, D. G., Caulfield, M., . . . ASCOT Investigators. (2005). Prevention of cardiovascular events with an antihypertensive regimen of amlodipine adding perindopril as required versus atenolol adding bendroflumethiazide as required, in the Anglo-Scandinavian Cardiac Outcomes Trial-Blood Pressure Lowering Arm (ASCOT-BPLA): a multicenter randomised controlled trial. *Lancet, 366*(9489), 895–906.

Donzé, J., Ruffieux, & C., Cornuz, J. (2007). Determinants of smoking and cessation in older women. *Age and Aging, 36*(1), 53–57.

Ferrier, I. N. (2001). Characterizing the ideal antidepressant therapy to achieve remission. *Journal of Clinical Psychiatry, 62*(S26), 10–15.

Fiore, M. C., Jaén, C. R., Baker, T. B., Bailey, W. C., Benowitz, N., Curry, S. J., . . . Healton, C. G. (2008). Treating tobacco use and dependence: 2008 update. *Clinical Practice Guideline. Executive Summary.* Rockville, MD: U.S. Department of Health and Human Services. Retrieved from: http://rc.rcjournal.com/content/53/9/1217.full.pdf

Franklin, S. S. (2005). Arterial stiffness and hypertension. A two-way street? *Hypertension, 45*(3), 349–351.

Gates, P. E., Tanaka, H., Hiatt, W. R., & Seals, D. R. (2004). Dietary sodium restriction rapidly improves large elastic artery compliance in older adults with systolic hypertension. *Hypertension, 44*(1), 35–41.

He, F. J., Markandu, N. D., & MacGregor, G. A. (2005). Modest salt reduction lowers blood pressure in isolated systolic hypertension and combined hypertension. *Hypertension, 46*(1), 66–70.

Jamerson, K., Weber, M. A., Bakris, G. L., Dahlöf, B., Pitt, B., Shi, V., . . . ACCOMPLISH Trial Investigators. (2008). Benazepril plus amlodipine or hydrochlorothiazide for hypertension in high-risk patients. *New England Journal of Medicine, 359*(23), 2417–2428. doi: 10.1056/NEJMoa0806182

Keenan, N. L., & Rosendorf, K. A. (2011). Prevalence of hypertension and controlled hypertension—United States, 2005–2008. National Center for Chronic Disease Prevention and Health Promotion (CDC PMD: 21430632). Retrieved from www.ncbi.nlm. nih.gov/pubmed?term=%22Rosendorf%20KA%22

Khan, N., & McAlister, F. A. (2006). Re-examining the efficacy of beta-blockers for the treatment of hypertension: a meta-analysis. *Canadian Medical Association Journal, 174*(12), 1737–1742.

Kithas, P. A., & Supiano, M. A. (2010). Practical recommendations for treatment of hypertension in older adults. *Vascular Health and Risk Management, 6,* 561–569.

Kjeldsen, S. E., Lyle, P. A., Kizer, J. R., Dahlöf, B., Devereux, R. B., Julius, S., . . . & LIFE Study Group. (2005). The effects of losartan compared to atenolol on stroke in patients with isolated systolic hypertension and left ventricular hypertrophy. The LIFE study. *Journal of Clinical Hypertension, 7*(3), 152–158.

Kojda, G., & Harrison, D. G. (1999). Interactions between NO and reactive oxygen species: pathophysiological importance in atherosclerosis, hypertension, diabetes and heart failure. *Cardiovascular Research, 43,* 562–571.

Lakatta, E. G. (2007). Central arterial aging and the epidemic of systolic hypertension and atherosclerosis. *Journal of the American Society of Hypertension, 1*(5), 302–340.

Lindholm, L. H., Carlberg, B., & Samuelsson, O. (2005). Should beta blockers remain first choice in the treatment of primary hypertension? A meta-analysis. *Lancet, 366*(9496), 1545–1553.

London, G., Schmieder, R., Calvo, C., & Asmar, R. (2006). Indapamide SR versus candesartan and amlodipine in hypertension: the X-CELLENT Study. *American Journal of Hypertension, 19*(1), 113–121.

Messeril, F. (1986). Osler's maneuver: pseudohypertension and true hypertension in the elderly. *American Journal of Medicine, 80*(5), 906–910.

Oberleithner, H., Riethmuller, C., Schillers, H., MacGregor, G. A., de Wardener, H. E., & Hausberg, M. (2007). Plasma sodium stiffens vascular endothelium and reduces nitric oxide release. *Proceedings of the National Academy of Sciences, 104*(41), 16281–16286. doi:10.1073/pnas.0707791104

Obisesan, T. O., Obisesan, O. A., Martins, S., Alangir, L., Bond, V., Maxwell, C., & Gillum, R. F. (2008). High blood pressure, hypertension and high pulse pressure are associated with poorer cognitive function in persons aged 60 and older: the third National Health and Nutrition Examination Survey. *Journal of the American Geriatrics Society, 56*(3), 501–509.

O'Rourke, N. (2005). Aortic diameter, aortic stiffness, and wave reflection increase with age and isolated systolic hypertension. *Hypertension, 45,* 652–658.

Redón, J., Cea-Calvo, L., Moreno, B., Monereo, S., Gil-Guillén, V., Lozano, J. V., . . . Fernández-Pérez, C. (on behalf of the investigators of the PREV-ICTUS Study), (2008). Independent impact of obesity and fat distribution in hypertension prevalence and control in the elderly. *Journal of Hypertension, 26*(9), 1757–1764.

Somes, G. W., Pahor, M., Shorr, R. I., Cushman, W. C., & Applegate, W. B. (1999). The role of diastolic blood pressure when treating isolated systolic hypertension. *Archives of Internal Medicine, 159*(17), 2004–2009.

Stewart, K. J., Bacher, A. C., Turner, K. L., Fleg, J. L., Hees, P. S., Shapiro, E. P., . . . Ouyang, P. (2005). Effect of exercise on blood pressure in older persons: a randomized controlled trial. *Archives of Internal Medicine, 165*(7), 756–762.

Stokes, G. S. (2006). Nitrates as adjunct hypertensive treatment. *Current Hypertension Report, 8*(1), 60–68.

Stokes, G. S. (2009). Management of hypertension in the elderly patient. *Clinical Interventions in Aging, 4,* 379–389.

Stokes, G. S., & Ryan, M. (1997). Can extended-release isosorbide mononitrate be used as adjunctive therapy for systolic hypertension? An open study employing pulse-wave analysis to determine effects of antihypertensive therapy. *American Journal of Geriatric Cardiology, 6*(4), 11–19.

Supiano, M. A., Hogikyan, R. V., Sidani, M. A., Galecki, A. T., & Krueger, J. L. (1999). Sympathetic nervous system activity and alpha-adrenergic responsiveness in older hypertensive humans. *American Journal of Physiology, 276,* (3 Pt. 1), E519–E528.

Suskin, N., Sheth, T., Negassa, A., & Yusuf, S. (2001). Relationship of current and past smoking to mortality and morbidity in patients with left ventricular dysfunction. *Journal of the American College of Cardiology, 37*(6), 1677–1682.

Tanaka, H., DeSouza, C. A., & Seals, D. R. (1998). Absence of age-related increase in central arterial stiffness in physically active women. *Arteriosclerosis, Thrombosis & Vascular Biology, 18*(1), 127–132.

U.S. Department of Health and Human Services, National Institutes of Health, National Heart, Lung and Blood Institute. (2004). *The seventh report of the Joint National Committee on Prevention, Detection, Evaluation, and Treatment of High Blood Pressure.* (NIH Publication No. 04-5230.) Retrieved from www.nhlbi.nih.gov/guidelines/hypertension/jnc7full.pdf

Vasan, R. S., Beiser, A., Seshadri, S., Larson, M. G., Kannel, W. B., D'Agostino, R. B., & Levy, D. (2002). Residual lifetime risk for developing hypertension in middle-aged women and men. The Framingham Heart Study. *Journal of the American Medical Association, 287*(8), 1003–1010.

Vasan, R. S., Larson, M. G., Leip, E. P., Evans, J. C., O'Donnell, C. J., Kannel, W. B. & Levy, D. (2001). Impact of high normal blood pressure on the risk of cardiovascular disease. *New England Journal of Medicine, 345*(18), 1291–1297.

Veria, A. J., Kshirsagar, A. V., & Hinderliter, A. L. (2008). Lifestyle modifications to lower or control high blood pressure: is advice associated with action? The behavioral risk factor surveillance survey. *Journal of Clinical Hypertension, 10*(2), 105–111.

Weinberger, M. H., Miller, J. Z., Luft, F. C., Grim, C. E., & Fineberg, N. S. (1986). Definitions and characteristics of sodium sensitivity and blood pressure resistance. *Hypertension, 8,* 127–134.

Whelton, S. P., Chin, A., Xin, X., & He, J. (2002). Effect of aerobic exercise on blood pressure: a meta-analysis of randomized, controlled trials. *Annals of Internal Medicine, 136*(7), 493–503.

World Health Organization, World Heart Federation, World Stroke Organization. (2011). Global atlas on cardiovascular disease prevention and control: policies, strategies. Geneva, Switzerland: World Health Organization.

Wright, J. M., & Musine, V. M. (2009). First-line drugs for hypertension. *Cochrane Database of Systematic Reviews, 3.* doi:10.1002/14651858.CD001841.pub2

Xin, X., He, J., Frontini, M. G., Ogden, L. G., Motsamai, O. I., & Whelton, P. K. (2001). Effects of alcohol reduction on blood pressure: a meta-analysis of randomized controlled trials. *Hypertension, 38*(5), 1112–1117.

Zhou, B., Wu, Y., Yang, J., Li, Y., Zhang, H., & Zhao, L. (2002). Overweight is an independent risk factor for cardiovascular disease in Chinese populations. *Obesity Reviews, 3*(3), 147–156.

Ischemic Heart Disease

Anderson, J. L., Adams, C. D., Antman, E. M., Bridges, C. R., Califf, R. M., Casey, D. E., Jr., . . . & ACCF/AHA Task Force Members. (2011). 2011 ACCF/AHA focused update incorporated into thr ACC/AHA 2007 guidelines for the management of patients with unstable angina/non-ST-elevation myocardial infarction: a report of the American College of Cardiology Foundation/American Heart Association Task Force on Practice Guidelines. *Circulation, 123*(18), E426–E579. doi:10.1161/CIR.0b013e318212bb8b

Braunwald, E., Antman, E. M., Beasley, J. W., Califf, R. M., Cheitlin, M. D., Hochman, J. S., . . . Smith, S. C., Jr. (2000). ACC/AHA guidelines for the management of patients with unstable angina and non ST-segment elevation myocardial infarction: executive summary and recommendations: a report of the American College of Cardiology/American Heart Association task force on practice guidelines (committee on the management of patients with unstable angina). *Circulation, 102*(10), 1193–1209. doi:10.1161/01.CIR.102.10.1193

Fraker, T. D., & Fihn, S. D. (2007). 2007 chronic angina focused update of the ACC/AHA 2002 guidelines for the management of patients with chronic stable angina: a report of the American College of Cardiology/American Heart Association Task Force on Practice Guidelines Writing Group to develop the focused update of the 2002 guidelines for the management of patients with chronic stable angina. *Circulation, 116*(23), 2762–2772.

Hillis, L. D., Smith, P. K., Anderson, J. L., Bittl, J. A., Bridges, R., Byrne, J. G., . . . Winniford, M. D. (2011). 2011 ACCF/AHA guideline for coronary artery bypass graft surgery. *Journal of the American College of Cardiology, 58*(24), 2584–2614.

Kushner, F. G, Hand, M., Smith, S. C., King, S. B., 3rd., Anderson, J. L., Antman, E. M., . . . Williams, D. O. (2009). 2009 focused updates: ACC/AHA guidelines for the management of patients with ST-elevation myocardial infarction: a report of the American College of Cardiology Foundation/American Heart Association Task Force on Practice Guidelines. *Journal of the American College of Cardiology, 54*(23), 2205–2241.

Lavie, C. J., & Milani, R. V. (2010). High dose atorvastatin in acute coronary and cerebrovascular syndromes. [Editorial.] *Journal of the American College of Cardiology, 3*(3), 340–342.

Mitchell, R. N. (2012). The heart. In V. Kumar, A. K. Abbas, & J. C. Aster (Eds.), *Basic pathology* (9th ed.). Philadelphia, PA: Saunders/Elsevier.

Roger, V. L., Go, A. S., Lloyd-Jones, D. M., Benjamin, E. J., Berry, J. D., Borden, W. B., & Bravata, D. M. (2012). AHA statistical update: heart disease and stroke statistics—2012 update. *Circulation, 125*(1), e2–e220.

Uphold, C. R., & Graham, M. V. (2003). *Clinical guidelines in family practice* (4th ed.). Barmarrae Books: Gainesville, FL.

Wright, R. S., Anderson, J. L., Adams, C. D., Bridges, C. R., Casey, D. E., Jr., Ettinger, S. M., . . . Wenger, N. K. (2011). 2011 ACCF/AHA focused update of the guidelines for the management of patients with unstable angina/non-ST-elevation myocardial infarction: a report of the American College of Cardiology Foundation/ American Heart Association Task Force on Practice Guidelines developed in collaboration with the American College of Emergency Physicians, Society for Cardiovascular Angiography and Interventions, and Society of Thoracic Surgeons. *Journal of the American College of Cardiology, 57*(19), 1920–1959.

Lung Cancer

Alberg, A. J., & Samet, J. M. (2010). Epidemiology of lung cancer. In R. J. Mason et al. (Eds.), *Murray and Nadel's textbook of respiratory medicine* (5th ed.). Philadelphia, PA: Saunders Elsevier.

Bach, P. B., Silvestri, G. A., Hanger, M., & Jett, J. R., American College of Chest Physicians. (2007). Screening for lung cancer: ACCP evidence-based clinical practice guidelines (2nd edition). *Chest, 132*(3 Suppl.), 69S–77S.

Boffa, D. J. (2011). The revised stage classification system for primary lung cancer. *Clinics in Chest Medicine, 32*(4), 741–748. doi:10.1016/j.ccm.2011.08.013

Bonanno, L., Favaretto, A., Rugge, M., Taron, M., & Rosell, R. (2011). Role of genotyping in non–small cell lung cancer treatment: current status. *Drugs, 71*(17), 2231–2234.

Cagle, P. T., & Chirieac, L. R. (2012). Advances in treatment of lung cancer with targeted therapy. *Archives of Pathology & Laboratory Medicine, 136*(5), 504–509. doi:10.5858/arpa.2011-0618-RA

Carr, L. L., Finigan, J. H., & Kern, J. A. (2011). Evaluation and treatment of patients with non–small cell lung cancer. *Medical Clinics of North America, 95*(6), 1041–1054. doi:10.1016/j.mcna.2011.08.001

Collins, L. G., Haines, C., Perkel, R., & Enck, R. E. (2007). Lung cancer: diagnosis and management. *American Family Physician, 75*(1), 56–63.

Edge, S. B., Byrd, D. R., Compton, C. C., Fritz, A. G., Greene, F. L., & Trotti, A. (Eds.). (2010). *AJCC cancer staging manual* (7th ed.). New York City, NY: Springer.

Gettinger, S., & Lynch, T. (2011). A decade of advances in treatment for advanced non–small cell lung cancer. *Clinics in Chest Medicine, 32*(4), 839–851. doi:10.1016/j.ccm.2011.08.017

Gray, J., Mao, J. T., Szabo, E., Kelley, M., Kurie, J., & Bepler, G. (2007). Lung cancer chemoprevention: ACCP evidence-based clinical practice guidelines (2nd edition). *Chest, 132*(3 Suppl.), 56S–68S.

Hosgood H. D. III, Boffetta, P., Greenland, S., Yuan-Chin, A. L., McLaughlin, J., Seow, A., . . . Lan, Q. (2010). In-home coal and wood use and lung cancer risk: a pooled analysis of the International Lung Cancer Consortium. *Environmental Health Perspectives, 118*(12), 1743–1747. doi:10.1289/ehp.1002217

Howlader, N., Noone, A. M., Krapcho, M., Neyman, N., Aminou, R., Altekruse, S. F., . . . Cronin, K. A. (Eds.). (2012). *SEER cancer statistics review, 1975–2009* (vintage 2009 populations). Bethesda, MD: National Cancer Institute. Retrieved from http://seer.cancer.gov/csr/1975_2009_pops09

Manser, R., Wright, G., Hart, D., Byrnes, G., Campbell, D., & Manser, R. (2009). Surgery for early stage non–small cell lung cancer (Cochrane Review). Retrieved from *The Cochrane Library*, Issue 2.

Massion, P. P., & Carbone, D. P. (2010). Biology of non–small cell lung cancer. In R. J. Mason et al. (Eds.), *Murray and Nadel's textbook of respiratory medicine* (5th ed.). Philadelphia, PA: Saunders Elsevier.

Midthun, D. E. (2012a). Overview of the initial evaluation, treatment and prognosis of lung cancer. *UpToDate*. Retrieved from www.uptodate.com

Midthun, D. E. (2012b). Overview of the risk factors, pathology, and clinical manifestations of lung cancer. *UpToDate*. Retrieved from www.uptodate.com

National Cancer Institute Fact Sheet. (2012). Radon and cancer. Retrieved from www.cancer.gov/cancertopics/factsheet/Risk/radon

National Cancer Institute SEER Stat Fact Sheets. (n.d.). Lung and bronchus. Retrieved from http://seer.cancer.gov/statfacts/html/lungb.html

National Comprehensive Cancer Network guidelines for non–small cell lung cancer. (2011). Retrieved September 25, 2009, from www.nccn.org

NCCN guidelines version 1.2013. Lung cancer screening. (2011). Retrieved from www.nccn.org/professionals/physician_gls/pdf/lung_screening.pdf

Neal, J. W., Gubens, M. A., & Wakelee, H. A. (2011). Current management of small cell lung cancer. *Clinics in Chest Medicine, 32*(4), 853–863. doi:10.1016/j.ccm.2011.07.002

Pijls-Johannesma, M., De Ruysscher, D. K. M., Lambin, P., Rutten, I., & Vansteenkiste, J. F. (2009). Early versus late chest radiotherapy in patients with limited stage small cell lung cancer (Cochrane Review). In *The Cochrane Library*, Issue 2.

Quoix, E. (2011). Optimal pharmacotherapeutic strategies for elderly patients with advanced non–small cell lung cancer. *Drugs & Aging, 28*(11), 885–894.

Rowell, N. P., Gleeson, F. V., & Rowell, N. (2008). Steroids, radiotherapy, chemotherapy and stents for superior vena caval obstruction in carcinoma of the bronchus (Cochrane Review). In *The Cochrane Library*, Issue 2.

Silvestri, G. A., & Jett, J. R. (2010). Clinical aspects of lung cancer. In R. J. Mason et al. (Eds.), *Murray and Nadel's textbook of respiratory medicine* (5th ed.). Philadelphia, PA: Saunders Elsevier.

Spiro, S. G., Gould, M. K., & Colice, G. L. (2007). Initial evaluation of the patient with lung cancer: symptoms, signs, laboratory tests, and paraneoplastic syndromes: ACCP evidence-based clinical practice guidelines (2nd edition). *Chest, 132*(3 Suppl.), 149S–160S.

Stewart, L. (2009). Chemotherapy for non–small cell lung cancer (Cochrane Review). In *The Cochrane Library*, Issue 2. Summary accessed at www.medscape.org/viewarticle/753395

Myocardial Infarction

Alpert, J. (2010). Managing myocardial infarction in the elderly: what should the clinician do? *American Journal of Medicine, 123*(11), 969.

Arnold, S. V., Alexander, K. P., Masoudi, F. A., Ho, P. M., Xiao, L., & Spertus, J. A. (2009). The effect of age on functional and mortality outcomes after acute myocardial infarction. *Journal of the American Geriatrics Society, 57*(2), 209–217.

Aronow, W. (2008). Optimal medical therapy after MI in the elderly. *Geriatrics, 63*(1), 24–30.

Centers for Disease Control and Prevention. (2007). Prevalence of heart disease—United States (2005). *Morbidity and Mortality Weekly Report, 56*(06), 113–118.

Crane, P. B., Oles, K., & Kennedy-Malone, L. (2006). Beta blocker medication usage in older women after myocardial infarction. *Journal of the American Academy of Nurse Practitioners, 18*(10), 463–470.

Davi, G., & Patrono, C. (2007). Platelet activation and atherothrombosis. *New England Journal of Medicine, 357*, 2482–2494.

de Lemos, J. A., Drazner, M. H., Omland, T., Ayers, C. R., Khera, A., Rohatgi, A., . . . McGuire, D. K. (2010). Association of troponin T detected with a highly sensitive assay and cardiac structure and mortality risk in the general population. *Journal of the American Medical Association, 304*(22), 2503–2512.

de Ruijter, W., Westendorp, R., Macfarlane, P., Jukema, J., Assendelft, W., & Gussekloo, J. (2007). The routine electrocardiogram for cardiovascular risk stratification in old age: the Lieden 85-Plus study. *Journal of the American Geriatrics Society, 55*(6), 872–877.

Data on acute coronary syndrome described by A. Docherty et al. Docherty, A. (2010). *Aging & Elder Health Week*, p. 346.

Heart attack: Research from Duke Clinical Research Institute provides new data about heart attack. (2010, October). *Obesity, Fitness & Wellness Week*, p. 2035.

Khot, U. N., Khot, M. B., Bajzer, C. T., Sapp, S. K., Ohman, E. M., Brener, S. J., . . . Topol, E. J. (2003). Prevalence of conventional risk factors in patients with coronary heart disease. *Journal of the American Medical Association, 290*(7), 898–904.

Krumholz, H. A. (2006). ACC/AHA clinical performance measures for adults with ST-elevation and non-ST elevation myocardial infarction: a report of the American College of Cardiology/American Heart Association Task Force on Performance Measures. *Circulation, 113*(5), 732–761.

Kushner, F. H., Hand, M., Smith, S. C., Jr., King S. B. III, Anderson, J. L., Antman, E. M., . . . Williams, D. O. (2009). 2009 focused updates: ACC/AHA guidelines for the management of patients with ST-elevation myocardial infarction (updating the 2004 guidelines and 2007 focused update) and ACC/AGA/SCAI guidelines on percutaneous coronary intervention. *Circulation, 120*(22), 2271–2306.

Kyriakides, Z., Kourouklis, S., & Kontaras, K. (2007). Acute coronary syndromes in the elderly. *Drugs & Aging, 24*(11), 901–912.

Lambert, L., Brown, K., Segal, E., Brophy, J., Rodes-Cabau, J., & Bogaty, M. (2010). Association between timeliness of reperfusion therapy and clinical outcomes in ST-elevation myocardial infarction. *Journal of the American Medical Association, 303*(21), 2148–2155.

Maroo, B. P., Lavie, C. J., & Milani, R. V. (2008). Secondary prevention of coronary heart disease in elderly patients following myocardial infarction. *Drugs & Aging, 25*(8), 649–664.

McPhee, S. J., & Papadakis, M. A. (2008). *Current medical diagnosis and treatment* (47th ed.). New York City, NY: McGraw-Hill.

Mehta, R. R. (2006). Recent trends in the care of patients with non-ST-segment elevation acute coronary syndromes: insights from the CRUSADE initiation. *Archives of Internal Medicine, 166*(18), 2027–2034.

Modern Medicine Network (2010). Heart disease trends: women are looking more like men. *Healthcare Traveler, 17*(10), 35–37.

Morse, M., Todd, J., & Stouffer, G. (2009). Optimizing the use of thrombolytics in ST-segment elevation myocardial infarction. *Drugs, 69*(14), 1945–1966.

Nathan, S. (2010). Management on non-ST-segment elevation acute coronary syndromes. *American Journal of Health-System Pharmacy, 67*(Suppl. 7), S3–S6.

O'Connor, R. E., Bossaert, L., Arntz, H. E., Brooks, S. C., Diercks, D., Fietosa-Filho, G., . . . Woolfree, K. (2010). Part 9: acute coronary syndromes: 2010 international consensus on cardiopulmonary resuscitation and emergency cardiovascular care science with treatment. *Circulation, 122*(16 Suppl. 2), S422–S465.

O'Rourke, M. F., & Hashimoto, J. (2007). Mechanical factors in arterial aging: a clinical perspective. *Journal of the American College of Cardiology, 50*(1), 1–13.

Saenger, A. K. (2010). A tale of two biomarkers: the use of troponin and CK-MB in contemporary practice. *Clinical Laboratory Science, 134*(23), 134–140.

Shishehbor, M. H., Bhatt, D. L., & Topol, E. J. (2003). Using C-reactive protein to assess cardiovascular disease risk. *Cleveland Clinical Journal of Medicine, 70*(7), 634–640.

Sonel, A. F., Good, C. B., Mulgund, J., Roe, M. T., Gibler, W. B., Smith, S. C., Jr., . . . Peterson, E. D. (for the CRUSADE Investigators). (2005). Racial variations in treatment and outcomes of black and white patients with high-risk non–ST-elevation acute coronary syndromes: insights from CRUSADE (can rapid risk stratification of unstable angina patients suppress adverse outcomes with early implementation of the ACC/AHA guidelines?). *Circulation, 111*(10), 1225–1232.

Spinler, S. A. (2010). Oral antiplatelet therapy after acute coronary syndrome and percutaneous coronary intervention: balancing efficacy and bleeding risk. *American Journal of Health-System Pharmacy, 67*(15), S7–S17.

Thygesen, K., Alpert, J. S., & White, H. D., Joint ESC/ACCF/AHA/WHF Task Force for the Redefinition of Myocardial Infarction. (2007). Universal definition of myocardial infarction. *Journal of the American College of Cardiology, 50*(22), 2173–2195.

Tullmann, D., Haugh, K., Dracup, K., & Bourguignon, C. (2007). A randomized controlled trial to reduce delay in older adults seeking help for symptoms of acute myocardial infarction. *Research in Nursing & Health, 30*(5), 485–497.

Venkatesan, S. (2008). Expressions in cardiology: is the terminology of "Non-q MI" obsolete or still relevant? Retrieved from http://drsvenkatesan.wordpress.com/2008/10/19/is-the-terminology-of-non-q-mi-is-obsolete-or-still-relevent

Wiener, R. S., Wiener, D. C., & Larson, R. J. (2008). Benefits and risks of tight glucose control in critically ill adults: a meta-analysis. *Journal of the American Medical Association, 300*(8), 933–944.

Pneumonia

American Thoracic Society Documents. (2005). Guidelines for the management of adults with hospital-acquired, ventilator-associated, and healthcare-associated pneumonia. *American Journal of Respiratory and Critical Care Medicine, 171*(4), 388–416. Retrieved from www.thoracic.org/statements/resources/mtpi/guide1-29.pdf

Augustyn, B. (2007). Ventilator-associated pneumonia: risk factors and prevention. *Critical Care Nurse, 27*(4), 32–39.

Bartlett, J. G. (2012a). Aspiration pneumonia in adults. *UpToDate.* Retrieved from http://www.uptodate.com

Bartlett, J. G. (2012b). Diagnostic approach to community-acquired pneumonia in adults. *UpToDate.* Retrieved from http://www.uptodate.com

Bartlett, J. G., Dowell, S. F., Mandell, L. A., File, T. M., Jr., Musher, D. M., & Fine, M. J. (2000). Practice guidelines for the management of community-acquired pneumonia in adults. Infectious Diseases Society of America. *Clinical Infectious Diseases, 31*(2), 347–382.

Bruns, A. H. W., Oosterheert, J. J., Prokop, M., Lammers, J.-W. J., Hak, E., & Hoepelman, A. I. M. (2007). Patterns of resolution of chest radiograph abnormalities in adults hospitalized with severe community-acquired pneumonia. *Clinical Infectious Diseases, 45*(8), 983–991.

Chastre, J., & Luyt, C.-E. (2010). Ventilator-associated pneumonia. In R. J. Mason et al. (Eds.), *Murray and Nadel's textbook of respiratory medicine* (5th ed.). Philadelphia, PA: Saunders Elsevier.

Craven, D. E., Hudcova, J., & Lei, Y. (2011). Diagnosis of ventilator-associated respiratory infections (VARI): microbiologic clues for tracheobronchitis (VAT) and pneumonia (VAP). *Clinics in Chest Medicine, 32*(3), 547–557. doi: 10.1016/j.ccm.2011.06.001

Detterline, S. A. (2010). Pneumonia (adult overview). *Essential Evidence.* Retrieved from http://essentialevidenceplus.com

Donowitz, G. R., & Cox, H. L. (2007). Bacterial community-acquired pneumonia in older patients. *Clinics in Geriatric Medicine, 23*(3), 515–534.

Donowitz, G. R. (2010). Acute pneumonia. In G. E. Mandell, J. E. Bennett, & R. Dolin (Eds.), *Mandell, Douglas, and Bennett's principles and practice of infectious diseases* (7th ed., pp. 891–916). Philadelphia, PA: Churchill-Livingstone/Elsevier.

Ferri, F. F. (2012). Bacterial pneumonia. In F. F. Ferri (Ed.), *Ferri's Clinical Advisor 2013* (1st ed.). Philadelphia, PA: Mosby/Elsevier.

File, T. M. (2011a). Treatment of community-acquired pneumonia in adults in the outpatient setting. *UpToDate.* Retrieved from http://www.uptodate.com

File, T. M. (2011b). Treatment of community-acquired pneumonia in adults who require hospitalization. *UpToDate.* Retrieved from http://www.uptodate.com

File, T. M. (2012). Treatment of hospital-acquired, ventilator-associated, and healthcare-associated pneumonia in adults. *UpToDate.* Retrieved from http://www.uptodate.com

Fine, M. J., Auble, T. E., Yealy, D. M., Hanusa, B. H., Weissfeld, L. A., Singer, D. E., . . . Kapoor, W. N. (1997). A prediction rule to identify low-risk patients with community-acquired pneumonia. *New England Journal of Medicine, 336*(4), 243–250.

Institute for Clinical Systems Improvement. (2011). *Prevention of ventilator-associated pneumonia. Health care protocol.* Bloomington, MN: Institute for Clinical Systems Improvement.

Mandell, L. A., Wunderink, R. G., Anzueto, A., Bartlett, J. G., Campbell, G. D., Dean, N. C., . . . Whitney, C. G. (2007). Infectious Diseases Society of America/American Thoracic Society consensus guidelines on the management of community-acquired pneumonia in adults. *Clinical Infectious Diseases, 44*(Suppl. 2), S27–S72. doi:10.1086/511159

Marrie, T. J., & Tuomanen, E. I. (2012). Pneumococcal pneumonia in adults. *UpToDate.* Retrieved from http://www.uptodate.com

Nair, G. B., & Niederman, M. S. (2011). Community-acquired pneumonia: an unfinished battle. *Medical Clinics of North America, 95*(6), 1143–1161. doi:10.1016/j.mcna.2011.08.007

Niederman, M. S., Craven, D. E., Bonten, M. J., & American Thoracic Society and Infectious Diseases Society of America (ATS/IDSA). (2005). Guidelines for the management of adults with hospital-acquired, ventilator-associated, and healthcare-associated pneumonia. *American Journal of Respiratory and Critical Care Medicine, 171*(4), 388–416.

Sordé, R., Falcó, V., Lowak, M., Domingo, E., Ferrer, A., Burgos, J., . . . Pahissa, A. (2011). Current and potential usefulness of pneumococcal urinary antigen detection in hospitalized patients with community-acquired pneumonia to guide antimicrobial therapy. *Archives of Internal Medicine, 171*(2), 166–172. doi:10.1001/archinternmed.2010.347

Tang, K. L., Eurich, D. T., Minhas-Sandhu, J. K., Marrie, T. J., & Majumdar, S. R. (2011). Incidence, correlates, and chest radiographic yield of new lung cancer diagnosis in 3398 patients with pneumonia. *Archives of Internal Medicine, 171*(13), 1193–1198. doi:10.1001/archinternmed.2011.155

Watkins, R. R., & Lemonovich, T. L. (2011). Diagnosis and management of community-acquired pneumonia in adults. *American Family Physician, 83*(11), 1299–1306.

Yealy, D. M. (2011). Community-acquired pneumonia in adults: risk stratification and the decision to admit. *UpToDate.* Retrieved from http://www.uptodate.com

Pulmonary Embolism

Bettmann, M. A., Baginski, S. G., White, R. D., Woodard, P. K., Abbara, S., Atalay, M. K., . . . Expert Panel on Cardiac Imaging. (2012). ACR Appropriateness Criteria® acute chest pain—suspected pulmonary embolism. *Journal of Thoracic Imaging, 27*(2), W28–W31.

Goldhaber, S. Z., & Bounameaux, H. (2012). Pulmonary embolism and deep vein thrombosis. *Lancet, 379*(9828), 1835–1846.

Gurza, E. J. (2011). Pulmonary embolism. *Essential Evidence Plus*

Gutterman, D. D., & Schünemann, H. J. (for the American College of Chest Physicians Antithrombotic Therapy and Prevention of Thrombosis Panel). (2012). Executive summary. Antithrombotic therapy and prevention of thrombosis, 9th ed: American College of Chest Physicians evidence-based clinical practice guidelines. *Chest, 141*(2 Suppl.), 7S–47S.

Guyatt, G. H., Akl, E. A., & Crowther, M. (2010). Deep venous thrombosis–pulmonary embolism. In P. E. Marik (Ed.), *Handbook of evidence-based critical care* (2nd ed., pp. 245–252). New York City, NY: Springer.

Guyatt, G. H., Akl, E. A., Crowther, M., Gutterman, D. D., Schunemann, H. J. (for the American College of Chest Physicians Antithrombotic Therapy and Prevention of Thrombosis Panel). (2012). Executive summary: antithrombotic therapy and prevention of thrombosis, 9th ed.: American College of Chest Physicians evidence-based clinical practice guidelines. *Chest, 141*(2 Suppl.), S7–S47.

Holbrook, A., Schulman, S., Witt, D. M., Vandvik, P. O., Fish, J., Kovacs, M. J., . . . Guyatt, G. H. (2012). Evidence-based management of anticoagulant therapy antithrombotic therapy and prevention of thrombosis, 9th ed: American College of Chest

Physicians evidence-based clinical practice guidelines. *Chest, 141*(2 Suppl.), e152S–e184S.

Hunt, J. M., & Bull, T. M. (2011). Clinical review of pulmonary embolism: diagnosis, prognosis, and treatment. *Medical Clinics of North America, 95*(6), 1203–1222. doi:10.1016/j.mcna.2011.08.003

Jankowich, M. D., & Ferri, F. F. (2012). Pulmonary embolism. In F.F. Ferri (Ed.), *Ferri's Clinical Advisor 2013* (1st ed.). Philadelphia, PA: Mosby/Elsevier.

Kearon, C., Akl, E. A., Comerota, A. J., Prandoni, P., Bounameaux, H., Goldhaber, S. Z., . . . Kahn, S. R. (2012). Antithrombotic therapy for VTE disease: antithrombotic therapy and prevention of thrombosis, 9th ed: American College of Chest Physicians evidence-based clinical practice guidelines. *Chest, 141*(2 Suppl.), e419S–e494S.

Le Gal, G., Righini, M., Roy, P.-M., Sanchez, O., Aujesky, D., Bounameaux, H., & Perrier, A. (2006). Prediction of pulmonary embolism in the emergency department: the revised Geneva Score. *Annals of Internal Medicine, 144*(3), 165–171.

Le Gal, G., Testuz, A., Righini, M., Bounameaux, H., & Perrier, A. (2005). Reproduction of chest pain by palpation: diagnostic accuracy in suspected pulmonary embolism. *British Medical Journal, 330*(7489), 452–453.

Meyer, G., Planquette, B., & Sanchez, O. (2008). Long-term outcome of pulmonary embolism. *Current Opinion in Hematology, 15*(5), 499–503.

Ouellette, D. R. (2012). Pulmonary embolism. Retrieved from http://emedicine.medscape.com/article/300901

Qaseem, A., Snow, V. Barry, P., Hornbake, E. R., Rodnick, J. E., Tobolic, T., . . . Joint American Academy of Family Physicians/American College of Physicians. (2007). Current diagnosis of venous thromboembolism in primary care: a clinical practice guideline from the American Academy of Family Physicians and the American College of Physicians. Panel on deep venous thrombosis/pulmonary embolism. *Annals of Internal Medicine, 146*(6), 454–458.

Righini, M., Le Gal, G., Perrier, A., & Bounameaux, H. (2005). The challenge of diagnosing pulmonary embolism in elderly patients: influence of age on commonly used diagnostic tests and strategies. *Journal of the American Geriatrics Society, 53*(6), 1039–1045.

Schaffer, A. C., & McKean, S. C. W. (2010). Deep vein thrombosis and pulmonary embolism. In P. P. Toth & P. E. Cannon (Eds.), *Comprehensive cardiovascular medicine in the primary care setting* (pp. 345–352). New York City, NY: Springer.

Schneider, D., Lilienfeld, D. E., & Im, W. (2006). The epidemiology of pulmonary embolism: racial contrasts in incidence and in-hospital case fatality. *Journal of the National Medical Association, 98*(12), 1967–1972.

Spurzem, J. R., & Geraci, S. A. (2010). Outpatient management of patients following pulmonary embolism. *American Journal of Medicine, 123*(11), 987–990.

Stein, P. B. (2007). *Pulmonary embolism* (2nd ed.). New York City, NY: Springer.

Stein, P. D., Beemath, A., Matta, F., Weg, J. G., Yusen, R. D., Hales, C. A., . . . Woodard, P. K. (2007). Clinical characteristics of patients with acute pulmonary embolism: Data from PIOPED II. *American Journal of Medicine, 120*(10), 871–879.

Stein, P. D., Matta, F., Musani, M. H., & Diaczok, B. (2010). Silent pulmonary embolism in patients with deep venous thrombosis: A systematic review. *American Journal of Medicine, 123*(5), 426–431.

Stein, P. D., Sostman, H. D., Bounameaux, H., Buller, H. R., Chenevert, T. L., Dalen, J. E., . . . Woodard, P. K. (2008). Challenges in the diagnosis acute pulmonary embolism. *American Journal of Medicine, 121*(7), 565–571.

Tapson, V. F. (2008). Acute pulmononary embolism. *New England Journal of Medicine, 358*(10), 1037–1052.

Tapson, V. F. (2012). Treatment of acute pulmonary embolism. *UpToDate.* Retrieved from http://www.uptodate.com

Thompson, B. T., & Hales, C. A. (2012). Overview of acute pulmonary embolism. *UpToDate.* Retrieved from http://www.uptodate.com

Valentine, K. A., & Hull, R. D. (2012). Anticoagulation in acute pulmonary embolism. *UpToDate.* Retrieved from http://www.uptodate.com

Pulmonary Tuberculosis

Basgoz, N. (2010). Clinical manifestations of pulmonary tuberculosis. *UpToDate.* Retrieved from http://www.uptodate.com

Catanzaro, A. (2010). Rapid diagnostic tests for tuberculosis. *UpToDate.* Retrieved from http://www.uptodate.com

Centers for Disease Control and Prevention. (2010). Updated guidelines for using Interferon Gamma Release Assays to detect *Mycobacterium tuberculosis* infection—United States, 2010. *MMWR Morbidity and Mortality Weekly Report, 59*(RR-5).

Centers for Disease Control and Prevention. (2011). Treatment for TB disease. Retrieved from www.cdc.gov/tb/topic/treatment/tbdisease.htm

Centers for Disease Control and Prevention. (2012). TB fact sheet. Treatment options for latent tuberculosis infection. Retrieved from www.cdc.gov/tb/publications/factsheets/treatment/LTBItreatmentoptions.htm

Centers for Disease Control and Prevention. (2012). Trends in Tuberculosis – United States, 2011. *Morbidity and Mortality Weekly Report, 61*(11);181–185.

Fort, G. G., & Mikolich, D. J. (2012). Tuberculosis, pulmonary. In F. F. Ferri (Ed.), *Ferri's Clinical Advisor 2013* (1st ed.). Philadelphia, PA: Mosby/Elsevier.

Herchline, T. E. (2012). Tuberculosis. *Medscape Reference.* Retrieved from http://emedicine.medscape.com/article/230802

Horsburgh, C. R., & Rubin, E. J. (2011). Clinical practice. Latent tuberculosis infection in the United States. *New England Journal of Medicine, 364*(15), 1441–1448.

Jacob, J. T., Mehta, A. K., & Leonard, M. K. (2009). Acute forms of tuberculosis in adults. *American Journal of Medicine, 122*(1) 12–17.

Jeong, Y. J., & Lee, K. S. (2008). Pulmonary tuberculosis: up-to-date imaging and management. *American Journal of Roentgenology, 191*(3), 834–844. doi:10.2214/AJR.07.3896

Kliiman, K., & Altraja, A. (2009). Predictors of extensively drug-resistant pulmonary tuberculosis. *Annals of Internal Medicine, 150*(11), 766–775.

Mazurek, G. H., Jereb, J., Vernon, A., LoBue, P., Goldberg, S., & Castro, K. (2010). Updated guidelines for using Interferon Gamma Release Assays to detect *Mycobacterium tuberculosis* infection—United States, 2010. *MMWR Recommendations and Reports, 59*(RR-5), 1–25.

Pai, M., & Menzies, D. (2012). Diagnosis of latent tuberculosis infection in HIV-negative adults. *UpToDate.* Retrieved from http://www.uptodate.com

Potter, B. E., & Acevedo, S. E. (2011). Tuberculosis. *Essential Evidence Plus.* Retrieved from http://www.essentialevidenceplus.com

Pratt, R. H., Winston, C. A., Kammerer, J. S., & Armstrong, L. R. (2011). Tuberculosis in older adults in the United States, 1993–2008. *Journal of the American Geriatrics Society, 59*(5), 851–857. doi:10.1111/j.1532-5415.2011.03369.x

Sterling, T. R., Villarino, M. E., Borisov, A. S., Shang, N., Gordin, F., Bliven-Sizemore, E., . . . TB Trials Consortium PREVENT TB Study Team. (2011). Three months of rifapentine and isoniazid for latent tuberculosis infection. *New England Journal of Medicine, 365*(23), 2155–2166.

World Health Organization. (2011). Global tuberculosis control 2011 report. Retrieved from www.who.int/tb/publications/global_report/en/

Restrictive Lung Disease

Alhamad, E. H., & Cosgrove, G. P. (2011). Interstitial lung disease: the initial approach. *Medical Clinics of North America, 95*(6), 1071–1093. doi:10.1016/j.mcna.2011.08.008

American Thoracic Society & European Respiratory Society. (2002). American Thoracic Society/European Respiratory Society international multidisciplinary consensus classification of the idiopathic interstitial pneumonias. *American Journal of Respiratory and Critical Care Medicine, 165*(2), 277–304.

Behr, J. (2012). Approach to the diagnosis of interstitial lung disease. *Clinics in Chest Medicine, 33*(1), 1–10. doi:10.1016/j.ccm.2011.12.002

Cerri, S., Spagnolo, P., Luppi, F., & Richeldi, L. (2012). Management of idiopathic pulmonary fibrosis. *Clinics in Chest Medicine, 33*(1), 85–94. doi:10.1016/j.ccm.2011.11.005

Davies, H. R., Richeldi, L., Walters, E. H., & Davies, H. R. (2007). Immunomodulatory agents for idiopathic pulmonary fibrosis (Cochrane review). In *The Cochrane Library 2007*, Issue 1. Chichester, UK: John Wiley & Sons.

Gulati, M. (2011). Diagnostic assessment of patients with interstitial lung disease. *Primary Care Respiratory Journal, 20*(2), 120–127.

Kanaparthi, L. K. (2012). Restrictive lung disease. In Z. Mosenifar (Ed.), *Medscape Reference: drugs, diseases, & procedures.* Retrieved from http://emedicine.medscape.com/article/301760

King, T. E. (2012). Approach to the adult with interstitial lung disease: clinical evaluation. *UpToDate.* Retrieved from http://www.uptodate.com

King, T. E., Jr., Pardo, A., & Selman, M. (2011). Idiopathic pulmonary fibrosis. *Lancet, 378*(9807), 1949–1961.

Raghu, G., Collard, H. R., Egan, J. J., Martinez, F. J., Behr, J., Brown, K. K., . . . ATS/ERS/JRS/ALAT Committee on Idiopathic Pulmonary Fibrosis. (2011). An official ATS/ERS/JRS/ALAT statement: idiopathic pulmonary fibrosis: evidence-based guidelines for diagnosis and management. *American Journal of Respiratory and Critical Care Medicine, 183*(6), 788–824. doi:10.1164/rccm.2009-040GL

Reust, C. M. (2011). Interstitial lung disease. *Essential Evidence Plus.* Retrieved from http://www.essentialevidenceplus.com

Richeldi, L., Davies, H. R., Spagnolo, P., & Luppi, F. (2010). Corticosteroids for idiopathic pulmonary fibrosis. *Cochrane Database of Systematic Reviews,* 2:CD002880.

Whelan, T. P. M. (2012). Lung transplantation for interstitial lung disease. *Clinics in Chest Medicine, 33*(1), 179–189. doi:10.1016/j.ccm.2011.12.003

Upper Respiratory Tract Infection

Chow, A. W., Benninger, M. S., Brook, I., Brozek, J. L., Goldstein, E. J., Hicks, L. A., . . . File, T. M., Jr. (2012). IDSA clinical practice guideline for acute bacterial rhinosinusitis in children and adults. *Clinical Infectious Diseases, 54*(8), e72–e112.

De Sutter, A. I. M., van Driel, M. L., Kumar, A. A., Lesslar, O., & Skrt, A. (2012). Oral antihistamine-decongestant-analgesic combinations for the common cold. (2012). Retrieved from *Cochrane Database of Systematic Reviews.* doi:10.1002/14651858.CD004976.pub3

Douglas, R. M., Hemilä, H., Chalker, E., & Treacy, B. (2007). Vitamin C for preventing and treating the common cold. *Cochrane Database of Systematic Reviews, 18*(3), CD000980.

Gill, J. M., Fleischut, P., Haas, S., Pellini, B., Crawford, A., & Nash, D. B. (2006). Use of antibiotics for adult upper respiratory infections in outpatient settings: a national ambulatory network study. *Family Medicine, 38*(5), 349–354.

High, K. P., Bradley, S. F., Gravenstein, S., Mehr, D. R., Quagliarello, V. J., Richards, C., & Yoshikawa, T. T. (2009). Clinical practice guideline for the evaluation of fever and infection in older adult residents of long-term care facilities: 2008 update by the Infectious Diseases Society of America. *Journal of the American Geriatrics Society, 57*(3), 375–394.

Hwang, P. H., & Getz, A. (2012). Acute sinusitis and rhinosinusitis in adults: treatment. *UpToDate.* Retrieved from http://www.uptodate.com

Institute for Clinical Systems Improvement. (2008). Health care guideline: diagnosis and treatment of respiratory illness in children and adults, 2008. Retrieved from www.icsi.org/guidelines_and_more/gl_os_prot/respiratory/respiratory_illness_in_children_and_adults__guideline_/respiratory_illness_in_children_and_adults__guideline__13110.html

Institute for Clinical Systems Improvement. (2011). *Diagnosis and treatment of respiratory illness in children and adults.* Bloomington, MN: Institute for Clinical Systems Improvement.

Kassel, J. C., King, D., & Spurling, G. K. (2010). Saline nasal irrigation for acute upper respiratory tract infections. *Cochrane Database of Systematic Reviews* (3):CD006821.

Khandelwal, C., Lathren, C., & Sloane, P. (2012). Ten clinical situations in long-term care for which antibiotics are often prescribed but rarely necessary. *Annals of Long-Term Care: Clinical Care and Aging, 20*(4), 23–29.

Lee, F. E., & Treanor, J. (2010). Viral infections. In R. J. Mason (Ed.), *Murray and Nadel's textbook of respiratory medicine* (5th ed.). Philadelphia, PA: Saunders Elsevier.

Linde, K., Barrett, B., Wölkart, K., Bauer, R., & Melchart, D. (2006). Echinacea for preventing and treating the common cold. *Cochrane Database of Systematic Reviews* (1):CD000530.

Marshall, I. (2006). Zinc for the common cold. *Cochrane Database of Systematic Reviews* (3):CD001364.

Matheï, C., Niclaes, L., Suetens, C., Jans, B., & Buntinx, F. (2007). Infections in residents in nursing homes. *Infectious Disease Clinics of North America, 21*(3), 761–772.

Meneghetti, A. (2012). Upper respiratory tract infection. Medscape reference. Retrieved from http://emedicine.medscape.com/article/302460

Rosenfeld, R. M., Andes, D., Bhattacharyya, N., Cheung, D., Eisenberg, S., Ganiats, T. G., . . . Witsell, D. L. (2007). Clinical practice guideline: adult sinusitis. *Otolaryngology—Head and Neck Surgery, 137*(3 Suppl.), S1–S31.

Sexton, D. J., & McClain, M. T. (2011). The common cold in adults: diagnosis and clinical features. *UpToDate.* Retrieved from http://www.uptodate.com

Spellberg, B., Blaser, M., Guidos, R. J., Boucher, H. W., Bradley, J. S., Eisenstein, B. I., . . . Infectious Diseases Society of America (IDSA). (2011). Combating antimicrobial resistance: policy recommendations to save lives. *Clinical Infectious Diseases, 52*(Suppl. 5), S397–S428.

University of Michigan Health System. (2011, August 9). *Acute rhinosinusitis in adults.* Ann Arbor, MI: University of Michigan Health System.

Wong, D. M. (2009). Common cold and acute upper respiratory tract infection. *Essential Evidence Plus.* Retrieved from http://www.essentialevidenceplus.com

Valvular Heart Disease

Adams, D. H., Rosenhek, R., & Volkmar, F. (2010). Degenerative mitral valve regurgitation: best practice revolution. *European Heart Journal, 31*(16), 1958–1967.

Aronow, W. S. (2007a). Recognition and management of aortic stenosis in the elderly. *Geriatrics, 62*(12), 23–32.

Aronow, W. S. (2007b). Valvular aortic stenosis in the elderly. *Cardiology in Review, 15*(5), 217–225.

Bekeredjian, R., & Grayburn, P. A. (2005). Valvular heart disease: aortic regurgitation. *Circulation, 112*(1), 125–134.

Bonow, R. O., Carabello, B. A., Chatterjee, K., de Leon, A. C., Jr., Faxon, D. P., Freed, M. D., . . . Shah, P. M. (2008). 2008 focused update incorporated into the ACC/AHA 2006 guidelines for the management of patients with valvular heart disease: a report of the American College of Cardiology/American Heart Association task force on practice guidelines (writing committee to revise the 1998 guidelines for the management of patients with valvular heart disease). *Journal of the American College of Cardiology, 52*(8), 676–685. doi:10.1016/j.jacc.2008.05.007

Buttaro, T. M., Trybulski, J., Bailey, P. P., & Sandberg-Cook, J. (2008). *Primary care: a collaborative practice* (3rd ed.). St. Louis, MO: Mosby-Elsevier.

Carabello, B. A. (2005). Modern management of mitral stenosis. *Circulation, 112*(3), 432–437.

Faggiano, P., Antonini-Canterin, F., Baldessin, F., Lorusso, R., D'Aloia A., & Cas, L. (2006). Epidemiology and cardiovascular risk factors of aortic stenosis. *Cardiovascular Ultrasound, 4,* 27. doi:10.1186/1476-7120-4-27

Gillinov, M. A. (2006). Is ischemic mitral regurgitation an indication for surgical repair or replacement? *Heart Failure Review, 11*(3), 231–239.

Halter, J. B., Ouslander, J. G., Tinetti, M. E., Studenski, S., High, K. P., & Asthana, S. (2009). *Hazzard's geriatric medicine and gerontology.* New York City, NY: McGraw-Hill.

Keong, K. Y., & Low, R. I. (2007). Aortic stenosis: assessment of the patient at risk. *Journal of Interventional Cardiology, 6*(20), 509–515.

Leon, M. B., Smith, C. R., Mack, M., Miller, C., Moses, J. W., Svensson, L. G., . . . Pocock, S. (2010). Transcatheter aortic valve implantation for aortic stenosis in patients who cannot undergo surgery. *New England Journal of Medicine, 363*(17), 1597–1607.

Maganti, K., Rigolin, V. H., Sarano, M. E., & Bonow, R. O. (2010). Valvular heart disease: diagnosis and management. *Mayo Clinic Proceedings: Symposium on Cardiovascular Diseases, 85*(5), 483–500.

Martínez-Sellés, M., García-Fernández, M. A., Larios, E., Moreno, M., Pinto, A., García-Robles, J. A., . . . Fernández-Avilés, F. (2009). Etiology and short-term prognosis of severe mitral regurgitation. *International Journal of Cardiovascular Imaging, 25*(2), 121–126.

Otto, C. M. (2006). Vavular aortic stenosis: disease severity and timing of intervention. *Journal of the American College of Cardiology, 11*(47), 2141–2151.

Picano, E., Pibarot, P., Lancellotti, P., Monin, J. L., & Bonow, R. O. (2009). The emerging role of exercise testing and stress echocardiography in valvular heart disease. *Journal of the American College of Cardiology, 24*(54), 2251–2260.

Pompilio, F., Francesco, A., Baldessin, F., Lorusso, R., D'Aloia, A., & DeiCas, L. (2006). Eidemiology and cardiovascular risk factors of aortic stenosis. *Cardiovascular Ultrasound, 4*(27), 1–5.

Qiu, Z., Chen, X., Xu, M., Jiang, Y., Xiao, L., Liu, L., & Wang, L. (2010). Is mitral valve repair superior to replacement for chronic ischemic mitral regurgitation with left ventricular dysfunction? *Journal of Cardiothoracic Surgery, 5*(107), 1–9.

Soriano, R. P., Fernandez, H. M., Cassel, C. K., & Leipzig, R. M. (2007). *Fundamentals of geriatric medicine.* New York City, NY: Springer.

Stout, K. K., & Verrier, E. D. (2009). Valvular heart disease: changing concepts in disease management. *Circulation, 119,* 3232–3241.

Task Force on the Management of Valvular Heart Disease of the European Society of Cardiology. (2007). Guidelines on the management of valvular heart disease. *European Heart Journal, 28,* 230–268.

Todd, B. A., & Higgins, K. (2005). Recognizing aortic and mitral valve disease. *Nursing 2005, 6*(35), 58–63.

U.S. Department of Health and Human Services, National Institutes of Health, National Heart, Lung and Blood Institute. (2005). *Report of the NHLBI working group on vavular heart disease.* Retrieved from www.nhlbi.nih.gov/meetings/workshops/valvular_wg.htm #workinggroupmembers

Vahanian, A., Alfieri, O., Andreotti, F., Antunes, M. J., Baron-Esquivias, G., Baumgartner, H., . . . European Association for Cardio-Thoracic Surgery (EACTS). (2012). Guidelines on the management of valvular heart disease (version 2012). *European Heart Journal, 33*(19), 2451–2496. doi:10.1093/eurheart/ejs109

Yeo, K. Y., & Low, R. I. (2007). Aortic stenosis: assessment of the patient at risk. *Journal of Interventional Cardiology, 6*(20), 509–515.

chapter 9

Peripheral Vascular Disorders

Catherine Ratliff and David Strider

ASSESSMENT

A comprehensive vascular assessment may be integrated into the general history and physical examination for the patient with vascular disease. A systematic head-to-toe examination, done consistently for each vascular patient, will minimize the chance of missing subtle signs related to vascular deficits.

The clinician should begin with auscultation of the carotid arteries bilaterally. Of note, cardiac murmurs will usually radiate into the carotid arteries, and an underlying bruit may not be discerned. The subclavian arteries should then be auscultated over the upper anteromedial chest area. During this phase of the examination, the jugular veins should be inspected for jugular vein distention. This can best be appreciated when the patient is lying down with the head of the bed elevated 15 degrees.

The clinician should proceed to the palpation of the brachial, radial, and ulnar arteries. Such palpation should be scored on a scale of 0 to 4 (4 = pulsatile, hyperdynamic; 3 = easily palpable with full triphasic pulse; 2 = biphasic pulse that may be a bit harder to locate initially; 1 = monophasic pulse that may come and go depending on position of fingertips; and 0 = absent pulse by palpation, which may be detected by Doppler ultrasound). All palpable pulses should be graded in the assessment and documented.

The clinician should evaluate any pain, coolness, paresthesias, motor weakness, discoloration, or tissue loss in the hands. Careful inspection of the distal fingers and the nail beds may reveal signs of end tissue malperfusion. The finger joints should be inspected for cyanosis and/or petechiae. The fingernails should be checked for clubbing, which portends chronic hypoxemia. Routinely in any patient confirmed or suspected to have vascular disease, blood pressure should be checked in both arms at this point.

The heart should then be auscultated to permit delineation of rhythm regularity, S_1, S_2, and any extrasystolic sounds such as S_3, S_4, or pericardial rub. Murmurs should be noted and classified as per the cardiac assessment guidelines. The abdomen should be auscultated for celiac artery, superior mesenteric artery, and renal artery bruits, which are best heard 4 to 8 cm above the umbilicus and 1 to 2 cm to the right and left of midline abdomen. Then the clinician should listen to the femoral artery in each groin for the presence of bruits. Following this, the abdomen should be lightly palpated just to the left of midline, approximately 4 cm above the umbilicus, to evaluate for a pulsatile abdominal aorta. In slender individuals, the abdominal aorta is often fairly easy to palpate. A hyperdynamic, pulsatile abdominal aorta in an individual may suggest aneurysmal formation. The clinician should note and document any tenderness or guarding associated with the abdominal palpation.

Once the abdominal examination is complete, the clinician should progress to the vascular assessment of the lower extremities. The femoral arteries should be palpated over the groin area and documented on the scale of 0 to 4. Any pulse deficits should be followed up with a Doppler examination. The popliteal fossa should be inspected and palpated bilaterally, in order to locate the popliteal artery and to assess for the possibility of popliteal artery aneurysms. The clinician should inspect the calves and feet for edema, skin turgor, and skin pigmentation. Thick, hyperpigmented skin in the lower calves and feet may portend chronic venous insufficiency, whereas thin, shiny, pale skin is more consistent with peripheral arterial insufficiency. The dorsalis pedis and posterior tibial pulses should be palpated. If such pulses are not noted, Doppler ultrasound should be used. Any Doppler signals should be located and identified with an indelible marker pen. At this time the heel, the medial and lateral malleoli, and the toes of each foot should be inspected for breakdown. As in the hands, any pedal pain, coolness, paresthesias, motor weakness, discoloration, or tissue loss should be documented. Dorsal and plantar flexion of the feet should be assessed and recorded with muscular strength graded on a scale of 1 to 5.

The vascular examination then turns to a careful evaluation of the cranial nerves (CNs), usually focusing on CN II to CN XII. Evaluation of pupillary light and accommodation response (CN II), following the eyes in a lateral, medial, superior, and inferior gaze (CNs III, IV, and VI), and evaluation of facial smile, scowl, and opening eyes against pressure (CNs V and VII) should be completed. Gross hearing assessment, with follow-up by Weber and Rinne testing, may ascertain any CN VIII deficits. Evaluating the tongue protrusion, uvula rise, cough reflex, gag reflex, and shoulder shrug will provide information on the integrity of CNs IX, X, XI, and XII. Document the conformation of the uvula, which may be bifid or singular (some connective tissue disorders have associated bifid uvula). Completion of the CN examination provides the health-care team with an excellent neurological baseline before interventions for carotid artery disease. Assessment findings related to vertebrobasilar insufficiency may include balance problems, dizziness, and coordination deficits.

Following the neurological examination, the clinician should ascertain any specific end organ perfusion deficits, as shown by the following signs and symptoms:

- Pain in the feet, calves, thighs, and or buttocks, either at rest or with ambulation (peripheral arterial disease [PAD])
- Any open wounds or blisters on the distal aspects of feet and/or hands (PAD or chronic venous stasis ulcers)
- Abdominal pain, nausea, vomiting, and/or diarrhea after a meal (mesenteric ischemia)
- Persistent abdominal/back pain (abdominal aortic aneurysms or dissection)
- Acute unilateral CN deficits (carotid artery disease)
- Acute balance/coordination deficits (possible vertebrobasilar malperfusion)
- Acute chest and/or back pain (after ruling out myocardial ischemia and pulmonary embolus, one needs to quickly and thoroughly evaluate the patient for thoracic aortic dissection and/or expanding aneurysm)

Once the focused vascular assessment and abbreviated history are completed, the clinician will have achieved a very sound baseline with which to guide future interventions to delineate and treat vascular lesions.

ABDOMINAL AORTIC ANEURYSM

Signal symptoms: Persistent or intermittent pain in the middle or lower abdomen, often radiating to the lower back, which is characteristic of a rapidly expanding, leaking, or ruptured abdominal aortic aneurysm (AAA). Most AAAs are asymptomatic.

Description: The abdominal aorta is the large artery that provides blood to the digestive organs, liver, kidneys, spleen, and lower extremities. It extends inferiorly from the descending aorta to the iliac arteries. An AAA is a dilation of the abdominal aorta that is 1.5 to 2 times greater than the size of the nondilated proximal or distal aorta. The AAA involves all three layers of the arterial wall.

Etiology: Most AAAs are atherosclerotic in nature; other causes include trauma, infection, and inflammation. Connective tissue disorders, such as Ehlers-Danlos syndrome and Marfan syndrome, predispose the patient to AAA formation. Most AAAs are infrarenal (65%), occurring below the renal arteries. Patients with AAAs are more likely to have arterial aneurysms in other locations such as the thoracic aorta, the common iliac arteries, the common femoral arteries, and the popliteal arteries.

Occurrence: AAAs are the 13th leading cause of death in the United States. Mortality rates for ruptured aneurysms are 70% to 90% compared with 5% operative mortality for elective open surgical repair and 2% to 3% for endovascular stent AAA exclusion.

Age: More frequent in adults over 50 years old; prevalence rate is 2% to 4%.

Gender: Onset occurs around age 50 for men and 60 for women. Incidence steadily increases with age and peaks at age 80. AAA is 5 times more likely in men than in women.

Ethnicity: There is no dominant ethnic group that develops AAA, but there is a familial history associated with AAA development.

Contributing factors: Risk factors for developing AAA include arteriosclerotic heart disease and arteriosclerotic changes of other vessels, smoking history, hypertension, chronic obstructive pulmonary disease, obesity, family history of AAA, diabetes mellitus, cystic medial necrosis, Marfan syndrome, and previous spinal cord injury (Ammash, Sundt, & Connolly, 2008; Gonzales, 2009). Other risk factors include tobacco abuse, mycotic processes, Ehlers-Danlos syndrome, aortic dissection, Takayasu's arteritis, and recent cardiac surgery (Castlemain, 2010; Mooney, et al., 2004). Aortic dissection involves a splitting apart of the aortic wall layers, such that two or more blood flow channels are created within the aorta. Acute aortic dissection may produce intimal flaps that occlude major takeoff vessels, leading to end-organ ischemia. Progressive dissection may lead to weakening of the entire aortic wall, resulting in aneurysm formation and possible rupture.

Signs and symptoms: Most patients with AAAs are asymptomatic (66% to 75%) except in the presence of dissection, rupture, or impending rupture. A pulsatile abdominal mass at or slightly above the umbilicus in the epigastrium, as noted by palpation of the abdomen, is consistent with but not conclusive for an AAA. These are easier to palpate in thin individuals; however, if noted in an obese individual, they are usually quite large. AAA should be suspected in individuals with a femoral or popliteal aneurysm, because 30% of individuals with a peripheral aneurysm also have an AAA. In patients with symptomatic AAAs, the complaints include mild-to-severe abdominal, flank, or lower back pain. Other symptoms may include nausea and vomiting, gastrointestinal bleeding, and lower extremity ischemia. Rupture is the most lethal clinical presentation, with symptoms including sudden onset of severe abdominal and back pain, hypotension, and the presence of a pulsatile, expanding mass. There is a high mortality rate associated with ruptured AAAs; therefore the possibility of ruptured AAA in the differential diagnosis should be considered in any adult patient with acute abdominal or flank pain.

Diagnostic tests: The best initial screening test is an ultrasound of the abdominal aorta. In cases where surgery is planned, angiography and computed tomography (CT) with IV contrast are indicated to size the aneurysm and diagnose any tears or perforations (Ferri, 2010).

Differential diagnosis: It is important to evaluate for and treat hypertension and heart disease, because basic and early steps in AAA management include blood pressure control and recognition or enhancement of cardiac function. An ectatic abdominal aorta without aneurysm may be palpated and confused with AAA. Other acute causes of abdominal and back pain may mimic a ruptured AAA and must be ruled out. Major imaging modalities for a patient with suspected or known AAA include abdominal ultrasound, CT, magnetic resonance angiogram (MRA), and angiogram.

Treatment: The rate of AAA growth for an individual is unpredictable. Some aneurysms may remain stable for long periods, whereas others may enlarge quickly. Medical management of an asymptomatic, small AAA should include blood pressure control, regulation of heart rate, and smoking cessation. Beta blockers have been shown to slow the long-term growth of aortic aneurysms. Angiotensin receptor blockers (ARBs), such as losartan, may also have a major role in critical blood pressure and heart rate control for patients with aortic aneurysms and/or dissections.

Initial treatment for symptomatic AAA, whether ruptured or not, involves aggressive blood pressure control. Mean arterial pressure should be maintained between 60 and 70 mm Hg, and systolic blood pressure should be kept between 100 and 120 mm Hg. Arterial pressure monitoring is recommended, and IV antihypertensive agents, such as esmolol, nicardipine, nitroprusside, labetalol, and/or nitroglycerin, should be used to rapidly and consistently maintain blood pressure in these ranges. Cardiology should be consulted, and a transthoracic echocardiogram should be done to assess heart function. If the patient is to be medically managed, transition to oral antihypertensive agents should begin, using beta blockers, calcium channel blockers, clonidine, ARBs, and labetalol as needed to maintain very tight blood pressure control.

The two invasive options for excluding an AAA when it becomes symptomatic or becomes more than 5 cm in diameter include open surgical repair and endovascular repair. Elective operative repair has a mortality rate of

2% to 5%. Urgent repair (where cardiac and other known risk factors have not been optimized) of an intact symptomatic AAA has a mortality rate of 15% to 20% (National Quality Measures Clearinghouse, 2008a, 2008b). In emergent repair in which the AAA has ruptured, there is a 50% mortality rate in patients who reach the hospital. Average postoperative length of stay for an elective AAA surgical repair is 5 days. The major cause of death after AAA repair is myocardial infarction. Other complications include renal failure, limb ischemia, ischemic colitis, hemorrhage, pneumonia with prolonged ventilator dependence, and paraplegia.

Endovascular grafts are a more recent addition to the treatment modalities for elective AAA repair. The graft is deployed through the femoral or the iliac artery. Not all AAAs are anatomically appropriate for stenting. Experimental AAA stent trials began in 1993 in the United States. Current success rates are higher than 90% with a mortality rate of less than 2% (Karnwal, Lippman, Julka, & White, 2009; National Quality Measures Clearinghouse, 2009). Most patients are discharged from the hospital in 1 to 2 days. Complications after endovascular treatment include arterial injury at site of access, arterial embolization, endoleak (blood flow outside the lumen of the graft but within the original aneurysmal sac), post-implant syndrome (back pain and fever without elevated white blood cell count or other signs of infection), and graft limb distal thrombosis.

Follow-up: Initial management of patients with small aneurysms (fewer than 4 cm) should include serial evaluation with ultrasound every 3 to 6 months. Any symptomatic AAA or any asymptomatic AAA larger than 5 cm in diameter should be repaired using either open surgical or endovascular technique.

Sequelae: The most common complication of AAA is rupture. Infrequent complications are thrombi to the lower extremities and preexisting infection of the aneurysm (referred to as a mycotic aneurysm), with *Salmonella* and *Staphylococcus aureus* being the most commonly identified organisms. Fungal infections of the aorta pose significant challenges and require long-term IV antimycotics, such as fluconazole after 6 weeks of an IV course of antifungal agents, until a definitive surgical repair is done.

Prevention/prophylaxis: Because most AAAs are atherosclerotic in nature, the same long-term preventive measures for reducing coronary artery disease should be applied. These include lifestyle modification, control of hypertension, beta blockade and/or ARB therapy, statin therapy, daily aspirin, and maintenance of euglycemia if diabetic (Cooper, King, & Earnshaw, 2009). Early abdominal ultrasonographic screening is recommended for first-degree relatives of individuals who already have been diagnosed with an AAA (Brannstrom, Bjorck, Strandberg, & Wanhainen, 2009; National Quality Measures Clearinghouse, 2007). The prevalence of AAA in the first-degree relatives of affected families is reported to be 15% to 33%. Large studies in Western Europe and North America support the selective ultrasonographic screening of men over age 65 for AAA and all women and men over the age of 50 if a first-degree relative has been diagnosed with an AAA (Alund, Mani, & Wanhainen, 2008; Bertero, Carlsson, & Lundgren, 2010; Bonamigo & Siqueira, 2003; Eckstein et al., 2009; Ehlers, Sorensen, Jensen, Bech, & Kjolby, 2008; National Quality Measures Clearinghouse, 2005; Ogata et al., 2006).

Referral: Referral to a vascular surgeon is essential for all patients with symptomatic AAAs. Furthermore, any patient with a known AAA, even if not symptomatic, should be screened with serial ultrasound imaging at least once a year (Birkmeyer & Upchurch,, 2007).

Education: Patients and their families should be taught the importance of follow-up; ways to manage hypertension, hypercholesterolemia, smoking, and other risk factors; and the signs and symptoms that should be reported to the physician immediately (sudden onset of abdominal or back pain, dizziness). The risks of operative versus nonoperative treatment should be explained thoroughly to the patient and his or her family.

CHRONIC LYMPHEDEMA

Signal symptoms: Swelling of the affected body part, usually the limb, because of impaired flow of lymph fluid.

Etiology: Lymphedema is swelling caused by impaired lymph transport, which results in an accumulation or pooling of protein-rich fluid in the interstitial space. Lymphedema is most commonly caused by surgery, radiation, or infection that damages the lymphatic system.

Occurrence: Lymphedema may be classified as primary (idiopathic) or secondary (acquired). Primary lymphedema is congenital, and it affects 1 to 2 million individuals in the United States. Secondary lymphedema affects 2 to 3 million individuals in the United States (Choi & Hector, 2012; Werchek, 2010). One of the most common causes of secondary lymphedema in the United States is related to treatment of cancer.

Age: Age has not been confirmed as a risk factor for lymphedema.

Gender: With primary or congenital lymphedema, females are affected twice as often as males. With secondary lymphedema in the United States, females may be affected more often, but that is because a common cause of secondary lymphedema is breast cancer, which is primarily a woman's disease.

Ethnicity: Ethnicity has not been shown to be a risk factor for lymphedema.

Contributing factors: Patients with a history of breast cancer with axillary node dissection or radiation, groin node dissection or radiation, and a postoperative infection have an increased risk for developing lymphedema.

Signs and symptoms: Swelling or edema is the characteristic symptom of lymphedema. Additional symptoms may include heaviness or tightness, aching and fatigue in the affected limb, restricted range of motion, recurring cellulitis in the affected extremity, and hardening and thickening of the skin. The Stemmer sign (or Kaposi-Stemmer's sign) is another clinical indication of lymphedema in which one is unable to pinch a fold of skin at the base of the second toe on the dorsal aspect of the foot or between the second and third finger. Skin that does not fold up into a pinch is considered a positive sign of lymphedema (Rasmussen et al., 2008; Sarvis, 2003).

Diagnostic tests: Diagnosis of lymphedema is typically made through clinical presentation and medical history such as a cancer diagnosis. Lymphoscintigraphy is the imaging gold standard for lymphedema (Ernst & Stanley, 2001; Lewis & Walsh, 2007; Rasmussen et al., 2008).

Differential diagnosis: Knowing if the patient had a prior history of comorbid conditions that can cause swelling of the extremities, such as cardiac disease, venous ulcer disease, renal disease, hepatic disease, trauma, and infection, is also important. Patients with rheumatoid arthritis, obesity, lipedema, and venous ulcer disease are at greater risk for lymphedema, because these conditions add additional stress to the impaired lymphatics. Lymph nodes are located around most joints, so patients undergoing such surgical procedures as total knee replacements may be at greater risk for developing lymphedema, because lymph nodes can become injured during the surgery. Also procedures such as vein stripping can exacerbate mild lymphedema (Lewis & Walsh, 2007).

Treatment: Complete decongestive physiotherapy (CDP) is the gold standard for lymphedema management. CDP is a specialized massage technique designed to stimulate the lymph vessels, break up subcutaneous fibrous tissue, and redirect the lymph fluid to areas where lymph flow is normal. It involves four steps: manual lymph drainage (MLD), compression bandaging, exercises, and skin care.

Conservative treatment: The use of multilayer compression bandages and/or compression stockings is an important component for all patients with lymphedema to prevent the reaccumulation of lymph fluid in the limb.

Pharmacological treatment: Diuretics are not beneficial with lymphedema, because they draw off excess water in the interstitial spaces but not the protein. Lymphedema is a high-protein edema, and the high osmotic pressure from the increased protein in the interstitial space causes rapid reaccumulation of edema. In addition, the higher concentration of protein in the edema fluid causes increased fibrosis and induration of the skin. Diuretics are not contraindicated for the treatment of other conditions in lymphedema patients, but they should not be used as primary treatment for lymphedema.

Surgical treatment: Surgery is reserved for individuals with a positive lymphoscintigram who do not respond to more conservative methods such as CDP. Reconstructive or restorative procedures create lymphvenous shunts or autologous vessel transplantations. Debulking procedures remove excess tissue to reduce the size and weight of the limb (Lewis & Walsh, 2007; Rasmussen et al., 2008).

Follow-up: Patients with lymphedema need regular follow-up by health-care providers to make sure that the CDP is effective and adequate, and if not, appropriate modifications can then be made to the care plan.

Sequelae: Lymphangitis and cellulitis are complications seen with lymphedema. Once patients develop these infections, they are at greater risk for developing them again.

Prevention/prophylaxis: Lifelong CDP is essential to prevent worsening of the lymphedema and to avoid complications.

Referral: Patients with lymphedema should be referred to a lymphedema specialist.

Education: It is important to teach patients with lymphedema about the disease process, its lifelong treatment with compression bandaging, the importance of avoiding complications such as lymphangitis, and about resources, such as the National Lymphedema Network, that are available to them.

PERIPHERAL VASCULAR DISEASE

Signal symptoms: Pain, intermittent claudication of the feet, tissue loss in affected leg/arm.

Description: Peripheral vascular disease (PVD) refers to a disease or process that alters blood flow to or from the extremities and vital organs other than the heart. These processes may involve the arterial, venous, or lymphatic systems but most often are due to enlarging atherosclerotic plaques in the distal aorta or in major bifurcations or areas of angulation in the iliac, femoral, and popliteal arteries. Most activity limitations and limb loss are associated with PAD.

Etiology: Atherosclerotic plaques may be fatty streaks, fibrous plaques, or complicated calcified lesions. Fatty streaks are early lesions that occur in the intima of arteries. Fibrous plaques and areas of intimal thickening are the most frequently occurring type of lesion. Complicated (heterogeneous) plaques as well as calcified fibrous plaques with potential for necrosis and thrombosis are associated most often with symptoms in PAD patients.

Occurrence: PAD is referred to as an age-related disease. More diabetics than nondiabetics are diagnosed with PAD. Nearly 30% of older adults in the general population have PAD. This percentage is expected to increase as the number of elderly individuals in the population increases.

Age: Nearly 20% of individuals who are more than 70 years old have PAD compared with less than 8% of individuals who are younger than 70.

Gender: Symptomatic PAD is 2 to 5 times more prevalent in men than in women.

Ethnicity: There are few available data to support an ethnic predisposition for the development of PAD.

Contributing factors: Smoking remains the most important risk factor, with up to 80% of cases of intermittent claudication associated with tobacco use. Diabetes mellitus is another important risk factor; more than 80% of diabetics surviving 20 years from the time of diagnosis have some type of arterial disease. Of patients with a gangrenous lesion of the feet requiring amputation, more than 50% are diabetic. Other associated risk factors include hypertension, high serum cholesterol, obesity, sedentary lifestyle, strong family history, vasculitis, and hypercoagulopathy.

Signs and symptoms: Intermittent claudication is the early symptom of PAD. It is described as a painful cramping of the muscles of the leg during walking. It goes away when the patient stops walking and resumes after the patient starts walking again. It also may be described as a sensation of tiredness or fatigue. One-third of patients with proven arterial stenosis report symptoms of claudication. Ischemic rest pain occurs constantly and is differentiated easily from claudication. It is described as a burning sensation and localizes to the metatarsal heads or to an ischemic ulcer. Pain is often worse at night when the leg is elevated. Relief may occur with dependency of the foot. Ischemic rest pain requires immediate attention. Ulceration or gangrene develops at an area of external pressure or at the site of a minor injury, with gangrene representing the end-stage of PAD. Acute arterial ischemia results from arterial thrombosis, embolism, or trauma, with symptoms that are sudden in onset. It often causes the five Ps: *pain, pallor, pulselessness, paresthesia,* and *paralysis.* Other symptoms may include decreased sensation and mottling of the extremity. Acute arterial ischemia may be due to thrombus from the left atrium, sudden onset of atrial fibrillation, dislodging of calcium plaque in the aorta, and/or intrinsic hypercoagulopathy. A thorough patient history and physical examination are essential to determine the stage and type of vascular disease.

Diagnostic tests: Ankle-brachial index and systolic arterial pressure measurement with continuous-wave Doppler are first-line tests. In cases where surgical intervention is being considered, angiography is indicated. Assessment of distal arterial system patency can be done by Doppler ultrasound, which can also detect and pinpoint occluded areas (Ferri, 2010).

Differential diagnosis: Buerger's disease and Raynaud's phenomenon also should be considered when diagnosing PAD. Buerger's disease may occur in individuals less than 35 years old who are smokers, and it may affect the upper as well as the lower extremities. Raynaud's phenomenon affects the fingertips, the tips of the ears and nose, and the feet. Patients with Raynaud's phenomenon have symptom exacerbation with any cold temperatures. Other diagnoses that mimic the symptoms of PAD include gout, arthritis, diabetic neuropathy, sciatica, and severe venous insufficiency.

Of note, the hallmark signs and symptoms of venous stasis ulcers include distal lower extremity edema; warmth of the foot; large, irregular, copiously draining ulcers in the distal calf or foot dorsum; and hyperpigmentation of the surrounding skin. Arterial insufficiency ulcers usually are found over the medial or lateral malleolus, heel, or the distal aspect of the toes. Wounds associated with arterial ischemia are small and drain minimally but are extremely painful.

Treatment: The main goal of PAD treatment is to slow the progression of the disease. Treatment may be conservative, pharmacological, operative, or endovascular. Risk factor recognition and lifestyle modification are the central tenets for managing patients with long-term PAD.

Conservative treatment: Conservative treatment involves modification of risk factors, including smoking, blood pressure control, and diet (Hirsch et al., 2005). Smoking is the number one modifiable risk factor, and there are numerous methods available to help individuals stop smoking (Langston & Appel, 2010). In addition, managing diabetes and hyperlipidemia are key measures (Carthron, Johnson, Hubbart, Strickland, & Nance, 2010; Dancer & Courtney, 2010; Hughes, 2009; Martin, 2010). Exercise is an essential element of PAD management, because collateral vessels are strengthened and stimulated to grow with the onset of an exercise program such as walking. Formalized vascular rehabilitation programs exist; however, they are not currently recognized by insurers and rarely are reimbursed. Home exercise programs should focus on exercising 3 or more times per week for at least 30 minutes per day. Patients should be instructed to walk until pain develops, walk a few steps more through the pain, rest until pain goes away, then resume walking. Over time, the patient should be able to walk farther with fewer rest breaks. Meticulous foot care is important to prevent complications of ulceration and gangrene. Patients should be instructed about wearing properly

fitted footwear, daily inspection of feet and legs, avoidance of walking barefoot, application of lotion on feet and legs, and meticulous toenail trimming. Podiatrist consultation is recommended for patients with fungal overgrowth and/or ingrown toenails.

Pharmacological treatment: Pharmacological treatment is provided with conservative treatment. Currently, aspirin (81 to 325 mg daily) is one of the mainstays for such treatment. Aspirin has been shown to prevent progression of disease in patients with claudication. Pentoxifylline (Trental) is available for treatment of claudication; however, studies have not shown significant improvement in claudication symptoms. Vasodilators and anticoagulants have not proved effective in relieving pain symptoms. Clopidogrel (Plavix) (75 mg daily) is an antiplatelet medication that helps reduce the risk of stroke, heart attack, and other atherosclerotic problems. Clopidogrel is frequently used for at least 3 months after peripheral arterial stents have been placed. Medications for the management of hypertension, diabetes, and hyperlipidemia should be used with the goals of euglycemia, normotension, and attainment of a healthy lipid profile. Most patients with cardiovascular disease benefit significantly from a statin, a beta blocker, an aspirin, daily multivitamins with B-complex vitamins, vitamin E, and calcium supplements.

Surgical treatment: Surgical treatment of PAD involves revascularization of the affected extremity. Surgical options should be considered when pain limits the patient's lifestyle or when ulceration or gangrene is present. Surgical options involve using vein graft or synthetic graft material. Long-term patency rate is dependent on smoking cessation, exercise, antiplatelet therapy, and vigilant diabetic control as well as the location, length, and diameter of the graft.

Endovascular treatment: Endovascular options for the treatment of PVD include balloon angioplasty and endoluminal stents, which are minimally invasive for the patient. Angioplasty involves inflating a balloon across a stenotic lesion. Stents are devices that are deployed in a stenotic lesion to keep the vessel open. Other interventions include thrombolysis with fibrin-degrading infusions, mechanical thrombectomy, atherectomy, and subintimal recanalization.

Follow-up: Follow-up should include evaluating the patient's response to pharmacological intervention and the progression of risk factor modification. Pulse volume recording should be done at least once a year to assess lower extremity perfusion.

Sequelae: A history of intermittent claudication approximately doubles the risk of mortality resulting from ischemic heart disease. In patients with claudication, 25% develop worsening symptoms, and 5% require an amputation over their lifetime.

Prevention/prophylaxis: Prevention of PAD focuses on slowing the progression of disease in patients with symptoms. This can be accomplished through risk factor modification as discussed earlier. Good foot care, in conjunction with exercise, smoking cessation, glucose management if diabetic, and lipid management, can prevent the development of tissue loss or gangrene.

Referral: Referral for surgical or endovascular treatment should occur when claudication becomes disabling to the patient, when ischemic rest pain or gangrene is present, or when nonhealing ulceration is present.

Education: Education needs to focus on proper follow-up and the modification of risk factors as discussed earlier; patients also need to be taught to report any new onset of symptoms, including nonhealing ulcers. Of note, there is a need for more research on the differences between the treatment for PAD in men and in women (Gleeson & Crabbe, 2009; Lindberg, 2009; Tomczyk & Treat-Jacobson, 2009).

VENOUS DISEASE (CHRONIC VENOUS INSUFFICIENCY)

Signal symptoms: May be asymptomatic but could also present with swelling that subsides with elevation of lower extremities, eczematous skin changes, dull ache in lower extremities, and presence of varicosities.

Description: Venous leg ulcers (also known as chronic venous insufficiency ulcers, venous stasis ulcers, lower extremity venous ulcers, or varicose ulcers) are the most common leg ulceration. They typically occur over the medial malleolus but can also occur over the lateral malleolus. The ulcers are irregular and shallow with granulation tissue and fibrin present in the wound bed. Exudate is moderate to heavy, but if there is an arterial component, the amount of exudate may be decreased. These wounds are often odoriferous as well. The periwound often presents with dermatitis from the increased permeability of the venous capillaries causing protein to leak into the interstitial space, becoming irritating to the epidermis and dermis. The loss of protein and red blood cells into the subcutaneous tissue results in a brownish discoloration of the skin referred to as hemosiderin staining. Over time, the induration and hyperpigmentation is associated with fibrosis of the adipose tissue of the leg, which is called lipodermatosclerosis.

Etiology: Venous disease is caused by ambulatory venous hypertension. Normally blood flows from the superficial veins to the deep veins. Unidirectional valves and contraction of the calf muscles assist in blood flowing from the superficial to the deep veins. If there are any abnormalities (i.e., valvular incompetence, deep vein thrombosis, and/or failure of calf muscle pump), the deep and superficial veins become distended, increasing venous pressures.

Occurrence: Venous ulcers are the most common leg ulcers, accounting for 70% to 90% of all leg ulcers (Wound, Ostomy and Continence Nurses Society Conference, 2005). In the United States, there are approximately 7 million people with venous disease, and about 3 million of these will develop ulcers (Sieggreen, 2007).

Age: As one ages, the incidence of venous ulcers increases (Rasmussen et al., 2008).

Gender: Women are affected more than men, with multiple pregnancies or pregnancies close together increasing the risk.

Ethnicity: There are no data to support an ethnic predisposition to venous disease.

Contributing factors: Risk factors for venous leg ulcers include family history, varicose veins, multiple pregnancies (especially close together), thrombophilia (protein S deficiency, protein C deficiency), anticardiolipin antibody, deep vein thrombosis/phlebitis, trauma to leg, pulmonary embolus, and sedentary lifestyle. The presence of comorbid conditions, such as cardiac disease, PAD, rheumatoid arthritis, lymphedema, obesity (body mass index of more than 30 kg/m^2), smoking, and use or former use of IV drugs (e.g., heroin), can also increase the risk of venous leg ulcers (Nunnelee, 2007; Rasmussen et al., 2008; Sieggreen, 2008).

Signs and symptoms: Edema that worsens with standing and decreases with leg elevation is the classic sign of venous leg ulcers. The edema may be pitting or nonpitting. Other signs include hemosiderosis (hemosiderin staining), venous dermatitis (manifested as erythematous, scaly, pruritic skin), ankle flaring (cluster of spider veins), varicose veins, scarring from previous ulcers, and lipodermatosclerosis.

Diagnostic tests: In many cases of venous ulcers, diagnosis may be made by clinical assessment alone. Duplex ultrasonography imaging with or without color has become the standard diagnostic tool for assessing venous disease. Duplex imaging produces images of blood flow and its direction through vessels, pinpointing the anatomical site of reflux or obstruction; thickened, abnormal vein walls; and the presence and age of a thrombus. Duplex scanning can be used to calculate the superficial venous pressures and allows for quantification of venous reflux and valve closure times. An ankle-brachial pressure index is also recommended to rule out PAD, especially before application of compression therapy.

Differential diagnosis: Lower leg edema, which is one of the classic signs of venous disease, is also seen with other diseases as well. Deep vein thrombosis usually presents with pain and the presence of a thrombus on ultrasound. Patients with congestive heart failure usually present with dyspnea, orthopnea, and a decreased ejection fraction. Patients with cirrhosis will have abnormal liver functions, and those in renal failure will have proteinuria. In addition, vasculitis, pyoderma gangrenosum, or malignancies may initially present with edema (Werchek, 2010).

Treatment: Treatment for venous ulcers includes management with compression therapy, leg elevation, medications, and surgery.

Conservative treatment: Compression therapy is the gold standard for venous ulcers and is used by those with chronic venous disease to manage the edema and increase venous return. A Cochrane review found that venous ulcers heal more quickly with compression than without compression (Choi & Hector, 2012). Adherence to compression may be limited by pain, application difficulty, and physical limitations such as obesity (Rasmussen et al., 2008). Not wearing compression after the venous ulcer has healed is associated with recurrence (Marston & Criado, 2001; Rasmussen et al., 2008). Methods of compression include inelastic, elastic, and intermittent pneumatic compression. For patients with arterial disease (ankle-brachial index of more than 0.6 and of less than 0.8) with venous leg ulcers, a trial of supervised reduced compression may help decrease edema and promote ulcer healing (Choi & Hector, 2012; Nunnelee, 2007; Sieggreen, 2007). Leg elevation above the heart for 30 minutes 3 or 4 times per day when used with compression can also help reduce edema (Nunnelee, 2007).

Pharmacological treatment: Horse chestnut seed extract in a dose of 50 to 75 mg twice daily may reduce edema and pain in venous leg ulcers (Nunnelee, 2007; Sieggreen, 2007; Zuran & Mees, 2008). However, there may be interactions with certain medications, such as lithium, diabetic drugs, and anticoagulants, that might result in low blood sugars and slower blood clotting (Zuran & Mees, 2008). Aspirin may be effective when used with compression therapy with the recommended dosage of 300 mg/day as long as there are no contraindications to its use (Connelly & Lovell, 2007). Pentoxifylline (Trental) 400 mg 3 times per day has been used to treat venous ulcers. It has been shown effective when used with compression and may be beneficial as monotherapy in those patients who cannot tolerate compression (Nunnelee, 2007; Rasmussen et al., 2008). Topical steroids may provide short term improvement of venous dermatitis. Oral antibiotics are only warranted in cases of suspected cellulitis (Sieggreen, 2007).

Surgical treatment: Surgical options to treat venous disease include ablation of the saphenous vein, interruption of the perforating veins with subfascial endoscopic surgery, vein stripping, sclerotherapy, or laser therapy (Sottiurai, 2001). Ulcers with duration of 3 months or less have an 80% chance of healing versus ulcers with greater than 6 months' duration, which have a 22% chance of healing, so surgery may be beneficial for these refractory cases (Choi & Hector, 2012). Human skin grafts may be used for those with large or refractory ulcers using autograft, allograft, or artificial skin, but skin grafts are not effective if there is persistent edema (Sieggreen, 2007).

Follow-up: The goals of care are to reduce edema, promote ulcer healing, and prevent reoccurrence of the ulcer (Sieggreen, 2007).

Sequelae: Compliance with compression, ulcer size, and duration of the ulcer affect ulcer healing. Ulcers larger than 5 cm^2 and present for more than 6 months are predictive for nonhealing, so early assessment and treatment with compression therapy is important to reduce complications such as infection from nonhealing ulcers (Nunnelee, 2007; Sieggreen, 2007).

Prevention/prophylaxis: The daily use of compression therapy for the rest of one's life is recommended to promote healing and reduce the chance of reoccurrence.

Referral: Patients with venous leg ulcer disease with impaired calf muscle pump function may benefit from physical therapy that includes isotonic and resistance exercises to improve calf muscle pump function (Rasmussen et al., 2008; Zuran & Mees, 2008).

Education: Patients with venous ulcer disease should be instructed to use compression stockings every day for the rest of their lives and replace these compression stockings at least every 6 months. They should elevate the affected leg or legs above the heart several times a day. Physical activity is recommended to increase venous return and should be performed based on the patient's medical condition but may include ankle flexion exercises, brisk walking, and sitting in a rocking chair and using the feet to push down to plantar flex the ankles.

CLINICAL RECOMMENDATION	EVIDENCE RATING	REFERENCES
Smoking cessation, dietary management, exercise, and diabetic management are key treatments to slow the progression of peripheral arterial disease.	A	Durham et al. (2010) Hirsch et al. (2005) Tomczyk & Treat-Jacobson (2009) Zakhari (2013)
Hypertension treatment is an essential treatment for patients with known abdominal aortic aneurysms.	A	Birkmeyer & Upchurch (2007) Cooper et al. (2009)
Patients with known abdominal aortic aneurysms should receive periodic ultrasound, magnetic resonance imaging, or CT-guided images at least once a year.	A	Birkmeyer & Upchurch (2007) Eckstein et al. (2009)
Endovascular grafts for complex aortic aneurysms permit a lower perioperative risk profile than does the open surgical procedure for such patients. After the procedure, nursing proficiency with aortic endograft is key to the patient's safe postoperative progression.	A	Birkmeyer & Upchurch (2007) Karnwal et al. (2009) National Quality Measures Clearinghouse (2009)
Aggressive compression therapy is still the mainstay for venous insufficiency. Modalities include elastic compression, intermittent pneumatic compression, and leg elevation.	A	Werchek (2010)
Clinicians should prescribe one or more of the following for patients diagnosed with peripheral arterial disease: aspirin, beta blocker, statin agent.	B	Hirsch et al. (2005)
The use of multilayer compression bandages and/or compression stockings is an important treatment strategy for all patients with lymphedema. Diuretics are not beneficial for lymphedema patients. Major complications with lymphedema patients include cellulitis, lymphangitis, and limited mobility.	A	Werchek (2010)

A = consistent, good-quality, patient-oriented evidence; B = inconsistent or limited-quality, patient-oriented evidence; C = consensus, disease-oriented evidence, usual practice, expert opinion, or case series. For information about the SORT evidence rating system, go to www.aafp.org/afpsort.xml.

CASE STUDY

M. J. is a 76-year-old woman who lives on the side of a very steep mountain. The home health nurse has visited her once a week for the last year. She has running water, electricity, and a coal stove with backup oil heat for very cold winter nights. She uses the telephone for communication. She has diabetes mellitus, hypertension, and hypothyroidism and is in atrial fibrillation. She has never been in the hospital before.

Her current medications include metformin (250 mg twice a day), losartan (50 mg/day), levothyroxine sodium (Synthroid) (50 mcg/day), digoxin (0.125 mg/day), furosemide (Lasix) (10 mg/day), aspirin (81 mg/day), simvastatin (20 mg/day), and warfarin (Coumadin) (4 mg/day, with 6 mg on Sundays). Allergies are to penicillin (hives) and to metoprolol (hypotension and dizziness). M. J. stopped smoking 5 years ago, but until then she smoked one-half pack a day.

Last laboratory test results (1 week ago) were as follows: hemoglobin A1C (HgbA1C) 8.3, international normalized ratio (INR) 1.7, sodium 129, potassium 5.8, chloride 102, CO_2 20, blood urea nitrogen (BUN) 45, creatinine 1.5, glucose 289, white blood cell (WBC) count 6.8, Hgb 10.1, hematocrit 30.2, platelets 215,000.

The home health nurse calls you from the patient's house, where she notes that the patient had a 5-minute spell of visual loss in her right eye. It has not recurred. During this period, M. J. noted that her left hand and left leg felt "funny," and her left foot and leg were so weak that she could not walk.

M. J. has a heart murmur, described by the home health nurse as loudest over the right sternal border and more prominent in the systolic phase. Furthermore, the home health nurse tells you that she hears bruits on both sides of the neck, with the right being louder than the left. The blood pressure in the right arm is 135/72 mm Hg and in the left arm is 110/66 mm Hg. Heart rate is irregular, at 75 to 90 beats per minute. The left hand and fingers have always been cooler than the right. Lungs are remarkable for wheezes. The patient has no fever. Oxygen saturations at room temperature are 90% to 92%, which has been her baseline.

1. What concerns do you have regarding M. J. at this point?

2. Do you need to see M. J. fairly soon, or can she come to see you at her regularly scheduled appointment in 3 weeks?

3. If you were to see M. J. in the next 24 hours, what additional tests would you perform?

4. Based on the above laboratory results, what changes would you make in her medication profile?

5. Which arm will you use for blood pressure recordings in the future?

6. What systolic blood pressure range would you order for M. J., as a general target?

7. If M. J. has a repeat episode of right eye blindness, lasting 30 minutes this time, what would you do?

REFERENCES

Alund, M., Mani, K., & Wanhainen, A. (2008). Selective screening for abdominal aortic aneurysm among patients referred to the vascular laboratory. *European Journal of Vascular and Endovascular Surgery, 35*(6), 669–674.

Ammash, N., Sundt, T., & Connolly, H. (2008). Marfan syndrome: diagnosis and management. *Current Problems in Cardiology, 33*(1), 7–39.

Bertero, C., Carlsson, P., & Lundgren, F. (2010). Screening for abdominal aortic aneurysms: a one year follow-up study. *Journal of Vascular Nursing, 28*(3), 97–101.

Birkmeyer, J., & Upchurch, G. (2007). Evidence-based screening and management of abdominal aortic aneurysms [Editorial]. *Annals of Internal Medicine, 146*(10), 749–750.

Blebea, J. & Kempczinski, R. F. (2001). Doppler pressure evaluation of infrainguinal occlusive disease. In C. B. Ernst & J. C. Stanely (Eds.), *Current therapy in vascular surgery* (4th ed.; pp. 447–451). St. Louis, MO: Mosby.

Bonamigo, T., & Siqueira, I. (2003). Screening for abdominal aortic aneurysms. *Revista do Hospital das Clinicas, 58*(2), 4–11.

Brannstrom, M., Bjorck, M., Strandberg, G., & Wanhainen, A. (2009). Patients' experiences of being informed about having an abdominal aortic aneurysm: a follow up case study five years after screening. *Journal of Vascular Nursing, 27*(3), 70–74.

Carthron, D., Johnson, T., Hubbart, T., Strickland, C., & Nance, K. (2010). The diabetes self-management activities of African-American primary caregiving grandmothers. *Journal of Nursing Scholarship, 42*(3), 330–337.

Castlemain, T. (2010). Takayasu's arteritis with associated aortic insufficiency and coronary artery obliteration. *Journal of the American Academy of Nurse Practitioners, 22*(6), 305–311.

Choi, M., & Hector, M. (2012). Management of venous thromboembolism for older adults in long-term care facilities. *Journal of the American Academy of Nurse Practitioners, 24*(6), 335–344. doi: 10.1111/j.1745-7599.2012.00733.x

Connelly, S., & Lovell, M. (2007). Medications used in patients with peripheral arterial disease. In P. A. Lewis, A. Aquila, M. E. Walsh, & Society for Vascular Nursing (Eds.), *Core curriculum for vascular nursing* (pp. 78–118). Beverly, MA: Society for Vascular Nursing.

Cooper, D. G., King, J. A., & Earnshaw, J. J. (2009). Role of medical intervention in slowing the growth of small abdominal aortic aneurysms. *Postgraduate Medical Journal, 85*(1010), 688–692.

Dancer, S., & Courtney, M. (2010). Improving diabetes patient outcomes. *Journal of the American Academy of Nurse Practitioners, 22*(11), 580–585.

Durham, C. A., Mohr, M. C., Parker, F. M., Bogey, W. M., Powell, C. S., & Stoner, M. C. (2010). The impact of socioeconomic factors on outcome and hospital costs associated with femoropopliteal revascularization. *Journal of Vascular Surgery, (52)*3, 600–606.

Eckstein, H.-H., Böckler, D., Flessenkämper, I., Schmitz-Rixen, T., Debus, S., & Lang, W. (2009). Ultrasonographic screening for the detection of abdominal aortic aneurysms. *Deutsches Arzteblatt International, 106*(41), 657–663.

Ehlers, L., Sorensen, J., Jensen, L., Bech, M., & Kjolby, M. (2008). Is population screening for abdominal aortic aneurysm cost-effective? *BMC Cardiovascular Disorders, 8*, 32–35.

Ferri, F. F. (2010). *Ferri's best test* (2nd ed.). St. Louis, MO: Mosby/Elsevier.

Gleeson, D., & Crabbe, D. L. (2009). Emerging concepts in cardiovascular disease risk assessment: where do women fit in? *Journal of the American Academy of Nurse Practitioners, 21*(9), 480–487.

Gonzales, E. A. (2009). Clinical practice: Marfan syndrome. *Journal of the American Academy of Nurse Practitioners, 21*(12), 663–670.

Hirsch, A., Haskai, Z., Hertzer, N., Bakal, C., Creager, M., Halhperin, J., . . . ACC/AHA Task Force on Practice Guidelines. (2005). *ACC/AHA 2005 guidelines for the management of patients with peripheral arterial disease* (pp. 1–192). Bethesda, MD: American College of Cardiology Foundation.

Hughes, S. (2009). On the road to better dyslipidemia outcomes. *Nurse Practitioner, 34*(2), 14–24.

Karnwal, A., Lippman, M., Julka, I., & White, R. (2009). Endovascular abdominal aortic aneurysm repair in nonagenarians. *Texas Heart Institute Journal, 36*(6), 632.

Langston, S., & Appel, S. (2010). Smoking cessation: snub out coronary artery disease. *Nurse Practitioner, 35*(4), 42–46.

Lewis, P., & Walsh E. (2007). Lymphedema. In P. A. Lewis, A. Aquila, M. E. Walsh, & Society for Vascular Nursing (Eds.), *Core curriculum for vascular nursing* (pp. 403–429). Beverly, MA: Society for Vascular Nursing.

Lindberg, D. (Ed.). (2009). Women and peripheral arterial disease. *NIH Medline Plus, 4*(3), 20–21.

Marston, W., & Criado, E. (2001). Nonoperative management of chronic venous insufficiency. In C. B. Ernst & J. C. Stanely (Eds.), *Current therapy in vascular surgery* (4th ed.; pp. 843–846). St. Louis, MO: Mosby.

Martin, C. (2010). DPP-4 inhibitors: a new option for diabetes management. *American Nurse Today, 5*(11), 29–31.

Mooney, P., Hayoz, D., Tinguely, F., Cornuz, J., Haesler, E., Mueller, X., . . . Tevaerai, H. T. (2004). High prevalence of unsuspected abdominal aortic aneurysms in patients hospitalized for coronary revascularization. *European Journal of Cardiothoracic Surgery, 25*(1), 65–68.

National Quality Measures Clearinghouse. (2005). Screening for abdominal aortic aneurysm: recommendation statement. *Annals of Internal Medicine, 142*(3), 198–202.

National Quality Measures Clearinghouse. (2007). Aortic aneurysm and dissection. In *EBM Guidelines: Evidence-Based Medicine.* Helsinki, Finland: Wiley & Sons.

National Quality Measures Clearinghouse. (2008a). Abdominal aortic aneurysm repair: mortality rate. Rockville, MD: Agency for Healthcare Research and Quality.

National Quality Measures Clearinghouse. (2008b). Percentage of patients having an elective abdominal aortic aneurysm repair, who die within the same admission during the six month time period. Australian Council on Healthcare Standards.

National Quality Measures Clearinghouse. (2009). *Endovascular stent grafts for the treatment of abdominal aortic aneurysms.* Technology appraisal guidance, no. 167. London, UK: National Institute for Health and Clinical Excellence.

Nunnelee, J. D. (2007). Superior vena cava syndrome. *Journal of Vascular Nursing, 25*(1), 2–5.

Ogata, T., Arrington, S., Davis, M., Jr., Sam, A. D., II, Hollier, L., Tromp, G., & Kuivaneimi, H. (2006). Community based, nonprofit organization sponsored ultrasonography screening program for abdominal aortic aneurysms is effective in identifying occult aneurysms. *Annals of Vascular Surgery, 20*(3), 312–316.

Rasmussen, T. E., Clouse, W. D., & Tonnessen, B. H. (2008). *Handbook of Patient Care in Vascular Diseases* (5th ed.). Philadelphia, PA: Lippincott Williams & Wilkins.

Sieggreen, M. (2007). Venous ulcers. In P. A. Lewis, A. Aquila, M. E. Walsh, & Society for Vascular Nursing (Eds.), *Core curriculum for vascular nursing* (pp. 375–381). Beverly, MA: Society for Vascular Nursing.

Sottiurai, V. S. (2001). Surgical management of chronic venous insufficiency. In C. Ernst & J. C. Stanley (Eds.), *Current therapy in vascular surgery* (4th ed.; pp. 853–859). St. Louis, MO: Mosby.

Tomczyk, S., & Treat-Jacobson, D. (2009). Claudication symptom experience in men and women: is there a difference? *Journal of Vascular Nursing, 27*(4), 92–97.

Werchek, S. (2010). Diagnosis and treatment of venous leg ulcers. *Nurse Practitioner, 35*(12), 46–53.

Weyland, P. (2009). Warfarin management. *Nurse Practitioner, 34*(3), 22–29.

Zakhari, R. (2013). Smoking: harm reduction versus abstinence. *Journal of the American Academy of Nurse Practitioners, 25*(1), 1–2.

chapter 10

Abdominal Disorders

Laurie Kennedy-Malone

ASSESSMENT

Accurate history taking of abdominal complaints is essential for completing an assessment of the older adult. The physical examination is often unremarkable, and laboratory findings may not provide diagnostic information, because the presentation of illness in an older adult is usually subdued.

Gathering the Abdominal History

Explore with the patient any episodes of anorexia, dyspepsia, dysphagia, heartburn, nausea, regurgitation, vomiting, diarrhea, tenesmus, or constipation. Determine the sequence of events that triggered each symptom. Inquire about precipitating factors such as a meal, position of the body, use of caffeine, or alcohol and smoking. Were any other symptoms present that can be clustered to form a differential diagnosis? It is important to discern from patients what therapeutic measures they have initiated to alleviate the symptoms. Determine if the treatment is a previously prescribed regimen, an over-the-counter (OTC) medication, or a home remedy. Ask the patient when the last time a fecal occult blood test was performed and if he or she has had a recent colonoscopy or sigmoidoscopy examination.

Abdominal Pain

Although abdominal pain is a common acute problem with which patients present to their health-care providers, older adults may not experience the typical symptoms of abdominal disorders that younger patients report. If patients present with abdominal pain, it is important to discern the characteristic of the pain. How quickly did the pain begin? Was the pain abrupt? Is the pain progressive or intermittent? Has the patient noted any improvements with self-treatment, positioning, vomiting, or defecation? What is the referral pattern? Is the pain worse at night or during the day? Is it relieved or aggravated by food? Does the patient have any associated symptoms of regurgitation, reflux, cough, nausea, vomiting, constipation, or diarrhea? Gather a history of previous abdominal surgeries. Inquire about alcohol use or drug abuse. Inquire about any history of jaundice, heart disease, or peripheral vascular disease. Review all current medications (Spirit, 2010).

Inspection

The physical examination of the abdomen begins with inspection. The practitioner can consider the abdomen to be divided into four quadrants, visualizing an imaginary vertical line from the sternum to the pubis passing though the umbilicus and a horizontal line drawn through the umbilicus. Carefully examine for scars, lesions, dilated veins, or other marks. Determine if the abdomen is concave or protuberant. Is an umbilical, abdominal wall, incisional, or inguinal hernia present? Is a lift noticeable? Is there abdominal distention? If so, is the distention local or generalized? Causes of generalized distention include abdominal fat, peritoneal fluid, or gaseous distention, whereas local distention often is indicative of obstruction or organ or structural enlargement. Examine the umbilicus. Signs of ascites include a flat or everted umbilicus (Williams, 2008).

Examine the skin of the abdomen for color, noting if there is any jaundice, bruising, or telangiectasias. Note if there are any pulsatile movements across the abdomen. If present, this sign may be indicative of a vascular aneurysm or a wide arterial pulse pressure (Williams, 2008).

Auscultation

Auscultations follow inspection of the abdomen. Using the diaphragm place the stethoscope lightly against the skin. Listen for bowel sounds, vascular bruits, and rubs. Bowel sounds are produced by peristalsis. A murmur heard in the abdomen may be an aortic aneurysm. A constant systolic-diastolic bruit may occur when the patient has an arteriovenous fistula in the renal vessels. Other sites to auscultate for bruits during abdominal examination include the iliac arteries and the femoral arteries. When auscultating bowel sounds, take the time to listen for presence of bowel sounds. Generally, people who are hungry have active bowel sounds. Bowel sounds described as high pitched, rumbling, or tinkling are known as borborygmi. A rushing sound is associated with bowel obstruction. If bowel sounds are absent, listen for 5 minutes; suspect peritonitis, mesenteric thrombosis, or advanced intestinal obstructions when bowel sounds are absent. Listen for a loud succussion splash over the abdomen of a patient in whom you suspect a gastric obstruction or dilations (Williams, 2008).

Percussion

Percussion of the abdomen is performed to determine the density of tissue of the abdominal organs by the sounds emitted when tapped (LeBlond, Brown, & DeGowin,

2009). It is normal to hear tympanic sounds over the stomach, whereas dullness is expected over a distended bladder. Dullness noted over other areas of the abdomen is a deviation from the norm. Definitive percussion is used to ascertain the size and shape of the liver and spleen. Because the liver decreases in size starting at about age 50, the normal range of the liver size in an older person is 6 to 12 cm (Williams 2008).

Palpation

Perform light palpation to discern abdominal masses, enlarged organs, and areas of tenderness. Using the palm and extended fingers of the right hand, press about 21 cm deep. If a patient has complained of abdominal pain, always palpate in a quadrant away from the identified location. Once you discover the tender area, maintain pressure over the area to determine the consistency of the pain. If the pain diminishes despite the applied pressure to the area, inflammation is unlikely. If you suspect intra-abdominal tenderness, proceed to deep palpation. Check for referred rebound tenderness by applying pressure with the tips of the fingers to a site distant from the areas of questionable tenderness, and then quickly remove them from the abdomen. If tenderness is elicited remote from the areas palpated after release of pressure, consider peritoneal irritation (LeBlond et al., 2009). A mass detected in the lower abdomen on palpation warrants further rectal and/or pelvic examination. Rectal examination includes determining presence or absence of stool, checking for presence of hemorrhoids, and testing sphincter tone and guaiac. Ask the patient to strain gently as if having a bowel movement to relax the anal sphincter.

ACUTE KIDNEY INJURY

Signal symptoms: Fatigue, altered mental status, anorexia, shortness of breath.

Description: Acute kidney injury (AKI), previously known as acute renal failure (ARF), is defined as the abrupt loss of kidney function over a period of hours to days (Palevsky, 2012). This decrease in renal function results in the inability to maintain fluid, electrolyte, and acid-base homeostasis (Palevsky, 2008). Although in many instances return to baseline kidney function is possible, there is also a risk of chronic renal disease after AKI. Because of the broad scope that the term *ARF* encompasses, the term *AKI* is being used increasingly to

replace *ARF*. In addition, the term *AKI* reflects smaller decreases in renal function that may not result in full loss of renal function (Palevsky, 2012).

Etiology: Renal function with urine formation is based on four steps that occur in specific areas of the kidney. First, blood from the renal arteries is delivered to the glomeruli. Blood is then filtered through the glomeruli, and ultrafiltrate is formed. The ultrafiltrate, free of protein and blood elements, then flows into the renal tubules. The tubules reabsorb and secrete solute and/or water from the ultrafiltrate. The final tubular fluid, urine, leaves the kidney, draining through the renal pelvis and ureter and into the bladder. It is then excreted from the body through the urethra. Any disruption in the process of urine formation can result in the deterioration of renal function and may cause AKI.

Once it is determined that AKI has occurred, the level or degree of the kidney injury is ascertained as well as the underlying cause. Progression of the AKI is evaluated while monitoring for signs of renal recovery. Assessment of renal function is made by estimation of the glomerular filtration rate (GFR). GFR is used to assess the degree of kidney impairment and to follow the course of the disease and is the most useful index of kidney function in health and disease (Palevsky, 2012). However, GFR does not provide information on the cause of the kidney injury; this is determined through serologies and diagnostic testing. Normal GFR varies according to age, sex, and body size. In young adults, it is 120 to 130 mL/min and declines with age. Although a serum creatinine level has been used in the past to determine kidney function, GFR is a more accurate indicator of kidney function. This is because serum creatinine reflects not only kidney function but also muscle mass. As the GFR may decline to almost one-half before an increase in the serum creatinine level is seen, AKI may occur before an indication is seen in laboratory values. The GFR is calculated using the Modification of Diet in Renal Disease (MDRD) Study equation, which takes into account body surface area, age, race, and gender:

$$GFR = 175 \times \text{standardized Scr} - 1.154 \times \text{age} - 0.203 \times 1.212$$
$$[\text{if black}] \times 0.742 \text{ [if female]}$$

Estimates of GFR in patients with AKI will be less accurate than in those patients who have chronic kidney disease (CKD) (Inker & Perrone, 2010). Patients who have extremes of muscle mass, such as the frail elderly, the critically ill, cancer patients, body builders, or those with unusual diets, will also have inaccurate GFR. In these patients, a creatinine clearance, where urine is collected over 24 hours and the amount of creatinine is measured, may be a more accurate indicator of GFR.

The causes of AKI can be grouped into three categories:

- Prerenal, caused by reduced renal perfusion
- Intrinsic, in which there is damage to the renal parenchyma
- Postrenal, where there is obstruction to the flow of urine

Furthermore, AKI can be characterized as follows:

- Oliguric, which is less than 400 mL urine output in 24 hours
- Nonoliguric, which is greater than 400 mL urine output in 24 hours
- Anuric, which is less than 100 mL urine output in 24 hours (Safirstein, 2005)

Anuria is uncommon and may be caused by complete obstruction or a major vascular event such as aortic dissection or ruptured aortic aneurysm. Prerenal, intrinsic, and postrenal all present clinically with either oliguria or nonoliguria. Nonoliguria is more common with intrinsic AKI, whereas oliguria is more common with prerenal and postrenal AKI (Safirstein, 2005). A nonoliguric state is associated with much better renal prognosis and recovery of renal function.

Occurrence: Hospital admissions solely for AKI have declined, but admissions for septicemia, which can lead to AKI, have increased (U.S. Renal Data System [USRDS], 2010). In 2008, incidence of AKI was greatest in the eastern half of the United States, along the Gulf coast, and in parts of Nevada and Utah (USRDS, 2010).

Age: Although AKI can occur at any age, its incidence is highly associated with older adults, most notably those ages 85 and older (USRDS, 2010). Adults older than 70 years of age have a 3.5 times greater prevalence of AKI, with nearly one-third unable to regain function after an AKI (Palevsky, 2012).

Gender: Across age groups, a higher percentage of men are affected by AKI than women (USRDS, 2010).

Ethnicity: AKI is associated with a higher incidence in African Americans and has steadily increased in this group since 2013 (USRDS, 2010).

Contributing factors: Certain conditions predispose patients to AKI. Advanced age and volume depletion are leading factors. In addition, history of previous cardiac or renal disease, diuretic use, diabetes mellitus, and proteinuria can predispose patients to AKI.

In prerenal AKI, any condition in which there is volume depletion can lead to renal hypoperfusion. This includes vomiting, diarrhea, dehydration, hemorrhage (either surgical or gastrointestinal), excessive diuresis, and burns. In addition, any condition leading to decreased cardiac output, such as cardiogenic shock, valvulopathy, myocarditis, myocardial infarction, arrhythmias, congestive heart failure, pulmonary emboli, and cardiac tamponade, causes hypoperfusion. Volume depletion and decreased cardiac output are the main causes of prerenal AKI and may not cause permanent damage to the kidneys unless there is prolonged hypoperfusion leading to acute tubular necrosis. Sepsis, hypoxemia, anaphylactic shock, pancreatic disease, and liver disease also cause AKI. In addition, any condition that affects the renal vascular system, such as renal artery stenosis, renal vein thrombosis, hepatorenal syndrome, NSAIDs, and angiotensin-converting enzyme (ACE) inhibitors/angiotensin blockers, also can induce AKI (Holley, 2005).

Conditions that cause intrinsic AKI are centered around the area of the kidney that is damaged. These include the glomeruli, tubules, and interstitium. The most common cause of damage to the structures of the kidney is prolonged hypoperfusion and nephrotoxins such as radiopaque contrast agents or certain medications. Vascular damage to the kidney from ischemia or vasculitis leads to glomerular AKI. Systemic lupus erythematosus, antineutrophil cytoplasmic antibody (ANCA)-associated granulomatous polyangiitis, Goodpasture's syndrome, cryoglobulinemia, postinfectious glomerulonephritis, polyarteris nodosa, hemolytic uremic syndrome, thrombotic thrombocytopenic purpura, hepatitis B virus, and HIV are all conditions that can lead to the development of glomerular AKI (Liano & Pascual, 1999). Tubules of the kidney may be damaged by ischemia, cellular edema, or interstitial edema or become obstructed by cellular debris. AKI in this area of the kidney is called acute tubular necrosis (ATN). Any severe and prolonged prerenal cause of AKI will cause ATN. In addition, cyclosporine, tacrolimus, amphotericin B, aminoglycosides, ethylene glycol, radiopaque contrast agents, high-dose vitamin C, and Fleet's Phosphosoda (a commonly used bowel prep) can lead to ATN. Rhabdomyolysis, in which there is muscle necrosis leading to the release of myoglobin, causes tubular damage by accumulation of a greater quantity of myoglobulin than can be filtered by the kidney. Interstitial inflammation or nephritis is usually caused by an immunologic or allergic reaction. Acute interstitial nephritis can be caused by certain medications, including penicillins, cephalosporins, NSAIDs, phenytoin, cimetidine, sulfonamides, and allopurinol (McMillan, 2007).

Postrenal causes of AKI include any condition in which there is an impediment of the excretion of urine anywhere from the collecting tubules to the urethra. In the tubules, crystal or protein particles can precipitate, causing obstruction. This is associated with tumor lysis, myeloma, and calcium oxalate from ethylene glycol (antifreeze) ingestion and myoglobin from rhabdomyolysis. Ureteral obstruction can be caused by calculi, clots, fungus balls, tumors, or trauma. Bladder obstruction is of two types, either mechanical or neurogenic. Examples of mechanical obstruction include benign prostatic hypertrophy, prostate cancer, bladder cancer, and phimosis. Anticholinergic medications or upper or lower motor neuron lesions are the most common types of neurogenic obstruction. Prostatic disease, either hypertrophy or cancer, is the most common type of postrenal AKI.

Signs and symptoms: Predominant symptoms are usually those of the underlying illness or injury, which then leads to AKI. The patient may have symptoms directly resulting from alterations in kidney function such as decreased to no urine output, flank pain, edema, or hypertension. The patient may have noticed a change in his or her urine consistency or color, such as foamy urine, which indicates proteinuria, or dark brown/red urine that could be indicative of red blood cells. Patients may have nausea, vomiting, and diarrhea leading to volume depletion. Specific questions regarding use of medications that can cause renal injury, including NSAIDs and antihypertensive medications, such as ACE inhibitors and angiotensin receptor blockers, as well as recent antibiotic use, need to be asked of the patient. Factors that predispose the patient to vascular disease and a detailed history of hypertension, diabetes mellitus, smoking, hyperlipidemia, claudication, stroke, myocardial infarction, and atrial fibrillation should be noted. In addition, ask patients whether they have experienced any fatigue, arthritis, weight loss, cough, hemoptysis, arthralgias, or sinus symptoms, which may indicate a systemic illness, such as vasculitis or systemic lupus erythematosus. Use of illicit drugs, such as cocaine, ecstasy, and heroin, can also cause AKI. In addition, ask about any past history of drug use, tattoos, and piercings, which increase the risk for hepatitis B and HIV and can cause glomerular disease. Any recent diagnostic testing, such as computed tomography (CT) scans and cardiac catheterization, would also be indicative of a possible kidney injury due to use of radiocontrast dye. Past history of cancer, specifically prostate, cervical, or bladder cancer, may be indicative of an obstruction. Any family history of kidney disease increases the risk of a patient developing kidney disease in his or her lifetime as well. Patients with signs and symptoms of renal failure, such as weakness, easy fatigability, anorexia, altered mental status, weight loss, dysgeusia, nausea, cold intolerance, neuropathy, tremor, asterixis, seizures, and uremic fetor, where the patient has an ammonia-like or urine-like odor to the breath, may be suffering from end-stage renal disease and need hospital admittance for further evaluation. Physical examination includes assessment of weight, orthostatic blood pressures, mucous membranes, and skin turgor and neck veins for the presence of volume depletion or overload. A funduscopic examination positive for atrioventricular nicking, exudates, or arterial narrowing is indicative of hypertension. Cardiac examination may reveal an S_3, indicative of volume overload or congestive heart failure, and the presence of a pericardial rub may indicate pericarditis, a late finding in end-stage renal disease. Lung assessment may reveal tachypnea and rales. Skin assessment should include inspection for any rash, skin lesions, livedo reticularis, or purpura that may indicate vasculitis or autoimmune disease. Periorbital, lower extremity or pretibial, and presacral edema can indicate advancing renal disease from any cause. Abdominal assessment should include auscultation for renal or abdominal bruits as well as evaluation for abdominal masses, costovertebral angle tenderness, and bladder distention. Assess for asterixis, a tremor of the wrist when it is extended, often seen in patients with end-stage renal disease.

Diagnostic tests: Urinalysis is a noninvasive tool that can provide some information regarding AKI. Urine is analyzed for sediment, specific gravity, urine sodium, urine protein, and urine creatinine levels. Urinary casts are cylindrical particles formed from coagulated proteins secreted by tubular cells (USRDS, 2010). They are only formed in tubules of the kidney and occur during low-flow urine conditions. Different types of cast cells are associated with certain diseases, assisting in determination of the cause of the AKI. Prerenal AKI will have normal sediment, whereas ATN will have renal tubular cells with muddy brown granular casts. Specific gravity reflects the ability of the kidney to concentrate urine and can reflect a patient's volume status. Patients who have impaired concentrating ability, such as those with ATN, will have low specific gravity. Urine sodium can assist in differentiating between ATN and volume depletion but can be falsely elevated in patients on diuretics. Further laboratory tests show hyperkalemia, hypocalcemia, hyponatremia, and acidosis. A complete blood count (CBC) should also be drawn to evaluate for leukocytosis and anemia.

Radiographic studies are performed to assist in the diagnosis and cause of AKI. The most common used technique is the renal ultrasound (Dwinnell & Anderson, 1999). Renal ultrasound can be used to assess kidney size, obstruction, and the presence of masses. In AKI,

kidneys will be of normal size, as compared to chronic kidney disease where they are small. CT scan without radiocontrast dye is used to further evaluate any masses found on ultrasound as well as to evaluate for calculi with the presence of flank pain. Renal biopsy is only performed when laboratory data have been unrevealing, and no reversible causes could be identified as to the cause of AKI. It is performed percutaneously, and the most common complication is bleeding. Assessment of the patient's activated partial thromboplastin time (aPTT), prothrombin time (PT)/international normalized ratio (INR), and platelet count must be performed before the kidney biopsy. Renal biopsy is avoided in patients who have a "solitary" kidney, either from congenital absence or acquired absence such as nephrectomy for renal cell carcinoma.

Differential diagnosis:
- ▨ Hypovolemia
- ▨ Low cardiac output
- ▨ Sepsis
- ▨ Glomerulonephritis
- ▨ Ischemic nephritis
- ▨ Urethral obstruction
- ▨ CKD

Treatment: Treatment is indicative of the cause of AKI. In volume depletion, fluid resuscitation with isotonic saline and/or packed red blood cells to reestablish circulating volume as well as use of pressors to maintain blood pressure may be needed. Withdrawal of the offending medication and avoidance of other nephrotoxic agents are of the utmost importance. Dose adjustment of renally metabolized medications is needed as well. Antihypertensive medications should be judiciously titrated to avoid any further renal hypoperfusion. In obstructive AKI, treatment of the obstruction often results in renal recovery. Usually, rapid correction of prerenal and postrenal causes leads to full recovery of kidney function. Correction of electrolyte and acid-base imbalances is important as well. Administration of sodium bicarbonate will correct acidosis. Avoidance of exogenous sources of potassium, such as nutritional supplementation and IV fluids, should be discontinued. Treatment of hyperkalemia includes administration of IV calcium gluconate, insulin, beta-2 agonists (albuterol), dextrose, and occasionally kayexalate. Hyperphosphatemia may also occur in AKI, and calcium acetate or calcium carbonate can be used to reduce absorption of phosphorus from the gastrointestinal tract. Platelets are often dysfunctional in AKI and may require use of DDAVP to attempt to activate platelets. Due to lower levels of circulating erythro-poietin and decreased bone marrow responsiveness, anemia is often found in AKI, requiring transfusion of red blood cells to increase oxygen-carrying capacity to the kidney as well as administration of recombinant human erythropoietin to stimulate the bone marrow to increase production of red blood cells (Cho & Chertow, 2005).

In the event that there is no recovery in kidney function after correction of the cause of the AKI, hemodialysis may need to be initiated. This is especially important in the face of continued acid-base disturbances, electrolyte abnormalities, volume overload, and uremia. The risk of developing end-stage renal disease is higher in patients who already have chronic kidney disease and sustain dialysis-requiring AKI.

Follow-up: Patients who are unable to fully recover to their previous level of kidney function will need to be closely monitored and followed by a nephrologist. Unfortunately, 35% of patients who have AKI and require dialysis while hospitalized do not follow up with a nephrologist 30 days after leaving the hospital, and 23% do not see a nephrologist for 1 year after the AKI (USRDS, 2010). African Americans have a greater percentage of compliance with follow-up with a nephrologist than whites. In addition, rates for testing for proteinuria following AKI are poor, less than 20% at the end of 1 year. Thus, follow-up with a nephrologist 3 to 4 weeks after discharge to evaluate serum creatinine is important. Patients who have a new diagnosis of CKD stage 1 through 5 will require follow-up with a nephrologist for the remainder of their lives.

Sequelae: CKD is a direct result of AKI if there is no return to previous level of function. Patients with CKD are at an increased risk for stroke and peripheral vascular disease. In addition, they are at an increased risk for cardiovascular death, left ventricular hypertrophy, coronary artery disease, and congestive heart failure. Management of CKD includes management of anemia of chronic disease, secondary hyperparathyroidism, cholesterol, and hypertension.

Prevention/prophylaxis: Prevention of AKI begins first with identifying those at risk for CKD. Close monitoring of GFR, especially in older adults, is paramount. When there is a decline in GFR, prompt referral to a nephrologist is of the utmost importance. Avoidance of nephrotoxic medications, such as NSAIDs, as well as polypharmacy will decrease risk of AKI. Recognition of medications that need adjustment for levels of kidney dysfunction is also very important in the prevention of episodes of AKI.

Referral: All patients who have AKI need to be hospitalized. Evaluation and management by a nephrologist is warranted. After resolution of the AKI and discharge from the hospital, follow-up with a nephrologist is needed in 2 to 4 weeks to evaluate serum creatinine and GFR until recovery or plateauing occurs. In the event that the AKI is postrenal, follow-up with urology is needed as well.

Education: Patients should be educated on signs of congestive heart failure as well as avoidance of certain OTC medications such as NSAIDs, cimetidine, and phosphate enemas. Patients should be instructed to avoid diets high in salt and to strive for less than 2 grams of sodium per day. In addition, tight glycemic control, with hemoglobin A1c (HgbA1c) of less than 7% as well as optimal blood pressure control of less than 130/80 mm Hg, is paramount. Smoking cessation and maintenance of healthy body weight are also important.

CLINICAL RECOMMENDATION	EVIDENCE RATING	REFERENCES
Glomerular filtration rate (GFR) is the best indicator of kidney function.	C	Palevsky (2012)
Estimates of GFR in patients with AKI will be less accurate than in patients with chronic kidney disease.	C	Inker & Perrone (2010)
Renal ultrasound is the most common radiographic study used to assist in the cause and diagnosis of AKI.	C	Dwinnell & Anderson (1999)
Certain medications can cause acute interstial nephritis, leading to AKI.	A	McMillan (2007)

Continued

CLINICAL RECOMMENDATION	EVIDENCE RATING	REFERENCES
Any condition or medication that affects the renal vascular system can cause AKI.	A	Holley (2005)
Serum creatinine alone should not be used to monitor kidney function. GFR should also be used.	C	Inker & Perrone (2010)

A = consistent, good-quality, patient-oriented evidence; B = inconsistent or limited-quality, patient-oriented evidence; C = consensus, disease-oriented evidence, usual practice, expert opinion, or case series. For information about the SORT evidence rating system, go to www.aafp.org/afpsort.xml.

BLADDER CANCER

Signal symptoms: Painless hematuria, urinary frequency or urgency, mild suprapubic pain; often asymptomatic.

Description: Of bladder cancers, 90% are transitional urothelial cell cancer; 8% are squamous cell cancer; and the rest are adenocarcinoma. In bladder cancer, the posterior and lateral walls of the bladder are involved more frequently than the superior wall. Bladder cancer can be categorized as *superficial*, *invasive*, and *metastatic*. Superficial, or early, bladder cancer occurs when the lesion is located on the surface of the mucosa or when the tumor penetrates the mucosa and submucosa only. Invasive bladder cancer develops when lesions pervade the bladder muscularis or the perivesical fat. Metastatic bladder cancer is characterized by lymph node, visceral, or bone tissue involvement.

Etiology: Because of suspected chemical carcinogens, occupational exposures to aniline dye, leather processing, paint, rubber, and possibly tobacco tars have been linked to the development of bladder cancer. Squamous cell bladder cancer has been linked to chronic infection with *Schistosoma haematobium*.

Occurrence: In the United States each year, more than 50,000 new cases of bladder cancer are diagnosed, and more than 12,000 deaths can be attributed to bladder cancer.

Age: The average age of onset is in the late sixties.

Ethnicity: *S. haematobium* infection is prevalent in Africa and the Middle East. The incidence of bladder cancer increases among people from the industrialized areas of the northeastern United States because of their high exposure to carcinogens.

Gender: Bladder cancer is 4 times more common in men than in women.

Contributing factors: History of smoking increases the risk of bladder cancer. Pelvic irradiation, certain drugs (e.g., cyclophosphamide), and abnormal tryptophan metabolism contribute to the development of bladder cancer. Excessive coffee consumption, use of some artificial sweeteners (e.g., saccharin sodium and cyclamate sodium), and overuse of phenacetin-containing analgesics have been suggested risk factors. Occupational exposure to dyes, rubber, and leather has been shown to increase the risk of developing bladder cancer. There also has been an association between developing bladder cancer and working as a hairdresser, machinist, printer, painter, or truck driver. Exfoliation of cancer cells by cystoscopy, brushing, or transurethral biopsy or resection may spread bladder cancer cells to other sites within the bladder or may cause irritation from instrumentation. Some association has been shown with developing bladder cancer and a long history of indwelling catheters and urinary calculi.

Signs and symptoms: Gross, painless hematuria, pyuria, burning, and urinary frequency are common in the presentation of bladder cancer. Symptoms of advanced cancer may include pelvic or flank pain and lower extremity edema, resulting from lymphatic or venous blockage. Patients also may complain of abdominal pain, anorexia, and bone pain.

The clinician should palpate and percuss for evidence of any kidney enlargement and perform a prostate examination on men and a pelvic examination on women. Additionally, the examination should be directed toward searching for possible sites of metastasis in the lungs, liver, bone, and lymph nodes.

Diagnostic tests: Cystoscopy is the gold standard for the initial diagnosis and staging of bladder cancer (Jimenez, Campbell, & Jones, 2011). Cystoscopy can miss tumors during the initial transurethral resection of bladder tumors (TURBT); therefore, a repeat cystoscopy is performed (Lotan & Choueiri, 2012). The procedure begins with a bimanual examination under anesthesia (EUA) to determine whether or not a palpable mass is present and, if present, whether or not it is mobile. An EUA during cystoscopy is effective at identifying locally advanced disease, which may present as gross extravesical extension, invasion of adjacent organs, or pelvic sidewall involvement. If a mass is felt, the bimanual examination is repeated after the resection to see if it is still present.

Imaging studies may be used to define the location and the extent of the tumor as well as to detect sites of multifocal disease. CT scan is replacing the IV pyelogram (IVP) as the procedure of choice, but IVP remains an appropriate alternative where CT is not readily available (Lotan & Choueiri, 2012). CT scans should include both the abdomen and pelvis; scans need to be done with and without contrast; and they should include delayed images to identify defects in the collecting system. Although CT provides better visualization of tumors than ultrasound, it may miss tumors less than 1 cm in size, particularly those in the bladder trigone or dome, and it cannot differentiate depth of bladder wall invasion (i.e., mucosal versus lamina propria or muscularis propria).

Urine dipstick, cytology, and screening for tumor-specific molecular markers in the urine have been used for screening but are not recommended for screening asymptomatic patients due to low specificity, low sensitivity, and cost, respectively.

Laboratory studies should include an alkaline phosphatase, CBC, and chemistry profile. If the alkaline phosphatase is elevated, a bone scan should be considered (National Comprehensive Cancer Network [NCCN], 2012).

Differential diagnosis:
- Neurogenic bladder
- Nephrolithiasis
- Urinary tract infection
- Benign prostatic hypertrophy
- Other genitourinary cancers

Treatment: Management of bladder cancer depends on the stage of the disease. Initially, surgical intervention to remove the bladder tumors is warranted. Some patients may require a cystectomy with a urostomy, continent urostomy, or a replacement bladder. For patients with multiple recurrent superficial bladder tumors, the urologist may request collaboration with an oncologist for chemotherapy after surgery. Advanced disease generally requires surgery, radiation, and chemotherapy with combination agents. The patient's age and health status at the time of diagnosis must be considered in the management of bladder cancer.

Follow-up: Patients with superficial low-grade bladder cancer require a cystoscopy at designated intervals, although the value of repeated testing has been questioned. The need for supplemental nutritional support, pain management, prevention of complications such as skin breakdown, and an advance directive should be discussed during future follow-up care. Patients with a urostomy may need assistance from an ostomy nurse.

Sequelae: Metastasis to other parts of the body can occur. Survival of the untreated patient may be less than 2 years.

Prevention/prophylaxis: Encourage patients who smoke to quit, and exhort all patients to decrease exposure to harmful chemicals.

Referral: Refer patients with clinically significant hematuria to a urologist. An oncologist also may be involved in the patient's management of the disease. Patient and family support is important at this time; information pertaining to hospice services should be provided. Patients with a urostomy may seek support from a local chapter of a urostomy association (UOA) at 1-800-826-0826 or at www.uoa.org.

Education: Older adults with bladder cancer may need to be educated about palliative support measures when the disease becomes terminal.

CLINICAL RECOMMENDATION	EVIDENCE RATING	REFERENCE
Urine dipstick is not recommended for screening of bladder cancer in the general population due to lack of specificity.	A	Messing et al. (2006)

Continued

CLINICAL RECOMMENDATION	EVIDENCE RATING	REFERENCE
Routine screening for bladder cancer is not recommended for the general population.	B	Jimenez, Campbell, & Jones (2012)
Patients should be counseled to eliminate active and passive smoking for prevention of bladder cancer.	C	Babjuk et al. (2011)
Cystoscopy is recommended in all patients with symptoms suggestive of bladder cancer. It cannot be replaced by cytology or by any other noninvasive test.	A	Babjuk et al. (2011)

A = consistent, good-quality, patient-oriented evidence; B = inconsistent or limited-quality, patient-oriented evidence; C = consensus, disease-oriented evidence, usual practice, expert opinion, or case series. For information about the SORT evidence rating system, go to www.aafp.org/afpsort.xml.

BOWEL OBSTRUCTION

Signal symptoms: Abdominal distention with cramping, absent or minimal peristalsis, obstipation.

Description: Bowel obstructions are classified as mechanical or nonmechanical and partial or complete (Kent, 2007). Bowel obstruction occurs in the large or small intestine. Absent or minimal peristalsis and abdominal distention with cramping are signs of bowel obstruction.

Etiology: Forward flow of gastric and intestinal contents is blocked (Letizia & Norton, 2003). A mechanical bowel obstruction results when there is a complete or partial blockage of the lumen of the bowel by an adhesion, tumor, or hernia (Ansari, 2007). Postoperative adhesions cause approximately 60% of small bowel obstruction (SBO) in industrialized countries (Nobie, 2011). Older adults who have had previous abdominal surgery have an SBO occurrence rate of 50% to 70% (Lyon & Clark, 2006). A simple mechanical obstruction occurs without insult to the vascular or neurological system (Ansari, 2007). Strangulation of the bowel in older adults happens with compromised blood flow to the bowel, resulting in ischemia of the bowel wall (Ansari, 2007). The bowel may become edematous and infarcted, leading to perforation and gangrene (Nobie, 2011).

Occurrence: An estimated 20% of all hospital admissions for acute abdominal conditions are for suspected bowel obstruction (Kent, 2009; Nobie, 2011). In 2004, bowel obstruction ranked among the top 10 most common gastrointestinal diseases, with 75% of emergency admissions related to bowel obstruction (Milenkovic, Russo, & Elixhauser, 2006).

Age: Bowel obstruction from all causes, except intussusception, is more prevalent in older adults.

Gender: Bowel obstruction occurs equally in men and women.

Ethnicity: No prevalence is known among ethnic groups.

Contributing factors: Patients with a history of abdominal surgery may develop adhesions that can cause an SBO (Ansari, 2007; Nobie, 2011). Neoplasms, hernias, inflammatory disease, diverticulitis, mesenteric ischemia, stricture formation, volvulus (especially of the sigmoid colon), gallstones, and fecal impactions can cause a mechanical bowel obstruction (Ansari, 2007).

Signs and symptoms: Clinical presentation of bowel obstruction depends on the level and cause of the obstruction. Pain, vomiting, obstipation, and distention are the four cardinal symptoms of bowel obstruction (Jackson & Raiji, 2011; Kulayat & Doerr, 2001). Presentation of a mechanical SBO includes abdominal cramps located in the epigastrium or around the umbilicus, with associated pain that can be more severe the higher the obstruction. Profuse vomiting occurs early with an SBO. The vomitus first may consist of mucus and bile in a high SBO. With a lower ileal obstruction, the vomitus becomes feculent. Diarrhea may occur in partial SBO. Obstipation exists with complete obstruction. The patient may have a low-grade fever (Ansari, 2007; Kulayat & Doerr, 2001).

Inspect the abdomen for evidence of surgical scars and external hernias. Borborygmi may be heard on auscultation; however, late in the presentation of a strangulated bowel, peristalsis may be minimal or absent. Abdominal distention is found; the abdomen may not be tender in the case of a strangulated bowel. With mechanical obstruction of the large bowel, symptoms are similar to a small bowel obstruction but appear more gradually. The patient complains of persistent constipation leading to abdominal distention. Vomiting may be absent if the ileocecal valve is functioning. Physical examination reveals loud borborygmi, no abdominal tenderness, and an empty rectal vault. Patients with a strangulating bowel may exhibit signs of shock late in the presentation of the obstruction (Ansari, 2007).

Diagnostic tests: Laboratory evaluation should include a CBC and a metabolic panel. Patients with severe emesis may be hypokalemic. Elevated blood urea nitrogen (BUN) levels indicate dehydration. An elevated white blood cell (WBC) count may indicate translocation of intestinal bacteria into the bloodstream. Bowel necrosis is suspected with elevation of WBC count to 15,000/mm³ or greater (National Cancer Institute, 2011). Increasing serum lactate levels along with metabolic acidosis may signal bowel ischemia (Jackson & Raiji, 2011).

The initial imaging of a patient with a suspected bowel obstruction should include plain abdominal radiography with flat and upright views. Radiography allows for quick determination of the presence of bowel perforation; free air can be seen above the liver in upright films or decubitus films (Jackson & Raiji, 2011). Typical findings are bowel distention proximal to the obstruction and collapsed bowel distal to the obstruction (Kent, 2007; Kulayat & Doerr, 2001; Moses, 2012). If radiographs do not show an obstruction and there is a high index of suspicion, CT should be used to further evaluate. CT scan is found to have as much as a 90% sensitivity in the presence of high-grade bowel obstruction. CT scan is also useful in determining the level of obstruction and identifying volvulus or intestinal strangulation, which require surgical intervention (Jackson & Raiji, 2011). Ultrasonography is also a useful tool to evaluate unstable patients for whom the diagnosis remains uncertain (Jackson & Raiji, 2011).

Patients with a malignant obstruction may be treated with primary resection and reconstruction or palliative diversion or with placement of venting and feeding tubes (Jackson & Raiji, 2011). Patients with venting gastrostomy tubes are able to achieve decompression and have a means of nutrition after resolution of the obstruction (Letizia & Norton, 2003).

Differential diagnosis:
■ Acute appendicitis
■ Cholecystitis
■ Acute pancreatitis
■ Diverticular disease
■ Peptic ulcer disease and perforation (Lyon & Clark, 2006)

Treatment: Initial treatment of a bowel obstruction consists of hospitalization for nasogastric suctioning, urinary catheter to monitor output, and fluid and electrolyte replacement with IV fluids (Ansari, 2007; Kent, 2009). Immediate surgical intervention is indicated for suspected vascular insufficiency, perforation, or strangulation of the bowel (Kent, 2007). Complete obstruction requires early surgical intervention for removal of the lesion (Ansari, 2007). Simple or partial obstruction can be conservatively managed for up to 3 days. Treatment involves fluid replacement, nasogastric suctioning for bowel decompression, and surgical consultation (Moses, 2012; Nobie, 2011). Resolution of the obstruction without surgical intervention is common in many patients within 48 to 72 hours (Moses, 2012; Nobie, 2011). Indications for surgery may include persistent symptoms lasting longer than 48 hours, abdominal sepsis, bowel ischemia, or bowel perforation (Moses, 2012).

Follow-up: Postoperative care of the patient with a surgically corrected bowel obstruction includes monitoring for return of bowel function, maintaining fluid and electrolyte balance with IV alimentation, and observing for signs of sepsis. After discharge from the hospital, the patient should return within 2 weeks for surveillance. Patients being treated nonsurgically also should be monitored accordingly; observe for signs of recurrence of the bowel obstruction. If an ileus persists for longer than 1 week, an underlying mechanical obstruction should be ruled out, and a laparotomy may be necessary.

Sequelae: After correction of a bowel obstruction, slow return of bowel function is an early complication. The possibility of ensuing bowel obstructions and sepsis needs to be monitored in all patients. For patients who are not surgical candidates, complications, such as perforation and peritonitis, should be considered.

Prevention/prophylaxis: Caregivers must understand the importance of avoiding fecal impactions in patients at risk for this condition.

Referral: Recommend a surgical consultation for patients with susceptible bowel obstruction.

Education: Inform older adults with diagnosed, untreated internal and external hernias of the possible complication of bowel obstruction.

CLINICAL RECOMMENDATION	EVIDENCE RATING	REFERENCE
Small bowel obstruction (SBO) is routinely diagnosed with plain film radiographs that show distended small bowel loops, air-fluid levels, and decreased large bowel air.	C	Lyon & Clark (2006)
Computed tomography should be done when radiography indicates high-grade intestinal obstruction.	C	Jackson & Raiji (2011)
Digital rectal examination appears to have little diagnostic value for SBO.	C	Moll van Charante & de Jongh (2011)

A = consistent, good-quality, patient-oriented evidence; B = inconsistent or limited-quality, patient-oriented evidence; C = consensus, disease-oriented evidence, usual practice, expert opinion, or case series. For information about the SORT evidence rating system, go to www.aafp.org/afpsort.xml.

CHOLECYSTITIS

Signal symptoms: Pain that may radiate to the back, especially shortly after eating fatty foods.

Description: Cholecystitis, an acute or chronic inflammation of the gallbladder, results from an obstruction of the cystic duct.

Etiology: The pathological origin of gallstones is unknown. Most gallstones are a result of cholesterol accumulation. Cholecystitis usually occurs when a gallstone obstructs the cystic duct, except in cases involving trauma, recent surgery, or sepsis. Trapped bile caused by the blockage of the gallstone leads to inflammation; often a secondary infection may follow. Infection from *Escherichia coli, Klebsiella, Pseudomonas,* and *Bacteroides fragilis* occurs in in approximately 45% to 100% of patients with cholecystitis (Claesson, 1986). The possibility of undetected gallbladder cancer needs to be considered in all older adults presenting with symptoms of cholelithiasis (Makino, Yamaguchi, Nariatsu, Toshiaki, & Ichiro, 2009).

Occurrence: Approximately 10% of the U.S. population of adults ages 40 years and older have gallstones; 90% of cases of cholecystitis are associated with gallstones. Each year in the United States, more than 800,000 people undergo a cholecystectomy after cholecystitis (Giger et al., 2006).

Age: Presentation commonly is in the fifties and sixties; however, 25% to 30% of those older than age 80 develop gallstones due to the lithogenicity of bile.

Gender: Twice as many women as men have cholecystitis.

Ethnicity: A high prevalence for cholecystitis exists in older Native Americans and whites; the disease is less prevalent in African Americans. The prevalence of gallbladder disease is highest in the Pima, Hopi, and Navajo groups; almost 75% of the population are known to develop gallstones.

Contributing factors: Nonmodifiable risk factors for cholecystitis include advancing age, female gender, and family history of gallbladder disease. Obesity is a known predisposing factor to cholecystitis (Lee, Han, & Min, 2009). Diabetes, inflammatory bowel disease, chronic hemolysis, pancreatic insufficiency, and hyperlipidemia predispose patients to gallstone development. The consumption of a large, fatty meal may result in cholecystitis. Gallstone formation may be attributed to use of exogenous estrogens, prescribed for postmenopausal hormone replacement, and clofibrate, used to treat hyperlipidemia. Either past or current use of thiazide diuretics is associated with a modest increase in the formation of gallstones (Gorroll, 2009). Gallbladder stasis, a precursor to gallstone formation, occurs with extended total parenteral nutrition. Patients who experience rapid weight loss are at high risk for the development of gallstones. Cholelithiasis is common in patients who have undergone bariatric surgery (Decker, Swain, Crowell, & Scolapio, 2007).

Signs and symptoms: One type of presentation of acute cholecystitis includes nausea, vomiting, malaise, fever (which may be low grade), and abdominal pain that radiates around the sides to the back, reaching to the tip of the scapula as in biliary colic (Bellows, Berger, & Crass, 2005). Another type is associated with an acute change in mental status as the only outward sign. Physical examination may reveal right upper quadrant subcostal tenderness and pain on inspiration (Murphy's sign) (Adedeji & McAdam, 1996; Ralls et al., 1982). Biliary colic pain, however, can localize to the midepigastric region; thus, it is important to question the patient about generalized upper abdominal pain (Trowbridge, Rutkowski, & Shojania, 2003). In a patient who has reported symptoms for days, rebound tenderness may suggest perforation. Abdominal tenderness may be absent, however. Jaundice is present in less than 50% of patients.

Diagnostic tests: A CBC with differential may show WBC counts of 12,000 to 15,000 with peripheral leukocytosis, although WBC counts may not be elevated in older adults. A WBC count greater than 15,000 cells/μL may indicate perforation or gangrene. C-reactive protein (more than 3 mg/dL) would be indicative of inflammation. Serum amylase generally is increased, even without evidence of pancreatitis. Serum bilirubin and alkaline phosphatase levels also may be elevated if biliary obstruction has occurred. In chronic cholecystitis, however, laboratory values may be normal.

Real-time ultrasonography of the gallbladder and biliary tree is the diagnostic procedure of choice for both acute and chronic cholecystitis, showing gallstones, thickening of the gallbladder wall, and if the common bile duct is obstructed, dilation of the biliary tract. An alternative to the ultrasound for the detection of acute cholecystitis is the cholescintigraphy with radionuclide (Gorroll, 2009). In patients in whom stones in the common bile duct are suspected, an endoscopic retrograde cholangiopancreatography (ERCP) has been the gold standard, because the stones can be removed during the procedure.

Differential diagnosis:

- Perforated peptic ulcer in older adults
- Appendicitis
- Liver abscess
- Diverticulitis
- Hepatitis
- Acute pyelonephritis
- Gastrointestinal carcinoma
- Acute pancreatitis
- Myocardial ischemia
- Herpes zoster
- Left lower lobe pneumonia
- Gastritis
- Cholangitis
- Irritable bowel syndrome
- Gastroesophageal reflux disease (Gorroll, 2009)

Treatment: Patients with acute cholecystitis require hospitalization. Nasogastric suctioning, IV fluids with electrolytes, and intramuscular analgesics for severe pain are ordered. In older adults with suspected infection, IV antibiotics should be given, adjusting the dosage for creatinine clearance. Effective single-agent antibiotics, such as ampicillin, cephalosporins, and penicillins, are recommended except in cases of extremely debilitated patients. Patients with signs of gram-negative sepsis may require combination antibiotic treatment. Laparoscopic or open cholecystectomy should be considered when the patient stabilizes (Cho, Han, Yoon, & Ahn, 2010; Riall, Zhang, Townsend, Kuo, & Goodwin, 2010). Percutaneous cholecystostomy has been found to be a low-mortality treatment modality for frail and critically ill patients (Macrì et al., 2006; Winbladh, Gullstrand, Svanvik, & Sandström, 2009). When surgery is contraindicated in patients with acute calculus cholecystitis, treatment with an ursodeoxycholic acid may be considered if an adequately functioning gallbladder is present, and gallstones are determined to be composed of cholesterol. Additional medical management for patients, not deemed surgical candidates includes lithotripsy with bile salts.

Follow-up: Postoperative management includes monitoring for impending infection, adverse drug reactions and interactions, and changes in functional and mental status. For the frail older adult who is not a surgical candidate, observation for complications is crucial. Ultrasound of the gallbladder at 6-month intervals is recommended. For older women still prone to cholelithiasis after surgery, dosages of estrogen preparations may need to be reduced if applicable.

Sequelae: Complications of acute cholecystitis may result from severe inflammation with necrosis to the gallbladder, abscess formation, and localized perforation. Patients may develop jaundice, cholangitis, or pancreatitis. The gallbladder could rupture, resulting in severe peritonitis. Stone formation may occur subsequently in the bile ducts. Patients could experience bacterial superinfection with cholangitis or sepsis. The mortality rate for patients with perforation is about 30%. Frail older adults, especially those who are diabetic, are at high risk for complications from cholecystitis (Gorroll, 2009).

Prevention/prophylaxis: The importance of resting and avoiding risk factors after acute cholecystitis or an exacerbation of chronic cholecystitis needs to be emphasized.

Referral: A surgical consultation is necessary if acute cholecystitis is suspected. A gastroenterologist should be consulted for the frail older adult who is not a surgical candidate. Biliary pain in patients with a prior history of a cholecystectomy should be evaluated for a retained common bile duct stone. Referral to a gastroenterologist for evaluation by ERCP, magnetic resonance imaging (MRI), or endoscopic ultrasonography is highly recommended (Agrawal, Morrissey, & Thakkar, 2012).

Education: To prevent complications, encourage patients with chronic cholecystitis and patients for whom surgery is contraindicated to report early signs and symptoms of an acute attack. Patients also should be educated that gallstones could reoccur in the common bile duct.

CLINICAL RECOMMENDATION	EVIDENCE RATING	REFERENCES
For patients with cumulative risk factors for cholecystitis, early cholecystectomy is recommended before there is a progression of the disease leading to complications of acute cholecystitis.	B	Cho, Han, Yoon, & Ahn (2010) Riall, Zhang, Townsend, Kuo, & Goodwin (2010)
A positive Murphy's sign is a useful diagnostic tool when examining older adults presenting with symptoms of acute cholecystitis; a negative sign, however, should be cautiously interpreted.	C	Adedeji & McAdam (1996)
Older adults who underwent ultrasonograpahic percutaneous cholecystostomy for the treatment of acute cholecystitis had complete resolution of symptoms within 48 hours.	B	Macrì et al. (2006)
There was a negative correlation between BMI and the severity of cholecystitis; more complicated disease was found in males who were not obese.	B	Hyeon Kook, Ho-Seong, & Seog Ki (2009)

A = consistent, good-quality, patient-oriented evidence; B = inconsistent or limited-quality, patient-oriented evidence; C = consensus, disease-oriented evidence, usual practice, expert opinion, or case series. For information about the SORT evidence rating system, go to www.aafp.org/afpsort.xml.

CHRONIC KIDNEY DISEASE

Signal symptoms: Fatigue, anorexia, altered mental status, weakness, dysgeusia, pruritus, nausea, vomiting, and edema.

Description: Chronic kidney disease (CKD) is a growing worldwide health problem. The prevalence of kidney disease has been steadily increasing since 2003. In the Medicare population, the prevalence has increased from 2.7% in 2000 to 8.5% in 2009 (National Institutes of Health, 2011). Patients with CKD have higher rates of hospitalization and mortality than those without CKD (National Institutes of Health, 2011). The cost to Medicare for enrollees with CKD is $3,547 per year (National Institutes of Health, 2011). The major goal of Healthy People 2020 is to attempt to reduce new cases, complications, and economic costs of CKD (National Institutes of Health, 2011). With the increased prevalence of diabetes, the incidence of CKD will continue to rise.

Etiology: *Chronic kidney disease* is defined as structural abnormalities that can lead to the deterioration of kidney function over time (National Kidney Foundation, 2002). GFR is the best overall indicator of level of function and disease (National Kidney Foundation, 2002). CKD can then be further classified into five stages based on GFR and/or the presence of renal abnormalities such as proteinuria, hematuria, or histological/radiographical abnormalities (National Kidney Foundation, 2002). Following are the stages of chronic kidney disease:

- Stage 1—GFR is greater than or equal to 90 mL/min with other evidence of chronic kidney disease damage
- Stage 2—GFR between 60 and 89 mL/min
- Stage 3a—GFR 45 to 59 mL/min
- Stage 3b—GFR 30 to 44 mL/min
- Stage 4—GFR 15 to 29 mL/min
- Stage 5—GFR less than 15 mL/min or on dialysis

Diabetes is the leading cause of kidney failure, followed by hypertension. Other causes of kidney disease include glomerulonephritis, inherited polycystic disease, autoimmune diseases, infections, and urological diseases. Kidney disease is present when urine contains more than 30 mg of albumin per gram of creatinine, with or without decreased GFR.

Occurrence: An estimated 31 million people in the United States have been diagnosed with CKD.

Age: Although CKD can affect any age group, incidence increases with age. According to USRDS data, Medicare recipients with the highest incidence of CKD are ages 75 to 84. The age group with the highest incidence in the private sector includes people ages 45 to 54 (National Institutes of Health, 2011).

Gender: Among Medicare recipients, women have a higher incidence of CKD at 53% compared to men at 47% (National Institutes of Health, 2011). In the private sector, it is the opposite. A higher percentage of men are affected by CKD than women (National Institutes of Health, 2011).

Ethnicity: African Americans have a higher prevalence of CKD than Caucasians according to USRDS data. This is closely followed by Hispanics/Mexican Americans (National Institutes of Health, 2011).

Contributing factors: Diabetes mellitus is the leading cause of CKD and is the leading risk factor in the development of CKD. This is followed closely by hypertension, both a cause and a consequence of renal disease. Inflammatory diseases, such as systemic lupus erythematosus, and malignancy, such as renal tumors or multiple myeloma, also increase the risk of kidney failure. Vascular disease, chronic pyelonephritis, urinary stones, systemic infections, certain medications, and radiopaque dye also heighten the risk of developing CKD. AKI often predisposes a patient to the development of CKD. A family history of renal disease is an important risk factor in the development of CKD as well. Racial and ethnic minorities have an increased risk of CKD, as do patients with lower socioeconomic status and education level. Specifically, minorities may be more likely to progress from CKD to end-stage renal disease and less likely to see a nephrologist than other individuals with CKD. A reduced number of glomeruli is also a predisposing factor to development of CKD and hypertension (Aschner, 2011). It has been found that the diet that an individual's mother consumes during her pregnancy, specifically the protein content, is indicative of the number of protons in the adult kidney. A mother who is undernourished during her pregnancy will have offspring with a smaller number of glomeruli and thus increased risk of hypertension and renal disease (Aschner, 2011). In addition, the presence of inherited disease, such as autosomal dominant polycystic kidney disease, will lead to development of CKD.

Exposure to toxins can also play a role in the development of CKD. Exposure can be occupational, environmental, or recreational. There is a strong association between smoking and development of CKD. Chronic smoking causes nephrosclerosis, which is caused by microvascular atherosclerosis. This then leads to hypertension, further hastening the progression of CKD. Illicit substances that have been associated with CKD include heroin and cocaine. Recently, methamphetamines and ecstasy have been reported to be associated with CKD. Cocaine use is associated with acute rises in blood pressure, leading to AKI from hypertension. Although heroin use was initially thought to cause focal glomerular sclerosis, it is now thought that substances mixed with the heroin or even transmittable diseases, such as hepatitis and HIV associated with IV injection of street drugs, are the cause of the CKD (Connor, 2011). Methamphetamines cause accelerated hypertension, leading to renal damage and/or progression of CKD. Ecstasy use has risen recently, particularly among young adults. It can lead to rhabdomyolysis, drug-induced vasculitis, and severe hyponatremia. Recurrent episodes of rhabdomyolysis injury could lead to CKD for the patient (Connor, 2011). Exposure to heavy metals, such as lead, cadmium, mercury, and organic solvents, has been strongly linked to CKD. Lead nephropathy can be caused by retained lead bullets in patients with prior gunshot wounds or by eating from lead-glazed pottery. Exposure to cadmium is often occupational, whereas mercury vapor is released in coal-burning power plants and municipal incinerators and returned to earth through rain. Organic solvents, such as those found in paint thinners and degreasers, are derived from hydrocarbons. Painters and factory workers are at greatest risk of occupational exposure to these chemicals.

Signs and symptoms: Unfortunately, CKD does not produce symptoms until renal injury is quite advanced. Many individuals are unaware that they have CKD until it progresses to stage 3 or stage 4. In stages 1 and 2, BUN and creatinine are normal or nearly normal, and acid-base, fluid, and electrolyte balances are maintained through the adaption of remaining nephrons. In stage 3, there is moderate impairment of GFR, and BUN and creatinine begin to increase. The patient usually remains asymptomatic, but levels of erythropoietin and parathyroid hormone are abnormal. Early symptoms of kidney disease, if any, may be similar to other illnesses. Only when the patient develops stage 4 or 5 kidney disease do more profound symptoms of CKD occur. These include fatigue, loss of appetite and weight loss, dyspnea, edema in upper and lower extremities, confusion and difficulty with concentration, pruritus, dysgeusia, and foul-smelling breath.

Although diagnosis of kidney disease is based heavily on laboratory data and diagnostic imaging, a careful history may lead to clues associated with the diagnosis of CKD. Careful review of any kidney disease in the family is important. In addition, specific questions relating to any hereditary diseases, such as autosomal dominant polycystic kidney disease, are imperative. Questions should be asked regarding any abnormal findings from past routine examinations such as those for school, military service, or insurance purposes. If the patient has a past history of pregnancy, ask whether there were any complications, including proteinuria or preeclampsia. Also ask if the patient has had any past urological examinations that were abnormal, which could indicate postrenal causes of CKD.

Any history of diabetes mellitus or hypertension should immediately raise a strong suspicion for the presence of CKD. In addition, ask the patient if he or she has any history of congestive heart failure, cirrhosis, or gastrointestinal symptoms that may cause prerenal CKD. Specific questions regarding any disorders of the urinary tract, such as frequent infections, stones or obstruction, recent systemic infections, unusual rashes or skin lesions, and use of illicit substances, should also raise suspicion of CKD. A number of medications can be associated with CKD, so a through medication review, including prescription medications, OTC medications, and supplements, should be completed.

Diagnostic tests: As stated previously, estimation of GFR is the best indicator to level of kidney function and functioning renal mass. Monitoring for changes in GFR can indicate progression of disease and allow for monitoring for any complication of kidney disease. Furthermore, it allows for proper dosing of medications to avoid drug toxicity (National Kidney Foundation, 2002). Serum creatinine alone is not an accurate indicator of the GFR, because the GFR may decline to almost one-half before an increase in the serum creatinine level is seen. Among adults, GFR is calculated using the MDRD Study equation, which takes into account body surface area, age, race, and gender.

$$GFR = 175 \times standardized\ Scr - 1.154 \times age - 0.203 \times 1.212 \text{ [if black]} \times 0.742 \text{ [if female]}$$

Estimates of GFR in CKD are more accurate than those in patients with AKI, because they are in steady state with their kidney function. Patients who have extremes of muscle mass, such as the frail elderly, the critically ill, cancer patients, body builders, or those with unusual diets, will also have inaccurate GFR. In these patients, a creatinine clearance, in which a volume of urine is collected over 24 hours and the amount of creatinine secreted is measured, is a more accurate indicator of GFR.

Level of proteinuria is another indicator to the severity of CKD. Urine normally contains small amounts of protein, usually less than 30 mg/day. A persistent increase in protein excretion is usually a sign of kidney damage. The type of protein that is excreted, usually either albumin or low-molecular-weight globulins, depends on the type of kidney disease. Increased excretion of protein is a marker of CKD related to diabetes mellitus, glomerular disease, or hypertension. Under National Kidney Foundation guidelines, the term *proteinuria* relates to increased urinary excretion of albumin, other specific proteins, or total protein (National Kidney Foundation, 2002). The term *albumineria*, on the other hand, refers only to the increased urinary excretion of albumin. *Microalbumineria* is the excretion of protein above the normal range but below the level detected by tests for normal protein excretion in the urine (National Kidney Foundation, 2002). Monitoring proteinuria in adults is performed by an untimed spot urine sample to detect and monitor proteinuria. In most patients, the urine dipstick test is acceptable for detecting proteinuria. Standard dipstick may be used to detect any increase in total urine protein excretion, and albumin-specific dipsticks are used to detect albuminuria. In screening patients for CKD, if a urine dipstick is positive, the proteinuria should be confirmed within 3 months, using a protein-to-creatinine ratio or albumin-to-creatinine ratio (National Kidney Foundation, 2002). If a patient has two or more quantitative positive tests performed 1 to 2 weeks apart with persistent proteinuria, the patient should be evaluated for CKD by a nephrologist (National Kidney Foundation, 2002). The American Diabetes Association (ADA) and the National Institutes of Health (NIH) recommend annual testing of urine albumin excretion to assess for kidney damage in people with diabetes. Adults with known CKD are monitored with the albumin-to-creatinine ratio.

In addition to proteinuria, there are other markers that indicate damage to the kidneys. These include abnormalities in urinary sediment and abnormal findings on imaging studies. Examination of the urinary sediment can be useful in diagnosing CKD and in identifying of the type of kidney disease. The presence of white blood cells, red blood cells, or casts may indicate the presence of acute or chronic kidney disease and requires further investigation. Imaging studies should also be performed to suggest the cause of CKD. Ultrasound examination may indicate the presence of kidney stones, hydronephrosis, cysts, or masses. Small kidneys on ultrasound suggest chronic kidney disease, whereas "large" kidneys may indicate tumors, cysts, or infiltrating diseases. CT may reveal tumors, obstructions, cysts, or calculi. IV pyelography may reveal asymmetry of kidney size, presence of obstructing stones, tumors, or dilated collecting ducts (National Kidney Foundation, 2002).

Further laboratory data that should be assessed in patients with possible CKD include CBC to evaluate for anemia, electrolytes, albumin, BUN, and creatinine. Fasting lipids and HgbA1c should also be evaluated in the diabetic patient. Serum calcium, phosphorus, parathyroid hormone, and vitamin D levels should be drawn to evaluate for the changes in mineral metabolism and bone structure that begin early in CKD. Iron studies, vitamin B_{12}, and folate should also be completed and replacement begun if warranted.

Differential diagnosis:
- Acute kidney injury
- Cirrhosis
- Uropathic obstruction
- Nephrotic syndrome
- Tubulointerstitial disease

Treatment: Referral to a nephrologist should occur if (1) GFR is less than 30 mL/min, (2) there is a decline in GFR greater than 3 mL/min, (3) albumin-to-creatinine ratio is greater than 30 mg/mmol or 300 mg/g, (4) hypertension is hard to get to target level despite three or more antihypertensive agents, and (5) there is unexplained anemia with GFR less than 60 mL/min (Johnson, 2011). Further investigation using the diagnostic tests above will assist the nephrologist in the determination of the cause of the CKD. Once the stage of CKD is identified, management of CKD is aimed primarily at preventing progression of the disease through medications, risk factor reduction, lifestyle changes, and education of the patient and family regarding kidney disease. Eventually there is decline in kidney function to end-stage renal disease. Patients then must decide between renal replacement therapy—hemodialysis or peritoneal dialysis—in order for the patient to survive, or opt for no renal replacement therapy and end-of-life care.

Patients with CKD have a greater risk for cardiovascular disease than those without. As stated previously, hypertension is both a cause and a sequela of kidney disease. It is associated with a faster decline in kidney function by increasing proteinuria and furthering the development of cardiovascular disease. Thus reducing risk of progression of CKD and advancement of cardiovascular disease is paramount. Reduction of blood pressure to target levels is the most important treatment step in managing CKD. The targeted blood pressure for patients with hypertension, as recommended by the Joint National Committee's seventh report (JNC-7), is less than or equal to 140/80 mm Hg. Over the past few years all major guidelines, including those from JNC-7 and the National Kidney Foundation–Kidney Disease Outcomes Quality Initiative (NKF-KDOQI), have recommended a lower blood pressure goal of less than 130/80 mm Hg for patients with CKD and/or diabetes (Kalitzidis, 2011). Furthermore, KDOQI recommends a target blood pressure of less than 125/75 mm Hg for CKD patients with proteinuria of greater than 300 mg per day (National Kidney Foundation, 2002). Patients who are at greatest risk for complications or already have evidence of cardiovascular disease may need more aggressive and earlier treatment of hypertension. Multiple medications are frequently required in CKD patients to achieve goal blood pressure. ACE inhibitors and angiotensin receptor blockers (ARBs) are first-line treatment as antihypertensive medications. These agents reduce proteinuria and slow the rate of decline in kidney function in both diabetic and nondiabetic kidney disease. When beginning a patient on an ACE inhibitor or ARB, serum creatinine and GFR should be measured at 1 week and 4 weeks after initiation of therapy. If the initial rise in creatinine is more than 30% above the baseline value, the ACE inhibitor or ARB should be discontinued. ACE inhibitors or ARBs should also be withdrawn if serum potassium concentration exceeds 6 mmol/L despite dose reduction, potassium diet restriction, and diuretic therapy. In addition, treatment response to ACE inhibitors or ARBs can be monitored by albuminuria. Reduction in urinary albumin excretion will decrease risk of development of end-stage kidney disease and cardiovascular disease. Furthermore, sodium restriction of less than 2.4 grams per day is recommended for blood pressure control. This is especially important in "salt sensitive" groups, for example, African Americans, older individuals, and those with diabetes, hypertension, and CKD. These groups are more salt sensitive and have a greater response in their blood pressure with increased intake of salt.

Because of the increased salt and water retention with CKD, use of a diuretic should be included in the antihypertensive regimen of the CKD patient. Thiazide diuretics often become less effective as GFR falls below 40 mL/min due to decreased renal blood flow. Usually a loop diuretic, such as furosemide, torsemide, or bumetanide, is used. Side effects of loop diuretics include hypokalemia and hypomagnesia, which can lead to increased cardiovascular risk of arrhythmias. Thus, serum electrolytes should be monitored, and the patient should be instructed to report any paresthesias, rash, or tinnitus. Beta blockers, such as carvedilol, metroprolol, or bisprolol, should be used in patients with CKD when a proper dose of ACE inhibitor, ARB, or diuretic is not enough to lower blood pressure. Although these agents do not provide any renoprotective effects, they do assist in reducing cardiovascular mortality in high-risk patients. Beta blockers should be avoided in patients with bradycardia or heart block. Calcium channel blockers (CCBs) are also effective agents that can be used to lower blood pressure in CKD patients. However, there are differences between these medications' effects on reducing proteinuria. Nondihydropyridine CCBs (verapamil, diltiazem) reduce proteinuria among patients with advanced nephropathy, whereas dihydropyridine CCBs (nifedipine, felodipine, amlodipine) will not have this effect unless coupled with an ACE inhibitor or ARB (Kalitzidis, 2011). They should not be used as monotherapy in CKD patients but in combination with an ACE inhibitor or ARB to achieve optimal blood pressure control. Central alpha-adrenergic agonists decrease the effects of sympathetic activity to lower blood pressure. Vasodilators, such as hydralazine and minoxidil, are often used as fourth-line agents when other antihypertensive treatments have failed. Vasodilator therapy does not reduce proteinuria and has not been shown to improve renal outcomes. Side effects of minoxidil include increased hair growth and risk of pericardial effusion. Hydralazine is the leading cause of drug-induced lupus syndrome and should be avoided in any patient with an autoimmune disease.

Tight glycemic control in CKD patients reduces cardiovascular disease and CKD progression risk in both type 1 and type 2 diabetes mellitus. An HgbA1c of less than 7.0% is the goal of patients with diabetes and CKD. Although achieving this can be difficult for some patients and is associated with increased risk of hypoglycemia, tight control reduces not only albuminuria but also retinopathy and neuropathy. Insulin can be used to treat diabetes in CKD, and doses should be tailored to attain the goal HgbA1c while avoiding hypoglycemia. Insulin types and doses should be individualized to each patient and to the patient's level of CKD. First-generation sulfonylureas are metabolized in the kidney and may lead to longer half-lives with greater risk of hypoglycemia and thus should be avoided in CKD. Metformin, a biguanide, is also metabolized in the kidney and increases risk for lactic acidosis and so should also be avoided. Exenatide (Byetta) is not recommended for use in patients with a GFR less than 30 mL/min and has actually been found to cause renal failure in a number of patients (Hahr, 2011).

Anemia is a common complication of CKD. It worsens as kidney function declines and becomes prevalent in CKD stage 3 and continues through stage 5 into end-stage renal disease. The primary cause of anemia is decreased secretion of erythropoietin from decreased functioning renal cells. The anemia results in fatigue, decreased exercise capacity, decreased cognition, and impaired immunity. This then leads to decreased quality of life. In addition, increased workload of the heart, due to the anemia, leads to left ventricular hypertrophy and cardiomyopathy. This increases the patient's risk of death from ischemic heart disease and heart failure. Target hemoglobin goals are 11 to 12 g/dL in patients with CKD (National Kidney Foundation, 2002). In addition, iron studies should be completed to evaluate for a true iron deficiency or functional iron deficiency. Iron replacement is given orally as ferrous sulfate. IV iron is usually reserved for those patients severely iron depleted or those patients on hemodialysis. Erythropoietin-stimulating agents can be given once iron deficiency is corrected; other causes of anemia have been excluded or treated; and hemoglobin is consistently below 10 g/dL. Epoetin alfa and darbepoetin alfa are two genetically engineered agents that can be administered to CKD patients to increase bone marrow production of red blood cells.

Changes in mineral metabolism and bone structure begin early in CKD. This not only encompasses bone disease but also vascular and soft tissue calcification. As kidney function worsens and GFR continues to decline, the kidney must work harder to excrete phosphorus. This then reduces the formation of the active form of vitamin D (1,25D). Low levels of 1,25D, coupled with low serum calcium levels from decreased gut absorption, lead to a rise in parathyroid hormone. This leads to secondary hyperparathyroidism due to hypocalcemia, hyperphosphatemia, and low 1,25D levels. The increased parathyroid hormone affects bone

metabolism and increased bone turnover, causing decreased cortical bone and bone strength. This increases risk of fracture and causes increased "bone pain" in CKD patients. Development of secondary hyperparathyroidism can be decreased by dietary restriction of high-phosphate foods such as nuts, beans, dairy products, colas, and processed food products. A phosphate binder, which binds to the phosphate in food and is eliminated in the bowel movement, is also prescribed. Calcium acetate, lanthanum carbonate, and sevelemer carbonate are the common phosphate binders used today. In addition, administration of vitamin D (Rocaltrol, Hectoral, and Zemplar) also helps to reduce parathyroid hormone secretion.

Patients with CKD are also at increased risk for malnutrition and hypoalbuminemia. These are associated with poor outcomes when the time comes for the patient to initiate dialysis. The restriction of protein in the CKD population has been a topic of ongoing debate. Current recommendations from the NKF/KDOQI (2002) include a protein intake of 0.8 to 1.0 g/kg per day in patients with CKD. Patients need to be monitored for malnutrition with serum albumin levels and body weight assessments.

Smoking cessation is strongly encouraged in patients with CKD. Smoking compounds the risk for cardiovascular mortality in patients with CKD and hastens progression of kidney disease. It should be addressed with each office visit and risks reviewed with the patient.

Unfortunately, despite optimal treatment and practices by the patient, kidney disease may continue to progress until kidney failure occurs. Patients then develop uremia, which is the accumulation of toxins within the blood. This leads to anorexia, nausea, vomiting, asterixis, muscle weakness, platelet dysfunction, pericarditis, mental status changes, and possibly coma. At this point, dialysis is initiated to "clean" the blood of these toxins and will need to continue throughout the patient's lifetime.

Follow-up: Care of the patient with CKD is in the hands of the nephrologist for the rest of the patient's life span. In the year following diagnosis of CKD, there is a greater likelihood of having seen a primary care provider than a cardiologist or nephrologist (National Institutes of Health, 2011). On the other hand, the severity of the CKD increases the likelihood that the patient will follow up with a nephrologist (National Institutes of Health, 2011). Among Medicare patients, African Americans are 15% more likely to see a nephrologist 12 months after diagnosis with CKD than Caucasians (National Institutes of Health, 2011). Those factors associated with increased likelihood of follow-up with a nephrologist among Medicare patients included African American race and patients with diabetes, hypertension, and cardiovascular disease (National Institutes of Health, 2011).

The nephrologist continues to manage the patient in an attempt to avoid any further progression of CKD. Tight glycemic control, optimal blood pressure control, dietary phosphate restriction, and management of anemia are paramount. Patient education of CKD continues with every office visit as well. In addition, once the patient reaches stage 4, "options classes" are held with the family and the patient to discuss dialysis modalities (i.e., peritoneal dialysis or hemodialysis). Referral for renal transplant should be made before the patient begins dialysis. If the patient chooses not to proceed with dialysis, referral should be made for palliative care to discuss end-of-life decisions.

Sequelae: The major sequela of CKD is end-stage renal disease. In addition, CKD is associated with an increased risk for cardiovascular disease. Thus, lifestyle changes, such as maintaining healthy body weight, restriction of salt and high-fat diet, active participation in an exercise program, smoking cessation, limited alcohol intake, and tight glycemic and blood pressure control, are important, not only to reduce cardiac risk but also to slow progression of kidney disease.

Prevention/prophylaxis: Early screening for proteinuria in patients at risk for CKD is paramount. Any patient who has diabetes or hypertension should be screened annually for proteinuria. Tight glycemic control, optimal blood pressure control, tobacco cessation, low-salt diet, avoidance of nephrotoxic medications, and optimal weight with healthy lifestyle all assist in reduction of risk of CKD.

Referral: In patients who have hereditary or autoimmune diseases associated with CKD, referral to a nephrologist for close monitoring of kidney function is important.

Education: Patients with CKD are educated regarding their disease and the manifestations of this disease. Continued education of low-sodium diet, compliance with medications, tight glycemic control, and avoidance of NSAIDs and contrast dye is important. Patients are encouraged to continue to follow up with their primary care physician for other aspects of their health care.

CLINICAL RECOMMENDATION	EVIDENCE RATING	REFERENCES
Glomerular filtration rate (GFR) is the best indicator of kidney function.	A	National Kidney Foundation (2002)
In screening patients for CKD, a urine dipstick for proteinuria should be confirmed within 3 months, utilizing a protein-to-creatinine ratio or albumin-to-creatinine ratio. If a patient has persistent proteinuria, referral should be made to a nephrologist.	A	National Kidney Foundation (2002)
Target blood pressure in both diabetic and nondiabetic kidney disease is <130/80 mm Hg, and patients should be treated with either an ACE inhibitor or angiotensin receptor blocker.	A	National Kidney Foundation (2002)
Target hemoglobin A1c for people with diabetes should be <7%, regardless of the presence of chronic kidney disease.	A	National Kidney Foundation (2002)
Utilization of a nondihydropyridine reduces proteinuria among patients with advanced nephropathy.	A	National Kidney Foundation (2002)

CLINICAL RECOMMENDATION	EVIDENCE RATING	REFERENCES
Both calcium-based and non–calcium-based binders are effective in lowering serum phosphorus levels in patients with CKD.	A	National Kidney Foundation (2002)
Serum creatinine alone should not be used to monitor kidney function. GFR should also be used.	C	Inker (2010) Johnson et al. (2004a, 2004b) Post (2011)
Optimal blood pressure control with either an ACE inhibitor or angiotensin blocker coupled with nondihydropyridine calcium channel blockers (CCBs) will also reduce proteinuria.	C	Aschner (2011) Kalitzidis (2011)

A = consistent, good-quality, patient-oriented evidence; B = inconsistent or limited-quality, patient-oriented evidence; C = consensus, disease-oriented evidence, usual practice, expert opinion, or case series. For information about the SORT evidence rating system, go to www.aafp.org/afpsort.xml.

CIRRHOSIS OF THE LIVER

Signal symptoms: Jaundice, fatigue, spider angiomas, palmar erythema, and nodular liver.

Description: Cirrhosis occurs when there is chronic insult to the liver, resulting in fibrous and nodular regeneration of the existing hepatocytes. Forty percent of patients are asymptomatic initially when cirrhosis is diagnosed as part of a routine examination (Heidelbaugh & Bruderly, 2006).

Etiology: Chronic alcoholism and viral hepatitis are the most common causes of cirrhosis in the United States. Nonalcoholic fatty liver disease (NAFLD) that leads to cryptogenic cirrhosis is on the rise (Clark & Diehl, 2003). The cause of primary biliary cirrhosis, a chronic inflammatory disease of the liver in which the intrahepatic bile duct is destroyed, is unknown.

Occurrence: In the United States, there are approximately 900,000 total individuals with cirrhosis (Cirrhosis of the liver, 2005).

Age: Cirrhosis, which has an increase in onset in older adults, is the 12th leading cause of death, predominantly in patients with alcoholic liver disease (Heidelbaugh & Bruderly, 2006; Starr & Raines, 2011). Onset of primary biliary cirrhosis usually occurs before age 65.

Gender: Cirrhosis of the liver is equally prevalent in men and women with chronic alcoholism.

Ethnicity: No known prevalence exists among groups.

Contributing factors: Chronic alcohol consumption, combined with a poor nutritional intake, contributes to cirrhosis. Drug-inducted cirrhosis can occur in patients taking large doses of vitamin A, aldomet, isoniazide, and methotrexate. Certain infectious diseases (tertiary syphilis, brucellosis, schistosomiasis) have predisposed patients to a risk of developing cirrhosis. Patients with Wilson's disease, sarcoidosis, heart failure, and hemochromatosis may go on to develop cirrhosis (Heidelbaugh & Bruderly, 2006). A history of the following chronic conditions can contribute to the development of biliary cirrhosis: biliary obstruction, cystic fibrosis, primary sclerosing cholangitis, and congenital biliary cysts (Heidelbaugh & Bruderly, 2006). Chronic hepatitis B and C viruses also place patients at risk for developing cirrhosis (Chen, Chu, Yeh, & Liaw, 2007; Starr & Raines, 2011). Risk factors for developing cryptogenic cirrhosis, which occurs in patients with NAFLD, include obesity, diabetes mellitus, hypertriglyceridemia, and significant weight loss in patients who have had jejunoileal bypass surgery (Gill & Wu, 2006; Riley, Taheri, & Schreibman, 2009).

Signs and symptoms: Patients report anorexia, fatigue, pruritus, jaundice, and easy bruising of the skin. When questioned, reports of weight loss, weakness, and gastrointestinal bleeding may be common. An assessment tool, such as the AUDIT (Alcohol Use Disorders Identification Test) or the CAGE Questionnaire (Ewing, 1984), is recommended to discern alcohol-related problems. It allows the practitioner to explore the patient's history of chronic alcohol use and the status of functional impairment. Physical examination may reveal evidence of scleral icterus, Kayser-Fleischer ring around the cornea of the eye, xanthoma, palmar erythema, spider angiomas, dilated abdominal veins, clubbing of fingers, changes in the nail bed (Terry's nails, with two-thirds of the nail bed appearing white), Dupuytren's contracture, asterixis, and in men, decreased body hair, gynecomastia, and testicular atrophy. Palpation of the liver may reveal a firm, nodular liver; splenomegaly; and ascites (Heidelbaugh & Bruderly, 2006; Starr & Raines, 2011).

Diagnostic tests: CBC with indices may reveal a macrocytic anemia caused by nutritional deficiencies of vitamin B_{12} and folic acid. A decreased serum albumin level and prolonged prothrombin time occur in cirrhosis. The serum aspartate aminotransferase (AST) level is elevated; the alanine aminotransferase (ALT) level is usually above normal but not to the degree of the AST. The ALT is a more specific test for recognizing liver disease than the AST (Duke, 2012). The ammonia level is elevated in patients with hepatic encephalopathy. The alpha-fetoprotein (AFP) level is elevated in patients with hepatitis C and is also a tumor marker for hepatocellular carcinoma (Duke, 2012; Starr & Raines, 2011). Abdominal ultrasound can be ordered initially when cirrhosis is suspected, given clinical symptom presentation and other diagnostic studies as surface nodularity, ascites, increased parenchymal echogenicity of the liver, and the direction of portal blood flow can be detected using Doppler scanning (Heidelbaugh & Bruderly, 2006). A percutaneous liver biopsy can establish the diagnosis of cirrhosis.

Differential diagnosis:
- Liver cancer
- Alcoholic hepatitis
- Congenital hepatic fibrosis
- Portal hypertension
- Schistosomiasis

Treatment: Treatment of cirrhosis is primarily dependent on the cause of the disease. Cessation of all alcohol intake is imperative in all cases (O'Shea, Dasarathy, & McCullough, 2010). Review the patient's immunizations, and determine the need for influenza,

hepatitis A and hepatitis B, and pneumococcal pneumonia vaccines. Since protein-calorie malnutrition and vitamin deficiencies are prevalent in patients with alcoholic liver disease, nutritional therapy is of the essence. Nutritional support includes at least 1 g protein/kg body weight and 2000 to 3000 kcal/day, unless contraindicated by the presence of hepatic encephalopathy or coma. It is highly recommended that patients with cirrhosis have small frequent nutritious feedings, including a small snack at bedtime and a small morning meal, to improve overall nitrogen balance (Swart et al., 1989). Multiple-vitamin supplements should be prescribed, including adequate intake of vitamins A, D, and K; it is recommended, however, that a multiple vitamin without iron be recommended unless iron-deficiency anemia is present (O'Shea et al., 2010).

Studies have indicated that a 4-week course of prednisolone (40 mg/day for 28 days, typically followed by discontinuation or a 2-week taper) is beneficial in patients with alcoholic liver disease unless steroid therapy is contraindicated (Uribe, Schalm, Summerskill, & Go, 1978). The use of pentoxifylline (400 mg orally 3 times daily for 4 weeks) is also recommended for treatment of alcoholic liver disease (Akriviadis et al., 2000). Treatment for complications of cirrhosis may include antibiotics for infections, diuretics and reduction of salt if the patient has ascites, beta blockers for portal hypertension, symptomatic relief of pruritus, and the use of lactulose in hepatic encephalopathy (Heidelbaugh & Bruderly, 2006).

Follow-up: Surveillance of the older adult with cirrhosis depends on the stability of the patient and the presence of complications. Stable older adults should have repeat liver function tests 6 months to 1 year after initial diagnosis. Unstable patients may need to be monitored monthly. Complications of cirrhosis, listed under Sequelae, require additional medical therapy. On return visits, observation and testing for changes in mental status and depression may be indicated.

Sequelae: Complications from cirrhosis include ascites, spontaneous bacterial peritonitis resulting from uncontrolled ascites, portal hypertension, hepatopulmonary syndrome, portopulmonary hypertension (Kochar, Nevah, Moises, & Fallon, 2011), esophageal variceal bleeding, renal failure, and hepatic encephalopathy and hepatorenal syndrome. Alcoholic hepatitis may occur with cirrhosis. Patients with ascites and cirrhosis are at risk for developing an umbilical hernia (Eker et al., 2011). The incidence of developing cholelithiasis increases in patients with cirrhosis (Pessaux & Lermite, 2008). There is a very high risk of developing hepatocellular carcinoma, which is the leading cause of death for patients with cirrhosis.

Prevention/prophylaxis: Cessation of alcohol consumption is crucial to the prognosis of cirrhosis. Avoidance of hepatotoxic medications, especially NSAIDs, is recommended for patients with cirrhosis. All patients with cirrhosis should be given the hepatitis A and B vaccine, unless they are shown to be immune to the diseases. The polyvalent pneumococcal vaccine and annual influenza vaccines also are recommended for these patients. Preventive strategies for patients with cirrhosis need to focus on the prevention of complications by instituting measures such as endoscopic screenings and secondary prophylaxis.

Referral: A gastroenterologist should be consulted when varices are suspected and variceal bleeding occurs. An esophagogastroduodenoscopy is performed to manage complicated patients. Patients presenting with a new onset of ascites need to be referred for consideration of diagnostic paracentesis (Starr & Raines, 2011). Referral to a hepatologist for patients with cirrhosis should be considered early on to plan management for complications and formulate plans for end-stage liver disease.

Education: Instruct patients to eliminate all alcohol consumption. Recommend an alcohol treatment program, and provide the telephone number for the nearest chapter of Alcoholics Anonymous. Patients should be requested not to self-medicate with OTC medications, including herbal products. Patients with cirrhosis should eat small frequent meals of a balanced diet containing 1 to 1.5 mg protein/kg body weight per day unless contraindicated by advanced disease. Patients with encephalopathy should not be driving. For patients with end-stage liver disease, palliative care measures should be initiated.

CLINICAL RECOMMENDATION	EVIDENCE RATING	REFERENCES
A thorough nutritional assessment is highly recommended for patients with alcoholic liver disease to screen for protein-calorie malnutrition as well as vitamin and mineral deficiencies. Those with severe disease should be treated aggressively with enteral nutritional therapy.	B	O'Shea, Dasarathy, & McCullough (2010)
Patients with severe alcoholic liver disease with or without hepatic encephalopathy and lacking contraindications to steroid use should be considered for a 4-week course of prednisolone (40 mg/day for 28 days, typically followed by discontinuation or a 2-week taper).	A	O'Shea et al. (2010) Uribe et al. (1978)
Patients should be highly encouraged to abstain from drinking al alcohol.	B	Borowsky, Strome, & Lott (1981) Pessione et al. (2003)
It is highly recommended that patients with cirrhosis have small, frequent, nutritious feedings, including a small snack at bedtime and a small morning meal, to improve overall nitrogen balance.	A	Swart et al. (1989)

A = consistent, good-quality, patient-oriented evidence; B = inconsistent or limited-quality, patient-oriented evidence; C = consensus, disease-oriented evidence, usual practice, expert opinion, or case series. For information about the SORT evidence rating system, go to www.aafp.org/afpsort.xml.

CLOSTRIDIUM DIFFICILE

Signal symptoms: Fever, nonbloody diarrhea, abdominal cramping.

Description: *Clostridium difficile*–associated diarrhea (CDAD) and colitis are a consequence of the colonization and subsequent infection of the colon by this organism following a disruption of the normal flora of the gut. Once established in the colon, *C. difficile* produces two potent toxins, termed *Toxin A* and *Toxin B,* that cause fluid secretion, inflammation, and injury that result in diarrhea and/or colitis. Intestinal colonization by toxigenic *C. difficile* strains does not always result in infection or clinical symptoms.

Most patients with *C. difficile* diarrhea who are examined by endoscopy with mucosal biopsy have either gross or microscopic colitis. Pseudomembranous colitis, a more advanced state of *C. difficile* diarrhea, is characterized by a colonic mucosa exhibiting adherent, white and yellowish plaques that may coalesce. Histology shows a neutrophilic inflammation of the mucosa with overlying exudates (Kee, 2012).

Clinical presentation of *C. difficile* diarrhea varies from diarrhea without colitis to colitis with or without pseudomembranes and more rarely, fulminant colitis. Mild cases may present with only crampy lower abdominal pain or an occasional watery stool. Moderate to severe cases present with profuse diarrhea (15 to 30 loose stools per day), abdominal pain, tenesmus, nausea, anorexia, fever, and malaise. In 1% to 3% of patients, fulminant colitis will develop with ileus, toxic megacolon, perforation, and, rarely, death. Other complications include chronic diarrhea, electrolyte imbalance, hypoalbuminemia with anasarca, and reactive arthritis (Kee, 2012).

Etiology: CDAD may occur in any person taking antibiotics, but it is most common in patients of hospitals or long-term care facilities where the organism may be endemic or epidemic. The organism and its spores survive well in these environments and are transmitted horizontally from colonized or infected patients to susceptible persons via fomites and the hands of physicians, health-care workers, and nursing home employees. Asymptomatic carriage of the organism by patients is not uncommon and may hinder adequate infection control measures. The transfer of patients harboring *C. difficile* infection (CDI) from one hospital or long-term care facility to another enables spread of the infection within geographical regions (Cohen et al., 2010; Kee, 2012).

Clostridium difficile causes diarrhea of colitis almost exclusively in persons exposed to oral or parenteral antibiotics. Almost all antibiotics, including metronidazole and vancomycin, have been found to cause CDAD, although the most frequent offending agents are clindamycin, ampicillin, amoxicillin, extended-spectrum penicillins, and cephalosporins (Martinez, Leffler, & Kelly, 2012). There appears to be less risk for fluoroquinolones, macrolides (including azithromycin, clarithromycin, and erythromycin), trimethoprim-sulfamethoxazole, rifampin, and tetracyclines. Rarely is infection due to exposure to vancomycin or metronidazole. Broad-spectrum fluoroquinolones that exhibit anti-anaerobic activity, such as gatifloxacin, may carry more risk for subsequent CDI than other fluoroquinolones (ciprofloxacin or levofloxacin). Other risk factors that predispose to CDAD include advanced age, severity and number of comorbid illnesses, recent bowel surgery, uremia, malnutrition, antineoplastic chemotherapy, and shock.

Occurrence: CDIs are affecting significant numbers of hospitalized older adults. It is estimated that 20% to 40% of hospitalized patients are colonized with *C. difficile* toxin as compared to 2% to 3% of healthy adults. The incidence in long-term care patients varies from 4% to 50% (Kee, 2012). Of patients with antibiotic-associated diarrhea, 15% to 25% and more than 95% with pseudomembranous colitis carry the *C. difficile* toxin (Barbut & Petit, 2001).

Age: Although the infection is difficult to manage in all ages, elderly *C. difficile* patients can be particularly challenging to treat. The advanced age of these individuals puts them at increased risk for *C. difficile*; this is compounded by other risk factors (Simor, 2010).

Gender: Occurs in both males and females equally.

Ethnicity: Occurs in all ethnic groups.

Contributing factors: The main contributing factor to the development of CDI is antibiotic exposure; all antibiotics have the potential to stimulate the development of CDI. Advancing age is a known risk factor. Patients with prolonged length of stay in a health-care facility can be exposed to CDI, especially if they share common toilets, have severe underlying disease (malignancies), use proton pump inhibitors and H_2 blockers, need tube feeding, and show poor host immune response

(Hessen, 2010). Patients with prior gastrointestinal surgeries are at risk. The use of perioperative antibiotic prophylaxis has been known to contribute to CDI (Carignan et al., 2008; Cohen et al., 2010).

Signs and symptoms: The incubation period has not been established. Symptoms can appear immediately after beginning antibiotic therapy, or they may not develop until several weeks after it is completed. Older adults can present atypically, with lack of fever. There may be noticeable weakness, weight loss, decrease in the ability to carry out activities of daily living (ADLs) and frequent falling. Alteration in mental status or confusion can be an early sign (Bartlett & Gerding, 2008; Crogan & Evans, 2007). Most often, CDAD presents as mild to moderate nonbloody, foul-smelling diarrhea, sometimes accompanied by lower abdominal cramping. Systemic symptoms are typically absent, and physical examination is remarkable only for mild abdominal tenderness.

Severe infection or colitis tends to present with more severe symptoms, including profuse watery diarrhea, abdominal pain, and distention. Fever, nausea, and dehydration are often present. The patients may become hypovolemic. There may be occult blood in the stool, but this is rare. Sigmoidoscopy reveals a characteristic membrane with adherent yellow plaques, usually in the distal colon.

Diagnostic tests: Obtain stools for *C. difficile* toxins using enzyme-linked immunosorbent assay (ELISA) Toxins A and B (Musher et al., 2007). In addition, obtain CBC with differential to determine presence or extent of infection; electrolytes and serum creatinine to rule out dehydration; thyroid panel; fasting blood sugar; cholesterol (decreased in malabsorption); vitamin B_{12} (decreased in ileal disease, pancreatic insufficiency, and bacterial overgrowth); blood cultures; stool for culture, ova, and parasites, and occult blood; fecal alpha-1 antitrypsin (increased in protein loss); stool for fat; 24-hour stool volume and weight; osmotic gap (differentiate between osmotic and secretory diarrhea); abdominal x-ray (colon distention); CT scan (may be normal); and colonoscopy or sigmoidoscopy.

Differential diagnosis:
- Acute diarrhea caused by salmonella
- *Shigella*
- *Campylobacter jejuni*
- *E. coli* 0157:H7
- *Cryptosporidium*
- *Giardia*
- *Microsporida*
- *Isospora*
- *Cyclospora*
- Diarrhea associated with hyperthyroidism or diabetic neuropathy
- Irritable bowel syndrome
- Dietary causes, including nonabsorbable carbohydrates, caffeine, lactose intolerance, and gluten sensitivity
- Microscopic and collagenous colitis
- Pancreatic insufficiency
- Antibiotic-induced chemical effects
- Known antibiotic effects of bacterial and fungal overgrowth
- Food poisoning
- Bacterial or viral gastroenteritis
- Inflammatory bowel disease (Yassin, Young-Fadok, Zein, & Pardi, 2001)

Treatment: Nonpharmacological—enteric isolation, oral replacement therapy, IV fluids for severe dehydration, and dietary consultation. Pharmacological—remove offending antibiotics, use antidiarrheals cautiously, and decrease narcotic analgesics. According to the latest clinical practice guideline from the Society for Healthcare Epidemiology of America and the Infectious Diseases Society of America, the patient's WBC count and serum creatinine level influence the treatment decisions for antibiotic selection (Cohen et al., 2010).

Treatment of choice is metronidazole 500 mg 3 times a day for 10 to 14 days for mild or moderate CDAD, which is defined as leukocytosis with a WBC count ≤15,000 and a serum creatine level <1.5 times the premorbid level. For severe infection (defined as leukocytosis with ≥15,000 or a serum creatinine level ≥1.5 times the premorbid level), administer vancomycin 125 mg qid for 10 to 14 days or vancomycin in a 6-week taper. Patients with severe complicated CDI cases will need IV metronidazole as well as either orally, via nasogastric tube, or rectally installed vancomycin. Clinical signs of complicated CDI include hypotension, ileus, megacolon, or hypovolemic shock (Cohen et al., 2010; Kee, 2012).

Follow-up: There is no universal agreement on how to clinically distinguish whether a second episode of CDI is a reinfection or a relapse. Relapse occurs in 15% to 30% of patients, generally 2 to 10 days after the end of antibiotic treatment for CDI (Kyne & Kelly, 2001). Risk factors for relapse following treatment for CDI include patients with low serum albumin levels (Nair, Yaday, Corpuz, & Pitchumoni, 1998) and a history of diabetes mellitus and sepsis (Jung et al., 2010). Therapeutic response should be based on clinical signs and symptoms, not repeat diagnostic testing. Current therapies are ineffective for eradicating asymptomatic colonization.

Sequelae: Chronic colonization, paralytic ileus, toxic megacolon and fulminating colitis, chronic diarrhea, electrolyte imbalances, hypoalbuminemia, and reactive arthritis are complications of CDI.

Prevention/prophylaxis: Infection control in healthcare settings and reducing the individual's risk factors. Patients with CDI should be in isolation in the acute care setting. The use of electronic rectal thermometers should be avoided (Cohen et al., 2010). A vaccine to prevent CDI is currently being tested (Kyne, 2010).

Referral: Signs and symptoms of ileus or fulminating colitis. Properly diagnosed disease fails to respond to conventional therapy. Unexplained diarrhea lasting longer than 2 weeks requires specific evaluation, testing, or an expanded differential diagnosis. Refer to a specialist for the management of bloody diarrhea, secretory diarrhea with dehydration, fecal incontinence, or irritable bowel syndrome.

Education: Avoid caffeine, alcohol, dairy products, sorbitol, gluten, and magnesium-containing antacids. Drink commercial electrolyte solutions. Avoid antidiarrheal agents, especially if a fever is present.

CLINICAL RECOMMENDATION	EVIDENCE RATING	REFERENCES
Reducing the frequency and duration of antimicrobial therapy can reduce the risk of recurrence of CDI.	A	Cohen et al. (2010)
Metronidazole is the drug of choice for initial episodes of mild-to-moderate cases of CDI.	A	Cohen et al. (2010)
Removing the provoking antimicrobial agent may reduce the rate of CDI recurrence.	A	Cohen et al. (2010)
Low serum albumin was found to be associated with relapse of *C. difficile* colitis following initial treatment.	B	Nair, Yaday, Corpuz, & Pitchumni (1998)
Diabetes mellitus and sepsis were identified as independent risk factors for metronidazole treatment failure in CDI.	B	Jung et al. (2010)
Removal of environmental sources (electronic thermometers with disposal covers) can reduce the spread of CDI.	B	Cohen et al. (2010)

A = consistent, good-quality, patient-oriented evidence; B = inconsistent or limited-quality, patient-oriented evidence; C = consensus, disease-oriented evidence, usual practice, expert opinion, or case series. For information about the SORT evidence rating system, go to www.aafp.org/afpsort.xml.

COLORECTAL CANCER

Signal symptoms: Persistent diarrhea, bleeding from the rectum, bloating, increased gas, abdominal distention, weight loss, persistent constipation, rectal pressure, rectal pain, and/or reduction in diameter of stool.

Description: Approximately 50% of neoplasms in the colon occur in the sigmoid and descending colon (54%) (Wasif, Etzioni, Maggard, Tomlinson, & Ko, 2011). Highest percentages of cancers are adenocarcinomas and account for over 90% of colon cancers

(Buetow & Buck, 2006). Leiomyosarcomas account for less than 2% (Sarcoma Alliance, 2006), lymphomas around 0.5% (ACS, 2007), and melanomas are rare, with incidence of less than 2% (Kayhan & Turan, 2003). Neuroendocrine tumors with subsets including aggressive and indolent are less than 2% (Bernick et al., 2004).

Etiology: The etiology of colorectal cancer is unknown; however, nutritional factors play an important role in its development. High-fat, high-carbohydrate diets with highly processed sugars and carbohydrates and high intakes of red meat, processed meats, and alcohol (which may block the absorption of folic acid) appear to be factors. Inactivity, obesity, high insulin levels, and excessive adipose tissue centrally located all appear to influence the risk of colon cancer (Giovannucci, 2003).

Occurrence: Colorectal cancer is the second most common malignancy in the United States, and it is associated with a 50% mortality rate. Worldwide, 917,000 deaths occur yearly from colon cancer (Jonker et al., 2007). Approximately 90% of all colorectal cancers occur after age 50 (American Cancer Institute, 2012). Cancer rates vary in levels of education (Albano et al., 2007).

Age: The incidence of colorectal cancer increases with age; 90% of the cases of colorectal cancer occur in people over 50 years old, with a peak incidence in the seventies (ACS, 2012).

Gender: Colorectal cancer occurs at a significantly higher rate in men than women (Regula et al., 2006).

Ethnicity: Blacks have a higher incidence and mortality of colorectal cancer than non-Hispanic whites, with American Indians and Latino/Americans below 2% (Agrawal et al., 2005).

Contributing factors: Lifestyle, education, and specific genetic disorders (familial adenomatous polyposis and hereditary nonpolyposis colorectal cancer) are associated with high risk of developing colorectal cancer (Lynch et al., 1993) and inflammatory bowel diseases.

Signs and symptoms: Clinical symptoms include rectal pressure, passing bright red blood, constipation, bloating, diarrhea, weight loss, melenonic stools, nausea, and loss of appetite. Patients presenting in the clinic with microcytic anemic should be evaluated for rectal bleeding and possible colorectal cancer.

Diagnostic tests: Initial tests include fecal occult blood tests (FOBTs) such as Hemocult II and HemocultSENSA (Smith, Kline and French, Sunnyvale, Ca.), digital rectal examination to palpate for any identifying masses, CBC with differential, chemistry panel, carcinoembryonic antigen (CEA), C-reactive protein (CRP), flexible sigmoidoscopy and colonoscopy for a biopsy and diagnosis, CT scan to determine metastases, and a positron emission tomography (PET) scan for staging purposes. A new screening method, CT colonography or virtual colonoscopy, is a procedure that allows imaging the colorectal region by CT radiographs.

Differential diagnosis:
■ Diverticulitis
■ Weight loss
■ Blood in the stool
■ Mass in the colon
■ Prostatic carcinoma
■ Sarcoma
■ Inflammatory bowel disease
■ Hemorrhoids
■ Benign colonic polyps
■ Peptic ulcer disease
■ Functional bowel disorders

Treatment: The extent of treatment for colorectal cancer depends on how invasive the cancer is in the colon and surrounding sites and the condition of the patient at the time of diagnosis. The prognosis of colorectal cancer is predicted using the Dukes staging method. Patients should be referred to a surgeon for consideration of a radical resection; presence of metastatic disease does not rule out surgery. The chemotherapeutic agent 5-fluorouracil combined with Avastin is an effective adjuvant therapy after a surgical resection of stage III colorectal cancer, even in older adults.

Follow-up: After curative surgery, the following are essential: oncology follow-up, which may include CT scan and CEA markers regularly depending on stage of cancer. Primary care providers will need to closely monitor for symptoms of fatigue, weight loss, and change in bowel habits with annual FOBTs, and colonoscopy within 1 year. Annual physical examinations are encouraged.

Sequelae: Complications of colorectal cancer include obstruction and perforation and possible colostomy. Postresection recurrence of colorectal cancer is common. Radiation proctitis with burning and diarrhea may occur. Bowel adhesions and chronic pain may also be a complication. The liver and bone are two sites known for metastasis after colorectal cancer.

Prevention/prophylaxis: The American Cancer Society recommends that beginning at age 50 all asymptomatic individuals with no risk factors should have an annual FOBT. The gold standard for screening is delineated in Table 10-1 (ACS, 2012). Prolonged prophylactic use of aspirin, calcium, and vitamin D supplementation may reduce the risk of colon cancer, as might weight loss and a diet high in fruits and vegetables.

Referral: A gastroenterologist should be consulted for colonoscopy, and a biopsy of the lesion should be obtained to determine the kind of cancer. A surgical consultation with a cancer surgeon, usually found at a major medical center, is advised. A team including a radiologist, oncologist, cancer surgeon, nutritionist, pharmacist, and nurse will develop a plan of care individualized to the patient and type of cancer. The team, along with valuable input from the patient and family, will then decide the treatment. Hospice may be a necessary choice and is available in all communities.

Education: Teach older adults about the importance of routine surveillance for rectal bleeding and to report any change in bowel habits.

TABLE 10-1	American Cancer Society Guidelines on Screening and Surveillance for the Early Detection of Colorectal Adenomas and Cancer—Women and Men at Increased Risk or at High Risk		
RISK CATEGORY	**AGE TO BEGIN**	**RECOMMENDATION**	**COMMENT**
Increased Risk People with a single small 1 (<1 cm) adenoma	3–6 years after the initial polypectomy	Colonoscopy	If the examination is normal, the patient can thereafter be screened as per average risk guidelines.
People with a large (1 cm+) adenoma, multiple adenomas, or adenomas with high-grade dysplasia or villous change	Within 3 years after the initial polypectomy	Colonoscopy	If normal, repeat examination in 3 years; if normal then, the patient can thereafter be screened as per average risk guidelines.
Personal history of curative-intent resection of colorectal cancer	Within 1 year after cancer resection	Colonoscopy	Every 5–10 years. Colorectal cancer in relative more distant than first-degree does not increase substantially above the average risk group.
Either colorectal cancer or adenomatous polyps, in any first-degree relative before age 60, or in two or more first-degree relatives at any age (if not a hereditary syndrome)	Age 40, or 10 years before the youngest case in the immediate family	Colonoscopy	Every 5–10 years. Colorectal cancer in relatives more distant than first-degree does not increase risk substantially above the average risk group.
High Risk Family history of familial adenomatous polyposis (FAP)	Puberty	Early surveillance with endoscopy, counseling to consider genetic testing	If the genetic test is positive, colectomy is indicated. These patients are best referred to a center with experience in the management of FAP.
Family history of hereditary nonpolyposis colon cancer (HNPCC)	Age 2	Colonoscopy and counseling to consider genetic testing	If the genetic test is positive or if the patient has not had genetic testing, every 1–2 years until age 40, then annually. These patients are best referred to a center with experience in the management of HNPCC.
Inflammatory bowel disease, chronic ulcerative colitis, Crohn's disease	Cancer risk begins to be significant 8 years after the onset of pancolitis or 12–15 years after the onset of left-sided colitis	Colonoscopy with biopsies for dysplasia	Every 1–2 years. These patients are best referred to a center with experience in the surveillance and management of inflammatory bowel disease.

CLINICAL RECOMMENDATION	EVIDENCE RATING	REFERENCES
Prevention of colorectal cancer by screening is cost effective, and if caught early, colorectal cancer is curable. Recommend annual FOBT; screening colonoscopy at age 50, based on meta-analysis of research studies involving colonoscopy and annual screenings; 75% of colorectal tumors do not appear to be due to inherited genetic mutations.	A	American Cancer Society (2012)
Adenomas of the colon can be without symptoms, are precursors to adenocarcinoma of the colon, and account for >90% of colorectal cancers. Many can be detected radiographically. Patients have many choices in deciding kinds and costs of screening tools; shared decisions should be made after appropriate counseling.	B	Buetow & Buck (2006)
Rare cancer (<2%). Routine screening recommended unless diagnosed, then annually.	A	Sarcoma Alliance (2006)
Colorectal cancer (advanced neoplasia) is significantly higher in men than in women. This could warrant refinement of the screening recommendations for colorectal cancer.	A	Regula et al. (2006)
Diet and body weight with hyperinsulinemia are important risk factors for colorectal cancer. The majority of colon cancers may be prevented by consuming foods that are higher in dietary fiber, such as fruits and vegetables; keeping BMI within normal ranges and avoiding smoking have been proven to reduce the incidence of colorectal cancer.	A	Giovannucci (2003)
The most modifiable determinants of cancer risks are weight control, dietary choices, and levels of activity. Recommendations are maintain a healthy weight, get regular physical activity, limit processed meat and red meat, and avoid alcohol and tobacco. Collaborative work in communities to promote healthy worksites, schools, and marketing of foods and beverages that have good nutritional value, particularly to youth, is advised.	A	American Cancer Institute (2012)
Appropriate staging of colorectal cancer improves outcomes and allows for appropriate follow-up. Established guidelines are correlated to the staging of colorectal cancer and provide practitioners a better prognostic picture.	A	Bernick et al. (2003)
Colorectal cancer mortality rate is declining, but incidence rates are increasing. Obesity, diabetes, and diets high in processed foods all seem to correlate to higher rates. Providing patients with facts on colorectal cancer risks and preventive measures may reduce the incidence.	A	Jonker et al. (2007)

Continued

CLINICAL RECOMMENDATION	EVIDENCE RATING	REFERENCES
Diagnosing colorectal cancer early with yearly FOBT screens and colonoscopy beginning at age 50 have improved mortality rates.		

A = consistent, good-quality, patient-oriented evidence; B = inconsistent or limited-quality, patient-oriented evidence; C = consensus, disease-oriented evidence, usual practice, expert opinion, or case series. For information about the SORT evidence rating system, go to www.aafp.org/afpsort.xml.

CYSTITIS

Signal symptoms: Dysuria, frequency, urgency, suprapubic tenderness, change in urine character (hematuria, color change, change in odor), mental status changes (Juthani-Mehta et al., 2009).

Description: Cystitis is a pathogenic invasion of the wall of the bladder, usually resulting from an ascending infection via the urethra, of bowel flora organisms from the perineum (Beveridge, Davey, Phillips, & McMurdo, 2011; Dielubanza & Schaffer, 2011). Cases of cystitis are classified as complicated or uncomplicated. Comorbidities and host anatomy form the basis of the categorical designation, although consensus does not exist on the classification of age within this delineation (Dielubanza & Schaffer, 2011; Nicolle, 2005). Bacteriuria is the main clinical manifestation of cystitis. Asymptomatic bacteriuria (a urinary culture with more than 10^5 colony-forming units) with no corresponding urinary tract symptoms is prevalent in the elderly (especially those residing in nursing homes) and is not diagnostic in itself (Juthani-Mehta et al., 2009; Schmiemann, Kniehl, Gebhardt, Matejczyk, & Hummers-Pradier, 2010). The U.S. Preventive Services Task Force has found that evidence does not support the routine screening of nonpregnant adults for asymptomatic bacteriuria and that no benefit is derived from it (Lin & Fajardo, 2008). Bacteriuria plus pyuria (a urinalysis with more than 10 WBCs) along with the new onset of urinary tract–specific clinical findings (see Signal symptoms above) are necessary for the diagnosis of cystitis in the elderly (Beveridge et al., 2011; Juthani-Mehta et al., 2009).

Etiology: The susceptibility to urinary tract infections increases in old age because the host defenses of the body, needed to prevent phagocytic bacteria from coming in contact with the bladder mucosa, are diminished or impaired. The host's compromised anatomical defenses allow unheeded bacterial ascent and colonization of pathogens (Dielubanza & Schaffer, 2011). The most common organism identified in the development of cystitis in adults of all ages is *E. coli* (Grabe et al., 2011).

Occurrence: Community-dwelling men 70 years of age and older have a prevalence rate of bacteriuria from 3.6% to 19%, whereas their institutionalized counterparts have a prevalence rate from 15% to 40% (Nicolle et al., 2005). Community-dwelling women 70 years of age and older have a prevalence rate of bacteriuria from 10.8% to 16%, whereas their institutionalized counterparts have a prevalence rate from 25% to 50% (Nicolle et al., 2005).

Age: The incidence of cystitis increases with age, especially for men and all institutionalized older adults (Dielubanza & Schaffer, 2011). Cystitis is one of the most common infections in the elderly in both the institutionalized and community-dwelling populations (Beveridge et al., 2011).

Gender: Cystitis is more prevalent in older women than in older men. After age 65, the rate of cystitis in men significantly increases, but is still approximately one-half that of women (Dielubanza & Schaffer, 2011). Cystitis in men is generally considered to be a complicated infection of the urinary tract (Schmiemann et al., 2010). When postmenopausal women have recurrent cystitis, they are considered to have features of both complicated and uncomplicated infections of the urinary tract (Nicolle, 2005).

Ethnicity: No known prevalence exists among ethnic groups.

Contributing factors: Benign prostatic hyperplasia, incontinence, urinary retention, and institutionalization are all contributing factors to the increase in the prevalence of cystitis in elderly men (Dielubanza & Schaffer, 2011). The woman's shorter urethra is an anatomical reason why women are more susceptible to urinary tract infections over their lifetime. Their urethra's proximity to rectal and vaginal bacteria significantly contributes to infection, also. The length of the male urethra provides a protective barrier against ascending bacterial infection (Dielubanza & Schaffer, 2011). The loss of estrogen in elderly women leads to increased infection through increased vaginal pH and the loss of protective lactobacillus. Predisposing factors to the development of cystitis in older adults include indwelling catheters, urethral or condom catheters, incontinence (urinary and fecal), cognitive impairment, neurological conditions that impair bladder emptying, and diabetes, which can lead to neurogenic bladder (Beveridge et al., 2011). Other predisposing factors to cystitis include sexual intercourse, functional disability, sickle cell disease, prior antibiotic therapy, genetic predisposition, and functional or structural genitourinary tract abnormalities (including urethral strictures, uterine or bladder prolapse, ureteral weakness, and vesicoureteral reflux or renal calculi) (Dielubanza & Schaffer, 2011; Nicolle, 2005; Schmiemann et al., 2010). Frail older adults in institutionalized settings are at additional risk due to lack of adequate fluids and immobility.

Signs and symptoms: Patients may report urgency, frequency, and dysuria. Gross hematuria is more common in younger women than in older adults with cystitis. An atypical presentation of mental confusion, anorexia, malaise, and incontinence may be the first symptoms of cystitis in an older patient, especially for patients with indwelling catheters or the frail elderly (Woodford & George, 2009). Caution must be exercised though, and the differential must be explored, before cystitis can be diagnosed in the absence of concurrent urinary-specific signs and symptoms (dysuria, change in urine character, etc.). Symptoms such as nonspecific functional decline, increased confusion, and other nonspecific signs and symptoms may be erroneously attributed to cystitis in the absence of key urinary tract symptoms and therefore should be thoroughly examined in the differential (Beveridge et al., 2011). Patients should be questioned about their sexual history, including about any use of spermicide (which can alter flora leading to increased uropathogen colonization) (Dielubanza & Schaffer, 2011). Women may report pelvic pain or vaginal or cervical discharge that may indicate an ascending infection. If fever, flank pain, and other systemic symptoms are reported, consider obstruction when ordering diagnostic tests.

Physical examination may reveal fever, tachypnea, and tachycardia. Suprapubic tenderness may be elicited on palpation. Percussion for costovertebral angle tenderness may be positive with reported flank pain (Beveridge et al., 2011).

Vaginal examination in women should rule out discharge, irritation, and erythema (Dason, Dason, & Kapoor, 2011). In men, the prostate gland should be examined gently to assess for enlargement, bogginess, and tenderness.

Diagnostic tests: A dipstick urinalysis for nitrate and leukocyte esterase shows a positive leukocyte esterase and positive nitrate with a gram-negative organism. Atypical organisms, such as gram-positive organisms and *Pseudomonas*, which can occur in the elderly population, would not be detected with this method (Woodford & George, 2009). A microscopic urinalysis in symptomatic bacteriuria shows pyuria and bacteria. Due to the prevalence of asymptomatic bacteriuria in institutionalized elders (15% to 50%) with concomitant pyuria (90%), bacteriuria plus pyuria in this population is not sufficient for diagnosis without additional genitourinary clinical symptoms (Juthani-Mehta et al., 2009). A bacteriological urine culture with pathogen identification, quantification, and sensitivity testing has traditionally been considered the gold standard for the diagnosis of cystitis (Schmiemann et al., 2010). The presence of greater than 10^5 colony-forming units/mL of a single bacterium in a culture of freshly voided urine is generally considered to be a significant bacteriuria (Beveridge et al., 2011). The most common organisms to cause urinary tract infections are anaerobes and gram-negative bacteria (Dielubanza & Schaffer, 2011). The most frequent causative pathogens of cystitis include *E. coli*, *Staphylococcus saprophyticus*, and *Enterobacteriaceae* species, including *Klebsiella* species and *Proteus mirabilis* (Dielubanza & Schaffer, 2011; Grabe et al., 2011). Additional radiographic testing may be necessary if obstruction is suspected or if an abnormal and persistent pattern of infection needs to be further explored (Dielubanza & Schaffer, 2011; Grabe et al., 2011).

Differential diagnosis:
- Urethritis
- Prostatitis
- Pyelonephritis
- Vaginitis

Treatment: Treatment recommendations have been changing to reflect trends in pathogen resistance, antibiotic adverse effects, and best evidence–based practice. Current recommendations include multiple treatment regimens based on the needs of the patient. Older women with symptomatic uncomplicated bacteriuria should be treated with oral trimethoprim-sulfamethoxazole (TMP-SMX) 160 mg/800 mg every 12 hours for 3 days (if local *E. coli* resistance to TMP-SMX is less than 20% and there is no existing allergy) or with nitrofurantoin 100 mg orally every 12 hours for 5 days or fosfomycin 3 grams orally in 1 dose (if sulfa allergy). If local *E. coli* resistance to TMP-SMX is more than 20% or there is an existing sulfa allergy, ciprofloxacin 250 mg can be given every 12 hours for 3 days. Pyridium 200 mg by mouth every 8 hours for 3 days can be added to these regimens for the relief of dysuria (Gilbert, Moellering, Eliopoulos, Chambers, & Saag, 2011). Based on expert consensus opinion, for cystitis, the optimal antimicrobials, dosages, and treatment durations appear to be similar for both premenopausal and postmenopausal women, but more high-quality research is needed to be done in the future to further explore this recommendation (Grabe et al., 2011). For acute, uncomplicated bacterial cystitis in all women (including those over 65 years old), a 3-day antimicrobial regimen is recommended by the American College of Obstetricians and Gynecologists (2008). A Cochrane review of the evidence supported short-course therapy (3 to 6 days) in this population (elderly women with uncomplicated cystitis) (Beveridge et al., 2011). Short-course therapy optimally balances pathogen eradication with minimizing adverse drug effects (including vaginal and bowel flora alterations) (Dielubanza & Schaffer, 2011). A regimen of 7 to 10 days of antibiotics is recommended for complicated cystitis (including functional or structural abnormalities of the urinary tract) (Nicolle, 2005).

Older men with uncomplicated cystitis require medication for 10 to 14 days. Longer treatments, for 4 to 6 weeks, may be necessary to sterilize the urinary tract in older men after an infection (Gilbert et al., 2011). Monitor renal function before dosing medications.

Patients with catheter-associated bacteriuria may require a two-drug combination owing to polymicrobial infection; the duration of antibiotic therapy for these patients should be 14 to 21 days (Gilbert et al., 2011). Second-generation or third-generation cephalosporins may be prescribed if there has been known resistance or the patient cannot tolerate the first-line medications.

Follow-up: Follow-up test-of-cure urinalysis and urine cultures are not indicted for uncomplicated cases of cystitis (Grabe et al., 2011; Nicolle et al., 2005). Relapse occurs when symptoms persist and the same organism is found in the culture specimen shortly after cessation of treatment. Cystitis treated with the correct antimicrobial therapy resolves 90% of the cases. Recurrence is not uncommon, though, and over 25% of the time another infection occurs within a year (Dielubanza & Schaffer, 2011). Change in treatment is warranted if the organisms are resistant to the original treatment.

Sequelae: Untreated symptomatic cystitis can lead to pyelonephritis, sepsis, shock, and death.

Prevention/prophylaxis: Prophylactic use of antibiotics by patients with indwelling catheters is not recommended (Woodford & George, 2009). For older adults who require frequent instrumentation of the lower genitourinary tract or who have frequent cystitis, suppressive antimicrobial therapy may be considered on an individual basis (Nicolle, 2005).

Referral: In complicated cystitis that has progressed to pyelonephritis or urosepsis, consultation with a specialist is recommended for hospitalization.

Education: Inform all patients receiving antimicrobial therapy for cystitis of the necessity of drinking at least 8 oz of water with each tablet. Encourage patients with recurrent cystitis to drink cranberry juice (or take cranberry capsules) as part of their daily routine. Cranberry products can be helpful to reduce recurrent cystitis (Epp et al., 2010).

CLINICAL RECOMMENDATION	EVIDENCE RATING	REFERENCES
Evidence does not support the routine screening of nonpregnant adults for asymptomatic bacteriuria. No benefit has been found to be derived from it.	A	Lin & Fajardo (2008) Nicolle et al. (2005)
Before the start of antimicrobial therapy, a urine specimen should be collected and cultured for bacterial	A	Epp et al. (2010) Nicolle (2005)

CLINICAL RECOMMENDATION	EVIDENCE RATING	REFERENCES
pathogen identification, quantification, and sensitivity testing, for every episode of complicated cystitis.		
The presence of $>10^5$ colony-forming units/mL of a single bacteria in a culture of freshly voided urine is consistent with significant bacteriuria in symptomatic subjects.	A	Beveridge et al. (2011) Juthani-Mehta et al. (2009) Nicolle (2005)
For acute, uncomplicated bacterial cystitis in all women (including those >65 years old), a short course of antimicrobial therapy (3–6 days) is recommended.	A	American College of Obstetricians and Gynecologists (2008) Beveridge et al. (2011) Dielubanza & Schaffer (2011)
Antimicrobial selection for empirical therapy should be based on the patient's individualized history and requirements (including prior antibiotic use, symptoms, urine culture results, and institutional susceptibilities). Treatment should be reevaluated and modified as appropriate.	A	Nicolle (2005)
Follow-up test-of-cure urinalysis and urine cultures are not indicted for uncomplicated cases of cystitis.	B	Grabe et al. (2011) Nicolle et al. (2005)
In patients with complicated, unresolved, recurrent, or worsening cystitis, specialist referral is recommended. In complicated cystitis that has progressed to pyelonephritis or urosepsis, urgent evaluation and consultation with a specialist is recommended for further testing and hospitalization as appropriate.	B	Nicolle (2005)
Cranberry products can be helpful to reduce recurrent cystitis.	B	Epp et al. (2010) Grabe et al. (2011)

A = consistent, good-quality, patient-oriented evidence; B = inconsistent or limited-quality, patient-oriented evidence; C = consensus, disease-oriented evidence, usual practice, expert opinion, or case series. For information about the SORT evidence rating system, go to www.aafp.org/afpsort.xml.

DIVERTICULITIS

Signal symptoms: Impaired cognitive status, lower quadrant pain.

Description: Diverticulitis is an inflammatory condition that involves perforation of one or more colonic diverticula, which are herniations of the mucosa through the muscularis of the colon. It usually occurs in the sigmoid or descending colon. Inflammation of the diverticulum begins at the apex when the narrow opening of the lumen is exposed to fecal residue. Mucosal erosion within the diverticulum also can occur, leading to diverticulitis.

Etiology: Diverticula are common in older adults. Age-related changes in the elastic matrix of the colon and the resulting sluggish fecal mass are thought to cause increased intraluminal pressure of the colon. Diverticular disease is rare in societies that consume high-fiber diets. It is thought that a low-fiber diet produces less bulky stool and increased intracolonic pressure. Diverticulitis is thought to develop when one or more diverticula are perforated (macroperforation or microperforation). A pseudodiverticulum occurs when only the mucosa and submucosa of the colon are affected (Sheth, Longo, & Floch, 2008). Approximately 85% of all cases of diverticulitis involve the left colon and sigmoid. Because this perforation is usually a localized process, free intraperitoneal air or diffuse peritoneal signs are usually not evident; their presence would indicate a more severe case and the possible need for surgical consultation.

Occurrence: An estimated 70% of older adults develop diverticulosis by age 85, with the prevalence rising to 80% for adults in their nineties. Approximately 10% to 25% of the population with diverticulosis goes on to develop symptoms of diverticulitis, which is usually most severe in older adults (Jacobs, 2007).

Age: Diverticulitis is found most commonly in older adults, most commonly in the sixties to eighties.

Gender: Diverticulitis occurs more commonly in women than men (Commane, Arasardnam, Mills, Mathers, & Bradburn, 2009).

Ethnicity: Diverticulitis is found almost exclusively in Westernized countries or populations that have begun to consume a refined Western diet. People of Asian descent are more likely to have *right-sided* diverticulitis (Jacobs, 2007).

Contributing factors: Advancing age is the primary nonmodifiable risk factor for developing diverticulitis (Commane et al., 2009). Chronic constipation and the need to strain to defecate contribute to diverticulitis. These two conditions lead to colonic wall weakness and raise the intraluminal pressure (Jacobs, 2007). Long-term use of NSAIDs and aspirin increases the incidence of diverticulitis (Strate, Liu, Huang, Giovannucci, & Chan, 2011). The development of diverticulitis also has been associated with chronic cigarette smoking, adult polycystic kidney disease, and use of immunosuppressant drugs. There

is a relationship between physical inactivity and the development of diverticulitis. A recent study also indicated a connection between increased body mass index (BMI) in men (over 30) and diverticulitis (Strate, Liu, Syngal, Aldoori, & Giovannucci, 2008). Similarly, patients with increased waist circumference have a tendency to develop diverticular disease (Strate et al., 2008).

Signs and symptoms: Clinical presentation of diverticulitis in an older adult may be suppressed despite the presence of severe disease. Mental confusion may be the first overt indication of diverticulitis in older adults with known diverticular disease. They may report a low-grade fever. History of left lower quadrant pain aggravated by movement and fever may be present. They may report that the pain is precipitated by eating and describe a colicky pain (Salzman & Lillie, 2005). Pain also may be reported in the flank, back, or right side of the abdomen. Patients may describe the pain as dull, aching, and intermittent. A sensation of "bloating" may be the initial complaint offered. Associated complaints of nausea and vomiting suggest obstruction (Wilkins, Embry, & George, 2013). Obstipation or constipation or diarrhea, abdominal cramping without the abdominal pain, and fever also may occur (McQuaid, 2010). Patients may experience abdominal or perirectal fullness. If the bowel is inflamed adjacent to the bladder, the presentation may mimic a urinary tract infection. Joint pain may be reported in the hip, knee, and/or thigh (Frattini & Longo, 2006). Acutely ill patients with a moderate-to-severe episode of diverticulitis may present with lethargy, reflecting signs of fluid depletion and sepsis.

Bowel sounds may be normal in mild disease; however, bowel sounds become hypoactive until there is an obstruction, when a tinkling sound may be heard. Hyperresonance may reflect intestinal obstruction. Localized tenderness is usually present in the left lower quadrant. Rebound tenderness, involuntary rigidity, and guarding are signs of peritonitis. A mass palpated in the left lower quadrant may indicate an abscess. Occult rectal bleeding occurs in about 25% of patients with diverticulitis. Tenderness may be elicited during the rectal examination. Patients in acute distress may have pyrexia, tachycardia, and impending signs of hypovolemia (Jacobs, 2007).

Diagnostic tests: A CBC, urinalysis, a basic metabolic panel, C-reactive protein, and plain abdominal radiographs can be initially ordered (Wilkins, Embry, & George, 2013). Leukocytosis may be present. Urinalysis may reveal sterile pyuria due to adjacent colonic irritation; however, if mixed colonic flora are present, consider the presence of a colovesical fistula (McQuaid, 2010). Abdominal x-rays may reveal perforation (free air) and bowel obstruction. Patients should be scheduled for a CT of the abdomen and pelvis. CTs performed with oral, IV, and rectal contrast can enhance the accuracy of the diagnostic image (Rafferty, Shellito, Hyman, & Buie, 2006). Sigmoidoscopy, colonoscopy, and barium enema are usually *avoided* during acute diverticulitis because these tests may cause further perforation or leakage of bowel contents (Jacobs, 2007). These tests may be performed several weeks after the resolution of the acute episode. Gram stain and testing for *C. difficile* should be considered in patients with diarrhea (Strate et al., 2008).

Differential diagnosis:
- Acute appendicitis—suspect if right lower quadrant symptoms or nonresolution with medical therapy
- Inflammatory bowel disease (Crohn's disease)
- Complicated peptic ulcer disease—suspect if pneumoperitoneum or peritonitis
- Ischemic colitis—suspect if high-risk patient, bloody diarrhea, or thumb printing
- Pseudomembranous colitis—suspect if antibiotic use or diarrhea
- Vascular ectasia—consider leaking abdominal aortic aneurysm
- Carcinoma of the colon—suspect if weight loss or bleeding
- Urological disorders, such as infection or ureteric colic
- Gynecological carcinomas or abscesses
- Pelvic inflammatory disease
- Infectious colitis
- Small bowel obstruction
- Endometriosis
- Ovarian cyst
- Testicular torsion
- Gastroenteritis
- Bowel obstruction
- Irritable bowel syndrome
- Kidney stone (Hall et al., 2011; Jacobs, 2007; McQuaid, 2010; Rafferty et al., 2006)

Treatment: Diverticulitis is found to be polymicrobial and results from bacteria normally found in the gastrointestinal tract (Spirit, 2010). The selection of antibiotics for the treatment of diverticulitis needs to consider the most common bacteria found in the colon, which are gram-negative aerobic rods and anaerobic microorganisms (Rafferty et al., 2006). For mild cases, use broad-spectrum antibiotics such as ciprofloxacin 250 to 500 mg every 12 hours *or* levofloxacin 500 mg *or* moxifloxacin 400 mg once a day, plus metronidazole 250 to 500 mg 3 times a day for 7 to 10 days. An alternative choice is amoxicillin and clavulanate potassium 875 mg twice a day for 7 to 10 days. It is important to follow up with the patient within 48 to 72 hours and inquire about pain, ability to tolerate clear liquid fluids, and if the patient has become febrile (McQuaid, 2010) because improvement should occur if a medication regimen such as this is followed (World Gastroenterology Organization, 2007). Before recommending outpatient treatment, ensure that there is reliable support system available. Patients treated at home should be able to tolerate oral fluids and lack peritoneal signs (Lutwak & Dill, 2013). The diet can be advanced if there has been improvement in symptoms during this time (Alonso et al., 2010).

Hospitalization may be necessary should be considered for older adults with diverticulitis, owing to the uncertainty of the severity of the disease because of possibly subdued presentation and comorbid diseases (Jacobs, 2007; Lutwak & Dill, 2013). Acute treatment for hospitalized patients consists of bedrest; restriction of any fluids by mouth; nasogastric suction if nausea, vomiting, or other indication of obstruction is present; and IV fluids and electrolytes. It is recommended to try a single-agent parenteral antibiotic for adequate coverage of bowel flora for the treatment of severe diverticulitis. Selection of antibiotics used in the treatment of acute diverticulitis includes the following:

- Ciprofloxacin 250 to 500 mg IV every 12 hours plus metronidazole 500 mg IV every 6 hours
- Ceftizoxime 2 g IV every 12 hours
- Cefoxitin 2 g IV every 8 hours plus metronidazole 500 mg IV every 6 hours
- Moxifloxacin 400 mg IV every 24 hours
- Ampicillin-sulbactam 3 g every 6 hours
- Piperacillin-tazobactam 3.375 g every 6 hours or 4.5 g every 8 hours
- Ticarcillin-clavulanate 3.1 g every 4 hours (Mazuski, 2007; McQuaid, 2010; Solomkin, Goldstein, Stollman, Barie, & Mazuski, 2007; Spirit, 2010)

Pay special attention to the patient's renal function and creatinine clearance level; aminoglycosides should only be considered in patients with normal renal function (Rafferty et al., 2006). Antibiotics may need to be adjusted following culture from any drainage or aspiration.

Follow-up: Older adults with mild cases treated at home with prescribed therapy should expect improvement by the third day. If, however, patients are not able to tolerate fluids and/or fail to respond to narcotic analgesics, refer for hospitalization. Hospitalized patients require daily monitoring for persistent signs and symptoms of diverticulitis, laboratory values, and response to treatment. Surgical consultation may be necessary if the patient does not respond to treatment and continues to have an elevated WBC count, fever, rebound tenderness, pain, and tachycardia; approximately 25% of patients with diverticulitis require surgical intervention. Once the acute diverticulitis has resolved, consider referring the patent for further diagnostic imaging studies such as colonoscopy or contrast enema x-ray (Lau et al., 2011; McQuaid, 2010; Rafferty et al., 2006).

Sequelae: Complications include anemia, bowel perforation, peritonitis, pericolonic or intramesenteric abscess, colovesical fistula (most common fistula in patients with diverticulitis), hemorrhage, and bowel obstruction. Of patients with diverticulitis, more than 50% eventually have bowel obstruction (Floch, 2006; Jacobs, 2007). Complications from diverticulitis tend to be most severe in patients who are immunocompromised, including those with diabetes, chronic kidney disease, cirrhosis, and on immunosuppressant therapies (Hall et al., 2011).

Prevention/prophylaxis: Recognition of early signs and symptoms of diverticulitis helps prevent severe cases (Maconi, Barbara, Bosetti, Cuomo & Annibale, 2011). The use of a symbiotic mixture was found to be beneficial in preventing recurrence of constipation-related abdominal pain in patients with diverticulum disease (Lamiki et al., 2009). Evidence does not support that the inclusion of nuts, seeds, corn, and popcorn in the diet contributes to the development of diverticulitis (Strate et al., 2008).

Referral: Severe episodes of diverticulitis require consultation with a gastroenterologist for hospitalization. Patients with localized abscesses need to be referred for consideration of a CT-guided percutaneous drainage (Jacobs, 2007). Repeated episodes may require surgical consultation for an elective sigmoid resection.

Education: Provide information on a high-fiber diet or fiber supplementation or both (Strate et al., 2008; Tarleton & DiBaise, 2011). Teach patients to increase their fluid intake unless otherwise cautioned, especially when taking fiber supplements. Diverticulitis recurs in approximately one-third of all patients who receive medical management only. Encourage obese older adults to consider weight reduction, as obesity has been found to be a contributing factor to complicated cases of diverticulitis (Wilkins, Embry, & George, 2013).

CLINICAL RECOMMENDATION	EVIDENCE RATING	REFERENCES
Despite long-time popular belief, current evidence is lacking to show that including nuts, seeds, corn, and popcorn in one's diet contributes to the development of diverticulitis.	B	Strate, Liu, Syngal, Aldoori, & Giovannucci (2008)
Regular intake of fiber may be beneficial in the prevention and recurrence of diverticular disease.	B	Tarleton & DiBaise (2011)
Patients with known diverticular disease benefited from taking a prescribed symbiotic mixture; recurrence of diverticular disease was prevented in patients with constipation-predominant symptoms.	B	Lamiki et al. (2009)
CT scan of the abdomen and pelvis is highly recommended as the imaging study of choice in patients with suspected acute diverticulitis.	A	Ambrosetti, Jenny, Becker, Terrier, & Morel (2000)

CLINICAL RECOMMENDATION	EVIDENCE RATING	REFERENCES
Regular use of NSAIDs or aspirin has been associated with an increased risk of developing diverticulitis and diverticular bleeding.	B	Strate, Liu, Huang, Giovannucci, & Chan (2011)

A = consistent, good-quality, patient-oriented evidence; B = inconsistent or limited-quality, patient-oriented evidence; C = consensus, disease-oriented evidence, usual practice, expert opinion, or case series. For information about the SORT evidence rating system, go to www.aafp.org/afpsort.xml.

ESOPHAGITIS

Signal symptoms: Dysphagia, regurgitation, pyrosis.

Description: Esophagitis is an inflammation of the lining of the esophagus.

Etiology: There are a number of different causes for esophagitis. Patients may develop esophagitis if they ingest medication improperly; have chronic medical conditions; ingest caustic chemicals; are exposed to radiation treatments; have a bacterial, viral, or fungal infection (especially those patients who are immunocompromised); or have a history of gastroesophageal reflux disease (GERD) (Aparanji, Annavarappu, Russell, & Dharmarajan, 2012). *Candida albicans* is the most common fungal infection (Kliemann, Pasqualotto, Falavigna, Giaretta, & Severo, 2008). The herpes simplex virus type 1 also can cause esophagitis, as does cytomegalovirus. Bacterial esophagitis is rare but can coincide with a fungal or viral infection, making it difficult to diagnose. In GERD, esophagitis is a common complication; older adults are found to have an increased prevalence of hiatal hernias than younger adults, which is an intrinsic factor to the development of reflux esophagitis (Pilotto et al., 2006). Eosinophilic esophagitis results from inflammation and is clinically evident by dense esophageal eosinophilia with severe squamous epithelial hyperplasia.

Occurrence: It is estimated that 30% to 44% of the general population experiences some symptoms of esophagitis monthly (Prasad et al., 2009).

Age: Esophagitis can occur at all ages.

Ethnicity: No known prevalence exists among ethnic groups.

Gender: Esophagitis occurs equally in men and women.

Contributing factors: In older adults, normal aging changes such as decreased salivation, gastric motility, and delayed gastric emptying can contribute to the development of esophagitis. Obesity and conditions that contribute to limited upper body mobility such as spinal cord injuries may increase the risk of esophagitis. Infectious agents are known to cause esophagitis in patients with certain viral, bacterial, parasitic, and fungal infections. Predisposing factors for patients who develop *Candida* esophagitis include radiation therapy, chemotherapy, certain hematological malignancies, AIDS, alcoholism, and malnutrition. Swallowing certain medications such as aspirin, antibiotics, ferrous sulfate, certain chemotherapeutic agents, NSAIDs, quinidine, steroids, alendronate, alprenolol, vitamin C, phenytoin, calcium preparations, theophylline, and potassium chloride contributes to pill esophagitis due to chemical irritation of the esophageal mucosa. Patients often report that insufficient fluid intake and not remaining upright after the medication is taken contributed to the symptoms of esophagitis (Aparanji et al., 2012). Substances that can weaken the lower esophageal sphincter (coffee, peppermint, alcohol, spicy foods, citric fruits, chocolate, nifedipine, verapamil, and progesterone) can contribute to esophagitis. Several systemic disorders place patients at risk for esophagitis, including pemphigus vulgaris, bullous pemphigoid, Stevens-Johnson syndrome, lichen planus, inflammatory bowel disease, sarcoidosis, scleroderma, chronic granulomatous disease, and motility disorders of the esophagus. Patients with left atrial enlargement may experience esophagitis due to the pressure of the left atrium exerted on the distal esophagus (Aparanji et al., 2012).

Signs and symptoms: A history of dysphagia and pain on swallowing is common. Associated pyrosis, regurgitation, coughing, wheezing, and progressive hoarseness may occur. A fever may be present in patients with an infectious process. Patients should be questioned about medication usage, history of radiation treatments, smoking, and intake of substances that weaken the lower esophageal sphincter; sleeping habits; and use of any tight or restrictive clothing. Review patient medical history for chronic conditions that can contribute to esophagitis.

Physical examination usually produces no positive findings. Oral thrush may be found in patients with *C. albicans*. Palpate for any upper abdominal masses or tenderness. Perform a rectal examination to detect any frank bleeding (Mukherjee, 2011).

Diagnostic tests: If suspicion was aroused on the physical examination, stool should be checked using the guaiac test to determine if there has been any intestinal bleeding. Laboratory studies are not required when antacids, position change, or both relieve pyrosis. For older adults who complain of persistent dysphagia or odynophagia with or without fever, a barium swallow or an endoscopy (with brush and biopsy if structural mucosal damage is suspected) or both are ordered. pH monitoring studies may be considered; however, in patients with eosinophilic esophagitis, the results are usually normal (Furuta et al., 2007).

Differential diagnosis:
- Esophageal stricture (upper gastrointestinal sinus)
- Esophageal carcinoma
- Cholecystitis
- Peptic ulcer disease (Mukherjee, 2011)

Treatment: For infectious esophagitis, temporary symptomatic relief can be obtained with sucralfate slurry, 1 g/10 mL orally 4 times daily. Viscous lidocaine (2%), 15 mL orally every 4 hours as needed to swish and swallow, can be used for short-term temporary relief, unless contraindicated by potential drug interactions or history of cardiac or hepatic disease. For mild cases of *C. albicans* infection, nystatin oral suspension, 400,000 to 600,000 units 4 times daily spaced evenly over 24 hours, is prescribed. Ketoconazole should not be given at the same time as antacids or H_2 blockers. For severe cases of herpes simplex virus–induced esophagitis, IV acyclovir may be given, adjusting the dosage for the patient's weight and creatinine clearance.

Esophagitis from radiation can be treated with viscous lidocaine. For erosive esophagitis, use of proton pump inhibitors (PPIs) is recommended for 4 weeks followed by reevaluation. In moderate to severe cases, esomeprazole magnesium, 20 to 40 mg daily, or pantoprazole sodium, 40 mg for 4 to 8 weeks, has been found to be effective in esophageal healing (McDonagh, Carson, & Thakurta, 2009).

Follow-up: Patients should report progress at least 1 week after treatment. An endoscopy may be repeated if the patient is still symptomatic but compliant after the initial treatment. Yearly endoscopy is recommended thereafter for patients with severe cases of esophagitis. Patients with eosinophilic esophagitis generally do not respond to treatment with PPIs (Furuta et al., 2007).

Sequelae: Ulceration and bleeding, if reflux esophagitis is present, can occur after esophagitis; Barrett's esophagus with possible adenocarcinoma may be a long-term complication (Erichsen et al., 2012).

Prevention/prophylaxis: Because of the high recurrence rate of esophagitis, patients should be instructed to follow all nonpharmacological measures unless otherwise instructed. Maintenance therapy for esophagitis may be prescribed for an extended time (Winstead & Bulat, 2004).

Referral: A gastroenterologist should be consulted for the endoscopy and for patients with severe or nonresponsive esophagitis.

Education: Patients with reflux esophagitis should be instructed to raise the head of the bed 4 to 6 in. with shock blocks. Factors that increase abdominal pressure, such as wearing tight restrictive clothing, should be avoided. The patient should avoid smoking and ingestion of fatty foods, coffee, chocolate, mints, citric juices, alcohol, and large quantities of fluids with meals. Remind patients not to break or crush extended-release or delayed-release tablets. Teach the patient the importance of swallowing medications with an adequate amount of fluids.

CLINICAL RECOMMENDATION	EVIDENCE RATING	REFERENCES
Patients with erosive reflux disease are at increased risk for developing adenocarcinoma.	B	Erichsen et al. (2012)
Older adults with reflux esophagitis had more atypical and nonspecific symptoms than younger patients.	B	Pilotto et al. (2006)

CLINICAL RECOMMENDATION	EVIDENCE RATING	REFERENCES
The incidence and size of hiatal hernia were also found to increase with age.		
Older adults had a significantly lower prevalence of heartburn or acid regurgitation than younger adults.	B	Pilotto et al. (2006)
In patients with moderate to severe esphagitis, esomeprazole (40 mg) was found to be more effective in healing at 4 and 8 weeks than was either omeprazole (20 mg) or lansoprazole (30 mg).	C	McDonagh, Carson, & Thakurta (2009)

A = consistent, good-quality, patient-oriented evidence; B = inconsistent or limited-quality, patient-oriented evidence; C = consensus, disease-oriented evidence, usual practice, expert opinion, or case series. For information about the SORT evidence rating system, go to www.aafp.org/afpsort.xml.

GASTRIC CANCER

Signal symptoms: Vague sense of fullness, dyspepsia, weight loss, palpable abdominal mass.

Description: Gastric cancer generally is classified as early or advanced carcinoma. Gastric cancer usually begins in the distal portion of the stomach and spreads via the lymph or circulatory system.

Etiology: The etiology of gastric cancer is multifactorial, with the leading risk factor being *Helicobacter pylori* (Wroblewski, Peek, & Wilson, 2010); however, several dietary risk factors are associated with the incidence of stomach cancer. Patients who regularly consume diets high in highly salted and preserved foods (salted, pickled, and/or smoked) and high in refined carbohydrates have an increased risk for gastric cancer (Compare et al., 2011; Tsugane & Sasazuki, 2007). Smoking is also a known risk factor. Adenocarcinoma accounts for 90% to 95% of all gastric malignancies. Additional types of gastric cancer include lymphoma, leiomyosarcoma, carcinoid, squamous cell carcinoma, and gastrointestinal stromal tumors. Gastric cancers are then further subdivided by histopathological and anatomical criteria. Recent work has identified that further subgroupings by gene expression exist and suggest a new classification of gastric tumors (Shah et al., 2011). Early gastric cancers generally are confined to the mucosa or submucosa; advanced gastric carcinomas penetrate the muscularis propria with lymph node involvement.

Occurrence: Each year in the United States, more than 20,000 new cases of gastric carcinoma are diagnosed. There are approximately 11,500 deaths a year from gastric cancer (Jemal et al., 2009). The incidence worldwide is much greater. With over 880,000 new cases a year and 650,000 deaths, gastric cancer is the most frequent cause of cancer death worldwide (Tsugane & Sasazuki, 2007).

Age: The average age at onset of gastric cancer is 65. Of patients with gastric cancer, more than 65% are over 50 years of age (Jemal et al., 2011).

Gender: Gastric cancer is found predominantly in men with a ratio of 3:2 (Jemal et al., 2011).

Ethnicity: A high incidence of gastric cancer has been found in Native Americans, African Americans, Asians, Hispanics, and Scandinavians and for Eastern Europeans (Jemal et al., 2011).

Contributing factors: Identified risk factors for the development of gastric cancer include the following: chronic *H. pylori* infection (associated with ingestion of spoiled food products) (Correia, Machado, & Ristimaki, 2009; Uemura et al., 2001); tobacco abuse and regular alcohol consumption; prolonged ingestion of food products that are high in salt and nitrates; and long-term, extensive exposure to heavy metals, rubber, asbestos, or polycyclic hydrocarbons (wood-burning stoves, charcoal-grilled meats). Gastric ulcers and adenomatous polyps are known precursors to gastric cancer. Patients with a history of atrophic gastritis resulting from pernicious anemia and who have had a partial gastrectomy (Billroth I or II) are at risk for developing gastric cancer. History of previous radiation has been shown to be a risk factor for developing gastric cancer. An association between the Epstein-Barr virus and gastric cancer has been noted. A family history of first-degree relatives with gastric cancer increases the risk to 2 to 3 times that of people without this history. There is an association of blood type A and developing gastric cancer. Finally, lower socioeconomic status has been shown to be a risk factor for stomach cancer (Bjelakovic, Nikolova, Simonetti, & Gluud, 2009; Joossens et al., 1996).

Signs and symptoms: Early detection of gastric cancer is often difficult because of the absence of clinical presentation. Patients often describe a vague sensation of fullness after a meal that is relieved by belching, nonspecific complaints of abdominal pain of varying intensities, nausea, anorexia, dyspepsia, vomiting and evidence of gastrointestinal blood (hematemesis and melena), and constipation. Epigastric discomfort is present in more than 75% of patients, and the presentation may be similar to that of a gastric ulcer.

Weight loss and pallor, if the patient is anemic, may be the only signs noted during physical examination. Examination of the skin may reveal diffuse seborrheic keratosis. A palpable mass in the abdomen may be felt in an advanced carcinoma. Patients with metastatic disease often have enlargement of the left supraclavicular lymph nodes (Virchow's node) and left axillary node (Irish node). In advanced disease, ascites may be present; an enlarged ovary may be detected in females (Krukenberg's tumor); or a rectal mass (Blumer's shelf) or periumbilical adenopathy (Sister Mary Joseph's node) may be present (Ioannidis et al., 2010).

Diagnostic tests: For patients presenting with symptoms of gastric cancer, the following laboratory studies should be considered: CBC with indices to determine presence of anemia, complete metabolic panel, and FOBT to detect bleeding in the intestinal tract. Patients will need to be referred for an endoscopy with a biopsy and cytological examination (Kapoor, Bassi, Sturgess, & Bodger, 2005; Lee et al., 2005). If there is suspicion of advanced disease state, imaging studies should be ordered, including abdominal CT scan if metastatic

disease is suspected (pelvic in females). Consider chest CT scan in patients with advanced cancer involving the esophagus (Lee et al., 2005).

Differential diagnosis:
- Chronic gastritis
- Functional dyspepsia
- Peptic ulcer disease
- Esophageal carcinoma
- Lymphoma
- Crohn's disease
- Sarcoidosis
- Mesenteric ischemia
- Gastroenteritis
- Irritable bowel syndrome
- Gastric ulcers
- Reflux esophagitis (McQuaid, 2009)

Treatment: A partial or complete gastric resection with adjacent lymph nodes is the treatment of choice for gastric cancer; the value of extended surgery to remove lymph nodes near to the tumor remains controversial. One systematic review found that extended surgery carries increased mortality risks associated with spleen and pancreas resection (McCulloch, Nita, Kazi, & Gama-Rodrigues, 2007). Extensive cancer or metastases negate the need for surgery. Chemotherapeutic agents (most commonly, 5-fluorouracil) have been used alone or in combination with other treatments such as radiation.

Follow-up: For the patient who has had gastric resection, continued surveillance every few months is necessary to check for weight loss, bleeding, and obstruction. Laboratory evaluation of CBC, routine liver tests, and measurement of serum CEA should occur at 3- to 6-month intervals for the first year after surgery. After the initial surveillance interval an annual endoscopy is recommended for the next 5 years (Dan, So, & Yeoh, 2006).

Sequelae: Malnutrition, hemorrhage, obstruction, possibly evasive cancer, and metastases are complications from gastric cancer.

Prevention/prophylaxis: Patients should eliminate the use of food products that contain nitrates and are highly salted. Screening for *H. pylori* in high-risk populations has been advocated (Tsugane & Sasazuki, 2007).

Referral: A gastroenterologist should be consulted for the endoscopy and complicated management problems, including annual follow-up endoscopy. For patients with advanced disease, referral for palliative care or local hospice should be made (Wöhrer, Raderer, & Hejna, 2004).

Education: After partial and complete gastrectomy, teach patients about the importance of adequate nutrition. Consuming six small meals a day may be necessary instead of the usual three. Supplementation with vitamins, especially vitamin B_{12}, and minerals, such as calcium and iron, should be prescribed. Patients may prefer taking nutritional supplements in place of one or more of the meals each day.

CLINICAL RECOMMENDATION	EVIDENCE RATING	REFERENCES
Extended surgery to remove lymph nodes near the tumor remains controversial. Increased mortality risk exists with surgery involving spleen and pancreas resection.	A	McCulloch, Nita, Kazi, & Gama-Rodrigues (2007)
Patients with metastatic or recurrent gastric cancer have a very poor prognosis and should be offered chemotherapy and/or palliative care.	B	Wöhrer, Raderer, & Hejna (2004)
Upper gastrointestinal endoscopy with biopsy is the recommended initial diagnostic test.	C	Lee et al. (2005)
Persons with diets high in salted and preserved foods (salted, pickled, and/or smoked) and in refined carbohydrates have an increased risk for gastric cancer.	C	Compare et al. (2011) Tsugane & Sasazuki (2007)

A = consistent, good-quality, patient-oriented evidence; B = inconsistent or limited-quality, patient-oriented evidence; C = consensus, disease-oriented evidence, usual practice, expert opinion, or case series. For information about the SORT evidence rating system, go to www.aafp.org/afpsort.xml.

GASTRITIS

Signal symptoms: Anorexia, nausea and vomiting, epigastric pain or discomfort with tenderness.

Description: Gastritis is an inflammation of the mucosal lining of the stomach. A number of conditions can cause gastritis, including infection, autoimmune, exogenous substances, and stress. Patients may be asymptomatic; however, dyspepsia and gastrointestinal bleeding are common findings in older adults.

Etiology: Gastritis represents a group of disorders characterized by inflammation of the stomach lining; each disorder has distinct clinical attributes, pathogeneses, and histological features. Gastritis is divided first into *erosive* and *nonerosive* types; a possible inflammatory process within each group may be categorized as acute or chronic. It is also classified according to the area of the stomach involved (i.e., cardia, body, antrum). Gastritis may be caused by infectious agents such as *H. pylori*, *E. coli*, *Staphylococcus aureus*, *Clostridium perfringens*, and *Streptococcus* and viruses such as cytomegalovirus (CMV), herpesvirus, and Epstein-Barr virus. *Candida* may be found in immunocompromised patients, but also in alcoholic patients or those who have ingested corrosive chemicals (Lauwers, Fujita, Nagata, & Shimizu, 2010). Acute erosive gastritis occurs when there is damage to the surface epithelium of the stomach. Erosion results from contact from exogenous agents such NSAIDs, acetylsalicylic acid, chemotherapeutic agents, and alcohol, infections, or bile secretions (Pilotto, Sancarlo, Addante, Scarcelli, & Franceschi, 2010). In the case of burns, trauma, sepsis, or prolonged hypotension, mucosal hypoxia occurs, leading to acute erosive gastritis (Pilotto et al., 2011).

Chronic gastritis can be classified further as nonatrophic, atrophic, and specific types related to precipitating factors, such as chemical or radiation gastritis. Chronic nonspecific gastritis results from ongoing injury to the gastric mucosa causing chronic inflammation and gastric atrophy (Sepulveda & Patil, 2008). It is estimated that 90% of patients with chronic gastritis have been exposed to *H. pylori* (Chey & Wong, 2007). There are a number of types of uncommon chronic gastritis. These include autoimmune, reactive chemical, noninfectious granulomatous, lymphocytic, eosinophilic, radiation, and ischemic gastritis (Franceschi, Di Mario, Leandro, Maggi, & Pilotto, 2009).

Occurrence: Exact incidence of gastritis is unknown.

Age: Although gastritis occurs in all ages, it is a common occurrence in older adults. Although patients of all ages can be infected with *H. pylori*, extensive atrophic damage generally occurs after age 50 (Weck, Gao, & Brenner, 2009). Pernicious anemia developed as a result of long-standing autoimmune atrophic gastritis often occurs around the sixth decade.

Gender: Atrophic gastritis occurs equally in men and women; autoimmune gastritis is more prevalent in females (3:1 ratio).

Ethnicity: Worldwide, the risk for developing *H. pylori* infection is greatest among Asian and Hispanic persons. Chronic gastritis resulting from *H. pylori* infection is higher in the United States among African Americans than Caucasians. Autoimmune atrophic gastritis occurs more frequently in individuals of northern European descent.

Contributing factors: Many factors can precipitate the development of gastritis. Acute gastritis can be caused by physiological stressors, hypovolemic shock, portal hypertension, aspirin, NSAIDs, alcohol, radiation, chemotherapy, gastric lymphoma, Crohn's disease, and *H. pylori* and other bacterial, viral, and fungal infections. Stress, trauma, and burns can trigger this acute condition. Patients on mechanical ventilation are at risk for developing acute gastritis. Chronic gastritis can develop because of gastric atrophy, *H. pylori* infection, bile and pancreatic secretions, and pernicious anemia. Exposure to long-term smoking makes the stomach lining more vulnerable to the development of chronic gastritis. Most patients who have had a previous gastrectomy develop gastritis.

Signs and symptoms: Anorexia, nausea (with or without vomiting), and epigastric distress aggravated by eating are common with gastritis. Halitosis may be noted. Patients may report a bloating sensation and early satiety. Physical examination may be unremarkable in cases of chronic gastritis. Palpate for abdominal masses and liver tenderness. Perform a rectal examination to test for occult blood. Any unexplained weight loss should be noted. Gastrointestinal bleeding may be exhibited by coffee-ground vomitus, melena, hematochezia, or the passing of bright red blood in a nasogastric tube. Any patient suspected of gastrointestinal bleeding should be examined for changes in mental status; coolness of the extremities; and pallor of the nail beds, mucous membranes, and conjunctivae. Assessment should include watching for any changes in cardiac output, such as decreasing blood pressure and increased heart rate.

Diagnostic tests: Diagnostic studies include CBC with indices to detect blood loss and anemia, stool guaiac test, and gastroscopy with a biopsy, which is the definitive diagnostic test for gastritis. If *H. pylori* is suspected, noninvasive testing includes antibody testing, urea breath tests (UBTs) ^{13}C and ^{14}C, and fecal antigen tests. Though more costly, UBTs and fecal antigen tests have excellent sensitivity and specificity (95%) and can be used for diagnosis and posttherapy evaluation. PPI use will need to be restricted 7 to 14 days and antibiotics for 28 days before UBT and fecal antigen testing (not serology) to ensure more accurate diagnosis (Chey & Wong, 2007). During endoscopy, a biopsy-based *H. pylori* test can be ordered.

Differential diagnosis:

- GERD
- Biliary tract disease
- Food poisoning
- Functional dyspepsia
- Peptic ulcer disease
- Perforated or penetrated ulcer
- Gastric carcinomas
- Pancretic disease
- Esophageal rupture
- Myocardial colic (McQuaid, 2009)

Treatment: Patients with acute gastritis should avoid offensive agents, such as alcohol, NSAIDs, aspirin, and cigarettes. Acute hemorrhagic gastritis requires hospitalization for IV fluids, IV PPIs, nasogastric aspiration, transfusion of blood products as necessary, and monitoring of vital signs. H_2 blockers, such as famotidine, ranitidine, or nizatidine, can be given for 6 to 8 weeks. An oral dose of ranitidine, 300 mg, or nizatidine, 300 mg, daily at bedtime can be ordered. The dosage of the H_2 blockers may have to be reduced, however, depending on renal status of the patient. If treatment for *H. pylori* is indicated, treatment options are delineated in Table 10-2.

Follow-up: A repeat endoscopy is advised after 6 weeks for patients who had severe gastritis or who

TABLE 10-2   *Helicobacter pylori* Regimens

Patients who are not allergic to penicillin and have not previously received a macrolide	Standard dose PPI twice daily (or esomeprazole 40 mg once daily) plus clarithromycin 500 mg twice daily, and amoxicillin 1000 mg twice daily for 10–14 days
Patients who are allergic to penicillin, and who have not previously received a macrolide or metronidazole or are unable to tolerate bismuth quadruple therapy	Standard dose PPI twice daily, clarithromycin 500 mg twice daily, metronidazole 500 mg twice daily for 10–14 days
Patients who are allergic to penicillin or failed one course (above) of *H. pylori* treatment	Bismuth subsalicylate 525 mg 4 times daily, metronidazole 250 mg 4 times daily, tetracycline 500 mg 4 times daily, standard dose PPI twice daily for 10–14 days OR Bismuth subcitrate 420 mg 4 times daily, metronidazole 375 mg 4 times daily, tetracycline 375 mg 4 times daily, standard dose PPI twice daily for 10–14 days

continue to have symptoms despite treatment. Obtain a CBC, and check stool for occult blood at subsequent office visits every 3 to 6 months after the diagnosis of gastritis. At each follow-up appointment, review all drugs, including OTC medications and home remedies.

Sequelae: Acute hemorrhagic gastritis has a high mortality rate in older adults. For the patients with *H. pylori*, there is a risk for developing gastric carcinoma; after eradication, the risk decreases (Leung et al., 2004; Malfertheiner et al., 2007). Patients with autoimmune gastritis may develop pernicious anemia given the loss of parietal cell mass and subsequently anti-intrinsic factor antibodies (Miceli et al., 2012). It is important to note that unexplained or refractory iron deficiency anemia can develop in patients with either *H. pylori*–associated atrophic gastritis or autoimmune atrophic gastritis.

Prevention/prophylaxis: Prophylaxis with acid-suppressive drugs can reduce the incidence of acute stress gastritis. Older adults who are high-risk intensive care unit patients, including those with severe burns, central nervous system trauma, coagulopathy, sepsis, shock, multiple trauma, mechanical ventilation for longer than 48 hours, hepatic or renal failure, and a history of peptic ulcer or gastrointestinal bleeding, benefit from prophylaxis medication to prevent acute gastritis. Critically ill older adults need to be monitored for signs and symptoms of hypovolemic shock secondary to acute gastric bleeding.

Alternative anti-inflammatory or nonnarcotic analgesics should be considered in the treatment of pain or inflammation in older adults with a history of gastritis, dyspepsia, or other upper gastrointestinal clinical events (Laine, Curtis, Cryer, Kaur, & Cannon, 2010).

Referral: Older patients with acute hemorrhagic gastritis require hospitalization, probably with intensive care unit admission. Consultation with a gastroenterologist for endoscopy and management of complicated cases of gastritis is recommended.

Education: Advise patients to report any black, tarlike stools or frank bleeding to the health-care practitioner immediately. All alcohol, caffeine, salicylates, tobacco, and NSAID product use should be discontinued.

CLINICAL RECOMMENDATION	EVIDENCE RATING	REFERENCES
A strong association between *H. pylori* and developing chronic atrophic gastritis exists.	B	Weck, Gao, & Brenner (2009)
Vitamin B_{12} deficiency was found in patients diagnosed with autoimmune atrophic gastritis.	B	Miceli et al. (2012)

Continued

CLINICAL RECOMMENDATION	EVIDENCE RATING	REFERENCES
Eradication of *H. pylori* is protective against progression of premalignant gastric lesions. Age was found to be an important factor in the progression of intestinal metaplasia compared to younger subjects.	B	Leung et al. (2004)
Advanced age (≥65), prior episodes of dyspepsia, and upper gastrointestinal clinical events increase the risk for severe dyspepsia and warrant the discontinuation of NSAIDs.	A	Laine, Curtis, Cryer, Kaur, & Cannon (2010)

A = consistent, good-quality, patient-oriented evidence; B = inconsistent or limited-quality, patient-oriented evidence; C = consensus, disease-oriented evidence, usual practice, expert opinion, or case series. For information about the SORT evidence rating system, go to www.aafp.org/afpsort.xml.

GASTROENTERITIS

Signal symptoms: Sudden onset of diarrhea, abdominal pain with distention, flatulence, vomiting.

Description: Gastroenteritis is an infectious response of the gastrointestinal tract to various microorganisms that can be viral, bacterial, or parasitic in origin.

Etiology: Gastroenteritis is caused by exposure to toxins and drugs or viruses, bacteria, and parasites:

- Viruses such as Norovirus, formerly called the Norwalk-like virus and astrovirus
- Bacteria such as *Salmonella, Campylobacter, Shigella, E. coli,* and *Vibrio cholerae*
- Parasites such as *Giardia lamblia*

Occurrence: Exact incidence of infectious gastroenteritis is unknown because of underreporting of symptoms. Noroviruses cause approximately 23 million cases of acute gastroenteritis each year and are the leading cause of outbreaks of gastroenteritis. Approximately 30% to 40% of gastroenteritis diarrhea in the United States is thought to be viral in origin, with more than 55% of the adult population exposed to a common enteric calicivirus, one of which is Norovirus. Norovirus caused about 800 deaths a year from 1999 to 2007.

Age: Gastroenteritis occurs at all ages, but its incidence and the mortality rate from infectious diarrhea are higher in older adults. Epidemic cases of gastroenteritis occur in nursing home populations. Adults over age 65 accounted for 83% of deaths from enteritis between 1999 and 2007 (Keuhn, 2012).

Gender: Gastroenteritis is equally prevalent in both sexes, although diarrhea is more common in women.

Contributing factors: Specific to the older adult population, age-related factors such as decreased motility, mucosal atrophy, and decreased gastric acidity inhibit natural defense mechanisms against infectious agents. The use of H_2 blockers, antacids, anticholinergic drugs, and narcotics increases the potential for developing gastroenteritis. Gastroenteritis also can be caused by emotional stress, viral or bacterial infection, food intolerance, and organic (shellfish, certain mushrooms) or inorganic (sodium nitrate) poisons. Travel to another country with a change in surroundings or to an area of poor sanitation standards and facilities can contribute to the development of gastroenteritis. Nursing home populations are susceptible to epidemics because of contact with health-care workers who may not use proper hand washing techniques. Some viruses, such as Norovirus, can be transmitted by an airborne route. Fecal-to-oral contact has been identified as a mode of transmission of organisms (Monroe, 2011).

Signs and symptoms: History of possible fecal-to-oral contact; exposure to other patients with gastroenteritis; and ingestion of certain food products such as mayonnaise, custards, fried rice, vegetables, beef, poultry, bean sprouts, or raw seafood should be explored. Try to estimate the length of time that has elapsed since the patient ingested the food product suspected of contamination. Travel to a foreign country or region that may have contaminated water should be recorded, as should any previous history of diarrhea and related symptoms and the duration of the current episode. A sudden onset of diarrhea, abdominal pain with distention, flatulence, and vomiting may be reported. Associated anorexia, headache, fatigue, dizziness, and myalgias are also symptoms of gastroenteritis. Fever may or may not occur in the older adult; mental confusion may result from dehydration. The stool's color, odor, amount, and frequency should be described, and the presence of any blood or mucus in the stool should be discerned. Patient use of prescription drugs, OTC medications, and home remedies needs to be included in the history.

In the physical examination, the skin is checked for signs of rashes or dehydration, and the lymph nodes are assessed for lymphadenopathy. Abdominal examination may reveal distention, hyperactive bowel sounds, and tenderness. Perform a rectal examination to note any bleeding and the color of the stool and to check for an impaction (Reuben et al., 2008).

Diagnostic tests: CBC with differential should be ordered. WBC shift to the left may suggest an infection, and a decreased hemoglobin value indicates anemia from probable blood loss. Serum electrolyte evaluation shows an increased sodium level in dehydrated patients and decreased potassium resulting from the diarrhea. Elevated serum creatinine and BUN levels also occur in dehydration. Stool samples for blood, ova and parasite, leukocytes, and bacteria are ordered to try to identify the microorganism. A stool culture positive for blood is found in bacterial infections and in inflammatory processes; the culture and sensitivity report may show Salmonella, Campylobacter, Shigella, and V. cholerae. Consider sigmoidoscopy for patients with bloody diarrhea (DuPont, 1997).

Differential diagnosis:
▪ Fecal impaction
▪ Fecal incontinence
▪ Colorectal cancers
▪ Adverse reaction to medications
▪ Diverticulitis
▪ Malabsorption
▪ Pseudomembranous colitis if the patient has been prescribed an antibiotic within 2 months of onset of symptoms

Treatment: Lost fluids and electrolytes must be replaced. Clear liquids and specially formulated rehydration liquids, such as Gatorade, should be given as tolerated. Clear broths and crackers may be added to the diet when diarrhea has ceased. Patients should avoid caffeine, dairy products, alcohol, fruits, bran, vegetables, and red meats. Solid foods should be added gradually, starting with rice or potatoes. When the patient no longer has loose stools, foods such as applesauce and bananas and skinless chicken can be added. Physical activity should be limited, to avoid unnecessary exertion. Care should be taken to prevent any skin excoriation or pressure sores. Patients with infectious diarrhea should avoid antidiarrheal medications. Antibiotic therapy is specific to the bacterial or parasitic organisms identified from the stool culture:

▪ Campylobacter infection is treated with erythromycin, 250 to 500 mg 4 times daily for 7 days, or, if sensitivity to erythromycin is present, ciprofloxacin, 500 mg twice daily for 7 days, adjusting the dose for renal function.
▪ G. lamblia infection is treated with metronidazole, 250 mg 3 times daily for 5 to 7 days.
▪ Severe cases of traveler's diarrhea (enterotoxigenic E. coli) can be treated with trimethoprim-sulfamethoxazole, 160/800 mg (double strength) orally twice daily for 5 days, or ciprofloxacin, 500 mg twice daily for 3 days (DuPont, 1997).

Follow-up: Contact outpatients 4 days after the onset of symptoms to determine progress. Request nursing home staff to provide a verbal report of the patient's condition on the third or fourth day; note any further outbreak of gastroenteritis. When contacting the patient at home, question if there have been any additional symptoms, including fever and neurological developments such as paresthesia, motor weakness, and cranial nerve palsies. For older adults with chronic diarrhea or other persistent gastrointestinal symptoms, refer to a gastroenterologist (Reuben et al., 2008).

Sequelae: Dehydration, anemia, metabolic acidosis, and hypovolemic shock could occur in untreated cases of severe infectious diarrhea.

Prevention/prophylaxis: Older adults with travel plans to foreign destinations should be urged to avoid contaminated water. Avoid ice cubes and brushing teeth with nonbottled water. Discard any foods that contain dairy or egg products that have not been refrigerated for an extended time or have been exposed to warm temperatures. Raw or undercooked meat and seafood should be avoided (Monroe, 2011).

Referral: Refer to a specialist when symptoms persist beyond 4 days, when severe dehydration develops, or when the patient has bloody stools.

Education: Gastroenteritis, although generally self-limiting, can be debilitating. Infections with some microorganisms, such as *G. lamblia*, can become chronic and result in lactose intolerance, which is common in older adults. Any new case of diarrhea not resolved in 3 to 4 days requires health-care provider intervention. Use of OTC antiperistaltic agents, such as loperamide, is contraindicated in infectious diarrhea.

CLINICAL RECOMMENDATION	EVIDENCE RATING	REFERENCES
Assess risk of dehydration on the basis of age and frequency of watery stools and vomiting.	B	Murphy (1998)
Assess presence/severity of dehydration on recent weight loss if possible and clinical examination.	A	Murphy (1998)
Most bacterial gastroenteritis does not require or benefit from antibiotic treatment. Antibiotic treatment may be indicated for *Shigella* gastroenteritis in the very young, in immunocompromised patients, and in those who are very ill. Patients with *Shigella* dysentery should receive antibiotic treatment.	A	Murphy (1998)
In the vast majority of cases, oral rehydration therapy (ORT) should be carried out.	A	Murphy (1998)
In hypernatremic dehydration, ORT is safer than IV rehydration.	B	Murphy (1998)
Probiotic products containing *Lactobacillus casei*, *Streptococcus thermophilus*, and *L. bulgaricus* have been shown to decrease the incidence of antibiotic-associated diarrhea and *C. difficile* diarrhea.	C	Reuben et al. (2008)

A = consistent, good-quality, patient-oriented evidence; B = inconsistent or limited-quality, patient-oriented evidence; C = consensus, disease-oriented evidence, usual practice, expert opinion, or case series. For information about the SORT evidence rating system, go to www.aafp.org/afpsort.xml.

GASTROESOPHAGEAL REFLUX DISEASE

Signal symptoms: Regurgitation, pyrosis, hoarseness, chronic cough, atypical chest pain.

Description: GERD is a common disorder characterized by various symptoms ranging from mild heartburn to more severe physical complaints, caused by the reflux of gastric contents into the esophagus. These symptoms may or may not occur in patients who present with laryngopharyngeal and/or respiratory symptoms. Influencing factors in the development of GERD include a weakened lower esophageal sphincter (LES) pressure, hiatal hernia, abnormal esophageal clearance, slowed esophageal peristalsis, esophageal mucosal resistance, and delayed gastric emptying (Vakil et al., 2006).

Etiology: The presentation of GERD is a complex problem than involves reduction in the tone of the lower esophageal sphincter, episodic relaxation of the lower esophageal sphincter at inappropriate times, decreased secondary peristalsis, and faulty mucosal resistance to caustic fluids.

Occurrence: GERD affects more than 20% of the U.S. population (Sandler et al., 2002).

Age: Approximately 10% to 30% of elderly individuals experience weekly symptoms of heartburn or regurgitation. Other studies have indicated a daily reporting of GERD symptoms in older adults to average around 12% for men and women (Shams, Siddiqui & Heif, 2009; Sharma, Wani, Romero, Johnson, & Hamilton, 2008).

Gender: The ratio of men to women with GERD is equal. Severe esophagitis is more common in men than in women (2:1). Barrett's esophagus is more common in men than in women (10:1) (Kubo et al., 2013).

Ethnicity: Severe esophagitis is more common in whites than in nonwhites.

Contributing factors: Intrinsic factors that contribute to the development of GERD include LES incompetence, hiatal hernia, esophageal motility disorders, delayed gastric emptying, and gastric distention. Certain medications can trigger GERD. Nitrates, CCBs, benzodiazepines, tricyclic antidepressants, beta agonists, and anticholinergics lower the LES tone. NSAIDs, aspirin, steroids, iron sulfates, gelatin capsules, antibiotics, potassium chloride tablets, vitamin C, quinidine, and bisphosphonates contribute to esophagitis, local erosions, or ulcers. Additional medications that contribute to GERD due to decreased esophageal motility include theophylline, sedatives, and narcotics. Substances that weaken the lower esophageal sphincter pressure include caffeine, mints, chocolate, alcohol, spicy foods (including yellow onions and garlic), and citrus fruits. Smoking, alcohol, obesity, and certain dietary products (food substances that contain lactose in some patients lead to gastric distention) may contribute to the development of the symptoms of GERD (Hart, 2013). There is an increased risk in developing nonerosive esophagitis in patients with metabolic syndrome. Patients with nasogastric tubes are known to be at risk for having symptoms of GERD. Patients with certain medical conditions that affect gastric motility such as stroke, diabetes, scleroderma, myasthenia gravis, and Parkinson's disease are at risk for developing GERD (Shams et al., 2009).

Signs and symptoms: Determine from patients precipitating factors related to the development of GERD, length of time they have been experiencing symptoms, and what regimens and/or lifestyle changes they have tried. Patients should be questioned about medication usage, smoking, and intake of substances that can weaken the lower esophageal sphincter; sleeping habits; and use of any tight or restrictive clothing. Determine if any activity triggers GERD such as bending over, exercise, or being recumbent. Review the patient's dietary habits and elicit if there are food products that the patient regularly ingests that aggravate symptoms of GERD. Question the patient about history of heartburn, pyrosis, belching, halitosis, regurgitation, nausea, atypical chest pain (radiation of pain to back, neck, and/or jaw), hoarseness, recurrent laryngitis, cough, choking, pharyngeal tightness, globus sensation, persistent clearing of the throat, sore throat, recent dental caries, dysphagia, odynophagia, anorexia, weight loss, vomiting, otitis media, bronchospasms, chronic bronchitis, and asthma (Richter, 1996). Determine if the patient's sleep is disturbed because of GERD symptoms. Review the medications the patient is taking to determine if any medications reduce the lower esophageal pressure, decrease the lower esophageal sphincter pressure, and/or irritate the esophageal mucosa. Question the patient about any previous history and/or treatment for *H. pylori*. Ask about any family history of esophageal cancer or hiatal hernia.

Physical examination usually produces no positive findings. Conduct a thorough examination of the oral cavity and a respiratory examination. Palpate for any upper abdominal masses or tenderness. Perform a rectal examination to detect any frank bleeding.

Diagnostic tests: If suspicion was aroused on the physical examination, stool should be checked using the guaiac test to determine if there has been any intestinal bleeding. Laboratory studies are not required when antacids, position change, or both relieve pyrosis. For older adults who complain of persistent dysphagia or odynophagia with or without fever, barium swallow or an endoscopy (with brush and biopsy if structural mucosal damage is suspected) or both are ordered. Any patient presenting with laryngopharyngeal symptoms of GERD should be considered for a laryngoscopy. A majority of GERD patients have a negative endoscopy.

Differential diagnosis:
- Nonulcer dyspepsia
- Esophageal spasms
- Esophagitis
- Esophageal stricture (upper gastrointestinal sinus)
- Esophageal carcinoma
- Cholecystitis
- Peptic ulcer disease (Hart, 2013)

Treatment: The goals for the treatment of GERD include eliminating symptoms, healing esophagitis, managing or preventing complications, and maintaining remission (Poh, Navarro-Rodriguez, & Fass, 2010). Important to the management of GERD are the lifestyle changes or nonpharmacological measures that patients need to incorporate along with the medication regimen; these include avoidance of smoking, alcohol, and food products such as chocolate, mints, spicy or acidic foods, caffeine. For older adults, PPIs remain the mainstay of treatment, given the rapid relief of GERD symptoms and esophageal healing that result from PPI treatment; once-a-day dosing is beneficial to aid in medication compliance. It is important to note that older adults will require long-term maintenance therapy for GERD. A step-down approach can be initiated in patients with GERD by reducing the dosage of the PPI or by adding an H_2 blocker in the evening. Another recommended approach for patients who have had symptomatic relief after 8 to 12 weeks of therapy is to recommend an H_2 blocker on demand or a PPI as needed (University of Michigan Health System, 2007). The use of prokinetic agents is not recommended in older adults given the serious side effects. Pharmacological recommendations are listed in Table 10-3.

Follow-up: Review lifestyle changes and the impact modifications have had on the patient's symptoms of GERD. Evaluate compliance with the medication regimen. Determine if the patient has experienced any complications or alarming changes in status since the last evaluation.

Sequelae: Ulceration and bleeding, if reflux esophagitis is present, can occur after esophagitis. In esophagitis with esophageal stricture, Barrett's esophagus with possible adenocarcinoma may be a long-term complication (Shams et al., 2009). Abdominal obesity, not specifically increased BMI, was found to be associated with the development of Barrett's esophagus in both men and women (Kubo et al., 2013). Older adults are also at risk for developing pulmonary complications of GERD such as chronic cough, recurrent pneumonitis, and aspiration pneumonia. Patients who present with otolaryngological symptoms of GERD may develop chronic laryngitis, laryngeal polyps, laryngotracheal stenosis, and laryngeal carcinoma (Patrick, 2011). Given the reflux of gastric content to the pharynx, dental erosions are also a common consequence of laryngopharyngeal reflux.

Prevention/prophylaxis: Prevention of GERD should be aimed at eliminating or at least modifying the extrinsic factors that contribute to the development of the condition. Patients should be encouraged to make lifestyle adjustments and avoid potentially harmful medications to prevent further complications.

Referral: A gastroenterologist should be consulted for the endoscopy and for patients with anemia, severe or nonresponsive reflux disease, dysphagia, odynophagia, unexplained weight loss, or evidence of hemorrhage. When a patient presents with laryngopharyngeal reflux, he or she should be referred for an indirect or direct laryngoscopy. If a patient presents with dysphagia, odynophagia, unexplained weight loss, or gastrointestinal bleeding or if a patient did not respond to initial therapy, refer to a gastroenterologist (Katz, Gerson, & Velva, 2012; Müller, Gockel, Konig, Kuhr, & Eckardt, 2011).

Education: Patients with reflux esophagitis should be instructed to raise the head of the bed 4 to 6 in. with shock blocks or foam wedge that can be placed at the head of the bed. While there has been limited evidence to suggest that making lifestyle changes to decrease abdominal pressure, such as avoiding tight, restrictive clothing, counteracts the symptoms of GERD, medical practitioners should encourage patients to adopt this strategy, especially given the small number of patients in studies that made this recommendation (Katz et al., 2012). The patient should avoid smoking and ingestion of fatty foods, coffee, chocolate, mints, citric juices, alcohol, and large quantities of fluids with meals.

TABLE 10-3	**Pharmacological Recommendations for Gastroesophageal Reflux Disease**

Treatment of erosive or nonerosive gastroesophageal reflux disease
Proton Pump Inhibitors

DRUG	DOSAGE
Dexlansoprazole	30 mg daily
Esomeprazole	20 mg daily
Lansoprazole	15 mg daily
Omeprazole	20 mg daily
Pantoprazole	40 mg daily
Rabeprazole	20 mg daily
H2-Receptor Antagonists	
Nizatidine	150 mg q12h
Famotidine	20 mg q12h
Ranitidine	150 mg q12h
Cimetidine*	400 or 800 mg q12h

*Cimetidine is not recommended for use in older adults.

Remind patients not to break or crush extended-release or delayed-release tablets. Patients should avoid eating a meal for at least 3 hours before becoming recumbent. Teach the patient the importance of swallowing medications with an adequate amount of fluids. An oral PPI needs to be ingested 60 minutes before a meal; it is suggested to then wait 30 minutes after the PPI has been taken before eating.

CLINICAL RECOMMENDATION	EVIDENCE RATING	REFERENCES
Older adults reported typical symptoms of GERD at postprandial times.	B	Furuta et al. (2012)
Despite negative results of pH monitoring indicating no evidence of GERD, patients were found to continue PPI use.	B	Gawron et al. (2012)
Endoscopy is recommended for patients >50 years with alarm symptoms or for those with prolonged symptoms despite medical treatment.	B	Müller et al. (2011)
Antisecretory therapy with H_2 blockers is effective for mild or intermittent GERD.	A	Kahrilas et al. (2008)

A = consistent, good-quality, patient-oriented evidence; B = inconsistent or limited-quality, patient-oriented evidence; C = consensus, disease-oriented evidence, usual practice, expert opinion, or case series. For information about the SORT evidence rating system, go to www.aafp.org/afpsort.xml.

HERNIA

Signal symptoms: A dual dragging sensation with an inguinal hernia; male patients may report pain and swelling in the scrotum; patients with strangulated abdominal hernia usually have a tender mass with associated fever, nausea, and vomiting.

Description: A hernia is the protrusion of tissue through a weakened section in the abdominal wall. Abdominal wall hernias usually occur at the groin (inguinal) and umbilicus. Hernias are classified by their severity as reducible, incarcerated, or strangulated. A *reducible hernia* moves easily through the anatomical defect. An *incarcerated hernia* does not return to a normal position automatically or when manipulated externally. A *strangulated hernia* results when an incarcerated hernia develops edema with ischemia to the entrapped bowel.

In addition to these classifications, inguinal hernias may be either direct or indirect. A direct inguinal hernia passes through the posterior inguinal wall, whereas an indirect or congenital inguinal hernia enters in through the internal abdominal inguinal ring along the spermatic cord through the inguinal passage, to exit out the external inguinal ring.

Etiology: Hernia development has been linked to recurrent Valsalva maneuvers and dysfunctional connective tissue resulting from malnutrition or long-term steroid use. In older women, a history of multiple pregnancies and relaxation of the pelvic musculature, combined with loss of extraperitoneal fat, are considered etiological factors in the development of an obturator hernia (Haraguchi et al., 2007).

Occurrence: In the United States, more than 700,000 herniorrhaphies are performed annually. The most common type of hernia is the inguinal hernia, which accounts for 80% of all cases, followed by the femoral hernia, which has been noted to be 5% of all hernias. The remaining 15% include umbilical, epigastric, obturator, and those resulting from a surgical incision (Greenfield, 2001).

Age: The incidence of femoral and obturator hernias in women increases with age (Haraguchi et al., 2007).

The incidence of male indirect (congenital) hernias decreases with age but that of direct inguinal hernias increases.

Gender: Indirect inguinal hernias are 8 to 10 times more common in men than in women, yet the indirect inguinal hernia is the most common type of hernia in women. Older women are 3 to 5 times more likely than men to develop a femoral hernia. The obturator hernia is a rare condition that occurs predominantly in women (Haraguchi et al., 2007).

Ethnicity: No known prevalence exists among ethnic groups.

Contributing factors: A chronic cough, ascites, abdominal surgery, obesity, and symptomatic prostatism can contribute to development of a hernia because of the associated risk factor of increased intra-abdominal or intrathoracic pressure. Chronic straining for bowel movements, straining to urinate, and lifting heavy objects may be precursors to hernia formation. For women, a weakened pelvic floor after childbirth can contribute to the development of femoral herniation. Older women who are underweight and have a history of chronic illness can develop obturator hernias (Haraguchi et al., 2007).

Hernias also may form at the site of a surgical incision or a large scar. Patients with known liver cirrhosis with ascites have a 20% chance of developing an umbilical hernia (Eker et al., 2011). Family history of organ herniation is also recognized as an intrinsic factor contributing to the development of hernias.

Signs and symptoms: Patients should be asked, How long has the discomfort (swelling, pain, and mass) been present? Is the pain aggravated by any activity such as heavy lifting or positioning? Inquire about abdominal surgical history. Question if there is a family history of hernias. Patients may report a dual dragging sensation with an inguinal hernia. Male patients may report pain and swelling in the scrotum. Hernias may be asymptomatic, only to be discovered as part of a routine physical examination. A reducible hernia presents as a nontender mass that becomes more pronounced after a Valsalva maneuver. An incarcerated hernia, also a nontender soft mass, is found in the abdominal, femoral, or inguinal area and remains even after gentle manipulation. Patients with strangulated abdominal hernia usually have a tender mass with associated fever, nausea, and vomiting. No attempt should be made to reduce a strangulated hernia.

Physical examination reveals decreased flatus, high-pitched or tinkling bowel sounds, abdominal distention, and tenderness of the mass. When examining a patient with a suspected hernia, assess the patient in both the supine and standing position, first observing the suspected mass before change in position. Have the patient also perform the Valsalva maneuver. If possible, attempt to identify the location of the hernia sac and the fascial opening of the hernia when palpating the abdomen. Identify the border of the suspected hernia (Goroll, 2009). For a suspected inguinal hernia, ask the patient to flex the leg on the side you will examine and then palpate gently the groin area. Then fingertips placed over the femoral area, external ring, and internal ring should be inserted up into the inguinal canal (LeBlanc, LeBlanc, & LeBlanc, 2013).

Gross screening for an inguinal hernia in a male patient is made easier with the patient coughing because "hernia bulges can be felt either against the examining finger (direct hernia) or at the tip of the finger, as it approaches the internal ring (indirect hernia)" (Amerson, 1990, p. 484). A femoral hernia can often be elicited by having a patient cough or strain; the bulge will be felt below the inguinal ligament (LeBlon et al., 2009). A positive Howship-Romberg sign along with intestinal obstruction has been found in 45% to 50% of patients diagnosed with an obturator hernia (Haraguchi et al., 2007). A mass is detected in the femoral triangle; patients experience pain down the medial aspect of the thigh all the way to the knee as a result of compression of the obturator nerve (LeBlond et al., 2009).

Diagnostic tests: In an uncomplicated asymptomatic hernia, laboratory and diagnostic tests are unwarranted. If there is questionable strangulation from a prolonged incarcerated hernia, laboratory studies for complications may reveal leukocytosis, elevated serum amylase, and guaiac-positive stool. The use of higher-resolution multidetector CT scan allows for a clearer image of the anatomy studied. Axial CT should be requested first if a hernia is suspected (Burkhardt, Arshanskiy, Munson, & Scholz, 2011). Abdominal series are done postoperatively to look for signs of perforation (free air) or obstruction of the bowel (multiple air-fluid levels). Ultrasonography may be ordered for a patient with a suspected recurring hernia or hydrocele (LeBlanc et al., 2013).

Differential diagnosis:
- Femoral lymphadenopathy
- Femoral artery aneurysm

■ Psoas abscess
■ Undescended testicle
■ Muscle strain (Goroll, 2009; LeBlanc et al., 2013)

Treatment: Surgical repair of strangulated inguinal, umbilical, and femoral hernias is recommended immediately unless the patient is a poor surgical risk. These patients need to be hospitalized, receive IV solutions, and remain on nothing-by-mouth (NPO) status. Small direct inguinal hernias and painless indirect inguinal hernias do not need immediate attention; however, surgery generally is recommended within 1 week of diagnosis. Patients who are not surgical candidates can be fitted for a truss and monitored for signs of prolonged incarceration. Patients with a small direct, nonpainful hernia should be observed for reduction of the hernia when supine.

Follow-up: For patients with reducible hernias, observation of the hernia during subsequent physical examination is recommended (Fitzgibbons et al., 2006). Patients suspected of having an incarcerated hernia should be followed up within 1 week to determine if they are experiencing any tenderness of the mass and if a general surgeon has seen them. For the postoperative patient who has had a herniorrhaphy, assess for wound healing and recurrence of the hernia. The mortality rate is increased for patients who have undergone an emergent hernia repair (Altom et al., 2011).

Sequelae: An untreated inguinal, umbilical, or femoral hernia may become incarcerated and strangulated, with subsequent intestinal gangrene; the likelihood of incarceration is greatest for femoral hernias. Postsurgical complications of a herniorrhaphy include wound hematomas and superficial wound infections. Nerve entrapment is a serious complication of an inguinal herniorraphy. Approximately 50% of hernia recurrence occurs within 5 years, and an additional 20% occur 15 to 20 years after surgical repair of a hernia (Sevonius, Gunnarsson, Nordin, Nilsson, & Sandblom, 2011).

Prevention/prophylaxis: Cessation of cigarette smoking is recommended to reduce intrathoracic pressure from chronic coughing. Encourage the use of fiber, fluids, and stool softeners for patients who strain with defecation. Patients should avoid lifting heavy objects without proper support.

Referral: Refer the patient to a general surgeon when a hernia is detected. A strangulated hernia requires immediate attention.

Education: Inform the patient with a reducible hernia of the potential complications of an untreated hernia and the importance of reporting immediately any new clinical signs and symptoms such as increase in pain, swelling, and/or fever. Teach patients to avoid straining to defecate or urinate. Encourage smoking cessation to reduce the probability of a chronic cough. Instruct the patients on proper techniques for lifting heavy objects. Weight reduction should be encouraged for obese patients. Patients also should be advised to discuss with their surgeon postoperative restrictions and plan for rehabilitation and home support given the probable restrictions to activity (Goroll, 2009).

CLINICAL RECOMMENDATION	EVIDENCE RATING	REFERENCES
CT scan of the pelvis is a useful diagnostic tool in diagnosing obturator hernias.	A	Haraguchi et al. (2007)
A positive Howship-Romberg sign is common in patients with an obturator hernia.	B	Haraguchi et al. (2007)
Patients with cirrhosis and ascites benefit from elective umbilical hernia repair.	B	Eker et al. (2011)
No significant difference was found in patients with inguinal hernias with mild symptoms who delayed surgical repair and those who did not.	B	Fitzgibbons et al. (2006)

A = consistent, good-quality, patient-oriented evidence; B = inconsistent or limited-quality, patient-oriented evidence; C = consensus, disease-oriented evidence, usual practice, expert opinion, or case series. For information about the SORT evidence rating system, go to www.aafp.org/afpsort.xml.

IRRITABLE BOWEL SYNDROME

Signal symptoms: Abdominal pain (may be described as colicky, pain relieved by defecation), abdominal distention, mucus in the stool, and the sensation of incomplete evacuation; patients often complain of associated symptoms such as fatigue, flatulence, headache, backache, and dyspepsia.

Description: Irritable bowel syndrome (IBS) is a chronic functional gastrointestinal disorder characterized by persistent abdominal pain and distressed defecation that has lasted for at least 3 months. The two major classifications of IBS are *spastic colon*, in which bowel movements are variable, alternating between periods of diarrhea and constipation, and *painless diarrhea* that occurs immediately after a meal or on rising (Furman & Cash, 2011).

Etiology: No anatomical or biochemical cause of IBS is known. This syndrome is a functional disorder of intestinal motility and altered visceral sensation, leading to constipation or diarrhea or both. Stressful and emotional life events often precede or coexist with the presentation of IBS.

Occurrence: A common presentation for patient referral, IBS accounts for almost 20% to 50% of all referrals to a gastroenterologist (Drossman et al., 2003). It is estimated that 10% to 15% of adults in the Western world have IBS (Kay, 1994).

Age: Of cases of IBS, 50% are diagnosed before age 35. Because most cases of IBS present by age 50, this syndrome is often a chronic condition in older adults.

Gender: Prevalence of IBS is twice as great in women as in men in the United States (Kay, 1994; Heitkemper et al., 2011).

Ethnicity: IBS has a higher prevalence among whites than among other ethnic groups (Minocha, 2008).

Contributing factors: Female gender and family history of IBS are associated with the development of IBS. Traumatic life events, such as physical or sexual abuse, may trigger the onset of IBS. Stressful psychosocial situations may hasten an exacerbation of IBS. Small bowel overgrowth is a common finding in older adults with IBS (Lin, 2004).

Certain food products, such as fructose, sorbitol, and lactose, have been known to alter bowel motor function. Review any new prescribed and OTC medications to determine if side effects include constipation or diarrhea. Given the increased prevalence of diverticulosis and intra-abdominal surgeries such as hysterectomy and cholecystectomy, it has been suggested that these conditions may cause or contribute to symptoms that occur in IBS in older adults. It is important to note that common medical conditions such as diabetes, stroke and Parkinson's disease are known to alter defecation patterns (Minocha, 2008).

Signs and symptoms: A thorough dietary history is essential to establish a differential diagnosis of IBS, ruling out the possibility of food intolerance. Review recent travel history with the patient. Explore the patient's psychosocial history to determine the relationships between stressful events and exacerbation of IBS. Determine the onset of symptoms, including the time of day when the pain and gastrointestinal disturbances usually occur. A report of postprandial abdominal pain suggests biliary tract disease, pancreatitis, or peptic ulcer disease. Patients often report loose and frequent stools or alternating constipation and diarrhea. Abdominal pain may be described as colicky. Pain often is relieved by defecation. Abdominal distention, mucus in the stool, and the sensation of incomplete evacuation are other presenting symptoms. Patients often complain of associated symptoms, such as fatigue, bloating, flatulence, headache, backache, and dyspepsia. It is common in older adults for them to present with nongastrointestinal-related symptoms such as lethargy, back pain, headache, or urinary frequency (Agrawal, Khan, & Whorwell, 2009). Older adults tend to have greater incidence of rectal urgency with fecal incontinence than younger patients (Minocha, 2008). If patients report fever, unexplained weight loss, dysphagia, or rectal bleeding, these are *not* symptoms of irritable bowel and should be evaluated closely, especially with a past personal history of any malignancy and a family history of colon cancer.

The physical examination is usually unremarkable. Abdominal tenderness may be elicited, especially in the left lower quadrant, but is not pronounced. Presence of an abdominal mass, lymphadenopathy, hepatosplenomegaly, or ascites in a patient with IBS should prompt further investigation. A routine digital rectal examination generally reveals a tender rectum that is either empty or full of hard firm feces. It is important to discern if there are any disorders that may contribute to difficult or painful defecation such as fissures, external hemorrhoids, or rectocele. A pelvic examination in women is recommended to rule out the presence of an ovarian neoplasm.

Diagnostic tests: The Rome III criteria for the diagnosis of irritable bowel has been simplified; it is important to discern from the patient the time frame of symptom presentation and duration to help distinguish IBS from other conditions that can mimic this chronic functional disorder of the bowel (Table 10-4). A new presentation of IBS in older adults is one of the alarm symptoms, so when ordering diagnostic tests in older adults, determine the length of time since the last evaluation and the nature of the current symptoms. There is no biological indicator for IBS. In general, a CBC and erythrocyte sedimentation rate can rule out anemia and inflammation (Furman & Cash, 2011). If diarrhea is the presenting symptom, stool culture and examination for occult blood, ova and parasites, bacteria, and celiac sprue in patients with diarrhea are recommended. For patient with constipation, plain abdomen x-ray series and colonic transit markers may be useful in determining functional causes (Minocha, 2008).

Patients with documented involuntary weight loss of ≥5% within a 6-month period or with signs of obstruction should have an abdominal CT scan and a small bowel series. Colonoscopy with biopsies may be considered in patients with diarrhea-predominant symptoms to rule out microscopic colitis (Furman & Cash, 2011).

Patients with persistent constipation should be evaluated for hypothyroidism. If the presenting symptoms are bloating and abdominal distention with cramping and diarrhea, a 3-week trial of a lactose-free diet is recommended to rule out lactose intolerance.

Differential diagnosis:

- Food intolerance
- Diverticular disease
- Parasitic diseases
- Biliary tract disease
- Colonic polyps
- Neoplasms
- Pancreatic disease
- Abuse of cathartics

TABLE 10-4	Rome III Criteria for the Diagnosis of Irritable Bowel Syndrome

Symptoms present for at least 3 days per month in the past 3 months (with symptom onset at least 6 months previously) with at least two of the following features:

- Pain improved with defecation
- Onset of pain associated with a change in stool frequency
- Onset of pain associated with a change in stool form

- Latent celiac disease
- Crohn's disease
- Ulcerative colitis
- Ischemic colitis
- Chronic prostatitis
- Thyroid dysfunction
- Lactose malabsorption (Furman & Cash, 2011; Minocha, 2008).

Treatment: The management of IBS depends on the presentation of the patient's condition. If the patient presents predominantly with constipation, prescribe psyllium preparation 1 tbsp twice a day or 2 tablets 1 to 4 times a day of calcium polycarbophil taken with two glasses of water. For patients who choose bulk-forming products, a total of 15 to 25 g/day is necessary to achieve results. Caution patients with diabetes about using any products that have high sugar content. Patients should be warned that increased bloating might occur initially with fiber products but usually resolves in 2 to 3 weeks.

Polyethylene glycol (PEG) 3350 is a Food and Drug Administration (FDA)–approved osmotic laxative used for short-term constipation; however, it has been recommended for patients with irritable bowel syndrome-constipation (IBS-C). Lubiprostone is a chloride channel activator used in the treatment of IBS-C; a dose of 8 to 24 mcg twice a day with food is recommended. Results of clinical trials show efficacy in reducing chronic constipation and abdominal pain with bloating in patients with IBS-C (Lembo et al., 2010).

Foods that may exacerbate irritable bowel syndrome-diarrhea (IBS-D) should be avoided (e.g., caffeinated beverages, histamine-releasing foods like wine and beer, sorbitol-containing candies or gums, citrus fruits for persons with fructose intolerance, and milk products for persons who have known lactose intolerance) (Bohn, Storsrud, Tornblom, Bengtsson, & Simren, 2013). Antispasmodics are not recommended for treatment of IBS-D in older adults because of the anticholinergic side effects of these medications. If diarrhea is severe, loperamide, 2 mg every 4 to 8 hours, can be taken, but antidiarrheal medications are not beneficial in treating global IBS-D symptoms. Early studies point to the use of rifaximin, an antibiotic, for consideration of the treatment of IBS without constipation (Menees, Maneerattannaporn, Kim, & Chey, 2012).

Follow-up: With chronic IBS patients, a positive relationship between the health-care provider and the patient is mutually beneficial. Dietary intervention and stress-reduction techniques should be reviewed and evaluated. In patients with newly diagnosed IBS, evaluation of persistent symptoms is necessary because IBS is a diagnosis of exclusion. Patients with IBS have been found to have multiple comorbidities that need to be considered. Functional dyspepsia and depression were the most common comorbidities in patients with chronic constipation (Nellesen, Chawla, Oh, Weissman, Lavins, Murray, 2013).

Sequelae: Older adults with a chronic history of IBS may have a concomitant illness, such as diverticulosis (Agrawal et al., 2009; Minocha, 2008). Complications may develop because of other pathological processes mistaken for IBS symptoms. Patients with uncontrollable diarrhea are at risk for dehydration because of fluid and electrolyte loss. Fecal impaction may result from chronic constipation, especially in an immobile, cognitively impaired older patient.

Prevention/prophylaxis: The patient should use stress-reduction techniques during emotionally stressful situations. Patients should avoid all food products that are known to irritate their bowels (Bohn et al., 2013).

Patients with known food intolerance must read nutrition labels and be informed of the inactive contents of medications, which may contain irritating substances.

Referral: Refer patients to a gastroenterologist for colonoscopic imaging. Refer again if patients exhibit persistent abdominal pain or uncontrollable diarrhea despite compliance with treatment and if signs of gastrointestinal bleeding are present. Patients may benefit from psychotherapy, biofeedback, or hypnosis. Women with severe diarrhea should be referred for consideration of treatment with alosetron, a serotonin type-3 receptor.

Education: Inform patients that because the increase of dietary fiber could aggravate their IBS symptoms, they should increase gradually to the recommended dose. It may take 3 to 4 weeks to reach a therapeutic level sufficient to produce results. Inform patients with chronic IBS that although the disease itself does not lead to a more serious illness, any change in symptoms should be reported to the health-care practitioner.

CLINICAL RECOMMENDATION	EVIDENCE RATING	REFERENCES
Patients with IBS without constipation treated for 2 weeks with rifaximin versus placebo experienced significantly less bloating and other global symptoms of IBS than before the treatment started.	A	Pimentel et al. (2011)
A systematic review and meta-analysis of randomized controlled trials (RCTs) that tested the use of rifaximin against placebo in patients with IBS without constipation showed the efficacy of rifaximin in reducing global symptoms of IBS, including bloating.	A	Menees et al. (2012)
Older adults diagnosed with IBS presented with noncolonic symptoms such as lethargy, headache, joint pain, and back pain.	B	Agrawal, Khan, & Whorwell (2009)
Women with IBS reported greater psychological stress with the increased severity of abdominal pain/discomfort regardless of the bowel pattern.	B	Heitkemper et al. (2011)
Lubiprostone has been well tolerated in patients with chronic constipation.	A	Drossman et al. (2009) Lembo et al. (2011)

A = consistent, good-quality, patient-oriented evidence; B = inconsistent or limited-quality, patient-oriented evidence; C = consensus, disease-oriented evidence, usual practice, expert opinion, or case series. For information about the SORT evidence rating system, go to www.aafp.org/afpsort.xml.

LIVER CANCER

Signal symptoms: Cachexia, jaundice.

Description: The liver is the most common organ in the body for metastasis from other cancers. Common sites of primary tumors that metastasize to the liver are the lungs, colon, pancreas, stomach, breast, and gallbladder. Hepatocellular cancer is associated with cirrhosis of the liver.

Etiology: The hepatic filtration of arterial and portal venous blood is a major reason for the high prevalence of metastases from primary cancerous sites in the body to the liver. Metastases also may result from an extension from an abdominal tumor or through the lymphatic system. Malignant tumors of the liver are primarily adenocarcinomas.

Occurrence: Primary liver cancer, rare in the United States, accounts for about 2% of all cancers. A malignant lesion is 20 times more likely to be from a metastatic source than from a primary lesion.

Age: Most common onset of disease is in the sixties to eighties.

Gender: Liver cancer is more prevalent in men than in women (3:1 to 4:1).

Ethnicity: Primary liver cancer is prevalent in people from Africa and Asia because of the widespread occurrence of hepatitis B virus and hepatitis C virus.

Contributing factors: The incidence of liver cancer increases for patients who have a history of cirrhosis of the liver, hepatitis B virus, and hepatitis C virus. Exposure to certain chemicals, such as vinyl chloride and arsenic, has been associated with the development of liver cancer.

Signs and symptoms: Complaints of weakness, malaise, weight loss, sweating, and anorexia may be reported. Pain associated with the cancer also may be reported.

Physical examination reveals cachexia. Auscultation may reveal a bruit over the tumor and tenderness of the liver. A mass may be palpable. In more advanced cases, jaundice may appear.

Diagnostic tests: Laboratory findings may be nonspecific and are related to the underlying liver disease. Findings may include thrombocytopenia, hypoalbuminemia, hyperbilirubinemia, and hypoprothrombinemia. Additionally, patients may have mild anemia and electrolyte disturbances (Schwartz & Carithers, 2012). Serum alkaline phosphatase, AST, ALT, and gamma-glutamyl transpeptidase (GGT) are often abnormal in a nonspecific pattern.

Patients at high risk for hepatocellular carcinoma (HCC) should be screened using ultrasound every 6 months (Bruix & Sherman, 2011). Identification of a liver nodule that is smaller than 1 cm should be reimaged with an ultrasound in 3 months. Nodules that are larger than 1 cm should be reimaged with contrast-enhanced MRI. Nodules that demonstrate arterial hypervascularity and venous or delayed phase washout are consistent with HCC. Those nodules that do not demonstrate arterial hypervascularity and venous or delayed phase washout should be reimaged with another contrast-enhanced study such as a CT scan. Lesions that demonstrate arterial hypervascularity and venous or delayed phase washout are diagnostic for HCC. Lesions that do not demonstrate arterial hypervascularity and venous or delayed phase washout should undergo percutaneous biopsy.

Elevated serum α-fetoprotein can be seen in patients without HCC (Sterling et al., 2012). A rise in the α-fetoprotein is concerning for the development of HCC in patients with cirrhosis. Elevated serum α-fetoprotein found at levels of more than 500 g/L in patients with cirrhosis is diagnostic for HCC. However, HCC is often found with lower levels of α-fetoprotein when high-risk patients are undergoing routine screening.

Differential diagnosis:
- Cirrhosis
- Chronic hepatitis B or C infection
- Metastatic malignancy of the liver

Treatment: Advancements in the surgical treatment of hepatic metastatic cancers include tumor ablation and microscopic glass beads containing a radioactive element. Surgical resection of the liver is beneficial only if the patient has a resectable tumor; even so, the survival rate remains low. Intrahepatic chemotherapeutic agents, such as 5-fluorouracil and floxuridine, may alter the growth of the tumor, but the prognosis remains the same. Older patients with known renal function impairment may require a reduced dosage of these agents compared with younger patients. Often the treatment is palliative at best, however.

Follow-up: Patients and family members should be given the opportunity to explore adjunctive methods of pain relief and relaxation. After diagnosis of liver cancer, the focus should be on holistic palliative care, including the intervention of a hospice and services provided by the American Cancer Society.

Sequelae: The prognosis is poor because the tumor grows rapidly and often metastasizes to the lungs or bones. The survival rate is only 4 to 6 months.

Prevention/prophylaxis: Hepatitis vaccine is recommended for high-risk patients. Avoidance of chemical exposure, as part of occupational safety, is suggested. Annual ultrasound screening for patients with chronic hepatitis B should be considered as a preventive measure for liver cancer.

Referral: Refer the patient to an oncologist when the diagnosis of liver cancer is suspected. Local hospice care services should be contacted for care for the patient and family.

Education: Although no further medical treatment is aimed at reversal of the disease, the patient needs to know that you will collaborate with the hospice nurses to provide for the patient's comfort throughout the disease process. The patient can be referred to www.livertumor.org for basic information about liver cancer.

CLINICAL RECOMMENDATION	EVIDENCE RATING	REFERENCES
Prevention of HCC should focus on preventing infection with hepatitis B virus (HBV) and hepatitis C virus (HCV), treating patients with viral hepatitis who are candidates for treatment, avoiding environmental toxins, and attempting to prevent the development of cirrhosis in patients with liver disease.	A	Sherman (2012)
Patients with chronic HBV infection who are at increased risk for HCC should undergo routine surveillance.	A	Bruix & Sherman (2011)
All patients with cirrhosis, regardless of etiology, should undergo surveillance for HCC.	B	Bruix & Sherman (2011) Sherman (2012)
Surveillance in high-risk patients should be performed with ultrasonography every 6 months rather than annually.	B	Bruix & Sherman (2011)
Surveillance should be carried out with ultrasonography rather than combined ultrasonography and serum AFP, because the combined use of AFP and ultrasonography increases detection rates but also increases costs and false-positive rates.	B	Sherman (2012)

A = consistent, good-quality, patient-oriented evidence; B = inconsistent or limited-quality, patient-oriented evidence; C = consensus, disease-oriented evidence, usual practice, expert opinion, or case series. For information about the SORT evidence rating system, go to www.aafp.org/afpsort.xml.

NEPHROLITHIASIS

Signal symptoms: Vague flank pain, hematuria, renal colic, abdominal pain.

Description: In the Western hemisphere, most cases of nephrolithiasis, or kidney stones, are

calcium salts, uric acid, cysteine, and struvite. These substances begin to form crystals and become attached to the kidney, eventually developing into stones. Calculi range in size from microscopic to several centimeters in diameter. Nephrolithiasis often attempt to travel through the urinary system and out in urine. Pain occurs when the calculi become lodged (Curhan, Aronson, & Preminger, 2011).

Etiology: Kidney stones develop from the supersaturation of urine with stone-forming salts that occurs either by overexcretion of salt or underexcretion of urine. Some preformed nuclei form to create a calculus. Abnormal crystal growth inhibitors are formed as well because of hypocitraturia or magnesium deficiency. Approximately 70% of diagnosed kidney stones contain calcium; 20% to 25% are struvite stones, resulting from urinary tract infections; 5% are uric acid calculi; and 2% contain cystine.

Occurrence: One out of 11 people had been diagnosed with a kidney stone in the years 2007–2010. Approximately 50% of patients who have had previous urinary calculi have a recurrence in 5 to 7 years.

Age: The average age of onset of patients with a kidney stone is in the thirties. The incidence of kidney stones for women peaks again at about age 55.

Gender: Men are more likely than women to form calcium stones; struvite stones are more common in women, however, because of the higher incidence of urinary tract infections. Cystine stone formation occurs equally in men and women (Wolf, 2012).

Ethnicity: The incidence of kidney stones in whites is 3 to 4 times greater than in African Americans.

Contributing factors: A major contributing factor to the development of calculi is decreased fluid intake leading to high concentration of urine. Certain food substances that augment the formation of kidney stones include dairy products, chocolate, green leafy vegetables (calcium oxalate stones) and eggs, fish, poultry, peanuts, and wheat (cystine stones). Certain medications, such as furosemide, nitrofurantoin, probenecid, silicates, theophylline, triamterene, indinavir, acetazolamide, and vitamins C and D, in a small percentage of cases can contribute to the development of nephrolithiasis (Brener, Winchester, Salman, & Bergman, 2011; Curhan et al., 2011). A history of hyperparathyroidism, sarcoidosis, Cushing's syndrome, Paget's disease, and immobilization may contribute to the development of calcium phosphate stones. Chronic urinary tract infections may be precursors to struvite stone formation. In patients with gout who are not adequately medicated with anti-gout therapy, approximately 20% develop uric acid nephrolithiasis (Becker, 2011).

Signs and symptoms: Patients may have abrupt, severe, colicky pain in either flank or pain that originates in the flank and radiates to the groin. The pain sensation can begin as vague flank pain. Pain spreading downward suggests movement of the stone along the ureter. Associated nausea and vomiting may occur. Hematuria may be reported (Curhan, 2009).

Physical examination may reveal local abdominal and costovertebral angle tenderness. Men complaining of groin pain should have a testicular examination to rule out testicular torsion, prostatitis, or epididymitis. Women with pain radiating to the labia should have a pelvic examination to rule out possible ovarian torsion, cysts, or tumors. A cursory physical examination for evidence of systemic diseases, such as sarcoidosis or cancer, should be conducted (Hall, 2009).

Diagnostic tests: For patients who have not yet passed a stone, urine collection for recovery of stones or gravel should be ordered. A urinalysis (UA) reveals the presence of leukocytes, bacteria, and blood, which can be indicative of a urinary tract infection. The presence of crystals in a UA can aid in the determination of the type of stone present. The urine pH, if acidic, indicates uric acid stones and if alkalitic, indicates struvite stones (Wolf, 2012). Although abdominal plain films are inexpensive and quick, they can fail to detect radiolucent stones, small stones, or obstructions (Curhan et al., 2011; Wolf, 2012). Ultrasonography is reserved for those patients who should avoid radiation exposure and may not reveal small stones or stones in the ureter (Curhan et al., 2011). The ability to view the entire urinary system is provided by IVP; however, there is a large amount of radiation exposure with IVP, and multiple films may be required over several hours (Brener et al., 2011; Curhan et al., 2011; Hall, 2009; Wolf, 2012). A noncontrast helical CT scan is the gold standard for nephrolithiasis detection. The helical scan is quick and often detects stones and obstructions not seen on other imaging studies (Brener et al., 2011; Curhan et al., 2011; Hall, 2009; Pietrow & Karellas, 2006; Wolf, 2012).

Differential diagnosis:
- Papillary necrosis
- Hydronephrosis
- Ileus
- Diverticulitis
- Appendicitis

- Bowel obstruction
- Mesenteric ischemia
- Ovarian cyst
- Testicular torsion
- Constipation
- Arterial aneurysms
- Cholecystitis
- Acute cystitis
- Pyelonephritis (Curhan, 2009; Wolf, 2012)

Treatment: Size and location of the stone, coupled with the length of time since the onset of symptoms, directs treatment. Stones ≤4 mm usually pass on their own; stones 4 to 5 mm have a 50% chance of passing without intervention. A stone of more than 5 mm requires *immediate* referral to a urologist for possible extracorporeal shock-wave lithotripsy. Unless contraindicated, IV normal saline can be administered, 125 to 150 mL/hr, to help flush out the stone. Instruct patients not in distress and without obstruction to drink at least 2 L of fluid daily and to strain the urine until a stone has passed (Hall, 2009). Oral analgesics can be prescribed: 1 tablet of acetaminophen, 300 mg, and codeine phosphate, 30 mg, or 1 or 2 tablets of acetaminophen, 300 mg, and codeine phosphate, 15 mg, every 4 hours, without exceeding 4 g of acetaminophen a day or 2.5 to 5 mg of hydrocodone component with acetaminophen every 4 to 6 hours. An adequate fluid intake should continue throughout the day as part of therapy (Brener et al., 2011; Hall, 2009; Pietrow & Karellas, 2006).

Follow-up: A 24-hour urine collection 6 months after treatment for nephrolithiasis is recommended. At this time, also review with the patient the need for compliance with dietary restrictions and fluid requirements.

Sequelae: Immediate complications of unresolved kidney stones include obstruction and urinary tract infection and sepsis. A high incidence of recurrence of kidney stone formation exists; metabolic causes of kidney stones need to be ruled out when dietary measures are unsuccessful. Additional complications of nephrolithiasis include renal failure, ureteral stricture, perinephric abscess, and pyelonephritis (Wolf, 2012).

Prevention/prophylaxis: An adequate daily fluid intake is essential. Patients should be encouraged to increase their fluid intake during heavy exercise or when traveling long distances. To prevent recurrent stones, review the patient's dietary habits to discern if there are any excessive food products that may be factors in kidney stone formation (calcium, purine, protein).

Referral: Refer the patient to a urologist when
- Obstruction is detected.
- The stone is more than 5 mm.
- The stone has not passed within 24 to 48 hours of the onset of pain.
- The patient has complicated diagnostic reports.
- The patient has urosepsis, anuria, or renal failure.

Education: Inform all patients with nephrolithiasis that there is a high probability of a second occurrence of a kidney stone. Advise the patient, if possible, to strain urine with the provided strainer when experiencing symptoms of kidney obstruction. A daily fluid intake of 10 large glasses of liquid per day is recommended. Explain to patients that fluid intake needs to be increased when urine appears dark yellow. Provide information about any food restrictions that may be deemed necessary to prevent specific stone formation (Brener et al., 2011; Curhan, 2009; Curhan et al., 2011; Wolf, 2012).

CLINICAL RECOMMENDATION	EVIDENCE RATING	REFERENCES
A noncontrast helical CT scan is the gold standard for nephrolithiasis detection. It is quick, is readily available, and can be completed without contrast.	B	Brener et al. (2011) Curhan (2009) Curhan et al. (2011) Hall (2009) Pietrow & Karellas (2006) Wolf (2012)
A urinalysis can provide an extensive amount of information that can be used to determine the type of renal calculi present. Information, such as the existence of leukocytes, bacteria, or crystals and the pH of the	B	Wolf (2012)

CLINICAL RECOMMENDATION	EVIDENCE RATING	REFERENCES
urine, aid the diagnosis of the current nephrolithiasis and prevention of further episodes.		
Increased urine flow accelerates the passage of renal calculi. Thus, it is recommended to increase the intake of fluid, which has also been found to aid in stone prevention.	B	Brener et al. (2011) Curhan (2009) Curhan et al. (2011) Hall (2009) Pietrow & Karellas (2006) Wolf (2012)
Severe complications of untreated renal calculi include acute kidney injury and sepsis.	B	Wolf (2010)

A = consistent, good-quality, patient-oriented evidence; B = inconsistent or limited-quality, patient-oriented evidence; C = consensus, disease-oriented evidence, usual practice, expert opinion, or case series. For information about the SORT evidence rating system, go to www.aafp.org/afpsort.xml.

NONALCOHOLIC FATTY LIVER DISEASE

Signal symptoms: Fatigue, right upper quadrant pain or fullness, hepatomegaly.

Description: Nonalcoholic fatty liver disease (NAFLD) is the most common liver disease in Western countries (Parrish, 2010). NAFLD refers to a spectrum of liver disorders that include simple steatosis (fatty liver) and nonalcoholic steatohepatitis (NASH). NASH is characterized by hepatocyte injury, inflammation, and fibrosis, which can ultimately lead to cirrhosis and end-stage liver disease. Risk factors for the development of NASH include elevated fasting blood glucose, low high-density lipoprotein (HDL), and elevated fasting cholesterol (Moore, 2010; Vernon, Baranova, & Younossi, 2011). It has been estimated that less than 10% of patients with NAFLD will develop cirrhosis, end-stage liver disease, and hepatocellular carcinoma. Alcohol use must be minimal to meet the criteria for NAFLD (Bayard, Holt, & Boroughs, 2006). The maximum intake of alcohol is two standard drinks a day for men and one for women. Nonalcoholic fatty liver disease is the most common reason for elevated transaminases (Vernon et al., 2011).

Etiology: Risk factors for the development of NAFLD include obesity, insulin resistance, hypertension, and dyslipidemia (Bayard et al., 2006). Insulin resistance is the most important risk factor for the development

of NAFLD (Moore, 2010; Vernon et al., 2011). Up to 90% of patients with NAFLD have at least one of these risk factors (Parrish, 2010). It has been suggested that there may be a genetic predisposition to NAFLD especially in patients who also develop metabolic syndrome (Croke & Sampson, 2012).

Occurrence: NAFLD is the most common liver disease in Western countries (Parrish, 2010). It is estimated that the prevalence of NAFLD ranges from 16% to 35% in the general population (Bayard et al., 2006; Caballería et al., 2010; Croke & Sampson, 2012).

Age: The incidence of NAFLD increases with age (Vernon et al., 2011). Older patients have more risk factors for NAFLD such as hypertension, obesity, and diabetes (Parrish, 2010). Older adults are also at an increased risk for developing hepatic fibrosis and hepatocellular carcinoma.

Gender: NAFLD is more common in men than women (Hamaguchi et al., 2012).

Ethnicity: The prevalence of NAFLD is highest in Hispanics, followed by non-Hispanic whites (Croke & Sampson, 2012). The prevalence of NAFLD is lowest in African Americans (Vernon et al., 2011).

Contributing factors: The risk factors for the development of NAFLD are obesity, diabetes and hypertriglyceridemia, metabolic syndrome, glucose intolerance, hypertension, and dyslipidemia (Croke & Sampson, 2012; Greenberger, Blumberg, & Burakoff, 2009; Wilkins, Tadkod, Hepbrun, & Schade, 2013). Aging was found to be a risk factor for developing NAFLD in premenopausal women, but the same could not be said for men with NAFLD (Hamaguchi et al., 2012). NAFLD has also been found in patients with elevated uric acid levels (Petta, Camma, Cabibi, Di Marco, & Craxi, 2011). Severe weight loss may place patients at risk for the development of NAFLD. NAFLD may present in patients who have had jejunoileal bypass or gastric bypass or who have experienced starvation and/or protein-energy malnutrition. Also at risk are patients on total parenteral nutrition (Bayard et al., 2006). Drug-induced NAFLD can be caused by methotrexate, griseofulvin, diltiazem, zidovudine, steroids, valproate, amiodarone, aspirin, tetracycline, estrogens, tamoxifen, and highly active antiretrovirals (Croke & Sampson, 2012). Certain metabolic conditions (hypopituitarism), infections (HIV, hepatitis C, bacterial overgrowth), and hemochromatosis are known risk factors for NAFLD (Adams & Angulo, 2006). In patients with coexisting conditions, such as ulcerative colitis, Graves' disease, or type 1 diabetes, consider an autoimmune cause for NAFLD (Croke & Sampson, 2012).

Signs and symptoms: Most patients with NAFLD are asymptomatic (Bayard et al., 2006). Some patients may complain of fatigue, pruritus, nausea, or right upper quadrant pain or fullness. Inquire about rapid weight loss. On examination, look for evidence of jaundice of the skin, scleral icterus, and spider angiomas. Patients may have unexplained abnormal liver blood tests as part of a routine physical or drug monitoring such as statins. It is estimated that 50% of patients with NAFLD have hepatomegaly on examination. Patients presenting with cirrhosis from NAFLD will have findings and symptoms similar to patients with cirrhosis from other causes. Measurement of BMI should be recorded (Croke & Sampson, 2012).

Diagnostic tests: NAFLD is a diagnosis of exclusion. The most common abnormal laboratory tests are elevated ALT and AST (Bayard et al., 2006). ALT and AST may be elevated 1 to 4 times the upper limits. It is important to exclude other causes of elevated transaminase levels. Hepatitis B and C need to be ruled out, as does autoimmune hepatitis. Serum albumin, bilirubin, and a prothrombin should be obtained. Hemochromatosis, thyroid disease, and drugs also need to be

excluded. It may be useful to rule out Wilson's disease and α_1-antitrypsin deficiency. A fasting lipid panel and glucose should also be obtained (Bayard et al., 2006; Greenberger et al., 2009). An ultrasonography of the liver will assist in the diagnosis of NAFLD by identifying fatty infiltration in the liver (Bayard et al., 2006; Wilkins, Tadkod, Hepbrun, & Schade, 2013). An ultrasonography of the liver has a sensitivity of 82% to 89% and a specificity of 93% for identifying a fatty liver. For patients suspected of liver fibrosis, commercially available serologic markers are available to order (Wilkins, Tadkod, Hepbrun, & Schade, 2013). A liver biopsy should be considered for patients who are likely to have a more advanced liver disease. The risk factors for advanced liver disease include morbid obesity, diabetes, advanced age, and an AST/ALT ratio greater than 1. Patients with persistent elevations in liver enzymes despite lifestyle changes may be considered for liver biopsy. Patients should be questioned carefully about alcohol use (Bayard et al., 2006).

Differential diagnosis:
- Alcoholic hepatitis
- Autoimmune hepatitis
- Viral hepatitis
- Thyroid disease
- α_1-Antitrypsin disease
- Medication-induced hepatitis
- Wilson's disease
- Hemochromatosis (Greenberger et al., 2009)

Treatment: Management of NAFLD should focus primarily on risk factors such as insulin resistance and hyperlipidemia (Moore, 2010). Overweight patients with NAFLD should consider a weight-loss program (Wilkins, Tadkod, Hepbrun, & Schade, 2013). It has been shown that weight loss and exercise reduce liver enzyme levels and steatosis (Greenberger et al., 2009). Weight loss should not exceed 1 to 2 lb per week (Farrell & Larter, 2006). Treatment for hyperlipidemia (atorvastatin, gemfibrozil) has been shown to improve liver enzymes and liver steatosis (Ghamar-Chehreh et al., 2012). Statin drugs should not be withheld due to mild elevation of liver enzymes. The initial dose of statin drugs should be low and liver enzymes checked in 2 weeks and then monthly for the first 3 months (Bayard et al., 2006). If there is an increase in transaminases of 2 times the baseline value, statin therapy should be discontinued. Medications for the treatment of insulin resistance (metformin, rosiglitazone, pioglitazone) have been shown to improve transaminases levels and decrease hepatitis steatosis (Kashi, Torres, & Harrison, 2008). Morbidly obese patients should be considered for bariatric surgery. Obese patients who are unable to lose weight with lifestyle changes should be considered for bariatric surgery; individual risk for complications from surgery need to first be evaluated (Greenberger et al., 2009). Betaine, a nutritional supplement, reduces steatosis and reduces ALT, AST, and GGT (Miglio, Rovati, Santoro, & Setnikar, 2000). Orlistat reduces the absorption of dietary triglycerides and has been shown to improve liver enzymes and steatosis in obese patients (Greenberger et al., 2009). Ursodeoxycholic acid has shown little efficacy in the treatment of NAFLD or NASH (Leuschner et al., 2010).

Follow-up: Patients on statin drugs should be monitored every 6 months. Liver enzymes should be monitored every 6 months. Patient should be monitored for weight loss. Patients with decompensated liver disease should be referred to a specialist.

Sequelae: Steatosis alone usually has a benign course (Bayard et al., 2006). It has been estimated that less than 10% of patients with NAFLD will develop cirrhosis, end-stage liver disease, and hepatocellular carcinoma (Parrish, 2010). Steatohepatitis can progress to cirrhosis. Morbidly obese patients, patients with diabetes, and older patients are at the greatest risk for progression to severe liver disease.

Prevention/prophylaxis: Weight loss should be encouraged in obese patients. Patients should be encouraged to exercise (Greenberger et al., 2009). Minimize alcohol intake to two standard drinks a day for men and one standard drink a day for women (Bayard et al., 2006). Patients with diabetes, hypertension, and hyperlipidemia should be closely monitored and managed to help prevent the progression of NAFLD.

Referral: Consider referral to a specialist when the clinical parameters are indicating a severe disease state. Patients whose liver enzymes remain elevated despite weight loss, those who are morbidly obese, those with AST/ALT greater than 1, and those with NASH whose clinical picture suggests the likelihood of fibrosis should be referred (Kashi et al., 2008).

Education: Patients should be advised that NAFLD is usually caused by the same conditions that cause an increased risk for heart disease and stroke (Greenberger et al., 2009). Most cases of NAFLD do not cause serious problems. The management of NAFLD is directed at risk factors, specifically, diabetes, elevated lipids, and obesity.

CLINICAL RECOMMENDATION	EVIDENCE RATING	REFERENCES
Orlistat reduces the absorption of dietary triglycerides and has been shown to improve liver enzymes and steatosis in obese patients.	C	Greenberger, Blumberg, & Burakoff (2009)
Ursodeoxycholic acid has shown little efficacy in the treatment of NAFLD or NASH.	C	Leuschner et al. (2010)
Treatment for hyperlipidemia has been shown to improve liver enzymes and liver steatosis.	C	Ghamar-Chehreh et al. (2012)
Obese patients should lose weight; however, it is not recommended to lose >1–2 lb per week. Rapid weight loss can worsen NAFLD, particularly after bariatric surgery.	C	Bayard, Holt, & Boroughs (2006)
Medications for the treatment resistance (metformin, rosiglitazone, pioglitazone) have been shown to improve transaminase levels and decrease hepatitis steatosis.	C	Kashi, Torres, & Harrison (2008)

Continued

CLINICAL RECOMMENDATION	EVIDENCE RATING	REFERENCES
Long-term use of statins in patients with NAFLD had a significant reduction in hepatic steatosis compared to patients not taking statins.	B	Ekstedt et al. (2007)

A = consistent, good-quality, patient-oriented evidence; B = inconsistent or limited-quality, patient-oriented evidence; C = consensus, disease-oriented evidence, usual practice, expert opinion, or case series. For information about the SORT evidence rating system, go to www.aafp.org/afpsort.xml.

PEPTIC ULCER DISEASE

Signal symptoms: Gastric ulcers: history of dyspepsia, epigastric pain, or right upper quadrant pain that radiates to the back after the ingestion of a meal. Duodenal ulcers: pain 1 to 3 hours after a meal (patients with gastric ulcers have pain immediately on eating). Nocturnal pain may occur in duodenal ulcers in the older adult; definitive symptoms may be absent, and vomiting and anorexia may be reported instead of epigastric pain.

Description: Peptic ulcer disease (PUD) involves ulcerations of the mucous membrane of the esophagus, stomach, or duodenum. The disease is classified according to the nature and anatomical location of the lesion. *Peptic ulcers* usually originate near mucosal transition zones in areas exposed to acid, pepsin, bile, and pancreatic enzymes. *Gastric ulcers* generally are found along the lesser curvature of the stomach between antral and acid-screening mucosa occurring anywhere in the stomach, from the cardia to the pylorus. *Duodenal ulcers* develop in the duodenal bulb or in the immediate postbulbar area (Barkun & Leontiadis, 2010).

Etiology: The etiology of PUD is characterized best as an imbalance between the noxious agents to which the gastrointestinal mucosa is exposed (primarily hydrochloric acid and pepsin) and the protective factors (mucus production, bicarbonate secretion) that the mucosa uses to resist destruction from such noxious agents. An increase in destructive influences (e.g., with NSAID use) can destroy the mucosa, leading to the dvelopment of an ulcer (Lockrey & St. Lim, 2011).

Occurrence: Approximately 25 million Americans have experienced PUD. Annually, more than 500,000 people are diagnosed with PUD (Barkun & Leontiadis, 2010).

Age: The predominant age range for gastric ulcers is 55 to 65, with rare occurrences in people under 40 years old. Duodenal ulcers can occur in adults ages 25 to 75. Middle-aged men (45 to 64 years old) and women more than 55 years old have the highest incidence of peptic duodenal disease.

Gender: Gastric ulcers are more prevalent in older women than in older men because of the increased use of NSAIDs. The occurrence of duodenal ulcers is twice as common in men as in women.

Ethnicity: Prevalence of PUD is higher in African Americans and Hispanics than in whites.

Contributing factors: *H. pylori* infection is a factor in more than 90% of duodenal ulcers and 80% of gastric ulcers (Chey & Wong, 2007). Use of aspirin and other NSAIDs because of their ability to inhibit prostaglandin synthesis has been shown to increase the risk of PUD (Laine et al., 2010). Spironolactone was found to increase the risk for GI bleeding in patients (Gulmez et al., 2008).

There has been some association with smoking, drinking alcohol, and the use of caffeine in contributing to PUD, although there is little evidence to support these risk factors. Certain infectious conditions and other comorbidities such as tuberculosis, Crohn's disease, hepatic cirrhosis, chronic renal failure, and sarcoidosis are associated with developing PUD (Crosby & Dexter, 2013). Patients who have critical illness, undergone major surgery, or experienced hypovolemic shock are at high risk for PUD (Ramakrishnan & Salinas, 2007). Question patients about a family history of PUD, as there is an increased likelihood of developing a duodenal ulcer if a first-degree relative has had one in the past (Crosby & Dexter, 2013).

Signs and symptoms: Older adults presenting with symptoms of PUD must be evaluated for alarm symptoms of upper gastrointestinal bleeding, anemia, fatigue, and melena (Chey & Wong, 2007). Persistent severe epigastric pain can be indicative of perforation. Patients with gastric ulcers have a history of dyspepsia, epigastric pain, or right upper quadrant pain that radiates to the back after the ingestion of a meal. Pain may be described as gnawing or burning. Patients with duodenal ulcer have pain 1 to 3 hours after a meal and pain may be relieved with eating food and/or taking antacids. The pain associated with gastric ulcers generally occurs immediately with eating. Nocturnal pain may occur. In older adults, definitive symptoms may be absent. Vomiting and anorexia may be reported instead of epigastric pain (Ramakrishnan & Salinas, 2007).

Physical examination of a patient with PUD may be normal. Palpation may reveal upper abdominal tenderness and guarding. Rigidity of the abdomen and absence of bowel sounds may suggest perforation. Patients with chronic duodenal ulcer disease may exhibit signs of dehydration if nausea and vomiting accompany the other symptoms. In patients with suspected gastrointestinal bleeding, signs of shock may be detected. Guaiac stool testing should be done.

Diagnostic tests: Endoscopic gastroduodenoscopy with a biopsy for the detection of peptic ulcer, malignancy, and *H. pylori* remains the gold standard in diagnostic testing for this disease. In the diagnostic breath test to detect the presence of *H. pylori*, patients are given C-13–labeled or C-14–labeled urea to drink. The marked carbon is absorbed and is measured as carbon dioxide in the patient's expired breath (Collazo, 2012). PPI use will need to be restricted for 7 to 14 days and antibiotics for 28 days before UBT and fecal antigen testing (not serology) to ensure more accurate diagnosis (Chey & Wong, 2007). Endoscopic gastroduodenoscopy with a biopsy for the detection of peptic ulcer, malignancy, and *H. pylori* remains the gold standard in diagnostic testing for this disease (Cohen et al., 2006; Crosby & Dexter, 2013).

Differential diagnosis:
- Angina
- Gastric carcinoma
- GERD
- Gallbladder disease
- Zollinger-Ellison disease
- Nonulcer dyspepsia
- IBS (Lockrey & St. Lim, 2011)

Treatment: The FDA-approved treatment options for *H. pylori*–induced peptic ulcers include the following:
- Lansoprazole, 30 mg twice daily, plus amoxicillin, 1 g twice daily, plus clarithromycin, 500 mg 3 times daily for 10 (or 14) days; *or*
- Omeprazole, 20 mg twice daily, plus clarithromycin, 500 mg twice daily, plus amoxicillin, 1 g twice daily for 10 days (Prevpac); *or*
- Omeprazole, 40 mg daily, plus clarithromycin, 500 mg 3 times daily for 2 weeks, then omeprazole, 20 mg daily for 2 weeks; *or*
- Lansoprazole, 30 mg 3 times daily, plus amoxicillin, 1 g twice daily for 2 weeks (only for persons allergic or intolerant to clarithromycin); *or*
- Ranitidine bismuth citrate, 400 mg twice daily, plus clarithromycin, 500 mg 3 times daily for 2 weeks, then ranitidine bismuth citrate, 400 mg twice daily for 2 weeks; *or*
- Ranitidine bismuth citrate, 400 mg twice daily, plus clarithromycin, 500 mg twice daily for 2 weeks, then ranitidine bismuth citrate, 400 mg twice daily for 2 weeks; *or*
- Bismuth subsalicylate, 525 mg 4 times daily (after meals and at bedtime), plus metronidazole, 250 mg 4 times daily, plus tetracycline, 500 mg 4 times daily for 2 weeks (Helidac), plus H_2-receptor antagonist therapy as directed for 4 weeks.

Encourage patients to complete the therapeutic regimen despite the cessation of pain. Eradication of *H. pylori* reduces the risk of recurrence of PUD (Collazo, 2012; Ford, Delaney, Forman, Moayyedi, & Ford, 2011). For PUD not related to *H. pylori* infection, treatment with PPIs should be scheduled for 4 weeks for duodenal ulcer and 8 weeks for gastric ulcer in cases of uncomplicated PUD. Complicated ulcers may require more extensive PPI treatment. Avoid the use of NSAIDs if possible (McQuaid, 2010).

Follow-up: If a gastric ulcer was detected on endoscopy and the patient continues to have symptoms after 8 weeks of treatment, referral for endoscopic examination with a biopsy is indicated. Periodic stool guaiac testing and blood counts can detect bleeding.

Sequelae: Complications originating from PUD in older adults include gastric bleeding, perforation, and gastric outlet obstruction (Lockrey & St. Lim, 2011).

Prevention/prophylaxis: Any patients with previous history of gastrointestinal bleeding, multiple and/or high NSAID use (including aspirin), over 70 years of age, on corticosteroids, and *H. pylori* infection are at risk for developing PUD (Laine et al., 2010; Lockrey & St. Lim, 2011). Signs and symptoms of impending recurrence of PUD, including epigastric pain, anorexia, and weight loss, should be identified early. Guaiac stool testing should be performed for all patients taking NSAIDs. Misoprostol has been approved as prophylaxis against NSAID-induced gastric ulcers.

Referral: Refer the patient to a gastroenterologist for initial endoscopy and for treatment of upper gastrointestinal bleeding. There is a decreased mortality rate from bleeding peptic ulcers when IV PPIs are used to manage upper gastrointestinal bleeding (Leontiadis et al., 2007).

Refer again if epigastric pain and dyspepsia persist despite treatment and if signs of gastrointestinal bleeding are present (Ramakrishnan & Salinas, 2007).

Education: Avoidance of aspirin and other NSAIDs and tobacco is essential. Reduction of stressful events, coffee (including decaffeinated forms) and other caffeine products, and alcohol is recommended. Caution patients about taking OTC medication preparations without professional advice. The Centers for Disease Control and Prevention has established an *H. pylori* information hotline for health-care providers and patients (888-MYULCER).

CLINICAL RECOMMENDATION	EVIDENCE RATING	REFERENCES
Assess patients for NSAID use if they are ≥65 years, for prior gastrointestinal (GI) clinical conditions including dyspepsia, and for low-dose aspirin use to determine if medication should be avoided or used with protective measures to reduce for GI bleeding.	B	Laine, Curtis, Cryer, Kaur, & Cannon (2010)
Spironolactone was found to increase the risk for GI bleeding in patients.	A	Gulmez et al. (2008)
There is a decreased mortality rate from bleeding peptic ulcers when IV PPIs are used to manage upper GI bleeding.	A	Leontiadis et al. (2007)
Treat patients with PUD symptoms and *H. pylori* infection with a PPI twice daily, clarithromycin 500 mg twice daily, and either amoxicillin 1 g or metronidazole 500 mg twice daily for at least 7 days.	A	Ford, Delaney, Forman, Moayyedi, & Ford (2011)

A = consistent, good-quality, patient-oriented evidence; B = inconsistent or limited-quality, patient-oriented evidence; C = consensus, disease-oriented evidence, usual practice, expert opinion, or case series. For information about the SORT evidence rating system, go to www.aafp.org/afpsort.xml.

CASE STUDY

A 71-year-old Hispanic woman presents with a 4-week history of dyspepsia and abdominal pain that she describes as gnawing. She states that for years she has had occasional heartburn, but she cannot recall having abdominal pain. She states that she also has arthritis and has taken Motrin every day for the past 2 years. For her stomach pains, she has been taking Tums extra strength a couple of times a day. She states that the pain began soon after visiting her sister, who is a nurse at a mission in Nicaragua.

Chief Complaint: "My stomach hurts and wakes me up from my sleep. I find myself belching after meals and I feel bloated."

CASE STUDY—cont'd

Objective: Blood pressure (BP) 118/70 mm Hg, heart rate (HR) 90 beats/min, respiratory rate 18 breaths/min, BMI 29.

1. How will you use this information to prepare for today's visit?

2. What additional subjective data are you seeking?

3. What additional objective data will you be assessing for?

4. What are the differential diagnoses that you are considering?

5. What laboratory tests will help you rule out some of the differential diagnoses?

6. What is your treatment and specific information on the prescription you will give to this patient?

7. What are the potential complications from the treatment ordered?

8. What additional specific laboratory tests will you consider ordering?

9. What additional patient teaching may be needed?

10. What type of specialist will you be consulting for this patient?

REFERENCES

Assessment

Gulmez, S. E., Lassen, A. T., Aalykke, C., Dall, M., Andries, A., Andersen, B. S., . . . Hallas, J. (2008). Spironolactone use and the risk of upper gastrointestinal bleeding: a population-based case-control study. *British Journal of Clinical Pharmacology,66*(2), 294–299. doi: 10.1111/j.1365-2125.2008.03205

Laine, L., Curtis, S. P., Cryer, B., Kaur, A., & Cannon C. P. (2010). Risk factors for NSAID-associated upper GI clinical events in a long-term prospective study of 34 701 arthritis patients. *Alimentary Pharmacology and Therapeutics, 32*(10), 1240–1248. doi: 10.1111/j.1365-2036.2010.04465.x

LeBlond, R. F., Brown, D. D., & DeGowin, R. L. (2009). *DeGowin's diagnostic examination* (9th ed.). New York City, NY: McGraw-Hill Medical.

Leontiadis, G. I., Sreedharan, A., Dorward, S., Barton, P., Delaney, P., Howden, C. W., . . . Forman, D. (2007). Systematic reviews of the clinical effectiveness and cost-effectiveness of proton pump inhibitors in acute upper gastrointestinal bleeding. *Health Technology Assessment, 11*(51), iii–iv, 1–164.

Leuschner, U. F., Lindenthal, B., Herrmann, G., Arnold, J. C., Rössle, M., Cordes, H. J., . . . NASH Study Group. (2010). High-dose ursodeoxycholic acid therapy for nonalcoholic steatohepatitis: a double-blind, randomized, placebo-controlled trial. *Hepatology, 52*(2), 472–479. doi: 10.1002/hep.23727

Spirit, M. J. (2010). Complicated intra-abdominal infections: a focus on appendicitis and diverticulitis. *Postgraduate Medicine, 122*(1), 39–51. doi:10.3810/pgm.2010.01.2098

Williams, M. (2008). *Geriatric physical diagnosis*. Jefferson, NC: McFarland & Co.

Acute Kidney Injury

Cho, K. C., & Chertow, G. M. (2005). Management of acute renal failure. In A. Greenberg (Ed.), *Primer on kidney diseases* (pp. 315–321). Philadelphia, PA: Saunders.

Dwinnell, B., & Anderson, R. J. (1999). Diagnostic evaluation of the patient with acute renal failure. In R. W. Schrier (Ed.), *Atlas of kidney disease*. Retrieved October 8, 2011, from http://www.kidneyatlas.org/

Holley, J. L. (2005). Clinical approach to the diagnosis of acute renal failure. In A. Greenberg (Ed.), *Primer on kidney diseases* (pp. 287–292). Philadelphia, PA: Saunders.

Inker, L., & Perrone, R. D. (2010). Assessment of kidney function: serum creatinine; BUN; and GFR. *UpToDate*. Retrieved October 5, 2011, from www.uptodate.com/contents/assessment-of-kidney-function-serum-creatinine-bun-GFR

Liano, F., & Pascual, J. (1999). Acute renal failure: causes and prognosis. In R. W. Schrier (Ed.), *Atlas of kidney disease*. Retrieved September 30, 2011, from www.kidneyatlas.org/book1/adk1_12.pdf

McMillan, J. I. (2007). Acute renal failure (AKI). In *Merck manual*. Retrieved September 28, 2011, from www.merckmanuals.com/professional/genitourinary_disorders/renal_failure/acute_renal_failure_arf.html?qt=acute kidney injury&alt=sh

Palevsky, P. M. (2008). Definition of acute kidney injury (acute renal failure). *UpToDate*. Retrieved October 5, 2011, from www.uptodate.com/contents/definition-of-acute-renal-failure?view

Palevsky, P. M. (2012). Epidemiology, etiology, pathophysiology and diagnosis of acute kidney injury. In E. V. Lerma & A. R. Nissenson, *Nephrology secrets* (pp. 43–50). Philadelphia, PA: Elsevier.

Safirstein, R. L. (2005). Pathophysiology of acute renal failure. In A. Greenberg (Ed.), *Primer on kidney diseases* (pp. 279–286). Philadelphia, PA: Saunders.

U.S. Renal Data System. (2010). USRDS 2010 annual data report: atlas of chronic kidney disease: end-stage renal disease in the United States. Retrieved October 4, 2011, from www.usrds.org/2010/view/v1_08.asp

Bladder Cancer

Babjuk, M., Oosterlinck, W., Sylvester, R., Kaasinen, E., Böhle, A., Palou-Redorta, J., . . . European Association of Urology (EAU). (2011). EAU guidelines on non-muscle-invasive urothelial carcinoma of the bladder, the 2011 update. *European Urology, 59*(6), 997–1008.

Jimenez, J. A., Campbell, S. C., & Jones, J. S. (2011). Screening for bladder cancer. *UpToDate*. Retrieved from www.uptodate.com

Lotan, Y., & Choueiri, T. K. (2012). Clinical presentation, diagnosis, and staging of bladder cancer. *UpToDate*. Retrieved from www.uptodate.com

Messing, E. M., Madeb, R., Young, T., Gilchrist, K. W., Bram, L., Greenberg, E. B., . . . Feng, C. (2006). Long-term outcome of hematuria home screening for bladder cancer in men. *Cancer, 107*(9), 2173–2179.

National Comprehensive Cancer Network. (2012). NCCN clinical practice guidelines in oncology (NCCN guidelines): bladder cancer: version 2.2012. Retrieved from www.nccn.org

Bowel Obstruction

Ansari, P. (2007). Intestinal obstruction. In *The Merck manual* (18th ed.). Retrieved from www.merckmanuals.com/professional/gastrointestinal_disorders/acute_abdomen_and_surgical_gastroenterology/intestinal_obstruction.html

Jackson, P. G., & Raiji, M. (2011). Evaluation and management of intestinal obstruction. *American Family Physician, 83*(2), 159–165.

Kent, V. P. (2007). Caring for a patient with a bowel obstruction. *LPN2007, 3*(5), 30–38.

Kent, V. P. (2009). Treating a patient with an intestinal obstruction. *Perspectives, 8*(1), 1, 7–11. Retrieved from www.perspectivesinnursing.org/pdfs/perspectives29.pdf

Kulayat, M. N., & Doerr, R. J. (2001). Small bowel obstruction. In R. G. Holzheimer & J. A. Mannick (Eds.), *Surgical treatment: evidence-based and problem-oriented*. Munich, Germany: Zuckschwerdt.

Letizia, M., & Norton, E. (2003). Successful management of malignant bowel obstruction. *Journal of Hospice and Palliative Nursing, 5*(3). Retrieved from www.medscape.com/viewarticle/459580

Lyon, C., & Clark, D. C. (2006). Diagnosis of acute abdominal pain in older adults. *American Family Physician, 74*(9), 1537–1544.

Milenkovic, M., Russo, A., & Elixhauser, A. (2006). Hospital stays for gastrointestinal diseases, 2004 (Healthcare Cost and Utilization Project Statistical Brief #12). Agency for Healthcare Research and Quality. Retrieved from www.hcup-us.ahrq.gov/reports/statbriefs/sb12.jsp

Moll van Charante, E., & de Jongh, T. O. (2011). Physical examination of patients with acute abdominal pain. *Nederlands Tijdschrift voor Geneeskunde, 155*, A2658.

Moses, S. (2012). Small bowel obstruction. *Family Practice Notebook*. Retrieved from www.fpnotebook.com/Surgery/GI/SmlBwl/Obstrctn.htm

National Cancer Institute. (2011). PDQ® gastrointestinal complications. Retrieved from http://cancer.gov/cancertopics/pdq/supportivecare/gastrontestinal complications/HealthProfessional

Nobie, B. A. (2011). Small-bowel obstruction. Retrieved from http://emedicine.medscape.com/article/774140-overview

Cholecystitis

Adedeji, O. A., & McAdam, W. A. (1996). Murphy's sign, acute cholecystitis and elderly people. *Journal of the Royal Colleges of Surgeons of Edinburgh, 41*(2), 88–89.

Agrawal, R. M., Morrissey, S., & Thakkar, S. (2012). Gall bladder disease. In C.S. Pitchumoni & T.S. Dharmarajan (Eds.), *Geriatric Gastroenterology.* New York City, NY: Springer. doi: 10.1007/978-1-4419-1623-5_42

Bellows, C. F., Berger, D. H., & Crass, R. A. (2005). Management of gallstones. *American Family Physician, 72*(4), 637–642.

Cho, J. Y., Han, H. S., Yoon, Y. S., & Ahn, K. S. (2010). Risk factors for acute cholecystitis and a complicated clinical course in patients with symptomatic cholelithiasis. *Archives of Surgery, 145*(4), 329–333; discussion 333. doi:10.1001/archsurg.2010.35

Claesson, B. (1986). Microflora of the biliary tree and liver—clinical correlates. *Digestive Diseases, 4*(2), 93–118.

Decker, G. A., Swain, J. M., Crowell, M. D., & Scolapio, J. S. (2007). Gastrointestinal and nutritional complications after bariatric surgery. *The American Journal of Gastroenterology, 102*(11), 2571–2580.

Giger, U. F., Michel, J. M., Opitz, I., Th Inderbitzin, D., Kocher, T., & Krahenbuhl, L. (2006). Risk factors for perioperative complications in patients undergoing laparoscopic cholecystectomy: analysis of 22,953 consecutive cases from the Swiss Association of Laparoscopic and Thoracoscopic Surgery database. *Journal of the American College of Surgeons, 203*(5), 723–728. doi:10.1016/j.jamcollsurg.2006.07.018

Goroll, A. (2009). Management of asymptomatic and symptomatic gallstones. In A. H. Goroll and A. G. Mulley (Eds.), *Primary care medicine: office evaluation and management of the adult* (6th ed.). Philadelphia, PA: Lippincott Williams & Wilkins.

Hyeon Kook, L., Ho-Seong, H., & Seog Ki, M. (2009). Clinical surgery—international: the association between body mass index and the severity of cholecystitis. *American Journal of Surgery, 197*, 455–458. doi:10.1016/j.amjsurg.2008.01.029

Lee, H. K., Han, H. S., & Min, S. K. (2009). Clinical surgery—international: the association between body mass index and the severity of cholecystitis. *The American Journal of Surgery, 197*, 455–458. doi: 10.1016/j.amjsurg.2008.01.029

Macrì, A., Scuderi, G., Saladino, E., Trimarchi, G., Terranova, M., Versaci, A., & Famulari, C. (2006). Acute gallstone cholecystitis in the elderly: treatment with emergency ultrasonographic percutaneous cholecystostomy and interval laparoscopic cholecystectomy. *Surgical Endosteroly, 20*(1), 88–91.

Makino, I., Yamaguchi, T., Nariatsu, S., Toshiaki, Y., & Ichiro, K. (2009). Xanthogranulomatous cholecystitis mimicking gallbladder carcinoma with a false-positive result on fluorodeoxyglucose PET. *World Journal of Gastroenteroly, 15*(29), 3691–3693.

Ralls, P. W., Halls, J., Lapin, S. A., Quinn, M. F., Morris, U. L., & Boswell, W. (1982). Prospective evaluation of the monographic Murphy sign in suspected acute cholecystitis. *Journal of Clinical Ultrasound, 10*(3), 113–115.

Riall, T. S., Zhang, D., Townsend, C. M., Jr., Kuo, Y. F., & Goodwin, J. S. (2010). Failure to perform cholecystectomy for acute cholecystitis in elderly patients is associated with increased morbidity, mortality, and cost. *Journal of the American College of Surgeons, 210*(5), 668. doi:10.1016/j.jamcollsurg.2009.12.031

Trowbridge, R. L., Rutkowski, N. K., & Shojania, K. G. (2003). Does this patient have acute cholecystitis? *Journal of the American Medical Association, 289*(1), 80–86.

Winbladh, A., Gullstrand, P., Svanvik, J., & Sandström, P. (2009). Systematic review of cholecystostomy as a treatment option in acute cholecystitis. *HPB: The International Journal of the Hepato Pancreato Biliary Association, 11*(3), 183–93. doi: 10.1111/j.1477-2574.2009.00052.x

Chronic Kidney Disease

Aschner, P. G. (2011). The global epidemic of obesity, diabetes, hypertension and chronic kidney disease. In J. Daugirdas (Ed.), *Handbook of chronic kidney disease management* (pp. 19–26). Philadelphia, PA: Lippincott Williams & Wilkins.

Connor, R. N. (2011). Smoking, substance abuse and environmenal hazards. In J. Daugirdas (Ed.), *Handbook of chronic kidney disease management* (pp. 44–51). Philadelphia, PA: Lippincott Williams & Wilkins.

Hahr, A. M. (2011). Glucose control in diabetes mellitus and kidney disease. In J. Daugirdas (Ed.), *Handbook of chronic kidney disease management* (pp. 207–223). Philadelphia, PA: Lippincott Williams & Wilkins.

Inker, L., & Perrone, R. D. (2010, October 5). Assessment of kidney function: Serum creatinine; BUN; and GFR. *UpToDate.* Retrieved October 5, 2011, from www.uptodate.com/contents/assessment-of-kidncy-function-serum-creatinine-bun-GFR

Johnson, C. A., Levey, A. S., Coresh, J., Levin, A., Lau, J., & Eknoyan, G. (2004a). Clinical practice guidelines for chronic kidney disease in adults: Part I. Definition, disease stages, evaluation, treatment, and risk factors. *American Family Physician, 70*(5), 869–876.

Johnson, C. A., Levey, A. S., Coresh, J., Levin, A., Lau, J., & Eknoyan, G. (2004b). Clinical practice guidelines for chronic kidney disease in adults: Part II. Glomerular filtration rate, proteinuria, and other markers. *American Family Physician, 70*(6), 1091–1097.

Johnson, D. W. (2011). Screening and management: overview. In J. T. Daugirdas (Ed.), *Handbook of chronic kidney disease management* (pp. 32–43). Philadelphia, PA: Lippincott Williams & Wilkins.

Kalitzidis, R. B. (2011). Optimizing blood pressure and reducing proteinuria. In J. T. Daugirdas (Ed.), *Handbook of chronic kidney disease management* (pp. 224–239). Philadelphia, PA: Lippincott Williams & Wilkins.

National Institutes of Health. (2011). USRDS 2009 annual data report: atlas of chronic kidney disease in the United States. U.S. Renal Data System. Retrieved October 4, 2011, from www.usrds.org/atlas.aspx

National Kidney Foundation. (2002). KDOQI clinical practice guidelines for chronic kidney disease: evaluation, classification and stratification. Retrieved October 4, 2011, from www.kidney.org/professionals/KDOQI/guidelines_ckd/p3_pubhealth.htm

Post, T. R. (2011). Diagnostic approach to the patient with acute or chronic kidney disease. *UpToDate.* Retrieved October 11, 2011, from www.uptodate.com.

Cirrhosis of the Liver

Akriviadis, E., Botla, R., Briggs, W., Han, S., Reynolds, T., & Shakil, O. (2000). Pentoxifylline improves short-term survival in severe alcoholic hepatitis: a double-blind, placebo-controlled trial. *Gastroenterology, 119*(6), 1637–1648.

Borowsky, S. A., Strome, S., & Lott, E. (1981). Continued heavy drinking and survival in alcoholic cirrhosis. *Gastroenterology, 80*(6), 1405–1409.

Chen, Y.-C., Chu, C.-M., Yeh, C.-T., & Liaw, Y.-F. (2007). Natural course following the onset of cirrhosis in patients with chronic hepatitis B: a long-term follow-up study. *Hepatology International, 1*(1), 267–273.

Cirrhosis of the liver (NIH Publication No. 06-5166). (2005, October). *National Digestive Diseases Information Clearinghouse.* National Institute of Diabetes and Digestive and Kidney Diseases. Retrieved from http://digestive.niddk.nih.gov/ddiseases/pubs/cirrhosis_ez

Clark, J. M., & Diehl, A. M. (2003). Nonalcoholic fatty liver disease: an underrecognized cause of cryptogenic cirrhosis. *Journal of the American Medical Association, 289*(22), 3000–3004.

Duke, R. (2012, February). Demystifying the liver and its diseases. *Clinical Advisor,* pp. 28–34.

Eker, H. H., vanRamshorst, G. H., deGoede, B., Tilanus, H. W., Metselaar, H. J., deMan, R. A., . . . Kazemier, G. (2011). A prospective study on elective umbilical hernia repair in patients with liver cirrhosis and ascites. *Surgery, 150*(3) 542–546. doi:10.1016/j.surg.2011.02.026

Ewing, J. A. (1984). Detecting alcoholism: the CAGE Questionnaire. *Journal of the American Medical Association, 252*(14), 1905–1907.

Gill, H. K., & Wu, G. Y. (2006). Non-alcoholic fatty liver disease and the metabolic syndrome: effects of weight loss and a review of popular diets. Are low carbohydrate diets the answer? *World Journal of Gastroenterology, 12*(3), 345–353.

Heidelbaugh, J. J., & Bruderly, M. (2006). Cirrhosis and chronic liver failure: Part I. Diagnosis and evaluation. *American Family Physician, 74*(5), 756–762.

Kochar, R., Nevah, R., Moises, I., & Fallon, M. B. (2011). Pulmonary complications of cirrhosis. *Current Gastroenterology Reports, 13*(1), 34–39.

O'Shea, R. S., Dasarathy, S., & McCullough, A. J. (2010). Alcoholic liver disease. *American Journal of Gastroenterology, 105*(1), 14–32; quiz 33.

Pessaux, P., & Lermite, E. (2008). Hepatic cirrhosis and biliary stones. In G. Borzellino & C. Cordiano (Eds.), *Biliary lithiasis: basic science, current diagnosis and management.* Milano: Springer Milan.

Riley, T. R., Taheri, M., & Schreibman, I. R. (2009). Does weight history affect fibrosis in the setting of chronic liver disease? *Journal of Gastrointestinal and Liver Disease, 18*(3), 299–302.

Starr, S. P., & Raines, D. (2011). Cirrhosis: diagnosis, management, and prevention. *American Family Physician, 84*(12), 1353–1359.

Swart, G. R., Zillikens, M. C., van Vuure, J. K., & van den Berg, J. W. (1989). Effect of a late evening meal on nitrogen balance in patients with cirrhosis of the liver. *British Medical Journal, 299*(6709), 1202–1203.

Uribe, M., Schalm, S. W., Summerskill, W. H., & Go, V. L. (1978). Oral prednisone for chronic active liver disease: dose responses and bioavailability studies. *Gut, 19*(12), 1131–1135.

Clostridium Difficile

Barbut, F., & Petit, J. C. (2001). Epidemiology of clostridium difficile-associated infections. *Clinical Microbiology Infection, 7*(8), 405–410.

Bartlett, J. G., & Gerding, D. N. (2008). Clinical recognition and diagnosis of *Clostridium difficile* infection. *Clinical Infectious Diseases, 46*(Suppl. 1), S12–S18.

Carignan, A., Allard, C., Pépin, J., Cossette, B., Nault, V., & Valiquette, L. (2008). Risk of clostridium difficile infection after perioperative antibacterial prophylaxis before and during an outbreak of infection due to a hypervirulent strain. *Clinical Infectious Diseases. 46*(12),1838–1843. doi: 10.1086/588291

Cohen, S. H., Gerding, D. N., Johnson, S., Kelly, C. P., Loo, V. G., McDonald, L. C., . . . Wilcox, M. H. (2010). Clinical practice guidelines for *Clostridium difficile* infection in adults: 2010 update by the Society for Healthcare Epidemiology of America (SHEA) and the Infectious Diseases Society of America (IDSA). *Infection Control and Hospital Epidemiology, 31*(5), 431–455. doi:10.1086/651706

Crogan, N. L., & Evans, B. C. (2007). *Clostridium difficile:* an emerging epidemic in nursing homes. *Geriatric Nursing, 28*(3), 161–164.

Hessen, M. T. (2010). In the clinic: clostridium difficile in the long term care setting. *Journal of the American Medical Director's Association, 153*(7), ITC4-1–ITC4-16. doi: 10.7326/0003-4819-153-7-201010050-01004

Jung, K. S., Park, J. J., Chon, Y. E., Jung, E. S., Lee, H. J., Jang, H. W., . . . Cheon, J. H. (2010). Risk factors for treatment failure and recurrence after metronidazole treatment for clostridium difficile-associated diarrhea. *Gut and Liver,4*(3), 332–3377. doi: 10.5009/gnl.2010.4.3.332

Kee, V. R. (2012). *Clostridium difficile* infection in older adults: a review and update on its management. *American Journal of Geriatric Pharmacotherapy, 10*(1), 14–24. doi:10.1016/j.amjopharm.2011.12.004

Kyne, L. (2010). *Clostridium difficile*—beyond antibiotics. *New England Journal of Medicine, 362*(3), 264–265.

Kyne, L., & Kelly, C. P. (2001). Recurrent clostridium difficile diarrhea. *Gut, 49*(1), 152–153.

Martinez, F. J., Leffler, D. A., & Kelly, C. P. (2012). Clostridium difficile outbreaks: prevention and treatment strategies. *Risk Management and Healthcare Policy, 5,* 55–64. doi:10.2147/RMHP.S13053. Retrieved from http://nrs.harvard.edu/urn-3:HUL.InstRepos: 10445587

Musher, D. M., Manhas, A., Jain, P., Nuila, F., Waqar, A., Logan, N., . . . Graviss E. A. (2007). Detection of clostridium difficile toxin:

comparison of enzyme immunoassay results with results obtained by cytotoxicity assay. *Journal of Clinical Microbiology, 5*(8), 2737–2739.

Nair, S., Yadav, D., Corpuz, M., & Pitchumoni, C. S. (1998). Clostridium difficile colitis: factors influencing treatment failure and relapse—a prospective evaluation. *The American Journal of Gastroenterology, 93*(10), 1873–1876.

Simor, A. E. (2010). Diagnosis, management, and prevention of clostridium difficile infection in long-term care facilities: a review. *Journal of the American Geriatrics Society, 58*(8), 1556–1564. doi:10.1111/j.1532-5415.2010.02958.x

Yassin, S. F., Young-Fadok, T. M., Zein, N. N., & Pardi, D. S. (2001). Clostridium difficile-associated diarrhea and colitis. *Mayo Clinic Proceedings, 76*(7), 725–730.

Colorectal Cancer

Agrawal, S., Bhupinderjit, A., Bhutani, M. S., Boardman, L., Nguyen, C., Romero, Y., . . . Figueroa-Moseley, C. (2005). Colorectal cancer in African Americans. *American Journal of Gastroenterology, 100*(3), 515–523.

Albano, J., Ward, E., Jemal, A., Anderson, R., Cokkinides, V., Murray, T., . . . Thuss, M. (2007). Cancer mortality in the United States by education and race. *Journal of the National Cancer Institute, 99*(18), 1384–1394.

American Cancer Institute. (2012). *Cancer prevention and early detection: facts and figures 2010.* Atlanta, GA: American Cancer Society.

American Cancer Society. (2012). American Cancer Society guidelines on nutrition and physical activity for cancer prevention. doi:10.3322/caac.20140

Bernick, P., Klimstra, D., Shia, J., Minsky, B., Saltz, L., Shi, W., . . . Wong, W. (2004). Neuroendocrine carcinoma. *Diseases of the Colon and Rectum, 47*(2), 163–169.

Buetow, P., & Buck, J. (2006). Adenocarcinoma of the colon and rectum. *Archives of Armed Forces Institute of Pathology, 15,* 1.

Giovannucci, E. (2003). Diet, body weight, and colorectal cancer: a summary of the epidemiologic evidence. *Journal of Women's Health, 12*(2), 173–182.

Jonker, D., O'Callaghan, C., Karapetis, C., Zakberg, J., Tu, D., Au, H., . . . Moore, A. (2007). Cetuximab for the treatment of colon and rectal cancer. *New England Journal of Medicine, 377*(10), 2040–2048.

Kayhan, B., & Turan, N. (2003). A rare entity in the rectum: malignant melanoma. *Turkish Journal of Gastroenterology, 14*(4), 273–275.

Lynch, H. T., Riley, B., Weissman, S., Coronel, S., Kinarsky, Y., Lynch, J., . . . Shaw, T. (1993). Hereditary nonpolyposis colorectal carcinoma (HNPCC) and HNPCC-like families: problems in diagnosis, surveillance, and management. *American Cancer Society, 100*(1), 53–65.

Regula, J., Rupinski, M., Kraszewska, E., Polkowski, M., Orlowska, J., Nowacki, M., & Butruk, E. (2006). Colonoscopy in colorectal-cancer screening for detection of advanced neoplasia. *New England Journal of Medicine, 355*(18), 1863–1872.

Sarcoma Alliance. (2006). What is sarcoma? Retrieved from www.sarcomaalliance.com/master.htm1?ArticleId=90

Wasif, N., Etzioni, D., Maggard, M. A, Tomlinson, J. S, & Ko, C. Y. (2011). Trends, patterns, and outcomes in the management of malignant colonic polyps in the general population of the United States. *Cancer, 117*(5),931–937. doi: 10.1002/cncr.25657

Cystitis

American College of Obstetricians and Gynecologists. (2008). *Treatment of urinary tract infections in nonpregnant women* (ACOG Practice Bulletin No. 91). Washington, DC: American College of Obstetricians and Gynecologists.

Beveridge, L. A., Davey, P. G., Phillips, G., & McMurdo, M. (2011). Optimal management of urinary tract infections in older people. *Clinical Interventions in Aging, 6,* 173–180.

Dason, S., Dason, J., & Kapoor, A. (2011). Guidelines for the diagnosis and management of recurrent urinary tract infection in women. *Canadian Urological Association Journal, 5*(5), 316–322. doi:10.5489/cuaj.11214

Dielubanza, E., & Schaffer, A. J. (2011). Urinary tract infections in women. *Medical Clinics of North America, 95*(1), 27–41. doi:10.1016/j.mcna.2010.08.023

Epp, A., Larochelle, A., Lovatsis, D., Walter, J. E., Easton, W. Farrell, S. A., . . . Marshall, C. (2010). Recurrent urinary tract infection. *Journal of Obstetrics and Gynecology Canada, 32*(11), 1082–1090.

Gilbert, D. N., Moellering, R. C., Eliopoulos, G. M., Chambers, H. F., & Saag, M. S. (2011). *The Sanford guide to antimicrobial therapy* (41st ed.). Westville, NJ: Royalty Press.

Grabe, M., Bjerklund-Johansen, T. E., Botto, H., Wullt, B., Cek, M., Naber, K. G., . . . Wagenlehner, F. (2011, March). *Uncomplicated UTIs in adults. Guidelines on urological infections* (pp. 15–27). Arnhem, The Netherlands: European Association of Urology.

Juthani-Mehta, M., Quagliarello, V., Perrelli, E., Towle, V., Van Ness, P. H., & Tinetti, M. (2009). Clinical features to identify urinary tract infections in nursing home residents: a cohort study. *Journal of the American Geriatrics Society, 57*(6), 963–970. doi:10.1111/j.1532-5415.2009.02227.x

Lin, K., & Fajardo, K. (2008). Screening for asymptomatic bacteriuria in adults: evidence for the U.S. Preventive Services Task Force reaffirmation recommendation statement. *Annals of Internal Medicine, 149*(1), W20–W24.

Nicolle, L. E. (2005). Complicated urinary tract infections in adults. *Canadian Journal of Infectious Diseases & Medical Microbiology, 16*(6), 349–360.

Nicolle, L. E., Bradley, S., Colgan, R., Rice, J. C., Schaeffer, A., & Hooton, T. M. (2005). Infectious Diseases Society of America guidelines for the diagnosis and treatment of asymptomatic bacteriuria in adults. *Clinical Infectious Diseases, 40*(5), 643–654.

Schmiemann, G., Kniehl, E., Gebhardt, K., Matejczyk, M. M., & Hummers-Pradier, E. (2010). The diagnosis of urinary tract infection: a systematic review. *Deutsches Aerzteblatt International, 107*(21), 361–367. doi:10.3238/arztebl.2010.0361

Woodford, H. J., & George, J. (2009). Diagnosis and management of urinary tract infection in hospitalized older people. *Journal of the American Geriatrics Society, 57*(1), 107–114. doi:10.1111/j.1532-5415.2008.02073.x

Diverticulitis

Alonso, S., Pera, M., Parés, D., Pascual, M., Gil, M. J., Courtier, R., & Grande, L. (2010). Outpatient treatment of patients with uncomplicated acute diverticulitis. *Colorectal Disease, 12*(10 Online), e278–e282.

Ambrosetti, P., Jenny, A., Becker, C., Terrier, T. F., & Morel, P. (2000). Acute left colonic diverticulitis—compared performance of computed tomography and water-soluble contrast enema: prospective evaluation of 420 patients. *Diseases of the Colon and Rectum, 43*(10), 1363–1367.

Commane, D. M., Arasaradnam, R. P., Mills, S., Mathers, J. C., & Bradburn, M. (2009). Diet, ageing and genetic factors in the pathogenesis of diverticular disease. *World Journal of Gastroenterology, 15*(20), 2479–2488.

Floch, C. L. (2006). Diagnosis and management of acute diverticulitis. *Journal of Clinical Gastroenterology, 40*(Suppl. 3), S136–S144.

Frattini, J., & Longo, W. E. (2006). Diagnosis and treatment of chronic and recurrent diverticulitis. *Journal of Clinical Gastroenterology, 40*(Suppl. 3), S145–S149.

Hall, J. F., Roberts, P. L., Ricciardi, R., Read, T., Scheirey, C., Wald, C., . . . Schoetz, D. J. (2011). Long-term follow-up after an initial episode of diverticulitis: what are the predictors of recurrence? *Diseases of the Colon and Rectum, 54*(3), 283–288.

Jacobs, D. O. (2007). Clinical practice. Diverticulitis. *New England Journal of Medicine, 357*(20), 2057–2066. doi:10.1056/NEJMcp073228

Lamiki, P., Tsuchiya, J., Pathak, S., Okura, R., Solimene, U., Jain, S., . . . Marotta, F. (2009). Probiotics in diverticular disease of the colon: an open label study. *Journal of Gastrointestinal and Liver Disease, 19*(1), 31–36.

Lau, K. C., Spilsbury, K., Farooque, Y., Kariyawasam, S. B., Owen, R. G., Wallace, M. H., & Makin, G. B. (2011). Is colonoscopy still mandatory after a CT diagnosis of left-sided diverticulitis: can colorectal cancer be confidently excluded? *Diseases of the Colon and Rectum, 54*(10), 1265–1270. doi:10.1097/DCR.0b013e31822899a2

Lutwak, N., & Dill, C. (2013). Mild to moderate diverticulitis: what's new in diagnositic approach, treatment, and prevention of recurrence? *Clinical Geriatrics, 21* (7). Retrieved from http://www.clinicalgeriatrics.com/articles/Mild-Moderate-Diverticulitis-Whats-New

Maconi, G., Barbara, G., Bosetti, C., Cuomo, R., & Annibale, B. (2011). Treatment of diverticular disease of the colon and prevention of acute diverticulitis: a systematic review. *Diseases of the Colon and Rectum, 54*(10), 1326–1338. doi:10.1097/DCR.0b013e318223cb2b

Mazuski, J. E. (2007). Antimicrobial treatment for intra-abdominal infections. *Expert Opinion on Pharmacotherapy, 8*(17), 2933–2945.

McQuaid, K. R. (2010). Gastrointestinal disorders. In S. J. McPhee & M. A. Papadakis (Eds.), *Current medical diagnosis and treatment* (49th ed.). New York City, NY: McGraw-Hill.

Rafferty, J., Shellito, P., Hyman, N. H., & Buie, W. D. (2006). Practice parameters for sigmoid diverticulitis. *Diseases of the Colon and Rectum, 49*(7), 939–944.

Salzman, H., & Lillie, D. (2005). Diverticular disease: diagnosis and treatment. *American Family Physician, 72*(7), 1229–1234.

Sheth, A. A., Longo, W., & Floch, M. H. (2008). Diverticular disease and diverticulitis. *The American Journal of Gastroenterogy, 103*(6), 1550–1556. doi: 10.1111/j.1572-0241.2008.01879.x

Solomkin, J. S., Goldstein, E. J. C., Stollman, N. H., Barie, P. S., & Mazuski, J. E. (2007). The role of moxifloxacin in the management of complicated intra-abdominal infections. *Infectious Disease Clinics of North America, 21*(Suppl. 1), 16–24.

Spirit, M. J. (2010). Complicated intra-abdominal infections: a focus on appendicitis and diverticulitis. *Postgraduate Medicine, 122*(1), 39–51. doi:10.3810/pgm.2010.01.2098

Strate, L. L., Liu, Y. L., Huang, E. S., Giovannucci, E. L., & Chan A. T. (2011). Use of aspirin or nonsteroidal anti-inflammatory drugs increases risk for diverticulitis and diverticular bleeding. *Gastrorenterology, 140*(5), 1427–1433. doi: 10.1053/j.gastro.2011.02.004

Strate, L. L., Liu, Y. L., Syngal, S., Aldoori, W. H., & Giovannucci, E. L. (2008). Nut, corn, and popcorn consumption and the incidence of diverticular disease. *Journal of the American Medical Association, 300*(8), 907–914. doi: 10.1001/jama.300.8.907

Tarleton, S., & DiBaise, J. K. (2011). Low-residue diet in diverticular disease: putting an end to a myth. *Nutrition Clinical Practice, 26*(2), 137–142. doi:10.1177/0884533611399774

Wilkins, T., Embry, K., & George, R. (2013). Diagnosis and management of acute diverticulitis. *American Family Physician, 87*(9) 612–620.

World Gastroenterology Organization. (2007). Practice guidelines 2007. Diverticular disease. Retrieved June 10, 2011, from www.worldgastroenterology.org/diverticular-disease.html

Esophagitis

Aparanji, K. P., Annavarappu, S., Russell, R. O., & Dharmarajan, T. S. (2012). Severe dysphagia from medication-induced esophagitis: a preventable disorder. *Clinical Geriatrics, 20*(2), 34–39.

Erichsen, R., Robertson, D., Farkas, D. K., Pedersen, L., Pohl, H., Baron, J. A., & Sorensen, H. T. (2012). Erosive reflux disease increases risk for esophageal adenocarcinoma, compared with nonerosive reflux. *Clinical Gastroenterology and Hepatology, 10*(5), 475–480.

Furuta, G .T., Liacouras, C. A., Collins, M. H., Gupta, C., Justinich, C., Putnam, P. E., . . . Rothenberg, M. E. (2007). Eosinophilic esophagitis in children and adults: a systematic review and consensus recommendations for diagnosis and treatment. *Gastroenterology, 133*(4), 1342–1363.

Kliemann, D. A., Pasqualotto, A. C., Falavigna, M., Giaretta, T., Severo, L. C. (2008). Candida esophagitis: species distribution and risk factors for infection. *Journal of the Institute of Tropical Medicine of São Paulo, 50*(5), 261–263.

McDonagh, M. S., Carson, S., & Thakurta, S. (2009). Drug class review: proton pump inhibitors: final report update 5. Portland, OR: Oregon Health and Science University. Retrieved from www.ncbi.nlm.nih.gov/books/NBK47260

Mukherjee, S. (2011). Esophagitis differential diagnoses. Retrieved from http://emedicine.medscape.com/article/174223-differential

Pilotto, A., Franceschi, M., Leandro, G., Scarcelli, C., D'Ambrosio, L. P., Seripa, D., . . . Di Mario, F. (2006). Clinical features of reflux esophagitis in older people: a study of 840 consecutive patients. *Journal of the American Geriatrics Society, 54*(10), 1537–1542.

Prasad, G. A., Alexander, J. A., Schleck, C. D., Zinsmeister, A. R., Smyrk, T. C., Elias, R. M., . . . Talley, N. J. (2009). Epidemiology of eosinophilic esophagitis over three decades in Olmsted County, Minnesota. *Clinical Gastroenterology and Hepatology, 7*(10), 1055–1061.

Winstead, N. S., & Bulat, R. (2004). Pill esophagitis. *Current Treatment Options in Gastroenterology, 7*(1), 71–76.

Gastric Cancer

Bjelakovic, G., Nikolova, D., Simonetti, R. G., & Gluud, C. (2009). Systematic review: primary and secondary prevention of gastrointestinal cancers with antioxidant supplements. *Alimentary Pharmacology and Therapeutics, 28*(6), 689–703.

Compare, D., Rocco, A., Liguori, E., D'Armiento, F. P., Persico, G., Masone, S., . . . Nardone, G. (2011). Global DNA hypomethylation is an early event in *Helicobacter pylori*–related gastric carcinogenesis. *Journal of Clinical Pathology, 64*(8), 677–682.

Correa, P., Piazuelo, M. B., & Wilson, K. T. (2010). Pathology of gastric intestinal metaplasia: clinical implications. *American Journal of Gastroenterology, 105*(3), 493–498.

Correia, M., Machado, J. C., & Ristimäki, A. (2009). Basic aspects of gastric cancer. *Helicobacter, 14*(Suppl. 1), 36–40. doi:10.1111/j.1523-5378.2009.00696.x

Dan, Y. Y., So, J. B., & Yeoh, K. G. (2006). Endoscopic screening for gastric cancer. *Clinical Gastroenterology and Hepatology, 4*(6), 709–716.

Ioannidis, O., Cheva, A., Stavrakis, T., Paraskevas, G., Papadimitriou, N., Kakoutis, E., & Makrantonakis, A. (2010). Sister Mary Joseph's nodule as the sole presenting sign of gastric signet ring cell adenocarcinoma. *Gastroenterologie Clinique et Biologique, 34*(10), 565–568.

Jemal, A., Bray, F., Center, M. M., Ferlay, J., Ward, E., & Forman, D. (2011). Global cancer statistics. *CA: A Journal for Clinicians, 61*(2), 69–90. doi:10.3322/caac.20107

Jemal, A., Siegel, R., Ward, E., Hao, Y., Xu, J., & Thun, M. J. (2009). Cancer statistics, 2009. *CA: A Cancer Journal for Clinicians, 59*(4):225–249. doi: 10.3322/caac.20006

Joossens, J. V., Hill, M. J., Elliott, P., Stamler, R., Stamler, J., Lesaffre, E., . . . Kesteloot, H., (on behalf of European Cancer Prevention (ECP) and the INTERSALT Cooperative Research Group). (1996). Dietary salt, nitrate and stomach cancer mortality in 24 countries. *International Journal of Epidemiology, 25*(3), 494–504.

Kapoor, N., Bassi, A., Sturgess, R., & Bodger, K. (2005). Predictive value of alarm features in a rapid access upper gastrointestinal cancer service. *Gut, 54*(1), 40–45.

Lee, Y. T., Ng, E. K., Hung, L. C., Chung, S. C., Ching, J. Y., Chan, W. Y., . . . Sung, J. J. (2005). Accuracy of endoscopic ultrasonography in diagnosing ascites and predicting peritoneal metastases in gastric cancer patients. *Gut, 54*(11), 1541–1545.

McCulloch, P., Nita, M. E., Kazi, H., & Gama-Rodrigues, J. (2007). Extended versus limited lymph nodes dissection technique for adenocarcinoma of the stomach (Cochrane review). In *The Cochrane Library 2007*, Issue 1. Chichester, UK: John Wiley & Sons, Ltd.

McQuaid, K. R. (2009). Gastrointestinal disorders. In S. J. McPhee & M. A. Papadakis (Eds.), *Current medical diagnosis and treatment 2010* (49th ed.). New York City, NY: McGraw-Hill.

Shah, M. A., Khanin, R., Tang, L., Janjigian, Y. Y., Klimstra, D. S., Gerdes, H., & Kelsen, D. P. (2011). Molecular classification of gastric cancer: a new paradigm. *Clinical Cancer Research, 17*(9), 2693–2701. doi:10.1158/1078-0432.CCR-10-2203

Tsugane, S., & Sasazuki, S. (2007). Diet and the risk of gastric cancer: review of epidemiological evidence. *Gastric Cancer, 10*(2), 75–83. doi:10.1007/s10120-007-0420-0

Uemura, N., Okamoto, S., Yamamoto, S., Matsumura, N., Yamaguchi, S., Yamakido, M., . . . & Schlemper, R. J. (2001). Helicobacter pylori infection and the development of gastric cancer. *New England Journal of Medicine, 345*(11), 784–789.

Wöhrer, S. S., Raderer, M., & Hejna, M. (2004). Palliative chemotherapy for advanced gastric cancer. *Annals of Oncology, 15*(11), 1585–1595.

Wroblewski, L. E., Peek, R. M., Jr., & Wilson, K. T. (2010). *Helicobacter pylori* and gastric cancer: factors that modulate disease risk. *Clinical Microbiology Reviews, 23*(4), 713–739.

Gastritis

Chey, W. D., & Wong, B. C. (2007). American College of Gastroenterology guideline on the management of *Helicobacter pylori* infection. *American Journal of Gastroenterology, 102*(8), 1808–1825.

Franceschi, M., Di Mario, F., Leandro, G., Maggi, S., & Pilotto, A. (2009). Acid-related disorders in the elderly. Best practice and research. *Clinical gastroenterology, 23*(6), 839–848. doi: 10.1016/j.bpg.2009.10.004

Lauwers, G., Fujita, H., Nagata, K., & Shimizu, M. (2010). Pathology of non–*Helicobacter pylori* gastritis: extending the histopathologic horizons. *Journal of Gastroenterology, 45*(2), 131–145. doi:http://dx.doi.org/10.1007/s00535-009-0146-3

Leung, W. K., Lin, S.-R., Ching, J. Y. L., To, K.-F., Ng, E. K. W., Chan, F. K. L., . . . Sung, J. J. Y. (2004). Factors predicting progression of gastric intestinal metaplasia: results of a randomised trial on *Helicobacter pylori* eradication. *Gut, 53*(9), 1244–1249.

Malfertheiner, P., Megraud, F., O'Morain, C., Bazzoli, F., El-Omar, E., Graham, D., . . . Kuipers, E. J. (2007). *Helicobacter pylori:* Current concepts in the management of *Helicobacter pylori* infection: the Maastricht III Consensus Report. *Gut, 56*(6), 772–781. doi: 10.1136/gut.2006.101634

McQuaid, K. R. (2009). Gastrointestinal disorders. In S. J. McPhee & M. A. Papadakis (Eds.), *Current medical diagnosis and treatment 2010* (49th ed.). New York City, NY: McGraw-Hill.

Miceli, E., Lenti, M. V., Padula, O., Luinetti, C., Vattiato, C., Monti, C. M., . . . Corrazza, G. R. (2012). Common features of patients with autoimmune atrophic gastritis. *Clinical Gastroenterology and Hepatology, 10*(7), 812–814. doi:10.1016/j.cgh.2012.02.018

Müller, M., Gockel, I., Konig, J., Kuhr, K., & Eckardt, V. F. (2011). Long-term recurrence rates following dilation of symptomatic Schatzki rings. *Digestive Diseases and Sciences, 56*(5), 1432–1437. doi:10.1007/s10620-010-1427-7

Pilotto, A., Maggi, S., Noale, M., Franceschi, M., Parisi, G., & Crepaldi, G. (2011). Association of upper gastrointestinal symptoms with functional and clinical characteristics in elderly. *World Journal of Gastroenterology, 17*(25), 3020–3026.

Pilotto, A., Sancarlo, D., Addante, F., Scarcelli, C., & Franceschi, M. (2010). Non-steroidal anti-inflammatory drug use in the elderly. *Surgical Oncology, 19*(3), 167–172.

Sepulveda, A. R., & Patil, M. (2008). Practical approach to the pathologic diagnosis of gastritis. *Archives of Pathology & Laboratory Medicine, 132*(10), 1586–1593.

Weck, M. N., Gao, L., & Brenner, H. (2009). *Helicobacter pylori* infection and chronic atrophic gastritis: associations according to severity of disease. *Epidemiology, 20*(4), 569–574.

Gastroenteritis

DuPont, H. L. (1997). Guidelines on acute infectious diarrhea in adults. The Practice Parameters Committee of the American College of Gastroenterology. *The American Journal of Gastroenterology. 92*(11), 1962–1975.

Keuhn, B. (2012). Gastroenteritis related deaths increase. *Journal of the American Medical Association, 307*(16), 1683–1683. doi: 10.1001/jama.2012.510

Monroe, S. S. (2011). Control and prevention of viral gastroenteritis. *Emerging Infectious Diseases, 17*(8), 1347–1348. doi:10.3201/eid1708.110824

Murphy, M. S. (1998). Guidelines for managing acute gastroenteritis based on a systematic review of published research. *Archives of Diseases in Childhood, 79*(3), 279–284.

Rueben, D., Herr, K., Pacala, J., Pollock, B., Potter, J., & Semla, T. (2008). Gastrointestinal diseases. In *Geriatrics at your fingertips* (10th ed., pp. 96–97). New York, City NY: American Geriatrics Society.

Gastroesophageal Reflux Disease

Furuta, K., Kushiyama, Y., Kawashima, K., Shibagaki, K., Komazawa, Y., Fujishiro, H., . . . Kinoshita, Y. (2012). Comparisons of symptoms reported by elderly and non-elderly patients with GERD. *Journal of Gastroenterology, 47*(2), 144–149. doi:10.1007/s00535-011-0476-9

Gawron, A. J., Rothe, J., Fought, A. J., Fareeduddin, A., Toto, E., Boris, L., . . . Pandolfino, J. E. (2012). Many patients continue using proton pump inhibitors after negative results from tests for reflux disease. *Clinical Gastroenterology and Hepatology, 10*(6), 620–625.

Hart, A. M. (2013). Evidence-based recommendations for GERD treatment. *Nurse Practitioner. 38*(8), 26–34. doi:10.1097/01.NPR.0000431881.25563.84

Kahrilas, P. J., Shaheen, N. J., Vaezi, M. F., Hiltz, S. W., Black, E., Modlin, I. M., . . . American Gastroenterological Association. (2008). American Gastroenterological Association Medical Position Statement on the management of gastroesophageal reflux disease. *Gastroenterology, 135*(4), 1383–1391, 1391.e1-5.

Katz, P. O., Gerson, L. B., & Vela, M. F. (2012). Guidelines for the diagnosis and management of gastroesophageal reflux disease. *The American Journal of Gastroenterology, 108*(3), 308–328. doi: 10.1038/ajg.2012.444. Retrieved from http://d2j7fjepcxuj0a.cloudfront.net/wp-content/uploads/2013/03/ACG_Guideline_GERD_March_2013.pdf

Kubo, A., Cook, M. B., Shaheen, N. J., Vaughan, T. L., Whiteman, D. C., Murray, L., & Corely, D. A. (2013). Sex-specific associations between body mass index, waist circumference and the risk of Barret's oesophagus: a pooled analysis from the international BEACON consortium. *Gut.* Published Online: January 26, 2013. doi: 10.1136/gutjnl-2012-303753

Müller, M., Gockel, I., Konig, J., Kuhr, K., & Eckardt, V. F. (2011). Long-term recurrence rates following dilation of symptomatic Schatzki rings. *Digestive Diseases and Sciences, 56*(5), 1432–1437. doi:10.1007/s10620-010-1427-7

Patrick, L. (2011). Gastroesophageal reflux disease (GERD): a review of conventional and alternative treatments. *Alternative Medicine Review, 16*(2), 116–133.

Poh, C., Navarro-Rodriguez, T., & Fass, R. (2010). Review: treatment of gastroesophageal reflux disease in the elderly. *American Journal of Medicine, 123*(6), 496–501. doi:http://dx.doi.org/10.1016/j.amjmed.2009.07.036

Richter, J. E. (1996). Typical and atypical presentations of gastroesophageal reflux disease. The role of esophageal testing in diagnosis and management. *Gastroenterology Clinics of North America, 25*(1), 75–102.

Sandler, R. S., Everhart, J. E., Donowitz, M., Adams, E., Cronin, K., Goodman, C., . . . Rubin R. (2002). The burden of selected digestive diseases in the United States. *Gastroenterology, 122*(5), 1500–1511.

Shams, D., Siddiqui, N. H., & Heif, M. N. (2009). Gastroesophageal reflux disease in older adults. *Clinical Geriatrics, 17*(3), 32–37.

Sharma, P., Wani, S., Romero, Y., Johnson, D., & Hamilton, F. (2008). Racial and geographic issues in gastroesophageal reflux disease. *The American Journal of Gastroenterology, 103*(11), 2669–2680. doi: 10.1111/j.1572-0241.2008.02089.x

University of Michigan Health System. (2007). UMHS GERD guideline (p. 10). Retrieved May 4, 2012, from www.med.umich.edu

University of Michigan Health System. (2012). Gastroesophageal reflux disease (GERD). Ann Arbor, MI: University of Michigan Health System.

Vakil, N., van Zanten, S. V., Kahrilas, P., Dent, J., Jones, R., & Global Consensus Group. (2006). The Montreal definition and classification of gastroesophageal reflux disease: a global evidence-based consensus. *American Journal of Gastroenterology, 101*(8), 1900–1920.

Hernia

Altom, L. K., Snyder, C. W., Gray, S. H., Graham, L. A., Vick, C. C., & Hawn, M. T. (2011). Outcomes of emergent incisional hernia repair. *The American Surgeon, 77*(8), 971–976.

Amerson, J. R. (1990). Inguinal canal and hernia examination. In H. K. Walker, W. D. Hall, & J. W. Hurst (Eds.), *Clinical methods: the history, physical, and laboratory examinations* (3rd ed., pp. 484–485). Boston, MA: Butterworths.

Burkhardt, J. H., Arshanskiy, Y., Munson, J. L., & Scholz, F. J. (2011). Diagnosis of inguinal region hernias with axial CT: the lateral crescent sign and other key findings. *Radiogrpahics, 31*(2), E1–E12. doi: 10.1148/rg.312105129

Eker, H. H., van Ramshorst, G. H., de Goede, B., Tilanus, H. W., Metselaar, H. J., deMan, R.A., . . . Kazemier, G. (2011). A prospective study on elective umbilical hernia repair in patients with liver cirrhosis and ascites. *Surgery, 150*(3), 542–546. doi:10.1016/j.surg.2011.02.026

Fitzgibbons, R. J., Jr., Giobbie-Hurder, A., Gibbs, J. O., Dunlop, D. D., Reda, D. J., McCarthy, M., Jr., . . Jonasson O. (2006). Watchful waiting vs. repair of inguinal hernia in minimally symptomatic men: a randomized clinical trial. *Journal of the American Medical Association, 295*(3), 285–292.

Goroll, A. H. G. (2009). Approach to the patient with an external hernia. In A. H. G. Goroll & A. G. Mulley (Eds.), *Primary care medicine: an office approach* (6th ed.). Philadelphia, PA: Lippincott Williams & Wilkins.

Greenfield, L. J. (2001). *Review for surgery: scientific principles and practice.* Philadelphia, PA: Lippincott Williams & Wilkins.

Haraguchi, M., Matsuo, S., Kanetaka, K., Tokai, H., Azuma, T., Yamaguchi, S., & Kanematsu, T. (2007). Obturator hernia in an ageing society. *Annals of Academy of Medicine of Singapore, 36*(6), 413–415.

LeBlond, R. F., Brown, D. D., & DeGowin, R. L. (2009). *DeGowin's diagnostic examination* (9th ed.). New York City, NY: McGraw-Hill Medical.

LeBlanc, K. E., LeBlanc, L. L., & LeBlanc, K. A. (2013). Inguinal hernias: diagnosis and management. *American Family Physician, 87*(12), 844–848.

Sevonius, D., Gunnarsson, U., Nordin, P., Nilsson, E., & Sandblom, G. (2011). Recurrent groin hernia surgery. *British Journal of Surgery, 98*(10), 1489–1494. doi:10.1002/bjs.7559

Irritable Bowel Syndrome

Agrawal, A., Khan, M. H., & Whorwell, P. J. (2009). Irritable bowel syndrome in the elderly: an overlooked problem? *Digestive and Liver Disease, 41*(10), 721–724. doi:10.1016/j.did.2009.03.011

Bohn, L., Storsrud, S., Tornblom, H., Bengtsson, U. & Simren, M. (2013). Self-reported food-related gastrointestinal symptoms in IBS are common and associated with more severe symptoms and reduced quality of life. *American Journal of Gastroenterology, 108*(5), 634–641. doi: 10.038/ajg.2013.105

Drossman, D. A., Chey, W. D., Johanson, J. F., Fass, R., Scott, C., Panas, R., & Ueno, R. (2009). Clinical trial: lubiprostone in patients with constipation-associated irritable bowel syndrome—results of two randomized, placebo-controlled studies. *Alimentary Pharmacology and Therapeutics, 29*(3), 329–341. doi: 10.1111/j.1365-2036.2008.03881.x

Drossman, D. A., Ringel, Y., Vogt, B. A., Leserman, J., Lin, W., Smith, J. K., & Whitehead, W. (2003). Alterations of brain activity associated with resolution of emotional distress and pain in a case of severe irritable bowel syndrome. *Gastroenterology, 124*(3), 754–761.

Furman, D. L., & Cash, B. D. (2011). The role of diagnostic testing in irritable bowel syndrome. *Gastroenterology Clinics of North America, 40*(1), 105–119.

Heitkemper, M., Cain, K. C., Shulman, R., Burr, R., Poppe, A., & Jarrett, M. (2011). Subtypes of irritable bowel syndrome based on abdominal pain/discomfort severity and bowel pattern. *Digestive Diseases and Sciences, 56*(7), 2050–2058. doi:10.1007/s10620-011-1567-4

Kay, L. (1994). Prevalence, incidence and prognosis of gastrointestinal symptoms in a random sample of an elderly population. *Age and Aging, 23*(2), 146–149.

Lembo, A. J., Johanson, J. F., Parkman, H. P., Rao, S. S., Miner, P. B., Jr., & Ueno, R. (2011). Long-term safety and effectiveness of lubiprostone, a chloride channel (ClC-2) activator, in patients with chronic idiopathic constipation. *Digestive Disease and Sciences, 56*(9), 2639–2645. doi: 10.1007/s10620-011-1801-0

Lin, H. C. (2004). Small intestine bacterial overgrowth: a framework for understanding irritable bowel syndrome. *Journal of the American Medical Association, 292*(7), 852–858.

Menees, S. B., Maneerattannaporn, M., Kim, H. M., & Chey, W. D. (2012). The efficacy and safety of rifaximin for the irritable bowel syndrome: a systematic review and meta-analysis. *American Journal of Gastroenterology, 107*(1), 28–35. doi:10.1038/ajg.2011.355

Minocha, A. (2008). Irritable bowel syndrome in the older patient. Retrieved May 13, 2012, from www.clinicalgeriatrics.com/articles/Irritable-Bowel-Syndrome-Older-Patient

Nellesen, D., Chawla, A., Oh, D. L., Weissman, T., Lavins, B. J., & Murray, C. W. (2013). Comorbidities in patients with irritable bowel syndrome with constipation or chronic idiopathic constipation: a review of the literature from the past decade. *Post Graduate Medicine,125*(2), 40–50. doi: 10.3810/pgm.2013.03.2640

Pimentel, M., Lembo, A., Chey, W. D., Zakko, S., Ringel, Y., Yu, J., . . . Forbes, W. P. (2011). Rifaximin therapy for patients with irritable bowel syndrome without constipation. *New England Journal of Medicine, 364*(1), 22–32.

Liver Cancer

Bruix, J., & Sherman, M. (2011). AASLD Practice Guideline, management of hepatocellular carcinoma: an update. *Hepatology, 53*(3), 1020–1022.

Schwartz, J. M., & Carithers, R. L. (2012). Clinical features and diagnosis of primary hepatocellular carcinoma. *UpToDate.* Retrieved from www.uptodate.com

Sherman, M. (2012). Prevention of hepatocellular carcinoma and recommendations for surveillance in adults with chronic liver disease. *UpToDate.* Retrieved from www.uptodate.com

Sterling, R. K., Wright, E. C., Morgan, T. R., Seeff, L. B., Hoefs, J. C., DiBisceglie, A. M., . . . Lok, A. S. (2012). Frequency of elevated hepatocellular carcinoma (HCC) biomarkers in patients with advanced hepatitis C. *American Journal of Gastroenterology, 107*(1), 64–74.

Nephrolithiasis

Becker, M. A. (2011). Clinical manifestations and diagnosis of gout. *UpToDate.* Retrieved from www.uptodate.com/contents/clinical-manifestations-and-diagnosis-of-gout?view

Brener, Z. Z., Winchester, J. F., Salman, H., & Bergman, M. (2011). Nephrolithiasis: evaluation and management. *Southern Medical Journal, 104*(2), 133–139.

Curhan, G. (2009). Nephrolithiasis. In A. Greenberg (Ed.), *Primer on kidney diseases* (5th ed., pp. 382–388). Philadelphia, PA: Saunders Elsevier.

Curhan, G. C., Aronson, M. D., & Preminger, G. M. (2011). Diagnosis and acute management of suspected nephrolithiasis in adults. *UpToDate.* Retrieved from www.uptodate.com/contents/diagnosis-and-acute-management-of-suspected-nephrolithiasis-in-adults?view

Hall, P. (2009). Nephrolithiasis: treatment, causes and prevention. *Cleveland Clinic Journal of Medicine, 76*(10), 583–591. Retrieved from www.ccjm.org/content/76/10/583.long

Pietrow, P. K., & Karellas, M. E. (2006). Medical management of common urinary calculi. *American Family Physician, 74*(1), 86–94. Retrieved from www.aafp.org/afp/2006/0701/p86.html?printable=afp

Wolf, J. S. (2012). Nephrolithiasis clinical presentation. *Medscape.* Retrieved from http://emedicine.medscape.com/article/437096-clinical

Nonalcoholic Fatty Liver Disease

Adams, L. A., & Angulo, P. (2006). Treatment of non-alcoholic fatty liver disease. *Postgraduate Medicine, 82*(967), 315–332. doi:10.1136/pgmj.2005.042200

Bayard, M., Holt, J., & Boroughs, E. (2006). Non-alcoholic fatty liver disease. *American Family Physician, 73*(11), 1962–1968.

Caballería, L., Pera, G., Auladell, M. A., Torán, P., Muñoz, L., Miranda, D., . . . Aizpurua, M. M. (2010). Prevalence and factors associated with the presence of nonalcoholic fatty liver disease in an adult population in Spain. *European Journal of Gastroenterology & Hepatology, 22*(1), 24–32. doi:10.1097/MEG.0b013e32832fcdf0

Croke, B., & Sampson, D. (2012). Nonalcoholic fatty liver disease: implications for clinical practice and health promotion. *Journal for Nurse Practitioners, 8*(1), 45–50.

Ekstedt, M., Franzén, L. F., Mathiesen, U. L., Holmqvist, M., Bodemar, G., & Kechagias, S. (2007). Statins in non-alcoholic fatty liver disease and chronically elevated enzymes: a histopathological follow-up study. *Journal of Hepatology, 47*(1), 135–141.

Farrell, G., & Larter, C. Z. (2006). Nonalcoholic fatty liver disease: from steatosis to cirrhosis. *Hepatology, 43*(2), 4999–5112.

Ghamar-Chehreh, M., Amini, M., Khedmat, H., Daraei, F., Mohtashami, R., & Karbasi, A. (2012). Comparative effectiveness of ezetimibe in improving lipid profile in non-alcoholic fatty liver disease patients: statins still rule. *International Journal of Biology, 4*(2), 184–190. doi:10.5539/ijb.v4n2p184

Greenberger, N. J., Blumberg, R. S., & Burakoff, R. (2009). *Current diagnosis and treatment: gastroenterology, hepatology, and endoscopy* (3rd ed.). New York City, NY: McGraw-Hill.

Hamaguchi, M., Kojima, T., Ohbora, A., Takeda, N., Fukui, M., & Kato, T. (2012). Aging is a risk factor of nonalcoholic fatty liver disease in premenopausal women. *World Journal of Gastroenterology, 18*(3), 237–243.

Kashi, M., Torres, D. M., & Harrison, S. A. (2008). Current and emerging therapies in nonalcoholic fatty liver disease. *Seminars in Liver Disease, 28*(4), 396–406. doi:10.1055/s-1091984

Miglio, F., Rovati, L. C., Santoro, A., & Setnikar, I. (2000). Efficacy and safety of oral betaine glucuronate in non-alcoholic steatohepatitis. A double-blind, randomized, parallel-group, placebo-controlled prospective clinical study. *Arzneimittelforschung, 50*(8), 722–727.

Moore, B. (2010). Symposium 1: overnutrition: consequences and solutions. Non-alcoholic fatty liver disease: the hepatic consequence of obesity and the metabolic syndrome. *Proceedings of the Nutrition Society, 69*(1), 211–220.

Parrish, C. R. (2010, February). Nutritional recommendations for patients with non-alcoholic fatty liver disease: an evidence based review. *Practical Gastroenterology,* pp. 8–16.

Petta, S., Camma, C., Cabibi, D., Di Marco, V., & Craxi, A. (2011). Hyperuricemia is associated with histological liver damage in patients with non-alcoholic fatty liver disease. *Alimentary Pharmacology & Therapeutic, 34*(7), 757–766. doi:10.1111/j.1365-2036.2011.04788

Vernon, G., Baranova, A., & Younossi, Z. M. (2011). Systematic review: the epidemiology and natural history of non-alcoholic fatty liver disease and non-alcoholic steatohepatitis in adults. *Alimentary Pharmacology & Therapeutics, 34*(3), 274–285.

Wilkins, T., Tadkod, A., Hepbrun, I., & Schade, R. E. (2013). Nonalcoholic fatty liver disease: diagnosis and management. *American Family Physician, 88*(1), 36–42.

Peptic Ulcer Disease

Barkun, A., & Leontiadis, G. (2010). Systematic review of the symptom burden, quality of life impairment and costs associated with peptic ulcer disease. *American Journal of Medicine, 123*(4), 358–366.

Chey, W., Wong, B. C., & Practice Parameters Committee of the American College of Gastroenterology. (2007). American College of Gastroenterology guideline on the management of helicobacter pylori infection. *American Journal of Gastroenterology, 102*(8), 1808–1825. doi:10.1111/j.1572-0241.2007.01393.x

Cohen, J., Safdi, M. A., Deal, S. E., Baron, T. H., Chak, A., Hoffman, B., . . . Pike, I. M. (2006). Quality indicators for esophagogastroduodenoscopy. *Gastrointestinal Endoscopy, 63*(Suppl. 4), S10–S15.

Collaza, S. (2012). Helicobacter pylori: toward effective eradication. *Clinical Advisor.* Retrieved from http://www.clinicaladvisor.com/helicobacter-pylori-toward-effective-eradication/article/231156/#

Crosby, K., & Dexter, K. (2013). Clinical evaluation of peptic ulcer disease. *The Clinical Advisor, 16*(6), 42–48.

Ford, A. C., Delaney, B., Forman, D., Moayyedi, P., & Ford, A. C. (2011). Eradication therapy for peptic ulcer disease in *Helicobacter pylori* positive patients (Cochrane review). In *The Cochrane Library 2011,* Issue 1. Chichester, UK: John Wiley & Sons, Ltd.

Lockrey, G., & St. Lim, L. (2011). Peptic ulcer disease in older people. *Journal of Pharmacy Practice & Research, 41*(1), 58–61.

McQuaid, K. R. (2010). Gastrointestinal disorders. In: S. J. McPhee & M. A. Papadakis (Eds.), *Current Medical Diagnosis & Treatment.* (49th ed.). New York City, NY: McGraw-Hill Companies.

Ramakrishnan, K., & Salinas, R. C. (2007). Peptic ulcer disease. *American Family Physician. 76*(7), 1005–1012.

chapter 11

Urological and Gynecological Disorders

Lori Martin-Plank

ASSESSMENT

Changes in the female reproductive system occur well before the life stage of older adulthood, considering that the average age of menopause is 51 years. A plethora of choices are now available to women in this age group for prevention and management of postmenopausal problems such as atrophic vaginitis, incontinence, osteoporosis, dyslipidemia, and cardiac problems. The nurse practitioner will likely encounter a variety of physical findings during assessment of the older female patient, based on these emerging choices. A comprehensive medication history is very important to identify medications or dietary supplements that affect the reproductive system, including hormone replacement therapy and vaginal applications. Equally important is a thorough history, including family history of breast or reproductive organ cancer in a first-degree family member or in the patient herself. The patient should be questioned about any prior breast surgery, including surgery for breast augmentation or reduction. History of mammograms and gynecological examination with a Papanicolaou (Pap) smear (unless the patient has had a total hysterectomy, including removal of the cervical cuff) should be included in the assessment process. Does the patient do breast self-examination? Has she ever discovered a lump or had a biopsy or ultrasound? The patient should also be questioned about breast pain, nipple discharge, rash, trauma, or swelling.

Normal aging changes in the female breast include the atrophy of glandular breast tissue and replacement with connective tissue. There may be a decrease in breast size or breasts may become pendulous and flabby owing to loss of elasticity. Areolar nipple ducts may be palpable, feeling stringy and firm. Nipple retraction may result from breast atrophy; however, the possibility of malignant changes causing nipple retraction must be ruled out. The inframammary ridge assumes more prominence. Axillary hair decreases.

Physical examination of the female breasts includes inspection for symmetry, lumps, dimpling, or nipple retraction. Optimally, the patient should be sitting, with her hands placed on her hips, raising them over her head during the inspection. Patients with large, pendulous breasts should lean forward, so the examiner can observe for attachment to chest wall or retraction; a bimanual hand technique can be used to examine their breasts at this time also. While the patient's arms are at her sides, the examiner palpates the axillary area for lymphadenopathy, probing deeply while manipulating the patient's arm for maximal access. The patient is then positioned supine with a small towel or pillow under the side to be examined and the corresponding arm placed over the head. Using the finger pads, the examiner palpates in one of three patterns:

- Concentrically from the nipple to the periphery, including the breast tail
- Extending out from the nipple in a pattern similar to spokes on a wheel
- In a linear pattern from top to bottom, starting medially, moving laterally with each line

Breast self-examination technique may also be taught at this time, if the patient desires.

Age-related changes in the male breast include gynecomastia in some patients. Examination of the male breast and axillary areas follows the same sequence as for the female breast but in an abbreviated format, because less breast tissue exists.

Assessment of the urogenital system of older men and women includes a complete sexual history. Sexual orientation, patterns of sexual expression, current or desired activity, protective practices to avoid transmission of sexually transmitted infections (STIs) including HIV, past or recent history of STIs, number of current partners, and problems with expression of sexuality should be explored. Review of the medication regimen for potential effects on libido and impotence is important.

If the patient is in a community living situation, are opportunities provided for privacy and intimacy? If medications or medical problems interfere with sexual expression, what interventions are possible? Age-related changes in the reproductive system of both sexes do not interfere with libido and sexual satisfaction, although physiological response time is slower and more prolonged, and orgasmic response is more generalized.

Assessment of the genitoreproductive system of the older female patient includes historical elements such as menarche, obstetrical history, menopause, history of STIs including herpes, condyloma, surgeries, or malignancies. Medication history and sexual history were discussed previously. The patient should be questioned about urinary symptoms and about any vulvovaginal itching, discharge, or bleeding.

Normal aging changes in the female genitoreproductive system include atrophic changes in most structures. Pubic hair becomes gray and sparse, and the labia flatten. Vaginal epithelium is thinner, drier, and itchy, with less rugae; decreased secretions and alkalinity predispose patients to painful intercourse, friability, and vaginitis. The vagina becomes shorter, narrower, and less elastic; tissue is pale pink and shiny. Sexual abstinence or infrequent intercourse intensifies atrophic changes. Undergarments often irritate sensitive external structures. The uterus shrinks, and the ovaries, which atrophy, are not palpable. The pelvic floor muscles, sacral ligaments, and other supporting structures relax, frequently leading to organ (bladder, rectum, uterus) prolapse.

Examination of the female genitoreproductive system is the same in older patients as in younger patients. With an older patient, before positioning her in the lithotomy position with stirrups, external inspection may be performed by having the patient flex one knee and abduct it. Patients with arthritis may be helped by taking pain medication before the examination. Equipment should be assembled and ready, to limit time spent in the stirrups. Lubrication of the speculum with water before insertion is important for comfort. The choice of speculum is an individual one; the Pederson speculum, with narrow blades, is frequently chosen for virginal or postmenopausal women with a narrow introitus. Examination may reveal relaxation of internal organs, including a cystocele or rectocele. The cervix, which appears pale and shiny, may be flush with the vaginal mucosa or may protrude into the vagina with uterine prolapse. On bimanual examination, the ovaries should not be palpable and the uterus is small and firm. Some patients may require local hormone application before examination. Pap smears are no longer recommended for women over 65 years who have had adequate prior screening and are not at high risk for cervical cancer (U.S. Preventive Services Task Force [USPSTF], 2012).

The genitourinary and reproductive systems of the older male patient undergo more gradual changes than those of the older female patient. Pubic hair turns gray and becomes sparse. Penile size decreases slightly. Scrotal contents hang lower; the testes decrease in size and firmness, and less sperm are produced owing to the increase in connective tissue in the tubules. Testosterone production declines slowly, resulting in slower arousal and more prolonged erection before ejaculation. Ejaculation is less intense and shorter, with less seminal fluid and rapid detumescence. Prostatic tissue enlargement is common, frequently resulting in nocturia, urinary hesitancy, decreased urine flow, retention (sometimes with overflow incontinence), and less forceful ejaculation.

When taking the history related to the genitourinary and reproductive systems of the older male patient, ask about difficulty urinating, hesitancy, decreased force of stream, frequency with decreased amount, dribbling, or nocturia. If nocturia is present, establish its onset and frequency, and explore possible contributing factors other than prostatic enlargement. These include diuretics, caffeine or alcohol ingestion, increased fluid consumption in the evening, habit of frequent urination, mild heart failure, or dependent edema. Other pertinent questions concern urinary symptoms such as frequency, urgency, dysuria, hematuria, or documented urinary tract infection (UTI).

Examination of the urogenital system of the older male patient is essentially the same as for a younger male patient. The normal changes of aging have been described earlier. Examination of the prostate is conducted with the rectal examination, which begins with inspection and palpation of the genitalia for lesions, proceeding to palpation of the inguinal canal for hernia and then to palpation of the inguinofemoral areas for lymphadenopathy. For examination of the prostate through the rectum, the patient is placed in the left lateral decubitus position, or standing and leaning forward over the examination table with toes pointed inward, for easier access to the anorectal area. The examiner uses a well-lubricated, gloved finger, advanced above the anal canal, to palpate the anterior wall of the rectum for the prostate gland. The gland is normally heart shaped with a central groove that can be felt. The normal surface is smooth, elastic, and nontender on palpation. Absence of the central groove in a smooth gland or protrusion of the gland more than 1 cm into the rectum is typical of benign prostatic hypertrophy. A hard, irregular nodule may indicate carcinoma. Either finding requires further workup.

ATROPHIC VAGINITIS

Signal symptoms: Vaginal dryness, dysuria, vulvar and vaginal itching, urinary frequency, blood-tinged vaginal discharge, dyspareunia.

Description: Atrophic vaginitis, also called vulvovaginal atrophy, urogenital atrophy, or adhesive vaginitis, is a noninfectious, sometimes inflammatory, postmenopausal process in which the female genital and urological tissue thins and becomes fragile. Changes in vaginal pH due to a hypoestrogenic state present a more favorable environment for bacterial invasion by trichomonas, candida, and bacterial vaginosis as well as by resident skin and rectal flora. Dysuria, increase in UTIs, and urinary frequency, as well as dyspareunia, are potential consequences (Bachmann & Santen, 2011a). Up to 70% of women do not address this issue with health-care providers due to its personal nature (Nappi & Kokot-Kierepa, 2010; Pearson, 2011; Reimer & Johnson, 2011).

Etiology: Estrogen deprivation leads to atrophy of the vaginal and vulvar epithelium. Atrophic vaginitis, a common disorder in postmenopausal women, can be surgically induced, created by the natural aging process, or brought on through primary ovarian failure.

Occurrence: This disorder affects all postmenopausal women, to some degree, unless estrogen replacement therapy is provided. Women who experience earlier menopause, have diabetes, or have lower body mass may experience more pronounced symptoms (Pearson, 2011).

Age: Atrophic vaginitis is predominantly a problem of postmenopausal women. The average age of natural menopause in the United States is 52.5 years.

Gender: Occurs in women only.

Ethnicity: Not significant.

Contributing factors: Estrogen-deficient states accompanying metabolic disorders and changes of normal aging create the risk of atrophic vaginitis. Changes in vaginal epithelium and pH caused by estrogen deficiency provide an environment in which pathogenic bacteria and fungi can flourish. Drugs also may alter vaginal secretions and clinical findings (Bachmann & Santen, 2011b).

Signs and symptoms: Itching, discomfort, burning, dyspareunia, and, at times, a thin blood-tinged vaginal discharge or bleeding after intercourse as the epithelium thins characterize atrophic vaginitis. As vaginal secretions decrease, vaginal dryness can be another bothersome symptom. Complaints of urinary frequency, urgency, and stress incontinence are common. On physical examination, signs include pale, dry, nonrugated vaginal walls with patches of erythema or petechiae or both. The vaginal canal is short and narrow. A watery white vaginal discharge without foul odor may be found. Estrogen deficiency can lead to loss of uterine support and subsequent uterine descensus (Tan, Bradshaw, & Carr, 2012).

Diagnostic tests:

Atrophic Vaginitis Diagnostic Tests	
TEST	**RESULTS INDICATING DISORDER**
Pelvic examination with speculum examination and Pap smear (may do wet mount and KOH preparation if infection is suspected)	Pale, dry, nonrugated vaginal mucosa; Pap smear results should be normal; vaginal pH by litmus paper will be ≥5.
Urinalysis to rule out UTI if symptoms	Variable; if dipstick is positive for white blood cells and nitrites, a culture and sensitivity should be done. If negative, UTI is not cause of symptoms.

KOH, potassium hydroxide; *Pap,* Papanicolaou; *UTI,* urinary tract infection.

Differential diagnosis:

- Malignancy—both atrophic vaginitis and malignancy such as cervical cancer can present with spotting. An endometrial biopsy and a Pap smear would be done if malignancy is suspected, and this would differentiate malignancy from atrophic vaginitis.
- Lichen sclerosus—whitish lesions on the vulva, squamous cells involved, may be immune mediated. Biopsy is needed to diagnose.
- Lichen simplex chronicus—pruritus results in scratching and thickened skin plaques or patches in the area (as opposed to thin skin in atrophic vaginitis). A potassium hydroxide (KOH) wet mount or fungal culture may be done to rule out candidiasis.
- Squamous cell hyperplasia—pruritus results in scratching and inflammatory changes in squamous cells of the vulvar area seen on biopsy.
- Lichen planus—papular, purple lesions that are pruritic; thought to be immunological in origin. Biopsy and direct immunofluorescence study show clumps of immunoglobulin M (IgM) and complement blended with dead keratinocytes.
- UTI.
- STIs and other infections, such as *Candida albicans* and bacterial vaginosis (Samra-Latif, 2012)—*Candida* is a fungal organism that presents as pruritis, burning, and with thick white discharge. Bacterial vaginosis is also pruritic with a thin, white, adherent discharge and may have a fishy odor when mixed with KOH, referred to as a whiff test. Wet mount with KOH will show clue cells in bacterial vaginosis and hyphae in candidiasis.

Treatment: First-line treatment of dryness and dyspareunia associated with atrophic vaginitis includes nonhormonal lubricants and moisturizers. Use of vaginal dilators and/or sexual activity also promotes a healthy vaginal epithelium (Bachmann & Santen, 2011b). If this is unsuccessful in providing symptom relief, low-dose vaginal estrogen in the form of tablets, cream, or vaginal ring is the preferred treatment. Vagifem is an estrogen-containing tablet that is inserted vaginally daily for 1 week, followed by maintenance dosing of twice weekly. Estring is an estrogen-containing vaginal ring that continuously releases small amounts of the hormone; it is used for a 90-day period and is left in place during sexual activity. Premarin vaginal cream is inserted every other day or daily for a 3-week cycle, then off for 1 week, then resumed again. This is done for 3 months, and the patient is then reevaluated.

Endometrial biopsy may be required periodically to detect hyperplasia (Samra-Latif, 2012). Hormonal modalities should only be used after careful evaluation of the patient for risks and benefits and discussion with the patient. Initial doses are higher, then taper off in frequency. Women requiring oral hormone replacement therapy should be referred for gynecological consultation. Women with a history of breast cancer should also be referred to a specialist. Most providers do not add an oral progestin for those treated with low-dose vaginal therapy (Bachmann & Santen, 2011b).

Follow-up: Expected response is quick, with resolution of symptoms within 2 to 3 months. If this does not occur, the patient should be reevaluated and reexamined for other causes of symptoms. Because topical estrogen is absorbed and can cause systemic effects, patients should have a follow-up visit 1 to 2 months after beginning vaginal drug therapy. Patients treated with continuous hormone replacement therapy need regular return visits every 3 months to check side effects, blood pressure, and response to therapy. When efficacy is achieved, treatment can be discontinued. If symptoms recur, reinstitute short-term treatment.

Sequelae: With changes in the vaginal pH of postmenopausal women (pH > 5.0) and this loss of normal acidity, bacterial species grow in the vagina that are not found there commonly. Infections can become frequent and chronic.

Prevention/prophylaxis: Recognition of early signs and symptoms of atrophic vaginitis can lead to the individual's seeking treatment to prevent atrophy, dryness, infections, urinary and urethral problems, and sexual dysfunction. Intermittent use of topical vaginal estrogen can prevent recurrence of atrophic vaginitis, provide adequate levels of hormone, and give soothing relief. Use of a vaginal lubricant in conjunction with a regular vaginal moisturizer also may be helpful, especially before coitus.

Referral: Gynecology referral is appropriate for patients who do not respond to treatment or have vaginal bleeding. Patients who present with severe estrogen depletion, evidenced by marked perineal and vaginal changes, along with pelvic floor relaxation, need gynecological referral before initiating topical treatment.

Education: Use water-soluble lubricants for patients with atrophic vaginitis. Counsel the patient regarding the benefits of regular sexual activity. Identify age-related difficulty associated with intravaginal application of creams and address these needs with sensitivity.

CLINICAL RECOMMENDATION	EVIDENCE RATING	REFERENCES
Daily and twice-weekly use of low-dose conjugated estrogens (CE) cream was equally effective in relieving symptoms of vulvovaginal atrophy. Both regimens showed endometrial safety and sustained efficacy during 1 year of therapy.	A	Bachmann et al. (2009)
Vaginal estrogen therapy can be recommended for the prevention of recurrent urinary tract infections in postmenopausal women.	A	Urogenital Health (2009)
Creams, pessaries, tablets, and the estradiol vaginal ring are equally effective for the symptoms of vaginal atrophy.	A	Suckling, Kennedy, Lethaby, & Roberts (2010)

A = consistent, good-quality, patient-oriented evidence; B = inconsistent or limited-quality, patient-oriented evidence; C = consensus, disease-oriented evidence, usual practice, expert opinion, or case series. For information about the SORT evidence rating system, go to www.aafp.org/afpsort.xml.

BREAST CANCER

Signal symptoms: None, breast mass.

Description: As of January 2009, approximately 2.7 million women had been diagnosed with breast cancer. In 2012, it was expected that over 229,060 new cases of breast cancer would be diagnosed. Males were expected to represent 2,190 of those new cases, with women representing 226,870. There were expected to be over 39,000 deaths in 2012 from breast cancer (National Cancer Institute, 2012). Over one-half of these cases were expected to occur in women over 65 years old. Breast cancer is estimated to be the leading cancer diagnosis and the second leading cause of cancer deaths in women (National Cancer Institute, 2012). Approximately 89% of women underestimate their risk of developing breast cancer (Katapodi, Dodd, Lee, & Facione, 2009).

Breast cancers are classified as a malignant, neoplastic tumor that starts in the tissue of the breast. The two most common types of breast cancer are lobular and ductal carcinomas, with ductal carcinomas having a higher prevalence; approximately one in five cases of new breast cancers are ductal carcinoma in situ (American Cancer Society, 2011–2012). Breast cancers may be invasive or non-invasive (also called in situ). Lobular carcinomas are considered the noninvasive type. In rare instances, breast cancers may form in other areas of the breast. Some types of these less commonly occurring breast cancers are categorized as inflammatory breast cancer, triple-negative breast cancer, Paget disease of the nipple, Phyllodes tumor, and angiosarcoma (American Cancer Society, 2011–2012). The exact cause of breast cancer is unknown, with environmental and genetic contributions.

Occurrence: One in eight women (12.38%) will develop breast cancer in their lifetime; 124.3 out of 100,000 women develop breast cancer (National Cancer Institute, 2012). Breast cancer was the second most prevalent cancer in females in the United States during 2011 and was predicted to be the most prevalent cancer in women in 2012 (Cancer stats, 2012). One in four cancers in women is breast cancer. There are over 2.6 million breast cancer survivors in the United States (American Cancer Society, 2011–2012). From 2005 to 2008 there was a 0.7% increase in the incidence of breast cancer by race (National Cancer Institute, 2012). Less than 1% of all breast cancers occur in men (Mattarella, 2010).

Age: The median age of diagnosis of cancer is 61 years of age with the median age of death being 68 years of age. An increase in age is directly proportional to an increase in breast cancer diagnosis. Based on data from 2005 to 2009, 0% of cancer diagnoses were in women under 20 years old, 1.8% were in women from 20 to 34 years old, 9.9% were in women from 35 to 44 years old, 22.5% were in women from 45 to 54 years old, 24.8% were in women from 55 to 64 years old, 20.0% were in women from 65 to 74 years old, 15.1% were in women from 75 to 84 years old, and 5.7% were in women 85 years and older (National Cancer Institute, 2012). Breast cancer diagnoses increased in women over 50 years, compared to data from 2000–2005. Older women have received less than standard therapy (National Cancer Institute, 2012). They are less likely to undergo measures to preserve the breast and undergo axillary lymph dissection, radiation therapy, and systemic therapy. Women over age 70 are less likely to be enrolled in controlled clinical trials, leading to a decrease in evidence-based guidelines in this age group. Older women have also been found to have higher rates of skin and bone metastasis (Holmes, 1994).

Gender: Being of the female gender is one of the two most significant risk factors for developing breast cancer. An estimated 2190 cases of invasive breast cancer will be diagnosed in men as opposed to 226,870 in women. Approximately 410 men in 2012 were predicted to die from breast cancer compared to 39,510 women. Breast cancer is 100% less likely in men than in women (National Cancer Institute, 2012).

Ethnicity: Breast cancer is slightly more prevalent in white women, yet African American women have a higher mortality rate. After 45 years of age, the higher prevalence shifts to African American women. Incidence data reveal that 127.3 white women, 121.2 black women, 94.5 Asian/Pacific Islander women, 80.6 American Indian women, and 92.7 Hispanic women out of 100,000 suffer from breast cancer. This reflects an increase in the prevalence among minority populations. Mortality data reveal that 23.0 whites, 31.6 blacks, 11.9 Asians/Pacific Islanders, 16.6 American Indians, and 14.9 Hispanics out of 100,000 will die of breast cancer (National Cancer Institute, 2012). This reflects a decrease in mortality rates across races.

Factors that contribute to health-care disparities that exist in cancer are socioeconomic status (education, income, and employment), age, access to and use of health-care services, behaviors, social environment, exposure to carcinogens, and treatment (U.S. Cancer Statistics Working Group, 2010). Breast cancer screenings have been found to be lower among minority, low-income, inner-city women (Smith-Bindman, et al., 2006).

Contributing factors: The major factors that affect cancer risks are age and gender. As age increases, so does cancer risk. Over 99% of new breast cancer diagnoses occur in women (National Cancer Institute, 2012). White women have an increased risk of developing breast cancer until age 45, when black women experience an increase in prevalence. Other contributing factors to the development of breast cancer are family history, accounting for 5% to 10% of breast cancers. Family history is inclusive of a first-degree relative with a diagnosis of breast cancer. It is important to note that risk increases with the number of first-degree relatives diagnosed and the diagnosis of bilateral breast cancer (American Cancer Society, 2011–2012; Henderson et al., 2010; Litton et al., 2009).

A previous diagnosis of breast cancer or atypical cells in the breast increases the probability of further development of breast cancer. These factors include proliferating lesions with and without atypia and lobular carcinoma in situ (Henderson et al., 2010; Litton, 2009).

Inherited genetic mutations increase the risk of breast cancer. Sixty-five percent of women with a BRCA1 mutation will have been diagnosed with breast cancer by age 70. Forty-five percent of women with a BRCA2 mutation will be diagnosed by age 70 (Anderson, 2010; Nattinger, 2010).

Dense breast tissue is another contributing factor to breast cancer. Dense breast tissue decreases the ability to detect masses early (Henderson et al., 2010; Katapodi et al., 2009). Previous chest radiation, for example, for treatment of other cancers, increases the risk of breast cancer (Henderson et al., 2010; Patterson, 2010).

Early menarche and/or late menopause also increases the risk of breast cancer. Nulliparity, childbirth delayed until after age 30, and lack of breastfeeding increase breast cancer risk. These findings are thought to be related to the number of menstrual cycles in the woman's lifetime (American Cancer Society, 2011–2012).

Factors such as alcohol consumption, obesity, inactivity, recent oral contraceptive use, and hormone replacement therapy after menopause, specifically combined hormone therapy, increase the risk of breast cancer (Wishart, 2010). Specific mutations of the BRCA1 and BRCA2 gene increase the risk of breast cancer.

Changes in other genes also increase breast cancer risk, such as the p53 gene, ATM gene, CHEK2, PTEN, CDH1, and STK11 genes, and genetic syndromes such as Peutz-Jeghers, Bannayan-Riley-Ruvalcaba, Cowden, and Li-Fraumeni (American Cancer Society, 2011–2012; Berg, 2009; Henderson et al., 2010; Nattinger, 2010).

Discussion on the association of diet, vitamins, antiperspirants, bras, breast implants, chemicals, induced abortions, tobacco smoke, and night work have not been thoroughly supported in the current research.

A women's risk increases by 50% if she has a first-degree relative diagnosed with breast cancer. Approximately 5% to 10% of breast cancers are linked to a genetic mutation. The most commonly occurring mutation is of the BRCA1 and BRCA2 genes, which are inherited from a parent. Women with these specific genetic mutations have an 80% probability of developing breast cancer during their lifetime. These individuals are diagnosed before menopause. From 70% to 80% of breast cancers in women have no family history of breast cancer. One in 10 men with breast cancer has a BRCA2 mutation, with fewer men having breast cancer as a result of the BRCA1 mutation (U.S. Cancer Statistics Working Group, 2010).

Signs and symptoms: Signs and symptoms of breast cancer range from nonexistent to obvious. Symptoms include a breast lump or mass, bloody nipple discharge, change in the size or shape of the breast, changes of the skin, inverting of the nipple, and changes in the skin texture (e.g., peeling or flaking or redness or pitting over the breast) (Watkins, 2009). Early symptoms of breast cancer are painless; symptoms are usually evident when the cancer grows. Irregularly shaped, painless, hard masses have an increased probability of being cancerous. Due to the spread of cancer to the lymphatic system, a lump or swelling in the axilla should be further evaluated (American Cancer Society, 2011–2012).

Diagnostic tests: A triple assessment is used in the diagnoses of breast cancer. The first stage is history taking and examination, followed by mammography or breast ultrasound. Confirmatory fine-needle aspiration for cytology and core biopsy is the final stage of the triple assessment (Foy & Blowers, 2009).

Mammography, which is a breast x-ray, can be used as a screening or diagnostic tool and has been found to be the most effective resource in diagnosis of breast cancer. This tool is able to diagnose breast cancer much earlier than obvious sign and symptoms. A diagnostic mammogram is used to determine breast disease in women who have breast symptoms or abnormal screening mammography. Screening mammography is used to evaluate women who are asymptomatic; this is done with a two-view x-ray. Women with breast implants need to have an increased number of x-rays to provide a thorough evaluation of the breast tissue. Mammography provides information on calcifications, micro or macro, or masses in the breast. Mammography cannot diagnose breast cancer. This type of screening is ineffective on younger women because the breast tissue is very dense and may obscure masses or tumors. Suspicious findings on mammography must be confirmed by biopsy.

Magnetic resonance imaging (MRI) is also used for women at high risk for cancer in conjunction with mammography. MRIs have an increased sensitivity to detecting breast cancer but also lead to an increase rate of false positives. Breast mass biopsy is used for confirmation.

Excisional biopsy or large core biopsy is recommended for all palpable, solid lesions. Image-guided large core breast biopsy is the choice for nonpalpable lesions and abnormal breast calcification (Agency for Healthcare Research and Quality [AHRQ], 2012)

Diagnostic criteria established by the American College of Radiology Breast Imaging Reporting and Data Systems categorizes imagining as follows: 0 = incomplete, 1 = negative, 2 = benign, 3 = probably benign, 4 = suspicious abnormality, 5 = highly suspicious of malignancy, and 6 = known biopsy-proven malignancy (American College of Radiology, 2004).

Differential diagnosis: Not all breast masses are cancerous. Certain benign breast conditions exist. These conditions must be evaluated and malignancy ruled out. These benign conditions are classified as nonproliferating lesions, proliferating lesions without atypia, and proliferating lesions with atypia.

- ▦ Benign nonproliferating breast mass—nonproliferating lesions do not seem to affect future cancer risk.
  - ▦ Adenosis
  - ▦ Fibroadenoma
  - ▦ Fibrosis
  - ▦ Fat necrosis
  - ▦ Duct ectasia
  - ▦ Lipomas
  - ▦ Neurofibromas
  - ▦ Mastitis
- ▦ Proliferating lesions without atypia—increase cancer risk by approximately 1 to 2 times normal.
  - ▦ Radial scar
  - ▦ Sclerosing adenosis
  - ▦ Ductal hyperplasia
  - ▦ Papillomas

- Proliferating lesions with atypia—increase cancer risk by 4 to 5 times normal (Ferrara, 2011).
  - Atypical ductal hyperplasia
  - Atypical lobular hyperplasia

Treatment: The treatment for breast cancer confirmed by biopsy includes neoadjuvant therapy, adjuvant therapy, chemotherapy, surgical therapy, and endocrine therapy.

Neoadjuvant therapies include the therapies given to reduce the size of the tumor, allowing for improvement of outcomes and breast conservation (Waljee & Newman, 2007).

Adjuvant therapy is administered after the primary therapy, which is surgical resection, to decrease the risk of metastasis and increase rates of remission (Muss et al., 2009; National Cancer Institute, 2012). Chemotherapeutic agents such as capecitabine are used as either neoadjuvant therapy or adjuvant therapy. The goal of chemotherapy is to destroy both malignant and nonmalignant cells and interrupt the corrupt reproduction cell cycle. Endocrine therapy is used with estrogen- or progesterone-dependent tumor cell growth. This treatment is preferred for these hormone-dependent tumors because it targets the tumor and has fewer side effects (Gibson, Lawrence, Dawson, & Bliss, 2009; Narayanan & Taylor, 2007). The drug of choice for endocrine therapy is tamoxifen for premenopausal and postmenopausal women.

The primary therapy for breast cancer is surgical treatment except in the case of primary endocrine tumor, metastatic breast cancer, or in the older frail patient. Surgical therapy is classified as breast conserving, skin sparing, or radical. Breast conserving surgery includes lumpectomies, partial mastectomy, and segmental mastectomy. This breast conserving type of surgery attempts to conserve breast while removing the tumor and normal tissue borders. This type of surgical resection is not recommended for women with inflammatory breast cancer (Baron, 2007).

Skin sparing mastectomy attempts to leave a flap of skin for future reconstruction, while sparing the nipple, areola, or both. This type of surgery is the surgical procedure of choice when breast reconstruction will be done immediately (Yi et al., 2011). In a modified skin sparing mastectomy, the entire breast or breast and axillary lymph nodes are removed. Radical mastectomies remove the entire breast, axillary lymph nodes, and underlying muscle.

Reconstructive surgery can occur immediately after surgery or be delayed. This may be done with implants, tissue expanders, or autologous reconstruction. Immediate reconstruction has been associated with improved outcomes. These findings may be attributed to socioeconomic status, diet, or activity levels (Bezuhly et al., 2009).

Radiation therapy is also used in the treatment of breast cancer. This can be neoadjuvant, to reduce the size of the tumor, or adjuvant, to destroy remaining cancer. Postmastectomy radiation treatments have been shown to reduce recurrence rates and decrease mortality rates due to disease (Deutsch & Flickinger, 2009; Jagsi & Pierce, 2009). Radiation therapy has been linked to a slight increase in mortality rate due to cardiac and vascular problems.

Follow-up: Follow-up of breast masses and breast cancer is based on the specific diagnosis, cancer staging, and treatment rendered.

Sequelae: Survival rates are calculated as relative survival. The relative survival rate for breast cancer from 2001 to 2010 was 89.1%. Relative survival during that time frame by race was 90.4% for whites and 77% for blacks (National Cancer Institute, 2012).

Prevention/prophylaxis: Routine risk assessments for breast cancer are recommended, and based on these screenings it would be determined if women should undergo additional screenings. Early detection and diagnosis improve women's survival rates (Gotzsche & Nielsen, 2009). The American Cancer Society recommends yearly mammography for women in good health from age 40. Clinical breast examinations should be done at least every 3 years for women in their twenties and thirties, then annually for women 40 and over. Breast self-examinations are an option for women starting in their twenties (American Cancer Society, 2011–2012). The U.S. Preventive Services Task Force (USPSTF) also issued recommendations in 2009. The USPSTF recommends biannual mammography for women ages 50 to 74 (USPSTF, 2009). The conduction of lifetime risk assessment should be done to discuss and determine screening options and potential side effects. Risk assessment categories can be determined with the utilization of risk assessment tools such as the Gail model, Claus model, or Tyrer-Cuzick model. Women at high risk should have an MRI and mammogram every year, and women with moderate risk should discuss the benefits of adding an MRI screen to their annual mammogram. Women at low risk (less than a 15% lifetime risk) should not obtain MRI screenings (American Cancer Society, 2011–2012).

Breast examinations and screening mammography remain the most effective means of breast cancer screening in women. It is no longer recommended to teach breast self-examination during health examinations for women between ages 40 and 69 due to potential overdiagnosis and overtreatment. Approximately one in three women will have a false-positive screening result (Hubbard et al., 2011). The age to discontinue screening mammography remains unclear.

Genetic testing is recommended for individuals with a mutation detection probability of at least 10%. Mammography, ultrasound, and MRIs are recommended for women with a lifetime risk greater than 29% or a heterozygous risk greater than 19% starting at age 25. Mutation carriers may obtain prophylactic surgery of a bilateral salpingo-oophorectomy or bilateral mastectomy (Metcalfe et al., 2008). These screening are currently not supported in the general population. Chemoprevention has been shown to decrease breast cancer risk in the context of risk factors (Kelly et al., 2010). Chemoprevention should be discussed with high-risk women; this has been associated with decreased breast cancer risk and death (Armstrong et al., 2007).

Lifestyle modification has been shown to have a positive impact on cancer diagnosis. These modifications include maintaining a healthy body mass index (BMI), increased physical activity, and improved general nutrition (Wishart, 2010). High soy intake and breastfeeding have been associated with a reduction in breast cancer risk (Schmitz et al., 2010; Trock, Hilakivi-Clarke, & Clarke, 2006).

Referral: All breast masses should be further evaluated for malignancy. Referrals to surgeons, oncologists, geneticists, genetic counselors, mental health services, and appropriate support groups are made as necessary. Negative mammography with a positive breast mass may need further evaluation, especially in young women with dense breast tissue.

Education: It is important to instruct patients on current breast screening recommendations. Currently, screening mammography is recommended every 2 years for women 50 years and older, with or without clinical breast examinations. The age to discontinue screening is unclear. It is not recommended to teach breast self-examination (USPSTF, 2009).

CLINICAL RECOMMENDATION	EVIDENCE RATING	REFERENCES
Screening mammography every 2 years for women 50–74 years old.	B	USPSTF (2009)
Breast cancer risk assessment by a clinician between ages 40 and 49 years.	B	American Cancer Society (2011–2012)
Age to discontinue screening mammography is uncertain.	B	Gotzsche & Nielsen (2009)
Chemoprevention should be discussed with high-risk women.	C	Armstrong, Moye, Williams, Berlin, & Reynolds (2007)
Clinical breast examination with annual mammography over age 40.	B	American Cancer Society (2011–2012)
Clinical breast examinations every 3 years for women in their twenties and thirties.	B	American Cancer Society (2011–2012)

A = consistent, good-quality, patient-oriented evidence; B = inconsistent or limited-quality, patient-oriented evidence; C = consensus, disease-oriented evidence, usual practice, expert opinion, or case series. For information about the SORT evidence rating system, go to www.aafp.org/afpsort.xml.

ENDOMETRIAL CANCER

Signal symptoms: Postmenopausal bleeding.

Description: Cancer of the endometrium is the most common gynecological malignancy in the United States. Endometrial cancer is an abnormal proliferation and neoplastic transformation of endometrial tissues.

Etiology: Adenocarcinoma of the endometrium of the uterus has a histological precursor of atypical endometrial hyperplasia. Type I tumors are grade 1 or 2 estrogen responsive, occur in endometroid tissue, and have a favorable response rate, accounting for 80% of endometrial cancers. Type II account for 10% to 20%, are grade 3, and include some endometroid and nonendometroid variants; they have a poorer prognosis (Chen & Berek, 2012). Uterine sarcomas, a third type, are unrelated to either of the others and occur very rarely.

Occurrence: Endometrial cancer, which is 3 times more prevalent than cervical cancer, represents 10% of all cancers in women; it is the most common gynecological cancer in developed countries. Although most women with endometrial cancer present with an early-stage disease and have an excellent chance of cure, in 2008 there were 8120 deaths from uterine cancer and approximately 46,470 new cases (Jemal et al., 2011; Siegel, Ward, Brawley, & Jemal, 2011). The lifetime probability of developing endometrial cancer for all American women is 3%.

Age: Advancing age is the most important risk factor for endometrial cancer; 5% of tumors occur in women younger than 40 years old. Most tumors occur in women their sixties and seventies, with 61 being the average age of diagnosis (Chen & Berek, 2012).

Gender: Endometrial cancer is limited to women.

Ethnicity: Incidence rates are higher in Caucasian women, but the mortality rate is almost twice as high in African Americans as it is in Caucasians; Asian women have the lowest rates of endometrial cancer (Allard & Maxwell, 2009; Yap & Matthews, 2006).

Contributing factors: Obesity and glucose intolerance have been correlated with endometrial carcinoma. Strong evidence exists that endogenous or exogenous estrogen has a role in the development of endometrial cancer. There is a high incidence of this cancer in women with polycystic ovarian syndrome. An association exists between menstrual abnormalities and infertility and endometrial cancer. Of women with endometrial cancer, 20% to 30% are nulliparous. The use of estrogen after menopause substantially increases the risk of endometrial cancer. A program of estrogen plus progesterone for postmenopausal therapy has not been associated with endometrial cancer. Low parity, early menarche, late menopause, obesity, hypertension, and diabetes have been associated with endometrial carcinoma. Use of tamoxifen in postmenopausal women is also a risk factor. Women who have Lynch syndrome, an autosomal dominant genetic condition causing hereditary nonpolyposis colorectal cancer, are at high risk for endometrial, ovarian, colon, and other malignancies (Heald et al., 2010; Ollikainen et al., 2005) and should be screened for endometrial cancer.

Use of hormonal contraception is a negative risk factor. Smoking is also a negative risk factor, although other health problems associated with smoking render it unacceptable (Zhou et al., 2008)

Signs and symptoms: Postmenopausal bleeding is the most common symptom associated with endometrial carcinoma. Occasionally an incidental finding of hyperplasia may be found on Pap testing or hysterectomy performed for other reasons.

Diagnostic tests: The diagnosis of endometrial cancer is a histological diagnosis; endometrial sampling, cytology after hysterectomy, or curettage sample are required to be examined for an accurate diagnosis. Transvaginal ultrasound to evaluate endometrial thickness is frequently used in postmenopausal women as an initial study. If the endometrial thickness or stripe is less than 4 mm, endometrial biopsy, the gold standard for diagnosis, may be deferred. Premenopausal women will need an endometrial biopsy; a pelvic ultrasound may be done to rule out other causes of abnormal bleeding such as uterine leiomyomas. A physical examination, including a pelvic examination, is essential to rule out pelvic masses and other urogenital causes of bleeding. A rectal examination should also be done to eliminate this as the bleeding source.

Differential diagnosis:
- Infection
- Atrophy
- Rectal bleeding
- Other causes of genital tract bleeding

Treatment: Surgical excision after pretreatment staging is the norm. Two stages are currently used:

- Stage IA: tumor is confined to endometrium or less than one-half of myometrium
- Stage IB: tumor encompasses greater than one-half of the myometrium (American Joint Committee on Cancer, 2010; Benedet, Bender, Jones, Ngan, & Pecorelli, 2000)

Follow-up: Operative and histological findings assign the risk for recurrence. Radiation therapy is used for women with intermediate or high risk. Hormonal therapy and chemotherapy may be used for advanced disease. Most episodes of recurrence are within 3 years of treatment; this can include vaginal/pelvic areas, abdomen, or chest. Posttreatment surveillance is by oncology or gynecology (Fung-Kee-Fung et al., 2006; Sartori et al., 2010).

Sequelae: Various factors influence the prognosis, including histological differentiation, depth of invasion, and lymph node metastases. Histological type also influences the outcome.

Prevention/prophylaxis: None; do not use estrogen therapy without progesterone in the presence of an intact uterus.

Referral: All cases of suspected endometrial cancer must be referred to a gynecologist for evaluation and treatment. Endometrial sampling should be discussed with a gynecologist for women at risk for endometrial cancer.

Education: Explain the significance of postmenopausal bleeding to every woman at the time of menopause. Estrogen should not be taken without progesterone in the postmenopausal period in the presence of an intact uterus.

CLINICAL RECOMMENDATION	EVIDENCE RATING	REFERENCES
The U.S. Preventive Services Task Force has no specific guidelines on screening for endometrial cancer, and the American Cancer Society does not recommend routine screening of asymptomatic women by ultrasound or endometrial biopsy.	C	Smith et al. (2001)
All women with postmenopausal bleeding or older than 35 years with abnormal uterine bleeding should be evaluated for endometrial cancer.	C	Bode & Seehusen (2011)
First-line treatment for most women is surgical total abdominal hysterectomy with bilateral salpingo-oophorectomy (TAH-BSO), which is both therapeutic and prognostic (allows staging).	B	American College of Obstetricians and Gynecologists (ACOG) (2005)
Prognosis is good for most patients with an overall 5-year survival rate of more than 80%; prognosis for uterine sarcoma is worse.	B	ACOG (2005)

A = consistent, good-quality, patient-oriented evidence; B = inconsistent or limited-quality, patient-oriented evidence; C = consensus, disease-oriented evidence, usual practice, expert opinion, or case series. For information about the SORT evidence rating system, go to www.aafp.org/afpsort.xml.

OVARIAN CANCER

Signal symptoms: None; most women are asymptomatic until the disease has metastasized. A group of four symptoms commonly found in women with ovar-

ian cancer has been identified and named the Ovarian Cancer Symptom Index (OCSI). These include (1) bloating, (2) pelvic or abdominal pain, (3) difficulty eating or feeling full quickly, and (4) urinary symptoms (i.e., urgency or frequency) (McLemore, Miaskowski, Aouizerat, Chen, & Dodd, 2009).

Description: Cancer of the ovary is the most lethal of pelvic malignancies in women. It is actually several different types of cancer, with epithelial ovarian cancer predominating (Murphy, 2012). Within epithelial ovarian cancer are several subtypes: serous, mucinous, endometroid, and clear cell adenocarcinomas; the rest are undifferentiated and mixed epithelial carcinomas. As histological and genetic mutations are studied further, it is anticipated that valuable clinical information will be uncovered to influence outcomes (McLemore et al., 2009; Vaughan et al., 2011). Serous malignancies are thought to arise in the fallopian tube fimbria; clear cell and endometroid tumors may develop from endometriosis and retrograde menstruation (Murphy, 2012).

Etiology: Unknown.

Occurrence: Each year, approximately 23,000 new cases of ovarian cancer are diagnosed, making ovarian cancer the fifth most common malignancy among U.S. women. For women in the United States, the overall risk for developing ovarian cancer is 1.4% to 1.8%. In 2012 it was estimated that 15,500 women would die of the disease (National Cancer Institute, 2012). The lifetime probability of developing the disease is 1 in 55 for American women (Murphy, 2012). Late diagnosis is the primary reason for the poor prognosis. Reliable screening for this disease is not available.

Age: Of ovarian cancers, 80% to 90% occur in women over 40 years old. Fewer than 1% of ovarian cancers occur in women less than 20 years old. The peak incidence of invasive ovarian cancer is age 63. Mortality peaks at age 71. Hereditary ovarian cancers occur approximately 10 years earlier (National Cancer Institute, 2012).

Gender: Ovarian cancer only occurs in women.

Ethnicity: The incidence of ovarian cancer is highest in the United States, Europe, and Israel and lowest in Japan and in developing countries. Ovarian cancer incidence is higher in white women than in African American, Hispanic, or Asian women (National Cancer Institute, 2012).

Contributing factors: Increasing age and family history are the most important risk factors for ovarian cancer. The most significant risk factor is family history of the disease (Fowler, 2011). The risk depends on the number of affected first-degree and second-degree relatives and their age at diagnosis with ovarian and breast cancer. This holds true for relatives on the maternal and paternal sides. Families with BRCA1 and BRCA2 mutations are at risk for breast and ovarian cancer. Overall lifetime risk for women with this genetic mutation for ovarian cancer is 30%. Some individuals are at risk for ovarian cancer as part of their colorectal cancer genetic risk. Late menopause may be associated with a slightly higher trend in ovarian cancer. An increase in ovarian cancer risk among nulliparas is reported.

Signs and symptoms: Ovarian cancer may be totally asymptomatic. The woman may experience pelvic or abdominal pain or pressure, bloating, early satiety, or urinary symptoms (frequency/urgency). Because many of these symptoms are nonspecific and occur with other health conditions, they are frequently overlooked by patient and health-care professional alike (Vaughan et al., 2011).

Diagnostic tests: Pelvic examination is recommended in all sexually active women on the schedule determined by the American College of Obstetricians and Gynecologists. Rectovaginal examination may be necessary to detect ovarian enlargement. Ovarian enlargement cannot always be palpated, making pelvic examination a limited diagnostic test.

Transvaginal ultrasonography is the best initial study; a mass of more than 4 cm is highly suspect; necrosis or hemorrhage, nodularity, or walls of more than 3 mm in thickness also raise the index of suspicion. Laparoscopy with subsequent confirmatory histopathological tissue report is the gold standard diagnostic tool for ovarian cancer (Fowler, 2011; Kim et al., 2004). A complete blood count (CBC), cancer antigen 125 (CA-125), chest x-ray, and liver function tests (LFTs) are also part of the initial evaluation (National Comprehensive Cancer Network [NCCN], 2012). The USPSTF recommends against screening for ovarian cancer in all women due to its low incidence. In women who have a family history of hereditary ovarian or breast cancer, the USPSTF recommends genetic counseling and BRCA testing (USPSTF, 2005).

Differential diagnosis:
- Stool-filled sigmoid colon
- Distended bladder
- Irritable bowel syndrome
- Benign ovarian mass
- Pelvic inflammatory disease
- Peritoneal tuberculosis
- Pelvic kidney, diverticular abscess
- Cysts (dermoid, functional, cystadenoma)
- Tubo-ovarian abscess (Fowler, 2011)

Treatment: Surgical excision; extent of surgery is specific to stage and if primary or metastatic. For advanced cases, debulking of the tumor is done. Chemotherapy with cisplatin and a taxane usually follows surgery, and there is a period of remission. Most cancers return within 1 to 4 years and eventually become resistant to the platinum-based chemotherapy. Palliative chemotherapy with gemcitabine, liposomal doxorubicin, and bevacizumab has yielded a more than 15% response (Seiden, 2012).

Follow-up: Surveillance includes regular office follow-up, usually every 2 to 4 months, pelvic examination, imaging, and CA-125 measurement (Fowler, 2011).

Sequelae: On diagnosis, three out of four cases of ovarian carcinoma have spread beyond the ovary. Ovarian cancer is less common than breast cancer but has the highest case-fatality rate. Ovarian cancer is the fifth leading cause of cancer mortality in women, with 14,000 deaths annually. More women die from ovarian cancer than from all the other gynecological malignancies combined.

Prevention/prophylaxis: Use of the oral contraceptive pill reduces the risk of ovarian cancer by 35% to 50%. Women reduce their risk of ovarian cancer by 40% to 60% by taking oral contraceptives for 4 to 8 years. Pregnancy reduces the risk by 50%; increasing the number of pregnancies further reduces the risk. In women who are high risk due to genetic mutations, risk-reducing bilateral salpingo-oophorectomy (RRSO) was carried out in four studies with a 90% risk reduction in ovarian cancer and 50% in breast cancer over a 5-year period of follow-up (Villella et al., 2006).

Referral: Women with a significant family history of ovarian cancer or breast cancer should be referred for genetic counseling. Women with a significant family history should be referred to a gynecological oncologist for discussion of prophylaxis.

Education: Routine screening for women without family history of ovarian cancer is not currently recommended. Stress the importance of an annual pelvic examination for all women. Women should also be aware of the Ovarian Cancer Symptom Index, a group of four symptoms that are more likely to occur in women with ovarian cancer: (1) bloating, (2) pelvic or abdominal pain, (3) difficulty eating or feeling full quickly, and (4) urinary symptoms (i.e., urgency or frequency) (McLemore et al., 2009).

CLINICAL RECOMMENDATION	EVIDENCE RATING	REFERENCES
Women with a family history of BRCA gene mutations should be referred for genetic counseling. They should be counseled on the risks, benefits, and limitations of genetic screening.	B	USPSTF (2005)
The best initial study for women with suspected ovarian cancer is transvaginal ultrasound.	C	Kim et al. (2004)
Surgery is required with histopathological evaluation for definitive diagnosis and staging.	A	National Comprehensive Cancer Network (NCCN) (2012)
Chemotherapy for ovarian cancer should include a platinum-based drug and a taxane-based drug.	A	NCCN (2012)
Women with early disease at diagnosis and absence of residual tumor after treatment have better prognosis and improved survival.	A	Fowler (2011)

A = consistent, good-quality, patient-oriented evidence; B = inconsistent or limited-quality, patient-oriented evidence; C = consensus, disease-oriented evidence, usual practice, expert opinion, or case series. For information about the SORT evidence rating system, go to www.aafp.org/afpsort.xml.

BENIGN PROSTATIC HYPERPLASIA (BENIGN PROSTATIC HYPERTROPHY)

Signal symptoms: Urinary frequency, nocturia, urgency hesitancy, weak or intermittent urine stream, straining to void, sensation of incomplete voiding, dysuria (with infection).

Description: Benign prostatic hyperplasia (BPH; also called benign prostatic hypertrophy) is the benign growth of the prostate that may lead to obstruction of the bladder outlet. Cellular elements of the prostate are involved, and dysfunction in normal cell apoptosis with excessive growth of epithelial and stromal cells occurs (Deters, Costabile, Leveillee, Moore, & Patel, 2012).

Etiology: BPH originates in the transitional and periurethral zones of the prostate and is hormonally influenced by testosterone and dihydrotestosterone (DHT) production. In younger males who have BPH, there may be a genetic component (Scher, 2012).

Occurrence: BPH occurs universally in older men; genetics is thought to play a part in males who develop it at a younger age.

Age: BPH is seen in 50% of men over 50 years old and in 90% of men by age 85.

Gender: BPH occurs in men only.

Ethnicity: Not significant; Asian males are less likely to require surgery than African American and Caucasians.

Contributing factors: Risk factors include male gender, age of more than 40 years, and intact testes. There is an association between obesity and diabetes and BPH (Parsons et al., 2006).

Signs and symptoms: Symptoms are lower urinary tract symptoms (LUTS), occur on a continuum, and do not necessarily reflect the degree of prostatic enlargement. The onset of symptoms is gradual and includes increased frequency of urination, nocturia, hesitancy, urgency, and weak urinary stream. These symptoms are not specific for BPH and progress gradually over a period of years.

The American Urological Association (AUA) has developed a self-administered symptom questionnaire that addresses the occurrence over the past month of the symptoms mentioned here. This questionnaire, contained in the Agency for Health Care Policy and Research guidelines, is helpful in quantifying symptoms, although not specific for BPH.

On physical examination, the prostate may be enlarged or normal sized. It should feel smooth, with a rubbery consistency. Nodularity or extreme hardness raises suspicions of malignancy. Prostate size does not correlate with degree of obstruction or severity of symptoms. The suggested rationale for this is that rectal examination is limited to palpation of the peripheral zone of the prostate and does not reach the periurethral zone where symptoms originate. In cases of advanced obstruction, the bladder may be palpated on examination. Focal neurological examination assessing the sacral nerve roots is also helpful.

Diagnostic tests: Urinalysis is recommended to rule out infection (pyuria or bacteriuria) or malignancy (suggested by hematuria). If the urinalysis is positive for bacteria, culture and sensitivity testing is indicated. Blood urea nitrogen and creatinine should be measured if renal insufficiency or obstructive uropathy is suspected. Optional testing includes serum prostate-specific antigen (PSA), postvoid residual measurement, and maximal urinary flow rate. PSA may be elevated in BPH, prostatitis, acute urinary retention, prostatic infarction, increased physical activity, ejaculation, and prostatic cancer; the test is used primarily to screen for prostate cancer (Cunningham & Kadmon, 2012a). Specialized tests, such as intravenous pyelogram, transrectal ultrasound, and cystourethroscopy, are not indicated routinely. In specific instances, they may be performed as a guide to therapy choices or to rule out other conditions.

Differential diagnosis:
  ▓ Prostate cancer (may coexist with BPH)
  ▓ Urethral stricture
  ▓ Neurogenic bladder
  ▓ UTI
  ▓ Prostatitis
  ▓ Detrusor muscle failure
  ▓ Infection
  ▓ Bladder neck contracture
  ▓ Bladder calculi
  ▓ Carcinoma of the bladder

Treatment: For patients with minimal symptoms, a program of watchful waiting, with instruction to avoid medications known to worsen symptoms, is prescribed (American Urological Association Education and Research, Inc., 2010; McVary et al., 2011). Medication groups to be avoided include decongestants and other sympathomimetics and anticholinergics (Cunningham & Kadmon, 2012b). Patients should also be instructed in lifestyle self-management such as limiting fluids in the evening and avoiding alcohol and caffeinated beverages, which act as mild diuretics, in addition to the drug categories mentioned above (McVary et al., 2011).

For mild-to-moderate symptoms, alpha-adrenergic blockers such as terazosin (Hytrin) and tamsulosin (Flomax) relax smooth muscle of the bladder neck and prostate and can increase peak urinary flow rate; all alpha-adrenergic blockers are equally effective (Cantrell, Bream-Rouwenhorst, Hemerson, & Magera, 2010; Wilt, Howe, Rutks, & MacDonald, 2007; Wilt, MacDonald, & Rutks, 2007). Taking the medication at bedtime minimizes hypotension, the primary side effect. Another medication frequently used is finasteride (Proscar), a 5-alpha reductase inhibitor that blocks the conversion of testosterone to dihydrotestosterone, the major intraprostatic androgen in men. Side effects include decreased libido, ejaculatory dysfunction, and impotence. Treatment for 6 months or longer is needed for maximal benefit. Long-term treatment has been associated with increased risk of high-grade prostate cancer (Thompson et al., 2003).

Finasteride and an alpha blocker used concurrently slow the progression of BPH; the greatest effect is seen in patients with significantly enlarged prostates (McConnell et al., 2003). Many patients prefer herbal products because of reduced side effects. Studies to date have found no difference between saw palmetto and placebo for treatment of BPH symptoms after 1 year (Bent et al., 2006). Serenoa repens was also deemed comparable to placebo for symptom management in a Cochrane review (Tacklind, MacDonald, Rutks, & Wilt, 2010). For severe BPH, surgical treatment may be the primary option. Patients with an AUA score >20, renal insufficiency secondary to obstruction, markedly large prostates, or acute urinary retention that must be treated with a catheter are prime candidates (Flannery, 2010). In recent years, many treatments have proliferated in this category. Transurethral resection of the prostate (TURP) has been the standard for years, with open prostatectomy for glands of >40 g. Newer treatments include transurethral incision of the prostate (TUIP) for gland enlargement of <30 g, transurethral needle-aspiration ablation of the prostate (TUNA), transurethral electrovaporization of the prostate (TVAP), transurethral or visual laser-assisted prostatectomy (TULIP/VLAP), insertion of a urethral stent, and transurethral microwave therapy (TUMT); stents are usually reserved for complex cases. Some of the newer laser/microwave procedures may need to be repeated after several years. A small longitudinal study with patients randomized to TURP, laser, or electrovaporization treatment demonstrated comparable outcomes in symptom relief, failure rates, and mortality (Hoekstra, Van Melick, Kok, & Ruud Bosch, 2010). Therapies including the injection of botulinum toxin, ethanol, and a luteinizing hormone–releasing receptor antagonist (cetrorelix pamoate) have shown promise for short-term symptom improvement, but further studies are needed (Debruyne, Tzvetkov, Altarac, & Geavlete, 2010; Kim, 2002; Smith & Chancellor, 2004).

Follow-up: Scheduling of follow-up depends on the course of treatment. Advise watchful waiting, and evaluate with the AUA symptoms index every 6 to 12 months. Patients receiving drug therapy should be evaluated for symptoms and side effects every 6 months. Annual digital rectal examination for prostate cancer is indicated, and usually PSA testing and urinalysis are done.

Sequelae: Complications of BPH include urinary retention and bladder outlet obstruction (BOO) requiring catheterization and/or surgery, renal insufficiency, UTIs, bladder stones, gross hematuria, prostatitis, treatment complications such as urethral stricture, treatment side effects, and possibly treatment-induced impotence.

Prevention/prophylaxis: No preventive measures are known; BPH occurs with aging.

Referral: Patients should be referred to a urologist if comorbid conditions exist, if there is repeated hematuria or UTIs, if surgical options are indicated, and to rule out acute prostatitis or prostate cancer. Patients with BPH symptoms that do not respond to medical management should be referred for evaluation (Kaplan, 2006). Consider collaborative management for drug therapy.

Education: Educate the patient about BPH and its treatment options and side effects. Instruct the patient to avoid any drugs that can increase retention or cause symptoms to flare up, including caffeine, alcohol, sedatives, over-the-counter (OTC) sleeping pills, and OTC cold and allergy remedies. Instruct the patient to report hematuria, UTI symptoms, or increased retention.

CLINICAL RECOMMENDATION	EVIDENCE RATING	REFERENCES
Watchful waiting is an option; the need for medical treatment is based on symptoms (American Urological Association [AUA] symptom score 3) and the degree of patient bother.	C	Flannery (2010)
Alpha-adrenergic antagonists are equally effective and work rapidly; patients can expect moderate improvement in symptoms.	A	Wilt, Howe, Rutks, & MacDonald (2007) Wilt, MacDonald, & Rutks (2007)
5-Alpha reductase inhibitors modestly improve AUA symptom score and reduce the risk of acute urinary retention or need for invasive surgery.	A	Wilt et al. (2007)
Combination therapy with an alpha blocker and a 5-alpha reductase inhibitor is superior to monotherapy, particularly in patients with higher prostate volumes and prostate-specific antigen (PSA) levels.	B	McConnell et al. (2003)

A = consistent, good-quality, patient-oriented evidence; B = inconsistent or limited-quality, patient-oriented evidence; C = consensus, disease-oriented evidence, usual practice, expert opinion, or case series. For information about the SORT evidence rating system, go to www.aafp.org/afpsort.xml.

DRUG-INDUCED IMPOTENCE

Signal symptoms: None; noncompliance with medication regimen, responses on sexual history query or questionnaire.

Description: Impotence, in the strictest sense of the word, is the consistent inability to achieve and maintain erection sufficient for sexual intercourse (*NIH Consensus Statement Online*, 1992); it is more commonly referred to as *erectile dysfunction (ED)*. In a broader sense, impotence encompasses problems with arousal, libido, orgasm, sensation, and relationships. Drug-induced impotence refers to that which is caused by a drug or drugs (Cunningham & Rosen, 2011; Hirsch & Birnbaum, 2009).

Etiology: Drug-induced impotence may be caused by many medications or medication interactions (see under Contributing factors).

Occurrence: An estimated 30 million American men experience impotence on a chronic basis.

Age: Incidence of ED increases with age. The prevalence is approximately 52% for men between age 40 and 70; in men over 70 years old, prevalence is increased further. Men over 70 years old with chronic medical problems, such as diabetes, have a prevalence of more than 90%. Because the condition frequently is underreported, the percentage is probably higher. Approximately 25% of erectile problems are related to drugs (McVary, 2012).

Gender: Men.

Ethnicity: Not significant.

Contributing factors: The following factors contribute to impotence (Heidelbaugh & Barry, 2011; Martin, 2012; Rudkin, Taylor, Hawton, & Taylor, 2009; Tacklind, Fink, MacDonald, Rutks, & Wilt, 2012).
- Stress
- Long-term alcohol use
- Tobacco use
- Recreational drug use (cocaine, marijuana, opiates)

- ▓ Antiandrogens
- ▓ Anticholinergics
- ▓ Anticonvulsants
- ▓ Antidepressants (including selective serotonin re-uptake inhibitors, monoamine oxidase inhibitors, tricyclic antidepressants)
- ▓ Antipsychotics
- ▓ Centrally acting depressants (sedatives/hypnotics, tranquilizers, opiates)
- ▓ H_2 blockers
- ▓ Levodopa
- ▓ Lithium
- ▓ Stimulants such as amphetamines
- ▓ Beta blockers
- ▓ Spironolactone
- ▓ Methadone
- ▓ Cytotoxic agents
- ▓ Antihypertensives (clonidine, methyldopa, thiazides, calcium channel blockers)
- ▓ Urologic drugs (alpha blockers)
- ▓ Anti-inflammatories (baclofen, naproxen)

Various processes are involved, including effect on libido, neurochemical mediation, and drug side effects.

Signs and symptoms: There may be no reported symptoms unless the provider includes a sexual history, is aware of the potential for impotence when prescribing certain medications, and asks about baseline sexual activity at that time, then periodically reassesses this during follow-up visits. The patient should be asked about sexual interest, sexual ability, and sexual activity. Also, if a provider detects noncompliance to a prescribed medication regimen in an otherwise cooperative patient, the provider should inquire whether impotence occurs when the medication is taken. Drug-induced impotence can be associated with starting a new medication.

Medication history including OTC remedies, alcohol use, tobacco use, and use of recreational drugs is also important. The CAGE test for alcoholism, a screening questionnaire for depression, or other psychological screens as needed may be included as part of the history. A history of surgical procedures, especially of procedures involving the prostate, bladder, or colorectal area and including the lymphatic channels, may reveal potential sources of impotence (Martin, 2012).

Physical examination is performed to rule out other causes of impotence; the cause may be multifactorial, especially in an older patient. Evaluate the patient's overall appearance and mobility, then assess the vital signs, specifically checking for orthostatic hypotension. Palpation of the thyroid may reveal a goiter.

Gynecomastia may be related to certain drugs, such as cimetidine. Abdominal or femoral bruits may highlight an abdominal aortic aneurysm or vascular obstruction at the bifurcation of the abdominal aorta.

Diminished peripheral pulses suggest a circulatory problem. Lack of sensation or inability to discriminate between sharp and dull may indicate peripheral neuropathy, especially if the history is positive for diabetes. Abnormal reflexes point to a neurological problem. Decreased mobility may indicate a neurological or musculoskeletal problem contributing to impotence. Examination of the genital area may reveal testicular atrophy or penile plaques, as seen in patients with Peyronie's disease, or an enlarged prostate. Assess for the bulbocavernosus reflex; absence of this reflex indicates penile neuropathy.

Diagnostic tests: Diagnostic testing is not indicated specifically for drug-induced impotence, but it is performed to eliminate other possible causes of impotence, especially vascular and neurological causes, which are the most common causes (McVary, 2007; Selvin, Burnett, & Platz, 2007).

Differential diagnosis:
- ▓ Vascular
- ▓ Endocrine
- ▓ Neurological
- ▓ Neurovascular
- ▓ Substance abuse
- ▓ End-organ disease
- ▓ Psychogenic
- ▓ Social causes

As stated previously, impotence in elderly persons is frequently multifactorial (Blanker et al., 2001; Rosen et al., 2003; Rowland et al., 2010).

Treatment: Whenever possible, decrease the dose, eliminate the medication, or substitute another medication from available drugs that do not cause impotence. If this is not possible or if the patient continues to experience the problem after these changes have been made, consider other treatment measures. Adding a second drug while continuing the original drug may be effective (Zisook, Rush, Haight, Clines, & Rockett, 2006). Counsel the patient regarding alcohol, recreational drug, and tobacco use (Hirsch & Birnbaum, 2009; Martin, 2012).

Sildenafil citrate (Viagra) is a selective inhibitor of cyclic guanosine monophosphate (cGMP)–specific phosphodiesterase type 5. During sexual stimulation, nitric acid is released into the corpus cavernosum, resulting in increased cGMP levels, which prevents smooth muscle relaxation and increases blood flow to the penis. Sildenafil enhances this effect by inhibiting an enzyme that degrades cGMP in the corpus cavernosum. It is contraindicated with nitrates and in advanced heart disease; cytochrome influences include increased plasma levels with inhibitors of CYP3A4 or CYP2D9 and decreased plasma levels with inducers of CYP3A4. Side effects include headache, flushing, UTI, abnormal vision (blue-green, blurring, photosensitivity), nasal congestion, diarrhea, dizziness, and rash. It is effective in treating drug-induced impotence in patients taking antidepressants/antipsychotics and antihypertensives/diuretics (Nurnberg et al., 2003). Sildenafil was also found to be effective in treating impotence related to prior cancer therapy (Miles et al., 2011). For other types of treatment, such as penile implants or injection, refer the patient to a urologist specializing in this area.

Follow-up: Individualize follow-up according to cause and treatment. Periodic reassessment of treatment for recurrence of the problem is helpful. For medication treatment, monitor for side effects and response.

Sequelae: Disruption of sexual function may result in depression or relationship problems. Complications may arise from treatment.

Prevention/prophylaxis: Whenever possible, avoid prescribing medications with a high risk for causing impotence, and include a sexual history in routine history and physical examination whenever prescribing a new medication with impotence as a potential side effect.

Referral: Refer patients to a urologist to evaluate for other causes or multifactorial causes of impotence. Refer to a support group patients who are experiencing the problem. Refer for psychological services when indicated.

Education: Teach the patient about medication side effects. Have the patient report sexual dysfunction. Educate the patient about normal age-related changes in sexual functioning and how to adapt. If sildenafil is prescribed, take as ordered and do not exceed prescribed dosage.

CLINICAL RECOMMENDATION	EVIDENCE RATING	REFERENCES
There is no recommended diagnostic testing to serve as a gold standard for ED; history and physical examination are sufficient in making an accurate diagnosis in the majority of cases.	C	Martin (2010)
The PDE5 inhibitors are the most effective drugs in the treatment of ED, including ED associated with diabetes and spinal cord injury, and in men with sexual dysfunction secondary to antidepressants.	A	Heidelbaugh & Barry (2011)
Eight of the 12 most commonly prescribed medication classes list ED as a side effect, and it is estimated that 25% of cases of ED are due to medications. Examples of medications that disrupt normal male sexual function include antidepressants, particularly selective serotonin reuptake inhibitors (SSRIs); spironolactone; sympathetic blockers such as clonidine, guanethidine, or methyldopa; thiazide diuretics; ketaconazole; cimetidine; and beta blockers.	C	Grimm et al. (1997) Slag et al. (1983) Veterans Administration Cooperative Study Group on Antihypertensive Agents (1982) Wein & Van Arsdalen (1988)

A = consistent, good-quality, patient-oriented evidence; B = inconsistent or limited-quality, patient-oriented evidence; C = consensus, disease-oriented evidence, usual practice, expert opinion, or case series. For information about the SORT evidence rating system, go to www.aafp.org/afpsort.xml.

PROSTATE CANCER

Signal symptoms: Early stage—often asymptomatic. Obstructive voiding symptoms (hesitancy, intermittent urinary stream, decreased force of stream) are generally indicative of advanced disease.

Description: Prostate cancer is a malignant neoplasm of the prostate, which is a male sex accessory gland. The prostate encircles the urethra like a doughnut. The role of the prostate is to secrete fluid into the ejaculate that accompanies sperm and seminal fluid to make up semen. Ninety-five percent of prostate cancers are adenocarcinomas.

Etiology: Approximately one-half of prostate cancers demonstrate a genetic component. Testosterone has been identified as a prerequisite for the development of prostate cancer. Prostate cancers exhibit high levels of androgen receptors (Small, 2012).

Occurrence: Prostate cancer is the second most common cause of cancer death in men (Small, 2012), second only to lung cancer (McCormick, Osman, & Pomerantz, 2010). Prostate cancer is the most common cancer in men, with approximately a 17% lifetime risk (Ali & Walsh, 2011). The elderly are more frequently affected, with 75% of cases diagnosed after age 65, and 90% of deaths in this age group (McCormick et al., 2010).

Age: Mean age at diagnosis is 71 years (Wilbur, 2008).

Gender: Prostate cancer is a disease confined to men.

Ethnicity: African Americans have the highest incidence of prostate cancer in the world, with Asian and Hispanic men at lower risk than white men (Wilbur, 2008). Diagnosis in African Americans tends to be at a more advanced stage, and disease-specific survival is lower in this group (Prostate cancer, 2012).

Contributing factors: Age greater than 50 years, African American race, diet high in fat. Family history appears significant with a 2.5-fold increased risk with a first-degree relative affected before age 50, and even greater if the affected relative is a brother rather than a father, if the affected relative is younger than 55 years, or if two or more first-degree relatives are affected (Wilbur, 2008). No link has been determined with prior vasectomy or benign prostatic hyperplasia (Prostate cancer, 2012).

Signs and symptoms: There are usually no symptoms with early disease. Symptoms generally occur in advanced stages, making early detection desirable. Obstructive voiding symptoms (hesitancy, intermittent urinary stream, decreased force of stream) generally reflect locally advanced disease with growth into the urethra or bladder neck. Locally advanced tumors may result in hematuria and hematospermia (Small, 2012). If rectal obstruction occurs, a large bowel obstruction or difficulty in defecation may be present (McCance, Huether, Brashers, & Rote, 2010). Prostate cancer that has spread to the regional pelvic lymph nodes occasionally causes edema of the lower extremities or discomfort in pelvic or perineal areas. Metastasis occurs most often to the bone, resulting in pain and pathological fractures (Small, 2012).

Differential diagnosis:
- Benign nodule prostate growth
- Subacute prostatitis
- Prostatic intraepithelial neoplasia
- Prostate stones (Prostate cancer, 2011)

Diagnostic tests: Digital rectal examination (DRE) is the only method for physically examining the prostate, with awareness that only part of the gland can be palpated, allowing for tumors to be missed. DRE is considered abnormal if the prostate is enlarged, asymmetrical, nodular, or tender (Wilbur, 2008). The effectiveness of DRE for prostate cancer screening is not well established (Wilbur, 2008); screening with prostate-specific antigen (PSA) and DRE may detect cancer at an earlier stage than if no screening is performed (Wolf et al., 2010). DRE alone has a low sensitivity and specificity for the diagnosis of prostate cancer. PSA is a glycoprotein expressed by normal and neoplastic prostate tissue (Wilbur, 2008) and is excreted in the ejaculate to liquefy semen (Gjertson & Albertsen, 2011). Screening, when completed, is recommended with PSA with or without DRE. PSA should be drawn before DRE is undertaken to avoid a false-positive result. Both the PSA and DRE may produce false-positive or false-negative results. Screening should be conducted yearly for men whose PSA levels are 2.5 ng/mL or greater (see note below regarding screening controversy). For men whose PSA is less than 2.5 ng/mL, screening intervals can be extended to every 2 years. A PSA level of 4.0 ng/mL or greater historically has been used to recommend referral for further evaluation or biopsy, which remains a reasonable approach for men at average risk for prostate cancer. For PSA levels between 2.5 and 4.0 ng/mL, health-care providers should consider an individual-ized risk assessment that incorporates other risk factors for prostate cancer (African American race, family history, increasing age, and abnormal DRE) (Wolf et al., 2010). Transurethral ultrasonography with biopsies is indicated when the PSA level is elevated, when the percentage of free PSA is less than 25%, or when an abnormality is noted on DRE. When biopsy is undertaken, up to six biopsies on each side are preferred for evaluation. Seminal vesi-cles may be sampled in high-risk patients (Small, 2012).

As of May 2012, the USPSTF recommended against PSA screening for prostate cancer. The AUA opposes this recommendation (AUA, 2012). The discussion in this section reflects current practice.

Treatment: Treatment depends on stage of the tumor, anticipated effects of treatment, and the age, general health, and life expectancy of the patient. The Gleason Score determines the grade of the prostate cancer. The Gleason Score grades tumors on a 1 to 5 range based on the degree of glandular differentiation and struc-tural architecture. Grade 1 represents the most well-differentiated appearance, and grade 5 represents the most poorly differentiated (Ali & Walsh, 2011). Treat-ment options include active surveillance for a tumor of incidental histological findings in 5% or less of re-sected tissue. Tumors with histological findings in greater than 5% of resected tissue or identified by fine-needle biopsy because of elevated PSA may be a can-didate for prostatectomy, external beam radiation, or brachytherapy. For tumors involving about one-half of one lobe, prostatectomy, external beam radiation, or brachytherapy may be considered. Tumors extending through the prostatic capsule, possibly invading the seminal vesicles, may require possible prostatectomy or possible radiation. A tumor that is fixed or invades adjacent structures other than seminal vesicles (blad-der neck, external sphincter, rectum, levator muscles, and/or pelvic wall) may require hormonal (androgen ablation) and/or radiation therapy. Chemotherapy is reserved for hormone-refractory disease (Ali & Walsh, 2011). Newer approaches are using immunotherapy (McCance et al., 2010). Medications may be consid-ered, and treatment can include reducing testosterone with gonadotropin-releasing hormone (GnRH) ago-nists (leuprolide or goserelin). Combined androgen blockade with GnRH agonist and antiandrogen is often a second-line choice.

Follow-up: Depends on current treatment and pa-tient-specific risk. If prostatectomy is completed,

PSA/DRE is recommended every 6 months for 5 years, then yearly thereafter. A PSA greater than 0.2 ng/mL after surgery is suggestive of recurrence. After external beam radiation, PSA/DRE is recom-mended every 3 months for 1 year, every 3 to 6 months for 4 years, then yearly thereafter. PSA greater than 2.0 ng/mL after external radiation is suggestive of recurrence (Ali & Walsh, 2011). A thor-ough review of systems and focused physical exami-nation should be done at the same intervals while evaluating the patient for new or recurrent symp-toms or treatment complications.

Sequelae: Complications of treatment may include incontinence, ED, mild colitis, and radiation cystitis. After nerve-sparing prostatectomy, urinary conti-nence returns in under 6 months in about 50% of men. The rate of ED after external beam radiation ranges from 10% to 80%, and with brachytherapy ap-proximately 15% to 60% (Ali & Walsh, 2011).

Prevention/prophylaxis: PSA screening remains controversial because many of the prostate cancers detected are low grade and slow growing (Gjertson & Albertsen, 2011). The USPSTF latest recommen-dation is against screening for prostate cancer (USPSTF, 2012), with the AUA opting for PSA test-ing (AUA, 2012). The American Cancer Society rec-ommends that asymptomatic men who have at least a 10-year life expectancy have an opportunity to make an informed decision with their health-care provider about whether to be screened for prostate cancer. Men at average risk should receive this first information beginning at age 50. Men at higher risk, including African Americans and men with a first-degree relative (father or brother) diagnosed with prostate cancer before age 65 years, should receive this information at age 45. Men with an appreciably higher risk (multiple family members diagnosed with prostate cancer before age 65) should receive this information at age 40. Asymptomatic men with less than a 10-year life expectancy based on age and health status should not be offered prostate cancer screening (Wolf et al., 2010). Screening, when com-pleted, is recommended with PSA with or without DRE. Screening should be conducted yearly for men whose PSA levels are 2.5 ng/mL or greater. For men whose PSA is less than 2.5 ng/mL, screening inter-vals can be extended to every 2 years. A PSA level of 4.0 ng/mL or greater historically has been used to recommend referral for further evaluation or biopsy, which remains a reasonable approach for men at average risk for prostate cancer. For PSA levels between 2.5 and 4.0 ng/mL, health-care providers should consider an individualized risk assessment that incorporates other risk factors for prostate cancer (African American race, family history, increasing age, and abnormal DRE) (Wolf et al., 2010).

Referral: Appropriate referral sources may include urology, oncology, and radiology.

Education: Review risk factors and significance of reporting family history. Encourage screening per health-care providers' recommendations and current guidelines.

CLINICAL RECOMMENDATION	EVIDENCE RATING	REFERENCES
Screening, when completed, is recommended with PSA with or without digital rectal examination.	A	Wolf et al. (2010)
Screening should be conducted yearly for men whose PSA levels are ≥2.5 ng/mL.	A	Wolf et al. (2010)
For men whose PSA is <2.5 ng/mL, screening intervals can be extended to every 2 years.	A	Wolf et al. (2010)
A PSA level of ≥4.0 ng/mL historically has been used to recommend referral for further evaluation or biopsy.	A	Wolf et al. (2010)
The USPSTF recommends against PSA screening for prostate cancer.	C	USPSTF (2012)

A = consistent, good-quality, patient-oriented evidence; B = inconsistent or limited-quality, patient-oriented evidence; C = consensus, disease-oriented evidence, usual practice, expert opinion, or case series. For information about the SORT evidence rating system, go to www.aafp.org/afpsort.xml.

PROSTATITIS

Signal symptoms: Pain at various locations and lower urinary tract symptoms such as frequent need to void, difficulty urinating, and pain on urination or pain that increases with urination (Grabe et al., 2009).

Description: Prostatitis includes both acute and chronic bacterial prostatitis and prostatitis syndrome, which has recently been termed *chronic pelvic pain syndrome* (CPPS). The National Institutes of Health Consensus Classification of Prostatitis identifies four syndrome types: type I, acute bacterial prostatitis; type II, chronic bacterial prostatitis; type III, CPPS with either type IIIA inflammatory components or type IIIB non-inflammatory components; and type IV, asymptomatic prostatitis. Acute bacterial prostatitis is an acute bacterial infection of the prostate, and if left untreated, it can progress to sepsis or development of prostatic abscess. By definition an organism must be identified on culture. Chronic prostatitis is defined by symptoms being present for at least 3 months and urine cultures obtained over the course of the illness repeatedly growing the same bacterial strain. CPPS is pelvic pain in the absence of bacteria localized to the prostate (Sharp, Takacs, & Powell, 2010).

Etiology: Most common pathogens in prostatitis include *Escherichia coli*, *Klebsiella*, *Proteus mirabilis*, *Enterococcus faecalis*, and *Pseudomonas aeruginosa* (Grabe et al., 2009). *E. coli* is the most commonly isolated organism in chronic prostatitis, and these strains have been found to have a higher virulence factor and greater degree of biofilm formation, making this form more difficult to treat (Sharp et al., 2010).

Occurrence: Prevalence of prostatitis is approximately 8.2% (Sharp et al., 2010), accounting for approximately 2 million outpatient visits per year (Schaeffer, 2006). Some degree of prostatic inflammation is present in 4% to 36% of the male population (McCance, Huether, Brashers, & Rote, 2010).

Age: Predominant age 30 to 50 years, with chronic prostatitis more common in men over the age of 50 (Prostatitis, 2011).

Gender: Prostatitis is a disease confined to men.

Ethnicity: No ethnic predisposition.

Contributing factors: History of UTIs, anal intercourse, urological procedures, long-term bladder catheterization, STIs.

Signs and symptoms: The predominant symptom is pain in the prostate, perineum, scrotum, testes, penis, urinary bladder, or lower back. Acute bacterial prostatitis frequently includes symptoms similar to acute cystitis or pyelonephritis and includes malaise, low back and perineal pain, high fever, chills, dysuria, inability to empty the bladder, nocturia, and urinary retention. Men are acutely ill and may look toxic (McCance et al., 2010). Chronic bacterial prostatitis is the most frequent cause of recurrent UTIs in men. Symptoms are variable and are similar to those of an acute bladder infection such as frequency, urgency, dysuria, perineal discomfort, low back pain, and urinary dysfunction (McCance et al., 2010). These men often do not appear ill looking but present with recurrent or relapsing UTIs, urethritis, or epididymitis with the same bacterial strain (Sharp et al., 2010).

Physical examination may reveal a tender, boggy prostate on rectal examination. The prostate gland may be warm, swollen, firm, or irregular (Prostatitis, 2011). Prostatic massage is contraindicated (Grabe et al., 2009). If abdominal examination reveals a palpable, distended bladder, urinary retention may be present (Sharp et al., 2010).

Patients may also complete the National Institutes of Health Chronic Prostatitis Symptom Index assessing pain, urination, impact of symptoms, and quality of life at www.prostatitis.org/symptomindex.html.

Diagnostic tests: Diagnosis of acute bacterial prostatitis is often done on report of symptoms. Suspected acute prostatitis diagnostics include urinalysis, urine and blood cultures, urine Gram stain, and CBC with differential. Urine should be a midstream collection, and the presence of more than 10 white blood cells (WBCs) per high-power field suggests a positive diagnosis (Sharp et al., 2010). Suspected chronic

prostatitis/CPPS tests include urinalysis, urine culture, and postvoid residual, if sensation of incomplete emptying of bladder. Suspected chronic bacterial prostatitis testing includes two-glass preprostatic and postprostatic massage test and a positive urine culture. In most cases imaging is not required. Order computed tomography or MRI if malignancy or abscess is suspected. Transrectal ultrasound is indicated if prostatic calculi or abscess is suspected (Prostatitis, 2011). Sexually active men younger than age 35 and older men who engage in high-risk sexual behavior should be tested for *Neisseria gonorrhoeae* and *Chlamydia trachomatis* (Sharp et al., 2010). Measurement of free and total PSA is of no diagnostic benefit (Grabe et al., 2009).

Differential diagnosis:
- Acute cystitis—rapid onset and rapid response to antimicrobial therapy
- Urethritis—clinical diagnosis, mucopurulent or purulent urethral discharge, Gram stain for WBC count
- Pyelonephritis—usually results from an inadequately treated ascending infection; positive costovertebral angle tenderness, may have hematuria, may have abdominal pain; more common in younger men and pregnant women
- Acute urinary retention—physical assessment of distended bladder, immediate catheterization to alleviate
- Benign prostatic hyperplasia (see BPH in this chapter)
- Urinary tract stones—acute, crampy pain on urination; sludge or gravel may be seen in urine specimen, especially if specimen is strained; may be accompanied by nausea, vomiting
- Bladder cancer
- Prostatic abscess
- Enterovesical fistula
- Foreign body within the urinary tract (see Urinary stones) (Bope & Kellerman, 2013)

Treatment: Antibiotics are lifesaving in acute bacterial prostatitis and recommended in chronic bacterial prostatitis (Grabe et al., 2009). If the patient is acutely ill with acute bacterial prostatitis, the health-care provider may need to consider hospitalization and parenteral antibiotics (Prostatitis, 2012). Fluoroquinolones such as ciprofloxacin (Cipro) 500 mg twice a day or levofloxacin (Levaquin) 500 mg daily are recommended. They offer good activity against typical and atypical bacterial strains in addition to *P. aeruginosa*, and both penetrate the prostate tissue well (Grabe et al., 2009; Sharp et al., 2010). Oral medications are recommended for 10 days for acute cases. Trimethoprim/sulfamethoxazole (Bactrim, Septra) may be considered, but drawbacks include no activity against *P. aeruginosa*, poorer tissue penetration, and increasing resistance in some geographical areas (Grabe et al., 2009; Sharp et al., 2010). In chronic cases antibiotics are given for 2 weeks, then the patient is reassessed and antibiotics continued only if cultures are positive or the patient reports positive effects from the treatment. A total treatment period of 4 to 6 weeks is recommended (Grabe et al., 2009), and a 6- to 12-week course may be needed to eradicate the causative organism and to prevent recurrence (Sharp et al., 2010). Second-line antibiotics include doxycycline, azithromycin, and clarithromycin (Sharp et al., 2010) and are usually reserved for special indications (Grabe et al., 2009). May need to evaluate the patient for need for stool softeners if painful or difficult defecation. Evaluate for the need for analgesics, antipyretics, or anti-inflammatory medications, and warm water baths.

Follow-up: For patients with acute bacterial prostatitis, a repeat urine culture after the treatment regimen is recommended. Patients with chronic prostatitis or relapse should receive extended antimicrobial therapy. Refer patients with symptoms of BPH, intractable infection, or prostatodynia to urology.

Sequelae: Unresolved acute prostatitis can lead to bacteremia or pyelonephritis. Prostatic abscess rarely occurs as a complication of acute bacterial prostatitis except in immunocompromised patients.

Prevention/prophylaxis: There are no prevention strategies for prostatitis (Prostatitis, 2012).

Referral: Refer patients with symptoms of BPH, intractable infection, or prostatodynia to a urologist.

Education: Educate the patient and family regarding the cause of symptoms and treatment. Explain the need for extended antibiotics and importance of adherence with treatment. Encourage follow-up appointments as recommended. Condoms should be worn to prevent reintroduction of bacteria into the urethra during sex, and anal intercourse should be avoided with acute bacterial prostatitis (Buttaro, Trybulski, Bailey, & Sandberg-Cook, 2008). Patients should be advised to avoid bladder irritants such as alcohol and caffeine. Emphasize that prostatitis can recur and to report symptoms at onset.

CLINICAL RECOMMENDATION	EVIDENCE RATING	REFERENCES
Optimal duration of antibiotic treatment for acute bacterial prostatitis is 6 weeks.	B	Sharp, Takacs, & Powell (2010)
To prevent symptom flare-up, suppressive low-dose antibiotics should be considered in men with chronic bacterial prostatitis with positive cultures.	C	Sharp et al. (2010)

A = consistent, good-quality, patient-oriented evidence; B = inconsistent or limited-quality, patient-oriented evidence; C = consensus, disease-oriented evidence, usual practice, expert opinion, or case series. For information about the SORT evidence rating system, go to www.aafp.org/afpsort.xml.

CASE STUDY

Mrs. C., a 66-year-old woman, presents to your practice with a complaint of recent onset of leaking urine. She has no prior history of this. On further questioning you discover that she is newly married, after being widowed for 15 years, during which she had no sexual partners. She and her new husband have just returned from a cruise, and she reports that he is a "passionate" lover and she is having difficulty meeting his needs for daily intercourse. Other symptoms that Mrs. C. reports are vaginal burning and general discomfort "down there."

Medications: takes fish oil at bedtime, vitamin D_3 1000 IU daily. No known drug allergies.

Vital signs: blood pressure (BP) 128/76 mm Hg, pulse 82 (regular), respiratory rate 16 breaths/min, temperature 98.2°F (oral), BMI 23.4.

CASE STUDY—cont'd

A staff member has obtained a urine specimen for dipstick. Findings are as follows:

Nitrite—negative

Leukocyte esterase—negative

Blood—trace

Protein—trace

Glucose—negative

Ketones—negative

Specific gravity—1.015

1. What additional subjective data are you seeking?

2. What additional objective data will you be assessing for?

3. What national guidelines are appropriate to consider?

4. What tests will you order?

5. Are there any screening tools that you want to use?

6. What are the differential diagnoses that you are considering?

7. What is your plan of care?

8. Are there any Healthy People 2020 objectives that you should consider?

9. What additional patient teaching may be needed?

10. Will you be looking for a consultation?

REFERENCES

Assessment

U.S. Preventive Services Task Force. (2012). Screening for cervical cancer. Retrieved from www.uspreventiveservicestaskforce.org/uspstf/uspscerv.htm

Atrophic Vaginitis

Bachmann, G., Bouchard, C., Hoppe, D., Ranganath, R., Altomare, C., Vieweg, A., . . . Helzner, E. (2009). Efficacy and safety of low-dose regimens of conjugated estrogens cream administered vaginally. *Menopause, 16*(4), 719–727.

Bachmann, G., & Santen, R. J. (2011a). Clinical manifestations and diagnosis of vaginal atrophy. *UpToDate.* Retrieved from www.uptodate.com

Bachmann, G., & Santen, R. J. (2011b). Treatment of vaginal atrophy. *UpToDate.* Retrieved from www.uptodate.com

Nappi, R. E., & Kokot-Kierepa, M. (2010). Women's voices in the menopause: results from an international survey on vaginal atrophy. *Maturitas, 67*(3), 233.

Pearson, T. (2011). Atrophic vaginitis. *Journal for Nurse Practitioners, 7*(6), 502–505.

Reimer, A., & Johnson, L. (2011). Atrophic vaginitis signs, symptoms, and better outcomes. *Nurse Practitioner, 36*(1), 22–28.

Samra-Latif, O. M. (2012). Vulvovaginitis. *Medscape Reference.* Retrieved from http://emedicine.medscape.com/article/270872-overview

Suckling, J., Kennedy, R., Lethaby, A., & Roberts, H. (2010). Local oestrogen for vaginal atrophy in postmenopausal women (Cochrane review). In *The Cochrane Library 2010,* Issue 11. Chichester, UK: John Wiley & Sons, Ltd.

Tan, O., Bradshaw, K., & Carr, B. R. (2012). Management of vulvovaginal atrophy–related sexual dysfunction in postmenopausal women. *Menopause, 19*(1), 109–117.

Urogenital health. (2009). In: Menopause and osteoporosis update 2009. *Journal of Obstetrics & Gynaecology Canada, 31*(Suppl. 1), S27–S30.

Benign Prostatic Hyperplasia (Benign Prostatic Hypertrophy)

American Urological Association Education and Research, Inc. (2010). *Guideline on the management of benign prostatic hyperplasia (BPH).* Linthicum, MD: American Urological Association Education and Research, Inc.

Bent, S., Kane, C., Shinohara, K., Neuhaus, J., Hudes, E. S., Goldberg, H., & Avins, A. L. (2006). Saw palmetto for benign prostatic hyperplasia. *New England Journal of Medicine, 354*(6), 557–566.

Cantrell, M. A., Bream-Rouwenhorst, H. R., Hemerson, P., & Magera, J. S. (2010). Silodosin for benign prostatic hyperplasia. *Annals of Pharmacotherapy, 44*(2), 302–310.

Cunningham, G. R., & Kadmon, D. (2012a). Clinical manifestations and diagnosis of benign prostatic hyperplasia. *UpToDate.* Retrieved from www.uptodate.com

Cunningham, G. R., & Kadmon, D. (2012b). Medical treatment of benign prostatic hyperplasia. *UpToDate.* Retrieved from www.uptodate.com

Debruyne, F., Tzvetkov, M., Altarac, S., & Geavlete, P. A. (2010). Dose-ranging study of the luteinizing hormone–releasing hormone receptor antagonist cetrorelix pamoate in the treatment of patients with symptomatic benign prostatic hyperplasia. *Urology, 76*(4), 927–933.

Deters, L. A., Costabile, R. A., Leveillee, R. J., Moore, C. R., & Patel, V. R. (2012). Benign prostatic hypertrophy. *Medscape.* Retrieved from http://emedicine.medscape.com/article/437359-overview

Flannery, M. T. (2010). Benign prostatic hyperplasia. *Essential Evidence.* John Wiley & Sons, Inc. Retrieved from www.essentialevidenceplus.com

Hoekstra, R. J., Van Melick, H. H., Kok, E. T., & Ruud Bosch, J. L. (2010). A 10-year follow-up after transurethral resection of the prostate, contact laser prostatectomy and electrovaporization in men with benign prostatic hyperplasia; long-term results of a randomized controlled trial. *BJU International, 106*(6), 822–826.

Kaplan, S. A. (2006). Update on the American Urological Association guidelines for the treatment of benign prostatic hyperplasia. *Reviews in Urology, 8* (Suppl. 4) S10–S17.

Kim, E. D. (2002). Ethanol injection for the treatment of benign prostatic hyperplasia. *Current Urology Reports, 3*(4), 276–279.

McConnell, J. D., Roehrborn, C. G., Bautista, O. M., Andriole, G. L., Jr., Dixon, C. M., Kusek, J. W., . . . Medical Therapy of Prostatic Symptoms (MTOPS) Research Group. (2003). The long-term effect of doxazosin, finasteride, and combination therapy on the clinical progression of benign prostatic hyperplasia. *New England Journal of Medicine, 349*(25), 2387–2398.

McVary, K. T., Roehrborn, C. G., Avins, A. L., Barry, M. J., Bruskewitz, R. C., Donnell, R. F., . . . Wei, J. T. (2011). Update on AUA guideline on the management of benign prostatic hyperplasia. *Journal of Urology, 185*(5), 1793–1803.

Parsons, J. K., Carter, H. B., Partin, A. W., Windham, B. G., Metter, E. J., Ferrucci, L., . . . Platz, E. A. (2006). Metabolic factors associated with benign prostatic hyperplasia. *Journal of Clinical Endocrinology and Metabolism, 91*(7), 2562–2568.

Scher, H. I. (2012). Benign and malignant diseases of the prostate. In D. L. Longo, A. S. Fauci, D. L. Kasper, S. L. Hauser, J. L. Jameson, & J. Loscalzo (Eds.), *Harrison's principles of internal medicine* (18th ed., pp. 796–805). New York City, NY: McGraw-Hill Medical.

Smith, C. P., & Chancellor, M. B. (2004). Emerging role of botulinum toxin in the management of voiding dysfunction. *Journal of Urology, 171*(Pt. 1), 2128–2137.

Tacklind, J., MacDonald, R., Rutks, I., & Wilt, T. J. (2010). Serenoa repens for benign prostatic hyperplasia (Cochrane review). In *The Cochrane Library 2010,* Issue 4. Chichester, UK: John Wiley & Sons, Ltd.

Thompson, I. M., Goodman, P. J., Tangen, C. M., Lucia, M. S., Miller, G. J., Ford, L. G., . . . Coltman, C. A., Jr. (2003). The influence of finasteride on the development of prostate cancer. *New England Journal of Medicine, 349*(3), 215–224.

Wilt, T., Howe, R. W., Rutks, I., & MacDonald, R. (2007). Terazosin for benign prostatic hyperplasia (Cochrane review). In *The Cochrane Library 2007,* Issue 1. Chichester, UK: John Wiley & Sons, Ltd.

Wilt, T., MacDonald, R., & Rutks, I. (2007). Tamsulosin for benign prostatic hyperplasia (Cochrane review). In *The Cochrane Library 2007,* Issue 1. Chichester, UK: John Wiley & Sons, Ltd.

Breast Cancer

Agency for Healthcare Research and Quality (AHRQ). (2012). ACR Appropriateness Criteria" palpable breast masses. Reston, VA: American College of Radiology. Retrieved from http://www.guideline.gov/content.aspx?id=43866

American Cancer Society. (2011–2012). Breast cancer facts & figures 2011–2012. Atlanta, GA: American Cancer Society, Inc. Retrieved from www.cancer.org/acs/groups/content/@epidemiologysurveilance/documents/document/acspc-030975.pdf

American College of Radiology. (2004). BI-RADS guidelines. Virginia: American College of Radiology. Retrieved from http://www.acr.org/Quality-Safety/Resources/BIRADS/Mammography

Anderson, R. (2010). Understanding breast cancer risk. *Radiologic Technology, 81*(5), 457–476.

Armstrong, K., Moye, E., Williams, S., Berlin, J., & Reynolds, E. (2007). Screening mammography in women 40–49 years of age: a systematic review for the American College of Physicians. *Annals of Internal Medicine, 146*(7), 516–526.

Baron, R. (2007). Surgical management of breast cancer. *Seminars in Oncology Nursing, 23*(1), 10–19.

Berg, W. (2009). Tailored supplemental screening for breast cancer: what now and what next? *AJR: American Journal of Roentgenology, 192*(2), 390–399.

Bezuhly, M., Temple, C., Sigurdson, L., Davis, R., Flowerdew, G., & Cook, E. (2009). Immediate postmastectomy reconstruction is associated with improved breast cancer–specific survival: evidence and new challenges from the surveillance, epidemiology and end result database. *Cancer, 115*(20), 4648–4654. doi:10.1002/cncr.24511

Deutsch, M., & Flickinger, J. (2009). Compliance with adjuvant radiotherapy after surgery for primary breast cancer. *Community Oncology, 6*(12), 547–550.

Ferrara, A. (2011). Benign breast disease. *Radiologic Technology, 82*(5), 447M–462M.

Foy, S., & Blowers, E. (2009). Breast cancer overview: diagnosis and staging. *Practice Nursing, 20*(6), 276–281.

Gibson, L., Lawrence, D., Dawson, C., & Bliss, J. (2009). Aromatase inhibitors for treatment of advanced breast cancer in postmenopausal women. *Cochrane Database of Systematic Reviews* (4). doi:10.1002/14651858.CD003370.pub2

Gotzsche, P., & Nielsen M. (2009). Screening for breast cancer with mammography. In *The Cochrane Library 2009,* Issue 2. Chichester, UK: John Wiley & Sons.

Henderson, T., Amsterdam, A., Bhatia, S., Hudson, M., Meadows, A., Neglia, J., . . . Oeffinger, K. (2010). Systematic review: surveillance for breast cancer in women treated with chest radiation for childhood, adolescent, or young adult cancer. *Annals of Internal Medicine, 152*(7), 444–455. doi:10.1059/0003-4819-152-7-201004060

Holmes, F. F. (1994). Clinical course of cancer in the elderly. *Cancer Control, 1*(2), 108–114.

Howlader, N., Noone, A. M., Krapcho, M., Garshell, J., Neyman, N., Altekruse, S. F., & Cronin, K. A. (Eds). *SEER Cancer Statistics Review, 1975-2010.* Retrieved from http://seer.cancer.gov/csr/1975_2010

Hubbard, R. A., Kerlikowske, K., Flowers, C. I., Yankaskas, B. C., Weiwei, Z., & Miglioretti, D. L. (2011). Cumulative probability of false-positive recall or biopsy recommendation after 10 years of screening mammography. *Annals of Internal Medicine, 155*(8), 481–492.

Jagsi, R., & Pierce, L. (2009). Postmastectomy radiation therapy for patients with locally advanced breast cancer. *Seminars in Radiation Oncology, 19*(4), 236–243. doi:10.1016/j.semradonc.2009.05.009

Katapodi, M., Dodd, M., Lee, K., & Facione, N. (2009). Underestimation of breast cancer risk: influence on screening behavior. *Oncology Nursing Forum, 36*(3), 306–314. doi:10.1188/09.ONF.306-314

Kelly, C. M., Juurlink, D. N., Gomes, T., Duong-Hua, M., Pritchard, K. I., Austin, P. C., & Paszat, L. F. (2010). Selective serotonin reuptake inhibitors and breast cancer mortality in women receiving tamoxifen: a population based cohort study. *BMJ, 340,* c693.

Litton, J. K., Westin, S. N., Ready, K., Sun, C. C., Peterson, S. K., Meric-Bernstam, F., . . . Arun, B. K. (2009). Perception of screening and risk reduction surgeries in patients tested for a BRCA deleterious mutation. *Cancer, 115*(8), 1598–1604. doi: 10.1002/cncr.24199

Mattarella, A. (2010). Breast cancer in men. *Radiologic Technology, 81*(4), 361M–378M.

Metcalfe, K., Lubinski, J., Ghadirian, P., Lynch, H., Kim-Sing, C., Friedman, E., . . . Narod, S. (2008). Predictors of contralateral prophylactic mastectomy in women with a BRCA1 or BRCA2 mutation: the Hereditary Breast Cancer Clinical Study Group. *Journal of Clinical Oncology, 26*(7), 1093–1097.

Muss, H., Berry, D., Cirrincione, C., Theodoulou, M., Mauer, A., Kornblith, A., . . . Winer, E. (2009). Adjuvant chemotherapy in older women with early-stage breast cancer. *New England Journal of Medicine, 360*(20), 2055–2065. doi:10.1056/NEJMoa0810266

Narayanan, S., & Taylor, I. (2007). Adjuvant systemic therapy for operable breast cancer. *Surgeon (Edinburgh University Press), 5*(2), 101.

National Cancer Institute. (2012). Breast cancer. Maryland: National Cancer Institute at the National Institutes of Health. Retrieved from www.cancer.gov/cancertopics/types/breast

Nattinger, A. (2010). In the clinic. Breast cancer screening and prevention. *Annals of Internal Medicine, 152*(7), ITC41. doi:10.1059/0003-4819-152-7-201004060-01004

Patterson, K. (2010). Should women under 50 hold off on breast cancer screening? *CURE: Cancer Updates, Research & Education, 9*(1), 43.

Schmitz, K. H., Ahmed, R. L., Troxel, A. B., Cheville, A., Lewis-Grant, L., Smith, R., . . . Chittams, J. (2010) Weight lifting for women at risk for breast cancer–related lymphedema: a randomized trial. *Journal of the American Medical Association, 304*(24), 2699–2705.

Smith-Bindman, R., Miglioretti, D., Lurie, N., Abraham, L., Barbash, R., Strzelczyk, J., . . . Kerlikowske, K. (2006). Does utilization of screening mammography explain racial and ethnic differences in breast cancer? *Annals of Internal Medicine, 144*(8), 541–553.

Trock, B. J., Hilakivi-Clarke, L., & Clarke, R. (2006). Meta-analysis of soy intake and breast cancer risk. *JNCI: Journal of the National Cancer Institute, 98*(7), 459–471.

U.S. Cancer Statistics Working Group. (2010). United States cancer statistics: 1999–2007. Incidence and mortality Web-based report. Atlanta, GA: Department of Health and Human Services, Centers for Disease Control and Prevention, and National Cancer Institute. Retrieved from www.cdc.gov/uscs

U.S. Preventive Services Task Force. (2009). Screening for breast cancer: U.S. Preventive Services Task Force recommendation statement. *Annals of Internal Medicine, 151*(10), 716–726.

Waljee, J., & Newman, L. (2007). Neoadjuvant systemic therapy and the surgical management of breast cancer. *Surgical Clinics of North America, 87*(2), 399–415.

Watkins, J. (2009). Skin manifestations of breast cancer. *Practice Nursing, 20*(3), 134–138.

Wishart, G. (2010). Breast cancer: advances in risk assessment. *Practice Nursing, 21*(10), 511–514.

Yi, M., Kronowitz, S. J., Meric-Bernstam, F., Feig, B. W., Symmans, W. F., Lucci, A., . . . Hunt, K. K. (2011). Local, regional, and systemic recurrence rates in patients undergoing skin-sparing mastectomy compared with conventional mastectomy. *Cancer, 117*(5), 916–924. doi:10.1002/cncr.25505

Drug-Induced Impotence

Blanker, M. H., Bosch, J. L., Groeneveld, F. P., Bohnen, A. M., Prins, A., Thomas, S., & Hop, W. C. (2001). Erectile and ejaculatory dysfunction in a community-based sample of men 50 to 78 years old: prevalence, concern, and relation to sexual activity. *Urology, 57*(4), 763–768.

Cunningham, G. R., & Rosen, R. C. (2011). Overview of male sexual dysfunction. *UpToDate.* Retrieved from www.uptodate.com

Grimm, R. H., Jr., Grandits, G. A., Prineas, R. J., McDonald, R. H., Lewis, C. E., Flack, J. M., . . . Elmer P. J. (1997). Long-term effects on sexual function of five antihypertensive drugs and nutritional hygienic treatment in hypertensive men and women. Treatment of Mild Hypertension Study (TOMHS). *Hypertension, 29*(1 Pt 1), 8–14.

Heidelbaugh, J., & Barry, H. (2011). Erectile dysfunction. *Essential Evidence Plus.* John Wiley & Sons, Inc. Retrieved from www.essentialevidenceplus.com

Hirsch, M., & Birnbaum, R. J. (2009). Sexual dysfunction associated with selective serotonin reuptake inhibitor (SSRI) antidepressants. *UpToDate.* Retrieved from www.uptodate.com

Martin, K. A. (2012). Treatment of male sexual dysfunction. *UpToDate.* Retrieved from www.uptodate.com

McVary, K. T. (2007). Clinical practice. Erectile dysfunction. *New England Journal of Medicine, 357*(24), 2472.

McVary, K. T. (2012). Sexual dysfunction. In D. L. Longo, A. S. Fauci, D. L. Kasper, S. L. Hauser, J. L. Jameson, & J. Loscalzo (Eds.), *Harrison's principles of internal medicine* (18th ed., pp. 374–377). New York City, NY: McGraw-Hill Medical.

Miles, C., Candy, B., Jones, L., Williams, R., Tookman, A., & King, M. (2011). Interventions for sexual dysfunction following treatments for cancer (Cochrane review). In *The Cochrane Library 2011,* Issue 3. Chichester, UK: John Wiley & Sons, Ltd.

NIH Consensus Statement Online. (1992, December 7–9). Impotence. *NIH Consensus Statement Online, 10*(4), 1–31.

Nurnberg, H. G., Hensley, P. L., Gelenberg, A. J., Fava, M., Lauriello, J., & Paine, S. (2003). Treatment of antidepressant-associated sexual dysfunction with sildenafil: a randomized controlled trial. *Journal of the American Medical Association, 289*(1), 56–64.

Rosen, R., Altwein, J., Boyle, P., Kirby, R. S., Lukacs, B., Meuleman, E., . . . Giuliano, F. (2003). Lower urinary tract symptoms and male sexual dysfunction: the multinational survey of the aging male (MSAM-7). *European Urology, 44*(6), 637–649.

Rowland, D., McMahon, C. G., Abdo, C., Chen, J., Jannini, E., Waldinger, M. D., & Ahn, T. Y. (2010). Disorders of orgasm and ejaculation in men. *Journal of Sexual Medicine, 7*(4 Pt 2), 1668–1686.

Rudkin, L., Taylor, M. J., Hawton, K. E., & Taylor, M. J. (2009). Strategies for managing sexual dysfunction induced by antidepressant medication (Cochrane review). In *The Cochrane Library 2009,* Issue 1. Chichester, UK: John Wiley & Sons, Ltd.

Selvin, E., Burnett, A. L., & Platz, E. A. (2007). Prevalence and risk factors for erectile dysfunction in the US. *American Journal of Medicine, 120*(2), 151–157.

Slag, M. F., Morley, J. E., Elson, M. K., Trence, D. L., Nelson, C. J., Nelson, A. E., . . . Shafer, R. B. (1983). Impotence in medical clinic outpatients. *Journal of the American Medical Association, 249*(13), 1736–1740.

Tacklind, J., Fink, H. A., MacDonald, R., Rutks, I., & Wilt, T. J. (2012). Finasteride for benign prostatic hyperplasia (Cochrane review). In *The Cochrane Library 2012,* Issue 2. Chichester, UK: John Wiley & Sons, Ltd.

Veterans Administration Cooperative Study Group on Antihypertensive Agents. (1982). Comparison of propranolol and hydrochlorothiazide for the initial treatment of hypertension. II. Results of long-term therapy. *Journal of the American Medical Association, 248*(16), 2004–2011.

Wein, A. J., & Van Arsdalen, K. N. (1988). Drug-induced male sexual dysfunction. *Urologic Clinics of North America, 15*(1), 23–31.

Zisook, S., Rush, A. J., Haight, B. R., Clines, D. C., & Rockett, C. B. (2006). Use of bupropion in combination with serotonin reuptake inhibitors. *Biological Psychiatry, 59*(3), 203–210.

Endometrial Cancer

Allard, J. E., & Maxwell, G. L. (2009). Race disparities between black and white women in the incidence, treatment, and prognosis of endometrial cancer. *Cancer Control, 16*(1), 53–56.

American College of Obstetricians and Gynecologists. (2005). ACOG practice bulletin, clinical management guidelines for obstetrician-gynecologists, number 65, August 2005: Management of endometrial cancer. *Obstetrics and Gynecology, 106*(2), 413–425.

American Joint Committee on Cancer. (2010). Corpus uteri. In *AJCC staging manual* (7th ed., p. 403). New York City, NY: Springer.

Benedet, J. L., Bender, H., Jones, H., 3rd, Ngan, H. Y., & Pecorelli, S. (2000). FIGO staging classifications and clinical practice guidelines in the management of gynecologic cancers. FIGO Committee on Gynecologic Oncology. *International Journal of Gynaecology and Obstetrics, 70*(2), 209–262.

Bode, D. V., & Seehusen, D. A. (2011). Uterine cancer. *Essential Evidence Plus.* Retrieved from www.essentialevidenceplus.com

Chen, L., & Berek, J. S. (2012). Endometrial carcinoma: epidemiology and risk factors. *UpToDate.* Retrieved from www.uptodate.com

Fung-Kee-Fung, M., Dodge, J., Elit, L., Lukka, H., Chambers, A., & Oliver, T. (2006). Follow-up after primary therapy for endometrial cancer: a systematic review. *Gynecologic Oncology, 101*(3), 520–529.

Heald, B., Mester, J., Rybicki, L., Orloff, M. S., Burke, C. A., & Eng, C. (2010). Frequent gastrointestinal polyps and colorectal adenocarcinomas in a prospective series of PTEN mutation carriers. *Gastroenterology, 139*(6), 1927–1933.

Jemal, A., Bray, F., Center, M. M., Ferlay, J., Ward, E., & Forman, D. (2011). Global cancer statistics. *CA: A Cancer Journal for Clinicians, 61*(2), 69–90.

Ollikainen, M., Abdel-Rahman, W. M., Moisio, A. L., Lindroos, A., Kariola, R., Järvelä, I., . . . Peltomäki, P. (2005). Molecular analysis of familial endometrial carcinoma: a manifestation of hereditary nonpolyposis colorectal cancer or a separate syndrome? *Journal of Clinical Oncology, 23*(21), 4609–4616.

Sartori, E., Pasinetti, B., Chiudinelli, F., Gadducci, A., Landoni, F., Maggino, T., . . . Zola, P. (2010). Surveillance procedures for patients treated for endometrial cancer: a review of the literature. *International Journal of Gynecological Cancer, 20*(6), 985–992.

Siegel, R., Ward, E., Brawley, O., & Jemal, A. (2011). Cancer statistics, 2011: the impact of eliminating socioeconomic and racial disparities on premature cancer deaths. *CA: A Cancer Journal for Clinicians, 61*(4), 212–236.

Smith, R. A., von Eschenbach, A. C., Wender, R., Levin, B., Byers, T., Rothenberger, D., . . . Eyre, H. (2001). American Cancer Society guidelines for the early detection of cancer: update of early detection guidelines for prostate, colorectal, and endometrial cancers: ALSO: Update 2001—testing for early lung cancer detection. *CA: A Cancer Journal for Clinicians, 51*(1), 38–75.

Yap, O. W. S., & Matthews, R. P. (2006). Racial and ethnic disparities in cancers of the uterine corpus. *Journal of the National Medical Association, 98*(12), 1930–1933.

Zhou, B., Yang, L., Sun, Q., Cong, R., Gu, H., Tang, N., . . . Wang, B. (2008). Cigarette smoking and the risk of endometrial cancer: a meta-analysis. *American Journal of Medicine, 121*(6), 501–508.

Ovarian Cancer

Fowler, J. R. (2011). Ovarian tumor (malignant). *Essential Evidence Plus.* Retrieved from www.essentialevidenceplus.com

Kim, K. A., Park, C. M., Lee, J. H., Kim, H. K., Cho, S. M., Kim, B., & Seol, H. Y. (2004). Benign ovarian tumors with solid and cystic components that mimic malignancy. *AJR: American Journal of Roentgenology, 182*(5), 1259–1265.

McLemore, M. R., Miaskowski, C., Aouizerat, B. E., Chen, L., & Dodd, M. J. (2009). Epidemiological and genetic factors associated with ovarian cancer. *Cancer Nursing, 32*(4), 281–288.

Murphy, S. K. (2012). Targeting the epigenome in ovarian cancer: potential for epigenetic therapies. *Medscape.* Retrieved from www.medscape.com/viewarticle/759027_4

National Cancer Institute. (2012). Ovarian cancer. Retrieved from http://seer.cancer.gov/statfacts/html/ovary.html

National Comprehensive Cancer Network (NCCN). (2012). NCCN Clinical Practice Guidelines in Oncology. Ovarian cancer guidelines, 2012. Retrieved from www.nccn.org

Seiden, M. V. (2012). Gynecologic malignancies. In D. L. Longo, A. S. Fauci, D. L. Kasper, S. L. Hauser, J. L. Jameson, & J. Loscalzo (Eds.), *Harrison's principles of internal medicine* (18th ed., pp. 810–813). New York City, NY: McGraw-Hill Medical.

U.S. Preventive Services Task Force. (2005). Genetic risk assessment and BRCA mutation testing for breast and ovarian cancer susceptibility: recommendation statement. *Annals of Internal Medicine, 143*(5), 355–361.

Vaughan, S., Coward, J. I., Bast, R. C., Berchuck, A., Berek, J. S., Brenton, J. D., . . . Balkwill, F. R. (2011). Rethinking ovarian cancer: recommendations to improve outcomes. *Nature Reviews Cancer, 11*(10), 719–725.

Villella, J. A., Parmar, M., Donohue, K., Fahey, C., Piver, M. S., & Rodabaugh, K. (2006). Role of prophylactic hysterectomy in patients at high risk for hereditary cancers. *Gynecologic Oncology, 102*(3), 475–479.

Prostate Cancer

Ali, T., & Walsh, W. (2011). Prostate cancer. In F. J. Domino (Ed.), *The 5 minute clinical consult 2011* (19th ed., pp. 1066–1067). Philadelphia, PA: Wolters Kluwer.

American Urological Association. (2012) American Urological Association speaks out against USPSTF recommendations. Retrieved from www.auanet.org/content/health-policy/government-relations-and-advocacy/in-the-news/uspstf-psa-recommendations.cfm

Gjertson, C. K., & Albertsen, P. C. (2011). Use and assessment of PSA in prostate cancer. *Medical Clinics of North America, 95*(1), 191–200.

McCance, K., Huether, S., Brashers, V., & Rote, N. (2010). *Pathophysiology. The biologic basis for disease in adults and children* (6th ed.). Maryland Heights, MO: Mosby.

McCormick, K., Osman, M., & Pomerantz, M. (2010). Update on prostate cancer screening. *Journal of Clinical Outcomes Management, 17*(10), 470–478.

Prostate cancer. (2011). In F. J. Domino (Ed.), *The 5 minute clinical consult 2011* (19th ed., pp. 1066–1067). Philadelphia, PA: Wolters Kluwer.

Prostate cancer. (2012). In L. Goldman & A. Schafer (Eds.), *Goldman's Cecil medicine* (24th ed., pp. 1322–1325). Philadelphia, PA: Elsevier.

Small, E. J. (2012). Prostate cancer. In L. Goldman & A. Schafer (Eds.), *Goldman's Cecil medicine* (24th ed., pp. 1322–1325). Philadelphia, PA: Elsevier.

U.S. Preventive Services Task Force. (2012). Screening for prostate cancer. Retrieved from www.uspreventiveservicestaskforce.org/prostatecancerscreening.htm

Wilbur, J. (2008). Prostate cancer screening: the continuing controversy. *American Family Physician, 28*(12), 1377–1384.

Wolf, A. M., Wender, R. C., Etzioni, R. B., Thompson, I. M., D'Amico, A. V., Volk, R. J., . . . Smith, R. A. (2010). American Cancer Society guideline for the early detection of prostate cancer. *CA: A Cancer Journal for Clinicians, 60*(2), 70–98.

Prostatitis

Bope, E. T., & Kellerman, R. D. (2013). The urogenital tract. In *Conn's current therapy 2013.* Philadelphia, PA: Saunders/Elsevier.

Buttaro, T. M., Trybulski, J., Bailey, P. P., & Sandberg-Cook, J. (2008). *Primary care. A collaborative practice* (3rd ed.). St. Louis, MO: Mosby.

Grabe, M., Bishop, M. C., Bjerklund-Johansen, T. E., Botto, H., Çek, M., Lobel, B., . . . Wagenlehner, F. (2009). Prostatitis and chronic pelvic pain syndrome. In *Guidelines on urological infections* (pp. 65–73). Arnhem, The Netherlands: European Association of Urology. Data from http://www.guideline.gov/content.aspx?id=14811

McCance, K., Huether, S., Brashers, V., & Rote, N. (2010). *Pathophysiology. The biologic basis for disease in adults and children* (6th ed.). Maryland Heights, MO: Mosby.

Prostatitis. (2011). In F. J. Domino (Ed.), *The 5 minute clinical consult 2011* (19th ed., pp. 1070–1071). Philadelphia, PA: Wolters Kluwer.

Prostatitis. (2012). In L. Goldman & A. Schafer (Eds.), *Goldman's Cecil medicine* (24th ed., pp. 808–810). Philadelphia, PA: Elsevier.

Schaeffer, A. J. (2006). Clinical practice. Chronic prostatitis and the chronic pelvic pain syndrome. *New England Journal of Medicine, 355*(16), 1690–1698.

Sharp, V. J., Takacs, E. B., & Powell, C. R. (2010). Prostatitis: diagnosis and treatment. *American Family Physician, 82*(4), 397–406.

chapter 12

Musculoskeletal Disorders

Laurie Kennedy-Malone

ASSESSMENT

To make an accurate assessment of the musculoskeletal system in the older adult, the nurse practitioner needs to be familiar with changes in the musculoskeletal system caused by aging. For example, aging often brings about a decrease in height, resulting from a decrease in the length of the trunk with respect to the length of the extremities. An older person may tilt the head backward to compensate for the bend in the thoracic spine, producing the typical posture of those in this age group. Because of the loss of subcutaneous fat caused by aging, bony prominences became more noticeable. Some absolute loss of muscle mass occurs, with some muscles diminishing and others atrophying. Without continued use, muscles stiffen and range of motion becomes impaired as an older person ages (Loeser & DelBono, 2009).

Often when an older person experiences a limitation in functional ability resulting from pain, weakness, or physical impairment, he or she seeks medical attention. To obtain an accurate history of musculoskeletal problems, question the patient about the following:

- Any pain, swelling, stiffness, change in temperature perception (hot or cold), limitation of movement, weakness, body deformity, or paralysis.
- Whether the symptoms are constant or intermittent.
- Determine the sequence of events that triggered the onset of each symptom and inquire about precipitating factors.

- Ask if there is a trigger to the complaint such as lack of mobility, temperature, or position (as in sleeping). Often the patient complains of one or more of these symptoms; however, the condition may actually be a neurological condition such as Parkinson's disease or a systemic disorder (e.g., thyroid disease). Additionally, patients may be experiencing a new musculoskeletal condition concomitant with an existing condition, such as a new onset of gout with preexisting osteoarthritis of the interphalangeal joints.
- Determine if the condition has been triggered by medications such as statins with the known side effect of myalgias (Gillet & Norrell, 2011).
- Be alert for other symptoms the patient may describe; for example, constitutional symptoms of fever and malaise may be clustered to form a differential diagnosis (Pacala & Sullivan, 2010).

Pain or Stiffness

When a patient complains of pain or stiffness with movement, the history of the complaint should be discerned. Ask if the patient has experienced any severe trauma in the past that may be now manifesting itself as an articular degeneration. Because patients who have had a structural deformity or amputation typically place excessive strain on the joints for years, as older individuals they may now experience degeneration of the bone and surrounding musculature. An overextension or a recent increase in activity may lead to muscle soreness, followed by disuse, atrophy, and chronic pain. Adhesive capsulitis or frozen shoulder is a common condition in patients experiencing pain in the shoulder and in turn limiting their range of motion. Knowing the history of the presenting symptom may help you distinguish between a local inflammation and a systemic problem. Questioning the patient about the time of day when the symptoms of pain and stiffness occur can be helpful too. Rheumatic disease, for example, is associated with pain on waking, whereas osteoarthritic pain and stiffness worsen as the day progresses. It is important to remember that within the current cohort of older adults a stoic attitude toward pain may be displayed despite the presence of an acute or chronic musculoskeletal condition (Abdulla et al., 2013).

Weakness and Paralysis

Patients with musculoskeletal problems often complain of weakness and paralysis. Determine whether the disability is local or generalized, constant or intermittent. Local weakness or paralysis may be due to disuse because of pain, trauma, or a neurological problem. Generalized weakness may indicate a systemic disorder or recent deconditioning related to extensive immobility or frailty as in the case of patients with sarcopenia (Brown & Peel, 2009). Patients with an underlying thyroid disorder may have constant weakness, whereas those with rheumatoid arthritis may experience weakness intermittently (Pacala & Sullivan, 2010). Muscular weakness should always be differentiated from subjective fatigue. Generally, proximal weakness results from a myopathy and distal weakness from a neuropathy. The patient should be asked about his or her ability to carry out certain activities of daily living, such as the following:

- Does the patient have difficulty combing his or her hair?
- Can he or she lift objects?
- Does the patient have any trouble standing up after sitting in a chair?

Patients with a proximal weakness of the upper extremities may have difficulty grooming the hair or lifting objects. Those with a proximal weakness of a lower extremity may have trouble crossing the legs at the knees or walking. If a patient reports difficulty fastening buttons or turning doorknobs, a neuropathy involving the upper extremity is likely.

Deformity

Another common complaint in patients with a musculoskeletal disorder is deformity. In obtaining the history from a patient with a deformity, the examiner needs to know how long the patient has noticed the deformity:

- Did it occur suddenly?
- Was it the result of trauma?
- Has there been any change in the deformity since its onset?

Physical Examination

GAIT

The overall physical examination of the musculoskeletal disorder begins with observing the patient's gait. Any gait abnormalities or problems in maintaining balance should be noted. In addition, the patient's ability to sit in and rise from a chair should be observed. More sophisticated testing is warranted if the patient demonstrates difficulty in performing this task, because he or she could be at a high risk for falling.

STANDING ERECT

Examine the patient while the patient is standing erect, to note any changes in the spinal curvature. In older adults, kyphosis of the thoracic spine is accentuated. While looking at the older person from the side, the examiner may note that the spine appears to form the number 3. If the curve appears more to be a sharp angle, this is called a gibbus. A gibbus resulting from a vertebral compression fracture may be the first evidence of osteoporosis (Williams, 2008).

RANGE OF MOTION

Patients presenting with a functional limitation should be asked to demonstrate active range of motion (ROM). Active ROM should be performed smoothly and effortlessly. Remember that joint movements include flexion, extension, abduction, adduction, and external rotation. If the patient has limited active ROM, passive ROM should be performed. If the passive range exceeds the active range, the limitation is due to a muscle weakness. Patients may resist passive ROM because of fear, a neurological disorder, or a joint abnormality.

JOINT PAIN

When patients complain of joint-related pain, the practitioner needs to determine if the underlying condition is articular, periarticular, or both. When examining the patient's joints, the joints should be inspected in a relaxed position and then in flexion and in extension. Abnormalities of the position or carrying angle, joint deformity, erythema, swellings, nodulation, and muscle changes should be assessed. In an older patient with muscle changes, the limb or portion of the body will appear thinner, which indicates atrophy. To determine whether bone structure changes have occurred, appearance and symmetry should be observed. Enlargement, excessive curvature, and irregularity may indicate sequelae of childhood rickets, osteoporotic fractures, Paget's disease, osteoarthritis, tophaceous gout, or bone tumors. Crepitation or a crackling noise may be heard when the joints are put through ROM. Crepitation is produced by the rubbing together of bone or irregular cartilage surfaces (LeBlond, Brown, & DeGowin, 2009).

Specific questions about the duration of any swelling, presence of pain, limitation of movement, evidence of erythema, and locking or buckling of the joint are important to assess. Erythema is usually associated with active inflammation and accompanied by swelling. Examples of joint nodulation are the nodules found in the interphalangeal joints in patients with rheumatoid arthritis and osteoarthritis. Heberden's nodes are nodules of the distal interphalangeal joints; Bouchard's nodes are nodules of the proximal joints. Both are found in patients with osteoarthritis. Rheumatoid nodules are described as firm, nontender nodules often found on the dorsum of the wrist, elbow, or metacarpophalangeal joint. Haygarth's nodes are spindle-shaped enlargements of the middle interphalangeal joints that occur in rheumatoid arthritis (LeBlond et al., 2009). Any joint deformity should be palpated to determine whether it fluctuates because of fluid or is firm because of a thickening or enlargement. If there is fluid, the cause may be recent trauma, inflammation, or joint infection. An articular enlargement of rheumatoid arthritis is usually soft, whereas a joint deformity found in osteoarthritis is usually firm. Erythema may also be indicative of septic arthritis. If the joint swelling persists for more than 3 days, this may indicate an arthritic condition. Also examine the bursal areas around the joints, palpating for swelling, tenderness, ganglions, and presence of nodules. Tophaceous gout appears as salmon-colored nodules that do not transilluminate, as is possible when examining a superficial inflamed bursa (Williams, 2008). A ganglion is usually a soft cystlike swelling, often found near joints. Swelling of the bursa is usually tender on palpation. All masses should be measured across their greatest diameter (LeBlond et al., 2009).

MUSCLE WEAKNESS

For the patient complaining of muscle weakness, inspect for evidence of muscle atrophy and palpate the muscles during contraction and rest. Any fluttering or fasciculations of the muscles should be noted. To determine if a patient is having true muscle weakness, the patient should perform against the examiner's resistance. One side should be compared with the other and a numerical value for tested muscle strength recorded. Flexor and extensor muscles should be tested for strength (LeBlond et al., 2009).

BURSITIS, TENDINITIS, SOFT TISSUE SYNDROMES

Signal symptoms: Pain, tenderness in soft tissue areas.

Etiology: Overuse and abuse, possible crystal or bacteria origin.

Occurrence: May occur anytime but increases after middle age.

Age: Range of 53 to 71 years old with a median age of 62 years old (Brown & Peel, 2009).

Gender: In studies, females outnumber males. This condition is dependent on use of work and hobbies.

Ethnicity: None known.

Contributing factors: Certain diseases and conditions increase the risk of developing soft tissue disorders, such as bursitis, rheumatoid arthritis, osteoarthritis, gout, thyroid disease, and diabetes (Omoigu, 2007).

Diagnostic tests: Although diagnostic imaging is not helpful for plantar fasciitis, heel spurs are frequently (50%) a comorbidity with this condition. Radiographs can show calcifications in the soft tissue. Thickened heel aponeurosis is identified by ultrasound. Radiology tests can also rule out fractures (Cole, Seto, & Gazewood, 2005).

Differential diagnosis:
- Fracture
- Infection
- Arthritis

Treatment: Bursitis, supraspinatus tendinitis, subacromial bursitis, nontraumatic rotator cuff tear, and plantar fasciitis treatments are discussed in the following passages. Bursitis is defined as an inflammation of the bursa, which is a soft sac surrounding and protective of the joints; it is a soft tissue disorder. Conservative treatment can include the PRICEMM mnemonic for pain control in bursitis conditions:

P—Protect with padding, braces, and changes in techniques.

R—Rest, avoid activities that exacerbate pain.

I—Ice; cryotherapy can relieve pain and decrease inflammation.

C—Compression; elastic dressings can ease pain in olecranon bursitis.

E—Elevation; raise the affected limb above the level of the heart.

M—Modalities; electrical stimulation or ultrasound.

M—Medications; NSAIDs, acetaminophen, and/or corticosteroid injection (Simpson & Howard, 2009).

Supraspinatus tendinitis or tenosynovitis and subacromial bursitis are the most common shoulder problems to be presented in practice. Patients with these conditions most often complain of pain located at the shoulder tip. On clinical examination, palpable tenderness is normally noted over the superior aspect of the shoulder, and, on testing shoulder movements, painful active abduction is typically found between 70 and 140 degrees for tendinitis (Barratt, 2009). In subacromial bursitis, on clinical examination localized tenderness at the shoulder tip and a soft feeling may also be noted at the humeral head. When patients' shoulder movements are tested, there is a complaint of superior shoulder pain on both active and passive abduction, but they experience minimal pain on resisted abduction because the supraspinatus muscle and tendon are not inflamed. Pain happens with passive abduction of glenohumeral joint due to the subacromial space becoming restricted, compressing the subdeltoid bursa, which is exhibited as shoulder tip pain (Barratt, 2009).

The inflammatory condition of a nontraumatic tear of one or more of the rotator cuff muscles usually occurs in patients over 50 years old, because people in this age group tend to develop muscle fibrosis or long-term tendinitis or bone spurs. These everyday conditions can lead to the rotator cuff muscles tearing. On testing patients' shoulder movements by either active abduction or lateral or medial rotation, pain and weakness are often noted. Patients may also be unable to abduct their shoulders or hold abduction at 90 degrees (Barratt, 2009).

Extracorporeal shock waves are focused, single-pressure pulses of microsecond duration. The Food and Drug Administration (FDA) gave permission for its use in the treatment of chronic proximal plantar fasciitis in 2000 (Cole et al., 2005). Side effects of high-energy pulses are petechiae and hematomas. Extracorporeal shock wave therapy is ineffective in chronic heel pain. Results of a Cochrane review exhibited that corticosteroid injections improved symptoms of plantar fasciitis at 1 month but not at 6 months. Limited evidence showed that casting or surgery may be effective when conservative measures fail.

Randomized and quasi-randomized controlled trials examining the effects of acupuncture on lateral epicondyle pain were selected from six studies. The majority of these studies, five out of six, expressed strong evidence suggesting that acupuncture is effective in the short-term relief of lateral epicondyle or tennis elbow pain (Bisset, Coombes, & Vicenzino, 2011).

The review for surgery of the rotator cuff has shown that it may not lead to any difference in pain compared with different exercise programs. Arthroscopic surgery showed no difference except in recovery time. Side effects that have occurred in the studies included pain, infection, difficulty moving the shoulder after the operation, wasting of the shoulder muscle, and the need to have another surgical procedure (Green, Johnston, & Bell, 2008). There were no differences in side effects between types of surgery.

Corticosteroid injection can be effective when other treatment fails. A mix of corticosteroids and local anesthetic is injected into the tender site. At times of suspected infection/sepsis, the bursa is aspirated for content, and no cortisone is injected. A 4-week course of sensitivity-susceptible antibiotics is advised. Outpatient treatment is effective in 40% to 50% of cases, with hospitalization advised for severe cases.

Indications for therapeutic injection for soft tissue conditions include bursitis, tendinitis, trigger points, ganglion cyst, neuromas, entrapment syndromes, and fasciitis (Cardone & Tallia, 2002). Absolute contraindications for therapeutic injection include cellulitis, acute fracture, history of allergy, and joint prosthesis. The effects of injection are inversely related to solubility of the agent; therefore, the less soluble, the longer acting the agent (Cardone & Tallia, 2002). When using anesthesia, obtain informed consent and assess for toxicity, which can include hives, flushing, nausea, and pain. Fat atrophy, changes in pigmentation, and tendon rupture can occur. It is important to remember that with the introduction of steroids comes hyperglycemia, occurring in patients with diabetes mellitus.

Follow-up: Generally an acute concern; however, aspiration or surgery as listed may be needed.

Sequelae: Referral to physical therapy after severe cases needing surgery.

Prevention/prophylaxis: None listed.

Referral: Referral to orthopedist for injections, surgery. In some cases in the literature, an acupuncturist has been shown to be effective (Bisset et al., 2011).

Education: Informed consent before injection. Methods of immediate overuse injury treatment. Presurgical education if needed.

CLINICAL RECOMMENDATION	EVIDENCE RATING	REFERENCE
Extracorporeal shock wave therapy is not recommended in plantar fasciitis outside of runners.	A	Cole, Seto, & Gazewood (2005)
Surgery for rotator cuff disease may not lead to any differences in pain compared to exercise.	A	Coghlan, Buchbinder, Green, Johnston, & Bell (2008)
Evidence-based strategies for injection therapy in soft tissue.	A	Speed & Hazleman (2004)
Adhesion of the subacromial bursa increases impingement between the acromion and the insertion of rotator cuff tendons.	A	Machida et al. (2004)
Most patients who respond to injections do so in the first session.	C	Cardone & Tallia (2002)
Expert opinion on quick assessment of shoulder examination for possible soft tissue conditions.	C	Barrett (2009)
Strong evidence suggesting acupuncture is effective.	A	Bisset, Coombes, & Vicenzino (2011) Rheumatology (2004)

A = consistent, good-quality, patient-oriented evidence; B = inconsistent or limited-quality, patient-oriented evidence; C = consensus, disease-oriented evidence, usual practice, expert opinion, or case series. For information about the SORT evidence rating system, go to www.aafp.org/afpsort.xml.

FRACTURES

Signal symptoms: Fractures are a common cause of disability in older adults. A compound fracture or open fracture occurs when fragments of the bone pierce the skin or mucosa; an impacted fracture occurs when fragments wedge together. Common sites for fractures include proximal humerus, distal radius, pelvic ramus, proximal femur, proximal tibia, and thoracic and lumbar vertebral bodies.

Etiology: Many fractures are due to an indirect or direct injury. Vertebral fractures may result from an activity such as heavy lifting or bending over that puts sudden stress on the spine. Compression fractures may not have an antecedent. Osteoporosis decreases the chance of sustaining a fall. When a fracture is caused by multiple myeloma, bone marrow is replaced by malignant plasma cells, and thus bone is destroyed.

Occurrence: More than 250,000 hip fractures occur in the United States each year. Estimates show that 30% of people age 65 years and older fall each year; in that group, 5% of those falls result in fractures. Most fractures in the United States have been associated with a diagnosis of a bone density disease such as osteoporosis.

Age: "Women older than fifty years of age have a fifteen percent chance of experiencing a hip fracture; by age ninety, one out of three women and one out of six men experience a hip fracture. About fifty-four percent of women age fifty years or older may have an osteoporotic fracture in their lifetime" (Rahmani & Morin, 2009, p. 815). Prevalence occurs in women who are older than menopausal age due to decreased protective benefits of estrogen to bone, causing some degree of osteoporosis.

Gender: Older females tend to outnumber males because the majority of fractures in this age group occur due to menopausal osteoporosis.

Ethnicity: Those at high risk for osteoporosis include Caucasians and Asian American women. These ethnic groups have a higher prevalence of fractures than African American women because of their increased risk of osteoporosis.

Contributing factors: Multiple factors exist that predispose the elderly to fractures. These include low vitamin D levels, osteoporosis, malnutrition, and sedentary lifestyle; medications such as long-term high steroid doses; and impaired vision, neurological disease, poor balance, orthostatic hypotension, and muscle atrophy (Rahmani & Morin, 2009). Patients with diagnosed diabetes have been found to be at increased risk for fractures (Schneider et al., 2013).

Signs and symptoms: Symptoms include soft tissue swelling, ecchymosis, local tenderness, and pain with any motion. Fractures often are a result of injury to the affected area. For vertebral compression fractures, however, trauma may not be the precipitating factor. An older adult may report pain, pressure, spasms, and swelling in the injured area. A patient with a femoral neck fracture may report groin pain. Physical examination will reveal soft tissue swelling, ecchymosis, local tenderness, and pain with motion (particularly in weight-bearing limbs).

Diagnostic tests: Recommend ordering radiographs of the affected area/injury to rule out and identify area and type of fracture. Radiographs of the affected area are needed in two and three views. Also important is a complete blood count (CBC) to determine if internal blood loss has occurred during an injury. Further laboratory studies include a Westergren erythrocyte sedimentation rate (ESR). An elevated ESR may indicate whether an infectious process was a cause of the fracture.

Differential diagnosis:
- An infectious process/osteomyelitis
- Neoplastic process/multiple myeloma
- Osteoporosis

Treatment: For the pain related to the fracture, narcotic analgesics and/or short-term NSAIDs, if not prohibited, are helpful. Depending on the site of the fracture, casting, walking boot, elastic wrapping, splints, immobilization, traction, or surgical intervention may be used. The most common surgical intervention for a fractured hip is the open reduction with internal rotation, especially for fractures of the intertrochanteric or subtrochanteric region.

The long-term management of a patient with a fracture depends not only on the location of the fracture but also on the etiology of the fracture, whether osteoporosis, an infectious process, or neoplasia. Adequate nutrition and wound care are important for proper healing. It is common in nursing homes to start patients on zinc and vitamin C supplements; however, no study is conclusive in this treatment modality. Patients should be questioned about any muscle weakness or paresthesia after the incident. Patients may have return appointments with an orthopedist, physical therapist, or both. The function of the affected area should be evaluated. Determine what impact the injury had on the patient's activities of daily living (ADLs) and instrumental ADLs. The complications resulting from a fracture depend on many factors, including comorbidities, health status of the patient before the injury, and the location of the fracture. Patients are susceptible to postoperative anemia, hypovolemic shock, infection, incontinence, decubiti, subdural hematoma, dehydration, electrolyte imbalance, hypothermia, and phlebitis after sustaining the injury and throughout the recovery period (Miller, Christmas, & Magaziner, 2009). For hip fractures, approximately 15% of patients are readmitted to the hospital during the first 6 months. There is also a high mortality rate associated with hip fractures. Loss of physical and social function also may follow an injury. Monitor for signs and symptoms of depression and lack of sleep.

Prevention/prophylaxis: Related to osteoporosis, estrogen and progestin replacement therapy reduces the incidence of hip fractures by 39% (National Institutes of Health, 2005). Cerebrovascular accident and cancer side effects are major risks of estrogen-only replacement at this writing. Vitamin D and calcium supplements in combination, dosed according to current serum vitamin D 25 hydroxyl total laboratory level, range 30 to 100 ng/mL, have proved to improve absorption of calcium to bones for those who have low sunlight exposure (Avenell, Gillespie, Gillespie, & O'Connell, 2009). Those with low levels of vitamin D, less than 30 ng/mL, currently are prescribed 50,000 IU of vitamin D_3 once a week for 8 weeks. Maintenance doses range from 1000 IU daily to twice daily for those individuals with laboratory levels above 30 ng/mL.

Those who currently have osteoporosis may benefit from bisphosphonate medications, which have been shown to prevent bone fractures. First-line treatments of bisphosphonate include alendronate 10 mg daily for primary prevention as well as secondary prevention of fractures (Wiley-Blackwell, 2008). Side effects of gastrointestinal ulcerations were reported.

Weight-bearing exercise programs and cataract surgery in patients whose vision is impaired reduce the number of fractures. The modification of the patient's environment, including removal of hazards such as throw rugs and small pieces of furniture; improvements in lighting; and installation of grab bars, raised toilet seats, and ramps, helps prevent injuries (Miller et al., 2009).

Referral: Rehabilitation needs will include an orthopedic specialist for complex casting and surgical needs. Physical therapist/occupational therapist referrals to further evaluate and treat functional physical impairments and to improve ADLs are in order to provide as much independent living as possible. Keep in mind that older patients may be hesitant to resume previous normal activities due to falls. This may be resolved by the involvement of a rehabilitation team.

CLINICAL RECOMMENDATION	EVIDENCE RATING	REFERENCE
Frail older people in nursing centers may have fewer hip and other nonvertebral fractures if given vitamin D with calcium supplements. The effectiveness of vitamin D alone in fracture prevention is not clear.	A	Avenell et al. (2009)
Vitamin D taken with additional calcium supplements does appear to reduce hip fracture, particularly in people living in institutional care.	A	Handoll (2000)
Good evidence suggests that alendronate, risedronate, and estrogen prevent hip fractures more than placebo.	A	MacLean et al. (2008)
Oral bisphosphonate therapy would be considered first-line therapy in the management of osteoporosis.	A	Rahmani & Morin (2009)
Giving 10 mg per day of the bisphosphonate drug alendronate to women after their menopause can help prevent loss of bone mass, reducing their risk of fractures.	A	Wiley-Blackwell (2008)

A = consistent, good-quality, patient-oriented evidence; B = inconsistent or limited-quality, patient-oriented evidence; C = consensus, disease-oriented evidence, usual practice, expert opinion, or case series. For information about the SORT evidence rating system, go to www.aafp.org/afpsort.xml.

GOUT

Signal symptoms: Polyarticular in older adults, soft tissue tenderness, tophi, podagra (metatarsophalangeal [MTP]).

Description: Gout, an inflammatory disease associated with malfunctioning metabolism of purine, leading to overproduction or underexcretion of uric acid, results in deposits of sodium urate crystals in the joints, periarticular tissues, subcutaneous tissues, and kidneys. Primary gout is the clinical disease caused by hyperuricemia; secondary gout usually occurs as a result of extended use of agents that decrease uric acid excretion. Gout is the most prevalent inflammatory condition occurring in older adults. Although it is a common presentation in older adults, the diagnosis of gout is less than routine because gout flares in older adults mimic other arthritic conditions such as septic arthritis and can coexist on the osteoarthritic growths of the distal and proximal interphalangeal joints (Ning & Keenan, 2011). Initial presentation of gout in older adults tends to be polyarticular and directly associated with chronic conditions such as hypertension and renal impairment and the specific treatments for these conditions, namely diuretic use (Roberts, 2010). Physiological stressors, common in older adulthood, can contribute to the rapid development of an acute gout attack, for example, gout beginning in a dehydrated patient or postsurgical procedure (Doherty, 2009). Additionally, adults with hypertension, diabetes, cardiovascular disease, and metabolic syndrome are at high risk for developing gout (Weaver, 2008).The deposition of monosodium urate crystals in synovial fluid and other tissues occurs or the formation of tophi or uric acid stones in the kidney occurs in patients with chronic gout.

Etiology: Clinically, hyperuricemia is defined when the serum urate level is >6.8 mg/dL (Fravel & Ernst, 2011). With levels >10 mg/dL, the chance of an acute attack of gout is >90%. In 70% to 90% of patients with diagnosed gout, underexcretion of urate rather than a metabolic overproduction causes elevation of the plasma urate level. Although hyperuricemia is a risk factor for gout, some patients with a normal serum acid level develop acute gouty arthritis. The mere presence of intrasynovial urate crystals is not sufficient to cause flares of gouty arthritis. The majority of the patients who develop gout have been hyperuricemic for about two decades.

Occurrence: For every 100,000 people in the United States, 100 cases of gout occur. It is estimated that 3.9% of U.S. adults (age 18 years or over) are affected by gout annually (approximately 8.3 million people) (Lawrence et al., 2008; Zhu, Pandya, & Choi, 2011). It is estimated that 1.3% of older adults are affected by gout; the incidence of gout continues to rise in older adults (Wallace, Riedel, Joseph-Ridge, & Wortmann, 2004).

Age: Primary gout usually begins in the forties to sixties, whereas a new presentation in older adult occurs in the sixties to seventies as a result of factors contributing to a cause of secondary gout. Prevalence of gout increases with advanced age in men, peaking at 75 to 84.

Ethnicity: There is a high prevalence in Pacific Islanders, people from Samoa and the Philippines. Limited data suggest an increased incidence of gout in American blacks as compared to whites; however, clinically recognized gout is extremely rare in blacks living in Africa. In England, gout affects 16.4 of every 1000 men and 2.9 of every 1000 women.

Gender: Primary gout is 20 times more prevalent in men than in women; however, among older adults, gout occurs predominantly in women after menopause due to the use of diuretics, prevalence of renal insufficiency, and longevity over males (Chen & Schumacher, 2008; Fravel& Ernst, 2011).

Contributing factors: Factors associated with primary gout in men include positive family history, obesity, trauma, hypertension, hyperlipidemia, hypertriglyceridemia, diets high in purine (especially organ meats, anchovies, sardines, scallops, oatmeal), alcohol consumption (especially beer and moonshine whiskey), dietary intake of high-fructose corn syrup products, lead intoxication, dehydration, fasting (which causes ketosis), binge eating, analgesic nephropathy, nephrolithiasis, urolithiasis, and polycystic kidney disease (Choi & Curhan, 2008; Neogi, 2011). Research data have indicated elevated risk for gout in connection with the following conditions: insulin resistance/diabetes mellitus, the metabolic syndrome, renal insufficiency, chronic kidney disease, hypertension, cardiovascular disease, heart failure, and organ transplantation (Neogi, 2011). Additionally, common causes of secondary gout include hypothyroidism and hyperparathyroidism (Khanna et al., 2012).

Drugs leading to increased risk for gout include thiazide and loop diuretics, low-dose aspirin (<1 g/day), ethambuthol, pyrazinamide, levodopa-carbidopa, nicotinic acid, tacrolimus, and cyclosporine (Choy, 2005; Neogi, 2011). Diuretics are the most common cause of secondary gout because they cause intravascular depletion, lower the glomerular filtration rate, and increase the reabsorption of urate.

Signs and symptoms: Review the patient's history for evidence of excessive alcohol consumption, dietary habits (including foods that are high in purine), medical diagnosis of gout, family history of gout, diabetes mellitus, increased body mass index (BMI), exposure to lead, consumption of illicit whiskey, consumption of high-fructose beverages and additional food products, trauma, and all medication use. The following questions are helpful to ask the patient, to understand the presentation of symptoms:

- Did the pain occur suddenly or become noticeable gradually?
- Is the pain dull, throbbing, or unbearable to touch?
- Has the pain ever occurred before?
- If so, how long did it last, and was the swelling in the same joint?
- How was the pain and swelling treated?

In middle-aged men, the classic presentation of an acute gout attack is a hot, swollen MTP joint of the great toe known as podagra. Podagra is not synonymous with gout; it can occur in pseudogout, sarcoidosis, and psoriatic arthritis (Roberts, 2010). Usually, in the first presentation of gout in middle-aged men, joint involvement is monarticular. In elderly women, joint involvement with gout is usually polyarticular and often occurs in joints above the waist. The proximal interphalangeal (PIP) joints and the distal interphalangeal (DIP) joints should be examined and the instep, heel, ankle, knee, wrist, and olecranon bursa palpated for signs of swelling and tenderness. An acute attack can escalate over a 6- to 12-hour time frame with pain and erythema in the affected joints (Ning & Kennan, 2011). Tophi, subcutaneous deposits of sodium urate, are common in chronic gout. Examine the helix of the ear, olecranon bursa, prepatellar bursa, Achilles tendon, over Heberden's nodes, and finger pads for signs of tophi. Fever may be present. Although rare, gout may be found in the spine (Roberts, 2010).

Diagnostic tests: The Gold standard for confirming the diagnosis of gout is the presence of monosodium urate (MSU) crystals in the synovial fluid. Arthrocentesis is indicated for every patient in whom a diagnosis has never been proven by joint aspiration and for those in whom a possibility of septic arthritis exists (Ning & Keenan, 2011; Zychowicz, Pope, & Graser, 2010). A prior history of gout or pseudogout does not rule out the possibility of acute septic arthritis. Joint aspiration will also rule out septic arthritis and pseudogout. Even in the presence of crystals in the joint fluid, blood cultures are indicated if any sign of systemic toxicity is present. Septic arthritis can occur in patients with active crystalline arthropathy.

Elevated serum uric acid level is indicative of hyperuricemia; however, patients with high uric acid levels may be asymptomatic. Check a CBC to determine if leukocytosis is present to rule out sepsis. Serum creatinine and blood urea nitrogen (BUN) should be ordered initially on patients with suspected gout to determine the presence of renal insufficiency. Elevated ESR or C-reactive protein will indicate an inflammatory process but will not distinguish one arthritic condition from another.

Differential diagnosis:
- Pseudogout
- Traumatic joint injury
- Septic arthritis
- Cellulitis
- Hemarthrosis
- Rheumatoid arthritis
- Osteoarthritis
- Seronegative spondyloarthopathies

Pseudogout (calcium pyrophosphate deposition disease [CPDD]) is caused by the deposition of calcium pyrophosphate rather than the deposition of uric acid derivatives that cause gout. Also, in pseudogout, synovial fluid samples obtained with aspiration have positive birefringence. This finding is in direct contrast to the negative birefringence in gout.

Treatment: NSAIDs, corticosteroids, and oral colchicine are acceptable first-line options for treatment of acute gout with treatment started within 24 hours of attack onset. Management of the older adult with gout requires careful monitoring. Older adults are susceptible to renal insufficiency, may have other concomitant diseases, and experience hypersensitivity to some of the medications used to treat younger patients with gout. NSAIDs should be used cautiously in the treatment of gout in older adults who have a history of heart failure, renal failure, and gastrointestinal conditions (Fravel & Ernst, 2011). As with any NSAID, renal function must be monitored. NSAIDs can endanger existing renal function, especially when the creatinine clearance is ≤30 mL/min. Additional concern with NSAID use in older adults is the potential for gastrointestinal bleeding due to NSAID-induced peptic ulcers. An exacerbation of hypertension can occur with excessive use of NSAIDs in older adults. Extensive use of NSAIDs can lead to fluid retention and antagonism of diuretic therapy, which may precipitate heart failure (Fravel & Ernst, 2011).

Indomethacin is effective in the treatment of acute gout; the usual dose is 25 to 50 mg orally 2 to 3 times daily until the symptoms cease, then begin to taper the dose for 5 to 7 days. Liquid indomethacin is available for patient use. Although indomethacin has been traditionally favored in the treatment of gout, there has been no research documenting the advantage to its use over other NSAIDs such as naproxen (Zychowicz et. al, 2010). As with any NSAID, renal function must be monitored. NSAIDs can endanger existing renal function, especially when the creatinine clearance is ≤30 mL/min. Cyclooxygenase-2 inhibitors may be better tolerated in older adults with history of peptic ulcer.

Colchicine can be given for acute gout attacks orally. It is most effective if given within 24 hours of an attack. The oral colchicine dose is 1.2 mg followed by a single 0.6 mg dose 1 hour later. Dose should not exceed 1.8 mg a day for an acute flare. Consensus guidelines indicate that colchicine is not to be used in patients with a creatinine clearance of <10 mL/min. (Hanlon et al., 2009).

Gastrointestinal toxicity commonly precedes a therapeutic response. Because oral colchicine is associated with side effects, it should not be administered to patients with impaired renal or hepatic function or gastrointestinal disease or to postoperative patients because of the potential for vomiting. Patients for whom colchicine and NSAIDs are contraindicated may be given intra-articular steroid injections for monarticular joint involvement. Short-term corticosteroids can be initiated in patients unable to tolerate NSAIDS or colchicine, used cautiously in patients who are diabetic or immunocompromised. Xanthine oxidase inhibitors and uricosuric agents should not be prescribed for an acute gout attack (Fravel & Ernst, 2011). However, ongoing pharmacological urate-lowering therapy should not be stopped during a gout flare.

Follow-up: Patients having a first acute attack of gout should be followed up 72 hours after initiating treatment to determine effectiveness and presence of any side effects. Patients who have more than three attacks

of gout in a year are considered to have chronic disease. Before initiating a long-term medication regimen, uric acid level, BUN, creatinine, serum lipid level, CBC, and urinalysis should be ordered.

For patients with chronic gout, urate-lowering therapy with xanthine oxidase inhibitors, such as allopurinol or febuxostat, is the first-line treatment option. The starting dose for allopurinol is recommended at no higher than 100 mg/day, to be increased until the desired uric acid level of <6 mg/dL at a minimum if not lower to <5 mg/day is achieved (Khanna et al., 2012). In patients with moderate to severe kidney disease, a lower starting dose should be considered (Khanna et al., 2012). Recommendations from the American College of Rheumatology found that monotherapy with allopurinol at doses of 300 mg could be raised to 300 mg daily even with renal impairment; patients, however, will need to be educated on side effects of drug toxicity (Khanna et al., 2012). In patient populations known for high risk for allopurinol hypersensitivity (Koreans with stage 3 or worse chronic kidney disease and Han Chinese and Thai), screening for HLA-B 5801 should be considered before prescribing this medication (Khanna et al., 2012). Febuxostate is available in 40 to 80 mg daily doses. Dose adjustment is not necessary in the elderly with stage 2 or 3 chronic kidney disease (30 to 89 mg/dL) or mild hepatic insufficiency. Allopurinol or febuxostate should not be discontinued during a gout flare. Alternative treatment to chronic gout is low-dose indomethacin 25 mg twice a day or another NSAID (Fravel & Ernst, 2011). Once medications are initiated for gout, target serum urate levels should be 6 mg/dL or less according to EULAR guidelines (Jordan et al., 2009).

For patients with chronic tophaceous gouty arthropathy, the American College of Rheumatology guidelines recommend combination therapy with one xanthine oxidase inhibitor (allopurinol or febuxostat) and one uricosuric agent when the target urate levels are not achieved (Khanna et al., 2012). The usefulness of probenecid in the older adult is limited because it is effective only when the creatinine clearance is <30 to 40 mL/min and is contraindicated in patients with renal insufficiency and on diuretics. Pegloticase can be used in patients with severe gout when they do not respond to standard treatment with urate-lowering therapy (Khanna et al., 2012).

Sequelae: Older adults who have preexisting hypertension or primary renal disease or who use NSAIDs and diuretics are at risk for developing renal insufficiency, chronic urate nephropathy, and acute hyperuricemia nephropathy. Uric acid nephrolithiasis is also a complication of gout. Untreated chronic gout may lead to multilobular, tender subcutaneous tophaceous gout, which can be deforming and impair ADLs. Progressive renal failure is common in patients with gout and has been known to contribute to up to 20% of deaths (Rosenberg, 2005). Left untreated, elevated uric acid levels have been shown to contribute to the development of cerebrovascular disease and vascular dementia (Feig, Kang, & Johnson, 2008). Patients with draining tophi are at risk for infection, and untreated chronic tophaceous gout can lead to severe joint destruction (Khanna et al., 2012). Given the complexity of comorbid conditions common in patients with gout, risk for polypharmacy and drug–drug interactions should be of great concern to primary care providers (Dalbeth, 2013).

Prevention/prophylaxis: Thiazide diuretics and salicylates should be avoided in patients with gout. Patients should be cautioned about the use of alcohol and to avoid foods high in purine, especially during an acute gout flare. For patients with an elevated BMI, weight reduction is recommended. Maintaining control of diabetes and hyperlipidemia can aid in the reduction of developing gout flares.

Referral: Patients may need a referral to a rheumatologist if they require intra-articular injections of steroids or joint aspiration, have complications from treatment, or have unusual presentation of the disease. A patient also may benefit from a referral to a dietitian for information on how to follow a low-purine diet.

Education: Patients need to be informed that during an acute attack they should rest the affected area and limit weight bearing if the first MTP joint is involved. Patients should be encouraged to be well hydrated with an intake of 3 L/day of fluids unless contraindicated. The use of alcohol should be discouraged. Smoking cessation, weight loss for obese patients, physical exercise, and overall healthy diet are recommended lifestyle changes for all patients with gout (Khanna et al., 2012). Patients should consult their primary healthcare provider regarding selection of any over-the-counter medications.

CLINICAL RECOMMENDATION	EVIDENCE RATING	REFERENCE
A presumptive diagnosis of gout can be determined in many cases based on history, clinical presentation, and use of the American College of Rheumatology's decision rule; however, if possible, joint aspiration and polarized light microscopy should be performed to verify diagnosis and rule out sepsis or pseudogout.	B	Ning & Keenan (2011) Zychowicz, Pope, & Graser (2010)
A diagnosis of gout should lead to an assessment of potentially modifiable risk factors (e.g., dietary patterns, alcohol intake, and obesity) and associated comorbidities (e.g., hypertension and dyslipidemia) that may need intervention to reduce gout risk.	B	Choi (2010) Neogi (2011)
Weight reduction with daily aerobic exercise and limiting the intake of red meat, alcohol, certain seafood, and sugar-sweetened beverages help to reduce serum uric acid levels and the risk of gout. Also, low-fat dairy products, vegetables, legumes, and whole grains may decrease the risk of gout by reducing insulin resistance.	C	Choi (2010)
NSAIDs and colchicine are the first-line agents for acute gout attacks. No particular NSAID has shown greater effectiveness (e.g., naproxen 500 mg twice a day for 7–10 days).	B	Neogi (2011) Ning & Keenan (2011) Terkeltaub et al. (2010)

Continued

CLINICAL RECOMMENDATION	EVIDENCE RATING	REFERENCE
In patients with renal/liver impairment, heart failure, anticoagulation, or gastrointestinal bleeding, NSAIDs and colchicine should be avoided and a 5-day course of oral glucocorticoids can be used.	A	Janssen et al. (2008) Man, Cheung, Cameron, & Rainer (2007) Neogi (2011)
Medications that increase serum urate levels (e.g., thiazide diuretics, low-dose aspirin, niacin, and cyclosporine) should be stopped, if feasible, and alternative medicines used.	B	Choi (2010) Ning & Keenan (2011)
Urate-lowering therapy should be considered in those with hyperuricemia (serum urate >7.0 mg/ dL) who have at least two gout attacks per year or tophi (target serum urate level of 6.0 mg/dL). Coexisting illnesses, such as nephrolithiasis, can also be considered. Initiate after acute flare resolution.	B	Neogi (2011) Ning & Keenan (2011) Zychowicz et al. (2010)
Allopurinol is the first-line treatment in urate-lowering therapy (50–300 mg daily with a maximum daily dose of 800 mg).	A	Becker, Schumacher, MacDonald, Lloyd, & Lademacher (2009) Burns & Wortmann (2011) Neogi (2011)
For those with allopurinol hypersensitivity or treatment failure, febuxostat therapy can be used effectively to reach target serum urate levels (40 mg daily with titration to 80 mg daily).	A	Becker, Schumacher, MacDonald, Lloyd, & Lademacher (2009) Burns & Wortmann (2011) Neogi (2011)
Uricosuric agents such as probenecid (250–500 mg twice a day titrated to a maximum dose of 3 g/day) can be effective second-line agents for those with allopurinol intolerance, but only for those with normal renal function.	B	Neogi (2011) Zychowicz et al. (2010)
For those with moderate-to-severe renal impairment, chronic kidney disease, and allopurinol intolerance, febuxostat (40 mg daily with titration to 80 mg daily) is the treatment of choice.	A	Becker, Schumacher, MacDonald, Lloyd, & Lademacher (2009) Burns & Wortmann (2011) Neogi (2011)

A = consistent, good-quality, patient-oriented evidence; B = inconsistent or limited-quality, patient-oriented evidence; C = consensus, disease-oriented evidence, usual practice, expert opinion, or case series. For information about the SORT evidence rating system, go to www.aafp.org/afpsort.xml.

HERNIATED NUCLEUS PULPOSUS

Signal symptoms: Paresthesias, sciatica.

Description: Herniated nucleus pulposus (HNP), also referred to as a herniated disk, is a common spine pathology that occurs approximately 95% of the time at the L4–L5 or L5–S1 level (Asch et al., 2002; Fisher et al., 2004). The majority of herniated discs occur in a posterolateral direction, compressing the ipsilateral nerve root as it exits from the dural sac. Thus, a left L5–S1 disc herniation compresses the left S1 nerve root. It is an inflamed condition of the nerve due to dislocation or rupture of an intervertebral disc. The escaping nucleus pulposus consists predominantly of type II collagen, proteoglycan, and hyaluronan long chains; these have regions with hydrophilic, branching side chains. The chains draw water molecules, thus hydrating the nucleus of the disc by osmosis (Foster, 2010).

Occurrence: Lumbar disc herniations are among the most common diagnoses of back issues. The incidence of lumbar disc herniations that are symptomatic in the American population has been estimated to be nearly 20%, for which approximately 200,000 lumbar discectomies are performed annually.

Age: Peak incidence of HNP is between 30 and 55 years of age (Foster, 2010). The risk of lumbago, lower back pain, does not increase in age. This suggests that other conditions cause low back pain.

Gender: Most articles reviewed state that HNP affects both genders equally. However, comorbidities exist with osteoporosis of women after menopause when bone density decreases.

Ethnicity: None given within the research.

Contributing factors: HNP generally occurs in patients taller and heavier than average; aging intervertebral disks begin deteriorating and growing thinner by age 30. One-third of adults over 20 years old show signs of herniated discs, although only 3% of these discs cause symptoms (Foster, 2010). As people continue to age and discs lose moisture and atrophy, the risk for spinal stenosis increases. The incidence of low back pain and sciatica increases in women at the time of menopause as they lose bone density. In older adults, osteoporosis and osteoarthritis are also common.

Signs and symptoms: HNP can be asymptomatic and may be discovered by magnetic resonance imaging (MRI) only. However, generally lower back pain at the L4–S1 level affects daily life. The nucleus pulposus first

tears within the annulus fibrosus. It may eventually break through enough of the annulus to cause bulging. If the process continues, disc material may separate. Radiculopathy is pain, paresthesias, or both in the distribution of a nerve root. In this case, it is caused by nerve root irritation from an HNP. Each nerve root has a specific area of motor and sensory distribution. The radicular pain is often described as shooting or stabbing. There may be paresthesias in the same distribution. Sciatica is radicular pain in L5 or S1 distribution. Patients typically describe deep buttock, posterior, or posterolateral thigh pain that may or may not extend below the knee, into the lower leg and lateral foot. The pain is often aggravated by coughing, sneezing, or straining. It may also be aggravated by certain positions, such as sitting or standing. The pain usually subsides with rest.

Diagnostic tests: The diagnostic tests include spinal x-ray series, myelogram, and computer MRI series. The myelogram utilizes a contrast medium with fluoroscopy to detect herniations that the MRI and radiographs might not detect otherwise.

Differential diagnosis:
- Slipped vertebral apophysis
- Spondylolisthesis
- Intraspinal tumor
- Ankylosing spondylitis
- Meningocele of the nerve root sheath
- Tumor
- Infection

Treatment: There are differing techniques of treatment available. These include epidural injections, discectomy, and observation only. The theory behind the use of epidural corticosteroids over systemic (oral, intramuscular, or intravenous) corticosteroids is that a higher concentration of the medication is delivered to the pathological area. This provides two potential benefits. First, since the local concentration is much higher, a lower overall dose of corticosteroid is employed and potential systemic side effects are reduced. However, epidural injection is more invasive, thus increasing risk of morbidity (Chou et al., 2009). Serious complications such as paraplegia are extremely rare but have been reported from lumbar epidural corticosteroid injections. Epidural corticosteroid injections under fluoroscopy are more effective than shown in previous investigations (Levin & Smuck, 2007).

Another treatment is the surgical procedure of removing the disc, or discectomy. This is a minimally invasive procedure. The origins of the modern era of lumbar disc surgery can be traced to the seminal work of Mixter and Barr, 70 years later. Those authors found that sciatic pain could be relieved by removing herniated disc material compressing a nerve root. Logically, the association was made between lumbar disc herniation and the clinical entity of sciatica. That finding led to the general assumption that mechanical compression of the nerve root is the primary pathogenic factor inducing radiculopathy. Several lines of evidence support this notion. First, the structure of the nerve root renders it relatively poorly resistant to compression. Like peripheral nerves, nerve roots have an endoneurium. However, the layers equivalent to the perineurium and epineurium are cerebrospinal fluid and dural lining, respectively. Thus, the nerve root is a comparatively delicate structure that is not well insulated to resist compressive forces. Second, because nerve roots are tethered to the vertebral body at their takeoff from the common dural sac and to the subjacent pedicle within the foramen by ligamentous attachments, a disc herniation ventral to the root is posed to generate high tensile forces. The situation is analogous to the tension generated in a bowstring by the pull of an archer's hand. Third, animal models of cauda equina compression have demonstrated that compression of a nerve root impairs its nutrition in a series of experiments. Olmarker, Rydevik, Nordborg (1993) showed that mechanical compression on nerve roots within the porcine cauda equina led to decreased nutrient delivery by reducing both blood flow and nutrient diffusion from cerebrospinal fluid. Histologically, compressed nerve roots demonstrate evidence of intraneural edema, which can directly lead to nerve fibrosis and injury. Alternately, intraneural edema secondarily leads to interneural compartment syndrome as pressures within the nerve root overcome perfusion pressures, resulting in nerve root ischemia and injury. Although the above and other studies suggest that the mechanical effect of a herniated disc is the main factor in the genesis of radiculopathy, other lines of evidence indicate that mechanical compression alone may not be a sufficient cause for the radiculopathy associated with herniated discs. First, MRI studies have shown that nerve root compression is often asymptomatic. Boden et al. (1996) found that in a group of people who had never had radicular pain, 20% of those under 60 years of age and 36% of those over 60 years of age had evidence of a herniated disc on MRI.

It is commonly agreed that lumbar disc herniation has a favorable natural history (i.e., the clinical course of the disease without therapeutic intervention). When a patient has incapacitating pain, a period of bedrest is often unavoidable. Immobilization presumably diminishes inflammation around an irritated nerve root. However, there are no data to suggest that bedrest alters the natural history of lumbar disc herniations or improves outcomes. Because of the potentially harmful effects of prolonged bedrest, it is best to advise patients to limit bedrest to a short-term period and to resume activities as soon as possible. Bracing is another method of immobilizing the lumbar spine, but there is a lack of good evidence to support the use of braces and corsets for patients with lumbar disc herniations. The Cochrane review found "limited" evidence favoring lumbar supports compared with no treatments.

The available literature indicates that effective nonoperative treatments for lumbar disc herniations include observation only, as the condition has a favorable natural history, and probably epidural steroid injection, at least for short-term relief. Intramuscular injections of steroids may provide some benefit. NSAIDs are effective for low back pain only, and traction is probably not effective. There are insufficient data to provide recommendations regarding the role of oral steroids, physical therapy, transcutaneous electrical stimulation, corsets, and manual therapy (Chou & Huffman, 2008).

Regardless of treatment, lumbar disc herniations usually have a favorable natural history with improvement over time, but it may take 1 or 2 years for functional improvement to plateau. In the absence of a cauda equina syndrome or progressive weakness, the best indication for surgical management is refractory radicular pain. Surgical decision making should not be based on the size of the disc herniation, because large extruded herniations tend to resolve more predictably, or on either stable motor weakness or numbness, because the ultimate resolution of weakness and sensory deficits is similar following either nonoperative or surgical management, although surgery hastens the process. When intractable radicular pain is the strict indication for surgery, surgical intervention provides substantial and more rapid pain relief than does nonoperative treatment. The specific method of surgical intervention probably contributes little to the overall success of the intervention as long as the root is properly decompressed. Health surveys can provide additional assessment of psychosocial comorbidities that are not otherwise evident during the usual clinical evaluation. Such comorbidities should be identified preoperatively because they are not likely to resolve with surgical intervention but may have greater impact than the discal pathoanatomy on the ultimate outcome (Zieger, Schwarz, Konig, Harter, & Riedel-Heller, 2010).

Epidural steroid injection was not as effective as discectomy with regard to reducing symptoms and disability associated with a large herniation of the lumbar disc. However, epidural steroid injection did have a role: it was found to be effective for up to 3 years by nearly one-half of the patients who had not had improvements with 6 or more weeks of noninvasive care.

Follow-up: The primary emphasis of treatment for radicular complaints should be conservative care, reassurance, and education to allow the patient time to improve without surgical intervention (Atlas & Deyo, 2001). The most frequently used nonsurgical treatments are back exercises, short-term rest, physical therapy, spinal manipulation, NSAIDs, muscle relaxants, opioid analgesics, and epidural steroids (Atlas, Keller, Robson, Deyo, & Singer, 2000).

A 5-year prospective-outcome study evaluating the surgical and nonsurgical outcomes of sciatica caused by HNP found that the least symptomatic patients at baseline did well regardless of initial treatment. For patients with moderate-to-severe sciatica, surgical treatment was associated with greater improvement at the end of the 5-year period (Atlas et al. 2000).

Sequelae: Abnormal gait, balance issues, decreased physical ability/debility, increased glucose, Cushing syndrome with steroid treatment possible, addiction to narcotics, depression, and anxiety.

Prevention/prophylaxis: Stretching, exercise, bending with knees.

Referral: Orthopedic surgeon/radiology interventionalist.

Education: American Academy of Orthopedic Surgeons (orthoinfo.org).

CLINICAL RECOMMENDATION	EVIDENCE RATING	REFERENCE
Microsurgical, endoscopic techniques are superior to classic techniques with regard to blood loss and overall systematic repercussions.	A	Gotfryd & Avanzi (2009)
Automated percutaneous lumbar discectomy for the contained herniated lumbar disc provides short-term/long-term relief.	A	Hirsch, Singh, Falco, Benyamin, & Manchikanti (2009)
Standing leg raise (SLR) showed high specificity with consistently low sensitivity in physical examination test for herniated disc within clinical settings.	A	Van de Windt et al. (2010)
Disc surgery patients—higher risk for suffering depression/anxiety.	A	Zieger et al. (2010)
Acute low back pain—the only therapy with good evidence of efficacy is superficial.	A	Chou & Huffman (2008)
Chemonucleolysis is moderately superior to placebo injection but inferior to surgery.	A	Chou, Atlas, Stamos, & Rosenquist (2009)
Epidural treatment: short-term relief—fair evidence.	A	Chou et al. (2009)

A = consistent, good-quality, patient-oriented evidence; B = inconsistent or limited-quality, patient-oriented evidence; C = consensus, disease-oriented evidence, usual practice, expert opinion, or case series. For information about the SORT evidence rating system, go to www.aafp.org/afpsort.xml.

OSTEOARTHRITIS

Signal symptoms: Morning stiffness lasting <30 minutes, stiffness that improves with activity, Bouchard's nodes (PIP joints), Heberden's nodes (DIP joints), and crepitus.

Description: *Osteoarthritis* (OA), still also referred to as *degenerative joint disease*, is a degenerative disease of the joint cartilage. It is the leading cause of disability in older adults in the United States (Lawrence et al., 2008). OA most commonly affects the hips, knees, and cervical and lumbar spine. Joint deformity with minimal pain is found in the DIP and PIP joints of the hand, the first carpometacarpal joint, and the first metatarsophalangeal joint (Shelton, 2013). OA is a complex active disease process involving the wearing away (degradation) and, to a lesser extent, the repair of the cartilage surface. It is now understood that there is both a mechanical (wearing away) and a biological (abnormal joint biology) part of the osteoarthritis (Ling & Rudolph, 2006). Besides the cartilage degeneration, patients often experience neurological and mechanical dysfunction (Chao & Kalunian, 2010).

Etiology: The etiology of OA is unknown; however, it is recognized that OA is not age dependent. The underlying pain experienced in osteoarthritis is related to increased vascular pressure in the subchondral bone, stretching of the joint capsule, pressure on the ligaments, reactive muscle spasm, bone spur formation, and inflammatory irritation of innervated tissue surrounding the affected joints (bursitis) or within the joints (synovitis) (Ling & Rudolph, 2006).

Occurrence: Approximately 26.9 million people in the United States have OA (Lawrence et al., 2008).

Age: OA is common in older adults. An estimated 33% to 90% of the population over 65 years old is thought to have OA.

Gender: Among people 55 years and older, women are affected more often than men.

Ethnicity: OA of the knee is more common in African American women than in white women. Also, the prevalence of OA in male and female Alaskan natives is considerably lower than in whites.

Contributing factors: Increasing age, female sex, obesity, previous joint injury (torn meniscus, intra-articular mechanical damage), prior surgeries, occupation, hobby, and prolonged sport activity involving the weight-bearing joints contribute to the development of OA. Family history is a known contributing factor for osteoarthritis of the hand (Chao & Kalunian, 2010; Ringdahl & Pandit, 2011). Other factors include calcium pyrophosphate or uric acid crystal deposits in the joints, Wilson's disease, acromegaly, hyperparathyroidism, and diabetes mellitus. Conditions that change joint mechanics, such as untreated hip dislocation, may predispose an individual to OA.

Signs and symptoms: Complaints of morning stiffness lasting <30 minutes or stiffness that improves with activity and accompanying muscle spasms may indicate OA. Persistent pain and limitation of motion in the affected joint may be reported. Bouchard's nodes (nontender nodules of the PIP joints), Heberden's nodes (nontender nodules of the DIP joints of the hands and feet), or both may be found (LeBlond, Brown, & DeGowin, 2009). The carpometacarpal joint located at the thumb base is often involved, and crepitus may be elicited; however, it is rare in OA that the metacarpophalangeal joints are involved (Zhang et al., 2009). Consider secondary causes of OA if these joints are involved such as gout, pseudogout, hemochromatosis, trauma, or occupational risk (Chao & Kalunian, 2010). In women, erosive OA often occurs in the PIP joints and DIP joints, manifesting red, tender joints that eventually result in joint erosion, extensive joint deformity, and subsequent ankylosis. Consider psoriatic arthritis (PA) in patients presenting with these symptoms because PA can mimic inflammatory OA. The MTP joints may also be involved in OA. Ask patients about presence of muscle spasms, and look for signs of tendon and capsular contractures (Swagerty & Hellinger, 2001).

Clinical criteria for patients with OA of the knee include having crepitus (a grinding sensation on movement of the joint) of the affected joint. In addition to pain and morning stiffness, patients with osteoarthritis of the knee often report limited ROM and bony enlargement of the knee (Zhang et al., 2010). Some patients may complain of knee locking and unsteadiness. On examination, patients with OA of the hip and knee may present with an antalgic gait; patients are limping to avoid pain on the affected hip and/or knee. Examine bilateral quadriceps muscles for signs of weakness.

Internal and external hip rotation may be reduced (Zhang et al., 2010).

Patients with OA of the cervical spine often complain of paresthesias and numbness in the arms waking them from their sleep; this sensation generally improves when the limb is lightly shaken. Examination of the cervical spine may show some restricted joint movement and muscle tenderness. When OA affects the lumbosacral spine, patients may report pain across the lower back with radiation to the buttocks and posterior thigh; if nerve root compression has occurred, patients may complain of pain in the lower leg, known as pseudoclaudication. It is important to assess the patient's current functional status and pain level initially and at every subsequent visit and determine if any adaptive equipment is necessary (Chao & Kalunian, 2010).

Diagnostic tests: Although the diagnosis of OA is often made without x-rays, results of bilateral standing radiographs of the affected areas with OA reveal joint space narrowing, subchondral cyst formation, subchondral bony sclerosis, and osteophytosis resulting in proliferative bone spurs. The narrowing of the joint space occurs due to the loss of cartilage. Bony spurs known as osteophytes develop at the margin of the joint as a protective measure for the damaged joint structure. The cyst formation can be seen on x-ray beneath the surface of the joints. Two views of the affected joint are recommended with the exception of the sacroiliac joint and the pelvis (Swagerty & Hellinger, 2001). Other types of imaging tests, such as ultrasound and MRI, may be used to detect damage to cartilage, ligaments, and tendons, which cannot be seen on x-ray. Arthrocentesis should be considered for joint effusions to rule out crystalline disease or infection. A needle is gently inserted into the joint to withdraw a small amount of synovial fluid from the joint. The specimen should be tested for chemistry, viscosity (thickness), blood cell counts, overall appearance, blood cultures for suspected microorganisms, and presence of crystals to exclude diagnosis of gout and calcium pyrophosphate crystals. The synovial fluid in OA is usually clear, is viscous, and has ≤2000 white blood cells (WBCs)/μL. Baseline laboratory studies (CBC, liver function tests [LFTs], BUN, and creatinine) should be obtained before initiating long-term drug therapy for monitoring purposes (Chao & Kalunian, 2010).

Differential diagnosis:
- Osteoporosis (radiographs)
- Metastatic disease (radiographs)
- Multiple myeloma (bone marrow is infiltrated; lytic lesions are common in the axial skeleton), anserine bursitis (knee involvement)
- Polymyalgia rheumatica
- Rheumatoid arthritis
- Crystalline disease
- Septic arthritis
- Reiter syndrome
- Bursitis (Shelton, 2013)

The presence of any systemic symptoms in patients with existing osteoarthritis should alert practitioners that the patients may have a developing concomitant inflammatory condition (e.g., polymyalgia rheumatica or rheumatoid arthritis), crystalline disease, or septic arthritis (Ling & Rudolph, 2006). When ruling out conditions that mimic OA in specific joints such as hips, knees, and spine, additional conditions must be considered when the presence of pain is described in the specific area. Radiculopathies and neuropathy must be considered in patients with referred pain. Conditions that involve soft tissue and joint support mechanism (e.g., bursitis, tendinitis, and ligament instability and meniscal pathology) should be included in the differential diagnosis. Bone tumors and avascular necrosis need to be considered in patients complaining of pain in the large joints of the body (Ringdahl & Pandit, 2011).

Treatment: A multifaceted approach to the treatment of OA remains the mainstay of therapy (Chao & Kalunian, 2010). The recommendation for nonpharmacological therapies such as walking can be beneficial and should be advocated (Chao & Kalunian, 2010). Water therapy has been shown to improve the function of patients with OA with no evidence of inflammation (Ringdahl & Pandit, 2011). In noninflammatory OA, acetaminophen is the medication of choice in doses of 2.6 to 4 g/day (Abdulla et al. 2013; Zhang, Markowitz, Nuke, Abramson, & Altman, 2008); acetaminophen toxicity has become a growing concern. Caution needs to be taken when recommending acetaminophen, and advise to avoid using multiple acetaminophen products and to restrict alcohol intake (Ali, 2011). For patients not getting relief from acetaminophen and exercise, the cyclooxygenase type 2 (COX-2) selective agents should be tried, especially in patients with a history of gastrointestinal bleeding and who are anticoagulated. Starting doses are celecoxib 50 to 100 mg twice daily. The lowest starting dose should be used in the elderly, especially in elderly patients weighing <50 kg. Selection of a nonselective

NSAID should be based on dosing frequency, toxicity potential, and cost to the patient (Ali, 2011). Older adults should be started on a low dose of an NSAID, increasing the dose gradually. Combination use with a proton-pump inhibitor is recommended (Ali, 2011; Shelton, 2013). The use of NSAIDs should be avoided in older adults with a calculated creatinine clearance <35 mL/min. Nonacetylated salicylates such as magnesium trisalicylate 500 to 750 mg 2 to 3 times daily have been found to be effective for osteoarthritic pain in patients who cannot afford COX-2 medications, though caution is recommended in patients who need cardioprotection (Ali, 2011). Tramadol can be given at 50 mg every 4 to 6 hours; maximum dose in patients age 75 years and older should not exceed 300 mg/day. Other opiates such as codeine and oxycodone can be used for patients with severe OA pain who cannot tolerate NSAIDS; however, serious addictions remain a possibility with all opiates including tramadol. A slow tapering schedule is recommended to avoid withdrawal symptoms (Barsotti, Mycyk, & Reyes, 2003). Reports have shown that glucosamine and chondroitin sulfate (1500 mg/1200 mg per day) may relieve the pain of OA (Sawitzke, Shi, & Finco, 2010). Selection of capsaicin cream 25%, applied twice daily to the affected joint, also has been shown to reduce pain (Reid, Shengelia, & Parker, 2013). When only one or a few joints are inflamed, intra-articular corticosteroid injections may be beneficial; however, use of these injections should be limited to only a couple of times each year (Ali, 2011). The use of topical diclofenac sodium gel (DSG) 1% for osteoarthritis of the hand was found to relieve the local arthritic pain (Altman et al., 2009). Applying 4 g of DSG 4 times a day to the knee was found to be effective when rescue acetaminophen was permitted as adjunct to the topical corticosteroid (Baraf, Gloth, Barthel, Gold, & Altman, 2011). A patch form of DSG is available with similar efficacy as the gel formulation (Ali, 2011). Viscosupplementation is another nonpharmacological option for patients with OA; an intra-articular injection of the highly viscous joint lubrication has been shown to be effective for 6 months (Abdulla et al., 2013). Patients with severe pain and restricted mobility may benefit from surgical intervention or reconstructive joint surgery (Ringdahl & Pandit, 2010).

Follow-up: Patients should be reevaluated in about 2 to 3 weeks initially, to determine the effectiveness of the treatment. At this time, the patient should be weighed if obesity is a contributing factor; diet and exercise should be reviewed. The patient should be asked about benefits received from heat, cold, and massage. Response to pharmacological measures can be reevaluated in patients who have been prescribed NSAIDs. A CBC, creatinine clearance, and LFTs should be ordered at this time, then every 3 months. Question the patient about any new onset of dyspepsia, abdominal pain, or bleeding related to medications for OA. Determine if patients are interested in referrals for orthotics and physical and occupational therapy (Shelton, 2013).

Sequelae: Because OA is a slowly progressive disease, joint deformity and functional disability may occur in individuals who have difficulty responding to the therapeutic regimen.

Prevention/prophylaxis: Weight reduction and avoidance of joint trauma may prevent further joint deformity in patients with OA.

Referral: Patients may need a referral to a rheumatologist if they have complications from treatment or an unusual presentation of the disease. Patients with involved joint deformities should be referred to an orthopedic surgeon for possible joint replacement (Chao & Kalunian, 2010; Musuku, Zirker, Srulevich, Kahn, & DeSimone, 2011). Referral for special orthotics and occupational therapist for special splitting is recommended (Chao & Kalunian, 2010).

Education: Patients need education on specific strategies for joint protection (Ringdahl & Pandit, 2010). Information in the treatment plan should include the importance of exercise, such as water exercise and aerobic and resistance exercises as tolerated. Other nonpharmacological therapies shown to be beneficial to patients with OA are scheduled rest periods, weight reduction, and the safe use of heat, cold, and medications to control or alleviate pain. Information should be provided about acquiring necessary assistive devices, such as walkers, canes, elevated toilet seats, and any orthotics (unloading knee braces, knee sleeves, hand splints, insoles, and special footwear) as needed (Beaudreuil et al., 2009; Chao & Kalunian, 2010). Patients may require instruction on how to use these devices safely and should be measured properly for walker and cane size. It is essential to review all medications, especially over-the-counter drugs, to avoid duplication of NSAIDs.

CLINICAL RECOMMENDATION	EVIDENCE RATING	REFERENCE
Topical diclofenac sodium gel (DSG) 1% as prescribed for OA of the hand has been found to relieve local arthritic pain.	A	Altman et al. (2009)
Topical diclofenac sodium gel (DSG) 4% as prescribed has been found to relieve arthritic pain to the knee.	A	Baraf, Gloth, Barthel, Gold, & Altman (2011)
Water therapy has been found to be an effective nonpharmacological therapy in patients with OA.	A	Ringdahl & Pandit (2010)
Viscosupplementation has been found to be effective for OA of the knee for 6 months.	A	Bellamy et al. (2006)

A = consistent, good-quality, patient-oriented evidence; B = inconsistent or limited-quality, patient-oriented evidence; C = consensus, disease-oriented evidence, usual practice, expert opinion, or case series. For information about the SORT evidence rating system, go to www.aafp.org/afpsort.xml.

POLYMYALGIA RHEUMATICA

Signal symptoms: New onset of stiffness and aching in neck, shoulders, pelvic girdle; unable to get out of bed in the morning without extreme difficulty, difficulty in lifting arms over one's head.

Description: Polymyalgia rheumatica (PMR) is a clinical inflammatory syndrome characterized by fatigue, aching, pain, and stiffness primarily in the neck, shoulders, hips, and pelvic girdle, occurring primarily in older adults. Initially patients may report unilateral stiffness, but eventually muscle aching with guarded ROM will affect both sides of the body. Musculoskeletal symptoms have been linked to nonerosive articular and extra-articular synovitis (Paget & Spiera, 2006). Systemic manifestations include low-grade fever, anorexia, depression, weight loss, and malaise (Hernández-Rodríguez, Cid, Lopez-Soto, Espigol-Frigole & Bosch, 2009). Round cell infiltration and synovial proliferation are found in patients with PMR. Patients are often found to have an elevated ESR and C-reactive protein level (Salvarani, Cantini, & Hunder, 2008); if both of these inflammatory markers are not elevated, the diagnosis of PMR cannot be discarded (Dasgupta et al., 2010). There is a close association with patients presenting with PMR developing giant cell arteritis (GCA), a common vascular condition in older adults. It has been suggested that, given the similar clinical pathology of these two conditions, they may actually be manifestations of the same disease (Unwin, Williams, & Gilliland, 2006).

Approximately 50% of patients with PMR go on to develop GCA. Assessing for signs and symptoms of vasculitis early is important to avoid the complications of GCA, namely, irreversible blindness (Salvarani et al., 2008).

Etiology: The etiology of PMR is unknown. A relationship between the presence of the HLA-DR4 haplotype and presentation of PMR has been suggested.

Occurrence: PMR affects 1 in 1000 individuals 50 years and older in the United States. The incidence of PMR increases in northern states that have populations with similar ethnic backgrounds to northern European countries (Soubrier, Dubost, & Ristori, 2006).

Age: This disease occurs predominantly in adults over 50 years old with an average age of presentation of 72 (Salvarani, Cantini, Boiardi, & Hunder, 2002). PMR and GCA occur 10 times more frequently in adults over 80 years old than in adults under 60 years old.

Gender: PMR occurs 2 to 3 times as often in women as in men (Salvarani et al., 2008).

Ethnicity: PMR is 6 times more common in whites than in African Americans. Patients who are descendants from northern European countries have the highest rate of PMR and GCA, whereas the lowest prevalence has been noted in the Japanese. A genetic factor, the HLA-DR4 haplotype, is found in patients with PMR (Pease et al., 2005; Salvarani et al., 2008; Soubrier et al., 2006).

Contributing factors: Advanced age and a possible genetic predisposition are thought to contribute to the development of PMR.

Signs and symptoms: Patients complain of fatigue and generalized malaise and may attribute the symptoms to influenza or the exacerbation of existing arthritic conditions such as OA. Patients are often febrile and may report night sweating. Additionally, patients usually have bilateral, proximal aching and stiffness in the neck, shoulders, upper arms, hips, thighs, and lower back. Stiffness occurs in the morning and may last >30 minutes; however, on exertion, fatigue and aching may return. Limiting mobility and/or positional changes may also exacerbate the musculoskeletal pain. Anorexia, weight loss, apathy, fear, and depression are also constitutional symptoms of PMR. Musculoskeletal pain and related symptoms may be present about 1 month before the diagnosis is made; however, sudden onset of PMR can occur as well in older adults (Salvarani et al., 2008).

Muscle weakness usually is not elicited on physical examination. Tenderness may be detected on palpation to the muscle groups mentioned earlier. Check for signs of carpal tunnel syndrome, such as paresthesia of the thumb and index and middle fingers due to flexor tenosynovitis. Patients may complain of numbness and tingling in the fingers and a decreased ability to grasp small objects. Distal extremity swelling with pitting edema may be present over the dorsum of hands, wrists, ankles, and tops of feet (Salvarani et al., 2008). Examine for evidence of claudication in the lower extremities (Kermani & Warrington, 2011).

Diagnostic studies may reveal anemia; checking for signs of pallor is important. Because GCA is associated with PMR, the workup should include questions to evaluate for this vasculitis, such as complaints of occipital or temporal headaches, visual disturbances (amaurosis fugax and transient diplopia), high fever, jaw and tongue pain, sore throat, hoarseness, choking, cough, ear pain, painful scalp, and limb claudication as a result of vascular occlusion (Ezeonyeji, Borg, & Dasgupta, 2011; Salvarani et al., 2008). Assess for tender temporal arteries and visual acuity. Funduscopic examination may reveal retinal hemorrhages, cotton-wool patches, and edema of the optic disc (Paget & Spiera, 2006). Neurological findings are also common in patients with GCA due to occlusion of internal carotid or vertebral arteries; neuropathies, transient ischemic attacks, and stroke have been known to occur in patients with extensive GCA (Salvarani et al., 2008).

Diagnostic tests: Although pending new clinical guidelines are indicating that no diagnostic studies confirm the diagnosis of PMR (Dasgupta et al., 2012), the following diagnostic tests are recommended in the workup for patients with suspected PMR who eventually are placed on corticosteroid therapy.

An elevated ESR (<40 mm/hr) and C-reactive protein are common findings in PMR. For patients with GCA, the ESR generally is found to be ≥100 mm/hr or greater. However, there have been cases of patients who had a positive biopsy for GCA with normal C-reactive protein (Parikh et al., 2006). Obtain CBC with indices to determine presence of normochromic, normocytic anemia and thrombocytosis, which are common in patients with PMR. For patients with symptoms of claudication, imaging studies can be beneficial in determining presence of lower extremity vasculitis (Kermani & Warrington, 2011). Liver enzyme tests often show elevated alkaline phosphate in patients with GCA (Salvarani et al., 2008). Patients with symptoms of GCA need to be referred for temporal artery biopsy. Considering the need for long-term corticosteroids, diagnostic studies should also include urea and electrolytes, thyroid-stimulating hormone and dipstick urinalysis, and bone density testing (Dasgupta et al., 2010).

Differential diagnosis: The following are differential diagnoses for polymyalgia rheumatica (Dasgupta et al., 2010; Pease et al., 2005; Salvarani et al., 2008; Soubrier et al., 2006).

- Late-onset rheumatoid arthritis (specifically, the absence of rheumatoid factor and normal anticitrullinated protein antibody [ACPA] can rule out initial diagnosis of late-onset rheumatoid arthritis)
- Polymyositis (patients who have demonstrated proximal weakness characteristic of polymyositis would have a positive muscle biopsy)
- Fibromyalgia (generally fibromyalgia begins in younger adulthood and the ESR is normal)
- Hypothyroidism (thyroid hormone is not elevated as a result of PMR)
- Hyperparathyroidism (parathyroid hormone level is not elevated as a result of PMR)

- Osteoarthritis (radiographic changes would demonstrate evidence of osteoarthritis and not PMR)
- Bursitis and tendinitis (constitutional symptoms generally are not evident in patients with bursitis and tendinitis)
- Carcinomatosis
- Chondrocalcinosis
- Systemic lupus erythematosus (antinuclear antibody [ANA] would not be significantly elevated in patients with PMR; slight ANA elevation can be expected in older adults absent of disease)
- Multiple myeloma (patients with multiple myeloma do not respond to corticosteroids)
- Infective endocarditis
- Vasculitis
- Parkinson's disease (ESR is not elevated in patients with Parkinson's disease [PD] and corticosteroid therapy would not produce a clinical response to the stiffness experienced in PD)
- Polyarticular calcium pyrophosphate deposition disease (arthrocentesis of affected joints would be negative for this condition)

In patients with symptoms typical of PMR and a normal ESR, consider also drug-induced myalgias from lipid-lowering agents, beta blockers, and dipyridamole (Goëb, Guillemant, Vittecoq, & Le Loët, 2004; Snyder, 1991).

Treatment: If the patient presents with signs and symptoms only of PMR, start low-dose prednisone (10 to 20 mg/day). Patient's weight should be considered when dosing prednisone (Cimmino, Parodi, Montecucco, & Caporali, 2011). Symptoms should begin to resolve after 24 hours, and the ESR, C-reactive protein, anemia, and thrombocytosis should begin to normalize in 7 to 10 days, taking often 1 month to return to normal when higher levels were present in patients with GCA. Prednisone is tapered off slowly, continuing over months, when the symptoms have resolved and the ESR returns to normal. A slow tapering plan of 1 mg every 4 to 8 weeks until discontinuation is recommended; however, consensus has not been reached as to a tapering schedule (Dasgupta et al., 2010). Patients presenting with visual disturbances or other symptoms of GCA need a higher dose of oral corticosteroids; prednisone 40 to 80 mg in divided daily doses is the suggested starting dose, again with a gradual tapering depending on symptoms and laboratory values. Treatment may last 2 to 3 years.

Follow-up: Assess the patient for proximal pain, morning stiffness, resolution of constitutional symptoms, and adverse reaction to corticosteroids (Dasgupta et al., 2010). For patients with PMR, the ESR and/or C-reactive protein need monitoring until the levels decrease and previously reported symptoms are alleviated. The CBC can be repeated to determine if the anemia has resolved. Initially, the patients will need to return every couple of weeks to evaluate the clinical response to therapy; this is followed by approximately an every-3-month surveillance to determine response to treatment and any adverse reactions to the long-term corticosteroids. Additional monitoring of urea and electrolytes and glucose should continue every 3 months while on corticosteroids (Dasgupta et al., 2010). Follow up on the results of the dual-energy x-ray absorptiometry scan. Consider prophylactic therapy to prevent osteoporosis with bisphosphonates with calcium and vitamin D supplementation. Patients also presenting with GCA need to be monitored in the same way, with repeated eye examinations as warranted, including examination for cataracts resulting from corticosteroid therapy (Paget & Spiera, 2006). Because patients with GCA are at risk for developing aortic aneurysm, follow-up abdominal examination for aortic aneurysm is needed. This complication is of great concern especially with patients who are at high risk for developing aortic aneurysms such as patients who smoke, are hypertensive, and have arteriosclerotic heart disease (Unwin et al., 2006).

Sequelae: The diagnosis of PMR is confirmed when a response to the corticosteroid is noted. Usually the patient begins to exhibit a reduction in symptoms within 24 hours after starting treatment. Patients should be alerted to the signs of GCA. Patients with untreated GCA are at risk for blindness. Patients should be informed that they must complete all of the prescribed medication to avoid a relapse. Despite the initial symptom relief, extended treatment with corticosteroids can be expected. Patients often relapse following an initial case of PMR; up to 25% to 50% of patients have a recurrence of PMR (Kremers et al., 2005). Patients with PMR may be at risk for developing vascular disorders; thus these patients should be screened carefully and advised that if a smoker, smoking cessation is recommended (Hancock, Mallen, Belcher, & Hider, 2012). Practitioners will need to continue to monitor patients for any new symptoms following treatment for PMR. When examining a national database of patients with PMR, Muller, Hider, Belcher, Helliwell, and Mallen (2013) found a trend of new cancer diagnoses in patients with PMR without pre-existing cancer 6 months after initial diagnosis.

Prevention/prophylaxis: No preventive measures exist for PMR, but because the disease can recur, patients should be advised to contact their health-care providers when any of the prevailing signs and symptoms reappears. Patients on long-term corticosteroids should be up to date on immunizations for influenza and pneumonia.

Referral: For patients with signs of visual disturbance, funduscopic changes, or both, referral to an ophthalmologist is warranted if the patient can be evaluated immediately. If not, these patients should be referred to an emergency department for immediate evaluation for probable temporal artery biopsy. Consultation with a rheumatologist is warranted for patients who have GCA or who do not respond initially to corticosteroid treatment or have prolonged duration of PMR (greater than 2 years) (Dasgupta et al., 2010). Consider also referring younger patients (under 60 years) with symptoms of PMR to a rheumatologist (Helliwell, Hider, & Mullen, 2013).

Education: Patients should be taught the precautions needed when steroids are being taken; in addition to being at risk for osteoporosis, the likelihood for developing infections, fractures, diabetes, peptic ulcers, cataracts, depression, and weight gain increases with steroids. Patients should be instructed to include an adequate amount of dietary calcium and vitamin D (Helliwell et al., 2013). Patients who do not have GCA should be alerted to potential symptoms, such as visual disturbance, headache, temporal and scalp tenderness, jaw pain (especially while chewing), and limb pain.

CLINICAL RECOMMENDATION	EVIDENCE RATING	REFERENCE
Careful consideration of the patient's weight must be taken into consideration when prescribing corticosteroids to patients with PMR.	A	Cimmino et al. (2011)
It is critical to ask patients about signs and symptoms of GCA in patients who present with PMR, given that 50% of patients with GCA have had PMR at one time.	C	Salvarani et al. (2008)
Twenty-five percent of patients with PMR experience a relapse.	B	Kremers et al. (2005)
Positive biopsy for GCA may occur in patients with a normal C-reactive protein.	A	Parikh et al. (2006)

A = consistent, good-quality, patient-oriented evidence; B = inconsistent or limited-quality, patient-oriented evidence; C = consensus, disease-oriented evidence, usual practice, expert opinion, or case series. For information about the SORT evidence rating system, go to www.aafp.org/afpsort.xml.

RHEUMATOID ARTHRITIS

Signal symptoms: Morning stiffness, joint deformities, rheumatoid nodules, and symmetrical inflammatory polyarthritis.

Description: Rheumatoid arthritis (RA) is a chronic systematic inflammatory process evidenced by symmetrical polyarthritis; it is the most common inflammatory arthropathy. Patients generally experience episodes of remission and acute exacerbations of this disease. It is an incurable autoimmune condition that affects synovial joints in the body. This ongoing synovial membrane attack results in synovial proliferation, pannus formation, and loss of joint space and its surrounding soft tissues (Manno & Bingham, 2011).

Pain and stiffness result from the damage of the joints and soft tissues. RA is associated with decreased physical function and overall diminished quality of life. Loss of functionality is the aftereffect of joint destruction. Extra-articular features can result in damage to the heart, lungs, and other vital organs. There are multiple presentations of RA, which can include vasculitis, rheumatoid nodules, scleritis, pericarditis, neuropathy, interstitial fibrosis, Sjögren's syndrome, and Felty's syndrome. RA has been shown to increase cardiovascular risk and reduce overall life expectancy (Manno & Bingham, 2011).

Older patients with RA have already sustained significant joint damage as well as multiple comorbidities. These comorbidities may be directly related to the RA or may be a result of long-term treatments. Osteoporosis may occur after long-term use of corticosteroids. Older people may be hesitant about asserting themselves when exacerbations of their condition occur. Some may find the current approach of self-empowerment difficult. As with all conditions affecting older adults, comorbid factors such as impaired mental, visual, and auditory faculties and muscle weakness must be factored into the patient's individual treatment plan (Olivieri, Pipitone, D'Angelo, Padula, & Salvarani, 2009).

Etiology: The exact cause of RA is unknown. There is a demonstrated relationship between the presence of class II human leukocyte antigen (HLA) gene and RA. This relationship has a familial component.

Occurrence: Approximately 1% of the population of the Western world has RA. Although the condition can affect all ages, elderly-onset RA has a sixfold greater occurrence than in someone aged 25 years. RA affects more women than men, in a 3:1 ratio. RA is a worldwide disease estimated to occur in 30 in 100,000 adults (MacGregor & Silman, 2008).

Age: RA affects all ages, including children and the elderly. The mean age of onset is 40 to 60 years. It has been estimated that 20% to 55% of adults with RA will develop the condition in old age. Studies have indicated that there is a correlation between the increase in incidence of RA and age; cases peak between ages 60 and 80 for patients developing late-onset RA (Doran, Pond, Crowson, O'Fallon, & Gabriel, 2002).

Gender: Prevalence is 2 to 3 times higher in women than men. This occurrence can range up to 5% in women over age 65. However, late-onset or elderly-onset RA tends to have a more equal gender distribution (Olivieri et al., 2009).

Ethnicity: Its prevalence is approximately 1% in Caucasians. There is a variance among races from 0.1% in rural Africans to 5% in Native American Indians.

Contributing factors: Risk factors for the development of RA include positive family history, female gender, and the presence of the HLA haplotype DR4 and DRB1 (Manno & Bingham, 2011; Orozco & Barton, 2010). For patients who smoke and have the identified haplotype DRB1, the risk increases (Bang et al., 2010).

Signs and symptoms: The clinical presentation for patients with longstanding RA before age 60 reflects the duration of the individual's disease and concomitant conditions. For patients with older adult–onset RA, the presentation may be gradual onset of morning stiffness, swelling, and pain in multiple joints. In others the attack may be more acute. In older adults, constitutional symptoms with RA may include low-grade fever, weight loss, malaise, and depression. Joint involvement is usually accompanied by pain and early morning stiffness that gradually improve during the day. This differs from the osteoarthritis type of stiffness that presents after prolonged inactivity. Pain is usually present regardless of weight bearing or movement (Manno & Bingham, 2011).

During examinations of the patient with known RA, the metacarpophalangeal, wrist, PIP, MTP, shoulder, ankle, and elbow joints should be examined for ROM, tenderness, erythema, warmth, and swelling. Clinical joint findings prevalent in patients with a chronic history of RA include hyperflexion of the PIP joints and flexion of the DIP joints (called swan neck deformities), flexion of the PIP joints and extension of the DIP joints (called boutonniere deformity), ulnar deviation of the metacarpophalangeal joint, and knee and ankle effusions (LeBlond, Brown, & DeGowin, 2009). A gentle squeeze test for tenderness of joints of hands and feet will vary on exacerbation of condition. The skin should be checked for subcutaneous nodules, which are generally less than 1 to 3 cm in diameter and feel firm and fixed on palpation; these often are found proximal to the elbow. Systemic evaluation also includes an eye examination to check for keratoconjunctivitis, scleritis, and corneal ulcers. Conditions of the lung may include pleuritis and pneumonitis. Pericarditis, a possible manifestation of RA, warrants a cardiac examination. The clinician also should examine the patient for evidence of nerve entrapment and sensory neuropathy. All patients should be questioned about the impact of RA on their lifestyle and current ability to carry out ADLs by using the revised

Arthritis Impact Measurement Scale Health Status Questionnaire (AIMS 2) (Meenan, Mason, Anderson, Guccione, & Kazis, 1992). The initial presentation is usually one of an inflammatory polyarthritis (many painful joints). Some simple rules will help you to identify patients who have an inflammatory polyarthritis, such as RA, who should be referred promptly to a specialist rheumatology team for diagnosis within 3 months. Erosions may be seen within a few years of disease onset, and even patients with less than 3 months' duration of symptoms may already have evidence of destruction (Olivieri et al., 2009). The American College of Rheumatology (ACR) jointly with the European League Against Rheumatism (EULAR) have established new classification criteria for RA (Aletaha et al., 2010).

Diagnostic tests: Blood tests such as rheumatoid factor (RF) and ESR or the C-reactive protein are useful in the presence of diagnostic indicators on physical examination. Erosive disease and a raised RF concentration indicate that a person has seropositive RA (Olivieri et al., 2009). The laboratory test anti-citrullinated peptic antibodies has been shown to be an important indicator for destructive disease when accompanied by a high RF titer. Testing for antibodies to cyclic citrullinated peptide (anti-CCP antibodies) is newer than the RF testing and is associated with higher sensitivity and specificity for RA. Anti-CCP antibodies may be detected before the RF develops and are found in up to 40% of RF-negative patients. Radiographs of the hands and feet are needed to look for early signs of erosions, which are an important factor indicating the need to start an aggressive treatment approach aimed at halting further joint damage progression. Additional radiographic findings in RA include soft tissue swelling, symmetrical joint space narrowing, and joint subluxations. A CBC may show normochromic, normocytic anemia, mild leukocytosis, and thrombocytosis (Lee, Beck, & Hall, 2008; Majithia, Peel, & Geraci, 2009; Manno & Bingham, 2011).

Differential diagnosis: Differential diagnoses for rheumatoid arthritis include the following (Matjithia et al., 2009; Manno & Bingham, 2011; Olivieri et al., 2009; Villa-Blanco & Calvo-Alen, 2009).

- Polymyalgia rheumatica (rapid response to corticosteroid therapy)
- Crystal arthropathies, including gout and pseudogout (joint aspiration would reveal monosodium urate crystal or calcium pyrophosphate rhomboidal crystals)
- Septic arthritis (Gram stain and culture from arthrocentesis)
- OA (can be ruled out with radiographs)
- Spondyloarthropathy
- Remitting seronegative symmetrical synovitis with pitting edema syndrome
- Arthritis related to connective tissue disease or systemic vasculitis
- Polymyositis (normal muscled enzymes and muscle biopsy would be expected in RA)
- Malignancy-related arthritis
- Hypertrophic osteoarthropathy
- Sarcoidosis
- Infectious arthritis (hepatitis B and C, HIV, and others)

Treatment: The drug management of RA is one of symptom and disease control. Symptom control includes corticosteroid treatment, analgesia, and NSAIDs. Disease control includes corticosteroids, which can be used in combination with traditional disease-modifying therapies. The early or long-term use of corticosteroids remains a controversial topic, chiefly because of their long-term side-effect profile. Traditional disease-modifying antirheumatic drugs (DMARDs), which suppress the immune response, include medications such as methotrexate and sulfasalazine. Biological DMARDs are used to treat the disease and are administered subcutaneously, intravenously, and by mouth.

When using NSAIDs to treat older adults with RA, the NSAID selection should be based on the shortest half-life and the lowest effective dose. Low-dose oral corticosteroids may provide relief. Starting doses of <10 mg and tapering to find the most effective dose is recommended (Manno & Bingham, 2011).

Disease control treatment approaches start with the prompt introduction of a "traditional" DMARD as a single therapy or a combination of two or more DMARDs. DMARDs suppress the immune response and prevent joint damage, although they may take up to 3 months to have an effect. Traditional DMARDs include the following:

- Methotrexate (oral, intramuscular, or rarely subcutaneous given as a once-weekly dose; co-prescribed with folic acid, usually 5 mg once a week when the weekly dose of methotrexate is administrated to decrease nausea, diarrhea, and other common side effects)
- Sulfasalazine
- Leflunomide

■ Hydroxychloroquine

■ Azathioprine

■ Cyclosporine

There are added risks and long-term consequences of immune suppression associated with drugs such as methotrexate. Tuberculosis testing is done before initiating the immune-suppressing medications. Often more than one DMARD is prescribed at a time for efficiency. Patients require close monitoring for potential toxic effects such as renal toxicity, NSAID-induced gastritis, and central nervous system toxicity. RA patients with comorbidities on combinations are at a risk for drug interaction. The new biological agents are used with close observation of benefit versus risk of cancer and fungal infections.

Biological agents include the following drugs: abatacept, adalimumab, etanercept, infliximab, rituximab, and anakinra. The latest consensus statement on biological agents for the treatment of rheumatic disease reported that there is evidence indicating that tumor necrosis factor (TNF) receptor antagonists are effective for the treatment of RA with methotrexate. There is, however, no evidence that any of the current TNF receptor antagonists are better than any others in its class, so if the first agent fails, another medication of this class can be tried. Severe events include infections, potential worsening of heart failure, and demyelinating disease. TNF receptor antagonists should not be prescribed to patients with current, active infection and should be used with caution in elderly patients with other immune-suppressing conditions. Recently, studies have concluded that anti-TNF agents could be administrated to elderly patients with RA with similar effectiveness and tolerability as in younger patients (Koller et al., 2009). Another cytokine is IL-6, which importantly, may be involved in the pathogenesis of RA. The blocking of this receptor with the biological agent tocilizumab has led to reduction of the acute-phase response of rheumatoid arthritis, with elevated cholesterol being the main side effect known at this time (Singh, Beg, & Lopez-Olivio, 2011). There are many unscientific claims to improving and curing RA in the general marketplace. Support groups and gentle exercise are recommended regardless of age. Cycles of exacerbations are common. RA is not a diagnosed condition that goes without need of support.

Follow-up: Routine evaluations for patients with RA should include the patient's response to the pharmacological and nonpharmacological therapy. Medications should be adjusted if the patient does not obtain symptomatic relief from the current therapy. Progression of the articular and extra-articular disease should be monitored through physical examination. Any change in the patient's ability to carry out ADLs, as well as his or her psychosocial status, should be evaluated at each visit using the Arthritis Impact Measurement Scale Health Status Questionnaire 2 (AIMS) or similar scale (Meenan et al., 1992).

Sequelae: Older adults who have had RA for years eventually experience more severe disease with increased joint deformities. Comorbidities such as septic arthritis, Sjögren's syndrome, Felty's syndrome, and pericarditis may exist in patients with a history of RA. Patients with elderly-onset RA may tend to have a milder course of the disease with periods of remission; however, patients experiencing a more rapid decline have also been reported. Complications from the medication regimen need to be considered and monitored.

Prevention/prophylaxis: Although RA cannot be prevented, a program of gentle ROM exercises can help maintain function and muscle strength. Water exercise programs have been shown to be an effective therapy for patients with RA (Eversden, Maggs, Nightingale & Jobanputra, 2007; Hall, Skevington, Maddison, & Chapman, 1996).

Referral: Patients experiencing a period of prolonged inflammation despite therapy or one of the comorbidities mentioned earlier should be referred to a rheumatologist (Wasserman, 2011). Patients can also benefit from referral to a physical therapist and an occupational therapist, to assist them in their exercise programs, splinting needs, additional orthotics, and adaptive equipment requirements, all aimed at maintaining function and independence for as long as possible.

Education: Patients should be taught the importance of incorporating periods of rest and exercise into their daily lives. Medication education is important in RA because of the potential for side effects associated with a complicated drug regimen. Because there is no cure for RA, patients must be skeptical about antidotes promised for RA and check with their health-care providers if they have any concerns about treatments. Patients can contact the Arthritis Foundation (800-282-7800) for information; a booklet, *Overcoming Rheumatoid Arthritis*, is available (Oliver, 2009).

CLINICAL RECOMMENDATION	EVIDENCE RATING	REFERENCE
Hydrotherapy has been shown to be effective in improving overall health in patients with RA.	A	Eversden et al. (2007) Hall et al. (1996)
Late-onset RA may progress slowly over several months or may occur suddenly, mimicking an acute crystalline arthritis.	C	Manno & Bingham (2011)
Mild anemia of chronic disease is a common clinical find in older adults with RA.	C	Wasserman (2011)
ACPAs, which include anti-cyclic citrullinated peptide antibodies (anti-CCP), are more specific for diagnosing RA in older adults than RF.	A	Palosuo, Tilvis, Strandberg, & Aho (2003)

A = consistent, good-quality, patient-oriented evidence; B = inconsistent or limited-quality, patient-oriented evidence; C = consensus, disease-oriented evidence, usual practice, expert opinion, or case series. For information about the SORT evidence rating system, go to www.aafp.org/afpsort.xml.

CASE STUDY

Ruby, an 86-year-old, Caucasian, thin, osteoporotic woman, gets up onto a stepstool to reach something on the top shelf of her cabinet. She loses her balance and falls onto her left side. She finds that she cannot sit up without pain. Her daughter later finds her and calls an ambulance to take her to the emergency department. Per radiograph, left femoral fracture is present. Surgery is scheduled for open reduction with internal fixation (ORIF). Blood clot prevention injections and pain medications are prescribed. Next, the patient is monitored for postoperative anemia and infection. After discharge, Ruby has rehabilitation for inpatient and then nursing home temporary care for 30 days. She is discharged to her daughter's home with home health and assistive equipment.

1. How will you use the information to prepare for today's visit?

   Today's visit:

   Chief complaint: "I am still recovering from my fall last month and now am staying at my daughter's but want to go home."

Objective: Blood pressure (BP) 100/60 mm Hg, pulse 87, respiratory rate 20 breaths/min

2. What additional subjective data are you seeking?

3. What additional subjective data will you be assessing for?

4. Are there any national guidelines you want to consult for the postoperative and rehabilitation care of this patient with an ORIF related to osteopenia of the left femur?

5. What tests will you want to order as part of this follow-up visit?

6. Are there any new differential diagnoses you need to consider?

7. What is your plan of care?

8. What additional patient teaching may be needed?

9. Are there additional community resources to consider?

10. Will you be looking to add any referrals for this patient?

REFERENCES

Assessment

Abdulla, A., Adams, N., Bone, M., Elliott, A. M., Gaffin, J., Jones, D., . . . Schofield, P. (2013). Guidance on the management of pain in older people. *Age and Aging, 42*(Suppl. 1), i1–i57. doi: 10.1093/ageing/afs200

Brown, C. J., & Peel, C. (2009). Rehabilitation. In J. Halter, J. Ouslander, M. Tinetti, S. Studenski, K. High, S. Asthana, & W. Hazzard (Eds.), *Principles of geriatric medicine and gerontology* (6th ed.). New York City, NY: McGraw-Hill Medical.

Gillet, C., & Norrell, A. A. (2011). Considerations for safe use of statins: liver enzyme abnormalities and muscle toxicity. *American Family Physician, 83*(6), 711–716.

LeBlond, R. F., Brown, D. D., & DeGowin, R. L. (2009). *DeGowin's diagnostic examination* (9th ed.). New York City, NY: McGraw-Hill Medical.

Loeser, R., & DelBono, O. (2009). Aging of the muscles and joints. In J. Halter, J. Ouslander, M. Tinetti, S. Studenski, K. High, S. Asthana, & W. Hazzard (Eds.), *Principles of geriatric medicine and gerontology* (6th ed.). New York City, NY: McGraw-Hill Medical.

Pacala, J. T., & Sullivan, G. S. (2010). *The geriatrics review syllabus: a core curriculum in geriatrics* (7th ed.). New York City, NY: American Geriatrics Society.

Williams, M. (2008). *Geriatric physical diagnosis.* Jefferson, NC: McFarland & Co.

Bursitis, Tendinitis, Soft Tissue Syndromes

Barratt, J. (2009). History taking and clinical examination of the shoulder. *Emergency Nurse, 17*(1), 26–33.

Bisset, L., Coombes, B., & Vicenzino, B. (2011). Tennis elbow. *Clinical Evidence (Online),* 1117.

Brown, C. J., & Peel, C. (2009). Rehabilitation. In J. Halter, J. Ouslander, M. Tinetti, S. Studenski, K. High, S. Asthana, & W. Hazzard (Eds.), *Principles of geriatric medicine and gerontology* (6th ed.). New York City, NY: McGraw-Hill Medical.

Cardone, D., & Tallia, A. F. (2002). Joint and soft tissue injection. *American Family Physician, 66*(2), 283–288.

Coghlan J. A., Buchbinder, R., Green, S., Johnston R. V., & Bell, S. N. (2008). Surgery for rotator cuff disease. *The Cochrane Database of Systematic Reviews, 23*(1), CD005619. doi: 10.1002/14651858.CD005619.pub2

Cole, C., Seto, C., & Gazewood, J. (2005). Plantar fasciitis: evidence-based review of diagnosis and therapy. *American Family Physician, 72*(11), 2237–2242.

Green, S., Johnston, R. V., & Bell, S. N. (2008). Surgery for rotator cuff disease. *Cochrane Database of Systematic Reviews, 23,* CD005619. doi: 10.1002/14651858.CD005619.pub2

Machida, A., Sugamoto, K., Miyamoto, T., Inui, H., Watanabe, T., & Yoshikawa, H. (2004). Adhesion of the subacromial bursa may cause subacromial impingement in patients with rotator cuff tears: pressure measurements in 18 patients. *Acta Orthoaedica Scandinavica, 75*(1), 109–113.

Omoigu, S. (2007). The biochemical origin of pain: the origin of all pain is inflammation and the inflammation response. Part 2 of 3-Inflammatory profile of pain syndromes. *Medical Hypothesis, 69*(6), 1169–1178.

Simpson, M., & Howard, T. M. (2009). Tendinopathies of the foot and ankle. *American Family Physician, 80*(10), 1107–1114.

Speed, C., & Hazleman, B. (2004). Shoulder pain. *Clinical Evidence (Online),* 1613–1632.

Fractures

Avenell, A., Gillespie, W. J., Gillespie, L. D., & O'Connell, D. (2009). Vitamin D and vitamin D analogues for preventing fractures associated with involutional and post-menopausal osteoporosis. *Cochrane Database of Systemic Reviews 2009, 15*(2). doi: 10.1002/14651858.CD000227.pub3

Handoll, H. (2000). Update of a systematic review of vitamin D for preventing osteoporotic fractures. *Injury Prevention, 15*(3), 213.

MacLean, C., Newberry, S., Maglione, M., Ranganath, V., Suttorp, M., Mojica, W., . . . Grossman, J. (2008). Systematic review: comparative effectiveness of treatments to prevent fracture in men and women with low bone density or osteoporosis. *Annals of Internal Medicine, 148*(3), 197–213.

Miller, R. R., Christmas, C., & Magaziner, J. (2009). Hip fractures. In J. Halter, J. Ouslander, M. Tinetti, S. Studenski, K. High, S. Asthana, & W. Hazzard (Eds.), *Principles of geriatric medicine and gerontology* (6th ed.). New York City, NY: McGraw-Hill Medical.

National Institutes of Health. (2005). Facts about menopausal hormonal therapy (pp. 1–24). National Heart, Lung, and Blood Institute, NIH Publication No. 05-5200.

Rahmani, P., & Morin, S. (2009). Prevention of osteoporotic-related fractures among postmenopausal women and older men. *Canadian Medical Association Journal, 181*(11), 815.

Schneider, A. L., Williams, E. K., Brancati, F. L., Blecker, S., Coresh, J., & Selvin, E. (2013). Diabetes and risk of fracture-related hospitalization: the atherosclerosis risk in communities study. *Diabetes Care, 36*(5), 1153–1158. doi:10.2337/dc12-1168

Wiley-Blackwell. (2008). Alendronate can help prevent bone fractures in many postmenopausal women. *Science Daily.* Retrieved September 25, 2010, from www.sciencedaily.com/releases/2008/01/080122203154.htm

Gout

Becker, M. A., Schumacher, H. R., MacDonald, P. A., Lloyd, E., & Lademacher, C. (2009). Clinical efficacy and safety of successful longterm urate lowering with febuxostat or allopurinol in subjects with gout. *The Journal of Rheumatology, 36*(6), 1273–1282. doi:10.3899/jrheum.080814

Burns, C. M., & Wortmann, R. L. (2011). Gout therapeutics: new drugs for an old disease. *Lancet, 377*(9760), 165–177. doi:10.1016/S0140-6736(10)60665-4

Chen, L. X., & Schumacher, H. R. (2008). Gout: an evidence-based review. *Journal of Clinical Rheumatology, 14*(Suppl. 5), S55–S62. doi: 10.1097/RHU.0b013e3181896921

Choi, H. K. (2010). A prescription for lifestyle change in patients with hyperuricemia and gout. *Current Opinion in Rheumatology, 22*(2), 165–172. doi:10.1097/BOR.0b013e328335ef38

Choi, H. K., & Curhan, G. (2008). Soft drinks, fructose consumption, and the risk of gout in men: prospective cohort study. *British Medical Journal, 336*(7639), 309–312. doi: 10.1136/bmj.39449.819271

Choy, G. (2005). An update on the treatment options for gout and calcium pyrophosphate deposition. *Expert Opinion in Pharmacotherapy, 6*(14), 2443–2453. doi:10.1517/14656566.6.14.2443

Dalbeth, N. (2013). Management of gout in primary care: challenges and potential solutions. *Rheumatology Advance Access* online publication. doi: 10.1093/rheumatology/ket215

Doherty, M. (2009). New insights into the epidemiology of gout. *Rheumatology, 48*(Suppl. 2), ii2–ii8. doi: 10.1093/rheumatology/kep086

Feig, D. I., Kang, D. H., & Johnson R. J. (2008). Uric acid and cardiovascular risk. *New England Journal of Medicine, 359*(17), 1811–1821. doi: 10.1056/NEJMra0800885

Fravel, M. A., & Ernst, M. E. (2011). Management of gout in the older adult. *The American Journal of Geriatric Pharmacology, 9*(5), 271–285. doi: 10.1016/j.amjopharm.2011.07.004

Hanlon, J. T., Aspinall, S. L., Semla, T. P., Weisbord, S. D., Fried, L. F., Good, C. B., . . . Handler, S. M. (2009). Consensus guidelines for oral dosing of primarily renally cleared medications in older adults. *Journal of the American Geriatrics Society, 57*(2), 335–340. doi: 10.1111/j.1532-5415.2008.02098.x

Janssen, H. J., Janssen, M., van de Lisdonk, E. H., van Riel, P. L., & van Weel, C. (2008). Use of oral prednisolone or naproxen for the treatment of gout arthritis: a double-blind, randomized equivalence trial. *Lancet, 371*(9627), 1854–1860.

Jordan, K. M., Cameron, J. S., Snaith, M., Zhang, W., Doherty, M., Seckl, J., . . . Nuki, G. (2009). British Society for Rheumatology and British Health Professionals in Rheumatology Standards, Guidelines and Audit Working Group (SGAWG). *Rheumatology, 46*(8), 1372–1374.

Lawrence, R. C., Felson, D. T., Helmick, C. G., Arnold, L. M., Choi, H., Deyo, R. A., . . . National Arthritis Data Workgroup (2008). Estimates of the prevalence of arthritis and other rheumatic conditions in the United States: Part II. *Arthritis and Rheumatism, 58*(1), 26–35. doi: 10.1002/art.23176

Khanna, D., Fitzgerald, J. D., Khanna, P. P., Bae, S., Singh, M. K., Neogi, T., . . . Terkeltaub, R. (2012). 2012 American College of Rheumatology guidelines for management of gout. Part 1: Systematic nonpharmacologic and pharmacologic therapeutic approaches to hyperuricemia. *Arthritis Care & Research, 64*(10), 1431–1446.

Man, C. Y., Cheung, I. T., Cameron, P. A., & Rainer, T. H. (2007). Comparison of oral prednisolone/paracetamol and oral indomethacin/paracetamol combination therapy in the treatment of acute gout-like arthritis: a double-blind, randomized, controlled trial. *Annals of Emergency Medicine, 49*(5), 670–677. doi:10.1016/j.annemergmed.2006.11.014

Neogi, T. (2011). Clinical practice: gout. *New England Journal of Medicine, 364*, 443–452. Retrieved from www.nejm.org

Ning, T. C., & Keenan, R. T. (2011). Gout in the elderly. *Clinical Geriatrics, 19*(1), 20–25. Retrieved from www.clinicalgeriatrics.com

Roberts, J. R. (2010). Diagnosing gout: the basics. *Emergency Medicine News.* Retrieved from http://journals.lww.com/emnews/Fulltext/2010/03000/Diagnosing_Gout__The_Basics.5.aspx. doi:10.1097/01.EEM.0000369231.25628.2b

Rosenberg, A. (2005). Bones, joints and soft tissue tumors. In V. Kumar, A. Abbas, & N. Fausto (Eds.), *Pathologic Basis of Disease.* (7th ed., pp. 1311–1314). Philadelphia, PA: Elsevier.

Terkeltaub, R. A., Furst, D. E., Bennett, K., Kook, K. A., Crockett, R. S., & Davis, M. W. (2010). High versus low dosing of oral colchicine for early acute gout flare: twenty-four hour outcome of the first multicenter, randomized, double-blind, placebo-controlled, parallel group, dose comparison colchicine study. *Arthritis and Rheumatism, 62*(4), 1060–1068.

Wallace, K. L., Riedel, A. A., Joseph-Ridge, N., & Wortmann, R. (2004). Increasing prevalence of gout and hyperuricemia over 10 years among older adults in a managed care population. *The Journal of Rheumatology, 31*(8), 1582–1587.

Weaver, A. L. (2008). Epidemiology of gout. *Cleveland Clinic Journal of Medicine, 75,* (Suppl. 5), S9–S12.

Zhang, W., Doherty, M., Bardin, T., Pascual, E., Barskova, V., Conaghan, P., . . . Zimmermann, I. (2006). EULAR evidence-based recommendations for gout. Part II: Management. Report of a task force of the EULAR Standing Committee for International Clinical Studies Including Therapeutics (ESCISIT). *Annals of Rheumatic Diseases, 65*(10), 1312–1324. doi:10.1136/ard.2006.055251

Zhang, W., Doherty, M., Pascual, E., Barskova, V., Guerne, P. A., Jansen, T. L., . . . Bardin, T. (2010). EULAR recommendations for calcium pyrophosphate deposition. Part II: Management. *Annals of Rheumatic Diseases.* Advance online publication. doi:10.1136/ard.2010.139360

Zhu, Y., Pandya, B. J., & Choi, H. K. (2011). Prevalence of gout and hyperuricemia in the US general population: the National Health and Nutrition Examination Survey 2007–2008. *Arthritis Rheumatism, 63*(31), 3136–3141.

Zychowicz, M. E., Pope, R. S., & Graser, E. (2010). The current state of care in gout: addressing the need for better understanding of an ancient disease. *Journal of the American Academy of Nurse Practitioners, 22*(Suppl. 1), 623–636. doi:10.1111/j.1745-7599.2010.00556.x

Herniated Nucleus Pulposus

Asch, H. L., Lewis, P. J., Moreland, D. B., Egnatchik, J. G., Yu, Y. J., Clabeaux, D. E., & Hyland, A. H. (2002). Prospective multiple outcomes study of outpatient lumbar microdiscectomy: should 75 to 80% success rates be the norm? *Journal of Neurosurgery, 96*(Suppl. 1), 34–44.

Atlas, S. J., & Deyo, R. A. (2001). Evaluating and managing acute low back pain in the primary care setting. *Journal of General Internal Medicine, 16*(2), 120–131.

Atlas, S. J., Keller, R. B., Robson, D., Deyo, R. A., & Singer, D. E. (2000). Surgical and nonsurgical management of lumbar spinal stenosis: four-year outcomes from the Maine lumbar spine study. *Spine, 25*(5), 556–562.

Boden, S. D., Riew, K. D., Yamaguchi, K., Branch, T. P., Schellinger, D., & Wiesel, S. W. (1996). Orientation of the lumbar facet joints: association with degenerative disc disease. *The Journal of Bone and Joint Surgery, 78*(3), 403–411.

Chou, R., Atlas, S. J., Stamos, S. P., & Rosenquist, R. W. (2009). Nonsurgical interventional therapies for low back pain: a review of the evidence for an American Pain Society clinical practice guideline. *Spine, 34*(10), 1078–1093.

Chou, R., Baisden, J., Carragee, E. J., Resnick, D. K., Shaffer, W. O., & Loeser, J. D. (2009). Surgery for low back pain: a review of the evidence for an American Pain Society clinical practice guideline. *Spine, 34*(10), 1094–1109.

Chou, R., & Huffman, L. H. (2008). Nonpharmacologic therapies for acute and chronic low back pain: a review of the evidence for an American Pain Society/American College of Physicians clinical practice guidelines. *Annals of Internal Medicine, 148*(3), 247–248.

Fisher, C., Noonan, V., Bishop, P., Boyd, M., Fairholm, D., Wing, P., & Dvorak, M. (2004). Outcome evaluation of the operative management of lumbar disc herniation causing sciatica. *Journal of Neurosurgery, 100*(Suppl. 4), 317–324.

Foster, M. R. (2010). Herniated nucleus pulposus. *Emedicine.* Retrieved January 8, 2010, from http://emedicine.medscape.com/article/1263961-overview

Gotfryd, A., & Avanzi, O. (2009). A systematic review of randomized clinical trials using posterior discectomy to treat lumbar disc herniations. *International Orthopaedics, 33*(1), 11–17.

Hirsch, J. A., Singh, V., Falco, F. J. E., Benyamin, R. M., & Manchikanti, L. (2009). Automated percutaneous lumbar discectomy for the contained herniated lumbar disc: a systematic assessment of evidence. *Pain Physician, 12*(3), 601–620.

Levin, J. H., & Smuck, M. W. (2007). Radiculopathy from herniation of the nucleus pulposus: the role of corticosteroids. *Journal of Back and Musculoskeletal Rehabilitation, 20*(2,3), 103–113.

Olmarker, K., Rydevik, B., & Nordborg, C. (1993). Autologous nucleus pulposus induces neurophysiologic and histologic changes in porcine cauda equina nerve roots. *Spine, 18*(11), 1425–1432.

van der Windt, D. A., Simons, E., Riphagen, I. I., Ammendolia, C., Verhagen, A. P., Laslett, M., . . . Aertgeerts, B. (2010). Physical examination for lumbar radiculopathy due to disc herniation in patients with low-back pain. *Cochrane Database of Systematic Reviews* (2):CD007431. doi:10.1002/14651858.CD007431.pub2

Zieger, M., Schwarz, R., Konig, H. H., Harter, M., & Riedel-Heller, S. G. (2010). Depression and anxiety in patients undergoing herniated disc surgery: relevant but underresearched: a systematic review. *Central European Neurosurgery, 71*(1), 26–34.

Osteoarthritis

Abdulla, A., Adams, N., Bone, M., Elliott, A. M., Gaffin, J., Jones, D., . . . Schofield, P. (2013). Guidance on the management of pain in older people. *Age and Aging, 42*(Suppl. 1), i1–i57. doi: 10.1093/ageing/afs200

Ali, Y. (2001). Pharmacological treatments for osteoarthritis. *Clinical Geriatrics, 19*(11), 34–39.

Altman, R. D., Dreiser, R. L., Fisher, C. L., Chase, W. F., Dreher, D. S., & Zacher, J. (2009). Diclofenac sodium gel in patients with primary hand osteoarthritis: a randomized, double-blind, placebo-controlled trial. *The Journal of Rheumatology, 36*(9), 1991–1999. doi: 10.3899/jrheum.081316

Baraf, H. S., Gloth, F. M., Barthel, H. R., Gold, M. S., & Altman R. D. (2011). Safety and efficacy of topical diclofenac sodium gel for knee osteoarthritis in elderly and younger patients: pooled data from three randomized, double-blind, parallel-group, placebo-controlled, multicentre trials. *Drugs and Aging, 28*(1), 27–40. doi: 10.2165/11584880-000000000-00000

Barsotti, C. E., Mycyk, M. B., & Reyes, J. (2003). Withdrawal syndrome from tramadol hydrochloride. *American Journal of Emergency Medicine, 21*(1), 87–88.

Beaudreuil, J., Bendaya, S., Faucher, M., Coudeyre, E., Ribinik, P., Revel, M., & Rannou, F. (2009). Clinical practice guidelines for rest orthosis, knee sleeves, and unloading knee braces in knee osteoarthritis. *Joint Bone Spine, 76*(6), 629–636.

Bellamy, N., Campbell, J., Welch, V., Gee, T. L., Bourne, R., & Wells, G. A. (2006). Viscosupplementation for the treatment of osteoarthritis of the knee. *Cochrane Database of Systematic Reviews,* Issue 2. Art. No.: CD005321. doi:10.1002/14651858.CD005321.pub2

Chao, J., & Kalunian, K. (2010). Managing osteoarthritis: a multidisciplinary approach. *Journal of Musculoskeletal Medicine, 27*(10). Retrieved from www.musculoskeletalnetwork.com/display/article/1145622/1692827

Lawrence, R. C., Felson, D. T., Helmick, C. G., Arnold, L. M., Choi, H., Deyo, R. A., . . . National Arthritis Data Workgroup. (2008). Estimates of the prevalence of arthritis and other rheumatic conditions in the United States. Part II. *Arthritis and Rheumatism, 58*(1), 26–35.

LeBlond, R. F., Brown, D. D., & DeGowin, R. L. (2009). *DeGowin's diagnostic examination* (9th ed.). New York City, NY: McGraw-Hill Medical.

Ling, S. M., & Rudolph, K. S. (2006). Osteoarthritis. In T. Stephen, S. T. Wegener, L. Basia, E. P. Gall (Eds.), *Clinical Care in the Rheumatic Diseases* (3rd ed.). Atlanta, GA: American College of Rheumatology.

Musuku, M., Zirker, W., Srulevich, M., Kahn, D., & DeSimone, E. A. (2011). Total knee replacement in the very elderly. *Clinical Geriatrics, 19*(9), 41–43.

Reid, M. C., Shengelia, R., & Parker, S. J. (2013). Pharmacologic management of osteoarthritis-related pain in older adults: a review shows that many drug therapies provide small-to-modest

pain relief. *The Musculoskeletal Journal of Hospital for Specialty Surgery, 8*(2), 159–164. doi: 10.1007/s11420-012-9273-0

Ringdahl, E., & Pandit, S. (2010). Treatment of osteoarthritis of the knee. *American Family Physician, 8*(11), 1287–1292.

Sawitzke, A. D., Shi, H., & Finco, M. F. (2010). Clinical efficacy and safety of glucosamine, chondroitin sulfate, their combination, celecoxib or placebo taken to treat osteoarthritis of the knee: 2 year results from GAIT. *Annuals of Rheumatic Diseases, 69*(8), 1459–1464.

Shelton, L. R. (2013). A closer look at osteoarthritis. *The Nurse Practitioner, 38*(7), 31–36.

Swagerty, D. L., & Hellinger, D. (2001). Radiographic assessment of osteoarthritis. *American Family Physician, 64*(2), 279–286.

Zhang, W., Doherty, M., Leeb, B. F., Alekseeva, L., Arden, N. K., Bijlsma, J. W., . . . ESCISIT. (2009). EULAR evidence-based recommendations for the diagnosis of hand osteoarthritis: report of a task force of ESCISIT. *Annals of the Rheumatic Diseases, 68*(1), 8–17.

Zhang, W., Doherty, M., Peat, G., Bierma-Zeinstra, M. A., Arden, N. K., Bresnihan, B., . . . Bijlsma, J. W. (2010). EULAR evidence-based recommendations for the diagnosis of knee osteoarthritis. *Annals of the Rheumatic Diseases 69*(3), 483–489.

Zhang, W., Markowitz, R. W., Nuke, G., Abramson, S., & Altman, R.D. (2008). OARSI recommendations for the management of hip and knee osteoarthritis, part II: OARSI evidence-based expert consensus guidelines. *Osteoarthritis Cartilage, 16*(2), 137–162.

Polymyalgia Rheumatica

Cimmino, M. A., Parodi, M., Montecucco, C., & Caporali, R. (2011). The correct prednisone starting dose in polymyalgia rheumatica is related to body weight but not to disease severity. *BMC Musculoskeletal Disorders, 12*(12), 94. doi:10.1186/1471-2474-12-94

Dasgupta, B., Borg, F. A., Hassan, N., Barraclough, K., Bourke, B., Fulcher, J., . . . Samanta, A. (2010). British Society for Rheumatology and British Health Professionals in Rheumatology guidelines for the management of polymyalgia rheumatica. *Rheumatology, 49*(1), 186–190. doi:10.1093/rheumatology/kep303a

Dasgupta, B., Cimmino, M. A., Kremers, H. M., Schmidt, W. A., Schirmer, M., Salvarani, C., . . . Matteson, E. L. (2012). 2012 provisional classification criteria for polymyalgia rheumatica: a European League Against Rheumatism/American College of Rheumatology collaborative initiative. *Arthritis and Rheumatism, 64*(4), 943–954. doi: 10.1002/art.34356

Ezeonyeji, A. N., Borg, F. A., & Dasgupta, B. (2011). Delays in recognition and management of giant cell arteritis: results from a retrospective audit. *Clinical Rheumatology, 30*(2), 259–262. doi:10.1007/s10067-010-1616-y

Goëb, V., Guillemant, N., Vittecoq, O., & Le Loët, X. (2004). Cerivastatin-induced polymyalgia rheumatica–like illness. *Clinical Rheumatology 23*(2), 179. doi:10.1007/s10067-003-0772-8

Hancock, A. T., Mallen, C. D., Belcher, J., & Hider, S. L. (2012). Association between polymyalgia rheumatica and vascular disease: a systematic review. *Arthritis Care & Research, 64*(9), 1301–1305.

Helliwell, T. B., Hider, S. L., & Mullen, C. D. (2013). Polymyalgia rheumatica: diagnosis, prescribing, and monitoring in general practice. *British Journal of General Practice, 63*(10), e361–e366.

Hernández-Rodríguez, J., Cid, M. C., Lopez-Soto, A., Espigol-Frigole, G., & Bosch, X. (2009). Treatment of polymyalgia rheumatica: a systematic review. *Archives of Internal Medicine, 169*(20), 1838–1850.

Kermani, T. Z., & Warrington, K. J. (2011). Lower extremity vasculitis in polymyalgia rheumatica and giant cell arteritis. *Current Opinion in Rheumatology, 23*(1), 38–42.

Kremers, H. M., Reinalda, M. S., Crowson, C. S., Zinsmeister, A. R., Hunder, G. G., & Gabriel, S. E. (2005). Relapse in a population based cohort of patients with polymyalgia rheumatica. *Journal of Rheumatology, 32*(1), 65.

Muller, S., Hider, S., Belcher, J., Helliwell, T., & Mallen, C. (2013). Is cancer associated with polymyalgia rheumatica? A cohort study in the General Practice Research Database. *Annual of the Rheumatic Diseases.* doi: 10.1136/annrheumdis-2013-203465

Paget, S. A., & Spiera, R. F. (2006). Polymyalgia rheumatica. In S. Bartlett (Ed.), *Clinical care in the rheumatic diseases* (5th ed., pp. 153–156). Atlanta, GA: Association of Rheumatology Health Professions.

Parikh, M., Miller, N. R., Lee, A. G., Savino, P. J., Vacarezza, M. N., Cornblath, W., . . . Wall, M. (2006). Prevalence of a normal C-reactive protein with an elevated erythrocyte sedimentation rate in biopsy-proven giant cell arteritis. *Ophthalmology, 113*(10), 1842–1845.

Pease, C. T., Haugeberg, G., Morgan, A. W., Montague, B., Hensor, E. M., & Bhakta, B. B. (2005). Diagnosing late onset rheumatoid arthritis, polymyalgia rheumatica and temporal arteritis in patients presenting with polymyalgic symptoms. A prospective longterm evaluation. *Journal of Rheumatology, 32*(6), 1043–1046.

Salvarani, C., Cantini, F., Boiardi, L., & Hunder, G. G. (2002). Polymyalgia rheumatica and giant-cell arteritis. *New England Journal of Medicine, 347*(4), 261–271.

Salvarani, C., Cantini, F., & Hunder, G. G. (2008). Polymyalgia rheumatica and giant-cell arteritis. *Lancet, 372*(9634), 234–245. doi:10.1016/S0140-6736(08)61077-6

Snyder, S. (1991). Metoprolol-induced polymyalgic like syndrome. *Annals of Internal Medicine, 114*(1), 96–97.

Soubrier, M., Dobost, J.-J., & Ristori, J.-M. (2006). Polymyalgia rheumatica: diagnosis and treatment. *Joint Bone Spine, 73*(6), 599–605. doi:10.1016/j.jbsin.2006.09.005

Unwin, B., Williams, C. M., & Gilliland, W. (2006). Polymyalgia rheumatica and giant cell arteritis. *American Family Physician, 74*(9), 1547–1554.

Rheumatoid Arthritis

Aletaha, D., Neogi, T., Silman, A. J., Funovits, J., Felson, D. T., Bingham, C. O., III, . . . Hawker, G. (2010). 2010 Rheumatoid arthritis classification criteria: an American College of Rheumatology/European League Against Rheumatism collaborative initiative. *Arthritis and Rheumatism, 62*(9), 2569–2581.

Bang, S. Y., Lee, K. H., Cho, . S. K., Lee, H. S., Lee, K. W., & Bae, S. C. (2010). Smoking increases rheumatoid arthritis susceptibility in individuals carrying the HLA-DRB1 shared epitope, regardless of rheumatoid factor or anti-cyclic citrullinated peptide antibody status. *Arthritis and Rheumatism, 62*(2), 369–377.

Doran, M. F., Pond, G. R., Crowson, C. S., O'Fallon, W. M., & Gabriel, S. E. (2002). Trends in incidence and mortality in rheumatoid arthritis in Rochester, Minnesota, over a forty-year period. *Arthritis and Rheumatism, 46*(3), 625–631.

Eversden, L., Maggs, F., Nightingale, P., & Jobanputra, P. (2007). A pragmatic randomised controlled trial of hydrotherapy and land exercises on overall well being and quality of life in rheumatoid arthritis. *BMC Musculoskeletal Disorders, 8*, (23). doi:10.1186/1471-2474-8-23

Hall, J., Skevington, S. M., Maddison, P. J., & Chapman, K. (1996). A randomized and controlled trial of hydrotherapy in rheumatoid arthritis. *Arthritis Care Research, 9*(3), 206–215.

Koller, M. D., Aletaha, D., Funovits, J., Pangan, A., Baker, D., & Smolen, J. S. (2009). Response of elderly patients with rheumatoid arthritis to methotrexate or TNF inhibitors compared with younger patients. *Rheumatology, 48*(12), 1575–1580.

LeBlond, R. F., Brown, D. D., & DeGowin, R. L. (2009). *DeGowin's diagnostic examination* (9th ed.). New York City, NY: McGraw-Hill Medical.

Lee, A. L., Beck, C. E., & Hall, M. (2008). Rheumatoid factor and anti-CCP autoantibodies in rheumatoid arthritis: a review. *Clinical Laboratory Science, 21*(1), 15.

MacGregor, A. J., & Silman, A. J. (2008). Classification and epidemiology: rheumatoid arthritis and other synovial disorders. In M. C. Hochberg, A. J. Silman, J. S. Smolen, M. E. Weinblatt, & M. H. Weisman (Eds.), *Rheumatology* (4th ed., vol. 1, pp. 755–761). Spain: Elsevier Limited.

Majithia, V., Peel, C., & Geraci, S. A. (2009). Rheumatoid arthritis in elderly patients. *Geriatrics, 64*(9), 22–28.

Manno, R. L., & Bingham, C. O. (2011). Rheumatoid arthritis in the older patient. *Clinical Geriatrics, 19*(6), 43–51.

Meenan, R. F., Mason, J. H., Anderson, J. J., Guccione, A. A., & Kazis, L. E. (1992). AIMS2. The content and properties of a revised and expanded Arthritis Impact Measurement Scales Health Status Questionnaire. *Arthritis and Rheumatism, 35*(1), 1–10.

Oliver, S. (2009). Understanding the needs of older people with rheumatoid arthritis: the role of the community nurse. *Nursing Older People, 21*(9), 30–37.

Olivieri, I., Pipitone, N., D'Angelo, S., Padula, A., & Salvarani, C. (2009). Late-onset rheumatoid arthritis and late-onset spondyloarthritis. *Clinical and Experimental Rheumatology, 27*(Suppl. 55), S139–S145.

Orozco, G., & Barton, A. (2010). Update on the genetic risk factors for rheumatoid arthritis. *Expert Review of Clinical Immunology, 6*(1), 61–75.

Palosuo, T., Tilvis, R., Strandberg, T., & Aho, K. (2003). Filaggrin related antibodies among the aged. *Annals of the Rheumatic Diseases, 62*(3): 261–263. doi:10.1136/ard.62.3.261

Singh, J. A., Beg, S., & Lopez-Olivo, M. A. (2011). Tocilizumab for rheumatoid arthritis: a Cochrane systematic review. *Journal of Rheumatology, 38*(1), 10–20. doi:10.3899/jrheum.100717

Villa-Blanco, J. I., & Calvo-Alén, J. (2009). Elderly onset rheumatoid arthritis: differential diagnosis and choice of first-line and subsequent therapy. *Drugs & Aging, 26*(9), 739–750.

Wasserman, A. (2011). Diagnosis and management of rheumatoid arthritis. *American Family Physician, 84*(11), 1245–1252.

chapter 13

Central and Peripheral Nervous System Disorders

Laurie Kennedy-Malone

ASSESSMENT

The neurological assessment of the older adult begins with assessment of mental status. The interview should begin with an assessment of level of consciousness, speech pattern, mood and affect, concentration ability, short-term memory, and orientation. This information can usually be obtained during the course of a standard interview. "The key to appreciating a memory impairment or subtle dementing illness is to perceive incongruities among the patient's appearance, dress, language or behavior" (Williams, 2009, p. 236). There are several short screening tools that can be administered to the patient to assess cognition:

- The Mini-Cog is a short dementia assessment that combines three-word recall with clock-drawing capability. Patients are given a total score reflecting accuracy in clock drawing and recollection of the given three words. A score of 0 to 2 is a positive screen for dementia (American Association of Neuroscience Nurses, 2009).
- The St. Louis University Mental Status Examination (SLUMS), a 12-item assessment, has been shown to detect mild neurocognitive disorders. A patient's level of high school is considered when interpreting the score. A score of 19 or below in any patient is indicative of dementia (Tariq, Tumosa, Chibnall, Perry, Mitchell, & Morely,

2006). If any questions regarding the mental status arise, family members may be asked for additional information to investigate the patient's cognitive abilities further.

- The Montreal Cognitive Assessment (MoCA Version 7.1) is a tool designed to measure the status of a patient's attention, concentration, executive function, memory, and orientation. It has been tested on patients with a variety of neurodegenerative conditions, as well as those with a history of substance abuse (Berstein, Lacritz, Barlow, Weiner, & DeFina, 2011). The score can be adjusted for patients with a lower level of education (Johns et al., 2010). A score of 26 or higher out of a possible score of 30 is considered normal cognition.

The focused interview for a neurological complaint should include asking about the following common signs and symptoms in older adults:

- Loss of consciousness or presyncope, including a full description of any episodes and their precipitating factors.
- Any episodes of seizures, "spells," shaking palsy, dizziness, weakness or paralysis, tremors, involuntary movements, pain, numbness, paresthesias, gait problems, or restlessness of the legs.
- Any speech or language disturbances or change in vision or hearing, including diplopia, ptosis, or tinnitus reported by the patient or family.

- Any mood swings, new onset of headaches, and change in level of awareness or reversal or alteration in judgment or memory.
- Pertinent family history of any acute neurological or neurodegenerative disease or unknown conditions with specific symptomatology.
- Information about previous occupations and hobbies that may have involved trauma or chemical exposure for each patient.
- All medications (including over-the-counter medications), diet, and sleep patterns.
- A careful assessment of social history, including any current or previous substance abuse.

The positive findings determined in the history of present illness and review of systems will guide the episodic neurological examination. A complete neurological examination, however, begins with testing of the cranial nerve function.

Cranial Nerve Function

CRANIAL NERVE I (OLFACTORY)

Make sure to test one nostril at a time using familiar scents. This sense may be lessened or absent because of nasal disease, head trauma, smoking, use of cocaine, or normal aging. It may also be congenitally absent.

Patients with hyposmia or anosmia are at risk for safety issues (rancid foods, inability to detect smoke, gas, or other noxious chemicals) and malnutrition (American Association of Neuroscience Nurses, 2009). A distorted sense of smell in both nostrils of familiar odors has been found in patients early on in the progression of neurodegenerative conditions such as Alzheimer's disease or Parkinsonism, whereas a unilateral, nonoccluded loss of smell can be indicative of frontal brain tumor (Williams, 2009).

CRANIAL NERVE II (OPTIC)

Funduscopic examination will reveal disc or small vessel abnormalities. Assess pupillary reactions to light and visual fields. Presbyopia, the loss of accommodation, is a normal aging change. Older adults experience difficulty with depth perception, and contrast sensitivity is reduced as one ages (American Association of Neuroscience Nurses, 2009).

CRANIAL NERVES III, IV, AND VI (OCULOMOTOR, TROCHLEAR, AND ABDUCENS)

These nerves may be examined together by testing extraocular movements and convergence. Inspect for ptosis. Generally, pupils are smaller in an older adult, a condition known as senile mitosis (Larner, 2006).

CRANIAL NERVE V (TRIGEMINAL)

The motor function of this nerve can be assessed by palpating the temporal and masseter muscles. If the patient has no teeth, this test may be difficult to interpret. The sensory function of this nerve should be tested with sharp and dull stimuli in all three branches: ophthalmic, maxillary, and mandibular. If any abnormalities are noted, light touch and temperature sensation should also be assessed. The corneal reflex should be assessed using a wisp of cotton. Patients who wear contact lenses may have diminished corneal reflexes. Older adults may naturally have decreased lacrimal secretions; certain medications, such as anticholinergics, may exacerbate this condition (American Association of Neuroscience Nurses, 2009).

CRANIAL NERVE VII (FACIAL)

Observe the patient's face at rest and continue to observe throughout the examination for any asymmetry. Motor function may be tested by asking the patient to smile, frown, raise both eyebrows, close eyes tightly and resist the examiner's attempts to open them, and puff out both cheeks. A peripheral injury to this nerve, such as Bell's palsy, may affect both the upper and the lower face, whereas a central lesion mainly affects the lower face.

CRANIAL NERVE VIII (ACOUSTIC)

Assess auditory acuity using the whisper test. If hearing loss is present, test for lateralization using the Weber test and for air versus bone conduction using the Rinne test. The ear canals should be checked for cerumen impaction, which is a leading cause of conductive hearing loss and could contribute to overall hearing loss. Presbycusis, a normal aging change, results in older adults losing the ability to hear at higher tones (Larner, 2006).

CRANIAL NERVES IX AND X (GLOSSOPHARYNGEAL AND VAGUS)

Observe the quality of the patient's voice. Hoarseness may indicate vocal cord paralysis; a nasal quality may indicate paralysis of the palate. Difficulty in swallowing could indicate palatal or pharyngeal weakness. Inspect movement of the palate and pharynx when the patient swallows. With a bilateral lesion of the nerve, the palate will fail to rise. With unilateral lesion, one side of the palate will fail to rise and will be pulled, along with the uvula, to the normal side. Test the gag reflex by stimulating the back of the throat on each side. Older adults experience a decrease in taste perception of saltiness, sweetness, sourness, and bitterness (American Association of Neuroscience Nurses, 2009)

CRANIAL NERVE XI (SPINAL ACCESSORY)

Observe for atrophy or fasciculations in the trapezius muscles. Test motor strength bilaterally with a shoulder shrug.

CRANIAL NERVE XII (HYPOGLOSSAL)

Inspect for fasciculations of the tongue at rest. Look for asymmetry of movement, atrophy, or deviation from midline. Atrophy or fasciculations suggest peripheral lesions. With unilateral lesions, the protruded tongue will deviate toward the affected side (LeBlond, Brown, & DeGowin, 2009).

Motor Function

Assessment of motor function should focus on inspection of body position and involuntary movements (tremors, tics, or fasciculations). Note that the incidence of benign essential tremor increases with aging. Inspect the patient's muscle bulk, comparing sizes and contours of muscles. Pay particular attention to the hands, shoulders, and thighs. Atrophy of the hand muscles may occur with normal aging. Muscular atrophy may also result from diseases of the peripheral nervous system, motor neuron disease, rheumatoid arthritis, muscle disuse, and malnutrition.

Motor assessment also includes inspection of muscle tone, best assessed by the patient's resistance to passive stretch. Inspect tone in all extremities during flexion and extension. Increased tone that is worst at extremes of the range is known as spasticity; resistance that persists throughout and in both directions is known as lead-pipe rigidity. Decreased resistance suggests peripheral nervous system disease, cerebellar disease, or the acute stage of spinal cord injury. In patients with Parkinson's disease, cogwheel rigidity, ratchet-like jerking movements, can be detected by the examiner on passive flexion and extension of the muscle.

Assess muscle strength against resistance in all major muscle groups and grade on a scale from 0 to 5, with 5 being active movement against full resistance. Test the biceps and triceps; grip strength; finger abductions; opposition of the thumb; trunk strength; flexion, extension, abduction, and adduction at the hip; flexion and extension at the knee; and dorsiflexion and plantarflexion of the foot during passive range-of-motion exercises. If you note weakness, assess strength against gravity alone or with gravity eliminated. Many clinicians make further distinctions by using plus or minus signs toward the stronger end of the scale (Williams, 2009).

It is critical to accurately assess the presentation of weakness in older adults because it is a common complaint. It is first important to determine if it is subjective weakness, which in actuality is found to be fatigue rather than the loss or alteration of normal strength. Patients, however, may experience both fatigue and true weakness. Differentiate between constant versus intermittent weakness, and establish the patterns of weakness:

■ Weak arm and leg (same side): hemiparesis or hemiplegia
■ Weak legs, normal arms: paraparesis
■ All four limbs weak: tetraparesis
■ One limb weak: monoparesis
■ Proximal muscle weakness (often from a myopathy)
■ Distal muscle weakness (often from a neuropathy)

Determining subjectively the patient's limitations in activities of daily living (ADLs) can further help the practitioner establish the severity of the weakness. Asking questions pertaining to function of the upper extremities (ability to lift one's arms over the head for grooming or dressing [proximal upper extremity weakness] versus the ability to use utensils or turn a door handle [distal upper extremity weakness]). For lower extremity, proximal weakness questions can be asked about the ability to climb stairs or cross one's legs.

An overall test of weakness and mobility is the Get Up and Go Test. It includes a number of tasks such as standing from a sitting position, walking, turning, stopping, and sitting down, all of which are important tasks needed for a person to be independently mobile, as well as to determine if the patient is having proximal weakness of the lower extremities (Williams, 2009).

Test coordination using rapid alternating movements of the hands, fingers, and feet and point-to-point movements. In some neurodegenerative conditions such as Parkinson's disease, movements may be slow and irregular with imprecise timing. The inability to perform repetitive movements in a rapid rhythmic method is called dysdiadochokinesia. Patients with appendicular ataxia may have difficulty with finger-to-nose testing. The examiner may note undershooting (hypometria) and overshooting (hypermetria) of a target (dysmetria) as well as the decomposition of a movement or the inability to complete a movement (LeBlond et al., 2009).

Gait function should be tested; assess tandem gait, walking on toes and heels, hopping in place, and shallow knee bends on each side. Romberg's test is to evaluate position sense and is performed with the patient's feet together and eyes closed for 20 to 30 seconds without support. Only minimal swaying should occur in patients with a normal finding. This test may be combined with the pronator drift test, in which the patient stands with eyes closed and both arms straight forward, palms up. Normally, this position may be held for 20 to 30 seconds. After instructing the patient to maintain this position, tap the patient's arms briskly downward. The arms should return smoothly to the horizontal position; a downward drift indicates muscle weakness. Allow extra time for the elderly patient to perform gait and coordination maneuvers (Williams, 2009).

Sensory Function

Assessment of sensory function helps to establish a lesion of the sensory cortex, the level of a spinal cord lesion, or the location of a peripheral lesion. Sensory function is tested using pain and temperature (spinothalamic tract), position and vibration (posterior column), and touch (posterior horn). When you locate an area of hypersensitivity or sensory loss, map out its boundaries in detail. Unilateral sensory loss suggests a lesion in the spinal cord or higher pathways; a symmetrical sensory loss suggests a neuropathy such as that experienced by persons with diabetes. Touch and vibratory sensations may diminish as a result of normal aging. Discriminative sensations test the ability of the sensory cortex to analyze and interpret stimuli. These techniques include stereognosis, number identification, two-point discrimination, point localization, and extinction.

Reflexes

During assessment of the reflexes, the patient should be relaxed, with limbs positioned symmetrically. Palpate the tendon to locate position, and make sure the tendon is slightly stretched. Strike the tendon briskly, and note the speed, force, and amplitude of response. Grade on a scale from 0 to 4 pluses, with the normal

response at 2 pluses. The older adult may have diminished or absent reflexes, usually affecting lower extremities before upper extremities.

If the response is asymmetrical, check the force and location of the strike. If the response is symmetrically diminished, the examiner may use reinforcement, in which isometric contraction of other muscles may increase reflex activity. Ask the patient to clench the teeth when testing upper extremities and to lock hands together and pull hands against each other when testing lower extremities.

Assess all reflexes: biceps (C5, C6); triceps (C6, C7); brachioradialis (C5, C6); patellar (L2, L3, L4); and ankle (S1). Assess the abdominal reflex by stroking each side of the abdomen both above (T8, T9, T10) and below (T10, T11, T12) the umbilicus. Evaluate the plantar response by stimulating the lateral aspect of the sole of the foot from the heel to the ball of the foot, curving medially across the ball. Look for flexion of the toes as a normal response. If dorsiflexion of the big toe and fanning of the other toes is noted, this constitutes a positive Babinski response, indicating a central nervous system (CNS) lesion. This response may also be noted in certain unconscious states (e.g., drug or alcohol intoxication, postictal state) (LeBlond et al., 2009).

Abnormal or Involuntary Movements

With the incidence of neurodegenerative conditions increasing with older adulthood, the practitioner needs to assess for any involuntary movements such as fasciculations, spasms, chorea, tremors, tics, and athetosis. Abnormal movements could also be a side effect of psychotropic medications that can cause extrapyramidal symptoms. Make sure to document completely all findings of the neurological examination, especially if additional diagnostic testing is indicated. The identification of subtle nervous system abnormalities has been shown to be associated with the risk of stroke and even death in healthy older adults (Inzitari et al., 2008). Nurse practitioners are in a position to distinguish pathology from age-related neurological changes.

BRAIN TUMOR

Signal symptoms: Headaches, with or without nausea and vomiting, seizures, changes in mental function or personality, motor or language deficits, visual problems.

Description: A brain tumor is a malignant or benign neoplasm of the brain or its supportive structures, which may arise from glial cells, blood vessels, connective tissue, meninges, pituitary, or pineal glands. The most common primary brain tumor in adults is neuroglial tumor, which accounts for more than 80% of primary brain tumors and which can derive from astrocytes, oligodendrocytes, or ependymal cells (Michaud, Schiff, & Batchelor, 2010; Wong & Wu, 2010). Other types of primary brain tumors include CNS lymphoma arising from lymphocytes, meningioma from the meninges, and ganglioma from the neurons (Behin, Hoang-Xuan, Carpentier, & Delattre, 2003; Michaud et al., 2010).

Etiology: The etiology of brain tumors is largely unknown. CNS tumors have been associated with rare genetic conditions, including Li-Fraumeni syndrome and neurofibromatosis 1 and 2 (Chandana, Movva, Arora, & Singh, 2008).

Occurrence: Malignant brain tumors are a rare cancer, but the incidence has been increasing over the past 50 years. According to the American Cancer Society, 2% of cancers are primary malignant brain tumors, which account for 18,000 new diagnoses annually and 12,000 deaths each year in the United States. The incidence of CNS lymphoma among adults is increasing (DeAngelis, 2001).

Age: The incidence of brain tumor peaks between ages 65 and 79 years (Chandana et al., 2008).

Gender: Brain tumors occur more commonly in males than females (7.6 versus 5.5 per 100,000 person-years) (Chandana et al., 2008).

Ethnicity: Caucasians and Hispanic Americans have a higher incidence compared to African Americans. Malignant brain tumors are less common among Asian and Native Americans (Chandana et al., 2008; Michaud et al., 2010).

Contributing factors: High-dose ionizing radiation is the only proven risk factor. The increase in CNS lymphoma is associated with the increase in immunocompromised persons. Prior radiation and chemotherapy are associated with brain tumors (Chandana et al., 2008; DeAngelis, 2001).

Signs and symptoms: Signs and symptoms are produced by tumor infiltration of nervous tissue, displacement of brain structures by tumor mass, or increased intracranial pressure (ICP) (DeAngelis, 2001; Wong & Wu, 2010).

Headaches occur more than one-half of the time and are often associated with seizures, visual disturbances, and persistent nausea with vomiting. In one study, 77% of patients described the headache as dull and tension type or bifrontal; the "classic" early morning headache of brain tumor is no longer believed to be common. Any headache that presents with a different pattern or is associated with prolonged nausea and vomiting, seizures, positional worsening, or neurological symptoms should be evaluated for brain tumor (Chandana et al., 2008). Generalized headache can be associated with increased ICP.

Memory loss, cognitive changes, and motor or language deficits are present in about 30% of brain tumor patients. Psychomotor function may slow in patients with primary brain tumors. Personality changes may be marked or subtle, including changes in mood, concentration, and intellectual functions (Chandana et al., 2008; Wong & Wu, 2010).

Partial motor, sensory, or grand mal seizures occur in slightly more than 30% of patients with brain tumors. New-onset focal seizures in individuals over 40 years old are suspicious for brain tumor until proved otherwise. Syncope due to an increase in ICP can mimic a seizure with a few tonic-clonic jerks. Papilledema may be present in increased ICP though less commonly in the elderly (Behin et al., 2003; Chandana et al., 2008; Wong & Wu, 2010).

Focal neurological changes are related to the area of the brain invaded by tumor. Frontal and parietal lobe tumors may cause changes in memory, behavior, and cognitive function. Memory, hearing, vision, and emotions are affected most often by temporal lobe tumors. Symptoms of temporal lobe tumors may mimic symptoms of affective or psychotic thought disorders. Visual changes can occur with occipital lobe tumors, in addition to speech, motor, and sensory changes for left-sided occipital masses and an inability to grasp abstract concepts for right-sided occipital masses. Lesions in the cerebellum affect balance and coordination. Pituitary tumors may present with the symptoms of hypothyroidism, hypercortisolism, diabetes insipidus, or visual changes (Chandana et al., 2008; Wong & Wu, 2010).

Diagnostic tests: The following tests are recommended for a person with suspected brain tumor:

- Complete blood count (CBC) to assess for anemia or infection.
- Thyroid-stimulating hormone (TSH) because hypothyroidism or hyperthyroidism can be associated with mental status changes or hypothyroidism with pituitary tumors.
- Venereal Disease Research Laboratory (VDRL) if neurosyphilis is a possibility.

- Chemistries to assess for electrolyte and chemical imbalances.
- Gadolinium-enhanced magnetic resonance imaging (MRI) of the brain is the preferred radiological examination for either brain tumor or suspected bleeding in the brain. Computed tomography (CT) scan with contrast enhancement is acceptable in special circumstances such as when a patient is uncooperative or when MRI is unavailable. Magnetic resonance spectroscopy (MRS) is used in specialized circumstances.
- Positron emission tomography is not used to diagnose tumors of the CNS but may have an ancillary role to examine for metastasis or after treatment.
- Electroencephalogram (EEG) is useful for evaluating possible seizure activity.
- Lumbar puncture should not be performed before MRI or CT scan because of the potential for fatal brain herniation to result. Lumbar puncture can yield pressure readings and cerebrospinal fluid for cytology, protein, glucose, and tumor markers.
- Testing blood for tumor markers, α-fetoprotein, or β–human chorionic gonadotropin is useful for the diagnosis of some brain tumors.
- Histological examination of a biopsy specimen of brain tissue may be preferred when feasible (Behin et al., 2003; Chandana et al., 2008; DeAngelis, 2001; Wong & Wu, 2010).

A careful history of symptoms is invaluable. Complete physical examination should include skin survey for stigmata of neurocutaneous syndromes or melanoma, lymph node examination, abdominal examination for hepatomegaly or splenomegaly, and rectal examination with guaiac stool testing. Breast and pelvic examinations in women and cardiopulmonary examination are recommended. The neurological evaluation should include a mental status evaluation, testing for cognitive deficits or memory loss, and assessment for personality changes. Family members may be able to provide clues about subtle personality changes. Ophthalmic examination is essential to assess for papilledema, although this may not be present in patients 55 years old and older. Test also for asymmetry of strength, sensation, visual fields, reflex activity, cranial nerve function, and radicular signs.

Differential diagnosis:
- *Stroke:* There is acute onset of headache with persistent focal neurological deficits for more than 24 hours. CT or MRI is diagnostic.
- *Aneurysm:* In acute rupture, there is a sudden intense headache, often with signs of meningeal irritation. MRI is preferred for diagnosis.
- *Arteriovenous malformation:* There is a chronic unilateral throbbing headache with no prodromal or associated symptoms. CT or MRI may be diagnostic.
- *Meningitis:* Headache usually is associated with fever and nuchal rigidity. Cerebrospinal fluid is obtained through a lumbar puncture for diagnosis.
- *Abscess:* This often is associated with fever or other signs of infection.
- *Syphilis:* Neurosyphilis may occur at any time during infection and up to 35 years later. Symptoms vary according to the area infected. Diagnosis is based on cerebrospinal fluid abnormalities and a reactive serological test for syphilis.
- *HIV:* Various neurological manifestations can be caused by the virus or opportunistic infections; the incidence of CNS lymphoma is increasing in these patients.
- *Subdural hematoma:* Persistent headache occurs after trauma, with poorly defined intellectual impairment. This may be ruled out by noncontrast CT or MRI.
- *Postconcussion syndrome:* A dull, constant headache occurs within 24 hours of trauma. The patient may complain of loss of concentration, giddiness, irritability, and anxiety.
- *Trauma:* History of injury to the head or neck is present.
- *Temporal arteritis:* This usually is characterized by a slow-onset headache that is worse at night, temporal in more than one-half of patients, often with jaw claudication and temporal artery tenderness as well as an elevated erythrocyte sedimentation rate (ESR).
- *Normal-pressure hydrocephalus:* This condition often presents with dementia, gait disturbances, and incontinence of bladder or bowel.
- *Multi-infarct dementia:* This may present with impaired cognition and symptoms of upper motor neuron disease in patients with a history of hypertension, atrial fibrillation, diabetes, carotid artery disease, or smoking.
- *Alzheimer's disease:* This presents with progressive dementia, memory disturbances, and behavioral changes, which are usually gradual over years.
- *Chemical poisoning:* History of exposure to chemicals, such as carbon monoxide, pesticides, or industrial materials, is present.

■ *Migraine:* Migraine is characterized by an often-unilateral headache with a pulsating quality, associated with nausea and vomiting, photophobia, or phonophobia; prodromal or aura symptoms may be present.

Treatment: Treatment of brain tumor includes surgery, radiation, chemotherapy, glucocorticoids, anticonvulsants, immunotherapy, and gene therapy (Behin et al., 2003).

Follow-up: Prognosis depends on the tumor type, patient age, functional neurological status, extent of resection, tumor location, and extent of metastasis at diagnosis. Recent data revealed that tumor grade, patient age, functional status, and complete surgical resection are the important prognostic factors for survival in people with malignant gliomas (Chandana et al., 2008). During the first year after treatment, the patient should have a focused history and physical examination, including a neurological and funduscopic examination every 3 months. MRI of the brain is recommended at the same intervals during the first year. The patient should be seen every 6 months during years 2 through 5, with yearly MRI. Patients receiving palliative care should be seen as necessary for pain and symptom control; hospice care is recommended for these patients.

Sequelae: Various neurological deficits, personality changes, seizure disorders, and chronic head pain can result from brain tumor. Paraplegia, hemiplegia, and quadriplegia are also consequences of brain tumor. Bradycardia, hypertension, and respiratory arrest can occur with increased ICP. Brain herniation is a life-threatening emergent complication.

Prevention/prophylaxis: Instruct patients to avoid radiation exposure.

Referral: Refer patients to a neurosurgeon, oncologist, radiation oncologist, and hospice, as appropriate.

Education: Genetic counseling is warranted in hereditary syndromes of brain tumor.

CLINICAL RECOMMENDATION	EVIDENCE RATING	REFERENCES
Gadolinium-enhanced MRI of the brain is the recommended diagnostic examination for suspected brain tumor.	A	Behin et al. (2003) Chandana et al. (2008) DeAngelis (2001) Wong & Wu (2010)
Patients with persistent headache that is different from their usual pattern with protracted nausea, vomiting, seizures, neurological symptoms, or positional worsening should be evaluated for brain tumor.	A	Chandana et al. (2008) Wong & Wu (2011)

A = consistent, good-quality, patient-oriented evidence; B = inconsistent or limited-quality, patient-oriented evidence; C = consensus, disease-oriented evidence, usual practice, expert opinion, or case series. For information about the SORT evidence rating system, go to www.aafp.org/afpsort.xml.

PARKINSON'S DISEASE

Signal symptoms: Tremor, rigidity, akinesia, impaired postural reflexes.

Description: Parkinson's disease (PD) is a chronic progressive neurodegenerative disorder resulting in the loss of dopamine-producing cells in the substantia nigra, located in the basal ganglia. The loss of the inhibitory neurotransmitter dopamine results in an imbalance with the neurotransmitter acetylcholine, which is primarily responsible for worsening symptoms leading to immobility. Symptoms of PD include resting tremor, rigidity, akinesia, bradykinesia, and impaired postural reflexes (resulting in postural instability) (Vernon, 2009). Subtle motor impairments may precede the development of overt clinical signs and symptoms by many years. The Braak hypothesis (Burke, Dauer, & Vonsattel, 2008) indicates six pathological stages of PD, but clinical symptoms do not appear until stage 4 to 6. This stage correlates with 60% to 80% loss of substantia nigra neurons and striatal dopamine. It is the second most common neurodegenerative disease. It affects motor and autonomic function, mood, and cognition.

Etiology: The cause of idiopathic primary PD is unknown. Genetic causes, viral causes, mitochondrial dysfunction, oxidative stress, and possibly chronic inflammation may cause PD, and these causes are being researched. Secondary PD (Parkinson syndrome) may be caused by head injury, toxins, heavy metals, herbicides, pesticides, dopamine-depleting drugs, encephalitis, hypoparathyroidism, and Wilson's disease. Parkinsonism (idiopathic PD is the most common form) includes known variants of PD, including multisystem atrophy (MSA), olivopontocerebellar atrophy (OPCA), Shy-Drager syndrome (SDS), progressive supranuclear palsy (PSP), corticobasal ganglionic degeneration (CBGD), Lewy body dementia (LBD), vascular parkinsonism, and neuroleptic-induced parkinsonism.

Occurrence: Approximately 1.6% of the population (100 to 150 cases in 100,000) is diagnosed with PD. In the United States, 60,000 people are diagnosed each year. A recent study suggests that this is an underestimate. The study identified a sharp rise in PD prevalence from 170 per 100,000 in 2000 to 256 per 100,000 in 2007 (Chillag-Talmor et al., 2011).

Age: Parkinson's disease is predominantly discovered in adults ages 55 to 69; however, 15% of newly diagnosed cases occur in persons younger than 49 years old.

Gender: The age-standardized prevalence and incidence of PD is greater in men than in women for all races, with a mean sex ratio of 155 men per 100 women (Wright-Willis, Evanoff, Lian, Criswell, & Racette, 2010).

Ethnicity: PD can be found in all cultures. The age- and gender-adjusted rates per 100,000 was highest among Hispanics (16.6), non-Hispanic whites (13.6), Asians (11.3), and blacks (10.2) (Van Den Eeden et al., 2003).

Contributing factors: Stress is not a direct causative factor in PD, but it may contribute to worsening symptoms. A major life stressor is often reported with diagnosis of PD (a move, retirement, loss of a job, a fire, or loss of a child). Carbon monoxide exposure, MPTP (an illicit drug), and a combination of genetic and environmental factors contribute to the diagnosis of PD. It is known that in certain families genetic factors do result in risk of developing PD.

Signs and symptoms: An initial clinical symptom of PD is a resting tremor, initially unilateral, that disappears with movement. Tremor also is noted in the lips, chin, and tongue. Patients may make a motion of the thumb and forefinger known as pill rolling. Although common, tremor is not present in every patient with PD. Occasionally, a symptom of internal tremor is reported but may not be observed. Rigidity, as shown by increased resistance to passive range of motion, is a classic sign and is known as cogwheel rigidity, which can be noted in the wrists and elbows. Patients experience a slowing of movements termed *bradykinesia*. Patients also report having difficulty initiating movement. Autonomic movements, such as the normal pattern of arm swinging during ambulation, are decreased. Symptoms have an asymmetrical onset.

Other associated manifestations include masked facial expression, decreased blinking, and delayed ability to show facial expressions. Patients also experience an associated softening of the voice, hypophonia, and drooling (due to less frequent swallowing). The size of the patient's handwriting often changes (micrographia). Flexed posture is common, with a bowed head, kyphotic back, and a trunk that leans forward. The gait may become faster with the body propelled forward (festination). Ask the patient about associated symptoms, such as shuffling gait, constipation, seborrhea, myalgia, impotence, and urinary incontinence. Depression is common and affects 30% to 40% of Parkinson's patients (Blonder & Slevin, 2011). Dementia may occur with or without associated Alzheimer's involvement in 20% to 30% of people with PD. Patients and family members may report mood swings, hallucinations, and insomnia. Executive function may be impaired (i.e., the ability to plan, organize, pay attention, remember details, strategize, and manage time and space). Nonmotor symptoms are common, including orthostasis, bladder and sexual dysfunction, sleep disorders, fatigue, and anorexia. Early in the diagnostic phase, the patient's cognitive status needs to be assessed given the prevalence of dementia developing in patients with PD. Assess the patient's mood as well.

The neurological examination will reveal most PD symptoms, and noting the patient's movement, coordination, and gait is crucial. Note any differences in speed in alternating simultaneous pronation and supination of the hands as well as in finger tapping. The pull test (Hunt & Sethi, 2006) is a physical test of postural stability (balance). The examiner stands behind the patient, informs the patient that he or she is going to be pulled with two hands on the shoulders backward, then the patient is pulled, and the recovery is documented. Note whether the postural reflexes are impaired or absent. Ask the patient to ambulate and observe gait, including arm swing, as well as tandem (heel-to-toe in a straight line) walking, turning abruptly, and walking on toes. Observe stature for kyphosis and forward bending of the head. Smell is commonly impaired (hyposmia) early in PD; therefore, evaluating cranial nerve I (olfactory nerve) could be useful (Ponsen, Stoffers, Wolters, Booij, & Berendse, 2010). Check the patient's ocular movements; impairment of upward or downward gaze is common in progressive supranuclear palsy but not in PD. Examine the patient's upper and lower extremities. Test for range of motion and strength, noting any cogwheel rigidity. Strength generally does not deteriorate despite the rigidity. Tendon reflexes are almost always normal. To test for tremor, have the patient rest the arms on the legs while seated. Note the frequency and amplitude of the tremor. Hypotension is common in patients with PD. An orthostatic blood pressure check with the patient lying, sitting, and standing is recommended at each visit (Sanchez-Ferro, Benito-Leon, & Gomez-Esteban, 2013). The presence of two cardinal signs—bradykinesia and resting tremor, rigidity, or postural instability—is essential to establishing the diagnosis of PD.

Diagnostic tests: Parkinson's disease is established by history and physical examination, including the neurological examination (Haerer, 1992). There is a growing interest in neuroprotection to slow disease progression, and there are developing technologies that may detect PD in first-degree relatives earlier. These patients may benefit from discoveries of effective neuroprotective therapies, including antioxidants and exercise. Histological markers are not widely used to establish the diagnosis of PD. A simple blood test detecting phosphorylated alpha-synuclein, which is common is people with PD, has been discovered, but it is not yet widely available. A DaTSCAN (ioflupane [^{123}I] injection, also known as phenyltropane) can indicate the presence of PD and is reimbursed by Medicare. An MRI may be ordered to rule out suspected brain lesions or abnormalities such as normal-pressure hydrocephalus.

Differential diagnosis: Olfactory dysfunction, rapid eye movement (REM) sleep behavior disorder, autonomic dysfunction (constipation), and depression are strongly linked to PD.

- *Drug-induced parkinsonism:* This is confirmed by withdrawal of suspected medication such as neuroleptics and metoclopramide.
- *Cortical basal ganglionic degeneration:* This is distinguished by unilateral coarse tremor, ideomotor ataxia, limb dystonia, and lack of response to levodopa.
- *Essential (benign familial) tremor:* Tremor is an action tremor 6 to 8 Hz compared with PD tremor, which is 3 to 6 Hz.
- *Huntington's disease:* This disorder is genetic in origin and characterized by chorea, clumsiness, and cognitive decline.
- *Shy-Drager syndrome:* This syndrome is distinguished by early and prominent autonomic nervous system dysfunction and poor response to dopamine.
- *Progressive supranuclear palsy:* Supranuclear gaze abnormality, facial spasticity, and axial rigidity are present; tremor is usually absent.
- *Creutzfeldt-Jakob disease:* This is a rapidly progressive syndrome of mental deterioration, lead-pipe rigidity, myoclonus, aphasia, apraxia, and hallucinations.
- *Normal-pressure hydrocephalus:* Gait apraxia, urinary incontinence, and dementia are present.
- *Striatal nigra degeneration:* Autonomic dysfunction and dystonia are present.
- *Olivopontocerebellar atrophy:* This condition is distinguished by inherited parkinsonism, progressive ataxia, dementia, difficulty with balance, and dysarthria.
- *Multisystem atrophy:* This includes olivopontocerebellar atrophy, striatal nigral degeneration, and Shy-Drager syndrome.

Treatment: Drug therapy focuses on correcting the imbalance of dopamine and acetylcholine.

- Patients with mild disease and no interference with ADLs may not require treatment.
- With tremors and rigidity causing impairment of the patient's ability to perform ADLs and a disability level that is mild-to-moderate, treatment may include amantadine, which is thought to augment dopamine release from presynaptic nerve terminals or to inhibit dopamine reuptake. Initial dose is usually 100 mg with breakfast. In 5 to 7 days, add amantadine 100 mg with lunch, then increase daily dose to 300 mg.

- Supplements are not prescribed but often used as self-treatment for PD symptoms, including co-enzyme Q10 (ubiquinone), vitamins D and E, fava beans, and S-adenosylmethionine (SAMe).
- Always start low and slow with all medications. Asses for and treat depression early because it is common in PD and can contribute to worsening of symptoms.
- Patients with disability require carbidopa and levodopa to replenish the depleted dopamine in the brain by increasing the dopamine precursor levodopa to stimulate dopamine receptors. Carbidopa and levodopa can be started using 25/100 (carbidopa 25 mg, levodopa 100 mg, Sinemet), 2 tablets once a day. The dosage can be increased by 2 tablets every 3 to 5 days until the total daily dose is 2 tablets of Sinemet 25/100 3 times a day.
- Dopamine agonists include ropinirole (Requip) 0.25 mg 3 times a day and pramipexole (Permax) 0.125 mg 3 times a day.
- Give the catechol-O-methyltransferase inhibitor (COMT) entacapone (Comtan) 200 mg with each dose of levodopa or 1600 mg daily. Blocking the 3-O-methylation of levodopa prolongs the action of the levodopa dose; thus this inhibitor allows a larger amount of levodopa to reach the brain. Tolcapone (Tasmar) 100 mg 3 times daily can cause fulminant liver failure (check liver function); unless it has been most effective (given with levodopa) within 3 weeks, it may be best to try another COMT inhibitor or Stalevo. Stalevo is a combination of carbidopa, levodopa, and entacapone. Stalevo dosages reflect the amount of levodopa (50, 75, 100, 125, 150, and 200) in each pill combined with carbidopa and Comtan 200 mg.
- When the dosage of levodopa reaches 600 to 1000 mg (1 g) per day, an adjunct medication is recommended. Large doses of levodopa over time can contribute to the on-off phenomenon and abnormal involuntary movements (AIMs). The agonists may be used alone or to extend the usefulness of levodopa. Taking medication on a consistent schedule lowers the likelihood of AIMs.
- Selegiline (Deprenyl, Eldepryl), a monoamine oxidase–B inhibitor, inhibits the enzyme responsible for inactivating dopamine. Adding selegiline 5 mg/day (increasing to 10 mg/day within 1 week) can improve the wearing-off effect of levodopa (doses to be given before lunch). Rasagiline (Azilect) is a monoamine oxidase–B inhibitor that can be used alone or with Sinemet. It is recommended once a day and is available in 0.5 mg or 1 mg doses. "The advantage of agonist therapy is the reduction in the prevalence of motor fluctuations" (Smith, Wichmann, Factor, & DeLong, 2011).
- Apomorphine (Apokyn) and carbidopa/levodopa (Parcopa) are "rescue" medications, which means they are used when a person "freezes," becoming unable to move. Apokyn is a subcutaneous injectable (2 to 4 mg), and Parcopa is an immediate-release formulation that dissolves on the tongue. Doses start with 25/100 and are also available in carbidopa/levodopa ratios 10/100 and 25/250.

Deep brain stimulation (DBS) has been approved for treatment of Parkinson's symptoms in the United States. Stimulation of the thalamus is used for tremor-predominant Parkinson's disease, and stimulation of the globus pallidum and subthalamic nucleus is used for bradykinesia, akinesia, dyskinesia, and rigidity. (DBS is not appropriate for those with profound depression and dementia.)

Treatment must include exercise. Exercise activity promotes neuroplasticity. Neuroplasticity is the brain's ability to reorganize and repair throughout a lifetime. All sustained enriched activity exerts an acute and sustained effect on neuroplasticity.

Follow-up: Ask the patient if any medication seems to be wearing off or if the patient has had any falls, because medication and surgery do not improve balance, and falls are associated with disease progression. Ask about sleep disturbances and constipation because they are linked to PD, increase stress, and compromise quality of life. Depression is common in Parkinson's patients, adversely affecting quality of life, and must be treated aggressively.

Sequelae: Parkinson's disease results in chronic and progressive immobility. As the disease advances, the patient is at risk of injury from falls due to postural instability. The hazards of immobility (Olson, Johnson, & Thompson, 1990) can prove deadly, including megacolon from constipation, aspiration pneumonia, pulmonary embolism, decreased appetite from inactivity (anemia), urinary tract infections, and sepsis from disruption in skin integrity. With medical therapies, surgery, and consistent exercise, a patient with PD can have a normal life expectancy.

Prevention/prophylaxis: No preventive measures exist for idiopathic PD, but exercise can promote neuroplasticity and is safe (Petzinger et al., 2010).

Referral: Refer to a neurologist patients with unusual presentation or bothersome complications and patients who do not respond to the initial medication regimen. Patients benefit from a physiatrist who can recommend therapy to address axial rigidity and postural instability as well as adaptive equipment (rolling walker). Home health-care nurses have techniques to enhance independence while maintaining a safe environment. Refer patients with voice changes or difficulty swallowing to a speech pathologist.

Education: Provide patients and family members with written information about PD, including information about local support groups. Contact the National Institute of Neurological Disorders and Stroke for educational resources (www.ninds.nih.gov/disorders/Parkinsons_disease/parkinsons_disease.htm). For care of patients with PD, contact the Beth Israel Medical Center Parkinson and Movement Disorders Center, New York City (212-844-8482).

CLINICAL RECOMMENDATION	EVIDENCE RATING	REFERENCES
All hyposmic individuals developing Parkinson's disease had an abnormal baseline DaTSCAN, demonstrating the value of olfactory testing as a preclinical marker in this neurodegenerative disease.	A	Ponsen et al. (2010)
Depression affects 30%–40% of patients with Parkinson's disease.	A	Blonder & Slevin (2011)
Regular participation in exercise has been shown to promote neuroplasticity in patients with Parkinson's disease.	A	Petzinger et al. (2010)
The pull test is used to measure postural instability in Parkinson's disease.	A	Hunt & Sethi (2006)

A = consistent, good-quality, patient-oriented evidence; B = inconsistent or limited-quality, patient-oriented evidence; C = consensus, disease-oriented evidence, usual practice, expert opinion, or case series. For information about the SORT evidence rating system, go to www.aafp.org/afpsort.xml.

PERIPHERAL NEUROPATHY

Signal symptoms: Paresthesia, allodynia, sensory ataxia, autonomic dysfunction, distal symmetrical sensorimotor dysfunction.

Description: Peripheral neuropathy is a syndrome commonly used to describe disorders of the peripheral nerves involving the dorsal, ventral spinal nerve roots, dorsal root ganglia, brachial, lumbosacral plexus, cranial nerves, sensory, motor, autonomic, or mixed nerves, producing variable signs and symptoms (Shy, 2007). The pathology and severity of the disease vary (Cacchione, 2010; Zaida & Alexander, 2001). Normal function of the nerve depends on intact axon and its myelin sheath. Damage by mechanical insult or nerve infarction to the axon distal to the site of injury results in degeneration of the axon and myelin sheath distally. This pathological response is called wallerian degeneration (Andreoli, Carpenter, Griggs, & Benjamin, 2007; Harati & Bosh, 2008). Nerve unexcitability distally will take approximately 3 to 9 days to occur after the insult. Within the 3 to 9 days, motor response amplitude decreases between the third and fifth day and sensory loss occurs around the second or third day after injury (Harati & Bosch, 2008).

The proximal axon survives and has the potential for regeneration depending on the quality of the Schwann cells and myelin sheath. Denervation changes are observed on electromyogram studies in the affected muscle 10 to 14 days after injury. These changes are usually length dependent, occurring in smaller nerve fibers (Harati & Bosch, 2008). When there is damage to the axon by toxins or by metabolic or hereditary diseases, degeneration of the axon's myelin sheath occurs in a distal-to-proximal gradient pattern. This pathological process is called axonal degeneration or a dying-back syndrome or length-dependent neuropathy (meaning there is breakdown of the myelin sheath of the axon beginning distally at the nerve fiber and progressing to the nerve cell body) (Andreoli et al., 2007; Harati & Bosch, 2008). Early signs and symptoms will be ankle areflexia and weakness, initially involving the intrinsic muscles of the feet, the extensors of the toes, and the dorsiflexors at the ankle. Motor signs include distal changes involving large sensory fibers with that of vibratory sensory loss at the toes (Harati & Bosch, 2008). With progression of time, this loss may proceed to the legs and arms, resulting in a stocking and glove pattern. Recovery from axonal degeneration may range from 2 to 3 years (Andreoli et al., 2007). Injury to the myelin sheath, Schwann cell, with sparing of the axon, results in a pathological response called segmental demyelination by nerve. This response is commonly seen in autoimmune or inflammatory neuropathies. Nerve conduction is blocked, resulting in functional deficits similar to those seen in axonal degeneration. Recovery from injury is rapid. Clinically, there will be muscle weakness, generalized loss of reflexes, and disproportionately mild muscle atrophy. Sensation to temperature and pin prick is intact. Contributing causes to this pathological process may be related to toxins, nerve compression, or mechanical insult. Often this condition coexists with axonal degeneration. On electromyogram studies, demyelination is present when both motor and sensory nerve velocities to the lower extremities are decreased to less than 70% of normal (Andreoli et al., 2007; Harati & Bosch, 2008). Autonomic dysfunction (dizziness or syncope, anhidrosis, bladder atony, constipation, dry eyes, dry mouth, erectile dysfunction, pupillary abnormalities, paroxysmal hypertension, tachycardia, bradycardia, diarrhea, hyperhidrosis) may also be seen in generalized polyneuropathy such as diabetic polyneuropathy or Guillain-Barré syndrome (England & Asbury, 2004). Peripheral neuropathy, especially polyneuropathy, is one of the most common neurological disorders encountered by primary care providers (Cacchione, 2010; Zaida & Alexander, 2001). Peripheral neuropathy is prevalent in the older adult population but is often underdiagnosed because some of the normal changes occurring with aging are similar to the pathological changes seen in peripheral neuropathy. These changes are a modest decline in sensory touch, two-point discrimination, vibratory sense, and a slow withdrawal response from painful stimuli (Cacchione, 2010) In the absence of disease, these changes are minor and present no negative impact on function (Mold, Vesely, Keyl, Schenk, & Roberts, 2004). Polyneuropathy is commonly encountered in the clinical setting. Chronic idiopathic axonal polyneuropathy is well recognized in the elderly (Lor et al., 2009). Vasculitic polyneuropathy is the most common disabling neuropathy found in the elderly, followed by paraneoplasia, diabetes, and idiopathic axonal neuropathy (Kararizou, Davaki, Karandreas, Davou, & Vassilopoulos, 2006).

Etiology: Peripheral neuropathy results from various causes affecting the sensory, motor, or autonomic fibers, contributing to a diverse host of signs and symptoms that may be acute (sudden onset) as seen with trauma or nerve infarction; subacute (existing over a period of months) as seen when the causative agent may be related to drugs, toxins, or metabolic diseases; or insidious/chronic (ongoing for years) as occurring with chronic inflammatory demyelinating neuropathies (Lor et al., 2009; Poncelet, 1998). Some symptoms may relapse and remit over the years (Lor et al., 2009). Common causes of peripheral neuropathy include nutritional deficiencies, metabolic diseases, inflammatory processes, hereditary processes, autoimmune diseases, toxins and drugs, and malignancies; approximately one-third of all peripheral neuropathy causes remain unknown (Azhary, Farooq, Bhanushali, Majid, & Kassab, 2010; Lor et al., 2009; Mold et al., 2004; Zaida & Alexander, 2001).

Occurrence: The prevalence of peripheral neuropathy increases with age for those without predisposing disease, and for those with predisposing diseases, they are twice as likely to have peripheral neuropathy (Mold et al., 2004). Older adults are at high risk for peripheral neuropathy due to the many diseases that contribute to this disorder, with the incidence increasing with age (Backon & Glanzman, 2003; Mold et al., 2004). Vasculitic polyneuropathy is the most common disabling neuropathy in the elderly followed by paraneoplasia, diabetic, and idiopathic axonal neuropathy (Kararizou et al., 2006). A majority of persons with symmetrical distal sensory neuropathy (loss of tendon reflexes, vibratory sensation, fine touch, position sense in the ankles and feet, sweating, and circulatory instability in the feet) have idiopathic peripheral neuropathy or associated peripheral neuropathy occurring after age 75 (England & Asbury, 2004; Mold, Lawler, & Roberts, 2008). The overall prevalence of peripheral neuropathy is approximately 2400 (2.4%) per 100,000 population in individuals 55 and older with the prevalence increasing to approximately 8000 (8%) per 100,000. Peripheral neuropathy exists in approximately 70% of persons with chronic diseases (Kararizou et al., 2006). Diffuse symmetrical distal sensorimotor neuropathy is the most common manifestation in diabetic peripheral neuropathy and is thought to affect about 34% of persons with diabetes (Marchettini, Teloni, Formaglio, & Lacerenza, 2004).

Age: The incidence of peripheral neuropathy increases with age as the incidence of comorbidities/chronic diseases increases, with the exception of traumatic nerve injuries. Most peripheral neuropathy occurs after age 55 (Kararizou et al., 2006; Mold et al., 2008).

Gender: A diagnosis of peripheral neuropathy is not gender specific (Mold et al., 2004). However, it is interesting to note that a study of 894 participants in the Women's Health and Aging survey revealed that 58% of women had evidence of neuropathy by age 65 (Cacchione, 2010).

Ethnicity: Although there is no specific ethnic group with a high prevalence rate for developing peripheral neuropathy, studies have indicated that persons living in Southeast Asia, India, Africa, Central America, and South America have a higher prevalence of leprosy neuritis. In developing countries, there is high general increase in prevalence of peripheral neuropathy due to the rising diagnosis of diabetes mellitus (England & Asbury, 2004).

Contributing factors: Predisposing factors of peripheral neuropathy are multiple (Zaida & Alexander, 2001). Peripheral neuropathy is more likely to develop in patients with diabetes mellitus, with poor blood glucose control causing blood vessel damage. Persons having cardiovascular disease or hypertension are at risk for idiopathic neuropathy (due possibly to damage to blood vessels and poor circulation depriving the nerves of oxygen) (Mold et al., 2004). Peripheral neuropathy is commonly associated with HIV and AIDS.

Polyneuropathy develops during the late stages of HIV infection. Alcoholism is a leading cause of neuropathy. Symptoms of numbness, abnormal or painful sensations, and muscular weakness are caused by the effect of alcohol on nerve tissue. Habitual heavy drinking or history of alcoholism increases the risk for peripheral neuropathy. Autoimmune diseases, such as Guillain-Barré syndrome, rheumatoid arthritis, and lupus, are associated with peripheral neuropathy. Exposures to toxic chemicals or drugs can cause neuropathy. Toxic chemicals include industrial agents such as solvents; heavy metals such as lead, arsenic, and mercury; pesticides; and nitrous oxide. Some drugs, such as amiodarone, hydralazine, vincristine, cisplatin, metronidazole, nitrofurantoin, thalidomide, isoniazid, emetine, chlorobutanol, sulfonamides, dapsone, phenytoin, disulfiram, and barbital, can cause neuropathy. Nutritional deficiencies such as thiamine and vitamin B_{12} deficiency can cause polyneuropathy (Chaudhry, 2008; Shy, 2007; Zaida & Alexander 2001).

Signs and symptoms:

- Review with patients if they have a history of exposure to toxins/chemicals, use of alcohol or illicit drugs, and use of any over-the-counter medications such as herbal products.
- Determine if there is a positive family history of foot disorders such as high arches, hammer toes, gait abnormalities, or muscle dystrophy that would suggest a hereditary neuropathy (Harati & Borsch, 2008; Poncelet, 1998).
- Conduct a nutritional assessment to note if there is a nutritional deficiency indicating a possible anemia.
- Inquire if the patient has a military background for possible exposure to neuropathic agents (Mold et al., 2004).
- Conduct a review of systems, inquiring about the overall functional ability to perform ADLs, clumsiness, any falls or injuries, gait disturbances, difficulty with eating, nausea, vomiting, anorexia, problems with bowel and bladder functions (e.g., constipation, diarrhea, incontinence), any sensory changes such as numbness, dysesthesias, pain, any incidence of burn injuries due to decreased ability to detect temperature changes/hot or cold, and skin or hair changes (Chaudhry, 2008; England & Asbury, 2004; Harati & Bosh, 2008; Shy, 2007).
- Ask about any recent viral or other infectious diseases, recent vaccinations, or new medications (England & Asbury, 2004).

- Asking the following questions will help guide in physical examination and diagnostic studies:
  - When was the onset?
  - Is it acute, subacute, or chronic?
  - What is the disease progression? (Rapid onset, slow progression, relapses?)
  - What is the distribution pattern? (Generalized, symmetrical, or asymmetrical?)
  - Is the neuropathy sensory, motor, or both?
  - Does the neuropathy involve large fibers, small fibers, or both?
  - Are autonomic nerve fibers involved? Is the neuropathy more demyelinating, axonal, or mixed? (Azhary et al., 2010; Pourmand, 2002.)

The earliest symptoms patients complain of are sensory related: numbness, burning, paresthesia, or dysesthesia in the feet or toes. These symptoms are usually distal and symmetrical. Symptomatic sensory symptoms (defined as bilateral neuropathic symptoms, loss of pinprick sensation, proprioception loss) include complaint of postural instability, dizziness, and distal weakness (especially in patients with diabetes mellitus). Restless legs syndrome and nonspecific leg pain are also a problem, affecting restful sleep and quality of life (Lor et al., 2009).

The physical examination of patients who present with neurological symptoms of distal paresthesias, pain, and/or weakness needs to focus on differentiating between peripheral neuropathy and a lesion in the CNS (Azhary et al., 2010). One positive finding to note in evaluation of vital signs would be the presence of orthostatic hypotension without a compensated pulse rate (suggesting autonomic dysfunction involving small nerve fibers) (Chaudhry, 2008; Pourmand, 2002; Zaida & Alexander 2001). Overall, observe for any of the following:

- Look for hair loss near the affected areas involved with trophic changes (pes cavus) suggests a long-standing chronic neuropathy.
- Observe nail bed for Mees' lines (white transverse nail band), commonly seen with arsenic and thallium toxins.
- Look for telangiectasia on the abdomen and buttocks, suggestive of Fabry's disease, and purpuric lesions on the leg, suggestive of cryoglobulinemia. A bluish discoloration of the feet, cool and erythematous in a stocking glove distribution pattern, is due to sensory loss in small and larger fiber nerves due to damage.
- Note if the patient has any foot deformities. Observe for claw toes, calluses, or depressed metatarsal head, which suggest intrinsic muscle atrophy and peripheral neuropathy.
- Observe for any vertebral skeletal changes such as kyphoscoliosis. Evaluation of gait and balance is important; observe for any balance or footdrop problems. Patients with peripheral neuropathy have difficulty with position sense and standing on one foot for more than 3 seconds (Chaudhry, 2008; Zaida & Alexander, 2001).

Palpation along a nerve may reveal hypertrophy of a single nerve, suggesting a neoplastic process such as a neurofibroma, schwannoma, or malignant nerve neuropathy or leprosy and amyloid neuropathy (Poncelet, 1998). Generalized multifocal nerve hypertrophy is found in disorders of leprosy, neurofibroma, and Charcot-Marie-Tooth disease (Zaida & Alexander, 2001). With inspection of the head, alopecia of the scalp may be a sign of thallium poisoning (tightly curled hair suggestive of axonal type neuropathy). Evaluation of cranial nerves V, VII, IX, X, and XII may reveal a subtle bilateral weakness, proximal or distal symmetrical or asymmetrical, which cannot be detected by observation (Poncelet, 1998). A funduscopic examination may reveal optic pallor, which can be present in leukodystrophies and vitamin B deficiency (Poncelet, 1998).

Check muscle tone and muscle strength, observing for weakness and atrophy of distal muscles, which are suggestive of neuropathy. Muscle atrophy is a prominent finding, occurring in the lower extremities in the tibialis anterior muscle and the upper extremities in the intrinsic hand muscle (front dorsal interossesus). Tone may be normal or decreased (Chaudhry, 2008; England & Asbury, 2004; Harati & Bosch 2008; Zaida & Alexander, 2001). Vibratory sensory impairment may also be present. The inability to feel the 5.07 Semmes-Weinstein monofilament on at least one point of the plantar service of the foot and on vibration perception threshold >25 V suggests the presence of peripheral neuropathy (Kanji, Anglin, Hunt, & Panju, 2010)Tuttle, Sinacore, Cade, & Walle, 2007). Vibratory and proprioception impairment are usually related to large fiber neuropathies, whereas pain and temperature abnormalities are related to small nerve fiber neuropathies. Sensory impairment as it relates to touch can be due to both small and large fiber neuropathies (Poncelet, 1998). Bilateral absence of the heel jerk is indicative of demyelinating peripheral neuropathy (Mold et al., 2004).

Some patients may present with weakness in the feet and distal legs. As the disease progresses in a centripetal fashion, sensory loss and dysesthesia radiate upward toward the legs, causing decreased ankle jerks and weakness of the foot and toe with dorsiflexion. As muscle weakness progresses, patients may experience difficulty walking on the heels but plantar flexion remains strong, resulting in the patients walking on the toes (Azhary et al., 2010). As sensory deficits proceed upward toward the shin, numbness or dysesthesia may occur at the fingertips. Around this time, there is significant gait instability due to extensor muscle weakness and loss of proprioception. When sensory loss progresses toward the mid thigh and forearm, the lower abdomen or umbilicus and manubrium may be involved. With severe neuropathies, there is hyporeflexia and difficulty in standing and ambulating. In advanced polyneuropathy, there is a stocking glove sensory loss (diffuse sensory loss in distal lower extremities and hands), distal muscle wasting and weakness, and absence of tendon reflexes (Azhary et al., 2010; England & Asbury, 2004; Harati & Bosch, 2008).

Combined with the history and examination, electrodiagnostic studies, and focused laboratory tests, an underlying cause can be identified in approximately 75% of neuropathies. Distal symmetrical polyneuropathy is the most common variety of neuropathy and tests of this disorder are not standardized (England et al., 2009).

Diagnostic tests: Although there is no consensus of standardized tests for peripheral neuropathy, all should have routine laboratory tests. These should include CBC, chemistry profile, TSH, ESR, serum B_{12} with methylmalonic acid with or without homocysteine, and serum protein electrophoresis (SPE). A chest x-ray should be ordered in elderly patients. Additional tests ordered should be based on initial test results (Azhary et al., 2010; England et al., 2009). Other diagnostic tests offering the highest yield of abnormalities include a urinalysis, heavy metal testing, fasting blood glucose, and hepatic and thyroid function tests (England et al., 2009; Zaida & Alexander, 2001). It is also important to remember that the history and physical examination and electromyogram study will guide the clinician in specific tests to order.

Electromyogram and nerve conduction studies are the most useful diagnostic tests for initial workup in evaluating patients with suspected peripheral neuropathy. These tests validate the presence of a neuropathy and specify what type of nerve fibers are involved (sensory, motor, or a combination) and help in establishing the differential diagnosis. It is important to keep in mind that nerve conduction studies may be normal in patients with small fiber neuropathy, and lower extremity sensory response may not be detected in normal geriatric patients.

Despite an extensive workup, at least 25% of patients with polyneuropathy will have an unknown etiology. When this occurs, a thorough assessment of the first-degree relatives will be beneficial in identifying an unrecognized disease process (England et al., 2009; Harati & Bosh, 2008; Pourmand, 2002; Shy, 2007).

Differential diagnosis:
- Diabetic polyneuropathy, type II
- Diabetic polyneuropathy, type I
- Alcoholic peripheral neuropathy
- Chronic progressive or relapsing polyneuropathy (symmetrical, acquired, metabolic/endocrine, paraneoplastic, nutritional, idiopathic)
- Congenital sensory neuropathy
- Polyneuropathy, drug induced
- Dejerine-Sottas
- Myelopathy
- Myasthenia gravis (neuromuscular disorders)
- Nerve entrapment
- Syringomyelia/dorsal column disorders (e.g., tabes dorsalis)
- Hysterical symptoms (Azhary et al., 2010; Poncelette, 1998)

Treatment: Treatment goals for peripheral neuropathy involve treating the identifiable underlying disease, improving function of the affected body part, and pain management. Treating the underlying cause first will help to reduce the severity of the neuropathy thereby improving function and quality of life. Lifestyle changes will be beneficial, especially if alcohol or nicotine use is involved. Pain (allodynia/hyperalgesia), one of the cardinal symptoms in peripheral neuropathy disorders, is the major focus of care. The goal of treating neuropathic pain should be improvement in functional status given the adverse effects neuropathic pain has on functioning older adults (Schmader et al., 2010). Neuropathic pain may be difficult to treat. Neuropathic pain typically does not respond to simple analgesia such as Tylenol, NSAIDs, or aspirin. Choices of pharmacological agents are tailored to each individual's case based on preexisting medical conditions for symptom management. Rarely is there complete relief of neuropathic pain; at best, pharmacological interventions may result in 30% to 50% reduction in pain intensity (Harati & Bosh, 2008).

There is no consensus on the most appropriate treatment. However, recommendations are proposed for the first-line, second-line, and third-line pharmacological treatment based on the level of evidence for the different treatment strategies (Vranken, 2009). First-line medications (level A) include tricyclic antidepressants (TCAs), selective serotonin-norepinephrine reuptake inhibitors (SSNRIs), calcium channel alpha-2-delta ligands (anticonvulsants gabapentin and pregabalin), and topical lidocaine patch 5%. The second-line medications include an opioid analgesic and tramadol; third-line medicines include antiepileptics, antidepressants, mexiletine, N-methyl-D-aspartate (NMDA) receptor antagonists, and topical capsaicin (Dworkin et al., 2007). Level A or level B clinical studies support the use of pregabalin and gabapentin, which are usually well tolerated with few drug interactions (Dworkin et al., 2007). Pregabalin is effective in reducing pain and improving quality of life in peripheral diabetic neuropathy. Gapabetin and sodium valproate are considered treatment for peripheral diabetic neuropathy but are classified as level B. There are insufficient data to support the use of topiramate for treatment of peripheral diabetic neuropathy, and it is classified as level U (data inadequate and unproven). Level B drugs oxcarbazepeine, lamotrigine, and lacosamide are not considered treatment for peripheral neuropathy in diabetics (Bril et al., 2011).

Opioids are associated with a high rate of adverse effects but with careful monitoring can be effective in treating resistant neuropathic pain (Dworkin et al., 2007). Dextromethorphan is effective in reducing pain of peripheral diabetic neuropathy and improving quality of life and is rated level A/class 1. Level B drugs morphine sulfate, tramadol, and oxycodone have moderate effect and reduce pain by at least 27% in peripheral diabetic neuropathy (Bril et al., 2011).

TCAs such as nortriptyline or desipramine are often used for nocturnal pain but require much caution in the elderly and for anyone with cardiac disease. Venlafaxine and duloxetine successfully treated neuropathic pain independently of their effect associated with depression (Zilliox & Russell, 2011). Duloxetine may be considered in patients with cardiovascular conditions for which TCAs are contraindicated. Additionally, it may be considered in patients in whom weight gain, sedation, and/or edema is of concern as as an alternative to gabapentin or pregabalin (Kajdasz et al., 2007). Venlafaxine and duloxetine, which are level B drugs, should be considered when treating neuropathy in diabetics. Venlafaxine may be added to gabapentin for a better response although this combination is recommended at level C. The Lidoderm patch is effective

in relieving pain associated with postherpetic neuralgia, but only class III/level C evidence supports its use for diabetic neuropathies. Capsaicin is effective topical treatment without systemic effects (Zilliox & Russell, 2011). However, capsaicin and isosorbide dinitrate spray are considered as level B in the treatment of diabetic peripheral neuropathy (Bril et al., 2011).

The second-line medications that can be used for first-line treatment with a level A recommendation are the opioid analgesics and tramadol. During titration of first-line medications to an efficacious dose, an opioid and tramadol may be used; they may also be used for episodic exacerbation of severe pain, acute neuropathic pain, and neuropathic cancer pain (Dworkin et al., 2007).

There is no evidence supporting the use of vitamins and alpha-lipoic acid in the treatment of diabetic peripheral neuropathy (Bril et al., 2011). However, it is worth noting that vitamin B_1 (Benfotiamine) and thiamine have been used clinically extensively, safely, and successfully in Japan since 1962 and in Europe since 1978 for patients with peripheral neuropathy. Benfotiamine has no known significant adverse effects or drug interactions. The efficacy of Benfotiamine in the treatment of neuropathy is noted by over 100 clinicians in the United States. Many clinicians report at least a 30% or higher successful rate of peripheral neuropathy symptom relief. Plasma thiamine by high-performance liquid chromatography (HPLC) (commonly used in most laboratories) should be ordered. The normal values are 58.5 to 69.7 nmol/L. If the level is below this range, Benfotiamine should be started at one or two 150 mcg capsules twice daily. Follow up in 2 weeks for evaluation of symptom improvement and/or adverse effects. Discontinue medicine if side effects occur. If after 6 to 8 weeks there is no improvement, discontinue the medication because there will be no improvement. Patients may have a period of regression because the medication is constantly renally excreted. Therapy is individualized for each patient (Mann, 2009). Table 13-1 lists pharmacological agents for neuropathic pain.

It may be necessary to use a combination of drugs to achieve optimal pain control. There are no evidence-based recommendations for other treatment modalities, including low-intensity transcutaneous electrical nerve stimulation, medical hypnosis, acupuncture, massage therapy, meditation, yoga, and tai chi. Whole body vibration, especially for type 2 diabetes with peripheral neuropathy, is currently undergoing studies for its effectiveness in reducing pain and improving gait (complementary and alternative to resistive training

TABLE 13-1 Pharmacological Agents for Neuropathic Pain	
Tricyclic antidepressants (TCAs; desipramine, nortriptyline)	TCAs are effective for constant and lancinating, paroxysmal pain. Treatment should be initiated at a low dose (10–25 mg) at bedtime and increased by similar increments no more than twice weekly. Usually 75–150 mg (less for elderly patients) is required for pain suppression. At higher doses, sedation, confusion, anticholinergic effects, and orthostatic hypotension are common, especially in the elderly. A baseline ECG is recommended before administration of a TCA. Use with caution in the elderly and in patients who have ischemic heart disease, narrow-angle glaucoma, or prostatism.
Norepinephrine and serotonin reuptake inhibitor (venlafaxine, duloxetine)	Venlafaxine has fewer side effects than TCAs. Usual dose range is 150–225 mg/day. Venlafaxine is less efficacious than imipramine. Duloxetine at a dose of 60–120 mg/day has a moderate effect in reducing pain by about 30%. Side effects include nausea, constipation, sweating, asthenia, and dry mouth. Of concern is the possibility of hyponatremia; thus sodium levels and blood pressure should be monitored.
Anticonvulsants (gabapentin, pregabalin)	Often given to suppress shooting or stabbing pain. Gabapentin: initiate 300 mg qhs. Titrate dose up by 300 mg increments every 3–5 days until adequate pain relief is achieve. The median effective dose ranges from 900 to 1600 mg, although some patients may require doses of 3600 mg/day. Effective ranges for pregabalin are 150–600 mg/day.
Tramadol (nonnarcotic centrally acting analgesia)	Dose: 200–400 mg/day. Well tolerated but transient nausea and constipation occur in about 20% of patients. Use with caution in patients with impaired hepatic or renal function and in patients taking other psychoactive medications.
Topical agents (capsaicin, 5% lidocaine patch)	Dose: 0.025%–0.075% applied to affected area tid-qid. May be useful in patients with painful, burning feet. Presumably produces pain relief through the depletion of substance P in unmyelinated nociceptive fibers. Intense burning sensation of the skin occurs after initial application before improvement is seen. Allow at least 4 weeks to determine efficacy. Even after 4 weeks the beneficial effect may be marginal. Some patients may have relief from burning feet and allodynia by topical application of 5% lidocaine patch.

Source: Adapted from Chaudhry (2008); Finnerup, Sindrup, & Jensen (2010); Harati & Bosch (2008); Mahmoud & Tampi (2011); Shy (2007).

after a failed trial of conventional drugs and interventional pain management) (Hong, 2011). Percutaneous electrical nerve stimulation is considered in the treatment of peripheral diabetic neuropathy (level B) (Bril et al., 2011).

Follow-up: Because peripheral neuropathy is a persistent disease process, patients should be followed periodically based on the underlying disease processes involved.

Sequelae: Peripheral neuropathy carries significant morbidity for the elderly. The association between peripheral neuropathy and balance problems and falls is well established (Mold et al., 2008). It is commonly overlooked as a contributing factor for falls. Falls limit activities thereby leading to premature functional decline and decreased quality of life. Approximately 30% of adults age 65 and older fall each year. Of these, 20% to 30% sustain injuries leading to loss of functional independence and mobility. The inability to recognize position sense or to ascertain where the feet are on the floor is a major reason for falls. Peripheral sensory impairment leads to imbalances thereby contributing to falls and injury (Chaudhry, 2008; Mold et al., 2004).

In peripheral neuropathy with the underlying disease process being diabetes, hypoglycemia must also be considered as a partial risk factor for falls in the elderly. The American Geriatric Society recommends a hemoglobin A1C (HgbA1C) of 8% for the frail elderly having a life expectancy of less than 5 years (Mold et al., 2008). A trophic change in an enervated immobile extremity combined with recurrent painless trauma predisposes the skin to ulceration and poor wound healing. Severe infections such as osteomyelitis or osteolysis may eventually result in limb amputation. This unfortunate sequence of events can be avoidable with proper care (Chaudhry, 2008; Mold et al., 2004).

Prevention/prophylaxis: There are several health-promoting activities patients can do prophylactically:

■ Avoid repetitive motions, cramped positions, constant exposure to offending toxins, and excessive alcohol consumption.

■ Meticulous foot care, ankle braces, foot orthosis, and proper shoes help to reduce the risk of falls and injury, the development of ulcers, or the worsening of slow-healing wounds due to sensory impairment.

■ Assistive walking devices used due to substantial leg weakness will help to ensure safety and reduction of falls and injury.

■ Hand or wrist splints will be helpful if the hands or wrists are involved.

■ Become involved and/or familiar with local support groups:
   ■ Guillain-Barré Syndrome Support Group
   ■ Hereditary Neuropathy Foundation
   ■ Peripheral Neuropathy Trust
   ■ The Neuropathy Association

Referral: Refer patients to a neurologist when the onset of the disease is rapid as well as for symmetrical and multifocal peripheral neuropathy and when electromyogram study reveals either axonal or demyelinating conditions. Patients who cannot complete the tandem stand should be referred to physical therapy for balance and gait training. Reconditioning and appropriate exercises can help with pain control and reduce the risk of falls and injuries (Cleveland Clinic, 2010). Refer patients to podiatry to ensure appropriate shoes for extra depth and special orthotics especially in patients with loss of proprioception or gait disturbances (Caçchione, 2010; Jeffrey, 2000). An ankle-foot orthosis may be effective in improving ambulation in persons with footdrop (Botek, Anderson, & Taylor, 2010). Refer to occupational therapy for appropriate assistive ambulation devices, splints, and braces (Shy, 2007). Referral for psychological counseling may be beneficial because the disease can have a disabling effect on one's quality of life (Pourmand, 2002). Refer patients to hematology/oncology when M-protein is present on SPE for possible lymphoproliferative disorder (Pourmand, 2002).

Education: Teach the patient, family, and/or caregivers about the disease process and its management, the role of common causes of the disease, the interventions for palliation, fall precautions, the need for good supportive shoes, foot care, and about healthy eating to ensure all vitamins and minerals are included in the daily diet. Advise patients of the need for regular follow-up visits, even if no symptoms are present. Instruct patients to avoid crossing the legs at the knee to avoid prolonged pressure or constriction and avoid further nerve damage.

CLINICAL RECOMMENDATION	EVIDENCE RATING	REFERENCES
Pregabalin, a first-line medication, was found to be effective in reducing pain and improving quality of life in patients with peripheral diabetic neuropathy.	A	Dworkin et al. (2007)
Opioids and tramadol can be used as second-line treatment for peripheral neuropathy.	B	Dworkin et al. (2007)
Percutaneous electrical nerve simulation can be considered for pain relief in patients with peripheral diabetic neuropathy.	B	Bril et al. (2011)
Capsaicin, isosorbide dinitrate spray, may be used to treat diabetic peripheral neuropathy.	B	Bril et al. (2011)

A = consistent, good-quality, patient-oriented evidence; B = inconsistent or limited-quality, patient-oriented evidence; C = consensus, disease-oriented evidence, usual practice, expert opinion, or case series. For information about the SORT evidence rating system, go to www.aafp.org/afpsort.xml.

RESTLESS LEGS SYNDROME

Signal symptoms: Urge to move legs when lying down.

Description: Restless legs syndrome (RLS) is a common neurological disorder characterized by an intense urge to move the legs (or sometimes the arms) associated with discomfort. Patients may not be able to resist the urge to move their legs. Symptoms are reported as a need to move due to sensations variously described as aching, burning, creeping, crawling, cramping, gnawing, pulling, painful, tense, throbbing, tingling, restlessness, itchy, tense, tearing, and tugging. Movement of affected limbs provides relief, but discomfort recurs unless the movement continues. RLS symptoms have circadian rhythmicity, peaking between midnight and 3 a.m. Symptoms are elicited by sitting or lying down. It is a common sleep disorder.

Etiology: The cause of RLS is unknown; however, RLS is found in families and may have a genetic component. There is an indication that the brains of patients with RLS have reduced relative availability of iron and that this contributes to the symptoms (Satija & Ondo, 2008).

Occurrence: It is estimated that 9% to 20% of elders are affected by RLS, with an estimated prevalence of 10% to 35% of individuals over 65 years of age.

Age: Average age of symptom onset is 42 years (range: 20 to 80 years and older).

Gender: Because women are more likely to be iron deficient than men, RLS is more common in women, with a female/male sex ratio of 5:1.

Ethnicity: RLS has a prevalence of 5% to 15% in the white population. It is less common in Asian and African populations. It is more common in white women than in women of African origin.

Contributing factors: Peripheral neuropathy (diabetes mellitus) is an assumed cause of secondary RLS. A positive family history of RLS is often noted in patients with this condition. Antidepressants, antipsychotics, antiemetics, and neuroleptics can aggravate RLS symptoms. Anemia, especially iron deficiency (there is a relationship between the dopaminergic system and iron), vitamin B_{12} deficiency, or folate deficiency can contribute to symptoms. Renal patients receiving dialysis are at risk for secondary RLS. Herbal and over-the-counter medications can worsen RLS symptoms. Medications for hypertension, nausea, cold, allergies (antihistamines), and depression can make RLS worse.

Patients diagnosed with attention-deficit disorder are known to have RLS.

Signs and symptoms: Symptoms are worse at night, and there is a strong need to move a limb or limbs, which may be associated with paresthesias or dysesthesias. An urge to move the legs is usually accompanied or caused by uncomfortable and unpleasant sensations in the legs (though sometimes the urge to move is present without the uncomfortable sensations, and sometimes the arms or other body parts are involved in addition to the legs). The urge to move or unpleasant sensations begin or worsen during periods of rest or inactivity such as lying or sitting. Akathisia is a major symptom of RLS.

- Ask about the urge to move or unpleasant sensations and if they are partially or totally relieved by movement such as walking or stretching.
- Ask if the urge to move or unpleasant sensations are worse in the evening or night than during the day, or if the urge to move only occurs in the evening or night (when symptoms are very severe, the worsening at night may not be noticeable but must have been previously present).
- Ask about sleep patterns; does the patient keep his or her partner awake?
- Does the patient have trouble sitting still and need to stand up and walk around?
- Is the patient tired during the day from an interrupted night of sleeping?

Diagnostic tests: A CBC to begin the workup of anemia followed by specific studies indicated by the results. A sleep study may be helpful to those who experience the symptoms mainly during the night.

Differential diagnosis: Differential diagnosis may be challenging unless the suspicion of RLS is considered. Patients may not associate restless legs with disturbed sleep. Common disorders to rule out are listed, but many disorders may masquerade as RLS. These multiple disorders can mimic RLS:

- Hypotensive akathisia
- Radiculopathy
- Vascular claudication
- Neurogenic claudication
- Neuroleptic-induced akathisia
- Neuropathy

- Chronic pain syndrome associated with (lumbar, cervical) positional discomfort
- Nocturnal leg cramps
- Hypnic jerks
- Depression with somatic syndrome
- Volitional movements
- Foot tapping
- Leg rocking
- Lower limb arthritis
- Fibromyalgia
- Varicose veins (Garcia-Borreguero et al., 2011).

Diabetic neuropathy is damage to the peripheral nerves (microvascular injury) due to diabetes (high blood sugar damages nerves) and is most common in legs and feet. Symptoms include numbness, tingling, hypersensitivity, muscle weakness, and sharp pain.

Leg cramps (at night) are sudden, painful, and involuntary contractions of the muscles of the legs; these may have no real cause and are just bothersome. If leg cramping is disturbing sleep, assess and consider these causes as possibilities: diuretics, Addison's and Parkinson's diseases, muscle overextension and overexercise, diabetes, hypoglycemia, hemodialysis, calcium channel blockers, peripheral artery disease, nerve compression, diabetes, and dehydration.

Periodic limb movements are repetitive cramping or jerking of the legs during sleep. It only occurs during sleep. It may be associated with RLS but is not the same thing. Periodic refers to the fact that the movements are repetitive and rhythmic, occurring about every 20 to 40 seconds. It is a sleep disorder and can disturb sleep and result in daytime sleepiness.

Radiculopathy refers to neuropathy, which occurs from compression on nerves in the spine, resulting in pain, tingling, numbness, and weakness. "Sciatica" pain radiating to the legs is an example. Pain can occur from a herniated disk, bone, spur, osteoarthritis, tumor, infection, scoliosis, and stenosis. Box 13-1 lists the essential diagnostic criteria for RLS.

Treatment: RLS is a lifelong condition for which there is no cure. Conservation therapy or complementary care may be enough to manage symptoms, including avoiding alcohol and caffeine, a trial of relaxation techniques, massage, acupuncture, daily exercise, stretching, application of heat or cold, good sleep hygiene and small doses of melatonin (3 mg) and vitamins needed to correct the specific anemia. Recommend to patients to find distractions while sitting if RLS occurs in this position. Recommend participation in support groups as well to learn of new

---

BOX 13-1

Essential Diagnostic Criteria for Restless Legs Syndrome

An urge to move the legs, usually accompanied or caused by uncomfortable and unpleasant sensations in the legs (sometimes the urge to move is present without the uncomfortable sensations, and sometimes the arms or other body parts are involved in addition to the legs)

The urge to move or unpleasant sensations begin or worsen during periods of rest or inactivity such as lying or sitting

The urge to move or unpleasant sensations are partially or totally relieved by movement, such as walking or stretching, at least as long as the activity continues

The urge to move or unpleasant sensations are worse in the evening or night than during the day, or only occur in the evening or night (when symptoms are very severe, the worsening at night may not be noticeable but must have been previously present)

SUPPORTIVE CRITERIA

Positive family history

Positive response to dopaminergic drugs

Periodic leg movement during wakefulness or sleep as assessed with polysomnography or leg activity

ASSOCIATED FEATURES

Natural clinical course of the disorder: RLS can begin at any age, but most patients seen in clinical practice are middle-aged or older. Most patients have a progressive clinical course, but a static clinical course is sometimes seen. Remissions of a month or more are sometimes reported.

Sleep disorders are a frequent but unspecific symptom of RLS.

Medical evaluation/physical examination: The neurological examination is usually normal. Probable causes for secondary RLS should be excluded. A low serum ferritin (<45–50 mcg/L) may be found in RLS patients (Benes, Walters, Allen, Hening, & Kohnen, 2007).

supportive measures (Mitchell, 2011). For patients who experience RLS at night, promote good sleep hygiene. For medical treatment of RLS, extensive data are available for levodopa and dopamine agonists, especially pramipexole and ropinirole and to a small extent cabergoline, pergolide, and rotigotine (Oertel et al., 2007). Medical treatment for RLS often starts at age 50 to 60 years old, though RLS may develop by age 40 and treatment may begin when symptoms are persistent and disturbing (Garcia-Borreguero et al., 2011). Sedatives (ramelteon [Rozerem]), anticonvulsants (neurontin [Gabapentin]), and pain relievers (opioids) may be beneficial and are drug options for treatment of RLS. Dopaminergic agents are used to treat RLS; start and use low doses and change doses slowly.

Follow-up: Ask about sleep, exercise, and relationships. Sleep disturbances can cause hypertension and tension in relationships. Check blood pressure at each visit.

Sequelae: RLS can cause difficulty in falling asleep or staying asleep. Sleep deprivation can cause relationship problems, hypertension, and daytime sleepiness that can contribute to motor vehicle accidents.

Prevention/prophylaxis: There is no prevention for RLS, but recommend daily exercise and review the tenets of sleep hygiene to improve sleep (sleep in cool, quiet, dark environment; go to bed and get up at the same time; get enough sleep to feel rested). Cognitive-behavioral therapy may be beneficial. Sequential compression devices have been used for treatment with complete resolution of symptoms in 3 of 10 patients (Eliasson & Lettieri, 2007).

Referral: Patients may benefit from participating in yoga, Qi Gong, or treatment by an acupuncturist. Refer to a neurologist or a sleep or movement disorders specialist if unusual case or nonresponse to treatment.

Education: Provide patient and families with written information about RLS, including support groups in the community. Contact the National Institute of Neurological Disorders and Stroke for educational resources (www.ninds.nih.gov/disorders/restless_legs/detail_restless_legs.htm) or the Restless Legs Syndrome Foundation, 1610 14th Street NW, Suite 300, Rochester, MN 55901 (phone: 507-297-6465; e-mail: rlsfoundation@rls.org; Web site: www.rls.org).

CLINICAL RECOMMENDATION	EVIDENCE RATING	REFERENCES
The European Restless Legs Syndrome Study Group (EURLSSG) Task Force reached a consensus and agreed on diagnostic and treatment algorithms.	C	Garcia-Borreguero et al. (2011)
Uncontrolled prospective interventional pilot study using sequential compression devices on a convenience sample of adults diagnosed with RLS.	B	Eliasson & Lettieri (2007)
There is a growing body of evidence demonstrating the effectiveness of nonpharmacological treatments, including lifestyle changes, physical activity programs, pneumatic compression, massage, near-infrared light therapy, and complementary therapy.	B	Mitchell (2011)
A Movement Disorder Society task force performed an evidence-based review of medical literature on treatment modalities used to manage patients with RLS.	A	Trenkwalder et al. (2008)

A = consistent, good-quality, patient-oriented evidence; B = inconsistent or limited-quality, patient-oriented evidence; C = consensus, disease-oriented evidence, usual practice, expert opinion, or case series. For information about the SORT evidence rating system, go to www.aafp.org/afpsort.xml.

SEIZURE DISORDERS

Signal symptoms: Confusion, loss of consciousness, bizarre behavior, memory changes, falls, cognitive changes, sleep disorders, twitching, and involuntary movements.

Description: The term *seizure* describes a variety of symptoms, ranging from momentary loss of consciousness to total loss of consciousness and motor and sensory changes.

Etiology: In older adults, cerebrovascular disease is the most common underlying cause of seizures; other known causes include neurodegenerative disorders, brain tumors, and head injuries (Brodie, Elder, & Kaw, 2009). It is estimated that up to one-half of new cases of seizures in older adults have no known cause (Martin, Vogtle, Gilliam, & Faught, 2005).

Occurrence: The prevalence of seizures (epilepsy) increases progressively after age 60. The annual incidence of epilepsy rises from 85.9 per 100,000 people in those between 65 and 80 years of age to more than 135 per 100,000 people for those older than 80 years of age compared with an overall incidence of 80.8 per 100,000 people across all age groups. The cumulative risk of epilepsy by 80 years of age ranges from 1.3% to 4%. More important, elderly people with epilepsy have a 2 to 3 times greater mortality rate than the general population. Approximately 30% of acute seizures in elderly people present as status epilepticus, which has a mortality rate of about 40%. Onset of seizures late in life is a predictor of subsequent stroke.

Age: Some elderly individuals may continue to experience seizures after age 60 due to the natural course of the disease. There is an increased incidence in new-onset seizures after age 60.

Gender: Does not appear to be related.

Ethnicity: Although there is no well understood difference in the incidence of seizures among various ethnic groups, there is a belief that the incidence of seizures among ethnic minorities may be underreported. In some ethnic groups (e.g., Hispanic) neurocysticercosis may be a possible cause for seizures, which is not seen in other ethnic groups.

Contributing factors: Multiple factors can contribute to the onset or worsening of seizures. A family history or previous history of seizures or epilepsy increases the likelihood of seizures. Head injury, predominantly due to falls, accounts for up to 20% of cases of epilepsy in the elderly. Brain contusion with subdural hematoma, skull fracture, loss of consciousness, or amnesia for more than 1 day and age 65 years or older have been identified as risk factors for subsequent epilepsy. Cardiovascular disease and the presence of other neurological diseases, including neurodegenerative and ischemic, may also contribute to the incidence of seizures. Alzheimer's disease, dementia, and neurodegenerative disorders are estimated to account for 10% to 20% of all epilepsies in older people. Seizures can occur in any stage of the degenerative process. A common cause of epilepsy in the elderly is stroke, which accounts for up to 50% of cases in whom a cause can be identified. The risk of epilepsy increases up to 20-fold in the first year after a stroke. Individuals with a brain tumor, bacterial meningitis, or Alzheimer's disease are up to 10 times more likely to develop epilepsy than those without the diseases. Multiple drugs have been shown to either cause seizures or potentially lower seizure threshold. These include psychotropic drugs, theophylline, narcotics, tramadol (Ultram), antimicrobials, chemotherapeutic agents (methotrexate, chlorambucil), general anesthetics (ketamine, enflurane), local anesthetics, stimulants, antiarrhythmics (verapamil, mexiletine, procainamide, and propranolol), diphenhydramine, baclofen, and chlorpromazine.

Signs and symptoms: Multiple types of seizures exist, although there are two major categories. Generalized seizures occur due to involvement of both sides of the brain. These may begin on one side of the brain but are quickly transmitted to the other side of the brain. This is referred to as a secondarily generalized seizure. A summary of the types and potential symptoms of generalized seizures is presented in Table 13-2. Partial seizures occur in a specific area of the brain and are localized. Due to the variety of types of partial seizures and their subtle presentation, partial seizures can sometimes go unrecognized. A summary of types of partial seizures and their symptoms is presented in Table 13-3.

Diagnostic tests: In the initial workup of a new-onset seizure in an elderly person, multiple diagnostic tests are needed. Blood tests include a CBC (including differential and platelet count); liver function tests, electrolytes, blood urea nitrogen, creatinine, glucose, calcium, and magnesium should also be obtained. These are needed to establish a baseline and to allow

TABLE 13-2	Generalized Seizures—Consciousness Is Impaired and There Are Symptoms of Motor Dysfunction Involving Both Sides of the Brain	
TYPE OF GENERALIZED SEIZURE	**DESCRIPTION**	**POSSIBLE SYMPTOMS**
Absence seizures	A momentary interruption of consciousness lasting from a few seconds to up to 30 seconds	Blank staring, eyes may roll upward, eyelid fluttering, objects are dropped
Myoclonic seizures	Sudden shock-like muscle contractions confined to one or more limbs, often occur while falling asleep or waking up	Sudden, unexpected jerking of the limbs; jerking is repetitive
Clonic seizures	Generalized convulsive seizure without the initial tonic phase	Repetitive muscle jerking
Generalized tonic-clonic seizures	Lost or impaired consciousness; the entire seizure, composed of tonic and clonic action, lasts for several minutes	Rigidity, person falls to the ground, a loud cry, loss of bladder or bowel function, breathing stops, followed by labored breathing
Atonic seizures	Causes a sudden loss of muscle tone, usually with a brief loss of consciousness	Head nods, eyelids droop, person may fall to the ground

TABLE 13-3	Partial Seizures*	
TYPE OF PARTIAL SEIZURE	**DESCRIPTION**	**POSSIBLE SYMPTOMS**
Simple partial seizures	Consciousness is not lost or impaired	Rhythmic twitching of a limb or part of a limb, unusual taste, smell, buzzing noise, feeling of falling, paresthesias
Complex partial seizures	Consciousness is lost or impaired	Loss of consciousness, change in awareness, automatisms such as fiddling with clothes or objects, wandering, making gestures, nonsensical talking
Secondarily generalized seizures	A simple or complex partial seizure that spreads to involve both cerebral hemispheres	Generalized tonic-clonic seizure

*An electrical disturbance in one area of a cerebral hemisphere

decisions to be made about potential medications. A thyroid screen (i.e., TSH) is done, because thyroid disorders are frequently associated with seizures. A rapid plasma reagin (RPR) is done to rule out the possibility of syphilis, which, in tertiary form, may present as a seizure disorder. A lumbar puncture for cell count, protein, glucose, and stains with cultures may be needed if an infectious process is suspected. A basic electrocardiogram (ECG) is needed to rule out any cardiac problems. In the event that there is an abnormal ECG, an echocardiogram may be required. Tilt-table testing can be useful to detect baroreceptor and vasopressor dysfunction or sympathetic failure due to autonomic neuropathy in older people. A brain MRI with and without contrast should be done to rule out old scar tissue, mesial temporal sclerosis, or other structural reasons for the seizures. Neuroimaging with contrast increases the ability to identify tumors, inflammatory disease, and abscesses. An EEG should be done. Be aware that a normal EEG does not rule out the possibility of epilepsy and is seen in about one-third of patients with epilepsy. An interictal EEG in the elderly person has limited utility, with low sensitivity and specificity for the diagnosis of epilepsy.

Differential diagnosis: The most common differential diagnoses for seizures include the following:

- Vasovagal syncope
- Tumors
- Meningitis
- Tertiary syphilis
- Transient ischemic attack
- Global amnesia
- Migraine
- Hypoglycemia
- Hyponatremia
- Hypokalemia
- Obstructive sleep apnea
- Hypnic jerks
- Psychogenic seizures

A thorough history is critical in the assessment of new-onset seizures. Obtain information concerning family history, any head injuries, and any past history of seizures. Information concerning whether the individual has lived outside of the United States (particularly in unincorporated areas with poor sanitation) can raise suspicion of neurocysticercosis. Obtain a complete description of the seizure, including any aura (a warning of the seizure), along with a complete description of the patient's behavior during the seizure and in the postictal period. An estimate of the time for each phase of the seizure is helpful. How the patient felt before and after the seizure can offer insight into the potential nature of the cause of the event. A thorough neurological examination is performed, with particular attention paid to any focal or localizing symptoms. If the individual is currently taking antiepileptic drugs (AEDs), screen for any symptoms of toxicity, including nystagmus, ataxia, and slurred or slowed speech.

Treatment: The goal of management should be the maintenance of a normal lifestyle with complete control of seizures with minimal side effects. Seizures in the elderly tend to respond better to AEDs than those in young individuals and can often be appropriately controlled with monotherapy. Pharmacotherapy continues to be the mainstay of treatment for seizures. AEDs are commonly prescribed to the elderly and to about 10% of nursing home residents for a variety of reasons, including migraine prophylaxis, psychiatric disorders, pain management, and seizures. AEDs are the fifth most common cause of drug side effects in the elderly and therefore need to be carefully prescribed and monitored. The pharmacokinetics and pharmacodynamics of AEDs are distinct in elderly patients. Multiple changes occur with aging, including alterations in oral absorption, plasma protein binding, absorption kinetics, and intestinal transport. Pharmacodynamic changes include alterations in receptor distribution and density, receptor affinity and function, neurotransmitter release, and autonomic and homeostatic function. Toxicity from medications is poorly recognized in the elderly and can be attributed to multiple causes. Elderly with multiple chronic illnesses are more likely to be taking medications that interfere with AEDs. Multiple types of anticonvulsants are available, and new medications are being released frequently. Each medication has a side-effect profile that needs to be considered, and the dosages may need some adjustment specific to the elderly. Table 13-4 includes a summary of important information concerning AEDs.

Benzodiazepines (diazepam, lorazepam) are most commonly used for rescue or only in the acute setting. Although these are generally considered CNS depressants, the elderly may experience idiosyncratic effects such as restlessness, hyperactivity, and psychosis. Phenobarbital has been used in the treatment of seizures since the 1950s. Some elderly patients may have been on the medication for many years and will continue to require consistent monitoring. Generally, the sedative effects of this medication preclude starting it for a patient with new-onset seizures. Phenytoin is highly protein bound and may lead to toxicity in the elderly. With renal insufficiency, phenytoin concentrations can be falsely elevated. Carbamazepine clearance is reduced by 30% to 40% in the elderly, leaving the unbound plasma concentration higher due to decreased serum albumin. This leads to the need for lower initial dosages. Valproic acid is highly protein bound and can lead to toxicity along with idiosyncratic effects in the elderly.

The newer AEDs offer some advantages in working with the elderly, including a better side-effect profile. However, they are also more expensive, and the name brands may not be covered by various insurance programs. Oxcarbazepine is a second-generation carbamazepine but with fewer side effects. This drug is only 38% protein bound and can be introduced more quickly in the elderly than carbamazepine. Lamotrigine is well absorbed orally by the elderly. Although the medication is eliminated by hepatic metabolism, then excreted renally, the drug is safely used in the elderly with renal failure. Side effects are minimal, and several studies have shown that it is well tolerated by the elderly. Lamotrigine has some

TABLE 13-4	Major Anticonvulsants				
BRAND NAME	GENERIC NAME	DOSAGE	INDICATIONS	SELECTED SIDE EFFECTS	COMMENTS
Phenobarbital	Phenobarbital	Usual starting dose in adults is 60 mg/day, with additional 30-mg increases every 2–4 weeks to a target dose of 90–120 mg/day, or higher if clinically tolerated	Partial, PGTC, Myoclonic	Sedation, altered sleep cycle, hyperactivity, osteoporosis	Once a day dosage
Mysoline	Primidone	100–125 mg daily in divided doses; up to 2000 mg daily	Partial, PGTC, Myoclonic	Same as Phenobarbital	Metabolizes to phenobarbital
Dilantin	Phenytoin	300 mg daily in divided doses; up to 600 mg daily; dose to saturation kinetics	Partial, PGTC	Osteoporosis Dizziness	Once a day dosage if tolerated Other forms: Phenytek
Tegretol	Carbamazepine	200–400 mg daily in divided doses; up to 1600 mg daily	Partial, PGTC	Hyponatremia Osteoporosis	Other forms: Tegretol XR Carbatrol
Neurontin	Gabapentin	900–1200 mg daily in divided doses; up to 3600 mg daily	Partial	Dizziness, diplopia	
Trileptal	Oxcarbazepine	300–600 mg daily in divided doses; up to 2400 mg daily	Partial	Hyponatremia, nausea	
Depakote	Valproic acid	500–1000 mg daily in divided doses; up to 60 mg/kg daily	Partial, PGTC, Absence	Weight gain, hair loss, tremor, easy bruising	Other forms: Depakote ER for once daily dosing
Lyrica	Pregabalin	150 mg daily in divided doses; up to 600 mg daily	Partial	Weight gain, dizziness, sedation	
Keppra	Levetiracetam	500–1000 mg daily; up to 3000 mg daily	Partial, PGTC, Myoclonic	Fatigue, anxiety, depression	Other Forms: Keppra XR – once daily
Vimpat	Lacosamide	100–200 mg daily in divided doses; up to 400 mg daily.	Partial	Fatigue, nausea, dizziness	No generic available
Lamictal	Lamotrigine	100–200 mg daily; initiated slowly according to titration schedule; up to 700 mg daily.	Partial, PGTC, Absence	Sedation, dizziness, dose-related rash	Requires careful titration Other forms: Lamictal XR –once daily
Zonegeran	Zonisamide	100–200 mg daily; up to 600 mg daily.	Partial,	Sedation, weight loss	Once daily dosage
Gabitril	Tiagabine	4–8 mg daily in divided doses; up to 56 mg daily.	Partial	Fatigue, tremor, problems concentrating	
Topamax	Topiramate	100–200 mg daily; initiate with titration schedule; up to 400 mg daily.	Partial, PGTC	Weight loss, renal stones, paresthesis cognitive decline; acute myopia and glaucoma	

mood-stabilizing effects, which may also help in treatment of the elderly. Levetiracetam is not metabolized by the P450 system and is entirely renally excreted. Dosage in renal failure may need adjustment. Gabapentin is also completely excreted unchanged in the urine. This drug is generally well tolerated in the elderly and is less likely to be involved in drug interactions. However, high dosages are often required for effective seizure control. Topiramate has demonstrated good efficacy in elderly patients but may interact with digoxin and warfarin. Pregabalin has oral bioavailability exceeding 90%, is not bound to plasma proteins, and readily crosses the blood-brain barrier. Dosage must be titrated slowly to avoid adverse cognitive effects. Felbamate is primarily metabolized by the liver and has a number of drug interactions. Used carefully, this can be a good choice in pharmacoresistant seizures. Tiagabine is also metabolized by the liver and has a drug interaction profile similar to carbamazepine. Zonisamide is 40% bound to protein and its major elimination pathway is hepatic, but can be safely used in the elderly.

Caution should be exercised in the use of generic medications, because these have been shown to not have the same efficacy as name-brand medications. A patient who is stable on generic medications can become toxic or have breakthrough seizures if switched to name-brand medications. Similarly, the patient who is stable on name-brand medications and is switched to generic may experience a significant decrease in serum levels, leading to breakthrough seizures.

Seizure surgery can be considered in the elderly if the seizures are medically intractable and the seizures are related to a focal structural lesion. Limited data are available on the outcomes from surgery in those over age 65. Patients would be referred to a comprehensive epilepsy center for evaluation.

Vagus nerve stimulation (VNS) has also been used in patients with refractory epilepsy. VNS is provided by a surgically implanted device programmed to deliver a brief electric stimulation on a schedule. The efficacy of this treatment has been established in general populations, but the data on the elderly are sparse. The results of one meta-analysis on the efficacy of vagus nerve stimulation showed that there is a decrease in seizure activity during the first 3 months (Englot, Chang, & Auguste, 2011).

Follow-up: Seizure management is a significant challenge, and the patient and any caretakers should be seen frequently. A seizure calendar is maintained by the patient and should be reviewed on each visit. Precipitating factors for an increase in seizures, such as stress, sleep deprivation, or viral illness, should be noted. Questions concerning potential medication side effects are asked on each visit. For some medications, periodic levels are monitored and adjusted to ensure therapeutic levels. The incidence of depression in adults with epilepsy has been reported as high as 50%. Causes of the depression include lifestyle changes and the biochemical alterations in the brain due to the seizures. The potential loss of freedom following a seizure is heightened by driving restrictions, which are based on the laws of the individual state and range from 6 months to at least 1 year seizure free.

Sequelae: Sudden unexpected death in epilepsy (SUDEP) is defined specifically as the sudden, unexpected, witnessed or unwitnessed, nontraumatic, and nondrowning death in patients with epilepsy with or without evidence for a seizure, and excluding documented status epilepticus, in which postmortem examination does not reveal a structural or toxicological cause for death. Individuals with epilepsy have a mortality rate 2 to 3 times greater than that of the population at large. SUDEP accounts for 8% to 17% of these deaths and is more likely to occur in those with frequent seizures. Patients and their families need to be warned of the potential for SUDEP and the importance of controlling the variables that can lead to SUDEP, such as abrupt cessation of AEDs.

Convulsive status epilepticus incidence is almost twice that of the general population. Associated mortality rate is also higher in older patients, 38% in those over 60 and over 50% in those over 80 years. Nonconvulsive status epilepticus (NCSE) is equally common in the elderly, but much more difficult to diagnose, because it can present with general symptoms such as confusion, psychosis, lethargy, or coma or a more focal cognitive disturbance with aphasia. These symptoms are very general and may not be associated with any observable seizure activity. Due to the nonspecific nature of the symptoms, the presence of seizures on the EEG is the most important diagnostic step. Incidence rate of all types of status epilepticus in the elderly is 54.2 per 100,000 people.

Prevention/prophylaxis: Prevention of potential causative factors such as stroke, meningitis, and active management of disease processes such as Alzheimer's disease and dementia is an important part of prevention of seizures. Care in preventing falls may also decrease the incidence of head injuries leading to seizures. Prophylactic use of AEDs following head injury and stroke remains controversial but may be indicated.

Referral: For new-onset seizures, referral to a neurologist or to a comprehensive epilepsy center would be in the best interest of the patient. If traditional medications become difficult to manage, the patient should be referred to a neurologist.

Education: Educating patients and their families about SUDEP, ascertaining seizure precipitants, and promoting compliance with treatment are important strategies. Very specific information should be provided to patients who are noncompliant with medications or appear to be in denial of the diagnosis. Patients should maintain a seizure calendar that chronicles seizures and all precipitants. Strategies to ensure compliance with daily medication include the use of medication boxes and telephone alarms. Patients should inform the provider of any changes in other medications to avoid potential interactions. Inform patients and family members that abrupt cessation of medications is very dangerous and that all AEDs should be carefully weaned.

CLINICAL RECOMMENDATION	EVIDENCE RATING	REFERENCES
Monitoring of AED serum concentration is helpful after the initiation of treatments or after dose adjustments to achieve a target concentration in specific patients. AED serum concentration can also be used to establish individual therapeutic ranges.	C	Devinsky (2011) Patsalos et al. (2008)
AED discontinuation results in seizures in approximately 33% of patients.	A	Devinsky (2011) Shih & Ochoa (2009)
Avoid the use of generic medications for anticonvulsants if possible. There is some evidence of harm related to this practice.	C	Fitzgerald & Jacobson (2011)
Switching from trade-name to generic AEDs and from generic to trade-name AEDs may cause fluctuation in serum levels.	C	Fitzgerald & Jacobson (2011)
Patients with epilepsy should be screened for depression.	A	Fiest et al. (2013)
Antidepressant drugs of the selective serotonin reuptake inhibitor (SSRI) and selective norepinephrine reuptake inhibitor (SNRI) families are safe in the treatment of depressive and anxiety disorders in epilepsy.	C	Devinsky (2011)
SUDEP is likely to be caused by a combination of variables, and currently no specific guidelines have been developed.	B	Devinsky (2011)

A = consistent, good-quality, patient-oriented evidence; B = inconsistent or limited-quality, patient-oriented evidence; C = consensus, disease-oriented evidence, usual practice, expert opinion, or case series. For information about the SORT evidence rating system, go to www.aafp.org/afpsort.xml.

STROKE

Signal symptoms: Weakness, paralysis, aphasia, visual disturbances, balance dysfunction.

Etiology: A stroke occurs when a disruption in blood flow to the brain leads to brain tissue ischemia and infarction. The consequent impairment depends on the location and extent of the infarction. There are two major types of strokes: ischemic, indicating blockage of an artery, and hemorrhagic, usually resulting from a tear in an artery wall. Ischemic events account for approximately 87% of all strokes (Roger et al., 2011) and generally are classified as one of three types: thrombotic, embolic, or lacunar. Thrombotic strokes occur when an artery in the brain is blocked by a blood clot that forms as a result of an inflammatory response to an unstable atherosclerotic plaque. Embolic strokes occur when a blood clot forms elsewhere in the body or an unstable plaque breaks, travels to the brain through the circulatory system, and becomes lodged in a brain artery. Embolic strokes are generally associated with atrial fibrillation, alular disorders, heart failure, and other states associated with thrombus formation. Lacunar infarcts are a subtype of thrombotic stroke that occur in the smaller arteries that branch from main cerebral arteries.

Hemorrhagic strokes usually result from trauma or a hypertensive episode when a weakened area of an artery in or around the brain ruptures. Arteriovenous malformations also may cause hemorrhagic strokes. *Hemorrhagic transformation* is a term that refers to bleeding in the area surrounding an embolic infarct.

Occurrence: Stroke is the leading neurological cause of death and disability in the United States, with an estimated 795,000 people each year suffering a new or recurrent stroke (Roger et al., 2011).

Age: The prevalence of silent cerebral infarction between 55 and 64 years of age is 11%. This prevalence increases to 22% between 65 and 69 years of age, 28% between 70 and 74 years of age, 32% between 75 and 79 years of age, 40% between 80 and 85 years of age, and 43% at 85 years of age (Roger et al., 2011).

Gender: The stroke incidence rate is higher for men compared with women at younger ages but not at older ages. The male-to-female incidence ratio is 1.25 in those 55 to 64 years of age, 1.50 in those 65 to 74 years of age, 1.07 in those 75 to 84 years of age, and 0.76 in those 85 years of age. Each year, approximately 55,000 more women than men have a stroke (Roger et al., 2011).

Ethnicity: Native Americans, Hispanics, and African Americans are at higher risk for stroke and stroke mortality than whites. Among middle-aged adults, African Americans are 2 to 3 more times likely to have a stroke than their white peers (Roger et al., 2011).

Contributing factors: Risk factors for stroke include advanced age, family history of stroke, prior history of transient ischemic attack (TIA) or stroke, hypertension, diabetes, carotid stenosis, atrial fibrillation, hyperlipidemia, heart disease, sedentary lifestyle, smoking, alcohol abuse, obesity, and some infections (respiratory tract, periodontal disease). Less well studied risk factors include sleep apnea, antiphospholipid antibody, hyperhomocystinemia, drug abuse, hypercoagulability disorders, hormone replacement therapy or oral contraceptive use, sickle cell anemia, and other inflammatory processes.

Signs and symptoms: History may indicate a prior TIA. Patients having an ischemic stroke may report any of the following symptoms, usually with a sudden onset: weakness, numbness, or paralysis in the face, arm, or leg (usually unilateral); difficulty speaking or understanding verbal communication; blurred or decreased monocular or binocular vision; loss of balance or coordination; and severe headache. Patients with a hemorrhagic stroke may report any of the aforementioned symptoms and nausea and vomiting, altered mental status, sensitivity to light, and neck stiffness. Physical signs may include one or more of the following: decreased visual acuity or field cut, diplopia, slurred speech, and hemiparesis or sensory changes of the face, arm, or leg. A decrease in coordination or balance can occur. Acute confusional state and elevated blood pressure are also common. Any other focal signs on neurological examination should be assessed carefully. Physical examination should include repeated measures of vital signs and examination of the head and neck for signs of trauma and infection, checks of the peripheral and carotid pulses, auscultation of the neck for bruits, and a complete neurological examination for focal abnormalities.

Diagnostic tests: All patients with symptoms consistent with stroke should be transported via emergency medical services (EMS) to the nearest certified stroke facility for comprehensive workup and treatment. Initial diagnostic tests will depend on judgment and resources of the evaluating clinician but may include a CT or MRI to evaluate for presence of hemorrhage, ECG, echocardiography, carotid duplex studies, and laboratory assessment (CBC, prothrombin time/partial thromboplastin time [PT/PTT], lipids, and complete blood chemistry). A head CT scan reveals 95% of hemorrhagic strokes immediately. Ischemic events may not be visible on CT scan for 24 to 48 hours and may be noted anywhere in the cerebral cortex, cerebellum, or brainstem. MRI is helpful in early diagnosis of ischemic or hemorrhagic strokes but may not be available in all areas. Magnetic resonance angiography is a noninvasive method of showing vascular occlusion in the head or neck. If a hemorrhagic stroke is confirmed, the patient should be referred to a neurosurgeon immediately. Further diagnostic and treatment choices will depend on results of initial assessments and time elapsed between onset of symptoms and confirmed diagnosis (Caplan, 2011).

Differential diagnosis:

- *Temporal arteritis:* This condition is ruled out based on history, physical examination, ultrasound of temporal arteries, and laboratory tests (elevated ESR, alkaline phosphatase) if indicated.
- *Vertebral disc disease:* This condition is ruled out based on history, physical examination, and x-rays as indicated.
- *Migraine:* This is ruled out based on history and physical examination.
- *Head trauma:* Trauma is ruled out based on history, physical examination, and brain imaging studies as indicated.
- *Brain tumor:* Tumor is ruled out based on history, physical examination, and brain imaging studies as indicated.
- *Meningeal infection:* This is ruled out based on history, physical examination, and lumbar puncture if indicated.
- *Seizure disorder:* Seizure disorder is ruled out based on history, physical examination, and brain imaging studies as indicated.
- *Hypoglycemia:* Hypoglycemia is ruled out based on history, physical examination, and laboratory assessment as indicated.

Treatment: Emergency transport should be initiated for patients with suspected stroke. Patients should be given nothing by mouth (NPO), and intravenous (IV) fluids (isotonic sodium chloride) should be started to maintain euvolemic status in most patients. Excessive IV fluid administration is to be avoided. Patients with fever may be treated with antipyretics, and an aggressive search for the source of fever should be initiated. Hypoglycemia and hyperglycemia should be identified and treated promptly. Both can produce symptoms that mimic ischemic stroke, and both may worsen neuronal injury. Administration of glucose in hypoglycemia produces a prompt improvement, and insulin may be started for patients with serum glucose >200 mg/dL. Optimal levels of glucose control are yet to be determined (Bruno et al., 2008). Supplemental oxygen is recommended when the patient has a documented oxygen requirement or SaO_2 <94%.

If the patient presents within 3 hours of the onset of symptoms and a hemorrhagic event is ruled out, IV tissue plasminogen activator (tPA), a thrombolytic agent, may help minimize the size of the infarct. Newer evidence suggests that some patients may still benefit from thrombolytic agents up to 4.5 hours after stroke onset (del Zoppo, Saver, Jauch, & Adams, 2009). Recommendations regarding the administration of thrombolytics, endovascular therapies, and surgical management may depend on available imaging and expertise in acute stroke management (Adams et al., 2007).

Hypertension associated with stroke usually resolves spontaneously over the first 24 hours; aggressive use of antihypertensives may reduce perfusion pressure and prolong or worsen ischemia. Rapid reduction of blood pressure regardless of the degree of hypertension may be harmful. The consensus recommendation is to lower the blood pressure only in the event the systolic pressure is >220 mm Hg or diastolic blood pressure is >120 mm Hg. However, a systolic pressure >185 mm Hg or a diastolic pressure >110 mm Hg is a contraindication for thrombolytic therapy. Therefore, the management of blood pressure in acute ischemic stroke will depend on whether the patient is a candidate for thrombolytic therapy.

Hemorrhagic events should be immediately referred for neurosurgical consultation. Control of any other comorbid disease also is indicated. Patients should be monitored at frequent intervals for signs of cerebral edema.

Follow-up: Indications for follow-up depend on the type and extent of the infarct. Rehabilitation should begin during the acute phase when possible, preferably in a stroke-specific rehabilitation environment if available. Use of standardized assessment instruments will be helpful in establishing baseline, setting goals, and tracking progress. Standardized stroke assessment instruments may be found in Box 13-2 (VA DoD, 2010). Whenever possible, the stroke survivor,

BOX 13-2

Standardized, Validated Instruments for Assessment of Stroke Survivors

Level-of-consciousness scale (Glasgow Coma Scale)
Stroke deficit scales (National Institutes of Health Stroke Scale [NIHSS]; Canadian Neurological Scale)
Global disability scale (Rankin Scale)
Measures of disability/activities of daily living (Barthel Index; Functional Independence Measure [FIM™])
Mental status screening (Folstein Mini-Mental State Examination; Neurobehavioral Cognition Status Exam [NCSE])
Assessment of motor function (Fugl-Meyer; Motor Assessment Scale; Motricity Index)
Balance assessment (Berg Balance Assessment)
Mobility assessment (Rivermead Mobility Index)

Assessment of speech and language functions (Boston Diagnostic Aphasia Examination; Porch Index of Communicative Ability [PICA]; Western Aphasia Battery)
Depression scales (Beck Depression Inventory [BDI]; Center for Epidemiologic Studies Depression [CES-D]; Geriatric Depression Scale [GDS])
Measures of instrumental ADL (PGC Instrumental Activities of Daily Living; Frenchay Activities Index)
Family Assessment Device (FAD)
Health status/quality of life measures (Medical Outcomes Study [MOS] Item Short-Form Health Survey; Sickness Impact Profile [SIP]

Source: Department of Veterans Affairs, Department of Defense, & the American Heart Association/American Stroke Association, 2010.

family, and caregivers should be involved in decision making regarding treatment and care planning. Education regarding stroke, rehabilitation, recovery, and what to expect are critical for the survivor, family, and caregivers. Rehabilitation targets should be designed around (1) recovery of function, (2) cardiovascular fitness, and (3) prevention of complications and deconditioning. Risk assessments should routinely be performed for the common complications following stroke, including swallowing disorders, malnutrition, bowel and bladder incontinence, skin breakdown, deep vein thrombosis, pain, falls, and osteoporosis. Assessment of cognition, communication abilities, and psychosocial status should be undertaken regularly in the subacute and chronic phases of stroke recovery. After a stroke, patients should be followed regularly by a primary care provider to assess periodically changes in level of function, monitor risk factors, control comorbid illnesses, and implement prevention strategies for secondary stroke prevention (VA DoD, 2010).

Sequelae: Stroke survivors are most commonly at high risk for complications related to immobility such as skin breakdown, loss of muscle strength, and pulmonary compromise. Speech and swallowing difficulties also may persist after a stroke. Depression and anxiety are also common consequences of stroke. Stroke survivors should be screened for depression regularly and treated as indicated. Monitor the physical and emotional well-being of patients and families. Finally, all stroke survivors are at risk for recurrent stroke and other cardiovascular events. Appropriate strategies should be implemented for prevention/prophylaxis.

Prevention/prophylaxis: Strategies to prevent stroke are similar to strategies used to prevent other cardiovascular diseases—control of hypertension, diabetes, hyperlipidemia, and cardiac disease through lifestyle and pharmacotherapeutic agents. Encourage patients to increase physical activity levels, exercise regularly, lose weight (if indicated), and stop smoking. Prophylactic treatment with antiplatelet agents is recommended for patients with prior TIA or stroke and/or identified carotid disease unless otherwise contraindicated. Many clinicians now use combinations of antiplatelet agents to inhibit platelet aggregation at multiple points on the clotting cascade. Prophylactic warfarin therapy is recommended in patients with known arrhythmias or hypercoagulation states, but the international normalized ratio (INR) must be monitored regularly and should be kept within the range of 2.0 to 3.0. Newer agents are available that are approved for eligible patients that may be preferable because they do not require INR monitoring, but long-term data on safety and efficacy are not available. Carotid endarterectomy may be considered for stenosis >50%.

Referral: Referrals depend on the type and severity of impairment from the stroke and the influence of any comorbid illnesses. Referrals to physiatry (rehabilitation medicine), neurology, psychiatry, and cardiology for consultation are common.

Education: Education for patients after a stroke should emphasize cause of the stroke, limitation of risk factors to prevent future events, and early identification and treatment of recurrent stroke. A home exercise program or other therapies to maintain or improve functional levels should be introduced and strongly encouraged. Exercise has been shown to improve functionality many years after the index stroke (Globas et al., 2011). Recommendations for physical activity following stroke have been published and suggest a combination of aerobic, strength, and flexibility exercise, but a specific exercise program must be tailored to the individual's neurological and functional deficit profile (Gordon et al., 2004). Motivation to exercise can be enhanced by bolstering self-efficacy for exercise activities (Shaughnessy, Resnick, & Macko, 2006). Access to support groups for patients and caregivers should be provided. The importance of periodic follow-up with the primary care provider for recovery monitoring, surveillance for complications, ongoing management of risk factors, and secondary prevention should be emphasized. The National Stroke Association can be contacted at www.stroke.org and 1-800-STROKES (1-800-787-6537).

CLINICAL RECOMMENDATION	EVIDENCE RATING	REFERENCES
Suspected stroke symptoms should trigger EMS, with a goal of door to treatment (tPA, if indicated) of 60 minutes.	A	Adams et al. (2007)
Expansion of the time to treatment window may extend to 4.5 hours following onset of symptoms for patients who meet identified criteria.	B	del Zoppo et al. (2009)
Appropriate management of medical comorbidities (hypoglycemia and hyperglycemia, hyperthermia, hypoxia, arrhythmias, etc.) during the acute, subacute and chronic phases of stroke recovery can significantly improve outcomes.	A	Adams et al. (2007) Bruno et al. (2008) Caplan (2011)
Treatment of stoke in a stroke-specialty or stroke-certified environment is associated with better outcomes.	A	VA/DoD (2010)
Initial assessment for rehabilitation should have special emphasis on medical status, risk of complications (swallowing disorders, malnutrition, bowel and bladder incontinence, skin breakdown, deep vein thrombosis, pain, falls, and osteoporosis) and function.	A	VA/DoD (2010)
Clinicians should use standardized, validated assessment instruments to evaluate the patient's stroke-related impairments, functional status, and participation in community and social activities. The NIH Stroke Scale is recommended for use as an initial assessment during acute stroke.	A	VA/DoD (2010)
Rehabilitation therapy should start as early as medical stability is reached and continue as needed and tolerated to reach premorbid or optimal levels of independence and to prevent cardiovascular deconditioning.	A	VA/DoD (2010)

Continued

CLINICAL RECOMMENDATION	EVIDENCE RATING	REFERENCES
Stroke survivors should be assessed for motor, sensory cognitive, ADL, instrumental ADL, activity, and psychosocial impairments from admission to discharge, and treatment plans should reflect individualized goals in these domains.	A	VA/DoD (2010)
Patients should be educated about stroke. Family, social support, and community resources should be identified early and included in the plan of care.	A	VA/DoD (2010)
Stroke survivors should be regularly screened for depression and treated accordingly throughout the subacute and chronic phases of stroke recovery.	A	VA/DoD (2010)
Stroke survivors may gain strength, mobility, and cardiovascular fitness following stroke with continued progressive aerobic exercise.	B	Globas et al. (2011) Gordon, et al (2004) Shaughnessy et al. (2006)

A = consistent, good-quality, patient-oriented evidence; B = inconsistent or limited-quality, patient-oriented evidence; C = consensus, disease-oriented evidence, usual practice, expert opinion, or case series. For information about the SORT evidence rating system, go to www.aafp.org/afpsort.xml.

TRANSIENT ISCHEMIC ATTACK

Signal symptoms: Temporary monocular blindness, weakness and numbness on one side of the body, speech impairment, impairments in balance and/or coordination.

Description: A transient ischemic attack (TIA) is a neurological impairment of presumed ischemic origin, lasting less than 24 hours. Attacks usually last less than 10 minutes.

Etiology: A TIA is a transient episode of neurological dysfunction caused by a focal brain, spinal cord, or retinal ischemia without acute infarction (Easton et al., 2009). Transient hypotension, in conjunction with significant carotid stenosis, also may cause a TIA. The primary significance of TIA lies in the heightened short-term risk of stroke, with most studies finding that one-quarter to one-half of the strokes that occur within the first 3 months following TIA occur within the first 2 days (Easton et al., 2009).

Occurrence: Between 200,000 and 500,000 TIAs are diagnosed annually in the United States. The overall race-, age-, and gender-adjusted incidence rate for TIA in the U.S. population was 83 per 100,000, with age, race, and gender adjusted to the 1990 U.S. population (Kleindorfer et al., 2005). Emergency department (ED) visits for TIAs occur at an approximate rate of 1.1 per 1000 in the U.S. population, and TIAs are diagnosed in 0.3% of ED visits (Edlow, Kim, Pelletier, & Camargo, 2006). TIA carries a particularly high short-term risk of stroke, and approximately 15% of diagnosed strokes are preceded by TIAs.

Age: The incidence of TIAs increases with age, from 1 to 3 cases per 100,000 in those younger than 35 years to up to 1500 cases per 100,000 in those older than 85 years (Kleindorfer et al., 2005). TIAs can occur at any age, but risk increases exponentially with age.

Gender: The incidence of TIAs in men, 101 cases per 100,000 people, is significantly higher than that in women, 70 cases per 100,000 people (Bots, van der Wilk, Koudstaal, Hofman, & Grobbee, 1997).

Ethnicity: The incidence of TIAs in blacks, 98 cases per 100,000 people, is higher than that in whites, 81 cases per 100,000 people. Controversy exists regarding whether race influences emergent workup following TIA (Jacobs et al., 2006; White et al., 2005). Blacks and men had significantly higher rates of TIA than whites and women. Risk of stroke after TIA was 14.6% at 3 months, and risk of TIA/stroke/death was 25.2%. Age, race, and sex were not associated with recurrent TIA or subsequent stroke in the U.S. population, but age was associated with mortality.

Contributing factors: Risk factors for TIAs include advanced age, hypertension, diabetes, carotid stenosis, atrial fibrillation, hyperlipidemia, heart disease, sedentary lifestyle, smoking, alcohol abuse, obesity, and some infections (respiratory tract, periodontal disease). Less well studied risk factors include antiphospholipid antibody, hyperhomocystinemia, drug abuse, and hypercoagulability disorders.

Signs and symptoms: TIAs often are diagnosed on the basis of history alone because symptoms often resolve before a patient can seek health care. Patients report a sudden onset of neurological symptoms that diminish or resolve spontaneously. Examples of such symptoms include monocular blindness, weakness or numbness on one side of the body, and disturbed speech. Other signs and symptoms may be more nonspecific in nature, such as dizziness, vertigo, nausea and vomiting, paresthesia, ataxia, diplopia, dysarthria, generalized weakness, or loss of consciousness. Complete neurological and cardiovascular examinations are indicated. Cardiac physical examination may reveal a carotid bruit, cardiac arrhythmia, or heart murmur during auscultation. Blood pressure may be elevated.

Diagnostic tests: Diagnostic evaluation should include brain imaging within 24 hours of symptom onset. Diffusion-weighted MRI is preferred if available. The goals of imaging are to obtain evidence of a vascular origin for symptoms; exclude an alternative, nonischemic origin; ascertain the underlying vascular nature of the event; and identify the prognostic outcome category (Easton et al., 2009). Carotid duplex ultrasound is the most common and widely available method for evaluating extracranial circulation, but CT angiography and magnetic resonance angiography are alternatives with comparable sensitivity and specificity, although they carry risks, especially if contrast is used. Noninvasive testing of the intracranial vasculature can reliably exclude intracranial stenosis, but for reliable diagnosis of the presence and degree of intracranial stenosis, catheter angiography is necessary to confirm abnormalities detected with noninvasive testing methods.

There are limited data to guide the recommendation of cardiac evaluation in patients with TIA alone. Cardiac tests commonly used in the evaluation of stroke include ECG, echocardiography, and Holter monitoring. No systematic studies have been performed to assess the value of blood test in patients with TIA, but routinely obtained laboratory tests in the case of suspected stroke include a CBC, a chemistry panel, basic coagulation studies, and a fasting lipid panel (Easton et al., 2009).

Differential diagnosis:
- *Focal seizures:* Seizures are ruled out based on history, physical examination, MRI, and EEG.
- *Migraine:* Migraine is ruled out based on history and physical examination.
- *Drug or alcohol intoxication:* Intoxication is ruled out based on history, physical examination, and toxicology screen.
- *Cervical disc osteophyte:* This is ruled out based on history, physical examination, and x-rays as indicated.
- *Hypoglycemia:* Hypoglycemia is ruled out based on history, physical examination, and metabolic panel.
- *Brain tumor:* Tumor is ruled out based on history, physical examination, and brain imaging.

Treatment: If a TIA is suspected based on history and neurological and cardiac examinations, an ABCD2 score should be calculated to assess risk for early stroke. Treatment for TIA focuses on a multifaceted approach to prevention of stroke. Identify and control all modifiable risk factors, and aggressive management of hypertension, diabetes, and hyperlipidemia is warranted. Simvastatin may be considered as an agent to reduce cholesterol if necessary, because it has demonstrated direct benefits in reducing the incidence of strokes in a high-risk population. Blood glucose for those with diabetes or insulin resistance should be managed closely.

Prevention of clot formation is a priority and can be accomplished through multiple means, depending on patient profile, risk factors, and history. Consideration of the underlying disease processes will dictate the selection of treatment and continued evaluation (see follow-up and referral).

Surgical management (carotid endarterectomy) may be recommended for patients who have stenosis of 70% to 99% and a history of at least one TIA or minor stroke. Clinical features that influence stroke risk should be considered in the decision to pursue surgical management for patients with a less severe stenosis (50% to 69%).

Follow-up: Monitor patients periodically for continuation of symptoms, adequacy of antithrombotic therapy, and control of any comorbid illnesses.

Sequelae: About one-third of patients who have a TIA go on to have a stroke. Of those, 50% have a stroke within 1 year after the TIA; 20% of strokes occur within 1 month. A higher risk of myocardial infarction also is noted in this population.

Prevention/prophylaxis: See under Treatment.

Referral: All patients with suspected TIA or stroke should be referred to EMS and evaluated in an emergency setting if presenting for care within 72 hours of symptom onset, because it is not possible to know if focal ischemia is infarction without imaging. Though hospitalization rates vary widely across geographical regions of the country, admission allows for close monitoring, rapid evaluation, and intervention, particularly in those at high risk of subsequent stroke. An ophthalmologist may be consulted for patients whose complaints include transient monocular blindness. Patients with any gross cardiac abnormalities should be referred to a cardiologist.

Education: Focus patient education on the cause of the TIA and explain the increased risk of stroke, appropriate prevention modalities, and modification of risk factors. The National Stroke Association has an informative website at www.stroke.org; the association also can be contacted at 1-800-STROKES (1-800-787-6537).

CLINICAL RECOMMENDATION	EVIDENCE RATING	REFERENCES
Patients with suspected TIA should be evaluated as soon as possible after an event.	B	Easton et al. (2009)
Patients with TIA should undergo neuroimaging evaluation within 24 hours of symptom onset. Diffusion-weighted MRI is the preferred brain diagnostic imaging modality, but if not available, head CT should be performed.	A	Easton et al. (2009)
Noninvasive imaging of cervicocephalic vessels should be performed routinely as part of the evaluation for patients with suspected TIA.	A	Easton et al. (2009)
Noninvasive testing of the intracranial vasculature reliably excludes intracranial stenosis. Reliable diagnosis of the presence and degree of intracranial stenosis requires catheter angiography to confirm abnormalities detected with noninvasive testing.	A	Easton et al. (2009)
Initial assessment of extracranial vasculature may involve any of the following: carotid ultrasound/transcranial Doppler, magnetic resonance angiography, or CT angiography, depending on local availability and expertise and characteristics of the patient.	B	Easton et al. (2009)

CLINICAL RECOMMENDATION	EVIDENCE RATING	REFERENCES
ECG should occur as soon as possible after TIA. Prolonged cardiac monitoring (inpatient or outpatient) is useful in patients with an unclear origin after initial brain imaging and ECG.	B	Easton et al. (2009)
Echocardiography (at least transthoracic echocardiography) is reasonable in the evaluation of patients with suspected TIAs in patients in whom no other cause has been identified. Transthoracic echocardiogram (TTE) is useful in identifying patent foramen ovale, aortic arch atherosclerosis, and valvular disease, and such knowledge may alter management.	B	Easton et al. (2009)
Routine blood tests (CBC, chemistry, coagulation studies, and fasting lipid panel) are reasonable in the evaluation of suspected TIA.	B	Easton et al. (2009)
It is reasonable to hospitalize patients with TIA if they present within 72 hours of the event and any of the following criteria are present: (a) ABCD2 score ≥3 (b) ABCD2 score 0–2 and uncertainty that a diagnostic workup can be completed within 2 days as an outpatient (c) ABCD2 score 0–2 and other evidence that indicates the patient's event was caused by focal ischemia	C	Easton et al. (2009)
Treatment for TIA is focused on prevention of stroke and aggressive management of persistent stroke risk factors.	A	Sacco et al. (2006)
For patients with recent TIA or ischemic stroke within the last 6 months and ipsilateral severe (70%–99%) carotid artery stenosis, carotid endarterectomy (CEA) by a surgeon with a perioperative morbidity and mortality of <6% is recommended. For patients with recent TIA or ischemic stroke and ipsilateral moderate (50%–69%) carotid stenosis, CEA is recommended, depending on patient-specific factors such as age, gender, comorbidities, and severity of initial symptoms. When the degree of stenosis is <50%, there is no indication for CEA.	A	Sacco et al. (2006)
For patients with ischemic stroke or TIA with persistent or paroxysmal (intermittent) atrial fibrillation, anticoagulation with adjusted-dose warfarin (target INR, 2.5; range, 2.0 to 3.0) is recommended. For patients unable to take warfarin, aspirin 325 mg/day is recommended.	A	Sacco et al. (2006)

Continued

CLINICAL RECOMMENDATION	EVIDENCE RATING	REFERENCES
For patients with an ischemic stroke or TIA caused by an acute myocardial infarction in whom left ventricular mural thrombus is identified by echocardiography or another form of cardiac imaging, oral anticoagulation is reasonable, aiming for an INR of 2.0 to 3.0 for at least 3 months and up to 1 year.	B	Sacco et al. (2006)
Aspirin should be used concurrently for ischemic coronary artery disease during oral anticoagulant therapy in doses up to 162 mg/day.	A	Sacco et al. (2006)
For patients with ischemic stroke or TIA who have dilated cardiomyopathy, either warfarin (INR, 2.0 to 3.0) or antiplatelet therapy may be considered for prevention of recurrent events.	C	Sacco et al. (2006)
For patients with ischemic stroke or TIA who have rheumatic mitral valve disease, whether or not atrial fibrillation is present, long-term warfarin therapy is reasonable, with a target INR of 2.5 (range 2.0 to 3.0). Antiplatelet agents should not routinely be added to warfarin to avoid the additional bleeding risk.	C	Sacco et al. (2006)
For patients with noncardioembolic ischemic stroke or TIA, antiplatelet agents rather than oral anticoagulation are recommended to reduce the risk of recurrent stroke and other cardiovascular events. Aspirin (50 to 325 mg/day), the combination of aspirin and extended-release dipyridamole, and clopidogrel are all acceptable options for initial therapy.	A	Sacco et al. (2006)
For patients with ischemic stroke or TIA with rheumatic mitral valve disease, whether or not atrial fibrillation is present, who have a recurrent embolism while receiving warfarin, adding aspirin (81 mg/day) is suggested.	C	Sacco et al. (2006)
The addition of aspirin to clopidogrel increases the risk of hemorrhage and is not routinely recommended for ischemic stroke or TIA patients.	A	Sacco et al. (2006)

A = consistent, good-quality, patient-oriented evidence; B = inconsistent or limited-quality, patient-oriented evidence; C = consensus, disease-oriented evidence, usual practice, expert opinion, or case series. For information about the SORT evidence rating system, go to www.aafp.org/afpsort.xml.

CASE STUDY

Sue is a 68-year-old healthy white woman with no significant medical history. She is in the office today with complaint of intractable nausea and vomiting for the past 5 weeks with an 11 lb weight loss. On review of systems she also has noted a dull, persistent headache, difficulty with concentration, and some blurred vision. She states these other problems are likely due to this gastrointestinal "bug" that will not go away. She denies similar symptoms in the past. Her mother died from complications of diabetes at 42 years old, her father died from a heart attack in his late fifties, one brother died in a car accident in his late teens, and the other died from complications of diabetes in his late teens. She is a nurse, married, with two adult children who are in good health. She drinks a beer or glass of wine on most days, sometimes two. She has never used tobacco products or illegal drugs.

1. What additional subjective data are you seeking?

2. What additional objective data will you be assessing for?

3. What are the differential diagnoses that you are considering?

4. What laboratory tests will help you rule out some of the differential diagnoses?

5. What radiological examinations would you order?

6. What is your treatment and specific information on the prescription you will give to this patient?

7. What are the potential complications from the treatment ordered?

8. What are the additional specific laboratory tests you may consider ordering?

9. What additional patient teaching may be needed?

10. Will you be looking for a consultation?

REFERENCES

Assessment

American Association of Neuroscience Nurses. (2009). *Neurologic assessment of the older adult. A guide for nurses.* Glenview, IL: American Association of Neuroscience Nurses.

Berstein, I. H., Lacritz, L., Barlow, C. F., Weiner, M. F., & DeFina, L. F. (2011). Psychometric evaluation of the Montreal Cognitive Assessment (MoCA) in three diverse samples. *Clinical Neuropsychologist, 25*(1), 119–126.

Inzitari, M., Pozzi, C., Ferrucci, L., Chiarantini, D., Rinaldi, L. A., Baccini, M., . . . Di Bari, M. (2008). Subtle neurological abnormalities as risk factors for cognitive and functional decline, cerebrovascular events, and mortality in older community dwelling older adults. *Archives of Internal Medicine, 168*(12), 1270–1276.

Johns, E., Phillips, N., Nasreddine, Z., Bergman, L., Solomon, S., Desormeau, J., . . . Chertkow, H. (2010, February). *Level of education and performance on the Montreal Cognitive Assessment (MoCA): new recommendations for education corrections.* Centre for Research in Human Development Annual Conference (CRDH), Montreal, QC. Retrieved from http://crdh.concordia.ca/about/presentations.html

Larner, A. J. (2006). Neurological signs of aging. In M. S. J. Pathy, A. J. Sinclair, & J. E. Morley (Eds.), *Principles and practice of geriatric medicine* (4th ed., pp. 743–750). Hoboken, NJ: John Wiley & Sons.

LeBlond, R. F., Brown, D. D., & DeGowin, R. L. (2009). *DeGowin's diagnostic examination* (9th ed.). New York City, NY: McGraw-Hill Medical.

Tariq, S. H., Tumosa, N., Chibnall, J. T, Perry, M. H., III, & Morley, J. E. (2006). Comparison of the Saint Louis University mental status examination and the mini-mental state examination for detecting dementia and mild neurocognitive disorder—a pilot study. *The American Journal of Geriatric Psychiatry, 14*(11), 900–910. doi: 10.1097/01.JGP.0000221510.33817.86

Williams, M. (2008). *Geriatric physical diagnosis.* Jefferson, NC: McFarland & Co.

Brain Tumor

Behin, A., Hoang-Xuan, K., Carpentier, A. F., & Delattre, J.-Y., (2003). Primary brain tumors in adults. *Lancet, 361*(9354), 323–331.

Chandana, S. R., Movva, S., Arora, M., & Singh, T. (2008). Primary brain tumors in adults. *American Academy of Family Physicians, 77*(10), 1423–1430.

DeAngelis, L. M. (2001). Brain tumors. *New England Journal of Medicine, 344,* 114–123.

Michaud, D., Schiff, D., & Batchelor, T. (2010). Incidence of primary brain tumors. *UpToDate.* Retrieved November 4, 2011, from www.uptodate.com

Wong, E. T., & Wu, J. (2010). Clinical presentation and diagnosis of brain tumors. *UpToDate.* Retrieved November 4, 2011, from www.uptodate.com

Parkinson's Disease

Blonder, L., & Slevin, J. (2011). Emotional dysfunction in Parkinson's disease. *Behavioral Neurology, 24*(3), 201–217.

Burke, R., Dauer, W., & Vonsattel, J. (2008). A critical evaluation of the Braak staging scheme for Parkinson's disease. *Annals of Neurology, 64*(5), 485–491.

Chillag-Talmor, O., Giladi, N., Linn, S., Gurevich, T., El-Ad, B., Silverman, B., . . . Peretz, C. (2011). Use of a refined drug tracer algorithm to estimate prevalence and incidence of Parkinson's disease in a large Israeli population. *Journal of Parkinson's Disease, 1*(1), 35–47.

Haerer, A. (1992). *The neurological exam.* Philadelphia, PA: J. B. Lippincott.

Hunt, A., & Sethi, K. (2006). The pull test. *Movement Disorders, 21*(7), 894–899.

Olson, E., Johnson, B., & Thompson, L. (1990). The hazards of immobility. *American Journal of Nursing, 90*(3), 43–44, 46–88.

Petzinger, G., Fisher, B., Van Leeuwen, J., Vukovic, M., Akopian, G., Meshul, C., . . . Jakowec, M. (2010). Enhancing neuroplasticity in the basal ganglia: the role of exercise in Parkinson's disease. *Movement Disorders, 25*(S1), S141–S145.

Ponsen, M., Stoffers, D., Wolters, E., Booij, J., & Berendse, H. (2010). Olfactory testing combined with dopamine transporter imaging as a method to detect prodromal Parkinson's disease. *Journal of Neurology, Neurosurgery & Psychiatry, 81*(4), 396–399.

Sanchez-Ferro, A., Benito-Leon, J., & Gomez-Esteban, J. C. (2013). The management of orthostatic hypotension in Parkinson's disease. *Frontiers in Neurology, 4*(64), 755–760.

Smith, Y., Wichmann, T., Factor, S. A., & DeLong, M. R. (2011). Parkinson's disease therapeutics: new developments and challenges since the introduction of levodopa. *Neuropsychopharmacology, 37*(1), 213–246. doi: 10.1038/npp.2011.212

Van Den Eeden, S., Tanner, C., Bernstein, A., Fross, R., Leimpeter, A., Bloch, D., & Nelson, L. (2003). Incidence of Parkinson's disease: variation by age, gender and race/ethnicity. *American Journal of Epidemiology, 157*(11), 1015–1022.

Vernon, G. M. (2009). Parkinson's disease and the nurse practitioner: diagnostic and management challenges. *The Journal for Nurse Practitioners, 5*(3), 195–206.

Wright-Willis, A., Evanoff, B., Lian, M., Criswell, S., & Racette, B. (2010). Geographic and ethnic variation in Parkinson disease: a population-based study of US Medicare beneficiaries. *Neuroepidemiology, 34*(3), 143–151.

Peripheral Neuropathy

Andreoli, T. E., Carpenter, C. J., Griggs, R. C., & Benjamin, I. J. (2007). *Cecil essentials of medicine* (7th ed.). Philadelphia, PA: Saunders/Elsevier.

Azhary, H., Farooq, M. U., Bhanushali, M., Majid, A., & Kassab, M. Y. (2010). Peripheral neuropathy: differential diagnosis and management. *American Family Physician, 81*(7), 887–892.

Backon, A. M., & Glanzman, R. L. (2003). Gabapentin: dosing for neuropathic pain: evidence from randomized, placebo controlled clinical trials. *Clinical Therapy, 25*(1), 81–104.

Botek, G., Anderson, M. A., & Taylor, R. (2010). Charcot neuroarthropathy: an often overlooked complication of diabetes. *Cleveland Clinic Journal of Medicine, 77*(9), 593–599.

Bril, V., England, J., Franklin, G. M., Backonja, M., Cohen, J., Del Toro, D., . . . Zochodne, D. (2011). Evidence-based guideline: treatment of painful diabetic neuropathy. Report of the American Academy of Neurology, the American Association of Neuromuscular and Electrodiagnostic Medicine, and the American Academy of Physical Medicine and Rehabilitation. *Neurology, 76*(20), 1758–1765.

Cacchione, P. Z. (2010). Sensory changes in peripheral neuropathy. Retrieved from http://consultgerirn.org/topics/sensory

Chaudhry, V. (2008). Peripheral neuropathy. In A. Fauci, E. Braunwald, D. Kasper, S. L. Hauser, D. L. Longo, J. L. Jameson, & J. Loscalzo (Eds.), *Principles of internal medicine* (17th ed., pp. 2651–2667). New York City, NY: McGraw-Hill.

Dworkin, R. H., O'Connor, A. B., Backonja, M., Farrar, J. T., Finnerup, N. B., Jensen, T. S., . . . Wallace, M. S. (2007). Pharmacologic management of neuropathic pain: evidence-based recommendations. *Pain, 132*(3), 237–251.

England, J. B., & Asbury, A. K. (2004). Peripheral neuropathy. *Lancet, 363*(9427), 2151–2161.

England, J. D., Gronseth, G. S., Franklin, G., Carter, G. T., Kinsella, L. J., Cohen, J. A., . . . Sumner, A. J. (2009). Practice parameter: evaluation of distal symmetric polyneuropathy: role of laboratory and genetic testing (an evidence-based review). Report of the American Academy of Neurology, American Association of Neuromuscular and Electrodiagnostic Medicine, and American Academy of Physical Medicine and Rehabilitation. *Neurology, 72*(2), 185–192.

Finnerup, N. B., Sindrup, S. H., & Jensen, T. S. (2010). The evidence for pharmacological treatment of neuropathic pain. *Pain, 150*(3), 573–581.

Harati, Y., & Bosch, E. P. (2008). Disorders of peripheral nerves. In W. G. Bradley, R. B. Daroff, G. M. Fenichel, & J. Jankovich (Eds.), *Neurology in clinical practice* (5th ed.). Philadelphia, PA: Elsevier.

Hong, J. (2011). Whole body vibration therapy for diabetic peripheral neuropathic pain: a case report. *Health Science Journal, 5*(1), 66–71.

Jeffrey, S. (2000). Neuropathy linked with loss of balance. *Neurology Reviews, 8*(8), 1–3.

Kajdasz, D. K., Iyengar, S., Desaiah, D., Backonja, M., Farrar, J. T., Fishbain, D. A., . . . McQuay, H. J. (2007). Duloxetine for the management of diabetic peripheral neuropathic pain: evidence-based findings from post hoc analysis of three multicenter, randomized, double-blind, placebo-controlled, parallel-group studies. *Clinical Therapeutics,* (Suppl. 29), S2536–S2546.

Kanji, J. N., Anglin, R. S., Hunt, D. L., & Panju, A. (2010). Does this patient with diabetes have large-fiber peripheral neuropathy? *Journal of the American Medical Association, 303*(15), 1526–1532. doi:10.1001/jama.2010.428

Kararizou, E., Davaki, P., Karandreas, N., Davou, R., & Vassilopoulos, D. (2006). Polyneuropathies in the elderly: a clinico pathological study of 74 cases. *International Journal of Neuroscience, 116*(5), 629–638. doi:10.1080/00207450600592180

Lor, T. L., Boon, K. Y., Cheo, F. F., Lau, S. C., Lee, G. W., Ng, B. H., & Goh, K. J. (2009). The frequency of symptomatic sensory polyneuropathy in the elderly in an urban Malaysian community. *Neurology Asia, 14*(2), 109–113.

Mahmoud, F., & Tampi, R. R. (2011). Pharmacotherapy for neuropathic pain in the elderly: focus painful diabetic peripheral neuropathy. *Clinical Geriatrics, 19*(12), 36–40.

Mann, R. H. (2009, March). Benfotiamine in the treatment of peripheral neuropathy. *Podiatry Management,* pp. 191–196.

Marchettini, P., Teloni, L., Formaglio, F., & Lacerenza, M. (2004). Pain in diabetic neuropathy case study: whole patient management. *European Journal of Neurology, 11*(Suppl. 1), S12–S21.

Mold, J. W., Lawler, F., & Roberts, M. (2008). The health consensus consequences of peripheral neurological deficits in an elderly cohort: an Oklahoma physician resource research network study. *Journal of the American Geriatrics Society, 56,* 1259–1268.

Mold, J. W., Vesely, S. K., Keyl, B. A., Schenk, J. B., & Roberts, M. (2004). The prevalence, predictors, and consequences of peripheral sensory neuropathy in older patients. *Journal of the American Board of Family Practice, 17*(5), 309–318.

Poncelet, A. N. (1998). An algorithm for the evaluation of peripheral neuropathy. *American Family Physician, 57*(4), 1–9.

Pourmand, R. (2002). Evaluating patients with suspected peripheral neuropathy: do the right thing, not everything. *Muscle and Nerve, 26*(2), 288–290.

Schmader, K. E., Baron, R., Haanpää, M. L., Mayer, J., O'Connor, A. B., Rice, A. S. C., & Stacey, B. (2010). Treatment considerations for elderly and frail patients with neuropathic pain. *Mayo Clinic Proceedings, 85*(Suppl. 3), S26–S32. doi:10.4065/mcp2009.0646

Shy, M. E. (2007). Peripheral neuropathies. In L. Goldman & D. Ausiello (Eds.), *Cecil medicine* (23rd ed.). Philadelphia, PA: Saunders Elsevier.

Vranken, J. H. (2009). Mechanisms and treatment of neuropathic pain. *Central Nervous System Agents in Medicinal Chemistry, 9*(1), 71–78.

Zaida, D., & Alexander, M. K. (2001). Falls in the elderly: identifying and managing peripheral neuropathy. *Nurse Practitioner, 26*(1), 86–88.

Zilliox, X. L., & Russell, J. W. (2011). Treatment of diabetic sensory polyneuropathy: current treatment options. *Neurology, 13*(2), 143–159.

Restless Legs Syndrome

Benes, H., Walters, A., Allen, R., Hening, W., & Kohnen, R. (2007). Definition of restless legs syndrome, how to diagnose it and how to differentiate it from RLS mimics. *Movement Disorders, 22*(Suppl. 18), S401–S408.

Eliasson, A., & Lettieri, C. (2007). Sequential compression devices for treatment of restless legs syndrome. *Medicine, 86*(6), 317–323.

Garcia-Borreguero, D., Stillman, P., Benes, H., Buschmann, H., Chaudhuri, K., Gonzalez Rodriguez, V., . . . Zucconi, M. (2011). Algorithms for the diagnosis and treatment of restless legs syndrome in primary care. *BMC Neurology, 11*, 11–28.

Mitchell, U. H. (2011). Nondrug-related aspect of treating Ekbom disease, formerly known as restless legs syndrome. *Neuropsychiatric Disease and Treatment, 7*, 251–257.

Oertel, W., Trenkwalder, C., Zucconi, M., Benes, H., Garcia-Borreguero, D., Bassetti, C., . . . Stiasny-Kolster, K. (2007). State of the art in restless legs syndrome therapy: practice recommendations for treating restless legs syndrome. *Movement Disorders, 22*(Suppl. 18) S466–S475.

Satija, P., & Ondo, W. G. (2008). Restless legs syndrome: pathophysiology, diagnosis and treatment. *CNS Drugs, 22*(6), 497–518.

Trenkwalder, C., Hening, W., Montagna, P., Oertel, W., Allen, R., Walters, A., . . . Samaio, C. (2008). Treatment of restless legs syndrome: an evidence-based review and implications for clinical practice. *Movement Disorders, 23*(16), 2267–2302.

Seizure Disorders

Brodie, M. J., Elder, A. T., & Kaw, P. (2009). Epilepsy in later life. *Lancet Neurology, 8*(11), 1019–1030.

Devinsky, O. (2011). Sudden unexpected death in epilepsy. *New England Journal of Medicine. 365*, 1801–1811.

Fiest, K. M., Dykeman, J., Patten, S. B., Wiebe, S., Kaplan, G. G, Maxwell, C. J., . . . Jette, N. (2013). Depression in epilepsy: a systematic review and meta-analysis. *Neurology, 80*(6), 590–9. doi: 10.1212/WNL.0b013e31827b1ae0

Fitzgerald, C. L., & Jacobson, M. P. (2011). Generic substitution of levetiracetam resulting in increased incidence of breakthrough seizures. *The Annals of Pharmacotherapy, 45*(5), e27.

Martin, R., Vogtle, L., Gilliam, F., & Faught, E. (2005). What are the concerns of older adults living with epilepsy? *Epilepsy & Behavior, 7*(2), 297–300.

Patsalos, P. N., Berry, D. J., Bourgeois, B. F. D., Cloyd, J. C., Glauser, T. A., Johannessen, S. I., . . . Perucca, E. (2008), Antiepileptic drugs—best practice guidelines for therapeutic drug monitoring: a position paper by the subcommission on therapeutic drug monitoring, ILAE Commission on Therapeutic Strategies. *Epilepsia, 49*(7), 1239–1276. doi: 10.1111/j.1528-1167.2008.01561.x

Shih, J. J., & Ochoa, J. G. (2009). A systematic review of antiepileptic drug initiation and withdrawal. *Neurologist, 15*(3), 122–131. doi: 10.1097/NRL.0b013e318190ad3

Stroke

Adams, H. P., del Zoppo, G., Alberts, M. J., Bhatt, D. L., Brass, L., Furlan, A., . . . Wijdicks, E. F. M. (2007). Guidelines for the early management of adults with ischemic stroke: a guideline from the American Heart Association/American Stroke Association Stroke Council, Clinical Cardiology Council, Cardiovascular Radiology and Intervention Council, and the Atherosclerotic Peripheral Vascular Disease and Quality of Care Outcomes in Research Interdisciplinary Working Groups. *Stroke, 38*(5), 1655–1711.

Bruno, A., Kent, T. A., Coull, B. M., Shankar, R. R., Saha, C., Becker, K. J., . . . Williams, L. S. (2008). Treatment of Hyperglycemia in Ischemic Stroke (THIS): a randomized pilot trial. *Stroke, 39*(2), 384–389.

Caplan, L. R. (2011). Overview of the evaluation of stroke. In S. E. Kasner (Ed.), *UpToDate*. Retrieved from wwwuptodate.com/contents/overview-of-the-evaluation-of-stroke

del Zoppo, G. J., Saver, J. L., Jauch, E. C., & Adams, H. P. (2009). Expansion of the time window for treatment of acute ischemic stroke with intravenous tissue plasminogen activator: a science advisory from the American Heart Association/American Stroke Association. *Stroke, 40*(8), 2945–2948.

Department of Veterans Affairs, Department of Defense, & the American Heart Association/American Stroke Association. (2010). VA/DoD clinical practice guideline for the management of stroke rehabilitation. Retrieved December 8, 2011, from www.queri.research.va.gov/tools/stroke-quality/VA_DoD-Mgmt-Stroke-Rehabilitation.pdf

Globas, C., Becker, C., Cerny, J., Lam, J. M., Lindemann, U., Forrester, L. W., . . . Luft, A. R. (2011). Chronic stroke survivors benefit from high-intensity aerobic treadmill exercise: a randomized controlled trial. *Neurorehabilitation and Neural Repair.* Published online before print, September 1, 2011. doi:10.1177/1545968311418675

Gordon, N. F., Gulanick, M., Costa, F., Fletcher, G., Franklin, B. A., Roth, E. J., & Shephard, T. (2004). Physical activity and exercise recommendations for stroke survivors: an American Heart Association scientific statement from the Council on Clinical Cardiology, Subcommittee on Exercise, Cardiac Rehabilitation, and Prevention; the Council on Cardiovascular Nursing; the Council on Nutrition, Physical Activity, and Metabolism; and the Stroke Council. *Circulation, 109*(16), 2031–2041.

Roger, V. L., Go, A. S., Lloyd-Jones, D. M., Adams, R. J., Berry, J. D., Brown, T. M., . . . Wylie-Rosett, J. (2011). AHA statistical update: heart disease and stroke statistics—2011 update: a report from the American Heart Association. *Circulation, 123*, e18–e209.

Shaughnessy, M., Resnick, B., & Macko, R. F. (2006). Testing of a model of exercise behavior following stroke. *Rehabilitation Nursing, 13*(1), 15–21.

Transient Ischemic Attack

Bots, M. L., van der Wilk, E. C., Koudstaal, P. J., Hofman, A., & Grobbee, D. E. (1997). Transient neurological attacks in the general population. Prevalence, risk factors, and clinical relevance. *Stroke, 28*(4), 768–773.

Easton, J. D., Saver, J. L., Albers, G. W., Alberts, M. J., Chaturvedi, S., Feldmann, E., . . . Sacco, R. (2009). Definition and evaluation of transient ischemic attack. *Stroke, 40*(6), 2276–2293.

Edlow, J. A., Kim, S., Pelletier, A. J., & Camargo, C. A., Jr. (2006). National study on emergency department visits for transient ischemic attack, 1992–2001. *Academic Emergency Medicine, 13*(6), 666–672.

Jacobs, B. S., Birbeck, G., Mullard, A. J., Hickenbottom, S., Kothari, R., Roberts, S., & Reeves, M. J. (2006). Quality of hospital care in African American and white patients with ischemic stroke and TIA. *Neurology, 66*(6), 809–814.

Kleindorfer, D., Panagos, P., Pancioli, A., Khoury, J., Kissela, B., Woo, D., . . . Broderick, J. P. (2005). Incidence and short-term prognosis of transient ischemic attack in a population-based study. *Stroke, 36*(4), 720–723.

Sacco, R. L., Adams, R., Albers, G., Alberts, M., Benavente, O., Furie, K., . . . Tomsick, T. (2006). Guidelines for prevention of stroke in patients with ischemic stroke or transient ischemic attack. A statement for healthcare professionals from the American Heart Association/American Stroke Association Council on Stroke: co-sponsored by the Council on Cardiovascular Radiology and Intervention. *Stroke, 37*, 577–617.

White, H., Boden-Albala, B., Wang, C., Elkind, M. S., Rundek, T., Wright, C. B., & Sacco, R. L. (2005). Ischemic stroke subtype incidence among whites, blacks, and Hispanics: the Northern Manhattan Study. *Circulation, 111*(10), 1327–1331.

Endocrine, Metabolic, and Nutritional Disorders

Laurie Kennedy-Malone

ASSESSMENT

Accurate history taking of complaints associated with endocrine, metabolic, and nutritional disorders is essential for completing the examination of the older adult. Recognizing that normal aging changes of the endocrine system primarily are related to a decrease in pancreatic function (inability to sufficiently secrete insulin) and alterations in thyroid function, the nurse practitioner needs to screen older adults periodically for diabetes mellitus and thyroid disease because the incidence of these conditions increases with age (Gruenewald & Matsumato, 2009). Overall the nurse practitioner managing the care of older adults needs to differentiate among four clinical states:

1. Endocrine function that is altered relative to that of younger patients but is an expected consequence of normal aging
2. Altered endocrine function secondary to coincident nonendocrine disease but is not of known pathologic significance
3. Iatrogenic changes in endocrine function that largely reflect the polypharmacy seen in the older adult population
4. Authentic endocrinopathy (Davis, Davis, & Leinung, 2007, p. 647)

Recognition of Endocrine, Metabolic, and Nutritional Disorders

Because changes in the endocrine system may appear subtle to the older person or atypical as compared to younger patients, it may be difficult to pinpoint the onset of the presentation. Reevaluate the patient's family history for endocrine and metabolic disease. Explore with the patient any difficulty with temperature regulation, changes in skin texture, or distribution of body hair. Review with the patient any episodes of unexplained weight loss or gain, new or increased fatigue, weakness, malaise, and recent infections (Gruenewald, Kenny, & Matsumato, 2010).

Focusing the Endocrine, Metabolic, and Nutritional Disorder Review of Systems

Given the vagueness or atypical presentation of endocrine, metabolic, and nutritional disorders in older adults, specific questions directed at these conditions are imperative during the review of systems.

- Any alteration in the ability to carry out activities of daily living (ADLs) or instrumental ADLs due to fatigue or subjective weakness?
- Ask the patient or significant other(s) if there have been any acute changes in memory or mood.
- Any decrease in appetite or reported change in weight?

- Has the patient noticed any excessive thirst, appetite, or urination?
- Is the patient experiencing incontinence for the first time?
- Has the patient experienced any repeated yeast infections?
- Has the patient had a skin ulcer that has failed to heal?
- Any mouth ulcerations?
- Any new episodes of chest pain, palpitations, tachycardia, dyspnea?
- Has the patient noticed a new onset of constipation or diarrhea?
- Has the patient noticed any complaints of paresthesias or carpal tunnel syndrome?
- Has the patient reported any hoarseness of the voice?
- Has the patient experienced vertigo or gait disturbances?
- Are there any other symptoms that could be clustered to form a differential diagnosis?
- Any changes in the color or texture of the skin?
- Any new presentation of abdominal pain and associated symptoms such as nausea or vomiting?

It is important to determine from the patient what therapeutic measures have been initiated or prescribed in the past to alleviate any of the symptoms and what response occurred following treatment (LeBlond, Brown, & DeGowin, 2009).

Approach to the Physical Examination

The physical examination should focus on the clinical signs of endocrine, metabolic, and nutritional disorders prevalent in older adults, recognizing, however, that they may present atypically. Evaluation of older vital signs and previous weight and height should be noted when recording current measures; note differences that could be indicative of unintentional weight loss (malnutrition and/or failure to thrive), vertebral fractures (reduction in inches), and alteration in temperature, pulse, respiration, and blood pressure (underlying thyroid disease).

Examine the skin for changes in texture, temperature, evidence of infection and/or rashes, or open, nonhealing wounds. Inspect the hair distribution and note any dryness, coarseness, or brittleness of hair. Has the hair distribution of the eyebrows changed? (This is a presentation found in hypothyroidism known as Queen Anne's sign.) Note any changes to the nail beds. Are they brittle, cracked, peeling, or discolored? Examination of the tongue and mouth could reveal signs of nutritional deficiencies (depapillated tongue and cheilitis caused by vitamin B_{12} deficiency). Perform a thyroid examination, looking for enlargement, tenderness, and evidence of goiter or nodularity. A thorough cardiac and respiratory examination is essential given the new manifestations of conditions such as atrial fibrillation, hypertension, or heart failure in patients with undiagnosed hyperthyroid disease. Examine the lower extremities for edema; nonpitting edema is a clinical sign of pretibial myxedema. Neurological examination in older patients with undiagnosed diabetes mellitus may reveal alterations in temperature, vibratory sense, and sensation. A fine tremor in the fingers and hands may be noted. Reflexes in an older adult may be altered by abnormal thyroid function. Testing the patient's proximal and distal strength is also important, because weakness can manifest in thyroid disease. As patients and/or their caregivers may report changes in cognition, an objective assessment of mental status is warranted in patients with untreated thyroid disease (Davis et al., 2007; Gruenewald & Matsumato, 2009).

Medication Review

A thorough review of all medications, including over-the-counter and home remedies, is important to discern if drug–drug interactions are responsible for alterations in the absorption of medications. Certain medications may be responsible for a new onset of anorexia, diarrhea, or constipation. Essential too is a thorough review of how the patient and/or medical facility is administering the medications (timing the doses to not conflict with food). Finally, review patient adherence and understanding of the medication regimen.

ACUTE PANCREATITIS

Signal symptoms: Mild-to-severe sharp pain in the upper abdomen with possible radiation to the back or chest with nausea and vomiting accompanying the pain in about 90% of patients.

Description: Acute pancreatitis is a reversible inflammation of the pancreas, an organ that produces enzymes that aid in digestion of food. The pancreas also produces the hormone insulin, which controls the level of glucose in the blood. It is located in the upper abdomen, behind the stomach. The enzymes are secreted into the duodenum through the pancreatic duct and join with bile produced by the liver to digest food. Generally these enzymes do not become active until they reach the small intestine; however, when the pancreas is inflamed, they attack and damage the tissues that produce them. It occurs suddenly and usually resolves in a few days with treatment. However, it can be a life-threatening illness with severe complications, one being chronic pancreatitis.

Etiology: The most common cause is gallstones, which block the common bile duct. Other gallbladder diseases (approximately 40%) and alcohol use (approximately 35%) are other common causes. If not due to gallstones or alcohol use, less common but useful to investigate in the older adult are drug-induced and hypertriglyceridemia-induced pancreatitis. The possible causes of acute pancreatitis are many and include viral infections (mumps, coxsackie B, mycoplasma pneumonia, and campylobacter), abnormalities of the pancreas itself, hereditary diseases such as cystic fibrosis, autoimmune disorders such as systemic lupus erythematosus, postprocedure endoscopic retrograde cholangiopancreatography (ERCP) (approximately 3%), and trauma to the abdomen. The list of drugs causing acute pancreatitis is long and includes sulfonamides, corticosteroids, thiazide diuretics, NSAIDs, estrogens, and antibiotics such as tetracycline, among others (Carroll, Herrick, Gipson, & Lee, 2007). Several studies have reported that smoking is a risk factor for acute pancreatitis, but the latest evidence suggests that it seems to be a greater risk for progression to chronic pancreatitis. Gardner and Berk (2010) recorded median ages of onset for various etiologies: alcohol related—39 years, biliary tract related—69 years, trauma related—66 years (1.5%), drug-induced etiology—42 years (2%), ERCP related—58 years, AIDS related—31 years, and vasculitis related—36 years. Other causes not given percentages are generally less than 1%.

Occurrence: In the United States, over 200,000 persons per year are admitted to hospitals for acute pancreatitis. Although mild pancreatitis has a very low mortality rate (less than 1%), for severe acute pancreatitis with organ failure, the death rate can be as high as 30%. The overall mortality rate is 10% to 15%. Eighty percent of pancreatitis is considered mild, and those persons generally recover without complication. The other 20% have severe disease with local and systemic complications.

Age: Acute pancreatitis in the older adult occurs in as many as 30% of those older than age 65 and is associated with a mortality rate as high as 20% to 25% in this population. The reasons are attributed to diminished organ function, comorbid illnesses, increased susceptibility to infection and ischemia, and age-associated changes in the pancreas and biliary system (Skolnick, Feller, & Nanda, 2008).

Gender: Acute pancreatitis affects males more than females. The cause for males is more often related to alcohol and for females it is biliary tract disease. Hospitalizations increase with age, doubling for males and quadrupling for females ages 35 to 75.

Ethnicity: African Americans have a higher risk than do Caucasians or Native Americans. The hospitalization rates of African Americans are 3 times higher than for whites and are more pronounced for males than females. For ages 35 to 64, African American hospitalization rates are 10 times higher than for any other group (Gardner & Berk, 2010).

Contributing factors: Biliary tract disease, binge alcohol use, recent surgery, family history of high triglycerides, and age 35 to 64 are some of the contributing factors.

Signs and symptoms: Examination findings will vary depending on severity of the attack. With a mild attack, the epigastric area may be minimally tender; however, with severe episodes, there may be abdominal distention, tenderness, and guarding. Respirations may be shallow due to diaphragmatic irritation. There may be ecchymotic discoloration of the flank (Grey-Turner's sign) or in the periumbilical area (Cullen's sign), which reflect intra-abdominal hemorrhage that occurs in about 1% of cases and is associated with a poor prognosis (Steven & Conwell, 2010).

Differential diagnosis:
- Cholangitis
- Cholecystitis
- Choledocholithiasis
- Cholelithiasis
- Colon cancer
- Colonic obstruction
- Duodenal or gastric ulcers
- Diverticulitis
- Dissecting aneurysm
- Gastric or pancreatic cancer
- Myocardial infarction
- Pneumonia

Diagnostic tests: Amylase is the most frequently ordered test, which rises within 6 to 12 hours of onset of pain and peaks around 24 hours and returns to normal within 3 to 7 days (Neoptolemos, 2009). Amylase and lipase amounts are generally 3 times the normal amount during acute pancreatitis and are the most common laboratory markers used to establish a diagnosis of acute pancreatitis, lipase being more specific for pancreatitis. However, they can both be nonspecific depending on the time the abdominal pain began, other possible intra-abdominal processes, and chronic comorbid diseases such as renal insufficiency. Amylase levels may be normal in an alcoholic, and plasma lipase becomes the more sensitive and specific test. But bear in mind that the level of the pancreatic enzyme does not correlate with the severity of the disease. Another potential marker of acute pancreatitis is trypsinogen activation peptide (TAP) that becomes markedly increased and may be useful in detection of early acute pancreatitis. Other laboratory tests are a metabolic panel to look at blood urea nitrogen (BUN), creatinine, glucose, and calcium levels, as well as liver function tests, triglycerides, a complete blood count (CBC), arterial blood gases (ABGs), and a urinalysis (Carroll et al., 2007).

Radiological evidence is used to confirm or exclude the clinical diagnosis, establish a cause, assess severity, and provide guidance for therapy. An abdominal x-ray is generally done first and helps to exclude other causes of abdominal pain such as an obstruction or bowel perforation. Findings in more severe disease is an ileus or "colon cutoff sign" reflecting paucity of air in the colon due to spasm of descending colon. This may be followed by an abdominal ultrasound, which is 87% to 98% sensitive for detection of gallstones as well as for showing a diffusely enlarged hypoechoic pancreas. Abdominal computed tomography (CT) with contrast is the standard imaging technique for detecting acute pancreatitis and for assessing severity (78% sensitive and 86% specific for severe acute pancreatitis) (Steven & Conwell, 2010). Endoscopic ultrasonography (EUS) is especially helpful in documenting stones and tumors and is useful in obese patients. It can also be useful in determining which patients with acute pancreatitis would benefit from a therapeutic ERCP (100% sensitive and 91% specific for gallstones) and should be done on every patient with a first attack of acute pancreatitis to search for gallstones. Magnetic resonance cholangiopancreatography (MRCP) may be ordered to assess for inflammation or calcium deposits or for changes in the ducts of the pancreas. MRCP has been found to be as accurate as CT in predicting severity of pancreatitis and identification of pancreatic necrosis. It is a newer, noninvasive technique but does not have the interventional capacity for stone extraction, stent insertion, or biopsy, as the ERCP does (81% to 100% sensitive for detecting common bile duct stones). ERCP may be used for the less common causes of pancreatitis such as sphincter of Oddi dysfunction or pancreatic duct strictures. It is indicated for those persons who have not passed a stone during the acute attack and those with evidence of sepsis, biliary obstruction, cholangitis, elevated bilirubin worsening, or persistent jaundice or worsening pain in the presence of an abnormal ultrasound (Carroll et al., 2007; Cherian, Slvaraj, Natrayan, & Venkataraman, 2007). An exploratory laparotomy may be done to confirm the diagnosis of acute pancreatitis and should be done on all patients with mild disease before discharge because these people run up to a 40% risk of recurrence within even weeks after the first episode.

Most patients will have mild disease, but it is important to know as early as possible whether the attack is mild or severe for purposes of management and use of resources. There are several scoring systems used to identify early prognostic signs to predict the severity of pancreatitis, including the Atlanta Classification of Severe Acute Pancreatitis, Ranson's criteria, the Imrie scoring system, the APACHE II scale (Acute Physiology and Chronic Health Evaluation), and the Computed Tomography Severity Index (CTSI). Each has its pros and cons. With all scoring systems, the higher the prognostic score, the poorer the clinical outcome.

The Atlanta classification is used to compare and standardize clinical trials. It defines severe disease as that which is associated with organ failure and/or local complications such as necrosis, abscess, or pseudocysts and is characterized by a 3 or over on the Ranson criteria and an 8 or over on the APACHE II (Alexakis & Neoptolemos, 2005).

The Ranson criteria was the first system and remains the best known and most widely used but has drawbacks in that it requires 2 days worth of objective measures for the total score, 5 to be obtained on the first day and 6 evaluated within 48 hours of the onset of pain, sensitivity being only 73% and 77% to predict mortality, and the threshold for abnormal values depends on whether the pancreatitis is caused by alcohol or gallstones (Balthazar, 2002). The criteria on admission or diagnosis include the following:

- Age of more than 55 years
- White blood cell count >16,000/mm³ $(16.0 \times 10^9/L)$
- Blood glucose >200 mg/dL (11.1 mmol/L)
- Serum lactate dehydrogenase >350 U/L
- Aspartate aminotransferase (AST) >250 U/L

During the initial 48 hours:

- Hematocrit decrease >10%
- BUN increases >5 mg/dL (1.8 mmol/L)
- Serum calcium <8 mg/dL (2 mmol/L)
- Base deficit >4 mmol/L (4 mEq/L)
- Fluid sequestration >6000/mL
- PaO_2 <60 mm Hg

Scoring: One point for each criterion met. The prognostic implication is as follows: 0 to 2 means 2% mortality; 3 to 4 means 15% mortality; 5 to 6 means 40% mortality; 7 to 8 means 100% mortality.

The APACHE score can be used to assess the patient at any point during the illness but is cumbersome to use; sensitivity is 77% and specificity is 84%. Equation includes the following factors: age, rectal temperature, mean arterial pressure, heart rate, PaO_2, arterial pH, serum potassium, serum sodium, serum creatinine, hematocrit, white blood cell count, Glasgow Coma Scale score, chronic health status. *Scoring:* Can be calculated at www.sfar.org/scores2/apache22.html#calcul.

The CT Severity Index developed by Balthazar (2002) is the only scoring system to use evidence of necrotic pancreas as criteria. A key criterion for identification of patients at higher risk for fatal pancreatitis is pancreatic necrosis.

CT grade:

- A is normal pancreas (0 points)
- B is edematous pancreas (1 point)
- C is B plus mild extrapancreatic changes (2 points)
- D is severe extrapancreatic changes plus one fluid collection (3 points)
- E is multiple or extensive fluid collections (4 points)

Necrosis score:

- None (0 points)
- Less than one-third (2 points)
- Greater than one-third but less than one-half (4 points)
- Greater than one-half (6 points)

Scoring: CT grade plus necrosis score. The maximum score is 10, and a score of 6 or higher is considered severe disease.

None of the above scales is currently recognized as a criterion standard (Carroll et al., 2007).

Treatment: For acute pancreatitis, a short stay in the hospital is generally required for intravenous (IV) fluid replacement and pain management. Fluid resuscitation of up to 8 L/day is essential in the management of acute pancreatitis. Antibiotics are generally not indicated for a mild case (Steven, Parsi, & Walsh, 2009). If the ultrasound shows gallstones, a cholecystectomy should be performed during the hospital stay, generally after at least 24 hours of treatment. Patients can begin on a low-fat/low-protein diet. Persons admitted with severe acute pancreatitis or certain high-risk patients (elderly, gross obesity, diabetes) may require intensive care because multiple complications can develop within hours or days. These patients are kept on nothing-by-mouth (NPO) status with aggressive fluid hydration; enteral nutrition is safer and more effective regarding the suppression of the immune-inflammatory response (Ioannidis, Lavrentieva, & Botsios, 2008). In rare cases, acute pancreatitis can cause hypoxia, and this is more common in the older adult. Antibiotics should be used if there is evidence of pancreatic necrosis. If there is vomiting, a nasogastric tube may be inserted to remove fluid and air (Neoptolemos, 2009). Clear liquids followed by a diet high in carbohydrates and low in fat will be instituted, and the patient will be advised to have more frequent but smaller meals.

Follow-up: Treatment of the patient must address underlying causes of pancreatitis. If it is alcohol consumption, treatment should go beyond just telling the patient to quit drinking. An endocrinology consultation may be assistive for those with hypertriglycerides or hypercalcemia-induced pancreatitis. Those with medication-induced pancreatitis may benefit from a pharmacology consultation. There is an acronym based on recent evidence-based medical findings spelling out PANCREAS: Perfusion, Analgesia, Nutrition, Clinical management, Radiology, ERCP, Antibiotics, and Surgery for remembrance of management particulars (Khaliq, Dutta, Kochhar, & Singh, 2010).

Sequelae: Gallstones may be the cause of acute pancreatitis and will need to be removed. Removal of the gallbladder may be done by cholecystectomy if the pancreatitis is mild. If the pancreatitis is more severe, the gallstones may be removed using ERCP. A cholecystectomy will be performed after a full recovery from acute pancreatitis. Other possible complications can be an abscess or pseudocysts. Newly diagnosed patients with acute pancreatitis are at risk for developing prediabetes or diabetes after their initial attack (Das et al., 2013). Acute pancreatitis can also cause kidney failure. Repeated episodes of acute pancreatitis can lead to chronic pancreatitis.

Prevention/prophylaxis: Depending on the cause of the acute pancreatitis episode, the person needs to be counseled on the cause such as medication-induced pancreatitis, alcoholism, or gallstone pancreatitis.

Referral: A dietary consultation may be helpful for the patient in order for changes to be made to lessen reoccurrence, especially if the acute pancreatitis is due to high triglycerides or calcium. A referral for behavior modification can be useful for the person who continues to drink alcohol.

Education: It is necessary for persons who have had an episode of acute pancreatitis to understand the mechanism behind the episode so if there are changes to be made, they understand the importance of them.

CLINICAL RECOMMENDATION	EVIDENCE RATING	REFERENCES
Total enteral nutrition is equal to or more effective than total parenteral nutrition for nutritional management of patients with severe pancreatitis.	A	Besselink, Santvoort, Buskens, & Gooszen (2006)
Evaluate for less common causes of pancreatitis (e.g., sphincter of Oddi dysfunction, pancreas divisum, and pancreatic duct strictures) with endoscopic retrograde cholangiopancreatography.	C	Carroll et al. (2007) Cherian et al. (2007)
Contrast-enhanced computed tomography is the standard imaging technique for detection of acute pancreatitis. Computed tomography is not generally indicated for patients with mild, uncomplicated pancreatitis but should be reserved for cases of clinical or biological worsening.	C	Steven & Conwell (2010)
It is controversial whether antibiotics reduce mortality in patients with necrotic pancreatitis.	B	Steven et al. (2009)
Urgent endoscopic retrograde cholangiopancreatography is indicated in patients with or at risk for biliary sepsis.	A	Kapetanos (2010)

A = consistent, good-quality, patient-oriented evidence; B = inconsistent or limited-quality, patient-oriented evidence; C = consensus, disease-oriented evidence, usual practice, expert opinion, or case series. For information about the SORT evidence rating system, go to www.aafp.org/afpsort.xml.

CHRONIC PANCREATITIS

Signal symptoms: From 50% to 80% of people experience upper abdominal pain, often in the mid or left upper region and radiating in a bandlike fashion to the midback, and it is usually dull or boring in quality. The pain may feel worse after eating or

drinking, and also become chronic and disabling. The pain is not fleeting or transient; it tends to last several hours and for some, several weeks. Most persons experience intermittent attacks of pain at unpredictable intervals over years.

Description: Chronic pancreatitis is inflammation of the pancreas that does not heal or improve and gets worse over time and leads to permanent damage. It occurs due to the same underlying causes as acute pancreatitis; the digestive enzymes attack the pancreas but it now leads to chronic and irreversible inflammation, leading to fibrosis and calcification. This in turn results in exocrine and endocrine insufficiency causing diabetes mellitus and steatorrhea and, often, chronic, disabling pain. The TIGAR-O classification system is based on risk factors for chronic pancreatitis. TIGAR-O stands for Toxic-metabolic, Idiopathic, Genetic, Autoimmune, Recurrent, Obstructive (Nair, Lawler, & Miller, 2007).

Etiology: Seventy percent is caused by heavy and prolonged alcohol use. The chronic form can be triggered by an acute attack that damages the pancreatic duct, which causes the pancreas to become inflamed and slowly destroyed. Other causes are hereditary disorders of the pancreas, cystic fibrosis, hypercalcemia, hyperlipidemia or hypertriglyceridemia, certain autoimmune disorders, obstruction by tumors, and some medications as well as some causes that are still unknown. Autoimmune pancreatitis is a recent entity and has been found in association with Sjögren's syndrome, primary biliary cirrhosis, and renal tubular acidosis. With this particular cause of chronic pancreatitis, other characteristics seen are diffuse enlargement of the pancreas, increased circulating levels of gamma globulin, and the presence of autoantibodies.

Occurrence: It affects approximately 87,000 persons per year. Alcohol is the most common etiology in approximately 60% to 70%, but up to 30% are idiopathic, and 10% are due to rare diseases (Huffman, 2011).

Age: The onset of chronic pancreatitis related to alcoholism occurs in patients in the late thirties to forties. Older adults may develop idiopathic or obstructive pancreatitis (Shah, Farah, Goldwasser, & Agrawal, 2008).

Gender: There is an almost 4:1 ratio of occurrence between men and women. Alcohol plays a larger role in male causes and idiopathic and hyperlipidemia for females.

Ethnicity: The hospitalization rate for African Americans is 3 times higher than for Caucasians.

Contributing factors: Alcohol use remains the greatest contributing factor, accounting for 85% of the disease; idiopathic "late-onset" pancreatitis is more common in older adults. Obstructive chronic pancreatitis is caused by an ampullary tumor or adenocarcinoma of the pancreas. Pancreatic stones also have been known to develop in older adults (Shah et al., 2008). Prolonged use of medications known to contribute to acute pancreatitis can lead to the development of drug-induced chronic pancreatitis (Shah et al., 2008).

Signs and symptoms: The most important clue to a proper diagnosis of chronic pancreatitis is an accurate medical history. Persistent pain is responsible for most hospitalizations related to chronic pancreatitis. Some have no pain at all (Steven & Conwell, 2010). The pancreatic enzymes that are grossly elevated in acute pancreatitis may be normal or only mildly elevated. At times the abdominal pain goes away as the condition worsens, because the pancreas is no longer making enzymes. Other symptoms include nausea and vomiting, weight loss, diarrhea, and oily stools. Even if one's appetite is good, many with chronic pancreatitis lose weight because the body does not secrete enough enzymes to digest food so nutrients are not absorbed properly. This poor digestion leads to malnutrition and the fat in stools. Steatorrhea is the name given for the oily, smelly stools of chronic pancreatitis. During an attack, patients may assume a position of lying on the left side and drawing the knees up toward the chest in an effort to relieve some of the pain. If hyperlipidemia is present, the funduscopic examination may reveal a milky white hue in the retinal blood vessels. Occasionally a tender fullness or mass may be palpated in the epigastric area, suggesting a pseudocyst or an inflammatory mass in the abdomen. Patients with advanced disease may exhibit decreased subcutaneous fat, temporal wasting, sunken supraclavicular fossa, and other signs of malnutrition. Severe or rapid weight loss should be a red flag for the health-care provider as it generally is pointing toward pancreatic cancer.

Diagnostic tests: Symptoms between acute and chronic pancreatitis can be similar. Serum amylase and lipase levels may be slightly elevated in chronic pancreatitis but may also be normal or even decreased with the atrophy of the gland itself. Low concentrations of serum trypsin are specific for advanced chronic pancreatitis; however, they are not sensitive enough for those in the mild-to-moderate stage. If there is obstruction of the biliary tract, one may see elevated bilirubin, serum alkaline phosphatase, and hepatic transaminase levels. In the more advanced stages of pancreatitis, when malabsorption is present, the health-care provider may order blood, urine, and stool tests (testing fecal fat content) to help diagnose and also monitor progression. However, maldigestion and malabsorption do not occur until more than 90% of the pancreas is destroyed. Pancreatic function tests at present are direct tests such as determining duodenal aspirates, but although they are sensitive, they are invasive and expensive. Generally x-rays of the abdomen are first, and contrast-enhanced CT is the radiographic test of choice for diagnosis if pancreatic calcifications are found on x-ray and is used to look for complications of the disease and is helpful in planning surgical or endoscopic intervention. CT has a sensitivity of 80% and a specificity of 85%. ERCP provides the most accurate visualization of the ductal system and is regarded as the standard for diagnosing chronic pancreatitis, but the quality of the MRCP is overtaking it, limiting the use of the ERCP to cases with potential need of therapeutic intervention. Unfortunately, ERCP is also one of the reasons for chronic pancreatitis, when used to extract gallstones during an acute attack. EUS has a sensitivity of 97% and specificity of 60% and has emerged as one of the first-line diagnostic tests for early pancreatitis (Nair et al., 2007). Although late-stage chronic pancreatitis is often readily apparent on imaging tests, the diagnosis of early ("minimal change") chronic pancreatitis is more challenging (Shah et al., 2008).

Differential diagnosis:
- Ampullary carcinoma
- Cholangitis
- Cholecystitis
- Crohn's disease
- Chronic gastritis
- Intestinal perforation
- Mesenteric artery ischemia
- Myocardial infarct
- Pancreatic cancer
- Peptic ulcer disease
- Pneumonia

Treatment: Optimal management of chronic pancreatitis includes pain management, improvement of maldigestion, and management of any complications (Steven & Conwell, 2010). The treatment also includes modifying behaviors that exacerbate the disease. Cessation of consumption of alcohol and tobacco, if part of a patient's history, is extremely important. Treatment is also directed toward pain relief and management of complications. In the beginning a person may require IV fluids for hydration and pain management as well as pancreatic enzymes taken with each meal to help the person digest food. The person will be advised to drink plenty of nutritional support. Nasogastric tube feedings may be necessary for a few weeks if the person continues to lose weight. Limiting caffeinated beverages and not smoking or consuming alcohol is strongly advised. The pancreas is the key player in the digestion of fat, so if the pancreas cannot properly digest fat, one can have fatty or oily stools. So giving up high-fat meals, such as fried foods or fatty meats and cheeses, may be in a person's best interest. Use low-fat or fat-free dairy products and meats, along with low-fat cooking methods. The pancreas may also be stimulated by large meals of any kind, so avoid overloading the pancreas with a large intake at any one time. Six to 10 meals throughout the day along with snacks are best. Oral supplementation of fat-soluble vitamins (A, D, E, and K) and vitamin B_{12} is recommended (Obideen & Wehbi, 2011). Pain relief treatment options consist of analgesics coupled with antidepressants; NSAIDs and acetaminophen are first-line agents with long- and short-acting narcotics such as Ultram. Narcotic addiction is a common consequence of treatment and should be closely monitored (Huffman, 2011). In the case of exocrine pancreatic insufficiency, supplementation with enzymes is the recommended therapy (Shah et al., 2008).

Follow-up: If alcohol and/or smoking are among the habits of the patient, these are best treated by a team approach using a chemical dependency counselor, psychologist, or mental health nurse practitioner. The patient will be seen back for a stool enzyme quantification assay.

Sequelae: Complications can occur if the person continues to consume large amounts of alcohol, which will cause sudden bouts of abdominal pain. Chronic pancreatitis can also lead to calcification of the pancreas, where the tissue hardens and surgery may be necessary to remove part of the pancreas. Longstanding inflammation in the pancreas caused by chronic pancreatitis is a risk factor for developing pancreatic cancer. Benign cysts, called pseudocysts, are formed of pancreatic fluid and surrounded by a fibrous wall. However, these cysts can also fill with fluid and debris, become infected, and rupture. Biliary obstruction and gastric outlet obstruction may occur because of compression of the bile duct. If the beta cells of the pancreas are destroyed, diabetes may develop, and insulin and diet will be recommended also with frequent blood glucose monitoring (Steven & Conwell, 2010). When medical management no longer relieves pain, when patients are significantly malnourished, or when quality of life is decreased greatly, surgical intervention should be considered. Patients with chronic pancreatitis are at risk for developing diabetes; caution is advised when regulating glycemic control in older adults to prevent episodes of hypoglycemia (Shah et al., 2008).

Prevention/prophylaxis: Once a normal diet is resumed (low in fat and high in protein and carbohydrates), the person will be placed on pancreatic enzymes (a minimum of 30,000 units of lipase) for treatment of the steatorrhea and malabsorption. The enzymes are taken with every meal and help digest food and help the person gain weight. Response to enzyme therapy is measured by a 72-hour stool fat quantification. A daily proton pump inhibitor may be added to those with refractory therapy because gastric acid may denature exogenous enzymes. Medium-chain triglycerides (MCTs), a form of dietary fat, are more easily digested and absorbed than the long-chain triglycerides found in most foods. MCTs are available as oil that can be mixed with fruit juice. MCTs are a good source of calories for people with chronic pancreatitis who have lost weight and who do not respond to dietary changes or pancreatic enzyme supplements (Freedman, 2010). Those persons with a known reason for chronic pancreatitis, other than smoking or alcohol, should have those reasons corrected if possible.

Referral: Surgical intervention is indicated when there is an anatomical complication correctable by mechanical intervention and includes an abscess, fistula, and fixed obstruction such as a stone, pseudocyst, stenosis, or a varietal hemorrhage due to splenic vein thrombosis. Pancreatic resection is reserved for those with small duct disease or pain unresponsive to medical management (Steven & Conwell, 2010).

Education: All persons with chronic pancreatitis should have a consultation with a dietitian concerning a diet low in fat. They should also have instruction on how to cook low in fat and how to portion out small, frequent meals.

CLINICAL RECOMMENDATION	EVIDENCE RATING	REFERENCES
Pancreatic enzyme supplementation is indicated for steatorrhea and malabsorption and may help relieve pain in patients with chronic pancreatitis.	B	Freedman (2010) Nair et al. (2007)
Contrast-enhanced computed tomography is the recommended initial imaging study in patients with suspected chronic pancreatitis.	C	Nair et al. (2007)
Magnetic resonance cholangiopancreatogaphy and endoscopic ultrasonography provide similar diagnostic performance as endoscopic retrograde cholangiopancreatography for evaluation of pancreatic parenchyma and the duct system.	C	Nair et al. (2007)

A = consistent, good-quality, patient-oriented evidence; B = inconsistent or limited-quality, patient-oriented evidence; C = consensus, disease-oriented evidence, usual practice, expert opinion, or case series. For information about the SORT evidence rating system, go to www.aafp.org/afpsort.xml.

DIABETES MELLITUS, TYPES 1 AND 2

Signal symptoms: Anorexia, paresthesias, proteinuria, chronic skin infections, blurred vision, nausea, gastroparesis, yeast vaginitis, impotence, fatigue, weight loss or gain, polydipsia, polyuria, and polyphagia.

Description: Diabetes mellitus is a chronic state of hyperglycemia that is divided primarily into two types: *type 1 diabetes* and *type 2 diabetes*. Formerly, type 1 diabetes was called *insulin-dependent diabetes* and type

2 diabetes was called *non–insulin-dependent diabetes*, primarily to signify the age of onset of disease and whether or not insulin therapy was the required treatment. Diabetes in the older adult is a different disease than in the younger adult. A decline in beta-cell function and blood insulin levels along with a decrease in physical activity and muscle mass are common changes with aging that increase the likelihood of impaired glucose tolerance or diabetes. Furthermore, older adults often do not have the increase in fasting hepatic glucose production that is seen in middle age, resulting in normal or near-normal fasting glucose with elevated postprandial glucose (Hornick & Aron, 2008). This combination of normal changes with aging and lack of typical presentation results in the underdiagnosis of diabetes in the older adult.

Etiology: Type 1 diabetes most often occurs in childhood and is characterized by low or absent levels of insulin, often resulting from an autoimmune response leading to pancreatic beta-cell antibodies. Individuals with type 1 diabetes require insulin therapy for survival. Type 2 diabetes usually occurs in adulthood and is thought to be the result of insulin resistance and deficiency. Genetic predisposition for developing diabetes is more evident in type 2 diabetes. Hyperglycemic states that have not reached levels that warrant a type 2 diabetes diagnosis are identified as impaired glucose tolerance. Evidence indicates that individuals with impaired glucose tolerance have an increased risk of developing type 2 diabetes within 5 to 10 years of onset.

Occurrence: According to the Centers for Disease Control and Prevention (CDC) and the American Diabetes Association (ADA), it is estimated that 23.6 million children and adults in the United States, or approximately 7.8% of the population, are affected by diabetes. Of those with diabetes, 17.9 million people have been diagnosed with the disease, leaving 5.7 million that have been undiagnosed. It is thought that 57 million people have pre-diabetes. Each year 1.6 million people ages 20 years and older are diagnosed with diabetes. Diabetes is the seventh leading cause of death, illness, and disability in the United States. Approximately 90% to 95% of individuals with diabetes have type 2 diabetes; nearly one-half of persons with type 2 diabetes are 60 years of age or older. Men are slightly more affected than women by type 2 diabetes. Type 2 diabetes is also more likely to occur among people of African American, Hispanic, Native American, Asian American, and Pacific Islander decent. Boyle, Thompson, Gregg, Barker, and Williamson (2010) project that annual diagnosed

diabetes incidence (new cases) will increase from about 8 cases per 1000 in 2008 to about 15 per 1000 in 2050. Assuming low incidence and relatively high diabetes mortality, total diabetes prevalence (diagnosed and undiagnosed cases) is projected to increase from 14% in 2010 to 21% of the U.S. adult population by 2050. Morbidity includes blindness, end-stage renal disease, and lower extremity amputations. Macrovascular complications from diabetes substantially increase the risk of morbidity and death from coronary artery disease, stroke, and peripheral vascular disease. Complications may result from either type 1 diabetes or type 2 diabetes. Evidence indicates that the degree of severity with respect to microvascular, neuropathic, and possibly macrovascular complications seems to be related to the number of years an individual has had hyperglycemia and the magnitude of the glucose elevation.

Gender: Type 1 diabetes affects men and women equally. Type 2 diabetes affects men more frequently than women.

Age: The onset of type 1 diabetes usually occurs in childhood, with the major incidence of disease occurring in individuals under 30 years old. The onset of type 2 diabetes usually occurs after age 40 years, with a mean age of 51. Age cannot be the only factor used to determine the classification of diabetes, however, because type 1 diabetes or type 2 diabetes can occur at any age.

Ethnicity: Type 1 diabetes primarily affects white Americans. The incidence of type 2 diabetes and subsequent microvascular and neuropathic complications are more prevalent among African Americans, Native Americans, Asian Americans, Pacific Islanders, and Hispanics.

Contributing factors: Although the exact cause of type 1 diabetes is unknown, it has been linked to environmental, autoimmune, and viral toxins. A predisposition for acquiring type 1 diabetes has not been identified. Contributing factors for the development of type 2 diabetes have strongly been associated with obesity, sedentary lifestyle, and familial history. The following risk factors have been identified as significantly increasing an individual's risk of developing type 2 diabetes: age 45 years and older, a positive family history (parents or siblings with diabetes), a high-density lipoprotein (HDL) cholesterol level ≤40 mg/dL and a triglyceride level ≥250 mg/dL, a history of gestational diabetes or women delivering infants weighing ≥9 lb, hypertension (blood pressure ≥140/90 mm Hg), obesity (≥20% above ideal body weight or body mass index [BMI] ≥27 kg/m²), and a history of impaired fasting glucose or impaired glucose tolerance. Carter and colleagues (2013) found an association between treatment with the higher potency statins atorvastatin and simvastatin and new onset of diabetes in older adults. The greater number of risk factors present increases the risk of development of the disease.

Signs and symptoms: Among adults 40 years and older, diabetes often is discovered as an incidental finding during the workup for cardiovascular, renal, neurological, or infectious diseases. The primary presentation may be due to complications of the underlying and undiagnosed hyperglycemia in conditions such as stroke, myocardial infarction and ischemia, intermittent claudication, impotence, peripheral neuropathy, proteinuria, retinopathy, slow-healing wound, and fatigue. Often the classic symptoms of polyuria, polydipsia, and polyphagia with weight loss are attributed to other disease entities and overlooked among older adults. It is prudent for the primary care practitioner periodically to screen for hyperglycemia among individuals over 45 years old and repeat at 3-year intervals, as recommended by the American Diabetes Association (2013). More frequent screening is recommended for individuals with several risk factors. Periodic screening among adults over 65 years old is warranted because these individuals rarely present with classic symptoms.

The determination of whether or not the diabetes is type 1 or type 2 is based on ketonuria, age of onset, and BMI. Other diagnostic tools include the use of antibody testing and testing C-peptide levels. These are a more definitive determination of whether the patient has type 1 or type 2 diabetes. C-peptide is a byproduct of insulin production, and extremely low levels are consistent with type 1 diabetes. Antibodies to islet cells and beta cells are present in 70% to 80% of type 1 diabetics and would not be present with type 2 diabetes. Primarily, type 2 diabetes occurs in individuals who are 40 years and older, have no or minimal ketonuria, and have a BMI of >27. However, in advanced age, frail individuals may present with type 2 diabetes and have few if any symptoms.

Diagnostic tests: The criterion for the diagnosis of diabetes is either two fasting blood glucose readings with results ≥126 mg/dL or two random blood glucose readings with values ≥200 mg/dL, if symptoms of diabetes are present. Oral glucose tolerance testing is no longer recommended in clinical practice. Hemoglobin A1C (HbA1C) measurement >6.5 is indicative of type 2 diabetes. An individual with casual plasma glucose level ≥200 mg/dL but without symptoms should have fasting plasma glucose measured. Fasting is defined as no caloric intake for at least 8 hours. In the absence of unequivocal disease, tests should be repeated at least once. Parameters for the estimated glucose levels based on HgbA1C levels can be found in Table 14-1.

When hyperglycemia has been established, fasting urine for ketones should be performed to help differentiate between type 1 diabetes and type 2 diabetes and the need for insulin therapy. Ordering C-peptide levels and antibodies to islet cells and beta cells, as indicated previously, will help to clarify any uncertainty.

Differential diagnosis:
- Includes drug toxicity and endocrine disorders that may affect glucose tolerance, interfere with insulin secretion, and induce insulin resistance.
- Drugs associated with hyperglycemia include alcohol, beta-adrenergic agents, calcium channel blockers, corticosteroids, lithium salts, pentamidine, rifampin, asparaginase, diazoxide, diuretics, glycerol, niacin, phenytoin, and sympathomimetics.
- Drugs associated with hypoglycemia include anabolic steroids, beta-adrenergic blockers, chloroquine, disopyramide, pentamidine, salicylates, chloramphenicol, warfarin, clofibrate, ethanol, phenylbutazone, and sulfonamide.
- Endocrine disorders that may induce hyperglycemia include Cushing's syndrome, glucagonoma, acromegaly, and pheochromocytoma.

TABLE 14-1	Comparison of HbA1C to Glucose
HbA1C (%)	GLUCOSE (mg/dL)
6	126
6.5	140
7.0	154
7.5	169
8.0	183
8.5	197
9.0	212
9.5	226
10.0	240

Source: Adapted from American Diabetes Association. (2010). Insulin basics. Retrieved from http://forecast.diabetes.org/files/images/InsulinChart_4.pdf

Treatment: Establishing treatment goals for patients with type 2 diabetes centers around glycemic control, nutritional status with weight management, and exercise. Evidence shows that patients with type 2 diabetes benefit from maintaining near-normal glucose levels. The ADA (2013) recommendations for fasting/ preprandial glucose range are 70 to 130 mg/dL. Targets for HgbA1C are ≤7%. For patients with decreased life expectancies, comorbidities, and advanced age, strict glucose control may be unattainable and unwarranted. The Analyses from the Action to Control Cardiovascular Risk in Diabetes (ACCORD) concluded that the risk of hypoglycemia and the morbidity resulting from those episodes may outweigh the microvasculature benefits of tighter control (ADA, 2013). Individualized treatment plans are advisable. Recent evidence from several clinical trials identified the benefits of the patient-centered approach (ADA, 2013; Inzucchi et al., 2012). Any treatment choice should be made after a careful assessment of the patient's health beliefs, comorbidities, life expectancy, functional status, economic situation, and availability of support services. Aggressive glycemic control compromising functional independence and quality of life as well as increasing the risk of hypoglycemic episodes would be counterproductive. Hornick and Aron (2008) note that the risk of severe or fatal hypoglycemia increases exponentially with aging.

Nonpharmacological Treatment: Nonpharmacological therapy is the recommended first-line therapy for newly diagnosed patients with mild-to-moderate hyperglycemia. Lifestyle modifications of weight loss and exercise are particularly important in lowering HgbA1C. Although weight loss in frail elders is not recommended due to the risk of sarcopenia, exercise of even a modest nature can be beneficial in decreasing insulin resistance. If after 3 to 6 months nonpharmacological treatment fails or the hyperglycemia is severe (fasting plasma glucose 200 to 300 mg/dL or casual plasma glucose 250 to 350 mg/dL), oral agents may be added to the treatment regimen.

Pharmacological Treatment: Pharmacological treatment options for diabetes include oral agents and injectables. There are six classes of oral glucose-lowering agents: biguanides, sulfonylureas, meglitinides, alpha-glucosidase inhibitors, thiazolidinediones, and dipeptidyl peptidase IV (DPP4) inhibitors. Other oral agents that may be used in the management of type 2 diabetes include the bile acid sequestrant and the dopamine-2 agonist. Injectables include insulin and the glucagon-like peptide–1 (GLP-1) receptor agonists.

Oral Agents: Metformin (Glucophage, Glucophage XR) is a biguanide that acts by decreasing hepatic glucose production, decreasing glucose intestinal absorption, and increasing insulin sensitivity. It is now considered first-line therapy in treating type 2 diabetes (ADA, 2013). This agent generally does not increase endogenous insulin production and has few hypoglycemic effects. In addition to glucose control, patients tend to lose weight and improve lipid profiles. Side effects include nausea, vomiting, diarrhea, abdominal pain, anorexia, and taste disturbances. A rare but potentially life-threatening reaction is the development of lactic acidosis. Metformin is contraindicated in patients with renal insufficiency (estimated Glomerular Filtration Rate [eGFR] <60), hepatic insufficiency, congestive heart failure, alcohol abuse, or patients 80 years and older. Care should be taken when patients who are taking metformin undergo IV contrast studies. It is important to withhold the medication for 1 to 2 days after the contrast agent has been administered to ensure normal renal function. Usually, metformin is started at 500 mg once a day given before the evening meal and increased gradually to a maximum dose of 2550 mg daily divided 2 to 3 times a day before meals. When given with food, the gastrointestinal (GI) side effects tend to be decreased. GI side effects can result in patient intolerance and are minimized with slow up-titration. An extended-release formulation is available and may be very useful for increasing adherence to therapy. Research has shown that the use of sulfonylureas and biguanides has similar or superior effects on glycemic control, lipids, and other intermediate endpoints when compared to the newer oral agents (Hornick & Aron, 2008). The ADA (2013) now has an indication for the use of metformin in the prevention or delay of type 2 diabetes.

Sulfonylureas are insulin secretagogues and act by increasing pancreatic insulin secretion. The second-generation sulfonylureas include glipizide (Glucotrol, Glucotrol XL), glimepiride (Amaryl), and glyburide (DiaBeta, Micronase, Glynase). The first-generation agents (chlorpropamide, tolazamide, and tolbutamide) are no longer recommended and should be continued only in patients who are already adequately controlled on those medications and not experiencing side effects. Sulfonylureas are renally cleared, and renal function declines with aging. Longstanding diabetes increases the likelihood of nephropathy, which will further decrease renal function. This may result in an increase of the level of sulfonylurea in the blood and increase the risk of hypoglycemia. An important key to the use of sulfonylureas is to choose ones with the shortest half-life (e.g., glimepiride or glipizide rather than glyburide). Side effects of this class of medications include weight gain, nausea, hypoglycemia, weakness, and photosensitivity. These agents should not be used in patients who have had diabetic ketoacidosis, and caution should be exercised in patients who are allergic to sulfonamides. The starting dose depends on the particular drug but should be a small dose and increased as tolerated. Some sources suggest that starting doses should be one-half of what one would use in younger adults (Hornick & Aron, 2008).

Meglitinides are the other class of insulin secretagogues and include nateglinide (Starlix) and repaglinide (Prandin). They act quickly to increase the endogenous release of insulin from the pancreas. They may be used as needed to treat episodes of hyperglycemia. Because of their short duration of action they need to be dosed more frequently. Though frequent dosing may be seen as a drawback, it can be an advantage in patients with irregular eating habits. Side effects include hypoglycemia, headache, upper respiratory infection, nausea, vomiting, constipation, diarrhea, muscle aches, and chest pain. Nateglinide and repaglinide are contraindicated in patients who have had ketoacidosis or renal insufficiency. All insulin secretagogues should be used with caution in those with hepatic insufficiency.

Acarbose (Precose) and miglitol (Glyset) are α-glucosidases that act to decrease or delay glucose absorption and lower blood glucose levels. Serum triglycerides tend to be lowered also and this may be their greatest benefit. Side effects include flatulence, diarrhea, abdominal pain, and rash. α-Glucosidases are contraindicated in patients who have had ketoacidosis, inflammatory bowel disease, or intestinal obstruction and in patients who have renal or hepatic impairment. Liver function tests should be done every 3 months for the first year. The patient should be instructed to take the medication with the first bite of each meal, and the medication tends to be better tolerated if titrated slowly. Patient lack of tolerance to the side effects of this class have resulted in it rarely being used. There is only a minor reduction in HgbA1C by these agents, which further contributes to their minor clinical usefulness.

Thiazolidinediones (TZDs), which include pioglitazone (Actos) and rosiglitazone (Avandia), are insulin sensitizers. They act by increasing sensitivity to insulin, decreasing hepatic glucose production, and increasing peripheral glucose uptake and use. The TZDs require the presence of insulin to work effectively, and their full effectiveness is not realized until 4 to 6 weeks after the onset of treatment. Side effects include headache, weight gain, edema, and anemia. Serious reactions include liver toxicity and worsening congestive heart failure. Liver function tests should be monitored every 2 months for the first year of therapy. Black box warnings have been issued, and rosiglitazone has restricted use in the United States due to the risk of myocardial infarction. Pioglitazone should also be used with caution because it has been linked to bladder cancer.

DPP-4 inhibitors include sitagliptin (Januvia), linigliptin (Tradjenta), and saxagliptin (Onglyza). All are once-daily oral medications that help the body to reduce its own blood sugar levels. They have a unique action by inhibiting the enzyme DPP-4, which breaks down GLP-1; they increase the bioavailability of GLP-1. GLP-1 is secreted by the intestinal L cell, and it is a potent antihyperglycemic hormone that works by glucose-dependent insulin stimulation (so the risk of hypoglycemia is low) and suppresses glucagon secretion, slows gastric emptying, and reduces food intake. When used as monotherapy, DPP-4 inhibitors have a low risk of hypoglycemia but may increase the risk of hypoglycemia when used with sulfonylureas. Side effects of DPP-4 inhibitors include upper respiratory tract infection, stuffy or runny nose, sore throat, and headache. Dose reduction is required with moderate to severe renal insufficiency and should be used with caution in patients with a past history of pancreatitis.

The choice of an appropriate oral agent is a complex clinical decision. Consider the severity of the hyperglycemia and the need for HgbA1C reduction. Most guidelines agree that a biguanide (metformin) should be the first-line agent. If there are contraindications to the use of metformin, a sulfonylurea would be an alternative choice keeping in mind that it carries the risk of hypoglycemia and often results in weight gain. DPP-4 inhibitors are another possibility for initial treatment, but they are expensive and currently not first tier for formulary drug coverage. If monotherapy with any of these agents is unsuccessful, combination therapy with the two oral agents together should be considered. The most common combinations are as follows: adding a sulfonylurea to metformin or adding metformin to a sulfonylurea, or adding metformin to a DPP-4 inhibitor. If irregular meals are an issue, adding a meglitinide to either metformin or a DPP-4 inhibitor may be a reasonable option. The injectable GLP-1 agonists (exenatide and liraglutide) are non-insulin options for combination therapy and have a side benefit of weight loss. Insulin therapy is a reasonable choice at any point in the patient diagnosed with type 2 diabetes, but it is usually reserved as second-line therapy when combination therapy fails. Insulin therapy may be required either as a single agent or in addition to a sulfonylurea, metformin, a DPP-4 inhibitor, or GLP-1 agonist.

Injectables: GLP-1 agonists are within the drug class called incretins. Exenatide (twice-daily Byetta or weekly Bydureon) and liraglutide (Victoza) are approved by the Food and Drug Administration (FDA) for patients with type 2 diabetes who have not achieved adequate blood glucose control while taking metformin or a combination of metformin and a sulfonylurea. Unlike endogenous GLP-1, exenatide and liraglutide are resistant to degradation by the DPP-4 enzyme, and they have a longer half-life than endogenous GLP-1. GLP-1 agonists are contraindicated for use in type 1 diabetes and patients with a history of diabetic ketoacidosis. A black box warning exists for patients with medullary thyroid carcinoma or a family history of that disease or with multiple endocrine neoplasia syndrome type 2 (MEN2). GLP-1 agonists should be used with caution in patients with a history of pancreatitis or gastroparesis. These drugs are effective in reducing glucose levels as well as inducing weight loss. They may be prescribed for patients with impaired fasting glucose to delay the onset of type 2 diabetes. Side effects include nausea and a feeling of fullness that may dissipate after a few weeks of treatment. Other common side effects include hypoglycemia when used with sulfonylureas or insulin, vomiting, diarrhea, headache, nervousness, and stomach discomfort. Patients may also experience decreased appetite, acid reflux, and increased sweating.

The exenatide Byetta is injected from a prefilled pen into the abdomen, thigh, or upper arm. The starting dose is 5 mcg twice a day taken 1 hour before morning and evening meals. If severe nausea is present it can be taken with a light snack. After 1 month of therapy the dose may be increased to 10 mcg twice daily. Byetta should be refrigerated and protected from light. The pen should only be used for 30 days after the first use. Bydureon is offered in one dose of 2 mg and is administered once weekly. It comes in a prefilled syringe that requires mixing. Once mixed it must be used immediately. Liraglutide (Victoza) is once-a-day dosing starting at 0.6 mg and increasing weekly to a maximum of 1.8 mg. It is also delivered in a prefilled pen. In choosing a GLP-1 agonist it is important to consider ease of administration, dosing frequency, side-effect profile, and patient preference. All of these drugs are expensive and are not tier one on formulary drug plans.

Insulin therapy: After many years of having type 2 diabetes, almost all patients will require insulin therapy due to the decline of beta cells in the pancreas and endogenous insulin supply. The body's normal production of insulin is biphasic, with about one-half slowly released around the clock to suppress glucagon release from the liver between meals and while we sleep and one-half released in response to a rise in blood sugar after food intake. Insulins are the most natural agents and are always effective in lowering blood sugar. They all work alike; the difference is in the onset and duration of action. Insulin therapy may be added when optimal glycemic control is not achieved with an oral regimen or the addition of a GLP-1 agonist. Recent guidelines from the ADA (2013) suggest initiating insulin earlier in the treatment plan. Every type 2 diabetic needs to understand that the longer they live with diabetes the more likely it is that they will need to use insulin. The ADA Standards of Medical Care 2013 emphasize the importance of introducing the role of insulin from the beginning to avoid the implication that insulin is punishment for poor diabetic control. Insulin always should be used as first-line therapy in type 1 diabetes or with patients who have had diabetic ketoacidosis. A variety of regimens are used in the administration of insulin based on the time of onset of action, time of peak effects, and the duration of action. Currently the most frequently used regimen is the basal/bolus insulin concept. This reflects the body's physiological insulin response. Basal insulins have an intermediate to long duration of action while bolus insulins, immediate or rapid in their action, provide postprandial coverage.

Basal Insulins: Basal insulins suppress glucose production between meals and overnight and provide nearly constant levels of insulin. Basal insulin includes insulin glargine (Lantus), insulin detemir (Levemir), and neutral protein Hagedorn (NPH). Head-to-head studies comparing insulin detemir and glargine to NPH found a higher incidence of hypoglycemia and increased weight gain with the NPH (Hamaty, 2011). Administration of insulin glargine and detemir in the morning had even less incidence of nighttime hypoglycemia. Whereas NPH insulin has a distinct peak of action at 4 to 12 hours, insulin glargine and detemir are considered to have no peak. NPH and insulin detemir both may be dosed twice a day.

Bolus Insulins: Mealtime bolus insulins include regular human insulin and the analogues: aspart (NovoLog), glulisine (Apidra), or lispro (Humalog). Regular insulin is considered fast acting with an onset and duration of action that exceeds that of the analogues. It is given 30 minutes before eating and has a peak in 2 to 4 hours. The analogues are considered immediate acting with an onset within 15 minutes and a peak in 1 to 2 hours. The analogues should not be given until the person is eating and may be given immediately after a meal if the injection was forgotten. Bolus insulins have the advantage of being adaptable to the day. Less can be given if the person is exercising after a meal, and they may not be given at all if a meal will be missed. It is important to understand how to adjust the dose of bolus insulin. It is not sliding scale adjusted in response to the fasting glucose but rather it should be adjusted based on the preprandial glucose of the next meal (so the dose given at breakfast would be changed based on the lunchtime preprandial glucose).

Premixed insulin combinations of long- and short-acting insulins are available and offer less control but more convenience than the basal/bolus concept. A classic mixture has been the combination of NPH and regular insulin 70/30, with the NPH being 70% of that mixture. By adding protamine to insulin aspart or insulin lispro the release of those insulins is delayed. Humalog mix is the delayed-acting insulin lispro protamine and the immediate-acting lispro and is available as 50/50 or 75/25. The protamine lispro is 75% of that mixture. Novolog mix 70/30 is the delayed-acting insulin aspart protamine with the immediate-acting aspart. The insulin protamine aspart is the 70% of that solution. These mixtures are often dosed twice a day before breakfast and again before dinner. Although the ability to control mealtime spikes in blood glucose is decreased, the fact that fewer injections are required may be more agreeable to the patient. The participation of the patient in decision making is an essential part of individualized care. To further improve convenience of administration, insulin pens are available for all of these mixtures. Insulin pens are not self-explanatory, however, and taking the time to demonstrate their use with the patient returning the demonstration is essential for accurate insulin administration. Insulin pumps are available and most often used for type 1 diabetics with documentation of very low C-peptide levels often required for coverage by insurance companies. The types of insulin, their onset, peak, and the duration of action and how the insulin is normally used are delineated in Table 14-2.

TABLE 14-2 Insulin Types—Onset, Peak, Duration of Action, and Typical Use				
TYPE OF INSULIN (INCLUDES BRAND NAMES)	**ONSET OF ACTION**	**PEAK ACTION**	**DURATION OF ACTION**	**ROLE OF INSULIN IN MEAL PLANS**
Rapid Acting				
Humalog or lispro	15–30 min	30–90 min	3–5 hr	Take at same time as meal along with longer-acting insulin.
Novolog or aspart	10–20 min	40–50 min	3–5 hr	
Apidra or glulisine	20–30 min	30–90 min	1–2.5 hr	
Short Acting				
Regular-humulin or Novolin	30 min–1 hr	2–5 hr	5–8 hr	Take within 30–60 min of eating along with longer-acting insulin.
		2–3 hr	2–3 hr	
Vesosulin (pump)				
Intermediate Acting				
NPH (N)	1–2 hr	4–12 hr	18–24 hr	Covers insulin needs for one-half day or overnight. Often combined with rapid- or short-acting insulin.
Lente (L)	1–2.5 hr	3–10 hr		
Long Acting				
Ultralente (U)	0.5–3 hr	10–20 hr	20–36 hr	Covers up to 1 full day. May be combined with short- or rapid-acting insulin.
Lantus	1–1.5 hr	No peak	20–24 hr	
Levemir or detemir	1–2 hr	6–8 hr	Up to 24 hr	

Continued

TABLE 14-2 Insulin Types—Onset, Peak, Duration of Action, and Typical Use—cont'd				
TYPE OF INSULIN (INCLUDES BRAND NAMES)	**ONSET OF ACTION**	**PEAK ACTION**	**DURATION OF ACTION**	**ROLE OF INSULIN IN MEAL PLANS**
Premixed				
Humulin 70/30	30 min	2–4 hr	16–24 hr	Usually taken twice a day before meals. Premixed are combination intermediate- and short-acting insulin. The numbers indicate how much of each type of insulin.
Novolin 70/30	30 min	2–12 hr	up to 24 hr	
Novolog 70/30	10–20 min	1–4 hr	up to 24 hr	
Humulin 50/50	30 min	2–5 hr	18–24 hr	
Humalog mix 75/25	15 min	0.5–2.5 hr	16–20 hr	

Source: Adapted from American Diabetes Association. (2010). Insulin basics. Retrieved from http://forecast.diabetes.org/files/images/InsulinChart_4.pdf

The frequency and timing of self-monitoring of blood glucose levels (SMBG) need to be individualized based on several factors, including age, ability to adhere, and oral versus insulin therapies. SMBG results in promoting glycemic control and reinforcing adherence to therapy. Even patients maintaining glucose levels by nonpharmacological means may benefit from intermittent either postprandial or fasting SMBG. Patients requiring oral medications who are capable of SMBG should test glucose levels 2 to 3 times per week, preferably alternating before breakfast, the evening meal, and at bedtime, as well as an occasional 2-hour postprandial measurement. The postprandial measurement is particularly important for older adults who may not have increased hepatic glucose production when in the fasting state. Patients receiving insulin therapy should perform SMBG at least 2 to 3 times daily. For all diabetics, SMBG monitoring should increase during illness, changes in diet and exercise, or a change in medications.

Follow-up: Patients with diabetes should be scheduled for appropriate follow-up to evaluate response, tolerability to therapy, goal reassessment, and management of acute and chronic complications. Response to treatment is judged based on home glucose monitoring results and HbgA1C. The HbgA1C reflects the average control over the past 3 months and is not useful for judging the response to recent treatment adjustments. Older patients and patients on insulin therapy may need to be seen every 3 months. When there is a sudden change in health status or treatment regimen, follow-up of 1 month or less may be indicated. For stable patients who are able to maintain treatment goals, follow-up may be every 3 to 6 months. The following evaluations are recommended at follow-up visits: glycemia, foot complications, annual eye examination including dilation, routine urinalysis including evaluation for albuminuria, blood pressure, serum creatinine levels, annual electrocardiogram and fasting lipid profile, HgbA1C every 3 to 6 months, evaluation for neurovascular complications, self-management education, immunization update including influenza and pneumococcal vaccines, and a biannual oral examination. A special nutritional benefit is available for diabetics from Medicare and should be taken advantage of yearly. Medicare also covers the yearly ophthalmological examination.

Sequelae: Acute complications requiring immediate attention include diabetic ketoacidosis, recurring fasting hyperglycemia of >300 mg/dL, HgBA1C of ≥13%, or severe hypoglycemia with changes in sensorium, altered behavior, seizures, or coma. Complications resulting from prolonged hyperglycemia include renal failure, blindness, coronary artery disease, stroke, peripheral vascular disease, slow-healing wounds, autonomic neuropathies, hypertension, sexual problems, and genitourinary system disorders. Macrovascular complications from diabetes substantially increase the risk of morbidity and death from coronary artery disease, stroke, and peripheral vascular disease. Complications may result from either type 1 diabetes or type 2 diabetes. Evidence indicates that the degree of severity with respect to microvascular, neuropathic, and possibly macrovascular complications seems to be related to the number of years a patient has had hyperglycemia and the magnitude of the glucose elevation.

Prevention/prophylaxis: The focus of prevention for developing type 2 diabetes is diet modification and exercise with subsequent weight loss. Weight loss of 10 to 20 lb can reduce glucose levels markedly. When a patient is diagnosed with type 2 diabetes, the maintenance of glucose levels at as near-normal levels as possible is extremely beneficial in preventing complications from the disease. Monitoring and controlling serum lipid levels and blood pressure can reduce greatly complications from coronary artery disease and stroke. The ADA recommends considering 75 to 162 mg per day aspirin therapy in men 50 years old or older and women 60 years old or older or in persons with one other risk factor such as hypertension, hyperlipidemia, or others at increased risk for cardiovascular disease. Equally important is maintaining routine examinations recommended by the primary care provider.

Referral: Patients with type 2 diabetes should be referred when acute complications requiring hospitalization develop, such as ketoacidosis, severe hyperglycemia, or hypoglycemia. Patients with fasting glucose levels that are consistently >300 mg/dL or HgBA1C of ≥13% also should be referred. Annual eye and oral examinations should be referred to appropriate providers. Patients with uncontrolled hypertension, hyperlipidemia, unmanageable skin disorders, or renal insufficiency should be referred to appropriate providers. Consider referring all patients interested in greater control of self-management of the disease to diabetes educators.

Education: The cornerstone of education for patients with diabetes is disease self-management. Assess the patient's knowledge and understanding of the disease, treatment goals, management, and response to complications. Include in the assessment barriers to treatment, which include cultural influences, health beliefs and behaviors, socioeconomic status, psychological factors, and education and skills deficits that may preclude the ability to self-manage diabetes adequately. Explicit instructions should be given to patients who participate in daily SMBG monitoring. For optimal results, families of patients with diabetes always should be included in the education and management of the disease. Information and helpful tools that may be printed pertaining to diabetes can be obtained from the American Diabetes Association, 1701 North Beauregard Street, Alexandria, VA 22311, 1-800-DIABETES (1-800-342-2383), www.diabetes.org.

CLINICAL RECOMMENDATION	EVIDENCE RATING	REFERENCES
Diagnosis of type 2 diabetes mellitus: two fasting blood glucoses ≥126 mg/dL or two random blood glucoses ≥200 mg/dL.	C	Nathan et al. (2008, 2009) Rodbard et al. (2009)
Counsel patients regarding lifestyle modification (weight loss, exercise) (expected decrease in A1C 1%–2%).	C	Nathan et al. (2008, 2009) Rodbard et al. (2009)
Begin metformin (Glucophage) 500 mg once or twice daily, then titrate to 850 to 1000 mg twice daily (expected decrease in A1C 1% to 2%).	C	Nathan et al. (2008, 2009) Rodbard et al. (2009)
If A1C is ≥7% 3 months later, add sulfonylurea (expected decrease in A1C 1%–2%). **OR**	C	Nathan et al. (2008, 2009) Rodbard et al. (2009)
Add basal insulin (bedtime intermediate-acting insulin or bedtime or morning long-acting insulin) (expected decrease in A1C 1.5%).	C	Nathan et al. (2008, 2009) Rodbard et al. (2009)
With caution may add pioglitazone (Actos) (expected decrease in A1C 0.5%–1.4%) (less evidence). **OR**	C	Nathan et al. (2008, 2009) Rodbard et al. (2009)

Continued

CLINICAL RECOMMENDATION	EVIDENCE RATING	REFERENCES
May add exenatide (Byetta) (expected decrease in A1C 0.5%–1%). Less confidence in safety than other methods widely approved; expensive.	C	Nathan et al. (2008, 2009) Rodbard et al. (2009)
A1C ≥7% 3 months later. In those receiving metformin and basal insulin or sulfonylurea, change to metformin plus intensive or basal insulin. **OR**	C	Nathan et al. (2008, 2009) Rodbard et al. (2009)
In those receiving metformin plus pioglitazone, add sulfonylurea or change to metformin plus basal insulin (less evidence). **OR**	C	Nathan et al. (2008, 2009) Rodbard et al. (2009)
In those receiving metformin plus exenatide, change to metformin plus pioglitazone and sulfonylurea. **OR** Metformin plus basal insulin (less evidence).	C	Nathan et al. (2008, 2009) Rodbard et al. (2009)
In patients not yet receiving metformin plus insulin, change to metformin plus basal insulin. **OR**	C	Nathan et al. (2008, 2009) Rodbard et al. (2009)
In those receiving metformin plus basal insulin, intensify insulin and continue to adjust.	C	Nathan et al. (2008, 2009) Rodbard et al. (2009)

A = consistent, good-quality, patient-oriented evidence; B = inconsistent or limited-quality, patient-oriented evidence; C = consensus, disease-oriented evidence, usual practice, expert opinion, or case series. For information about the SORT evidence rating system, go to www.aafp.org/afpsort.xml.

FAILURE TO THRIVE

Signal symptoms: Weight loss of greater than 5% of baseline, decreased appetite, inactivity, impaired immune function, low cholesterol.

Description: Adult failure to thrive (FTT) is not considered a normal part of aging. The patient undergoes a process of functional decline, progressive apathy, and a loss of willingness to eat or drink that culminates in death. FTT is associated with increased infections, diminished cell-mediated immunity, hip fractures, decubitus ulcers, and increased surgical mortality (Dorner, 2010). This population of gravely ill and impaired older adult patients has experienced multiple hospitalizations, has multiple diagnoses, and can be viewed as a paradigm of the very sick and frail elders (Kumeliauskas, Fruetel, & Holroyd-Leduc, 2013). It can be concluded that patients given a diagnosis of FTT present with a complex picture of multifaceted problems across a spectrum of physiological ailments, psychological deficits, and social and environmental needs (Rocchiccioli & Sanford, 2009).

Early assessment of the elderly patient is necessary to improve functioning or prevent further decline. The goal of early assessment is to identify the precise needs of the patient in determining appropriate intervention strategies, providing necessary supports, and optimizing rehabilitation (Dorner, 2010; Hollinger-Smith & Buschmann, 2000).

Etiology: FTT is associated with medical conditions that include cancer, heart failure, chronic obstructive pulmonary disease, chronic renal insufficiency, chronic steroid use, cirrhosis, stroke, depression, diabetes, hepatitis, hip or large bone fractures, inflammatory bowel disease, GI surgery, myocardial infarction, recurrent urinary tract infections, recurrent pneumonia, rheumatoid arthritis, lupus, systemic infections, and tuberculosis.

Medications associated with FTT include anticholinergics, antiepileptics, benzodiazepines, beta blockers, central alpha antagonists, diuretics in high-potency combinations, glucocorticoids, neuroleptics, opioids, serotonin reuptake inhibitors, tricyclic antidepressants, and any combination of more than four medications.

Associated issues can be alcohol and substance abuse, cognitive impairment, functional impairment, social isolation, and nutritional problems. Nutritional marasmus decreases body fat stores indicated by a 75% fat loss and a 25% lean tissue loss. General catabolic responses are indicated by a 75% lean tissue loss and a 25% fat loss (Dorner, 2010; Moses, 2008).

Occurrence: Occurs in 5% to 35% of community-dwelling elderly and 25% to 40% of nursing home residents. Hospitalized veterans have an incidence rate of 50% to 60%. Greater than 50% of hospitalized elders with preexisting weight loss continue to lose weight after hospitalization, and 75% of those patients with irreversible weight loss will die within a year of diagnosis (Dorner, 2010).

Age: Incidence increases with age.

Gender: Occurs equally in males and females.

Ethnicity: Occurs in all ethnic groups.

Contributing factors: Unintentional weight loss, decreased appetite, poor nutrition, inactivity, dehydration, depression, impaired function, and cognitive impairment have been shown to contribute to the development of FTT in older adults. Patients with both acute conditions (infections, electrolyte and metabolic disorders) and exacerbations of chronic (cardiac or respiratory) and terminal diseases (cancers and neurodegenerative conditions) can develop the clinical characteristics of FTT (Moses, 2008). A rare but curable cause of FTT in older adults is chronic mesenteric ischemia (Snyder & Baum, 2011).

Signs and symptoms: Fever, orthostatic changes, weight loss, BMI less than 22, evidence of neglect, inability to transfer independently, temporal wasting, dry mucosa, cheilosis, glossitis, dysphagia, palpable lymph nodes, loss of subcutaneous fat, dehydration, venous distention, osteoporosis, decreased breath sounds, signs of heart failure, organomegaly, ascites, abdominal masses, muscle wasting, peripheral edema, joint inflammation, focal neurological symptoms, depression, and decreased mental status. Diminished scores on the Karnofsky Performance Scale (Schag, Heinrich, & Ganz, 1984) and Mini Nutritional Assessment (Morely, 2011) can also point to FTT (Robertson & Montagnini, 2004).

Diagnostic tests: Consider ordering a CBC, serum albumin level and thyroid-stimulating hormone (TSH), cholesterol, and comprehensive metabolic panel, initially in patients presenting with signs of malnutrition over time. For patients with suspected infection or inflammation associated with malnutrition, consider blood cultures, chest x-ray, CT or magnetic resonance imaging (MRI) if injury, malignancy, or infection is suspected, sedimentation rate or C-reactive protein, growth hormone for patients with suspected endocrine disorder, HIV, rapid plasma reagin (RPR), purified protein derivative (PPD), or urinalysis for specific infection (Moses, 2008). Assess function using the Karnofsky Performance Scale; a score of ≤50 indicates the need for considerable assistance and disability (Schag, Heinrich, & Ganz, 1984). Conduct a nutritional assessment with the Mini Nutritional Assessment (score of ≤17 indicates malnutrition). Depression screening with the Geriatric Depression Scale should be included with a score of 5 to 9 suggestive of depression and ≥10 significant for depression. St. Louis University Mental Status Exam should be administered if you suspect cognitive decline; an obtained score of 1 to 20 is indicative of dementia.

Differential diagnosis: The differential diagnosis for failure to thrive includes environmental and socioeconomic burdens as well as underlying or concomitant psychological and debilitating conditions that can lead to frailty if left undetected. It is important to note that if any of the conditions listed below are not recognized and treated or if the patient is nonadherent, FTT may ultimately develop.

- Poor living conditions
- Lack of caregiver
- Social isolation
- Inability to obtain prescription medications
- Alcohol and/or substance abuse (cirrhosis)

- Physical abuse and neglect
- Underlying medical conditions
- Malabsorption syndrome
- Endocrine deficiency
- Anemia
- Infections (urinary tract infection, chronic obstructive pulmonary disease exacerbation, pneumonia, cellulitis)
- Dementia (Moses, 2008)

Treatment: Treat underlying medical conditions. Review medication list to determine if any drugs contribute to anorexia, delayed gastric emptying, and altered taste perception (Evans, 2005). With positive scores on depression scale, consider antidepressants (with underlying benefit of increase in appetite), psychotherapy, and environmental modification. For patients with malnutrition, evaluate the need for a speech therapy assessment if dysphagia is present. Treat oral pathologies with regular and/or specialized oral hygiene measures as needed. Review dietary restrictions and adjust as needed. Increase frequency of feedings with smaller meals, and add nutritional supplements. For patients with cognitive impairment, optimize living conditions, treat infections, and administer anticholinesterase inhibitors. For patients with functional impairment, refer to physical and occupational therapy, modify environment, and provide assistive devices. Optimize chronic disease management and manage medications. Address advance directives and contingency planning (Robertson & Montagnini, 2004; Rocchiccioli & Sanford, 2009).

General recommendations for calorie needs: healthy maintenance for women—25 to 30 kcal/kg/day and for men 30 to 40 kcal/kg/day. Patients who are under physiological stress with pressure ulcers—30 to 35 kcal/kg/day. For obese and critically ill patients, consider 21 kcal/kg/day. Protein recommendations: 1 to 1.2 g/kg in healthy older adults, 1.25 to 1.5 g/kg/day for those under stress and with pressure ulcers, and 0.8 g/kg/day for those with renal failure (Dorner, 2010). While treatment with megestrol acetate did show improvement with appetite and small increase in body weight, no improvement was noted in quality of life. There remains limited data on the efficacy of megestrol acetate in the long-term care setting (Ruiz, Lopez-Briz, Carbonnell, Gonzalvez, & Borr-Marti, 2013). The use of Megace and Marinol to stimulate appetite has not shown any significant effect in treating failure to thrive. High-resistance exercise training counteracts muscle weakness and physical frailty (Robertson & Montagnini, 2004).

Follow-up: The multidimensional causes of FTT in the elderly speak to the importance of coordinated efforts by all health-care professionals in the care of elderly patients. Interdisciplinary assessments of the complex etiology related to age, disease, and reversibility of the syndrome provide the data needed to establish baselines and needs for follow-up (Evans, 2005).

Sequelae: Increased infections, decreased immunity, fractures, decubitus ulcers, muscle wasting, malnutrition, and increased mortality.

Prevention/prophylaxis: Early assessment of functional and cognitive decline in patients at risk. Close management of chronic illness and medications. Avoid restrictive diets in patients with unintentional weight loss.

Referral: Further workup of potential causes or for treatment of underlying conditions is warranted. Consider referral to hospice for patients with a BMI below 22 kg/m² and the patient with family refusing a feeding tube or IV nutritional support or who has not responded to nutritional support despite adequate caloric intake (Rocchiccioli & Sanford, 2009).

Education: Early signs and symptoms of decline, appropriate muscle strengthening exercises (Daniels, van Rossum, de Witte, Kempen, & van den Heuvel, 2008), environmental modifications to enhance socialization and stimulate appetite, end-of-life decisions, and caregiver support.

CLINICAL RECOMMENDATION	EVIDENCE RATING	REFERENCES
High-resistance exercise programs have been shown to positively affect both ADLs and instrumental ADLs of frail community-dwelling older adults.	A	Daniels et al. (2008)

CLINICAL RECOMMENDATION	EVIDENCE RATING	REFERENCES
Consider referral to hospice if a patient with a BMI <22 kg/m² is not responding to nutritional support despite adequate caloric intake or refuses any enteral nutrition.	C	Rocchiccioli & Sanford (2009)
Chronic mesenteric ischemia, which often leads to significant weight loss in patients left untreated, can lead to malnutrition and eventually failure to thrive.	C	Snyder & Baum (2011)
Depression, which has been found as one of the components of the failure to thrive syndrome, was found in up to 48% of community-dwelling older adults.	B	Dozeman et al. (2010)
Patients' nutritional health after hospitalization is often affected by functional status, evidence of depression, increased use of medication, decreased cognition, and poor oral health.	A	Chen, Tang, Wang, & Huang (2009)

A = consistent, good-quality, patient-oriented evidence; B = inconsistent or limited-quality, patient-oriented evidence; C = consensus, disease-oriented evidence, usual practice, expert opinion, or case series. For information about the SORT evidence rating system, go to www.aafp.org/afpsort.xml.

HYPERLIPIDEMIA

Signal symptoms: Severe obesity, central obesity, xanthelasma, xanthoma, and corneal arcus.

Description: Elevated levels of circulating lipoproteins, or hyperlipidemia, can result from an increase in their synthesis owing to a diet high in saturated fats or from a genetically determined reduction in the amount removed from the circulation. This situation causes an increase in the concentration of cholesterol or triglycerides or both in the plasma. Reductions in lipid levels have been shown to be effective in primary and secondary prevention of cardiovascular disease.

The Adult Treatment Panel III (ATP III) of the National Cholesterol Education Program (NCEP) published a set of evidence-based guidelines on cholesterol management in 2001. Since then, five large major clinical trials of statin therapy have been published involving clinical endpoints not examined in previous clinical trials of cholesterol-lowering therapy. The results from these trials have enhanced and improved the NCEP–ATP III guidelines for the treatment of high cholesterol (National Institutes of Health [NIH], 2002).

According to ATP III, therapeutic lifestyle changes (TLC) remain the most critical element, and first step, in the clinical management of hyperlipidemia. The primary target of therapy, in general, is lowering low-density lipoprotein (LDL) cholesterol. Emphasis should be placed on identifying patients with multiple risk factors (e.g., the metabolic syndrome; see section on Obesity). Risk factor determination should be made for the presence of cardiovascular diseases or diabetes, targeting these patients for intensive lifestyle changes along with the possible use of lipid-lowering agents. Diabetes now is viewed as a risk equivalent to known coronary heart disease; optimal LDL levels in diabetics should be <100 mg/dL, although levels <70 are now recommended (NIH, 2002).

Etiology: Cholesterol and other lipoproteins are normal and essential components of cell membranes and are metabolic precursors for the formation of bile acids and steroid hormones. Cholesterol is obtained from the diet, absorbed in the GI tract, and transported via the bloodstream for synthesis in the liver, intestinal mucosa, and other cells where they are either used or stored. Cholesterol and other lipids such as triglycerides are transported in systemic circulation as a constituent of lipoproteins because they are insoluble in water. Lipoproteins contain the hydrophobic core of cholesterol and triglycerides as well as a hydrophilic outer layer containing phospholipids and specialized proteins called apolipoproteins. Apolipoproteins give the lipoproteins structural stability and play a crucial role for the enzymes and receptors that regulate lipid transport and metabolism (Chase, 2002; Reiss & Glass, 2006).

Lipoproteins are characterized by their densities, which include chylomicrons, very-low-density lipoproteins (VLDLs), intermediate-density lipoproteins (IDLs), low-density lipoproteins (LDLs), and high-density lipoproteins (HDLs). Chylomicrons transport fatty acids and cholesterol from the intestines to the liver. LDL particles contain 60% to 70% of the total serum cholesterol and are the cause of the atherogenic changes involved in the development of cardiovascular disease (CVD) (Reiss & Glass, 2006). VLDL particles, containing only 10% to 15% of the total serum cholesterol, transport cholesterol to the peripheral tissues when the particles enter the bloodstream and eventually are converted to IDL and LDL through enzyme activity (Chase, 2002). HDL particles contain 20% to 30% of the total serum cholesterol. When cholesterol is released from peripheral cells into the plasma, it binds to the HDL particles and is transported to the liver where it is converted to bile acids, excreted into bile, or reprocessed (Reiss & Glass, 2006). This process is known as reverse cholesterol transport. Therefore, high HDL levels have a protective effect and help to promote the removal of cholesterol from the tissues. HDL levels >60 mg/dL are now considered a negative risk factor for cardiovascular disease (NIH, 2002).

The pathological process of atherosclerosis occurs when cholesterol deposits form in the arterial walls and lumen. This process is influenced by a number of different factors, including age, genetic abnormalities in lipoprotein metabolism, toxins and inflammatory processes occurring at the blood vessel walls and in the bloodstream, and the concentrations and characteristics of the various lipoproteins. Lifestyle factors such as physical inactivity, dietary intake of saturated fats and cholesterol, and high alcohol intake can also promote the atherosclerotic process (Chase, 2002; Reiss & Glass, 2006). Secondary causes of hyperlipidemia include hypothyroidism, poorly controlled diabetes mellitus, nephrotic syndrome, certain drug therapy such as glucocorticoids, and liver disease (Chase, 2002).

Occurrence: The American Heart Association (AHA) updated the heart disease and stroke statistics in 2010. It estimates that 102.2 million American adults have a serum total cholesterol (TC) level of ≥200 mg/dL. It has been estimated further that about 35.7 million American adults fall into the high-risk category, having a serum total cholesterol level of ≥240 mg/dL (AHA, 2010).

Age: Hyperlipidemia may be present in children and young adults but generally develops later in life. The proportion of American adults ages 20 to 39 with hyperlipidemia is roughly 7.1%, compared to 30.3% of those ages 40 to 59, and increasing further with advancing age (Crawford et al., 2010).

Gender: This condition is more prevalent in men than in women until menopause, or until women reach age 55. Once this occurs, the disease is more prevalent in women than in men (AHA, 2010; CDC, 2010).

Ethnicity: In the United States, hyperlipidemia is more common in Mexican Americans and Caucasians than in African Americans (AHA, 2010; CDC, 2010).

Contributing factors: Factors contributing to the development of hyperlipidemia are a high-fat diet, nephrotic syndrome, hypothyroidism, severe obesity (BMI ≥30 kg/m^2), central obesity (defined as a waist circumference ≥40 inches in men or ≥35 inches in women), diabetes mellitus, pancreatitis, hypertension, systemic lupus erythematosus, obstructive liver disease, excessive alcohol intake, renal failure, smoking, certain diuretics, anabolic steroids, sedentary lifestyle, and family history of coronary heart disease. The oils in caffeine called terpenes, which are present only in unfiltered coffees such as French press coffee and espresso, can also raise blood cholesterol levels (Rickets et al., 2007).

Signs and symptoms: Most patients do not present with physical complaints. Routine physical examination may reveal xanthoma, xanthelasma, arterial bruits, or evidence of claudication. Corneal arcus found in patients under 50 years old often indicates hyperlipidemia. Very high triglyceride (TG) levels can also be associated with pancreatitis. Because hyperlipidemia accelerates the atherosclerotic process, a cardiovascular or cerebrovascular event may be the first indication for the disorder.

Diagnostic tests: ATP III now recommends that in all adults ages 20 years or older, a complete lipoprotein profile (TC, TG, HDL, and LDL) be obtained every 5 years as the preferred initial test, rather than a screening test of TC and HDL. A fasting state for a minimum of 10 to 12 hours is essential for accurate results. If the opportunity for testing is limited to non-fasting, the total cholesterol and HDL cholesterol are acceptable. In such a case, if the TC is ≥200 mg/dL or the HDL is <40 mg/dL, a follow-up complete lipid profile is needed for appropriate management based on LDL results. TSH level should be measured, as should a fasting blood glucose level, if hypothyroidism or diabetes is suspected as contributing factors for hyperlipidemia.

TC of 200 to 239 mg/dL is considered borderline high, and ≥240 mg/dL is considered high. HDL level of ≤40 mg/dL is considered low and is of itself considered an independent risk factor for CVD (Grundy et al., 2004; Menown et al., 2009). TG levels of ≤150 mg/dL are what are desirable. Levels of 150 to 199 mg/dL are considered borderline high, 200 to 499 mg/dL are considered high, and levels of ≥500 mg/dL are considered very high. LDL levels of <100 mg/dL are optimal. Levels of 100 to 129 mg/dL are near optimal, 130 to 159 mg/dL are borderline high, 160 to 189 mg/dL are high, and levels of ≥190 mg/dL are considered very high (NIH, 2002).

Decisions on how to treat an abnormal lipid profile must involve a comprehensive assessment of an individual's risk for coronary heart disease (CHD). ATP III bases this on both the short-term (10 years or less) and long-term (10 years or more) risk of developing CHD. ATP III established three categories of risk that modify goals and treatment modalities for lowering LDL: established CHD and CHD equivalents, multiple (2+) risk factors for CHD, and 0 to 1 risk factor. Persons with established CHD are at very high risk for future CHD events and include those who have had a myocardial infarction (MI), myocardial ischemia and/or angina, or any type of coronary artery procedure such as angioplasty or bypass surgery. CHD risk equivalents are categorized as having diabetes or other atherosclerotic diseases such as renal artery disease, peripheral artery disease, abdominal aortic aneurysm, and carotid artery disease that is documented by >50% stenosis on angiography or ultrasound or from resulting stroke or transient ischemic attack of a carotid source. In addition, persons with multiple risk factors and a 10-year risk for developing CHD of >20% (based on the Framingham score) are considered having a CHD risk equivalent (Grundy et al., 2004).

For those who do not have CHD or CHD risk equivalents, the number of major risk factors for CHD is counted. Specific independent factors have been identified that increase the risk for developing CHD. These include smoking, age (men 45 years and older, women 55 years and older), family history of premature CHD (first-degree relative male under 55 years, female under 65 years), low HDL (40 mg/dL), and hypertension (≥140/90 or already taking an antihypertensive medication). An HDL of ≥60 mg/dL is considered a negative risk factor, resulting in 1 risk factor deducted from the total risk factor count. Persons with multiple risk factors are placed into one of three groups based on their calculated 10-year risk of CHD development by the Framingham risk score. The risk factors included in this calculation include age, smoking, systolic blood pressure, TC, and HDL. Each risk factor has an independent score, and the overall sum of the scores indicates the 10-year projected risk of MI and CHD death: >20%, 10% to 20%, and <10% (Grundy et al., 2004). Calculation of the 10-year risk is used by ATP III to group patients into categories for specific LDL treatment goals. Those with established CHD or CHD equivalents or with a 10-year risk of >20% are considered the highest risk and need the most aggressive treatment. The intermediate risk category consists of those with 2+ risk factors and a 10-year risk of 20% or less. The low-risk category consists of those with 0 to 1 risk factor and a 10-year risk of 10% or less (Grundy et al., 2004).

In addition to the risks identified by the Framingham risk score, clinical indications for the metabolic syndrome should also be assessed. Metabolic syndrome has become more prevalent in the United States and is the most frequent cause of dyslipidemia. The constellation of findings of abdominal obesity (waist circumference: men >40 inches, women >35 inches), blood pressure >130/85 mm Hg, low HDL (<40 in men, <50 in women), TG >150 mg/dL, and insulin resistance with or without glucose intolerance (>100 mg/dL) constitute the major components of metabolic syndrome and has been shown to promote significant contribution for the development of premature CHD regardless of LDL level (Alwaili, Alrasadi, Awan, & Genest, 2009; Grundy et al., 2004). A clinical diagnosis of metabolic syndrome involves identification of three or more of the above characteristics.

One additional diagnostic study has emerged as supporting the role of inflammation in promoting dyslipidemia and the metabolic syndrome. C-reactive protein (CRP), a serum inflammatory marker, has received increasing attention as a predictive marker for coronary events. High-sensitivity (hs) CRP is presently the most reliable marker. There has been growing recognition that the inflammation in growing coronary artery plaques makes them more susceptible to plaque rupture. Several theories suggest that an elevated hs-CRP represents existence of unstable plaques (Alwaili et al., 2009; Grundy et al., 2004). ATP III states that more aggressive LDL-lowering could be considered for those with an elevated hs-CRP (Grundy et al., 2004; Rubenfire, Brook, & Rosenson, 2009).

Differential diagnosis: Hyperlipidemia can be classified as a primary or a secondary disorder. Familial hypercholesterolemia (primary) is a genetic disorder that is usually characterized by very high LDL levels and early cardiovascular disease. It involves single or multiple mutations that cause either the overproduction of or the inability to get rid of TG or LDL cholesterol or the underproduction of or extreme clearance of HDL cholesterol (Hopkins, Toth, Ballantyne, & Rader, 2011). Secondary causes contribute to the majority of cases of dyslipidemia, the most prevalent being that of a sedentary lifestyle and a diet with a high caloric, fat, and cholesterol intake. Several other factors can influence lipid metabolism and must be taken into consideration when evidence presents an abnormal lipid panel. Alcohol abuse can cause an elevation in triglycerides. Anorexia nervosa and other starvation states can raise total cholesterol. Many medications can alter lipid levels. Beta blockers can increase TG and decrease HDL. Thiazide diuretics have been known to increase TC, TG, and LDL. Estrogens and glucocorticoids have been shown to increase HDL and TG levels; however, anabolic steroids can drastically decrease HDL. Metabolic disorders, especially diabetes, obesity, and hypothyroidism, are also related to lipid abnormalities. In addition, obstructive liver diseases and nephritic syndrome can cause lipid abnormalities.

Treatment: Life expectancy is increasing in most industrialized countries and particularly in the United States. As age increases, so does the incidence and prevalence of CVD and CHD. According to data from NCEP, approximately two-thirds of all new major cardiovascular events occur in persons 65 years or older (Grundy et al., 2004). Moreover, many older adults have advanced CVD but remain asymptomatic. Cholesterol-lowering therapy in older adults is clinically imperative for not only decreasing fatal cardiovascular events but also for decreasing other nonfatal events that may contribute to further morbidity and loss of autonomy (Roberts, Guallar, & Rodriguez, 2007).

Changing lifestyle and dietary habits is essential to lowering cholesterol levels. Dietary restrictions of cholesterol (200 mg) and a restriction of foods with saturated fats to <7% of total calories daily are recommended to reduce LDL cholesterol. For the frail older adult, secondary measures, such as smoking cessation and control of diabetes and hypertension, may be more advantageous because malnutrition may occur inadvertently if certain foods are restricted, which is often a problem in older adults with limited resources. Weight loss, increased regular physical activity, and stress reduction are also recommended for the stable, ambulatory older adult. Diet therapy with exercise and stress reduction should be initiated first for a 3- to 6-month trial before starting medications. However, these lifestyle changes should continue throughout a person's life span, regardless of age or treatment modalities.

Many large randomized placebo-controlled trials have documented proven benefit from aggressive LDL-lowering treatment in reducing the risk for CHD events. The only published trial to date that specifically targeted older adults with statin use is the PROspective Study of Pravastatin in the Elderly at Risk (PROSPER), which showed that statin therapy significantly reduced diverse cardiovascular events and CHD death in the elderly (Roberts et al., 2007; Wenger, Lewis, Herrington, Bittner, & Welty, 2007). Based on data from these trials, ATP III has recommended that the advantages of lipid-lowering medications not be withheld from persons 65 years and older (Grundy et al., 2004; Roberts et al., 2007; Wenger et al., 2007). It can be somewhat difficult to determine whether an older person needs pharmacotherapy based on assessment of risk factors alone. As age increases, the predictive power of LDL decreases, and thus can make the Framingham scoring less reliable. A partial solution suggested by ATP III is to perform noninvasive diagnostic studies, such as coronary nuclear imaging, Doppler studies, or ultrasound, to look for subclinical atherosclerosis. If the person is found to have advanced CHD or systemic vascular disease, it is reasonable to intensify LDL-lowering therapy even in the absence of clinical symptoms (Grundy et al., 2004).

ATP III bases LDL-lowering therapies on risk factors and baseline LDL. For persons with established CHD and CHD risk equivalents, the LDL goal is <100 mg/dL. If the baseline LDL is ≥130 mg/dL, drug therapy is generally started at the same time that TLC are implemented. If the baseline LDL is 100 to 129 mg/dL, drug options can be considered (i.e., LDL-lowering medications or drugs that modify other lipoprotein abnormalities). If the baseline LDL is <100 mg/dL, TLC are emphasized and no medications are required; see Table 14-3 (Grundy et al., 2004).

TABLE 14-3	ATP III LDL-Lowering Therapies Based on RF and Baseline LDL

Established CHD and CHD risk equivalents
LDL goal: <100 mg/dL

BASELINE LDL	TREATMENT
>130 mg/dL	TLC Drug therapy
100–129 mg/dL	TLC Consider drug therapy, such as lipid-lowering medications or other drugs that modify lipoprotein abnormalities
<100 mg/dL	TLC No medications required

Abbreviations: CHD = coronary heart disease; LDL = low-density lipoprotein; RF = Risk Factor; TLC = therapeutic lifestyle changes.

For persons with multiple (2+) risk factors, therapy is based on 10-year risk and LDL level. Persons in this category with a 10-year risk >20% are considered to have a CHD risk equivalent and are treated as outlined above; see Table 14-4.

Persons with multiple risk factors and a 10-year risk of 10% to 20% have an LDL goal of <130 mg/dL. If the baseline LDL is <130 mg/dL, TLC are emphasized, and the patient is reevaluated in 1 year. If the baseline LDL is ≥130 mg/dL, TLC are emphasized, and the patient is reevaluated in 3 months. If, at that time, the LDL is <130 mg/dL, TLC are continued. If the LDL remains ≥130 mg/dL, LDL-lowering therapy should be considered. Persons with multiple risk factors and a 10-year risk of <10% also have an LDL goal of <130 mg/dL. TLC are also initiated for a baseline LDL of <130 mg/dL, with reevaluation in 1 year. If the LDL is ≥130 mg/dL, TLC are emphasized, with reevaluation in 3 months. If, at that time,

TABLE 14-4	ATP III LDL-Lowering Therapies Based on RF and Baseline LDL

Multiple risk factors (2+)—therapy is based on 10-year risk and LDL level
LDL goal: <100 mg/dL

10-YEAR RISK	TREATMENT
>20% is considered a CHD risk equivalent	As shown in Table 14-3

Abbreviations: CHD = coronary heart disease; LDL = low-density lipoprotein; RF = Risk Factor.

LDL is <160 mg/dL, TLC are continued. If the LDL is ≥160 mg/dL, LDL-lowering therapy should be considered; see Table 14-5.

Persons with 0 to 1 risk factor generally have a 10-year risk <10%. The LDL goal for this category is <160 mg/dL. TLC are initiated when LDL exceeds this goal, and drug therapy should be considered when LDL is ≥190 mg/dL; see Table 14-6 (Grundy et al., 2004).

Cholesterol-lowering medications have been used to treat several hundred million patients over the last 20+ years, and have been proven to be relatively safe (Scirica & Cannon, 2005). However, it may be necessary to impart individual clinical judgment when deciding on treatment modalities for an older adult. Financial cost, functional and cognitive ability, social situation, and comorbid diseases should all be taken into consideration when evaluating treatment options. Additionally, the potential for medication side effects and drug interactions should be taken into account.

The general categories of cholesterol-lowering agents include 5-hydroxy-3-methylglutaryl-coenzyme A reductase inhibitors (HMG CoA) or statin medications, bile acid sequestrants, nicotinic acid, fibrates, and cholesterol absorption inhibitors. Statins have become standard treatment due to their superior efficacy in lowering LDL over other classes of cholesterol-lowering medications. They block the synthesis of cholesterol, particularly VLDL and LDL, and increase the uptake of LDL by receptor-mediated endocytosis (Alwaili et al., 2009). They can reduce LDL by 18% to 55%, reduce TG by 7% to 30%, and increase HDL by 5% to 15% (NIH, 2002). Medications currently available include atorvastatin, 20 to 80 mg/day; simvastatin, 10 to 80 mg/day; fluvastatin, 20 to 80 mg/day; lovastatin, 20 to 80 mg/day; pravastatin, 20 to 40 mg/day; and rosuvastatin, 5 to 40 mg/day. Statins are generally well tolerated, but they are not without the potential for side effects. Hepatic changes and myalgias are the most frequently reported (Law & Rudnicka, 2006; Scirica & Cannon, 2005). Most statins are metabolized through the CYP3A4 pathway in the liver. Polypharmacy is not uncommon in older adults, and statins may affect other drugs that are also metabolized through this same pathway, setting up the potential for drug side effects. Moreover, many older people already suffer from arthritis and may not recognize that an increase in muscle aches may actually be the result of a cholesterol medicine. Failure to evaluate

TABLE 14-5 ATP III LDL-Lowering Therapies Based on RF and Baseline LDL

Multiple risk factors (2+)—therapy is based on 10-year risk and LDL level
LDL goal: <130 mg/dL

10-YEAR RISK	BASELINE LDL	TREATMENT	EVALUATION	REEVALUATION LDL	TREATMENT
10%–20%	<130 mg/dL	TLC	1 year		
				<130 mg/dL	Continue TLC
	≥130 mg/dL	TLC	3 months		Continue TLC
				≥130 mg/dL	Consider drug therapy
<10%	≥130 mg/dL	TLC	1 year		
				<160 mg/dL	Continue TLC
	≥130 mg/dL	TLC	3 months		Continue TLC
				≥160 mg/dL	Consider drug therapy

Abbreviations: LDL = low-density lipoprotein; RF = Risk Factor ; TLC = therapeutic lifestyle changes.

TABLE 14-6 ATP III LDL-Lowering Therapies Based on RF and Baseline LDL

0–1 risk factors
LDL goal: <160 mg/dL

10-YEAR RISK	BASELINE LDL	TREATMENT	EVALUATION
<10%	>160 mg/dL	TLC	1 year
	≥190 mg/dL	TLC Consider drug therapy	3 months

Abbreviations: LDL = low-density lipoprotein; RF = Risk Factor ; TLC = therapeutic lifestyle changes.

these complaints could lead to serious muscle damage, which can become a significant problem due to increased muscle and bone loss and increased fall risk in the elderly.

Bile acid sequestrants lower LDL by interrupting the circulation of bile acids through the hepatic system due to reabsorption inhibition in the intestines. They can lower LDL by 15% to 30% and raise HDL by 3% to 5% (NIH, 2002). They are generally used as adjunct therapy for significantly elevated LDL or when statins are not well tolerated. Drugs currently available include cholestyramine, 4 to 16 g/day; colestipol, 5 to 20 g/day; and colesevelam, 1.5 to 3.75 g/day. Because these drugs are not absorbed as they pass through the GI tract, they can cause the GI side effects of bloating, flatulence, and constipation. They require multiple dosing throughout the day and can decrease the absorption of other drugs taken concomitantly,

making administration of these and other medications a potential problem.

Nicotinic acid (niacin, 2 to 3 g/day) decreases both LDL and TG and is the most effective agent for raising HDL. It lowers LDL by blocking the breakdown of adipose tissue and decreasing serum free fatty acids, resulting in decreased secretion of cholesterol by the liver. It raises HDL by reducing the transfer of HDL to VLDL and by delaying the clearance of HDL from the kidney (Alwaili et al., 2009). Lipoprotein-lowering effects include decreasing LDL by 5% to 25% and TG by 20% to 50% and increasing HDL by 15% to 35% (NIH, 2002). Niacin involves multiple dosing throughout the day, making it problematic for older adults with multiple medications. It can cause unpleasant GI side effects, hepatotoxicity, hyperglycemia, and hyperuricemia. It can also cause flushing and itching of the skin, although the extended-release form, Niapsan, is reported to cause less flushing. Flushing can also be decreased by taking the medication during or after meals, at bedtime, or by taking an aspirin before its ingestion.

Fibric acids are used primarily for the treatment of hypertriglyceridemia when TLC have not been effective. They increase the catabolism of TG and decrease the secretion of VLDL (Alwaili et al., 2009). They can lower LDL by 5% to 20% and TG by 20% to 50%, and raise HDL by 10% to 20%. Gemfibrozil (600 to 1200 mg/day), fenofibrate (48 mg/day or 145 mg/day), and fenofibric acid (35 to 105 mg/day) are the agents currently available. Because of the need for multiple dosing throughout the day and an increased risk of myopathy, these drugs are not used as first-line therapy in the elderly unless TG are >1000 mg/dL (Rubenfire et al., 2009). Other potential side effects include abdominal discomfort, gallstones, and liver enzyme abnormalities.

Cholesterol absorption inhibitors are used to lower LDL but are generally used as adjunct therapy with a statin due to a decrease in drug response when used as monotherapy. They lower LDL by inhibiting cholesterol absorption from the intestine and by working with the biliary system in removing cholesterol by keeping it in the intestinal lumen for excretion (Davis & Veltri, 2007). LDL can be lowered an average of 18%, and when used in combination with a statin, can lower LDL an additional 25% (Drexel, 2009). Ezetimibe (10 mg/day) is the only agent currently available. Potential side effects include myalgias, arthralgias, and diarrhea.

Supplements such as omega-3 fatty acids or fish oils can also be useful in lowering TG levels in patients who are refractory to conventional drug therapy. They work by decreasing the synthesis of VLDL. In addition to lowering TG levels, they also have antithrombotic properties. Lipoprotein response tends to be dose dependent, sometimes requiring a daily dose of up to 10 g/day. This can be problematic for some older adults, as are the side effects of burping and a fishy taste with some drug preparations.

Follow-up: Inform patients and family members that medication therapy, laboratory testing, and lifestyle changes become a way of life after the diagnosis of hyperlipidemia. TLC should be monitored after 6 weeks by evaluating LDL response. If the LDL goal has not been achieved, LDL-lowering treatment should be intensified by reinforcing the reduction in saturated fats and cholesterol, increasing fiber

intake, increasing exercise, consideration of adding plant stanols/sterols, and consideration of referral to a dietitian. The LDL response should again be evaluated in 6 weeks. If no improvement is found, drug therapy should be added. The patient's response should be monitored about 6 weeks after starting the medication. If the LDL goal has been achieved, the current dose can be maintained. If the goal has not been achieved, therapy can be intensified either by increasing the dose of the current medication or by using combination therapy. LDL response and liver function tests (LFTs) should be monitored after 6 weeks of starting a new cholesterol-lowering medication or after a dose adjustment. Once the LDL goal has been achieved, patients can be monitored every 4 to 6 months.

Sequelae: The major sequelae of hyperlipidemia are hypertension, atherosclerosis, ischemic events (e.g., myocardial infarction, cerebrovascular accident, and organ insufficiency), and thrombosis. If dietary and lifestyle changes are made and adhered to, prognosis is good for reduction of serum cholesterol. If drug therapy is employed, results are just as good, if not more promising.

Prevention/prophylaxis: Positive lifestyle choices involving diet and weight management, stress reduction, smoking cessation, and following a moderate exercise regimen are the preventive foundations for the treatment of hyperlipidemia. Risk reduction should persist even for the elderly. The need for monitoring TC levels throughout the patient's adult life span is emphasized.

Referral: Treating lipid disorders in most patients will not require referral to a specialist. However, many patients may benefit from a self-help group for dietary guidance, such as Weight Watchers, or from advice and education from a certified nutritionist. Others may benefit from referrals to community resources related to stress reduction and exercise guidelines. Patients with diabetes who have suffered a major cardiovascular event (e.g., myocardial infarction or stroke) are at extremely high risk for death and may benefit from being referred to a lipid management clinic.

Education: The patient and family require dietary instruction, exercise parameters, and stress reduction information. In addition, if medical therapy is prescribed, education about the potential side effects will help to increase adherence to treatment plans.

CLINICAL RECOMMENDATION	EVIDENCE RATING	REFERENCES
Because there continues to be a strong causal relationship between elevated LDL and CHD, LDL should continue to be the primary target of cholesterol-lowering therapy.	A	Grundy et al. (2004) NIH (2002)
TLC should be initiated in all persons at risk for CHD.	A	Chase (2002) Grundy et al. (2004) NIH (2002)
Routine cholesterol testing should begin in young adulthood (≥20 years of age).	A	NIH (2002)
Older persons with established CVD should receive intensive LDL-lowering therapy.	A	Grundy et al. (2004)
Elevated serum TG levels are associated with increased risk for CHD and should be a secondary target of therapy in addition to lowering LDL.	C	Grundy et al. (2004) NIH (2002)
A low HDL is strongly associated with risk for CHD.	C	NIH (2002)
Statins should be considered as first-line agents when LDL-lowering drugs are indicated to achieve LDL treatment goals.	A	Grundy et al. (2004) NIH (2002)
Bile acid sequestrants achieve moderate reductions in LDL and should be used for persons with moderate elevation of LDL or in combination with statins for those with very high LDL.	A	Grundy et al. (2004) NIH (2002)
Nicotinic acid produces a moderate reduction in CHD risk when used alone or in combination with other lipid-lowering medications by lowering TG and transforming small LDL particles into normal-sized LDL, and it is the most effective HDL-raising drug.	A, C	Grundy et al. (2004) NIH (2002)
Fibrates are effective in lowering serum TG and moderately reduce the risk for CHD.	B	NIH (2002)
Weight reduction and reducing intake of saturated fatty acids and cholesterol lowers LDL.	A	NIH (2002)

A = consistent, good-quality, patient-oriented evidence; B = inconsistent or limited-quality, patient-oriented evidence; C = consensus, disease-oriented evidence, usual practice, expert opinion, or case series. For information about the SORT evidence rating system, go to www.aafp.org/afpsort.xml.

HYPERTHYROIDISM

Signal symptoms: Apathy, heat intolerance, insomnia, palpitations, and lid lag.

Description: Hyperthyroidism occurs when there is an excessive synthesis and secretion of thyroid hormone by the thyroid (Bahn et al., 2011). Whereas the clinical signs and symptoms of hyperthyroidism are generally well recognized in younger patients, older adults present atypically, often with new cardiac arrhythmias and apathetic mood changes (Mooradian, 2008).

Etiology: The most common cause of hyperthyroidism in adults is Graves' disease; however, the proportion of patients with toxic multinodular goiter (Plummer's disease) and toxic adenoma increases with age. Graves' disease is a familial autoimmune disorder of unknown origin in which thyrotropin receptor antibodies stimulate the TSH receptor, resulting in increased thyroid hormone production (Bahn et al., 2011). It is thought to be an HLA-related, organ-specific defect in suppressing T-lymphocyte function (Lee et al., 2010). The multiple nodules of a toxic multinodular goiter are thought to produce thyroid hormone without TSH, resulting in thyrotoxicosis.

Occurrence: Less than 5% of people in the United States have hyperthyroidism.

Age: Of all cases of hyperthyroidism, 15% to 25% occur in people 60 and older (Gruenewald, Kenny, & Matsumoto, 2010).

Gender: Women develop Graves' disease more frequently than men, although it has been shown that by age 70, the prevalence of the disease among men and women is almost equal (Lee et al., 2010).

Ethnicity: Autoimmune thyroid disease occurs equally among Caucasians, Hispanics, and Asians. African Americans are less likely to develop hyperthyroidism (Lee et al., 2010).

Contributing factors: Toxic multinodular goiter occurs in a small percentage of people with hyperthyroidism in the United States; the number increases in countries known for iodine deficiency. Patients with other autoimmune problems such as diabetes, rheumatoid arthritis, and myasthenia gravis are at risk for developing hyperthyroidism. A familial tendency for developing hyperthyroidism exists. Patients taking amiodarone or radiographic contrast media can develop iodine-induced hyperthyroidism. Hyperthyroidism can occur in patients with metastatic thyroid cancer, certain ovarian tumors, and TSH-secreting pituitary tumors. Patients who are known to consume diets high in excess iodine or who consume large amounts of thyroid hormones are at risk for developing hyperthyroidism (Bahn et al., 2011; Reid & Wheeler, 2005).

Signs and symptoms: Older patients may report anorexia, weight loss, apathy, depression, heat intolerance, weakness, insomnia, palpitations, dyspnea, tremor, nervousness, and anxiety. Known as apathetic hyperthyroidism, patients and/or caregivers may report that the patient is withdrawn, anorexic, and experiencing new onset of muscle weakness, all contributing to inactivity. Patients may report a new onset of angina (Mooradian, 2008). Known smokers have been found to have increased symptom presentation of hyperthyroidism (Boelaert, Torlinska, Holder, & Franklin, 2010). When questioned about their bowel habits, patients may report that they are no longer constipated. Constipation, however, may occur in older patients with hyperthyroidism. A reduction or increase in appetite may be revealed; patients with severe hyperthyroidism may become cachectic. Photophobia and blurred and/or double vision may be noted. Onset of hyperthyroidism in the older adult often has a very subtle presentation, referred to as apathetic hyperthyroidism. Lethargy is more common than hyperactivity (Cooper, 2003).

Older patients with untreated hyperthyroidism may exhibit a cachectic or a chronically ill overall appearance. On physical examination, ophthalmological changes in the elderly such as exophthalmos are not as common. Lid lag is a more common finding. When tested, extraocular muscle palsy may be evident. An enlarged thyroid occurs in 20% to 40% of patients age 70 and older. The examiner needs to remember that the thyroid is found lower in the neck and substernal area in older adults than in a younger person. Palpate the thyroid to determine presence or absence of tenderness. Because cardiac findings are very prevalent in older adults with hyperthyroidism, a thorough examination is essential. Accurate measurement of pulse and blood pressure is important for the initial workup and ongoing surveillance of patients with hyperthyroidism. Tachycardia, new onset of atrial fibrillation, and heart failure are common manifestations of untreated hyperthyroidism (Bahn et al., 2011). A reduction in muscle mass may be detected (proximal weakness is common in hyperthyroidism), so muscle strength should be tested. Ask patients to demonstrate their ability to stand up from a seated position. Look for evidence of peripheral nonpitting edema with asymmetrical plaques or nodules (pretibial myxedema). A coarse tremor may be evident; note for presence in outstretched fingers. You may note brisk tendon reflexes; however, these are less common in older adults. Assess for signs of anemia such as pallor.

Diagnostic tests: The TSH level is decreased in patients with hyperthyroidism. If the T_4 result is normal following a decreased TSH, a serum T_3 test should be ordered (Gunder & Haddow, 2009). This value is sometimes increased, indicating T_3 toxicosis (Shivaraj et al., 2009). If the T_3 result is also normal, the patient is said to have subclinical disease (Cooper & Biondi, 2012). Radioactive iodide uptake (RAIU) is ordered to differentiate the cause of the thyrotoxicosis; this test is usually elevated in the presence of hyperthyroidism. There is a diffuse uptake of RAIU in Graves' disease, whereas there is focal uptake in toxic nodular thyroiditis. In older adults, an electrocardiograph (ECG) is warranted with associate cardiac arrhythmias.

Differential diagnosis:

- Anxiety
- Diabetes mellitus (normal fasting blood sugar)
- Severe anemia
- Leukemia
- Atrial fibrillation
- Certain endocrine malignancies (thyroid function studies are generally normal; fine-needle aspiration of nodule confirms diagnosis of malignancy) (Fitzgerald, 2009)

Treatment: Hyperthyroidism needs immediate attention in older adults because it is usually associated with involvement of other organ systems, especially cardiac. Radioisotope therapy is the treatment of choice for toxic thyroid nodules and Graves' disease; however, patients should be in a euthyroid state before receiving radioactive iodine treatment (Bahn et al., 2011). Patients may be treated with antithyroid agents, initially with methimazole or propylthiouracil. Beta blockers are indicated in the early treatment of hyperthyroidism to control the cardiac symptoms of palpitations and tachycardia unless contraindicated by other concomitant conditions (Bahn et al., 2011).

Follow-up: Patients with hyperthyroidism require monitoring during the course of treatment, including thyroid studies, cardiac status, and changes in mental status. The patient must be aware of changes to note impending hypothyroidism once treatment has been initiated. Diagnostic studies, usually ordered by the patient's endocrinologist, include free T_4 and serum T_3 monitored every 6 to 8 weeks until a euthyroid state is achieved, and then TSH levels every 3 months for the first year and twice yearly thereafter until the patient's condition is stable and he or she is asymptomatic for thyroid disease (Bahn et al., 2011). Underlying anemia diagnosed at the same time the hyperthyroidism was diagnosed needs reevaluation. With the hyperthyroidism resolved, adjustment of certain medications such as anticonvulsants and digoxin may need to be made (Gruenewald, Kenny, & Matsumoto, 2010).

Sequelae: Complications that can develop in patients with hyperthyroidism include ischemic heart disease, angina, cardiac arrhythmia, myocardial infarction, and congestive heart failure. Bone density may decrease also, rendering the patient susceptible to the development of osteoporosis (Bahn et al., 2011; Cooper, 2003)

Prevention/prophylaxis: Hyperthyroidism is not known to be preventable. However, because thyroid disease is prevalent in the elderly, regular screening for signs and symptoms of hyperthyroidism in patients with a history of rheumatoid arthritis and other collagen diseases, diabetes mellitus, and family history of thyroid disease should be considered.

Referral: Patients need to be referred to a radiotherapist for calculation of the dose of [131]I. Patients with complicated hyperthyroidism should be treated by an endocrinologist, especially in the presence of atrial fibrillation and thyroid storm; these patients usually require hospitalization.

Education: Patients should note a change in their overall behavior following the initial treatment. Thus, patients must realize that they will need to take the prescribed medication daily and to continue with the radioactive iodine treatment. After patients have achieved the euthyroid state and received the radioactive iodine treatment, have them report to their health-care provider if they experience signs and symptoms of hypothyroidism or hyperthyroidism.

CLINICAL RECOMMENDATION	EVIDENCE RATING	REFERENCES
Older patients tend to present with atypical or subtle symptoms of hyperthyroidism, with atrial fibrillation a common finding. Older patients with new cases of atrial fibrillation may be found to have subclinical hyperthyroidism.	A	Boelaert et al. (2010)
The use of beta-adrenergic blockade agents should be prescribed for older adults with symptomatic thyrotoxicosis, presenting with heart rates over 90 beats/min.	A	Bahn et al. (2011)
Atrial fibrillation was found in older patients with subclinical hyperthyroidism.	B	Cappola et al. (2006)
Older men with subclinical hyperthyroidism were found to be at a slightly higher risk for hip fracture than men who were found to be euthyroid.	B	Lee et al. (2010)

A = consistent, good-quality, patient-oriented evidence; B = inconsistent or limited-quality, patient-oriented evidence; C = consensus, disease-oriented evidence, usual practice, expert opinion, or case series. For information about the SORT evidence rating system, go to www.aafp.org/afpsort.xml.

HYPOTHYROIDISM

Signal symptoms: Weakness, cold intolerance, myalgias, depression, apathy, impaired memory, fatigue.

Description: Hypothyroidism occurs when the body tissues are subjected to subnormal amounts of thyroid hormone. Hypothyroidism is further classified as primary hypothyroidism, which is the failure of the thyroid gland to produce hormones; secondary hypothyroidism, which occurs when the pituitary gland fails to secrete adequate amounts of thyrotropin; and tertiary hypothyroidism, which is the failure of the thyroid to secrete thyrotropin-releasing hormone. It is a challenging disorder at times to recognize, given the often nonspecific symptoms the patients report. Progression is often slow and insidious.

Etiology: Autoimmune thyroiditis is the most common cause of hypothyroidism in older adults. Persons who have had prior thyroid surgery or ablation of the thyroid are also susceptible to hypothyroidism. Rarely, infection or infiltration of the thyroid will cause hypothyroidism (Guha, Krishnaswamy, & Peiris, 2002).

Occurrence: Approximately 11 million people in the United States have hypothyroidism. Around 10% are adults 65 and older (Mauk, 2005); however, up to 10% of patients ages 80 or older have subclinical hypothyroidism (Surks & Hollowell, 2007).

Age: Hypothyroidism predominantly begins at age 40, although the age of onset can continue through old age.

Gender: Hypothyroidism is more prevalent in women than in men; women are up to 10 times as likely to be diagnosed with the condition (Mauk, 2005). Women with small body frames and low BMI during childhood are at the highest risk (Kajantie et al., 2006).

Ethnicity: Hypothyroidism is most common in Caucasians; Mexican Americans have a higher incidence of hypothyroidism than African Americans (Aoki et al., 2007).

Contributing factors: Increased age and female gender are risk factors for developing hypothyroidism.

Patients with previous thyroid dysfunctions, Hashimoto's thyroiditis, and goiter may develop hypothyroidism. There is an association between leukotrichia and also vitiligo and developing hypothyroidism. Patients who have had extensive neck surgery or radiation or prior thyroid surgery without proper follow-up often develop hypothyroidism. Hypothyroidism can also result from pituitary disease and certain infiltrative diseases such as sarcoidosis and scleroderma (Guha et al., 2002). A relationship exists between contact with some environmental pollutants (e.g., fire retardation materials), fungicides, and coal conversion products and the development of hypothyroidism. Long-term lithium use can also be a contributor to the disease, as can taking amiodarone (Bharaktiya et al., 2011). Patients with first-degree relatives with thyroid disease are also at risk. Patients with type 1 and type 2 diabetes mellitus (Duntas, Orgiazzi, & Brabant, 2011), rheumatoid arthritis, pseudogout, or Addison's disease should be routinely screened for thyroid disease (Wilson & Curry, 2005). In patients with elevated lipids, consider hypothyroidism as an underlying condition. Practitioners should suspect underlying hypothyroidism in patients who are difficult to wean off of mechanical ventilation (Guha et al., 2002).

Signs and symptoms: Patients often present with weakness, myalgias, arthralgias, fatigue, urticaria, decreased perspiration, cold intolerance, constipation, hair loss, leg cramps, hoarseness, tinnitus with decreased hearing reported, snoring, paresthesias, numbness, stiffness, headaches, and reported weight changes. Patients or family members may report depression, impaired memory, changes in personality, or the inability to concentrate. If the disease has progressed untreated, patients appear apathetic and debilitated, with possible frank psychosis (Guha et al., 2002). Additionally, patients with undiagnosed hypothyroidism may begin to experience dyspnea and sleep apnea (Bharaktiya et al., 2011).

On physical examination, the overall appearance of the patient may reveal brittle nails, puffiness of the face and eyelids, thinning of the outer halves of the eyebrows, and xerosis. During the thyroid examination, the examiner should first observe the thyroid while the patient swallows and then proceed to the hands-on examination. If the thyroid gland is very tender to touch, the patient may have thyroiditis. A goiter may be present that feels rubbery, is not tender, and is possibly nodular. Thyroid nodules, which are very common in older adults, are benign if they feel smooth and easy to manipulate, whereas malignant nodules are hard, irregular, fixed, and tender on palpation. Physical examination may also reveal macroglossia (Bharaktiya et al., 2011). Bradycardia and cardiac enlargement may be detected during the cardiac examination; the diastolic blood pressure may be elevated (Mauk, 2005). Bowel sounds may be diminished. A change in reflexes may be present, notably normal upstroke with a delay in the relaxation phase. Nonpitting edema may be found in the lower extremities (pretibial myxedema). Patients should be examined for signs of carpal tunnel disease (often bilaterally) (Guha et al., 2002) and cerebellar dysfunction to check for ataxia. Myopathy may be a dominant presenting clinical sign in hypothyroidism; on physical examination, proximal weakness is noted (Madhu, Jain, Kant, Prakash, & Kumar, 2010). Signs of peripheral neuropathy may present in patients with hypothyroidism. Patients with secondary hypothyroidism may have diminished body hair and postural hypotension. A screening mental status examination should be performed.

Diagnostic tests: Patients may be asymptomatic, with hypothyroidism discovered only during diagnostic testing. Elevation of TSH and decreased free T_4 is indicative of hypothyroidism. An elevated TSH and a normal free T_4 occurs in subclinical hypothyroidism (Gaitonde, Rowley, & Sweeney, 2012). The presence of thyroid antibodies is useful in the diagnoses of subclinical hypothyroidism or goiter and Hashimoto's thyroiditis. If a recent CBC with indices has not been checked, evaluation for an underlying anemia is warranted (Vitale et al., 2010). A creatine kinase level would be elevated in patients with hypothyroid myopathy, but the level should return to normal once treated for the hypothyroidism (Madhu et al., 2010). In patients with subclinical hypothyroidism, review the patient's last lipid levels because it is common to see an increase in LDL cholesterol levels (Fenstemacher & Winn, 2011). In one study of thyroid patients, patients with elevated TSH also had elevated triglyceride levels (Wang et al., 2010). An ECG typically shows sinus bradycardia, prolonged QT intervals, and possibly atrioventricular block and conduction disturbances (Bharaktiya et al., 2011). A thyroid ultrasound is warranted in patients with thyroid nodule(s) or goiter (Fenstemacher & Winn, 2011).

Differential diagnosis: In determining whether or not a patient has hypothyroidism, the first thing to consider is whether the disease is primary or secondary hypothyroidism. Hashimoto's thyroiditis, post-irradiation disease, subacute thyroiditis, iodide deficiency, and subtotal thyroidectomy can cause primary hypothyroidism. People who have pituitary hyposecretion, pituitary tumors, and some infiltrative diseases (e.g., sarcoidosis) are susceptible to secondary hypothyroidism. In the older adult, when there are numerous signs and symptoms of hypothyroidism, an increased number of these clinical findings point to thyroid disease.

- Dementia
- Anemia
- Depression
- Chronic fatigue syndrome
- Fibromyalgia
- Sleep disorder
- Chronic megacolon (Bharaktiya et al., 2011; Gaitonde et al., 2012)

Treatment: Older adults with an underactive thyroid are prescribed levothyroxine for lifelong treatment. The starting dose in older adults is 25 to 50 mcg/day (Gaitonde et al., 2012). However, patients with severe coronary artery disease may need to be started on a lower dose of 12.5 mcg. Patients should then be reevaluated in 4 to 6 weeks for assessment of clinical presentation and TSH level. The dose can then be adjusted upward by 12.5- to 25-mcg intervals every 4 to 6 weeks. Usual replacement dose for older adults in the absence of cardiac disease eventually reach 100 to 125 mcg/day. Clinical presentation of hypothyroidism in older adults often mimics normal aging changes. Patients may continue to have increased TSH levels yet show signs of clinical improvement. Excessive doses of levothyroxine induce osteoporosis. Older adults with cardiac disease should receive no more than 0.025 mg/day; evaluate blood pressure and pulse before increasing dose (Fenstemacher & Winn, 2011). A thorough medication history is necessary when prescribing levothyroxine, cholestyramine, ferrous sulfate, and sucralfate, and antacids containing aluminum hydroxide can reduce the effectiveness of this medication. Phenytoin, carbamazepine, rifampin, and anticoagulants may increase the drug metabolism. Patients taking any of these medications with levothyroxine should allow a 4- to 6-hour interval between the medications (Bharaktiya et al., 2011). Dietary fiber and soy can also interfere with absorption, so suggest taking the levothyroxine on an empty stomach in the morning. Older patients who have lower serum protein levels may require reductions in their maintenance dosage over time, given the protein-bound nature of levothyroxine.

Follow-up: Patients should have a routine TSH evaluation every 6 to 12 months after stabilization. Patients with secondary hypothyroidism need a free T_4 test. Monitor clinical signs in all patients. Patients found to have subclinical hypothyroidism (TSH between 5 and 10 mU/L) should be reevaluated every 3 to 6 months to determine if hypothyroidism is clinically indicated at this time.

Sequelae: Patients with untreated hypothyroidism may develop coronary artery disease because of the increase in LDL and triglyceride levels associated with this disorder. Megacolon may occur in patients with a long history of untreated hypothyroidism. Myxedema coma with hypothermia and hypotension is a complication of severe untreated hypothyroidism (Bharaktiya et al., 2011).

Prevention/prophylaxis: Although the value of regular screening for thyroid disease has been debated, it is advocated for older adults with insulin-dependent diabetes, hyperlipidemia, chronic kidney disease, unexplained depression, rheumatoid arthritis and other collagen-related disorders, and a family history of thyroid disease and any other condition that is known to contribute to the development of hypothyroidism (Fenstemacher & Winn, 2011).

Referral: If the patient has numerous complications or is not responding to treatment despite compliance, refer him or her to an endocrinologist.

Education: Remind patients about the potential for drug interactions that have been shown to interfere with L-thyroxine absorption, including over-the-counter products that contain iron supplements, aluminum-containing antacids, and calcium carbonate. Tell patients not to increase their dosage even if they are experiencing symptoms of hypothyroidism; instead, they should contact their health-care provider. Any unexplained weight gain of 5 lb or more should be reported. Encourage patients to increase their activity level. Alert patients to contact their health-care provider if they experience signs and symptoms of hypothyroidism or hyperthyroidism.

CLINICAL RECOMMENDATION	EVIDENCE RATING	REFERENCES
Well-functioning older adults with subclinical hypothyroidism are not at risk for mobility problems or decline in function.	A	Simonsick et al. (2009)
Older hospitalized patients found to be anemic should be screened for hypothyroidism.	A	Vitale et al. (2010)
There is a positive relationship noted between elevated TSH levels and triglyceride levels.	B	Wang et al. (2010)

A = consistent, good-quality, patient-oriented evidence; B = inconsistent or limited-quality, patient-oriented evidence; C = consensus, disease-oriented evidence, usual practice, expert opinion, or case series. For information about the SORT evidence rating system, go to www.aafp.org/afpsort.xml.

MALNUTRITION

Signal symptoms: Deficit in muscle mass, depleted visceral protein.

Description: Malnutrition is defined in terms of nutritional imbalance, thus patients are categorized first as either undernutrition or overnutrition (White, Guenter, Jensen, Malone, & Schofield, 2012). Overnutrition is discussed later in the obesity section in this chapter. Although undernutrition and malnutrition are often used interchangeably and represent the same nutritional deficit, there are varying types of malnutrition depending on the initial insult. In recent years, the role of inflammation has been identified as a key component of malnutrition. Starvation-related malnutrition is a result of chronic starvation but lacks an inflammatory component (e.g., anorexia nervosa); chronic disease-related malnutrition is a result of the presence of mild to moderate chronic inflammation (e.g., organ failure or rheumatoid arthritis); and acute disease/injury-related malnutrition is attributed to acute and severe inflammation (e.g., burns, trauma, or acute systemic infection) (Jensen et al., 2010; White et al., 2012). Protein-calorie malnutrition is diagnosed by a combination of clinical factors. Generally an unexplained involuntary weight loss and a drop in the serum albumin level to less than 3.5 g/dL may be indicative of a nutritional deficit. A decrease in serum albumin and prealbumin levels is also understood to be a reflection of the inflammatory response (White et al., 2012). Undernutrition in older adults is multifactorial: age-related organ changes; psychosocial factors such as depression, social isolation, and poverty; and functional decline pose risks for developing this often underrecognized medical condition (Hajjar, Kamel, & Denson, 2004). Despite the increased prevalence of malnutrition in older adults, it often remains underdiagnosed (Loreck, Chimakurthi, & Steinle, 2012; White et al., 2012).

Etiology: Although a number of factors can lead to malnutrition in older adults, certain age-associated factors are precursors to malnutrition, including reduced food and micronutrient intake, decreased absorption of ingested food, and the increased bodily demands for protein, calories, or micronutrients because of physiological stressors (Duffy, 2008; Zeanandin et al., 2012). Decreases in metabolic rate, physical activity, and sensory input can also contribute to malnutrition, often referred to as the anorexia of aging (Hajjar et al., 2004). The relationship between inflammation and nutritional deficits has only recently been studied and is identified as a risk factor for malnutrition due to the metabolic stressors on the body during an inflammatory state. Inflammation in response to acute injury or illness hinders nutritional interventions in the healing process, contributing to the development or worsening of malnutrition (White et al., 2012).

Occurrence: More than 6 million older adults are at high risk for malnutrition. Reports indicate that approximately 16% of community-dwelling elderly,

17% to 65% of acute care hospital patients, and 20% to 54% of nursing home residents experience protein energy malnutrition (Kaiser et al., 2010).

Age: Malnutrition can occur at any age. Frail older adults and people over age 80 are at the highest risk for malnutrition.

Gender: Malnutrition in people age 85 and over is more prevalent in women because of the higher number of women than men in this age bracket.

Ethnicity: Because the reasons for malnutrition vary, no specific ethnic prevalence is known.

Contributing factors: Any of several factors may contribute to malnutrition in older adults: decreased olfactory sensitivity, loss of taste buds, being edentulous, gastroesophageal reflux disease, dysphagia, poor dietary habits, certain chronic diseases with or without an inflammatory component such as intestinal ischemia, hyperthyroidism, depression, chronic pain, chronic obstructive pulmonary disease, stroke, alcoholism, constipation, chronic impaction, malabsorption syndromes, dementia, obesity, and cholelithiasis (Kagansky et al., 2005). One study confirmed that patients requiring walking aids and patients with urinary incontinence, depression, and lower educational preparation were found to be malnourished compared with patients who had higher scores on the Mini Nutritional Assessment scale (vanBokhorst-de van der Schueren, 2013). Review medications because a number of medications can decrease appetite (digoxin), alter taste and smell (antibiotics, antihistamines, antifungals, chemotherapeutic agents), decrease salivary gland production contributing to dry mouth (anticholinergic agents), and cause malabsorption of nutrients (colchicine, neomycin, methotrexate, methyldopa, allopurinol) (Loreck et al., 2012). Patients who are less educated, exhibit more depressive symptoms, and have lower cognitive and functional status are at risk to be malnourished (Feldblum et al., 2007). Older adults who have difficulty with chewing and frequent episodes of nausea and vomiting are at risk for malnutrition. Limitations in the ability to not only prepare food but also to eat due to tremors and arthritic upper extremity conditions can lead to malnutrition. Hospitalization with a restricted diet, drug-nutrient interactions related to polypharmacy, and social isolation and ultimately, poverty also may contribute to malnutrition (Duffy, 2008; Zeanandin et al., 2012).

Signs and symptoms: Identification of elders at risk for malnutrition is a complex process; however, unexplained weight loss is identified as the best factor for predicting increased risk of malnutrition. Assessment of malnutrition is complex because it involves investigation of physiological, psychological, pathological, functional, and financial parameters to determine the possible causes of the malnutrition. Comprehensive assessment of the following diagnostic characteristics is essential in identifying at-risk and presently malnourished patients: history and clinical diagnoses, physical examination/clinical signs, anthropometric data, laboratory data, food/nutrient intake, and functional assessment (White et al., 2012). In patients with suspected malnutrition, all risk factors for poor nutritional status should be assessed using objective measures as indicated (i.e., depression scales, mental status scales, functional status tests) (Morely, 2011). Two screening tools have been validated as nutritional screening devices for the elderly; the Mini Nutritional Assessment and the SCALES screening device (Sadness, Cholesterol, Albumin, Loss of weight, Eating problems, and Shopping) (Table 14-7) have been cross validated for use in the outpatient setting (Morley & Silver, 1995). The SCALES assessment tool does not include a functional assessment, thus it would be beneficial to include a functional assessment tool or refer to a current evaluation of function (see Table 14-7) (Hajjar et al., 2004).

A thorough review of prescribed and over-the-counter medications is indicated in order to determine if the patient is taking any substance that can cause anorexia such as digoxin, quinidine, hydralazine, amiodarone, levodopa, fluoxetine, lithium, colchicine, NSAIDs, proton-pump inhibitors, and many of the chemotherapeutic agents (Ahmed & Haboubi, 2010). During the physical examination, determine if the malnutrition is related to cardiac, respiratory, intestinal, endocrine, hepatic, neurological, or renal impairment. Look for specific signs of nutritional deficiencies such as nail abnormalities, brittle hair, bruises, skin color (jaundice, pallor), cheilosis, glossitis, loss of subcutaneous body fat, muscle wasting, and edema (Duffy, 2008). Explore any unexplained weight loss to rule out treatable causes of malnutrition. If a patient is found to be 15% or more below ideal body weight or had a recent loss of 10% under baseline weight, consider protein-calorie malnutrition (although dehydration should be ruled out). BMI is calculated using the formula weight in kilograms divided by height in meters squared. BMI is an effective measurement for obesity but is generally not as sensitive in indicating malnutrition (Kaiser et al., 2010). In the normal healthy older adult, the BMI should range from 18.5 to 24.9 kg/m^2; BMI <18.5 kg/m^2 generally

TABLE 14-7	Scales Protocol for Evaluation Risk of Malnutrition in the Elderly	
ITEM EVALUATED	**ASSIGN 1 POINT**	**ASSIGN 2 POINTS**
Sadness (as measured by the Geriatric Depression Scale)	10–14	≥15
Cholesterol level	<160 mg/dL (<4.15 mmol/L)	—
Albumin level	3.5–4 g/dL	<3.5 g/dL
Loss of weight	1 kg (or ¼-inch midarm circumference) in 1 month	—
Eating problems	Patient needs assistance	—
Shopping and food preparation problems	Patient needs assistance	—

A total score ≥3 indicates that the patient is at risk of malnutrition.

Modified from Morely, J. E., & Miller, D. K. (1992). Malnutrition in the elderly. *Hospital Practice, 27,* 95–116. From Beers, M. H., & Berkow, R. (2000). *The Merck manual of geriatrics* (3rd ed.). Whitehouse Station, NJ: Merck & Co., Inc. Copyright 2000 by Merck & Co., Inc.

indicates a weight deficit and is an indication that nutritional intervention is required. In older adults, mid–upper arm circumference (MUAC) and triceps skinfold (TSF) measurement is not an accurate means for testing for malnutrition; however, as an estimate, an MUAC or TSF measurement below the 10th percentile indicates poor nutritional status (<17.2 cm in women and <19.6 cm in men) (Loreck et al., 2012). Hand grip strength should also be assessed over time; a decrease in strength can indicate nutritional deficits related to the loss of muscle function. Clinical signs of inflammation such as fever, hypothermia, or tachycardia should also be considered when evaluating the patient at risk for malnutrition (White et al., 2012).

Diagnostic tests: There is no gold standard test for diagnosis of malnutrition. Diagnostic studies help identify the severity and define the type of malnutrition. In screening for malnutrition, laboratory values should be considered only as an indirect measurement or as a tool to evaluate treatment. A CBC should be ordered to determine anemia and to rule out infection and immunocompromised status. Inflammatory markers such as leukocytosis, elevated blood glucose, or C-reactive protein level may be indicators of a nutritional deficit; however, they are not yet considered diagnostically specific for malnutrition (White et al., 2012). Total lymphocyte counts <1500 cells/mm^3 are found in mild-to-moderate malnutrition; a total of <1000 cells/mm^3 is associated with immune paralysis. Protein, iron, folate, and/or vitamin B$_{12}$ deficiencies should be assessed for to further identify deficiencies. A serum albumin level <3.5 mg/dL and especially <3.0 mg/dL predicts protein depletion and in the past has been the most common biochemical parameter indicated when considering malnutrition (Hajjar et al., 2004). However, serum albumin levels can be skewed in patients experiencing urinary loss from nephrotic syndrome or in those receiving IV fluids. A dilutional effect on albumin is also seen when the patient is bedridden, which can produce up to a 0.5 mg/dL decrease. Because the half-life of albumin is 21 days, serum albumin levels rise slowly following nutritional supplementation. Prealbumin with an average life span of 2 to 3 days is highly dependent on iron levels and is not indicated as an evaluation tool unless the individual is hospitalized. A decrease in the serum transferrin levels also points to malnutrition. In patients with coexisting iron-deficiency anemia, however, the results will be misleading (normal to elevated serum transferrin). If the elderly individual is not on a lipid-lowering agent, TC level <150 mg/dL is also considered a marker for malnutrition and has been associated with increased mortality (Loreck et al., 2012).

Differential diagnosis: When determining if a person is suffering from malnutrition, discern if any of the following conditions coexist:

- Anorexia
- Dehydration
- Dementia—Alzheimer's related
- Dementia—alcohol related
- Depression—major
- Dysphagia
- Eating disorder

- Failure to thrive
- Feeding problem/elderly
- Nutritional deficiency not otherwise specified (NOS)

Treatment: Identifying the contributing factors to malnutrition in each individual patient is essential to treating this condition. When possible, a 3-day diet intake should be obtained to determine the severity of the nutritional deprivation. All medications that can cause drug-induced malnutrition should be discontinued or reconsidered or an alternative should be used (Duffy, 2008). Any fecal impaction should be identified and removed. Because not all factors, such as alterations in sensory input, can be treated, dietary consultation should be ordered to assist in the diagnosis of malnutrition and planning of diet supplementation. Any older person experiencing a physiological stressor such as surgery, infection, or trauma requires an increase in protein, calories, and micronutrients. If the patient is diagnosed with protein-energy malnutrition (PEM), nutritional support will depend on the patient's medical condition and the degree of the PEM. Enteral nutritional support is considered when the patient's nutritional intake is inadequate to meet physiological requirements for >7 days or when the weight loss is >10% of the patient's pre-illness weight (McClave et al., 2009). A recent study by Lee et al. (2013) found that a soy-based nutritional supplement provided to patients with MNA scores of ≤24 and BMI scores of ≤24 kg/m^2 resulted in significant improvements in body weight, BMI, and clinical markers of malnutrition, serum albumin, and cholesterol (Lee et al., 2013).

Follow-up: Patients who are hospitalized for malnutrition or who develop malnutrition secondary to an acute-care hospitalization should be monitored daily for response to the nutritional supplementation. The patient's weight should be monitored weekly until the malnutrition has been corrected (Wernette, White, & Zizza, 2011). If a psychosocial factor contributed to the malnutrition, periodic review of the patient's improvement is warranted. Community-dwelling older adults may benefit from a nurse case manager to follow their progress in the home (Izawa et al., 2007; Vischer et al., 2012).

Sequelae: An older person's initial reaction to prescribed nutrient supplements may result in electrolyte abnormalities, hyperglycemia, hypotension, and aspiration pneumonia (Kagansky et al., 2005). Patients who are malnourished can develop sarcopenia and/or cachexia. Sarcopenia, defined as the progressive and generalized loss of skeletal muscle mass and function (Fielding et al., 2011, p. 249), has been associated with inadequate intake of protein from a variety of sources (Loreck et al., 2012). Cachexia is defined as "a complex metabolic syndrome associated with underlying illness and characterized by loss of muscle with or without loss of fat mass . . . clinical feature of cachexia is weight loss" (Evans et al., 2008, p. 793). Long-term malnutrition increases the risk of morbidity and mortality. Careful assessment is necessary to determine if a patient is suffering from failure to thrive (Feldblum et al., 2007).

Prevention/prophylaxis: Given the number of older adults who are at risk for malnutrition, the health-care provider must periodically screen patients for nutritional deficits. A two-step approach for identifying malnutrition is suggested using the Mini Nutritional Assessment (MNA). A shortened version of the MNA (MNA-SF) has been studied and approved as an initial screening tool when undernutrition is suspected in the geriatric population. The MNA-SF is highly correlated with the MNA with a diagnostic accuracy of 98.7% for predicting undernutrition. The six-item MNA-SF can be easily used in the first step of the process, because it does not require anthropometric testing. For the second level of screening, the MNA is considered the most reliable and validated nutritional tool. It is appropriate for use in the outpatient and nursing home settings. It does not require invasive laboratory testing and is cost-effective. The tool consists of an anthropometric assessment, general assessment, dietary assessment, and a self-assessment that engages the elderly person to assess his or her nutritional status. International studies have validated that an MNA score between 17 and 23.5 indicates risk of malnutrition and intervention is indicated. Soderstrom and colleagues (2013) found that the MNA is a useful tool for screening for nutritional status and predicting preterm death in older adults. The MNA-SF contains six questions; a score between 8 and 11 points indicates risk for malnutrition (Loreck et al., 2012).

Referral: Referring patients who are malnourished to a specialist depends on the identifiable cause of the nutrition depletion. A dietitian should be consulted for a nutritional support evaluation. Refer patients who need long-term enteral support to a gastroenterologist for consideration of a percutaneous endoscopic gastrostomy or, in some cases, a feeding jejunostomy. Arrangements can be made for the community-dwelling older adult to receive Meals on Wheels or attend a Title III meal site (Kamp, Wellman, & Russell, 2010). Provide information on the location of centers for congregate meals sites. Patients with swallowing difficulties need to be referred to a speech therapist, and those with difficulty with food preparation or eating can be referred to an occupational therapist for evaluation for adaptive equipment and retraining. For the patient diagnosed with a terminal illness, discuss the patient's and family's decision on nutritional support before beginning any intervention. If social isolation, low income, and/or functional status contributed to the development of malnutrition, the patient should be referred for social services and/or discharge planning. Patients with financial needs should be evaluated to see if they can qualify for food assistance and could be enrolled in the Supplemental Nutrition Assistance Program (SNAP) and/or participate in community-based food bank programs (Kamp et al., 2010).

Education: For the alert ambulatory older adult, review the Dietary Guidelines for Americans and My Plate guidelines (www.choosemyplate.gov/dietary-guidelines.html). Teach family members caring for cognitively impaired or physically disabled older adults about dietary requirements and nutritional supplementation. Caregivers and elderly persons can improve nutritional status by simple measures such as preparation of an adequate diet, hand feeding, adequate-fitting dentures and oral hygiene, and adding liquid nutritional supplements between meals.

CLINICAL RECOMMENDATION	EVIDENCE RATING	REFERENCES
The Mini Nutritional Assessment (MNA) tool has been used successfully globally to assess for malnutrition risk in older adults.	B	Kaiser et al. (2010)
Malnutrition as measured by the MNA was found in men with symptoms of depression and low self-perception of health.	B	Johansson, Bachrach-Lindstrom, Carstensen, & Ek (2010)
Community-dwelling older adults prescribed restrictive diets are at risk for developing undernutrition.	A	Zeanandin et al. (2012)
Social isolation was found to be associated with malnutrition in community-dwelling older adults.	A	Lee & Berthelot (2010)

A = consistent, good-quality, patient-oriented evidence; B = inconsistent or limited-quality, patient-oriented evidence; C = consensus, disease-oriented evidence, usual practice, expert opinion, or case series. For information about the SORT evidence rating system, go to www.aafp.org/afpsort.xml.

OBESITY

Signal symptoms: Elevated BMI, central obesity, generalized obesity.

Description: Obesity can be defined as the acquisition of enough body fat such that there is a negative effect on health. There are a variety of methods to determine if an individual is obese. Simply weighing a patient does not distinguish the effect of muscle versus body fat on weight. That is, a very muscular patient may weigh the same as a very obese patient. Also, taller patients will have a higher normal weight than shorter patients. The use of height to weight tables may be problematic in that there are many different tables in use with many different acceptable weight ranges. Although none of these methods distinguishes the effects of fat versus muscle, the most practical and accurate method is the measurement of the body mass index, or BMI, shown in Box 14-1 (CDC, 2011a; American College of Physicians [ACP], 2011).

BOX 14-1
Body Mass Index

$$BMI = (Weight\ in\ pounds/Height\ in\ inches\ squared) \times 703$$

Obesity is defined as a BMI >30 with morbid obesity as a BMI >40. Overweight is defined as a BMI of 25 to 29. The Centers for Disease Control and Prevention provide a BMI calculator on their Healthy Weight Web site (CDC, 2011b).

BMI	DEFINITION
<18.5	Underweight
18.5–24.9	Normal
25.0–29.9	Overweight
30.0–34.9	Class I obesity
35.0–39.9	Class II obesity
>40.0	Class III extreme obesity

In addition, the distribution of body fat is important as well. Central obesity, in which there is an increase in abdominal fat, appears to be a risk factor in the development of diabetes mellitus, hypertension, and the metabolic syndrome. A female patient with a waist measurement of >35 inches or a male patient with a waist measurement of >40 inches is defined as having central obesity. The National Heart, Lung, and Blood Institute (NHLBI, 2011) recommends waist circumference as a comparable measurement of central obesity. Taken with the subject standing, waist circumference is measured from the uppermost lateral border of the iliac crest. Adults over 18 years old are considered to have central obesity if waist circumference is >102 cm (40 inches) for men and 88 cm (35 inches) for women (NHLBI, 2011). Waist circumference cut points can be standardized across all adult ethnic populations except for individuals <5 feet tall or individuals with a BMI >35. The NHLBI (2011) recommends that waist circumference in these cases be adjusted by age and BMI (Klein et al., 2007; Rosenzweig et al., 2008).

Etiology: Obesity occurs when an individual consumes more calories than they expend. Genetics appear to play a role in that obese patients tend to have obese parents. However, it is difficult to separate the influence of genetics versus the influence of similar lifestyle habits that families share. Certainly,

environmental, social, and cultural influences also determine the risk of obesity. Obesity tends to occur more often when individuals eat high-calorie, high-fat, processed foods or are unable to participate in enough physical activity or exercise. Certain diseases, such as hypothyroidism, Cushing's syndrome, polycystic ovary disease, or obstructive sleep apnea, may increase the risk of obesity. Medications such as steroids, certain antidepressants, certain epileptic drugs, and some antipsychotic medications will increase the risk of weight gain. Often, weight gain is seen as patients quit smoking. Recently, a lack of sleep has been associated with the development of obesity (Mendes, 2010; Rosenzweig et al., 2008).

Occurrence: According to the CDC (2011a), obesity occurs in approximately 33.8% of the older adult population in the United States, with the South having the highest prevalence at 29.4%. According to the American College of Physicians (2011), 100 million Americans are overweight or obese.

Age: According to the Gallup-Healthways Well-Being Index report, the highest rate of obesity occurs in the 45 to 64 year age group (30.8%) followed by the 30 to 44 year age group (28.3%), the 65 or older age group (24.7%), and the 18 to 29 year age group (18.2%) (Mendes, 2010). From these data, it would seem that obesity peaks in the middle age group.

Gender: The overall rate for obesity is similar in men and women, but the rate of obesity in women ages 65 to 74 is higher than in women ages 75 and older in all racial and ethnic groups except for those indicating non-Hispanic black (Fakhouri, Ogden, Carroll, Kit, & Flegal, 2012).

Ethnicity: According to the CDC (2011a), the highest rate of obesity occurs in the African American population (44.1%) followed by Mexican Americans (39.9%), all Hispanics (37.9%), and whites (32.6%).

Contributing factors: Many factors contribute to the development of obesity. These factors include genetic makeup, environmental and social factors, cultural factors, psychological factors, and certain medical conditions. There is a 75% chance of obesity occurring in a patient if the patient's biological mother was also obese. Environmental factors that result in a lack of exercise or the increase in the use of a high-fat, high-calorie diet will result in the increased chance of obesity. Psychological influences such as depression, anger, or boredom may result in an unhealthy eating response such as binge eating, which contributes to an increase in calories (Brown et al., 2009; *Medical News Today*, 2011).

Signs and symptoms: Usually, obesity can be recognized by the initial physical examination and the appearance of the obese patient. A height and weight measurement should be obtained at each visit to the care provider. The use of any number of standardized height to weight tables can distinguish the normal-weight patient from the overweight patient or the obese patient. The use of the BMI is the most practical and accurate method to quantify obesity in the office setting. Measurement of waist circumference can predict the development of the metabolic syndrome. The use of calipers to measure skin folds can be used to determine the percent of body fat (ACP, 2011; Klein et al., 2007; Rosenzweig et al., 2008; WebMD, 2011).

Associated symptoms that older adults with obesity often present with include feelings of worthlessness, sadness, and hopelessness (Center on an Aging Society, 2003). Obese older adults should be questioned on associated functional limitations, joint pain, decreased mobility, and activity intolerance (Newman, 2009). Evidence of loss of muscle strength due to sarcopenia in sedentary older obese adults should be assessed; functional ability to perform ADLs should be measured (Benton, Whyte, & Dyal, 2011). Skin conditions prevalent in obese older adults include perspiration and friction; assess for areas of skin excoriation and pressure ulcers (Flood & Newman, 2007).

Diagnostic tests: Lipid profile and fasting glucose levels should be obtained in all obese patients. If an endocrine disorder is suspected, TSH levels should be ordered to rule out hypothyroidism. Dexamethasone suppression testing is suggested to determine presence of Cushing's syndrome.

Differential diagnosis: Determine the ideal body weight (IBW) for height. Patients 20% above are considered obese; those 40% above IBW are morbidly obese.

Treatment: The basic treatment for obesity involves a reduction of caloric intake while increasing physical activity. The goal of a standard weight loss regimen should be about 1 to 2 lb per week. Initially, patients should undergo a complete history and physical for screening of complicating diseases such as hypothyroidism, sleep apnea, Cushing's disease, or polycystic ovary disease. Social and psychiatric problems including eating disorders should be addressed as well. It is also important to have a clear understanding of a patient's expectations and degree of motivation (ACP, 2011; CDC, 2011a, 2011b; Hamdy, Citkowitz, Uwaifo, & Oral, 2011).

The initial diet should aim at reducing the caloric intake for the female patient to 1200 to 1500 calories per day and the male patient to 1500 to 1800 calories per day. This goal of caloric reduction can often be obtained by decreasing portion size and limiting high-calorie but poorly nutritious foods. Keeping a daily food diary and counting calories will often help patients to see how much they really consume each day. Other commercial programs such as Weight Watchers, Jenny Craig, or Take Off Pounds Sensibly involve prepackaged meals or meal replacement entities with a calorie count that has been predetermined. Very low calorie diets that reduce the caloric intake to less than 800 to 1200 calories per day require strict medical monitoring through a structured program. There are few data to support the use of low-carbohydrate diets such as Atkins or South Beach over the typical balanced but calorie-restricted diet in terms of safety or efficacy (ACP, 2011; Brown et al., 2009; CDC, 2011a, 2011b; Hamdy et al., 2011). In patients with sarcopenic obesity, an increase in dietary protein and protein supplements should be encouraged unless contraindicated by other concomitant conditions that restrict protein intake (Benton et al., 2011). Weight loss therapy in an older patient with sarcopenic obesity should be tailored to minimize loss to bone and muscle mass (Mathus-Vliegen et al., 2012).

In addition to dieting, exercising to increase caloric expenditure should also occur. It is important that the patient undergo cardiovascular and pulmonary evaluation for safety before starting an exercise program. A typical goal should be to achieve 30 to 60 minutes of aerobic exercise at least 5 to 7 days a week (ACP, 2011; Brown et al., 2009; CDC, 2011a, 2011b; Hamdy et al., 2011). For patients with sarcopenic obesity, resistance training is highly encouraged, even in frail older adults (Benton et al., 2011). Han and colleagues (2011) recommend modest calorie restriction combined with exercise for patients with sarcopenic obesity.

The only FDA-approved drug to treat obesity is orlistat (Xenical), which acts to inhibit the action of pancreatic lipase, which reduces triglyceride break-down and prevents absorption. The dose is 120 mg 3 times a day before a fat-containing meal and should be used in conjunction with a nutritionally balanced, calorie-reduced meal that contains about 30% fat. The major side effects relate to GI complaints such as abdominal pain, gas, fecal urgency, or diarrhea. It should not be used in patients with malabsorption syndrome or cholestasis. The patient should also take a fat-soluble vitamin supplement before the dose of orlistat.

Bariatric surgery may be recommended to patients who fail the typical diet and who have a BMI >40 along with the presence of other comorbid conditions (Hamdy et al., 2011).

Follow-up: The treatment of obesity should focus on the short-term weight loss phase and the long-term maintenance phase. Patients should be followed closely as the diet and exercise program is begun. As patients lose weight, there should be close monitoring of potentially harmful side effects of weight loss, including cardiac arrhythmias, exacerbation of gout, electrolyte abnormalities such as hypokalemia, development of gallstones, depression, or eating disorders such as binge eating or induced vomiting. The goal is to promote the long-term management of weight with a healthy lifestyle (Brown et al., 2009; Hamdy et al., 2011; *Medical News Today*, 2011).

Sequelae: Obesity is considered a risk factor for the development of a number of illnesses or diseases. The obese patient is more likely to develop coronary artery disease, hypertension, and hyperlipidemia. There is an increased risk of developing type 2 diabetes mellitus and cerebrovascular disease (Chung, Kang, Lee, Lee, & Lee, 2012). Additionally, in obese older adults, there is an increased risk for physical disability, sexual dysfunction, lower urinary tract symptoms, and impaired cognitive function and dementia (Hans, Tajar, & Lean, 2011). Certain types of cancer such as endometrial cancer, breast cancer, prostate cancer, and colon cancer are also associated with obesity (Houston, Nicklas, & Zizza, 2009). The obese patient is more likely to develop obstructive sleep apnea, gallbladder disease, fatty liver disease, and osteoarthritis. Often, the obese patient will have symptomatic varicose veins or reflux (Brown et al., 2009; Klein et al., 2007). In older adults who experience the loss of muscle mass combined with the increase in body fat, the loss of muscle strength contributes to reduction in function and overall quality of life (Benton et al., 2011).

Prevention/prophylaxis: Prevention of obesity must start in childhood with the promotion of a nutritionally balanced diet and proper exercise. Weight should be monitored at each visit to the primary care provider and education provided to support a healthy lifestyle with proper exercise (CDC, 2011b; Klein et al., 2007; U.S. Department of Health and Human Services, National Institutes of Health [NIDDK NIH], 2011). Medicare patients are now eligible to receive counseling services for obesity in patients with a BMI >30 (DiSantostefano, 2012).

Referral: Patients who fail the typical diets can often be referred to more structured programs such as Weight Watchers or Jenny Craig. The use of very low calorie diets must be monitored by specially trained providers. Referral to an endocrinologist is appropriate when dealing with such illnesses as Cushing's disease. Finally, a bariatric surgeon may be considered in the morbidly obese patient with a BMI >40 and other comorbid conditions (ACP, 2011; Brown et al., 2009; Klein et al., 2007).

Education: Teach patients and significant others meal preparation, calorie counts, and fat gram calculation. There are commercial weight programs that are available for individuals who prefer individualized, group, or online methods to assist with weight loss. They range in costs such that everyone should be able to find a weight loss program that suits their individual needs. To sustain the clinical benefits of weight loss (improved insulin sensitivity), exercise training needs to be added to the weight loss intervention (Bouchonville et al., 2013). Older adults are encouraged to include resistance, flexibility, and strength training in their aerobic exercise programs (Bocalini et al., 2012) Encourage patients to begin a safe exercise regimen. Walking is the most recommended exercise program (CDC, 2011b; NIDDK NIH, 2011; WebMD, 2011). One study found that older women benefit from participation in exercise programs; however, the participants in the study experienced some musculoskeletal injuries while exercising (Rossen, Milsom, Middleton, Daniels, & Perri, 2013). Practitioners should provide the older adult with numerous safe options for exercising. Older adults need to be educated on the importance of including micronutrients, including vitamins D and B_{12}, as well as dietary fiber in their diet (Houston et al., 2009).

CLINICAL RECOMMENDATION	EVIDENCE RATING	REFERENCES
Caloric restriction combined with exercise.	A	ACP (2011) Brown et al. (2009) CDC (2011a, 2011b) Hamdy et al. (2011) Laddu et al. (2011)
High-protein, low-carbohydrate diets are more effective at weight loss than low-fat diets.	A	ACP (2011) Brown et al. (2009) CDC (2011a, 2011b) Hamdy et al. (2011) Laddu et al. (2011)
Mediterranean diets consisting of increased fruits and vegetables are more effective at weight loss than low-fat diets.	A	Laddu et al. (2011)
Evidence suggests that commercial weight loss programs that require attendance are more effective in weight loss than the usual do-it-yourself programs.	A	ACP (2011) Brown et al. (2009) CDC (2011a, 2011b) Hamdy et al. (2011) Laddu et al. (2011)
Evidence suggests that Internet weight loss programs combined with personalized feedback from a therapist were more effective in weight loss than Internet programs that did not provide personal feedback.	A	Laddu et al. (2011)
Current physical activity recommendations call for approximately 30 minutes of moderate activity 5–7 days per week. For weight loss without calorie restriction, 1 hour of moderate activity is required.	A	ACP (2011) Brown et al. (2009) CDC (2011a, 2011b) Hamdy et al. (2011) Laddu et al. (2011)
Regular exercise is the primary predictor of maintenance of weight after weight loss.	A	Laddu et al. (2011)
Maintenance-tailored therapy uses a six-phase program each lasting 8 weeks with a 4-week break in between each phase. (Promising data; more research is needed.)	B	Laddu et al. (2011)
Those receiving motivational interviewing lost more weight and had less attrition than those receiving guided self-help without motivational counseling.	A	Laddu et al. (2011)

CLINICAL RECOMMENDATION	EVIDENCE RATING	REFERENCES
Weight reduction supplements usually resulted in repeated, unsuccessful attempts at weight loss.	A	ACP (2011) Brown et al. (2009) CDC (2011a, 2011b) Hamdy et al. (2011) Laddu et al. (2011)
Fat-blocking pharmaceuticals such as orlistat (Xenical) (prescription) and the over-the-counter version Alli work best with other behavior modification techniques. Can be used long term (without studies past 2 years).	A	ACP (2011) Brown et al. (2009) CDC (2011a, 2011b) Hamdy et al. (2011) Laddu et al. (2011)
Roux-en-y-gastric bypass (RYGB), most often used in the United States, causes 50%–80% loss of excess weight and improves glucose control outside of normal weight loss. May be used to normalize glucose in non–insulin-dependent diabetics.	A	Hamdy et al. (2011) Laddu et al. (2011)

A = consistent, good-quality, patient-oriented evidence; B = inconsistent or limited-quality, patient-oriented evidence; C = consensus, disease-oriented evidence, usual practice, expert opinion, or case series. For information about the SORT evidence rating system, go to www.aafp.org/afpsort.xml.

OSTEOPOROSIS

Signal symptoms: Kyphosis, decreased height, vertebral fractures, severe back pain.

Description: Osteoporosis is defined as a metabolic skeletal disease characterized by a decrease in bone mass and microarchitectural deterioration of bone tissue with a consequent increase in bone fragility and susceptibility to fracture (Kanis, 1994). The World Health Organization (WHO) defines osteoporosis as a bone mineral density (BMD) less than 2.5 standard deviations (SD) or more below the mean of the young adult (T-score of less than -2.5). When bone density is between 1 and 2.5 SD below the mean the patient is said to have osteopenia. Decreased bone density increases the risk of fractures. With every 1 SD decrease in bone density of the spine, the risk of vertebral fracture increases by a factor of 2.0 to 2.4 (Wasnich, 1993). Although osteoporosis has been called the silent disease because fractures, occurring late in the disease process, are often the first symptoms, an increase in screening has resulted in earlier diagnosis and treatment to prevent or minimize fractures. The primary health risk regarding osteoporosis is fractures.

Etiology: Bone mineral density results from both the peak bone mass achieved in adolescence and the amount of bone loss after maturity. Although osteoporosis is considered a disease of older adults, the origins of the disease begin in adolescence when there is a failure to achieve a high quality of bone. Healthy bone is maintained by the bone remodeling unit's (basic multicellular unit [BMU]) removal of old bone and replacement with new bone. This action repairs microdamage to maintain strength and also maintains serum calcium. Osteocytes, osteoblasts, and osteoclasts make up the BMU. Osteocytes make up 95% of the total bone cell number and trigger the remodeling sequence. Osteoblasts are the bone-forming units, and osteoclasts are responsible for bone resorption. Recently, RANK ligand (RANKL) has been identified as the cytokine responsible for the components of the BMU. This has resulted in the development of new treatment options. Remodeling is regulated by hormones, including estrogen, androgen, vitamin D, parathyroid hormone, locally produced growth factors, and immunoreactive growth hormone. Estrogen loss effects trabecular bone in preference to cortical bone. The loss of estrogen increases RANKL. Vitamin D plays a crucial role in calcium homeostasis. It acts on the kidney to decrease calcium and phosphorus excretion. Vitamin D works with parathyroid hormone to regulate the release of calcium from the bone. Approximately 99% of calcium is found in the skeleton. Calcium absorption is affected by age as well as by a decline in estrogen. When calcium is low it results in an increase in parathyroid hormonal activity, which increases bone remodeling in order to maintain serum calcium levels. Secondary hyperparathyroidism results from low levels of either calcium or vitamin D. Osteoporosis results from an imbalance between bone resorption and bone formation, causing a reduction in bone tissue. Fractures occur as a result of both the qualitative and quantitative character of bone. The quality of bone is not measurable by current screening techniques; it encompasses the microstructure and macrostructure, biochemical composition, distribution and integrity of material components within the bone, turnover, and microdamage accumulation. The importance of bone quality explains the fact that a 50-year-old woman with the same measured BMD as an 80-year-old woman has a much lower risk of fracture (Kolata, 2003). That BMD is not the only factor is also illustrated in the statistic that more than one-half of hip fractures occur in patients with BMD above 2.5 SD below the mean (the WHO definition of osteoporosis). Primary osteoporosis is a decrease in BMD unrelated to other diseases. It occurs with aging in both men and women as well as with the decline in hormones after menopause in women. Secondary osteoporosis may result from the use of systemic steroids, phenytoin, and diseases that cause malabsorption of calcium and vitamin D, chronic diseases such as rheumatoid arthritis, hyperparathyroidism, hyperthyroidism, overmedication of hypothyroidism, and celiac disease. Approximately 15% of those with celiac disease have osteoporosis as their only clinical sign (Stenson, Newberry, Lorenz, Baldus, & Civitelli, 2005).

Occurrence: In the United States, more than 10 million people have osteoporosis, with an additional 33.6 million experiencing low bone density of the hip (osteopenia) (National Osteoporosis Foundation [NOF], 2010). Of the 10 million, 8 million are female and 2 million are male. The National Osteoporosis Foundation (2010) estimates that 50% of women and 25% of men will suffer an osteoporosis-related fracture in their lifetime, costing an estimated $17 billion in direct expenditures. Each year in the United States, there are about 1.5 million osteoporotic fractures, approximately 350,000 hip fractures, close to 1 million vertebral fractures, and 200,000 wrist fractures. The occurrence of fractures has an interesting distribution with Colles (wrist) fractures peaking at age 60, while the risk for hip fracture doubles every 5 years after age 70. A 50-year-old woman has a risk of death from a hip fracture that is equal to her risk of death from breast cancer (Strom et al., 2011). Although the statistics on fractures are sobering, they do not define the whole problem; the IOF notes that in North America it is likely that 45% of vertebral fractures go unnoticed.

Age: Age is as great a risk factor for osteoporosis as low BMD. Osteoporosis is due to age-related changes as well as extrinsic and intrinsic factors. Osteoporosis is estimated to affect 200 million women worldwide, approximately one-tenth of women age 60, one-fifth of women age 70, two-fifths of women age 80, and two-thirds of women age 90 (Strom et al., 2011). With the increasing number of older adults in the United States the prevalence of osteoporosis is also expected to increase. When an adult over age 50 suffers any fracture the possibility of the diagnosis of osteoporosis should be considered.

Gender: Women have a lower peak bone mass and an increased rate of bone loss after menopause and an increased risk of falling. In the United States the risk of fracture in women is twice that in men, but the mortality rate after a fracture is higher in men. This disparity between women and men seen with regard to fracture risk in the United States is not the same in cultures where both sexes primarily engage in manual labor. Incidence of hip fracture increases in both men and women with age, but in men the incidence occurs 5 to 10 years later than in women. The incidences of osteoporotic fractures resulting from secondary osteoporosis differ in men and women, causing few of the fractures that occur in women and more than 50% of vertebral fractures in men.

Ethnicity: Peak bone mass and bone density are influenced by diet and lifestyle but primarily by genetics. From 3.9% of Caucasian American women 50 to 59 years old to 47.5% of those older than 80 years suffer from osteoporosis (WHO, 2003). The risk for osteoporosis is twice as great in white women compared with African American women. Asian American women are also at a high risk, and about 10% of Hispanic women have osteoporosis while 49% have osteopenia. White men are at greater risk for developing osteoporosis than African American men. Although African Americans have a lower rate of osteoporosis, their risk of fracture is equal to their Caucasian counterparts when they have a decreased BMD, and African

American women are more likely than white women to die after a hip fracture.

Contributing factors: Many risk factors predispose individuals to osteoporosis. Some of these risk factors cannot be changed, including age, family history of the disease, low peak bone mass, female gender, white or Asian race, small body structure, light hair and complexion, certain chronic disease states, and history of medication use. Chronic diseases that increase risk include hyperthyroidism, type 1 diabetes mellitus, rheumatoid arthritis, chronic kidney disease, past or present history of Cushing's syndrome, previous gastric surgery, major organ transplantation, liver disease, epilepsy, alcoholism, malabsorption states, anorexia nervosa, hyperparathyroidism, and women having menopause before age 40 without hormonal replacement. A history of fracture after age 50 or a history of falling puts a person at increased risk for sustaining an osteoporotic fracture. Medications may be an unmodifiable as well as a modifiable risk factor. Patients taking medications, such as corticosteroids, thyroid hormones, anticonvulsants (e.g., phenytoin), anticoagulants, lithium, chemotherapeutic agents, aluminum antacids, and tetracycline, are at increased risk, and these need to be reviewed to determine if alternatives are possible.

Other modifiable risk factors are tobacco use, excessive alcohol use, sedentary lifestyle, low gonadal hormone levels, and diet. The relationship of fat to osteoporosis is complex. Low BMI is known to increase risk of osteoporosis; this is assumed to be a result of less insulation in the event of a fall as well as decreased peripheral conversion of testosterone to estrogen, which depends on fat deposits. A recent study of weight loss in elderly men found that when at least 2% of weight was lost there was a decline in BMD, concluding that maintaining weight is important for bone health in elderly men (Bleicher et al., 2011). Diet is a key with calcium and vitamin D supporting good bone health, but large quantities of protein and sources of phosphorus such as carbonated sodas (due to their high phosphate content, which results in excessive urinary excretion of calcium) contributing to bone loss. Vitamin D deficiency in adults results in osteomalacia, a failure to mineralize the bone matrix. Those at highest risk are the elderly; those living in the northern latitudes; those suffering from poor nutrition, malabsorption, and chronic liver or kidney disease; and dark-skinned individuals.

Signs and symptoms: Patients with osteoporosis may be asymptomatic. All patients over age 50 should be screened for fracture risk. Patients need to be questioned about all of the risk factors for osteoporosis. Inquire about family history of fractures and obtain a thorough menstrual history in women; questions about libido and potency in men are important to determine secondary gonadal issues. After a vertebral fracture there may be acute pain that may resolve or may become chronic. There may be side pain due to iliocostalis syndrome, resulting from vertebral fractures that result in the lower ribs rubbing against the iliac crest.

Two new clinical tools have been developed to estimate the 10-year risk of fracture. The most widely used is the FRAX: WHO Fracture Risk Assessment Tool, accessible at www.shef.ac.uk/FRAX/tool.jsp. The tool is intended to screen patients who are not currently receiving treatment to help determine need for treatment. Japanese women were evaluated with the FRAX, and their fracture rate after 10 years was the same as the rate predicted by the FRAX (Tamaki et al., 2011). The more recent Q-fracture developed in the United Kingdom is accessible at www.qfracture. org; it includes additional factors intended to improve the estimate of risk. The FRAX is recommended for screening in most of the current clinical guidelines.

Physical examination may reveal loss of height with associated kyphosis of the spine. Height should be measured at the initial visit and yearly. Many patients are uncertain of what their normal height was. The arm span measurement is known to be a fairly close equivalent to adult height. Gait should be assessed, and the patient's body mechanics should be observed at the same time. The mouth should be examined to assess dentition and any evidence of oral bone loss. The thyroid gland should be palpated. Observe for restrictive respiratory problems due to decreased volume of the thoracic cage and poor expansion with breathing. The spine should be examined in detail, including configuration. The most common site for vertebral fractures in patients with osteoporosis is the lower thoracic (T12) or upper lumbar (L1) region. Any tenderness to palpation over the spinous processes and evidence of swelling, tenderness, and ecchymosis present at the sight of an injury should be noted. Range of motion should be determined, noting limitations or painful movement. An abdominal examination reveals whether the abdomen is protuberant from spinal changes. The distance between the rib cage and the anterior iliac crest should be recorded.

Diagnostic tests: Osteoporosis is defined based on the BMD measurement. BMD can be measured by several methods, including dual-energy x-ray absorptiometry (DEXA or DXA), quantitative computed tomography (QCT), and ultrasound. The results of the DEXA are reported as T and Z scores. The T score compares the bone mass of the patient to the mean of a young adult, and the Z score is a comparison with an age-matched individual. A Z score of (2.0 or more may indicate more serious causes of bone loss. QCT is three-dimensional and provides a true density measurement. It can also determine trabecular and cortical bone separately. It is used less often due to the increased expense, greater exposure to radiation, and less reproducibility (meaning difficulty comparing results over time). Ultrasound of the heel is FDA approved for screening, but positive results should be confirmed with DEXA. The reproducibility of the DEXA makes it the test of choice to follow up on response to treatment.

Signs and symptoms identified on physical examination should guide which tests to include. Currently there is investigation into the use of serum markers of bone turnover to help guide treatment of osteoporosis, but they are not recommended as a substitute for BMD measurement in diagnosis. Other tests are useful in determining secondary causes of osteoporosis. Vitamin D levels should be at least 77 μmol/L or 30 ng/mL because lower levels can result in secondary hyperparathyroidism and have been linked to an increase in other chronic diseases. When interpreting serum calcium level in older adults it is important to correct for albumin level because 30% to 55% of calcium is bound to albumin. A falsely low measurement results when albumin is low. Every 1 g/dL of albumin binds 0.8 mg/dL of calcium. The correction adds 0.8 mg/dL for every 1 g/dL decrease in albumin. Ionized calcium measures free calcium, but it is an expensive test that is difficult to interpret; consultation before requesting may be helpful.

Differential diagnosis:

- Multiple myeloma (bone marrow infiltrated; lytic lesions common in the axial skeleton)
- Hyperparathyroidism (serum calcium >10.5 mg/dL, intact PTH)
- Osteomalacia (abnormal serum calcium, alkaline phosphatase, and phosphate levels)
- Hyperthyroidism (decreased TSH levels, T_3, T_4, and the Free Thyroxine Index (FTI)
- Cushing's syndrome (serum cortisol levels >7.5 g/dL, 24-hour free urine cortisol)
- Paget's disease (serum alkaline phosphate is distinctly elevated)
- Hypogonadism (testosterone in men; estradiol, luteinizing hormone, follicle-stimulating hormone in women)

Treatment: Good management of osteoporosis requires a comprehensive approach. The goal of treatment is to prevent fractures. The basic level of prevention and treatment includes diet, exercise, and fall prevention strategies. Adequate intake of calcium and vitamin D is essential to decrease bone loss and bone turnover. After age 50 adults need 1200 mg of calcium a day to maintain bone health. When used as treatment for osteoporosis, 1500 mg a day is recommended. There is limited benefit in increasing calcium intake above 1500 mg, and the risk of renal stones or coronary artery disease is increased. Older women treated with calcium tablets have been shown to be at risk for hypercalcemia. In order to avoid overtreatment but reach the required amount of daily calcium, all sources should be evaluated. Food sources are preferable because they provide other nutrients as well. When supplements are prescribed, they should not exceed 600 mg in a single dose because absorption is decreased at higher doses. Several formulations of calcium are available: tablets and chews, with and without vitamin D. Calcium carbonate is 40% elemental calcium by weight, but it should be taken with food because stomach acid is required to increase the solubility. Side effects include intestinal gas and constipation. Calcium citrate, which is 21% elemental calcium by weight, is better absorbed and has fewer GI side effects. Tribasic calcium phosphate offers a third option with 39% elemental calcium by weight; absorption is similar to calcium citrate, with a price point between calcium carbonate and calcium citrate. Options for calcium treatment are identified in Table 14-8.

Vitamin D replacement is available in two forms, ergocalciferol (vitamin D_2) or cholecalciferol (vitamin D_3). Ergocalciferol is a prescription preparation and carries the potential advantage of coverage by insurance plans; cholecalciferol is over the counter. In a head-to-head comparison of the two forms of vitamin D, cholecalciferol was more effective in increasing serum 25-hydroxy vitamin D (25 OH D) than the same dose of ergocalciferol (Glendenning et al., 2009). However, there was no difference in the effect on parathyroid hormone, so the authors question the clinical significance of the difference between the two forms. The choice of which to recommend remains unclear, and both are effective in raising the level of serum vitamin D.

Lifestyle recommendations include the elimination of tobacco, excessive alcohol, and caffeine and a reduction in the amount of high-phosphorus foods and carbonated beverages. Patients should engage in regular

TABLE 14-8	Calcium Treatment		
FORM OF CALCIUM	**ELEMENTAL CALCIUM**	**PROS/CONS**	**BRAND NAMES**
Carbonate	40%	Cheap Readily available May not be as readily absorbed, take with food GI side effects include gas, bloating, constipation Tablet, liquid, chewable	Tums, Rolaids, Caltrate, Viactiv
Citrate	21%	Better absorbed May be taken on empty stomach Less GI upset Tablet and liquid	Citracal
Tribasic calcium phosphate	39%	Better absorbed Less expensive than calcium citrate	Posture
Food sources	1 cup milk 330 mg 1 oz cheese 100–200 mg ½ cup broccoli 50 mg ½ cup beans 100 mg	Include other nutrients Have the most bioavailable source of calcium	

Abbreviation: GI = gastrointestinal.

weight-bearing exercises, which help to reduce the rate of bone loss and increase strength. Muscle strengthening exercises improve strength, balance, and flexibility, which are important in preventing falls. The National Osteoporosis Foundation offers advice on exercise at www.nof.org/node/54. Measures to enhance safety in the home and environment should be emphasized. Personal risk factors should be minimized, such as compromised vision, orthostatic blood pressure drop, and drug or alcohol use. Consider a referral to physical or occupational therapy to improve gait and strength and instruct the patient on proper body mechanics to prevent fractures.

The National Osteoporosis Foundation's (2010) *Clinicians Guide to Prevention and Treatment of Osteoporosis* recommends pharmacological treatment for postmenopausal women and men with a hip or vertebral fracture, a T-score of −2.5 or less or a T-score between −1.0 and −2.5, and high 10-year risk of fracture as indicated by the score on the FRAX. Pharmacological measures to treat osteoporosis in postmenopausal women include antiresorptives, which decrease bone resorption, and anabolic therapy, which promotes bone formation. Antiresorptives include bisphosphonates, a RANKL antibody, a selective estrogen receptor modulator (SERM), calcitonin, and estrogen/hormone therapy. Recent clinical guidelines from the American Association of Clinical Endocrinologists (AACE) include the newest antiresorptive treatment, denosumab, a

monoclonal antibody that targets RANKL (Watts et al., 2010). The parathyroid hormone, teriparatide, is approved for the highest-risk individuals (both postmenopausal women and men). Bisphosphonates require adequate calcium in order to be affective. The AACE guidelines recommend for first-line treatment one of these bisphosphonates: alendronate, risedronate, zoledronic acid, or the RANKL antibody denosumab. Second-line therapies include the bisphosphonate ibandronate and the SERM raloxifine, which can also be used as third-line therapy. Because of the risk of hypersensitivity, calcitonin, available as an injection or a nasal spray, is recommended as the last line of therapy. Some of the available therapies are also a possibility for use in prevention. The details regarding their use are outlined in Table 14-9.

Follow-up: For persons at risk for osteoporosis or those already diagnosed, follow-up should include monitoring of height, exercise recommendations, lifestyle concerns, and diet, including intake of calcium and vitamin D. Safety measures for the home and proper body mechanics should be reviewed and the need for adaptive equipment should be reassessed. The timing of repeat DEXA has recently been better defined by results from a longitudinal study. The conclusions of the study were that women with normal bone density or mild osteopenia should be rescreened in 15 years. Those with moderate osteopenia should be rescreened in 5 years, and with advanced osteopenia yearly screening is recommended

TABLE 14-9 Pharmaceutical Prevention and Treatment

MEDICATION	ROUTE	DOSE	TREATMENT/PREVENTION	EFFECTIVENESS
ANTIRESORPTIVES *Bisphosphonates*				
Alendronate	PO	5 mg qd or 35 mg qwk / 10 mg qd or 70 mg qwk	Prevention / Treatment	Increase spine and hip BMD. Reduce fractures of spine, hip, and wrist by 50%.
Risedronate	PO	5 mg qd or 35 mg qwk	Both	Reduce fractures of spine by 41%. Others: 39%.
Zoledronic acid	IV	5 mg every 2 years / 5 mg yearly	Prevention / Treatment	Increase BMD spine and hip. Reduce fractures of spine by 70%, hip 41%, others 25%.
Ibandronate	PO / IV	150 mg monthly / 3 mg q3mo	Both / Treatment	Reduce fractures of spine by 40%. Not effective in reducing others.
SERM Raloxifene	PO	60 mg qd	Both	Increase BMD. Reduce fractures of spine by 35%. Reduce invasive breast cancer.
RANKL antibody Denosumab	SC	60 mg q6mo	Both	Increase BMD in the spine, hip, and forearm. Reduce fractures of the spine by 70%, hip 40%, others 20%.
Calcium metabolism modifier Calcitonin salmon	SC/IM / Nasal	100 U qod / 1 spray (200 U) qd	Treatment	Small increase in BMD. Small reduction in spine fractures. Not effective in reducing others. May reduce bone pain.
ANABOLIC **Parathyroid Hormone** Teriparatide	SC	20 mcg qd	Treatment Maximum 2 years	Increase in BMD. Reduce fractures of spine by 77%, others by 68%.

Abbreviations: BMD = bone mineral density; IM = intramuscular; IV = intravenous; PO = per os (by mouth); qd = every day; qod = every other day; qwk = every week; RANKL = RANK ligand; SC = subcutaneous; SERM = selective estrogen receptor modulator.

(Gourlay et al., 2012). For patients receiving pharmacological therapy, review the medication regimen, assess for side effects, and repeat laboratory tests as indicated. Repeating the DEXA in 2 years may be useful to monitor response to treatment, although the true measure of success is the prevention of fractures. Serum and urinary markers of bone turnover are being investigated for monitoring of response to treatment, and clear guidelines regarding their use are likely to be available soon. The patient should also be assessed for fractures and the need for analgesics. Patients with osteoporosis should be enrolled in a fall prevention program.

Sequelae: Osteoporosis-related fractures are major complications. The majority of fractures resulting from osteoporosis are fractures of the spine. Many of these are asymptomatic but may result in chronic pain and decline in function. By far the most devastating consequence of osteoporosis is a hip fracture. Of the

250,000 people who sustain a hip fracture yearly, 12% to 20% die within the first year after the injury, and >50% of patients require long-term care. The importance of exercise and continued mobility needs to be emphasized, because patients often have a fear of falling and injury. In an attempt to protect themselves from injury, a loss of social and physical function may occur.

Prevention/prophylaxis: As an adolescent disease with geriatric consequences, prevention needs to begin at an early age. All older adults need to be screened to determine their level of risk for the development of osteoporosis and, using the FRAX, determine the 10-year likelihood of fracture. Dietary history, exercise patterns, and habits should be reviewed with patients. A measurement of height should be recorded at least yearly for all adults. The benefits of changing lifestyle patterns should be emphasized to patients even in advanced age. The U.S. Preventive Services Task Force (USPSTF) recommends screening women over age 65 and women under age 65 who have a 10-year fracture risk equal to that of a woman 65 years of age. The USPSTF indicated there were insufficient data to make a recommendation for screening men. The NOF recommends screening men over age 70 regardless of risk factors.

Referral: Women who will be beginning hormone replacement therapy may be referred to a gynecologist. For patients who have sustained a fracture, depending on its location, an immediate referral to an orthopedist is recommended. Patients may require referral for physical therapy to be evaluated for weight-bearing exercises and for demonstration of safe transferring, lifting, and bending. Patients with functional limitations need instruction on the use of adaptive equipment (e.g., walkers, grabbers).

Education: Patients can contact the NOF at 1232 22nd Street NW, Washington, DC 20037 (202-223-2226), www.nof.org, for educational materials. Patients also should be given information about local support groups for persons with osteoporosis, senior exercise classes, and dietary counseling.

CLINICAL RECOMMENDATION	EVIDENCE RATING	REFERENCES
In a population-based study, CHAMP, of 1705 men ages 70–97 years, 368 subjects lost at least 2% of their body weight. Weight loss was associated with a decline in BMD. Conclusions from the results of the study were that maintaining body weight is important for bone health in elderly men.	A	Bleicher et al. (2011)
A study to determine if cholecalciferol and ergocalciferol were equally effective in treating vitamin D deficiency included 95 hip fracture inpatients of whom 70 completed the study. They were randomized to treatment with either cholecalciferol or ergocalciferol, and both 25 OH D levels and intact parathyroid hormone (iPTH) levels were used as outcome measures. Although the cholecalciferol group had a significantly greater increase in 25OH D than the group taking ergocalciferol, both increased to therapeutic levels. Because there was not a significant difference in measured iPTH, the authors questioned the biological importance of the finding that cholecalciferol was more effective in increasing vitamin D.	B	Glendenning et al. (2009)
Denosumab was studied in 7686 women with WHO-defined osteoporosis. The double-blind, placebo-controlled trial recorded new vertebral fractures as the primary endpoint but also evaluated hip and other fractures. Overall, the denosumab arm experienced 68% fewer spine fractures, 40% fewer hip fractures, and 20% fewer nonvertebral fractures. There were no significant adverse events in the patients treated with denosumab.	A	Cummings et al. (2009)

A = consistent, good-quality, patient-oriented evidence; B = inconsistent or limited-quality, patient-oriented evidence; C = consensus, disease-oriented evidence, usual practice, expert opinion, or case series. For information about the SORT evidence rating system, go to www.aafp.org/afpsort.xml.

PANCREATIC CANCER

Signal symptoms: Pancreatic cancer is called the "silent disease" because often the disease is advanced before any symptoms begin. Symptoms include weight loss, pain in the upper abdomen spreading to the back that may come and go and be worse after eating and at night, jaundice of the skin or eyes, dark urine and light-colored stools, bowel movements that look greasy and float in the toilet, weakness, loss of appetite, and nausea and vomiting.

Description: Pancreatic cancer is the fourth leading cause of cancer deaths in the United States, comprising 6% of all cancers. It is difficult to detect, hard to diagnose, early to metastasize, and resistant to treatment. At the time of diagnosis, over one-half of all patients have distant disease and 26% have regional spread of the disease (Freelove & Walling, 2006). The relative 1-year survival rate is 24%, and the 5-year survival rate is 5%; this has not improved in the last 25 years (Freelove & Walling, 2006). Cancers can arise from both exocrine and endocrine portions of the pancreas, though 95% develop in the exocrine portion. Approximately 75% of pancreatic cancers occur within the head or neck, 20% in the body, and 5% to 10% in the tail of the pancreas. The most common type of pancreatic cancer is pancreatic duct adenocarcinoma. Generally it metastasizes to regional lymph nodes, then to the liver or, less commonly, the lungs. In 2009 over 42,000 new cases were diagnosed and over 35,000 patients died (Kang & Saif, 2010). It is rarely found in persons younger than 50, and the risk increases as one ages.

It is as the cancer grows and metastasizes that symptoms begin. Presentation initially varies according to location of the tumor. Tumors that are in the pancreatic body or tail generally present with pain and weight loss, and those in the head of the pancreas typically present with steatorrhea, weight loss, and diarrhea (Freelove & Walling, 2006). In a large number of cases, new onset of glucose intolerance precedes the diagnosis of pancreatic cancer. The diagnosis of pancreatic cancer should be thought of with a patient older than 70 years old with a new diagnosis of diabetes and no diabetic risk factors (Dragovich, Erickson, & Larson, 2011).

Etiology: Pancreatic cancer is fundamentally a disease caused by damage to the DNA. These mutations can be inherited, or they can be acquired as one ages. DNA can also be damaged by certain behaviors, such as alcohol or smoking, or simply by chance (American Cancer Society, 2011).

Occurrence: There are approximately 32,000 new cases of pancreatic cancer per year, making it about 2% of new cancers, yet it is the fourth leading cause of cancer deaths in the United States.

Age: Increases with age; most occur in persons over age 60, peaking from age 70 to 79. Without predisposing factors, pancreatic cancer is unusual in those younger than 45 (Shah, Farah, Goldwasser, & Agrawal, 2008).

Gender: Since 1994, slightly more women than men have been diagnosed each year but slightly more men than women die. Slightly more men have pancreatic cancer than women.

Ethnicity: African Americans are more likely to have pancreatic cancer than Asians, Hispanics, or Caucasians.

Contributing factors: Smokers are 2 to 3 times more likely than nonsmokers to develop pancreatic cancer. Consumption of red and processed meats has been associated with the development of pancreatic cancer (Larsson & Wolk, 2012). It occurs more in those with diabetes. Having a family history increases one's risk for pancreatic cancer. Chronic inflammation may be a predisposing factor in developing pancreatic cancer. Chronic pancreatitis due to alcohol is associated with a higher incidence and earlier onset of pancreatic carcinoma. A recent study by Gapturn and colleagues (2011) found that death from pancreatic cancer in patients who consumed alcohol, especially liquor, was independent of cigarette smoking. Certain hereditary conditions are associated with pancreatic cancer: hereditary pancreatitis, hereditary nonpolyposis colon cancer, von Hippel–Lindau syndrome, ataxia-telangiectasia syndrome, familial atypical multiple mole melanoma, and familial breast-ovarian cancer (BRCA1 and BRCA2 mutations), among others (Larghi, Verna, Lecca, & Costamagna, 2009). Long-term occupational exposure to DDT, benzidine, and dry cleaning agents has been associated with the development of pancreatic cancer (Robinson, 2012).

Signs and symptoms: Patients should be questioned about abdominal and midback pain, anorexia, depression, nausea, vomiting, and changes in bowel movements. Along with significant weight loss and moderate epigastric tenderness, the patient may have a palpable gallbladder (Courvoisier sign) and skin excoriation from pruritus. One of the most characteristic signs of pancreatic cancer of the head of the pancreas is painless obstructive jaundice. However, patients may notice a darkening of the urine and lightening of stools before the jaundice is visually evident. When questioned, they may indicate that their stools float (Robinson, 2012). They may also have ascites, and an abdominal mass may be noted in those with advanced pancreatic cancer. Left supraclavicular lymphadenopathy (Virchow's node) may be palpated in some patients with widespread disease. Many patients with advanced disease have Trousseau's syndrome (a hypercoagulable state) and there is a high incidence of thromboembolic events as well (Dragovich et al., 2011; Robinson, 2012).

Diagnostic tests: Liver function testing may show an elevated bilirubin and alkaline phosphatase. Bilirubin may be noted in urine and stool samples as well. There are several tumor markers being evaluated for pancreatic cancer, the most useful being antigen 19-9; the reported sensitivity and specificity are 80% to 90%. The imaging studies that can be done include the following: contrast-enhanced multislice helical CT is the preferred method to diagnose and stage pancreatic cancer where available; CT scan, transcutaneous ultrasonography, EUS, MRI, ERCP, or positron emission tomography may also be used to look at the structures and vessels in the abdomen. Percutaneous transhepatic cholangiography can also be done, in which dye is injected into the liver and shows the bile ducts so they can be seen to detect a blockage. A biopsy will be done using fine-needle aspiration after a CT or EUS is done. Where expert EUS is available, it has proven to be the most specific and sensitive diagnostic test, with detection rates of 99% to 100%. The most difficult clinical situation to diagnose pancreatic cancer is the person with underlying chronic pancreatitis because all of the above imaging studies may show abnormalities and may not help differentiate between carcinoma and chronic pancreatitis.

Differential diagnosis:
- Aortic aneurysm
- Duodenal or gastric ulcers
- Ampullary carcinoma
- Bile duct strictures or tumors
- Cholangitis
- Cholecystitis
- Choledocholithiasis
- Cholelithiasis

Treatment: The extent of surgery depends on the location and size of the tumor, the stage of the disease, and the patient's general health. The Whipple procedure is the most common surgery for pancreatic cancer, especially if the tumor is in the head of the pancreas. A distal pancreatectomy removes the body and the tail of the pancreas, and a total pancreatectomy removes the entire pancreas, part of the small intestine, a portion of the stomach, the common bile duct, the gallbladder, the spleen, and nearby lymph nodes. After surgery one may have radiation therapy, chemotherapy, or a combination of both. Gemcitabine remains the standard of care for the disease, either alone or in conjunction with other drugs (Li & Saif, 2009). Pain relief is crucial in palliative care. This can be done with narcotic analgesics alone or by combining them with tricyclic antidepressants or antiemetics. Radiation therapy can also palliate pain but does not affect patient survival. Obstructive jaundice warrants relief if the patient has pruritus or right upper quadrant pain. Anorexia may also improve after relief of biliary obstruction. Pancreatic insufficiency and subsequent malabsorption is treated with pancreatic enzyme replacement.

Follow-up: Follow-up after surgery and/or treatment modalities is important to ensure that any changes are seen and dealt with as early as possible. This will include visits to the primary care provider, surgeon if surgery was done, and oncologist if that treatment modality was selected.

Sequelae: Patients with pancreatic carcinoma are often anorexic. Patients with malabsorption diarrhea and weight loss may benefit from pancreatic enzyme supplementation. Visits to a dietitian may also be useful for nutritional assistance.

Prevention/prophylaxis: Although pancreatic cancer is not completely preventable, patients need to be aware of probable modifiable risks associated with the development of pancreatic cancer, such as smoking and excessive alcohol intake (a contributor to chronic pancreatitis). A recent meta-analysis revealed a positive association between red meat and processed meats and the development of pancreatic cancer (Larsson & Wolk, 2012). It remains controversial whether people with given risk factors should be screened for pancreatic cancer. Practice recommendations by the Fourth International Symposium of Inherited Diseases of the Pancreas made a threshold of >10-fold increased risk for developing pancreatic cancer who might benefit from screening by an endoscopic ultrasound (Larghi et al., 2009)

Referral: The National Comprehensive Cancer Network's 2011 guidelines recommend that decisions about treatment and resectability involve input from a multidisciplinary group of specialists. Patients selected for surgery should be based on the probability of cure.

Other factors include comorbidities, overall performance, and age (Dragovich et al., 2011). A recent study found that age alone should not preclude pancreatic resection (Oliveira-Cunha, 2013). Melis and colleagues (2012) reported that the 30-day survival rate of patients over the age of 80 who had a pancreaticoduodenectomy was similar to younger patients who underwent the same procedure. In advanced pancreatic cancer, patients and family should be informed of availability of palliative care measures and hospice as indicated by the patient's progression of disease (Shah et al., 2008).

Education: The best decisions are made with a solid knowledge base, so one needs to learn as much about pancreatic cancer as possible. The patient and family will need end-of-life education. Although some patients may live up to 2 years or more, most with advanced pancreatic cancer die within months of diagnosis. There are support groups that can give one information on possible clinical trials pertinent to the patient's condition.

CLINICAL RECOMMENDATION	EVIDENCE RATING	REFERENCES
Gemcitabine is recommended as first-line chemotherapy for patients with metastatic pancreatic cancer.	B	Freelove & Walling (2006) Li & Saif (2009)
Dual-phase helical computed tomography is the best initial imaging test for diagnosis and staging of suspected pancreatic cancer.	C	Freelove & Walling (2006)

A = consistent, good-quality, patient-oriented evidence; B = inconsistent or limited-quality, patient-oriented evidence; C = consensus, disease-oriented evidence, usual practice, expert opinion, or case series. For information about the SORT evidence rating system, go to www.aafp.org/afpsort.xml.

CASE STUDY

A 65-year-old white man presents with pain in the left-upper quadrant and epigastric area of his abdomen. He states that he had an episode of acute pancreatitis 10 years ago without any real sequelae. He does say that he has had episodes of abdominal pain in the epigastric and upper abdominal area over the years but generally over time it goes away within hours or days and he does not seek medical care.

On further questioning, he admits to drinking anywhere from two to six beers at least 3 days a week. He does not feel this is a problem; he does remember being told to watch his alcohol intake when he had acute pancreatitis but after several years without pain, he decided that alcohol must not be a factor in his abdominal pain. Further questioning about his symptoms has him telling you that his pain radiates to the left scapular area of his back. He admits to being thirstier recently and has been urinating more frequently as well. He has had to notch his belt two holes within the last year. He has not been trying to lose weight. He denies diarrhea but has had nausea without vomiting. Eating aggravates the pain but bending over at the waist helps the pain lessen.

Objective: Blood pressure (BP) 135/80 mm Hg, heart rate (HR) 80 beats/min, BMI 21.

1. What additional subjective data are you seeking?
2. What additional objective data will you be assessing for?
3. What are the differential diagnoses that you are considering?
4. What laboratory tests will help you rule out some of the differential diagnoses?
5. What imaging studies are generally ordered for a patient with these symptoms?
6. What is your treatment plan for this patient?
7. Will you be looking for a consultation?

REFERENCES

Assessment

Davis, P. J., Davis, F. B., & Leinung, M. C. (2007). In E. D. Duthie, P. R. Katz, & M. L. Malone (Eds.), *Practice of geriatrics* (4th ed.). Philadelphia, PA: Saunders/Elsevier.

Gruenewald, D. A., Kenny, A., & Matsumato, A. M. (2010). In J. T. Pacala & G. S. Sullivan (Eds.), *The geriatrics review syllabus: a core curriculum in geriatrics* (7th ed.). New York City, NY: American Geriatrics Society.

Gruenewald, D. A., & Matsumato, A. M. (2009). In J. Halter, J. Ouslander, M. Tinetti, S. Studenski, K. High, S. Asthana, & W. Hazzard (Eds.), *Principles of geriatric medicine and gerontology* (6th ed.). New York City, NY: McGraw-Hill Medical.

LeBlond, R. F., Brown, D. D., & DeGowin, R. L. (2009). *DeGowin's diagnostic examination* (9th ed.). New York City, NY: McGraw-Hill Medical.

Acute Pancreatitis

Alexakis, N., & Neoptolemos, J. (2005). Algorithm for the diagnosis and treatment of acute biliary pancreatitis. *Scandinavian Journal of Surgery, 94*, 124–129.

Balthazar, E. (2002). Acute pancreatitis: assessment of severity with clinical and CT evaluation. *Radiology, 223*, 603–613.

Besselink, M., Santvoort, H., Buskens, E., & Gooszen, H. (2006). Evidence based treatment of acute pancreatitis: antibiotic prophylaxis in necrotizing pancreatitis. *Annals of Surgery, 244*(4), 637–638.

Carroll, J. K., Herrick, B., Gipson, T., & Lee, S. P. (2007). Acute pancreatitis: diagnosis, prognosis, and treatment. *American Family Physician, 75*(10), 1513–1520.

Cherian, J., Slvaraj, V., Natrayan, R., & Venkataraman, J. (2007). ERCP in acute pancreatitis. *Hepatobiliary Pancreatic Disease International, 6*, 233–240.

Das, S. L., Singh, P. P., Phillips, A. R., Murphy, R., Windsor, J. A., & Petrov, M. S. (2013). Newly diagnosed diabetes mellitus after acute pancreatitis: a systematic review and meta-analysis. *Gut*. doi: 10.1136/gutjnl-2013-305062

Gardner, T., & Berk, B. (2010). Acute pancreatitis. Retrieved from http://emedicine.medscape.com/article/181364

Ioannidis, O., Lavrentieva, A., & Botsios, D. (2008). Nutrition support in acute pancreatitis. *Journal of the Pancreas, 9*(4), 375–390.

Kapetanos, D. (2010). Endoscopic management of acute recurrent pancreatitis. *Annals of Gastroenterology, 23*(1), 31–37.

Khaliq, A., Dutta, U., Kochhar, R., & Singh, K. (2010). Management of acute pancreatitis: "PANCREAS" contains eight easy steps to remember the treatment. *Journal of the Pancreas, 11*(5), 492–493.

Neoptolemos, N. A. (2009). Algorithm for the diagnosis and treatment of acute biliary pancreatitis. *Scandinavian Journal of Surgery, 94*, 124–129.

Skolnick, A., Feller, E., & Nanda, A. (2008). Evaluation of acute pancreatitis in the older patient. *Annals of Long-Term Care, 16*(5), 30–35.

Steven, T., & Conwell, D. (2010). Chronic pancreatitis. Cleveland Clinic: Disease Management Project: Pancreatic Disorders. Retrieved from www.clevelandclinicmeded.com/medicalpubs. diseasemanagementproject

Steven, T., Parsi, M., & Walsh, R. (2009). Acute pancreatitis: problems in adherence to guidelines. *Cleveland Clinic Journal of Medicine, 76*(12), 697–704.

Chronic Pancreatitis

American Cancer Society. (2011). Pancreatic cancer. Retrieved from www.cancer.org/Cancer/PancreaticCancer/DetailedGuide/index

Freedman, S. D. (2010). Clinical manifestations and diagnosis, treatment and complications of chronic pancreatitis in adults. *UpToDate*. Retrieved from www.uptodate.com/contents/clinical-manifestations-and-diagnosis-of-chronic-pancreatitis-in-adults

Huffman, J. L. (2011). Chronic pancreatitis treatment and management. Retrieved from http://emedicine.medscape.com/article/181554

Nair, R. J., Lawler, L., & Miller, M. R. (2007). Chronic pancreatitis. *American Family Physician, 76*(11), 1679–1688.

Obideen, K., & Wehbi, M. (2011). Chronic pancreatitis. Retrieved from http://emedicine.medscape.com/article/181554

Shah, B. B., Farah, K. F., Goldwasser, B., & Agrawal, R. A. (2008). Pancreatic diseases in the elderly. *Practical Gastroenterology, 18*, 21–32.

Steven, T., & Conwell, D. (2010). Chronic pancreatitis. Cleveland Clinic: Disease Management Project: Pancreatic Disorders. Retrieved from www.clevelandclinicmeded.com/medicalpubs. diseasemanagementproject

Diabetes Mellitus, Types 1 and 2

Ackermann, R. T., Finch, E. A., Brizendine, E., Zhou, H., & Marrero, D. G. (2008). Translating the Diabetes Prevention Program into the community: the DEPLOY Pilot Study. *American Journal of Preventive Medicine, 35*, 357–363.

American Diabetes Association. (2007). Diabetes statistics. Retrieved from www.diabetes.org/diabetes-basics/diabetes-statistics

American Diabetes Association. (2010). Insulin basics. Retrieved from http://forecast.diabetes.org/files/images/InsulinChart_4.pdf

American Diabetes Association. (2013). Standards of medical care in diabetes—2013. *Diabetes Care, 36*(Suppl 1), S11–S66.

Boyle, J. P., Thompson T. J., Gregg, E. W., Barker, L. E., & Williamson, D. F. (2010). Projection of the year 2050 burden of diabetes in the US adult population: dynamic modeling of incidence, mortality, and prediabetes prevalence. *Population Health Metrics, 8*(29). doi:10.1186/1478-7954-8-29. Retrieved from www.pophealthmetrics.com/content/8/1/29

Carter, A. A., Gomes, T., Camacho, X., Juurlink, D. N., Shah, B. R., & Mamdani, M. M. (2013). Risk of incident diabetes among patients treated with statins: population based study. *British Medical Journal, 346*. doi: 10.1136/bmj.f2610

Centers for Disease Control and Prevention. (2008). *National diabetes fact sheet: general information and national estimates on diabetes in the United States*. Atlanta, GA: U.S. Department of Health and Human Services, Centers for Disease Control and Prevention. Retrieved from www.cdc.gov/diabetes/pubs/pdf/ndfs_2007.pdf

Gregg, E. W., & Albright, A. L. (2009). The public health response to diabetes—two steps forward, one step back. *Journal of the American Medical Association, 301*, 1596–1598.

Hamaty, M. (2011). Insulin treatment for type 2 diabetes: when to start, which to use. *Cleveland Clinic Journal of Medicine, 78*(5), 332–342.

Hornick, T., & Aron, D. (2008). Managing diabetes in the elderly: go easy, individualize. *Cleveland Clinic Journal of Medicine, 75*(1), 70–78.

Inzucchi, S. E., Bergenstal, R. M., Buse, J. B., Diamant, M., Ferrannini, E., Nauck, M., . . . Matthews, D. R. (2012). Management of hyperglycemia in type 2 diabetes: a patient-centered approach. *Diabetes Care, 35*(6), 1364–1379.

Nathan, D. M., Buse, J. B., Davidson, M. B., Ferrannini, E., Holman, R. R., Sherwin, R., & Zinman, B. (2009). Medical management of hyperglycemia in type 2 diabetes: a consensus algorithm for the initiation and adjustment of therapy. A consensus statement of the American Diabetes Association and the European Association for the Study of Diabetes. *Diabetes Care, 32*(1), 193–203.

Nathan, D. M., Kuenen, J., Borg, R., Zheng, H., Schoenfeld, D., & Heine, R. J. (2008). Translating the A1C assay into estimated average glucose values. *Diabetes Care, 31*(8), 1473–1478.

Rodbard, H. W., Jellinger, P. S., Davidson, J. A., Einhorn, D., Garber, A. J., Grunberger, G., . . . Schwartz, S. S. (2009). AACE/ACE consensus statement: statement by an American Association of Clinical Endocrinologists/American College of Endocrinology consensus panel on type 2 diabetes mellitus: an algorithm for glycemic control. *Endocrine Practice, 15*(6), 540–559. Retrieved from www.projectinform.org/pdf/diabetes_aace.pdf

Failure to Thrive

Chen, C. C., Tang, S. T., Wang, C., & Huang, G. H. (2009). Trajectory and determinants of nutritional health in older patients during and six-month post-hospitalisation. *Journal of Clinical Nursing, 8*(23), 3299–3307. doi:10.1111/j.1365-2702.2009.02932.x

Daniels, R., van Rossum, E., de Witte, L., Kempen, G. I., & van den Heuvel, W. (2008). Interventions to prevent disability in frail community-dwelling elderly: a systematic review. *BMC Health Services Research, 8,* 278.

Dorner, B. (2010, Fall). Creative nutrition: solutions for failure to thrive patients. *Aging Well,* pp. 8–11.

Dozeman, E., van Marwijk, H. W. van Schaik, D. J., Stek, M. L., van der Horst, H. E., Beekman, A. T., & van Hout, H. P. (2010). High incidence of clinically relevant depressive symptoms in vulnerable persons of 75 years or older living in the community. *Aging and Mental Health, 4*(7), 828–833. doi:10.1080/13607861003781817

Evans, C. (2005). Malnutrition in the elderly: a multifactorial failure to thrive. *Permanente Journal, 9*(3), 38–41.

Hollinger-Smith, L., & Buschmann, M. (2000). Failure to thrive syndrome. *Clinical Gerontologist, 20*(4), 65–88.

Kumeliauskas, L., Fruetel, K., & Holroyd-Leduc, J. M. (2013). Evaluation of older adults hospitalized with a diagnosis of failure to thrive. *Canadian Geriatrics Journal, 16*(2), 49. doi:10.5770/cgi.16.64

Morely, J. E. (2011). Assessment of malnutrition in older persons: a focus on the Mini Nutritional Assessment. *Journal of Nutrition, Health & Aging, 15*(2), 87–90.

Moses, S. (2008). Failure to thrive in the elderly. Retrieved November 10, 2010, from www.fpnotebook.com/Geri/Prevent?FlrThrvInTheElderly.htm

Robertson, R. G., & Montagnini, M. (2004). Geriatric failure to thrive. *American Family Physician, 70*(2), 343–350. Retrieved November 10, 2010, from www.aafp.org/afp/2004/0715/p343.html

Rocchiccioli, J. T., & Sanford, J. T. (2009). Revisiting geriatric failure to thrive: a complex and compelling clinical condition. *Journal of Gerontological Nursing, 35*(1), 18–25.

Ruiz, G. V., Lopez-Briz, E., Carbonnell, S. R., Gonzalvez, P. J. L., & Borr-Marti, S. (2013). Megestrol acetate for treatment of anorexia-cachexia syndrome. *Cochrane Database of Systematic Reviews, 3,* CD004310. doi:10.1002/14651858.CD004310

Schag, C. C., Heinrich, R. L., & Ganz, P. A. (1984). Karnofsky performance status revisited: reliability, validity, and guidance. *Journal of Clinical Oncology, 2*(3), 187–193.

Shivaraj, G., Prakash, B. D., Sonal, V., Shruthi, K., Vinayak, H. & Avinash, H. (2009). Thyroid function tests: a review. *European Review for Medical and Pharmacological Sciences, 13*(5) 341–349.

Snyder, S., & Baum, E. (2011). Chronic mesenteric ischemia: a curable case of failure to thrive. *Annals of Long-Term Care, 19*(12), 34–38.

Hyperlipidemia

Alwaili, K., Alrasadi, K., Awan, Z., & Genest, J. (2009). Approach to the diagnosis and management of lipoprotein disorders. *Current Opinion in Endocrinology, Diabetes and Obesity, 16*(2), 132–140. doi:10.1097/MED.0b013e328329135a

American Heart Association. (2010). Heart disease and stroke statistics: 2010 update. Retrieved from www.americanheart.org/downloadable/heart/1265665152970DS-3241%20Heart-StrokeUpdate_2010.pdf

Centers for Disease Control and Prevention. (2010). Cholesterol facts. Retrieved from www.cdc.gov/cholesterol/facts.htm

Chase, S. L. (2002). New lipid guidelines recommend tighter control. *Topics in Advanced Practice Nursing eJournal, 2*(3). Retrieved from www.medscape.com/viewarticle/438573_2

Crawford, A. G., Cote, C., Couto, J., Daskiran, M., Gunnarsson, C., Haas, K., . . . Schuette, R. (2010). Prevalence of obesity, type II diabetes mellitus, hyperlipidemia, and hypertension in the United States: findings from the GE centricity electronic medical record database. *Population Health Management, 13*(3), 151–161. doi:10.1089/pop.2009.0039

Davis, H. R., & Veltri, E. P. (2007). Zetia: inhibition of Niemann-Pick C1 Like 1 (NPC1L1) to reduce intestinal cholesterol absorption and treat hyperlipidemia. *Journal of Atherosclerosis and Thrombosis, 14*(3), 99–108. doi:10.5551/jat.14.99

Drexel, H. (2009). Statins, fibrates, nicotinic acid, cholesterol absorption inhibitors, anion- exchange resins, omega-3 fatty acids: which drugs for which patients? *Fundamental & Clinical Pharmacology, 23*(6), 687–692. doi:10.1111/j.1472-8206.2009.00745.x

Grundy, S. M., Cleeman, J. I., Bairey Merz, C. N., Brewer, H. B., Jr., Clark, L. T., Hunninghake, D. B., . . . Stone, N .J. (2004). Implications of recent clinical trials for the National Cholesterol Education Program Adult Treatment Panel III guidelines. *Circulation, 110,* 227–239. doi:10.1161/01.CIR.0000133317.49796.0E

Hopkins, P. N., Toth, P. P., Ballantyne, C. M., & Rader, D. J. (2011). Familial hypercholesterolemias: prevalence, genetics, diagnosis and screening recommendations from the national lipid association expert panel on familial hypercholesterolemia. *Journal of Clinical Lipidology, 5*(3, Suppl 1), S9–S17. doi:10.1016/j.jacl.2011.03.452

Law, M., & Rudnicka, A. (2006). Statin safety: a systematic review [Supplemental material]. *American Journal of Cardiology, 97*(8A), S52C–S60. doi:10.1016/j.amjcard.2005.12.010

Menown, I., Murtagh, G., Maher, V., Cooney, M., Graham, I., & Tomkin, G. (2009). Dyslipidemia update: the importance of full lipid profile assessment. *Advances in Therapy, 26*(7), 711–718. doi:10.1007/s12325-009-0052-3

National Institutes of Health. (2002). Third report of the Expert Panel on Detection, Evaluation, and Treatment of High Blood Cholesterol in Adults (Adult Treatment Panel III). (NIH Pub. No. 02-5215.) Retrieved from www.nhlbi.nih.gov/guidelines/cholesterol

Reiss, A., & Glass, A. (2006). Atherosclerosis: immune and inflammatory aspects. *Journal of Investigative Medicine, 54*(3), 123–131. doi:10.2310/6650.2006.05051

Rickets, M. L., Boekschoten, M. V., Kreeft, A. J., Hooiveld, G. J., Moen, C. J., Muller, M., . . . Moore, D. D. (2007). The cholesterol-raising factor from coffee beans, cafestol, as an antagonist ligand for the farnesoid and pregnane X receptors. *Molecular Endocrinology, 21*(7), 1603–1616. doi:10.1210/me.2007-0133

Roberts, C., Guallar, E., & Rodriguez, A. (2007). Efficacy and safety of statin monotherapy in older adults: a meta-analysis. *Journal of Gerontology: Medical Sciences, 62A*(8), 879–887. Retrieved from http://libproxy.uncg.edu:6292/content/62/8/879.full.pdf+html

Rubenfire, M., Brook, R. D., & Rosenson, R. S. (2009). Treating mixed hyperlipidemia and the atherogenic lipid phenotype for prevention of cardiovascular events. *American Journal of Medicine, 16*(2), 132–140. doi:10.1016/j.amjmed.2010.03.024

Scirica, B. M., & Cannon, C. P. (2005). Treatment of elevated cholesterol. *Circulation, 111*(21), e360–e363. doi:10.1161/CIRCULATIONAHA.105.539106

Wenger, N. K., Lewis, S. J., Herrington, D. M., Bittner, V., & Welty, F. K. (2007). Outcomes of using high- or low-dose atorvastatin in patients 65 years of age or older with stable coronary heart disease. *Annals of Internal Medicine, 147*(1), 1–9. Retrieved from www.annals.org/content/147/1/1.full.pdf+html

Hyperthyroidism

Bahn, R. S., Burch, H. B., Cooper, D. S., Garber, J. R., Greenlee, M. C., Klein, I., . . . Stan, M. N. (2011). Hyperthyroidism and other causes of thyrotoxicosis: management guidelines of the American Thyroid Association of Clinical Endocrinologists. *Endocrine Practice, 17*(3), 466–520.

Boelaert, K., Torlinska, B., Holder, R. L., & Franklin, J. A. (2010). Older subjects with hyperthyroidism present with a paucity of symptoms and signs: a large cross sectional study. *Journal of Clinical Endocrinology and Metabolism, 95*(6), 2715–2726.

Cappola, A. R., Fried, L. P., Arnold, A. M., Danese, M. D., Kuller, L. H., Burke, G. L., . . . Ladenson, P. W. (2006). Thyroid status, cardiovascular risk, and mortality in older adults: the Cardiovascular Health Study. *Journal of the American Medical Association, 295*(9), 1033–1041.

Cooper, D. S. (2003). Hyperthyroidism. *Lancet, 362*(9382), 459–468.

Cooper, D. S., & Biondi, B. (2012). Subclinical thyroid disease. *Lancet, 379*(9821), 1142–1154. doi:10.1016/S0140-6736(11)60276-6

Fitzgerald, P. A. (2009). Endocrine disorders. In S. J. McPhee & M. A. Papadakis (Eds.), *Current medical diagnosis and treatment 2009* (48th ed.). New York City, NY: McGraw-Hill.

Gruenewald, D., Kenny, A. M., & Matsumoto, A. M. (2010). Endocrine and metabolic disorders. In J. Pacala & G. Sullivan (Eds.), *Geriatrics review syllabus* (7th ed.). American Geriatrics Society. Mechanicsburg, PA: Fry Communications.

Gunder, L. H., & Haddow, S. (2009). Laboratory evaluation of thyroid function. *Clinical Advisor*. Retrieved from www.clinicaladvisor.com/laboratory-evaluation-of-thyroid-function/article/158683

Lee, J. S., Bůžková, P., Fink, H. A., Vu, J., Carbone, L., Chen, Z., . . . Robbins, J. (2010). Subclinical thyroid dysfunction and incident hip fracture in older adults. *Archives of Internal Medicine, 170*(21), 1876–1883.

Mooradian, A. D. (2008). Asymptomatic hyperthyroidism in older adults: is it a distinct clinical and laboratory entity? *Drugs & Aging, 25*(5), 371–380.

Reid, J. R., & Wheeler, S. F. (2005). Hyperthyroidism: diagnosis and treatment. *American Family Physician, 72*(4), 623–630.

Hypothyroidism

Aoki, Y., Belin, R. M., Clickner, R., Jeffries, R., Phillips, L., & Mahaffey, K. R. (2007). Serum TSH and T4 in the United States population and their association with participant characteristics: National Health and Nutrition Examination Survey (NHANES 1999–2002). *Thyroid, 17*(12), 1211–1223.

Bharaktiya, S., Orlander, P., Woodhouse, W., Davis, A. B., Ziel, F. H., Talavera, F., . . . Griffing, G. T. (2011). Hypothyroidism. *Endocrinology*. Retrieved from http://emedicine.medscape.com/article/122393-overview

Duntas, L., Orgiazzi, J., & Brabant, G. (2011). The interface between thyroid and diabetes mellitus. *Clinical Endocrinology, 75*(1), 1–9.

Fenstemacher, P. A., & Winn, P. (Eds.). (2011). *Long-term care medicine: a pocket guide.* New York City, NY: Humana Press.

Gaitonde, D. Y., Rowley, K. D., & Sweeney, L. B. (2012). Hypothyroidism: an update. *South African Family Practice, 54*(5), 384–390.

Guha, B., Krishnaswamy, G., & Peiris, A. (2002). The diagnosis and management of hypothyroidism. *Southern Medical Journal, 95*(5), 475–480.

Kajantie, E., Phillips, D. I., Osmond, C., Barker D. J., Forsen, T., & Eriksson, J. G. (2006). Spontaneous hypothyroidism in adult women is predicted by small body size at birth and during childhood. *Journal of Clinical Endocrinology and Metabolism, 91*(12), 4953–4956.

Madhu, S. V., Jain, R., Kant, S., Prakash, V., & Kumar, V. (2010). Myopathy presenting as a sole manifestation of hypothyroidism. *Journal of the Association of Physicians of India, 58*, 569–570.

Mauk, K. L. (2005). Rooting out hypothyroidism in the elderly. *Nursing, 35*(12), 65–66.

Simonsick, E. M., Newman, A. B., Ferrucci, L., Satterfield, S., Harris, T. B., Rodondi, N., . . . Health ABC Study. (2009). Subclinical hypothyroidism and functional mobility in older adults. *Archives of Internal Medicine, 169*(21), 2011–2017.

Surks, M. L., & Hollowell, J. G. (2007). Age-specific distribution of serum thyrotropin and antithyroid antibodies in the U.S. population: implications for the prevalence of subclinical hypothyroidism. *The Journal of Clinical Endocrinology & Metabolism, 92*(12), 4575–4582. doi: 10.1210/jc.2007-1499

Vitale, G., Fatti, L. M., Prolo, S., Girola, A., Caraglia, M., Marra, M., . . . Mari, D. (2010). Screening for hypothyroidism in older hospitalized patients with anemia: a new insight into an old disease. *Journal of the American Geriatrics Society, 58*(9), 1825–1827.

Wang, J. Y., Wang, C. Y., Pei, D., Lai, C. C., Chen, Y. L., Wu, C. Z., . . . Tang, S. H. (2010). Association between thyroid function and metabolic syndrome in elderly subjects. *Journal of the American Geriatrics Society, 58*(8), 1613–1614.

Wilson, G., & Curry, R. W. (2005). Subclinical thyroid disease. *American Family Physician, 72*(8), 1517–1524.

Malnutrition

Ahmed, T., & Haboubi, N. (2010). Assessment and management of nutrition in older people and its importance to health. *Clinical Interventions in Aging, 5*, 207–216.

American Medical Directors Association. (2011). *Clinical practice guideline (CPG): altered nutritional status (ANS).* Columbia, MD: American Medical Directors Association.

Duffy, E. G. (2008). Malnutrition in older adults: deciphering a complex syndrome. *Advance for Nurse Practitioners and Physician Assistants, 16*(9), 28–33.

Evan, W. J., Morely, J. E., Argiles, J., Bales, C., Baracos, V., Guttridge, D., . . . Anker, S. D. (2008). Cachexia: a new definition. *Clinical Nutrition, 27*(6), 793–799.

Feldblum, I., German, L., Castel, H., Harman-Boehm, I., Bilenko, N., Eisinger, M., . . . Shahar, D. R. (2007). Characteristics of undernourished older medical patients and the identification of predictors for undernutrition status. *Nutrition Journal, 6*, 37–45. doi:10.1186/1475-2891-6-37

Fielding, R. A., Vellas, B., Evans, W. J., Bhasin, S., Morley, J. E., Newman, A. B., . . . Zamboni, M. (2011). Sarcopenia: an undiagnosed condition in older adults. Current consensus definition: prevalence, etiology, and consequences. International working group on sarcopenia. *Journal of the American Medical Directors Association, 12*(4), 249–256.

Hajjar, R. R., Kamel, H. K., & Denson, K. (2004). Malnutrition in aging. *Internet Journal of Geriatrics and Gerontology, 1*(1). doi:10.5580/765

Izawa, S., Enoki, H., Hirakawa, Y., Masuda, Y., Iwat, M., Hasegawa, J., . . . Kuzuya, M. (2007). Lack of body weight measurement is associated with mortality and hospitalization in community-dwelling frail elderly. *Clinical Nutrition, 26*(6), 764–770.

Jensen, G. L., Mirtallo, J., Compher, C., Dhaliwal, R., Forbes, A., Grijalba, R. F., . . . Waitzberg, D. (2010). Adult starvation and disease-related malnutrition: a proposal for etiology-based diagnosis in the clinical practice setting from the International Consensus Guideline Committee. *Clinical Nutrition, 29*(2), 151–153.

Johansson, Y., Bachrach-Lindström, M., Carstensen, J., & Ek, A. C. (2010). Malnutrition in a home-living older population: prevalence, incidence and risk factors. A prospective study. *Journal of Clinical Nursing. 8*(9), 1354–1364. doi:10.1111/j.1365-2702.2008.02552.x

Kagansky, N., Berner, Y., Koren-Morag, N., Perelman, L., Knobler, H., & Levy, S. (2005). Poor nutritional habits are predictors of poor outcome in very old hospitalized patients. *American Journal of Clinical Nutrition, 82*(4), 784–791; quiz 913–914.

Kaiser, M. J., Bauer, J. M., Rämsch, C., Uter, W., Guigoz, Y., Cederholm, T., . . . Mini Nutritional Assessment International Group. (2010). Frequency of malnutrition in older adults: a multinational perspective using the Mini Nutritional Assessment. *Journal of the American Geriatrics Society, 58*(9), 1734–1738.

Kamp, B., Wellman, N. S., & Russell, C. (2010). Position of the American Dietetic Association, American Society for Nutrition, and Society for Nutrition Education: food and nutrition programs for community-residing older adults. *Journal of Nutrition Education and Behavior, 42*(2), 72–82.

Lee, L.-C., Tsai, A. C., Wang, J.-Y., Hurng, B.-S., Hsu, H.-C., & Tsai, H.-J. (2013). Need-based intervention is an effective strategy for improving the nutritional status of older people living in a nursing home: a randomized controlled trial. *International Journal of Nursing Studies.* doi:10.1016/j.ijnurst.2013.04.004

Lee, M. R., & Berthelot. E. R. (2010). Community covariates of malnutrition based mortality among older adults. *Annals of Epidemiology, 20*(5), 371. doi:10.1016/j.annepidem.2010.01.008

Loreck, E., Chimakurthi, R., & Steinle, N. I. (2012). Nutritional assessment of the geriatric patient: a comprehensive approach toward evaluating and managing nutrition. *Clinical Geriatrics, 20*(4), 20–26.

McClave, S. A., Martindale, R. G., Vanek, V. W., McCarthy, M., Roberts, P., Taylor, B., . . . Cresci, G. (2009). Guidelines for the provision and assessment of nutrition support therapy in the adult critically ill patient: Society of Critical Care Medicine (SCCM) and American Society for Parenteral and Enteral Nutrition (A.S.P.E.N). *JPEN: Journal of Parenteral and Enteral Nutrition, 33*(3), 277–316.

Morely, J. E. (2011). Assessment of malnutrition in older persons: a focus on the Mini Nutritional Assessment. *Journal of Nutrition, Health & Aging, 15*(2), 87–90.

Morley, J. E. & Silver, A. J. (1995). Nutritional issues in nursing home care. *Annals of Internal Medicine, 123*(11), 850–859.

Soderstrom, L., Rosenblad, A., Adolfsson, E. T., Saletti, A., & Bergkvist, L. (2013). Nutritional status predicts preterm death in older people: a prospective cohort study. *Clinical Nutrition.* doi:10.1016/j.clnu.2013.06.004

van Bokhorst-de van der Schueren, M. A., Lonterman-Monasch, S., de Vries, O. J., Danner, S. A., Kramer, M. H., & Muller, M. (2013). Prevalence and determinants for malnutrition in geriatric outpatients. *Clinical Nutrition.* doi:10.1016/j.clnu.2013.05.007

Vischer, U. M., Frangos, E., Graf, C., Gold, G., Weiss, L., Herrmann, F. R., & Zerky, D. (2012). The prognostic significance of malnutrition as assessed by the Mini Nutritional Assessment (MNA) in older hospitalized patients with heavy disease burden. *Clinical Nutrition, 31*(1), 113–117. doi:10.1016/j.clnu.2011.09.010

Wernette, C., White, D., & Zizza, C. A. (2011). Signaling proteins that influence energy intake may affect unintentional weight loss in elderly persons. *Journal of the American Dietetic Association, 111*(6), 864–873.

White, J. V., Guenter, P., Jensen, G., Malone, A., & Schofield, M. (2012). Consensus statement of the Academy of Nutrition and Dietetics/American Society for Parenteral and Enteral Nutrition: characteristics recommended for the identification and documentation of adult malnutrition (undernutrition). *Journal of the Academy of Nutrition and Dietetics, 112*(5), 730–738. doi:10.1016/jjand2012.03.012

Zeanandin, G., Molato, O., LeDuff, F., Guerin, O., Hebuteme, X., & Schneider, S. M. (2012). Impact of restrictive diets on the risk of undernutrition in a free-living elderly population. *Clinical Nutrition, 31*(1), 69–73.

Obesity

American College of Physicians. (2011). *Overweight/Obesity and Weight Control* [Entire issue]. Retrieved from www.acponline.org/patients_families/diseases_conditions/obesity

Benton, M. J., Whyte, M. D., & Dyal, B. W. (2001). Sarcopenic obesity: strategies for management. *American Journal of Nursing, 111*(12), 38–44.

Bocalini, D. S., Lima, L. S., de Andrade, S., Madureira, A., Rica, R. L., dos Santos, R. N., . . . Pontes, F. L., Jr. (2012). Effects of circuit-based exercise programs on the body composition of elderly obese women. *Clinical Interventions in Aging, 7*, 551–556.

Bouchonville, M., Armamento-Villareal, R., Shah, K., Napoli, N., Sinacore, D. R., Qualls, C., & Villareal, D. T. (2013). Weight loss, exercise or both and cardiometabolic risk factors in obese older adults: results of a randomized controlled trial. *International Journal of Obesity.* doi:10.1038/ijo.2013.122

Brown, T., Avenell, A., Edmonds, L. D., Moore, H., Whittaker, V., Avery, L., & Summerbell, C. (2009). Systematic review of long-term lifestyle interventions to prevent weight gain and morbidity in adults. *Obesity Reviews, 10*(6), 627–638. doi:10.1111/j.1467-789x.2009.00641.x

Center on an Aging Society. (2003). Obesity among older Americans. Retrieved January 7, 2013, from http://ihcrp.georgetown.edu/agingsociety/pdfs/obesity2.pdf

Centers for Disease Control and Prevention. (2011a). Defining overweight and obesity (Issue Brief 24/7). Retrieved from www.cdc.gov/obesity/defining.html

Centers for Disease Control and Prevention. (2011b). Healthy weight (Fact Sheet). Retrieved from www.cdc.gov/healthyweight/assessing/bmi/

Chung, J. Y., Kang, H. T., Lee, D. C., Lee, H. R., & Lee, Y. J. (2012). Body composition and its association with cardiometabolic risk factors in the elderly: a focus on sarcopenic obesity. *Archives of Gerontology and Geriatrics, 56*(1), 270–278. doi:10.1016/j.archer.2012.09.007

DiSantostefano, J. (2012). New Medicare preventive care offerings. *Journal for Nurse Practitioners, 8*(5), 410.

Fakhouri, T. H., Ogden, C. L., Carroll, M. D., Kit, B. K., & Flegal, K. M. (2012). Prevalence of obesity among older adults in the United States, 2007–2010. *NCHS Data Brief,* no. 106, pp. 1–8. Hyattsville, MD: National Center for Health Statistics.

Flood, M., & Newman, A. (2007). Obesity in older adults: synthesis of findings and recommendations for clinical practice. *Journal of Gerontological Nursing, 33*(12), 19–35.

Hamdy, O., Citkowitz, E., Uwaifo, G. I., & Oral, E. A. (2011). Obesity treatment and management [Special issue]. *EMedicine Medscape.* Retrieved from http://emedicine.medscape.com/article/123702-treatment

Han, T. S., Tajar, A., & Lean, M. E. J. (2011). Obesity and weight management in the elderly. *British Medical Bulletin, 97*(1), 169–196.

Houston, D. K., Nicklas, B. J., & Zizza, C. A. (2009). Weighty concerns: the growing prevalence of obesity among older adults. *Journal of the American Dietetic Association, 109*(11), 1886–1895. doi:10.1016/j.jada.2009.08.014

Klein, S., Allison, D. B., Heymsfield, S. B., Kelley, D. E., Leibel, R. L., & Nonas, C. (2007). Waist circumference and cardiometabolic risk: a consensus statement from Shaping America's Health: Association for Weight Management and Obesity Prevention; NAASO, the Obesity Society; the American Society for Nutrition; and the American Diabetes Association [Special issue]. *American Journal of Clinical Nutrition, 85*(5), 1197–1202.

Laddu, D., Dow, C., Hingle, M., Thomson, C., & Going, S. (2011). A review of evidence based strategies to treat obesity in adults. *Nutrition in Clinical Practice, 26*(5), 512–525.

Mathus-Vliegen, E. M., Basdevant, A., Finer, N., Hainer, V., Hauner, H., Micic, D., . . . Zahorska-Markiewicz, B. (2012). Prevalence, pathophysiology, health consequences and treatment options of obesity in the elderly: a guideline. *Obesity Facts, 5*(3), 460–483.

Medical News Today. (2011). *All about Obesity* [Entire issue]. Retrieved from www.medicalnewstoday.com/info/obesity

Mendes, E. (2010, August 31). In U.S. obesity peaks in middle age. (Issue Brief). *GALLUP® Wellbeing.* Retrieved from www.gallup.com/poll/142736/obesity-peaks-middle-age.aspx

National Heart, Lung, and Blood Institute. (2011). Aim for a healthy weight. (Issue Brief.) Retrieved from www.nhlbi.nih.gov/health/public/heart/obesity/lose_wt/risk.htm

Newman, A. (2009). Obesity in older adults. *OJIN: The Online Journal of Issues in Nursing, 14*(1), Manuscript 3. doi:10.3912/OJIN.Vol14No1Man03

Rosenzweig, J. L., Ferrannini, E., Grundy, S. M., Haffner, S. M., Heine, R. J., Horton, E. S., & Kawamori, R. (2008). Primary prevention of cardiovascular disease and type 2 diabetes in patients at metabolic risk: an Endocrine Society clinical practice guideline. *Journal of Clinical Endocrinology & Metabolism, 93*(10), 3671–3689.

Rossen, L. M., Milsom, V. A., Middleton, K. R., Daniels, M. J., & Perri, M. G. (2013). Benefits and risks of weight-loss treatment for older, obese women. *Clinical Interventions in Aging, 8,* 157–166.

U.S. Department of Health and Human Services, National Institutes of Health (NIDDK NIH). (2011). Understanding adult overweight and obesity. Retrieved from http://win.niddk.nih.gov/publications/understanding.htm

WebMD Medical Reference. (2011). *Obesity Facts, Causes, Emotional Aspects and When to Seek Help* [Entire issue]. Retrieved from www.webmd.com/diet/guide/what-is-obesity

Osteoporosis

Bleicher, K., Cumming, R. G., Naganathan, V., Travison, T. G., Sambrook, P. N., Blyth, F. M., & Seibel, M. J. (2011). The role of fat and lean mass in bone loss in older men: findings from the CHAMP study. *Bone, 49*(6), 1299–1305. doi:10.1016/j.bone.2011.08.026

Cummings, S. R., Martin, J. S., McClung, M. R., Siris, E. S., Eastell, R., Reid, I. R., . . . Christiansen, C. (2009). Denosumab for prevention of fractures in postmenopausal women with osteoporosis. *New England Journal of Medicine, 361*(8), 756–765.

Glendenning, P., Chew, G. T., Seymour, H. M., Gillett, M. J., Goldswain, P. R., Inderjeeth, C. A., & Fraser, W. D. (2009). Serum 25-hydroxyvitamin D levels in vitamin D–insufficient hip fracture patients after supplementation with ergocalciferol and cholecalciferol. *Bone, 45*(5), 870–875. doi:10.1016/j.bone.2009.07.015

Gourlay, M. L., Fine, J. P., Preisser, J. S., May, R. C., Li, C., Lui, L. Y., & Ensrud, K. E. (2012). Bone-density testing interval and transition to osteoporosis in older women. *New England Journal of Medicine, 366*(3), 225–233. doi:10.1056/NEJMoa1107142

Kanis, J. A. (1994). Assessment of fracture risk and its application to screening for postmenopausal osteoporosis: synopsis of a WHO report. *WHO Study Group. Osteoporosis International, 4*(6), 368–381.

Kolata, G. (2003, September 28). Bone diagnosis gives new data but no answers. *New York Times.* http://www.nytimes.com/2003/09/28/us/bone-diagnosis-gives-new-data-but-no-answers.html

National Osteoporosis Foundation (2010) *Clinician's guide to prevention and treatment of osteoporosis.* Washington, DC: National Osteoporosis Foundation.

Stenson, W. F., Newberry, R., Lorenz, R., Baldus, C., & Civitelli, R. (2005). Increased prevalence of celiac disease and need for routine screening among patients with osteoporosis. *Archives of Internal Medicine, 165*(4), 393–399. doi:10.1001/archinte.165.4.393

Strom, O., Borgstrom, F., Kanis, J. A., Compston, J., Cooper, C., McCloskey, E. V., & Jonsson, B. (2011). Osteoporosis: burden, health care provision and opportunities in the EU: a report prepared in collaboration with the International Osteoporosis Foundation (IOF) and the European Federation of Pharmaceutical Industry Associations (EFPIA). *Archives of Osteoporosis, 6*(1–2), 59–155.

Tamaki, J., Iki, M., Kadowaki, E., Sato, Y., Kajita, E., Kagamimori, S., & Yoneshima, H. (2011). Fracture risk prediction using FRAX®: a 10-year follow-up survey of the Japanese Population-Based Osteoporosis (JPOS) Cohort Study. *Osteoporosis International, 22*(12), 3037–3045. doi:10.1007/s00198-011-1537-x

Wasnich, R. (1993). Bone mass measurement: prediction of risk. *American Journal of Medicine, 95*(5A), 6S–10S.

Watts, N. B., Bilezikian, J. P., Camacho, P. M., Greenspan, S. L., Harris, S. T., Hodgson, S. F., & Petak, S. M. (2010). American Association of Clinical Endocrinologists medical guidelines for clinical practice for the diagnosis and treatment of postmenopausal osteoporosis. *Endocrine Practitioner, 16*(Suppl. 3), S1–S37.

World Health Organization. (2003). *Scientific group on the prevention and management of osteoporosis. Prevention and management of osteoporosis: report of a WHO scientific group.* Singapore: WHO.

Pancreatic Cancer

American Cancer Society. (2011). Pancreatic cancer. Retrieved from www.cancer.org/Cancer/PancreaticCancer/DetailedGuide/index

Dragovich, T., Erickson, R. A., & Larson, C. R. (2011). Pancreatic cancer. Retrieved from http://emedicine.medscape.com/article/280605

Freelove, R., & Walling, A. (2006). Pancreatic cancer: diagnosis and management. *American Family Physician, 73*(3), 485–492.

Gapstur, S. M., Jacobs, E. J., Deka, A., McCullough, M. L., Patel, A. V., & Thun, M. J. (2011). Association of alcohol intake with pancreatic cancer mortality in never smokers. *Archives of Internal Medicine, 171*(5), 444.

Kang, S. P., & Saif, M. W. (2010). Clinical outcome of pancreatic cancer patients with diabetes mellitus: is diabetes a poor prognostic factor? *Journal of the Pancreas, 11*(4), 334–335.

Larghi, A., Verna, E. C., Lecca, P. G., & Costamagna, G. (2009). Screening for pancreatic cancer in high-risk individuals: a call for endoscopic ultrasound. *Clinical Cancer Research, 15*(6), 1907–1914.

Larsson, S. C., & Wolk, A. W. (2012). Red and processed meat consumption and risks of pancreatic cancer: meta-analysis of prospective studies. *British Journal of Cancer.* doi:10.1038/bjc. 2011.585. Retrieved from http://ki.se/content/1/c6/13/59/26/ Larsson%20SC%20Publication.pdf

Li, J., & Saif, M. W. (2009). Advancements in the management of pancreatic cancer. *Journal of the Pancreas, 10*(2), 109–117.

Melis, M., Marcon, F., Masi, A., Pinna, A., Sarpel, U., Miller, G., . . . Newman, E. (2012). The safety of a pancreaticoduodenectomy in patients older than 80 years: risk vs. benefits. *Americas Hepato-Pancreato-Biliary Association, 14*(9), 583–588.

Oliveira-Cunha, M., Malde, D. J., Aldouri, A., Morris-Stiff, G., Menon, K. V., & Smith, A. M. (2013). Results of pancreatic surgery in the elderly: is age a barrier? *Americas Hepato-Pancreato-Biliary Association, 15*(1), 24–30.

Robinson, R. (2012). Early identification of pancreatic cancer. *Clinician Reviews, 22*(4), 27–33.

Shah, B. B., Farah, K. F., Goldwasser, B., & Agrawal, R. A. (2008). Pancreatic diseases in the elderly. *Practical Gastroenterology, 18*, 21–32.

chapter 15

Hematological and Immune System Disorders

Lori Martin-Plank

Many factors affect patients' hematological and immune status, and because blood and lymph circulate throughout the body, manifestations of these disorders may appear in different organ systems.

ASSESSMENT

The assessment process includes a detailed history, physical examination, and diagnostic testing. The presenting symptoms of hematological deficiency can include excessive bruising, petechiae, unexplained bleeding, epistaxis, or inflamed lymph nodes. Elderly patients with severe anemia may complain of fatigue, dizziness, heart palpitations, headache, shortness of breath with exertion, and exercise intolerance. Confusion, depression, and cold intolerance are also common. In many cases, symptoms are absent, subtle, or erroneously attributed to the aging process.

The medical history obtained from the patient should include past history of anemia, hemoglobin abnormalities (thalassemia), vitamin C or K deficiency, recent surgery or blood transfusion, lymphadenopathy, and clotting disorders. Also inquire about any occupational or other known exposure to toxic agents or radiation, family history of anemia, current medications, and history of chronic disease. Some of the most common causes of hematological disease in the elderly include iron-deficiency anemia (IDA), anemia of chronic disease, and pernicious anemia, which has an increased incidence in patients over the age of 60. Myelodysplastic syndromes and leukemias also are becoming more common. Systemic disease and severe clotting disorders need to be included in the differential diagnosis.

Physical Examination and Diagnostics

The physical examination should be complete and thorough. Assess the eyes for pale conjunctivae and icteric sclera, which occur with some anemias. Inspect the color of the skin, noting any ashen or yellow changes; pallor is difficult to assess in older adults. Check for petechiae, bruising, and pale mucous membranes. Assess the nails for the presence of concave spoon nails, seen with iron deficiency. A red, painful, beefy tongue can be present with pernicious anemia. Oral lesions may occur. Palpate the abdomen for any splenomegaly or tenderness. Tachypnea and tachycardia can be seen with severe anemia. Auscultate the heart for any systolic murmurs. If blood loss is suspected—and the history warrants—a rectal examination to assess for guaiac-positive stools is performed. Finally, determine whether any mental status changes have occurred; do a complete neurological examination, checking cranial nerve function and deep tendon reflexes. The absence or presence of physical findings on examination helps to narrow the clinical diagnosis.

Diagnostic tests done to complete the hematological assessment include the following:

- Complete blood count (CBC) with differential; check red blood cells (RBCs), hemoglobin (Hgb), hematocrit (Hct), mean corpuscular volume (MCV), and mean corpuscular hemoglobin concentration (MCHC)
- Iron, total iron-binding capacity (TIBC)
- Ferritin if iron-deficiency or microcytic anemia is considered
- Reticulocyte count to assess for blood loss or blood cell destruction
- Hemoglobin electrophoresis to assess for hemoglobin abnormalities or thalassemia
- Vitamin B_{12} and folate levels to rule out pernicious anemia

The general physical examination should note any weight loss or wasting, skin changes, or lymphadenopathy. The history and physical examination provide the baseline for the plan of care and necessary diagnostic testing.

The general laboratory tests ordered should include the following:

- CBC with differential (platelet count)
- Urinalysis
- Electrolyte panel with HgA1C or fasting glucose levels to assess for diabetes

- Erythrocyte sedimentation rate (ESR)
- Rapid plasma reagin (RPR)

Tests to rule out more specific disease include titers for HIV, Lyme disease, Epstein-Barr virus (EBV), toxoplasmosis, and cytomegalovirus (CMV). Clinical consultation or referral to a specialty physician or nurse practitioner may be necessary to work up the elderly patient with suspected immunological suppression or disease and to ensure that the appropriate diagnosis is made.

Immunological Assessment

The presentation or complaints of immunological disease may be vague and nonspecific. Elderly patients may present with chronic fatigue, frequent or recurrent illness, weight loss, lymphadenopathy, depression, or recurrent infections. As stated earlier, a complete medical history should be obtained. A complete sexual history also should be obtained with specific focus on the number of partners the patient has had in the past 6 months; encounters with men, women, or both; any history of sex with prostitutes; sexually transmitted infections; and protection used by the patient or his or her partners. Inquire about recent travel, tick bites, risk factors for HIV, recent immunization or surgery, and medication use. Ask about illicit or recreational drug use, including IV drug use.

ANEMIA OF CHRONIC DISEASE

Signal symptoms: Minimal to none; nonspecific fatigue.

Description: Anemia of chronic disease (ACD) is the most common form of anemia in the older adult, followed by IDA. The percentage of anemia in noninstitutionalized persons 65 and older, with respect to ACD, is 19.7% compared to 16.6% with IDA (Bross, Soch, & Smith-Knuppel, 2010). ACD has been described in the literature as "infection anemia," "anemia of chronic inflammation," and "anemia of chronic disorders," alluding to its etiology.

ACD has an insidious onset. Signs and symptoms can be vague or absent, and laboratory data can present an even more daunting challenge. It is generally normocytic and normochromic, although about 25% to 35% may be microcytic in advanced stages; it coexists with IDA in some older persons. Anemia in patients with renal, hepatic, or endocrine disorder is categorized

separately, because it manifests with a different hematological profile (Price & Schrier, 2011).

Anemias of any form in the elderly must never be attributed to old age and should be recognized as a sign of physiological decline. ACD in particular must be differentiated from IDA, because their treatments vary significantly.

Etiology: ACD, as its name implies, is associated with a chronic disorder, usually infection, inflammation, malignancy, or trauma, and in many cases, the cause is unknown. ACD can be classified as a normochromic, normocytic anemia, but approximately one-third of patients with ACD have microcytosis. The pathophysiological hallmark of ACD is a disregulation of iron homeostasis, characterized by an increased uptake and retention of iron within the cells of the reticuloendothelial system (liver/spleen), resulting in decreased RBC production. Essentially, iron is present but inaccessible for use in the production of Hgb with the erythrocytes (Bross et al., 2010). A shortened RBC survival is also a contributing factor to ACD.

Occurrence: Due in part to the fact that elderly persons frequently encounter multiple chronic comorbidities, ACD is a common cause of geriatric anemia, accounting for more than 30% of the cases.

Age: Although anemia can be present in all age groups, ACD is seen mostly in the older adult.

Gender: Sex distribution varies based on the underlying cause of anemias. In contrast to anemia in younger people, anemia in elderly persons is more common in men than in women (National Anemia Action Council [NAAC], 2009).

Ethnicity: Not significant.

Contributing factors: The presence of one or more chronic conditions, such as cancer, chronic infection, chronic inflammation, or autoimmune conditions, is a contributing factor to the development of ACD.

Signs and symptoms: Onset of signs and symptoms in ACD can be confounding and is usually masqueraded by the underlying conditions. The typical symptoms of anemia, such as fatigue, weakness, dyspnea, and palpitations, may be present but are nonspecific and in elderly patients tend to be attributed to the aging process. Additionally, many older patients adjust their activities as their bodies make physiological adaptations for the underlying disease. Although

it may be difficult to assess in the geriatric population, conjunctival pallor is a reliable sign. Its absence, however, cannot exclude anemia. Other signs may be discovered through incidental laboratory testing. Cognitive decline, depression, and decreased quality of life may also accompany ACD. The clinician should have a high index of suspicion of ACD in elderly patients with chronic conditions, and any presentation of the above symptoms should prompt further evaluation.

Diagnostic tests: In discussing diagnostic testing for ACD, it is important to reiterate that ACD is classified as a normocytic, normochromic anemia with one-third presenting with microcytosis. This is important to consider when interpreting laboratory tests to determine whether there is a coexisting IDA.

In ACD, serum ferritin is the most useful test. Recall that serum ferritin is a measure of iron stores and that the main abnormality in ACD is the impaired ability to use iron stores in the reticuloendothelial system (liver/spleen). This is reflected in a normal to high ferritin level (i.e., iron is present but inaccessible for use). Ferritin levels in IDA are low.

Other laboratory tests include CBC, RBC indices, serum iron, TIBC, transferrin saturation, reticulocyte count, peripheral blood smear, and reticulocyte production index (RPI), which corrects for the degree of anemia. Table 15-1 compares the laboratory data in ACD and IDA.

TABLE 15-1 Laboratory Data in ACD and IDA		
LABORATORY TEST	**ACD**	**IDA**
CBC	Hemoglobin (Hgb): <12 g/dL (120 g/L) women <13 g/dL (130 g/L) men Rarely <10 g/dL (100 g/L) Mean corpuscular volume: 80–96 mcm^3 (normocytic) Mean corpuscular hemoglobin Normochromic (normal color) RBC distribution width: normal	Hemoglobin (Hgb): <12 g/dL (120 g/L) women <13 g/dL (130 g/L) men Mean corpuscular volume: 70–80 mcm^3 (microcytic) Mean corpuscular hemoglobin Hypochromic (pale color) RBC distribution width: increased
Serum ferritin	Normal or high	Low
Serum iron	Low	Low
Total iron-binding capacity	Low	High
Transferrin saturation	Low	Low
Reticulocyte production index	Low	Low
Reticulocyte count	Low	Low
Peripheral smear	Nearly normal	Microcytosis, hypochromia

Abbreviations: ACD = anemia of chronic disease; CBC = complete blood count; IDA = iron deficiency anemia; RBC = red blood cell.

Differential diagnosis: Early or partially treated IDA is the main differential diagnosis for ACD, because microcytosis may be present or absent in either disorder. Hypoproliferative anemias (e.g., renal disease, endocrine disorders) and thalassemia are also considerations (Schrier & Camaschella, 2011).

Treatment: Treatment of ACD focuses on management of the underlying disorder. Iron supplementation is of no benefit in ACD, except in cases of coexisting IDA. A therapeutic trial of iron supplementation of no longer than 1 month may be useful in delineating between ACD and IDA. In ACD, there would be no hematological response to iron therapy (Chen & Gandhi, 2004).

Although there is no specific treatment for ACD, if anemia is severe or underlying disease is resistant to treatment, use of erythropoiesis-stimulating agents (ESAs; Epogen, Procrit) or transfusions may be indicated (Bross et al., 2010; Spivak, 2005). A recent warning from FDA Medwatch (2011) urged caution in using ESAs in patients with renal disease due to the potential for cardiovascular events. Dosage should be individualized and should be as low as possible while reducing the need for transfusion.

Follow-up: Follow-up is individualized depending on underlying cause and extent of anemia.

Sequelae: Variable depending on the underlying condition.

Prevention/prophylaxis: Early education in healthy lifestyle may prevent or delay onset of some chronic conditions.

Referral: Referral is indicated for progression of anemia and/or resistance to treatment of underlying condition.

Education: Teach the patient and his or her family the importance of lifestyle modifications and adherence to a treatment plan for management of underlying conditions.

CLINICAL RECOMMENDATION	EVIDENCE RATING	REFERENCES
Anemia is an independent risk factor for increased morbidity and mortality and decreased quality of life in community-dwelling older persons.	B	Bross et al. (2010)
Erythropoiesis-stimulating agents (ESAs) improve anemia, exercise tolerance, and quality of life and reduce symptoms in heart failure patients with mild anemia. More research is needed to clarify the full effects and safety of ESAs as a treatment for anemia in these patients.	B	Ngo et al. (2010)
When possible, treatment of the underlying disease is the therapeutic approach of choice for anemia of chronic disease.	B	Weiss & Goodnough (2005)

A = consistent, good-quality, patient-oriented evidence; B = inconsistent or limited-quality, patient-oriented evidence; C = consensus, disease-oriented evidence, usual practice, expert opinion, or case series. For information about the SORT evidence rating system, go to www.aafp.org/afpsort.xml.

ANEMIA, IRON DEFICIENCY

Signal symptoms: Minimal to none; nonspecific fatigue.
Description: IDA is classified as a microcytic, hypochromic anemia and is the second most common anemia in the elderly, preceded by ACD. Anemia is defined by the World Health Organization (WHO) as an Hgb concentration of <12 g/dL for women and

<13 g/dL for men (de Benoit, 2005). IDA can be acute (i.e., from rapid blood loss as in hemorrhage) or chronic, reflecting occult blood loss or poor nutrition.

Etiology: Multifactorial; in the United States, IDA in this population is rarely the result of dietary deficiency. The majority of elderly patients with IDA have an underlying gastrointestinal (GI) tract abnormality (NAAC, 2009).

Occurrence: IDA affects 30% of the population worldwide. IDA accounts for nearly 20% of all geriatric anemias, with the highest prevalence in men 85 years and older (Zuh, Kaneshiro, & Kaunitz, 2010).

Age: Most common in children; in older adults, increases with age; elderly males account for 4.4% (Ofran, 2011).

Gender: In ages 65 and older, IDA affects more men than women.

Ethnicity: Not significant; certain cultural groups may have underlying genetic factors predisposing to anemias, such as thalassemia.

Contributing factors: In the older adult patient, decreased oral intake, partial gastrectomy, malabsorption syndromes, low socioeconomic status, medications, combination of medication and alcohol, and chronic blood loss, most frequently from the GI tract, are contributing factors for IDA. Some GI causes include peptic ulcer disease, gastritis, hiatal hernia with mucosal ulceration, neoplasms, diverticular disease, or bleeding caused by inflammatory bowel disease (Zuh et al., 2010). In patients with prosthetic heart valves, intravascular hemolysis may lead to IDA related to increased hemosiderin loss in the urine. Epistaxis, hematuria, uterine bleeding, and bleeding diathesis are other possible contributing factors.

Signs and symptoms: Clinical presentation of IDA can be vague, unreliable, and in many cases asymptomatic. In the older adult, symptoms may be incorrectly attributed to the aging process. Diagnosis of IDA may be the result of an incidental blood study finding, requiring further investigation. Fatigue, weakness, lethargy, tachycardia, palpitations, dyspnea on exertion, headache, irritability, inability to concentrate, neuralgia, sore tongue, paresthesias, and susceptibility to infection are possible symptoms. Dizziness, faintness, claudication, exercise intolerance, or angina also may be present. In some cases, symptoms may reflect the underlying cause, for example, stomach discomfort with peptic ulcer disease (Ofran, 2011). Medication history, including over-the-counter (OTC) drugs, is especially important to rule out NSAID-induced bleeding. Dietary history also may be key to diagnosis.

Physical examination may be unremarkable. Pallor, common in patients with significant anemia, is also common in aging and may be discounted as a normal age-related finding. Conjunctival pallor, bluish discoloration of the sclera, cheilosis, glossitis, brittle ridged nails, or "spoon" nails (koilonychia) may also be present. Cardiovascular and respiratory examination may reveal tachycardia, systolic murmur, or signs of congestive heart failure (CHF). In some patients, splenomegaly may be present, owing to hemolysis of iron-deficient RBCs. Lymphadenopathy, weight loss, bruising, and jaundice are physical signs that require further evaluation (Ofran, 2011).

Diagnostic tests:

- CBC will reveal Hgb of <12 g/dL. Note that patients who are smokers and those with chronic hypoxemia have a higher premorbid Hgb and therefore can be anemic at higher hemoglobin levels.
- RBC indices reveal an MCV (mean corpuscular volume/RBC size) that will be decreased to <80 fL in adults; MCH (mean corpuscular hemoglobin/RBC color) will show hypochromia or pale cells; RBC distribution width (RDW)/volume variation will be increased.
- Serum ferritin level is the most accurate initial test for IDA; patients with IDA will test with low levels. A ferritin level of <25 ng/mL is highly predicative of IDA, whereas a level of >100 ng/mL indicates adequate iron stores with a decreased likelihood of IDA. Note that, in some patients, deficiency may be missed, because ferritin is an acute-phase reactant and ferritin levels may be falsely elevated in inflammatory conditions. The abnormal laboratory cutoff may be higher in these situations.
- TIBC: increased
- Serum iron: decreased
- Tranferrin saturation: decreased. This indicates that there is a decreased amount of iron available to bind to transferrin, which is an iron-carrying protein.
- Peripheral smear: reveals microcytosis, hypochromia, and poikilocytosis
- Bone marrow iron stain: usually not necessary

Once IDA is confirmed, further diagnostic studies to determine the cause must be undertaken. The presence of IDA in adults is presumed to be the result of blood loss in the GI tract, and the possibility of malignancy in the system must be ruled out. Endoscopic evaluation beginning with colonoscopy is indicated if the patient is 50 years or older (Zuh et al., 2010).

Differential diagnosis: Differential diagnosis for microcytic, hypochromic anemias by etiology includes the following:

- Defective iron utilization: thalassemia trait, sideroblastosis, G6PD deficiency
- Defective iron reutilization: infection, inflammation, cancer, and other chronic diseases
- Hypoproliferation: decreased erythropoietin from renal failure, hypothyroidism, and other hyporoliferative states

In adult men and nonmenstruating women, differential diagnosis for IDA includes the following in decreasing order of frequency: ACD, unexplained anemias, and thalassemia trait (Van Vranken, 2010).

Treatment: Oral iron therapy is usually first-line treatment for patients with IDA. Drug of choice is ferrous sulfate 325 mg (65 mg of elemental iron) bid-tid. Depending on the severity of the anemia, adults will usually require a dose of 80 to 200 mg of elemental iron daily (NAAC, 2008). In a study of hospitalized older adults, lower doses achieved the same results as higher doses with significantly fewer side effects (Rimon et al., 2005).

Ideally, a dose is administered on an empty stomach, 1 hour before meals. Absorption of iron is enhanced with ascorbic acid (vitamin C). Other measures to improve iron absorption include avoidance of foods high in tannate (tea, bran, cereal) and medications that increase gastric pH (milk, antacids, proton-pump inhibitors, H_2-histamine blockers, quinolones, and tetracycline). Liquid iron preparations are recommended for those who are unable to dissolve the coating of iron pills, which leads to decreased iron absorption. Avoid sustained-release formulations of iron for initial therapy, because they reduce the amount of iron presented for absorption by the GI tract (Dambro, 2003; Killip, Bennett, & Chambers, 2007). Dietary sources of iron include meat, fish, poultry, fruits, green leafy vegetables, beans, nuts, and grain products.

Oral iron therapy may cause significant GI side effects, including constipation, diarrhea, nausea, and abdominal cramping. Interventions to reduce GI symptoms include dose reduction of iron or starting with one-half the dose and gradually increasing; switching to ferrous gluconate 325 mg (35 mg of elemental iron) or ferrous fumarate 325 mg (99 to 108 mg of elemental iron), because these preparations may be better tolerated; or taking the iron with food, which may reduce absorption by 50% but may increase patient compliance with therapy. Measures to alleviate constipating effects of iron therapy include laxatives, stool softeners, fiber, and adequate liquid intake (NAAC, 2008). Medication effect should be demonstrated after 3 weeks of therapy.

Parenteral iron therapy is indicated in the following situations: chronic uncorrectable bleeding, intestinal malabsorption, intolerance to oral therapy, nonadherence, or Hgb level <6 g/dL with signs of poor perfusion in those who would otherwise receive transfusions (e.g., those with religious objections). Parenteral preparations available in the United States include iron dextran (Dexferrum), sodium ferric gluconate (Ferrlecrit), and iron sucrose (Venofer) (Killip et al., 2007).

Blood transfusions may be necessary initially and should always be considered for patients who are symptomatic (i.e., fatigue, dyspnea on exertion) as well as for asymptomatic cardiac patients with Hgb <10 g/dL (Killip et al., 2007).

Follow-up: The restoration of iron stores is the primary goal of treatment. The Hgb level should increase by 1 g/dL every 2 to 3 weeks, but restoration of iron stores may take up to 3 to 6 months *after* hemoglobin is corrected, during which time iron therapy should be continued. The patient should be seen at regular intervals to reassess symptoms or side effects from the treatment plan. Patients should be evaluated in 3 to 4 weeks for examination and Hgb after the initiation of therapy. Subsequent evaluations are at the discretion of the health-care provider but should be conducted at no later than 3 months (McPhee & Papadakis , 2010).

Sequelae: Possible complications include failure to identify an occult bleeding source, particularly one related to malignancy.

Prevention/prophylaxis: IDA can be prevented by promoting proper nutrition with adequate iron intake, identifying those at high risk, and prompt evaluation and treatment of any symptoms or bleeding.

Referral: Refer patients to a specialist in the area where anemia is suspected to originate (e.g., a gastroenterologist for diagnostic studies, an oncologist if malignancy is suspected). Collaborative management is appropriate for complex cases. Refer patients to a nutritionist for evaluation of dietary inadequacies and assistance with meal planning or with congregate or home-delivered meals.

Education: Educate the patient about the mechanism of anemia, the expected course of therapy with respect to frequency of office visits and blood tests, the importance of adhering to the treatment regimen, and the need to notify the patient's health-care provider about problems with the regimen. Provide patients with a guide to the dietary sources of iron to supplement oral iron medication.

CLINICAL RECOMMENDATION	EVIDENCE RATING	REFERENCES
Serum ferritin is the best test for iron deficiency anemia.	B	Ofran (2011)
Patients >65 years with iron deficiency anemia should be screened for gastrointestinal malignancy.	B	Wadland & Krishnamani (2011)
Treatment of iron deficiency once per day is as efficacious as a thrice-per-day regimen.	B	Wadland & Krishnamani (2011)

A = consistent, good-quality, patient-oriented evidence; B = inconsistent or limited-quality, patient-oriented evidence; C = consensus, disease-oriented evidence, usual practice, expert opinion, or case series. For information about the SORT evidence rating system, go to www.aafp.org/afpsort.xml.

HUMAN IMMUNODEFICIENCY VIRUS (HIV)

Signal symptoms: The initial HIV infection is characterized by mononucleosis-like illness with fever, sore throat, lymphadenopathy, headache, and fatigue. A roseola-like rash may also develop. These initial symptoms are followed by an asymptomatic phase, which may last 10 years or more. Later, if untreated, lymphadenopathy, weight loss, myalgias, and diarrhea may develop (Cohen, Kuritzkes, & Sax, 2011). In advanced disease, malignancies and opportunistic infections occur. Co-infection with hepatitis B or C is common (25% to 30%) in IV drug users, so hepatitis symptoms may also appear (Centers for Disease Control and Prevention [CDC], 2010a).

Description: HIV, a human RNA retrovirus, is the infectious agent that causes AIDS. The primary target of the virus is the CD4 lymphocyte. Two types of HIV have been identified: HIV-1 and HIV-2. Although the viruses share similar epidemiological traits, they are serologically and geographically distinct. HIV-1, the more pathogenic of the two viruses, is found worldwide, with infection being most prevalent in the sub-Saharan regions of Africa, the Americas, Western Europe, and Southeast Asia. HIV-1 was probably derived from transmission from chimpanzees in Central Africa. The HIV-2 virus resides primarily in West Africa, and cases in other geographical areas have been linked epidemiologically to West Africa. HIV-2 was derived from the Sooty Mangabey monkeys in West Africa (Gaitanis & Mikolich, 2011; Katz & Zolopa, 2011).

Etiology: HIV is spread by contact with parenteral and body fluids. Primary modes of HIV transmission include the following:

■ Contact with blood and blood products: needle sharing/injection, crack cocaine, blood transfusions
■ Sexual transmission: anal, vaginal, or (infrequently) oral intercourse
■ Maternal-fetus (perinatal) transmission: in utero, during delivery, or through breastfeeding

The primary mode of transmission (53%) in the United States is men having sex with men (MSM); however, heterosexual contact is the most rapidly increasing mode of transmission. In the United States, 16% of AIDS cases in people over age 50 are related to needle sharing (CDC, 2010c). The highest-risk behaviors for transmission with sexual intercourse are as follows: anal intercourse, due to mucosal tearing;

unprotected receptive vaginal intercourse, especially during menses; and unprotected rectal/vaginal intercourse in the presence of genital herpes, chancroid, or primary syphilis. About 55% of U.S. adults ages 18 to 64 have never been tested for HIV (CDC, 2010b).

Occurrence: HIV occurs worldwide; however, not all countries report their data. The WHO estimates that more than 40 million people have HIV. At the end of 2006, the United States had approximately 1,106,400 people living with HIV. There are approximately 56,300 new cases annually, one every 9.5 minutes (CDC, 2010a).

Age: The peak age group for new infections in 2006 was people ages 25 to 44. In the 50-year-old and older category, 35% have died from AIDS (CDC, 2010c). Since 1981, an estimated 15% of all new HIV/AIDS cases reported to the CDC involve patients who are more than 50 years old. The number of people age 50 and older living with HIV is increasing due to improved treatment with highly active antiretroviral therapy (HAART) and increased case reports of newly diagnosed infections.

Based on 2005 data the CDC gathered from 33 reporting states, 24% of persons living with HIV/AIDS are over the age of 50. In 2007, more than 800 new cases were ages 65 and over (Kearney, Moore, Donegan, & Lambert, 2010). Older patients with HIV/AIDS are likely to age more rapidly than noninfected patients and to die sooner from the disease. One-third or more of these deaths are due to comorbid conditions that may be exacerbated by HIV (Project INFORM, 2010). Thirty-seven percent of individuals 80 years and older have been reported to die within a month of HIV diagnosis (Zelenetz & Epstein, 1998). Despite an increased death rate in those over 80, the overall mortality rate has decreased from 40.8%, before the introduction of HAART, to 6.1% in 2004 to 2006 (Kearney et al., 2010).

Gender: In 2006, men accounted for 73% of new HIV cases. Women comprise a higher proportion of AIDS cases as age increases: 6.1% of AIDS patients 50 to 59 years old, 13.2% of AIDS patients 60 to 69 years old, and a total of 28.7% of AIDS patients over the age of 65 (DeCarol & Linsk, 2010).

Ethnicity: Blacks/African Americans have the highest rate of HIV/AIDS (51.2%). Hispanics have the second highest rate. In people 50 and older, HIV rates in blacks/African Americans are 12 times higher than rates in whites, and Hispanic HIV rates are 5 times higher than rates in whites (CDC, 2010a).

Blacks/African Americans represent 12% of the U.S. population but account for 46% of HIV/AIDS cases (CDC, 2010a).

Contributing factors: Because older adults perceive themselves at lower risk, they are also less likely to be tested. The older adult is much less likely to use a condom, because there is no fear of pregnancy. Some older adults may have lower educational levels and less responsive attitudes about HIV/AIDS than younger adults (Cichocki, 2010; Jacquescoley, 2008) and therefore are less likely to protect themselves (Ruiz, Cefalu, & Ogbuokiri, 2010). Health professionals may also perceive their older patients as less likely to be at risk and may not offer HIV testing (CDC, 2010c). Health-care providers do not routinely ask older patients about sexual behaviors and HIV risk factors; this leads to a delay in detection and treatment. HIV symptoms may be misdiagnosed as "normal" aging. For example, weight loss and mental confusion are part of the aging process. Because of this perceived lack of a need to target the older adult, few prevention programs have been developed for adults over the age of 50 (DeCarol & Linsk, 2010).

Cognitive impairment in the older adult puts them at an increased risk for HIV risk-taking behaviors and suboptimal adherence to medications. Cognitive impairment may be further compromised with the use of opioids, cocaine, methamphetamines, alcohol, and mental illness. Having hepatitis C as a co-infection also has been shown to compromise cognitive impairment (CDC, 2010c).

A recent survey showed that 73% of persons ages 57 to 64, 53% of persons 65 to 74, and 26% of persons 75 to 85 had intercourse during the past year (CDC, 2010c). Almost 60% of older single women engage in sex without using a condom (CDC, 2010c; Zelenetz & Epstein, 1998). Older women have a higher risk of contracting HIV due to the thinning of the vaginal and anal mucosa. The frequency of sexual contact and number of sexual partners affect an individual's risk for getting HIV. Social practices, such as divorce and impotence therapies, provide opportunities for more sexual relationships in older adults (Kearney et al., 2010). Older adults have fewer surviving friends for support and are even more isolated when they develop HIV (Anand, Springer, Copenhaver, & Altice, 2010).

Immune system changes that occur with aging may render older patients more susceptible to contracting HIV. Aging and disease-enhancing factors associated with HIV in the older adult include decline in both B-cell and T-cell functions, hyporesponsive T cells, age-related thymic involution, and depletion of naive CD4 and T cells. Drug metabolism is affected due to a decline in liver and renal function. The incidence of kidney disease increases with the type of HAART therapy. Liver volume, blood flow, drug metabolism, and hepatoregenerative capacity decrease with normal aging and are further compromised by HIV and HAART therapy (Kearney et al., 2010). Vascular age in the HIV-positive older adult has been found to be approximately 15 years older than chronological age (CDC, 2010c).

Elderly prisoners are at high risk for HIV due to sexual abuse within the prison system by younger inmates. Clinical research in this population is limited due to federal regulations.

All of the above factors contribute to at least 50% of older adults entering treatment too late to achieve the best results.

Signs and symptoms: In the acute phase of infection, the person often presents with a self-limited, mononucleosis-like infection characterized by fever, sore throat, lymphadenopathy, headache, and a rash resembling roseola. The acute phase is followed by an asymptomatic phase of viral replication. Untreated, the asymptomatic phase lasts approximately 10 years from the time of exposure to the virus (Katz & Zolopa, 2011).

In the older patient, the first sign of HIV may be confusion or AIDS-related dementia (CDC, 2010c). Weight loss, dehydration, fatigue, or withdrawal may go unnoticed or may be attributed to other illnesses. Fatigue is one of the most common and debilitating symptoms of HIV. Individuals at high risk for fatigue are unemployed/retired, are not on antiretroviral therapy, have fewer years since HIV diagnosis, and have a history of more childhood trauma, more stressful life events, less social support, and more psychological distress (Guaraldi et al., 2009).

In the advanced disease state, weight loss, lymphadenopathy, diarrhea, and skin changes such as seborrhea dermatitis, herpes zoster, or fungal infections develop (Gaitanis & Mikolich, 2011). The presence of disseminated herpes zoster, vaginal or oral candidiasis, tuberculosis, or pneumonia should raise the index of suspicion for HIV.

Advanced disease accompanied by low CD4 counts and elevated viral loads is characterized by opportunistic infections, such as *Pneumocystis jiroveci* pneumonia; bacterial, viral, and mycobacterial pneumonias; sinusitis; and malignancies (Kaposi sarcoma and non-Hodgkin's lymphoma). Other problems that may occur in advanced HIV/AIDS are pleural effusions, interstitial pneumonitis, toxoplasmosis, AIDS dementia complex, cryptococcal meningitis, HIV myelopathy, progressive multifocal leukoencephalopathy, inflammatory polyneuropathies, and myopathies. Rheumatological manifestations include joint effusions, Reiter syndrome, psoriatic arthritis, Sicca syndrome, and systemic lupus erythematosus. Oral candidiasis and oral hairy leukoplakia are suggestive of HIV infection. Other oral manifestations are angular chelitis, gingival disease, and aphthous ulcers. For the numerous other clinical manifestations seen in advanced disease, refer to www.CDC.gov/HIV.

Because the index of suspicion for HIV is generally low in the older patient, the diagnosis may be missed. A sexual history is crucial in exposing risk factors. When the possibility of HIV infection has been established, permission for diagnostic testing should be obtained.

TEST	SIGNIFICANCE
HIV enzyme-linked immunosorbent assay (ELISA)	Screening test for HIV. Positive within 22 days of exposure in 50% of patients. Sensitivity 99.9%, confirm with Western blot.
Confirmatory Western blot	Positive with HIV. Sensitivity when combined with ELISA is greater than 99.99%.
Absolute CD4 lymphocyte count	Low; levels with advanced disease <500/mm^3 is one factor used to consider initiating HAART therapy. Risk of malignances increases with counts <200/mm^3
Plasma HIV RNA test (viral load)	High; levels with advanced disease >100,000 copies/mL is one factor used to consider HAART therapy. This is the best test in the acute phase of the infection, before seroconversion. The level correlates with disease progress and response to HAART therapy.

Source: Adapted from Barroso et al. (2010) and Lundgren & Phillips (2010).

Diagnostic tests: HIV diagnosis requires a positive ELISA test result, followed by a confirmatory positive Western blot test. The CD4 count and HIV RNA polymerase chain reaction (viral load) should be measured in all HIV-positive patients. Rapid serological tests are increasingly useful in settings of high prevalence. Results from blood or saliva can be reported in 20 minutes.

Differential diagnosis: Differential diagnosis in the older adult with HIV can be divided into three categories:

- Acute infection presents as mononucleosis-like symptoms or viral respiratory infections.
- Late symptoms present as wasting illnesses, such as neoplasms, tuberculosis, pneumonias, disseminated fungal infections, malabsorption, depression, dementia, endocarditis, thyroid disease, or kidney dysfunction.
- Advanced disease presents as HIV-related encephalopathy, confusion or Alzheimer's disease, myelopathy, and neuropathy (Gaitanis & Mikolich, 2011; Katz & Zolopa, 2011).

Treatment: For best practice outcomes, patients should be referred to an HIV specialty center or HIV specialists for management. Every new HIV infection averted saves approximately $367,000 (in 2009 dollar prices) in lifetime medical costs (CDC, 2010a). Although there is a lack of clear guidelines for treatment specific to older adults with HIV, issues of older adults with HIV are beginning to be addressed (AIDsInfo, 2012). The primary goal of treatment is to reduce the risk of a detectable viral load and maintain the CD4 count at more than $500/mm^3$ while promoting health to the maximum possible (Sengupta, Lo, Strauss, Eron, & Gifford, 2010). Risk of transmission from a viral-suppressed HIV-positive individual to a negative partner is less likely due to effective HAART therapy.

The critical issues associated with development of HIV in older adults are ignorance of risk, attributing symptoms to age or comorbidities, delay in seeking care, and advanced disease before treatment is sought. Older adults with less effective immune systems develop a faster progression of HIV to AIDS, variable response to HAART therapy, and increasing comorbidities that may affect toxicity and effectiveness of therapy (Kearney et al., 2010; Project INFORM, 2010). The national guideline recommendation is to start treatment with a combination of drug therapies, with three or more HIV drugs (HAART), maintaining adequate nutrition, and treating comorbidities. Despite HAART therapy, there remains a low viral level

(nondetectable) that leads to inflammation and non-AIDS events such as heart disease. Other non-AIDS events that are higher in the older HIV population than in the general population include cancers (non-Hodgkin's lymphoma, anal, throat, liver, and head and neck), liver disease, cognitive impairment, and osteoporosis. Although inflammatory processes decrease with HAART therapy, they never return to normal. These non-AIDS events are due in part to the inflammatory process and the adverse effects of HAART therapy (Kearney et al., 2010; Project INFORM, 2010). National guidelines as of December 2009 recommend starting therapy when the CD4 count falls below $350/mm^3$ (Project INFORM, 2010). A more recent update advises starting HAART therapy in all older patients with HIV, regardless of CD4 count, because of increased risk of non-AIDS complications. A second concern is the risk of reduced immunologic response in older HIV patients. Evidence levels in this model are classified based on the CD4 count prior to initiating therapy (AIDS Info, 2012). The benefits of starting at this level are lower rates of non-AIDS conditions, better overall health, longer survival rates, and lower rates of passing HIV to others. The risks of starting therapy at $500/mm^3$ are drug complications, drug resistance, and the availability of fewer drug options later in treatment. HAART therapy is most effective when initiated during the asymptomatic period. In 2007, 32.3% of newly diagnosed patients were in the late phase of diagnosis (CDC, 2008). The ultimate decision on when to initiate HAART therapy is based on Panel recommendations, clinician knowledge of the patient, patient input, and resource availability (AIDsInfo, 2012).

During the initial acute phase of the HIV infection, no definitive treatment is required. Symptoms of fever, sore throat, and headache are self-limiting. During the asymptomatic phase, CD4 counts and viral load levels should be monitored every 3 months. Antiretroviral therapy (ART) or HAART should be initiated when the CD4 count falls below $500/mm^3$ or the patient has rapidly declining CD4 counts or very high viral loads (>100,000/mcL). If the patient has concomitant hepatitis B or C, therapy should be initiated. Patients at increased risk for heart disease and/or cancer also should be considered for early initiation of ART. Patients who lack the CCR5 gene are considered nonprogressors. They are typically monitored annually and do not require therapy. All patients with symptomatic disease should be offered antiretroviral therapy and treated for opportunistic diseases.

Studies have shown that antiretroviral therapy is clinically beneficial to HIV-infected patients with advanced disease and immunosuppression (AIDSInfo, 2012; Kearney et al., 2010; Project INFORM, 2010). The treatment options that offer the maximum benefit are medically complex and accompanied by adverse effects, drug interactions, and potential drug resistance. The challenge is achieving patient adherence to therapy, especially when some therapies make the person feel worse. A knowledgeable and experienced provider, who is a specialist in HIV treatment, should be managing the disease and its complications. (Complete guidelines can be found at www.CDC.gov or www.aidsinfo.nih.gov/ContentFiles/AdultandAdolescentGL.pdf.)

Before initiation of therapy, a general health work-up should be completed. This baseline work-up should include—but should not be limited to—the following:

- Complete history and physical examination
- CBC with differential and platelets, complete metabolic profile, fasting lipid profile
- CD4 cell count
- Plasma HIV RNA test (viral load)
- HIV resistance genotype (optional, but recommended by some experts)

Routine studies pertinent to prevention of opportunistic infections include the following:

- Syphilis serology: Venereal Disease Research Laboratory (VDRL) test or rapid plasma reagin (RPR)
- Tuberculin skin test (purified protein derivative) or QuantiFERON-TB Gold (QFT-G) test
- Toxoplasma serology immunoglobulin G (IgG)
- Cytomegalovirus—CMV serology (IgG)
- Varicella zoster virus—VZV serology (IgG)
- Hepatitis C virus (HCV) serology (anti-HCV)
- Hepatitis B virus (HBV) serologies (HBsAb, HBcAb, HBsAG)
- Hepatitis A virus (HAV) serology (anti-HAV)
- Papanicolaou (Pap) smear and gynecological examination for women

Other tests as clinically indicated may include the following:

- Chest x-ray examination
- G6PD screen if dapsone or primaquine is planned in the therapy regimen
- HLA-B 5701 if abacavir is planned in the therapy regimen
- Ophthalmological examination

For older persons, creatinine clearance studies are recommended.

Due to new research and new medications being developed annually, health-care providers should seek the latest guidelines before initiating antiretroviral therapy. The primary goal of therapy is complete suppression of the viral replication as measured by a nondetectable viral load. Depending on the laboratory test used for determining viral load, nondetectable means a viral load of <25 to 50 copies/mL. Recommended therapy includes three drugs from at least two different classes of antiretroviral agents. Currently, there are six classes of antiretroviral agents:

1. Nucleoside reverse transcriptase inhibitors (NRTIs): zidovudine (AZT or Retrovir), didanosine (ddI or Videx), zalcitabine (ddC or Hivid), stavudine (d4T or Zerit), lamivudine (3TC or Epivir), emtricitabine (Emtriva), or abacavir (Ziagen)
2. Nucleotide reverse transcriptase inhibitor: tenofovir (Viread)
3. Protease inhibitors (PIs): indinavir (Crixivan), saquinavir (Invirase), ritonivir (Norvir), nelfinavir, (Viracept), fosamprenavir (Lexiva), lopinivir/ritonavir (Kaletra), atazanavir (Reyataz), tipranavir/ritonaviro (Aptivus/Norvir), and darunavir/ritonavir (Prezista/Norvir)
4. Nonnucleoside reverse transcriptase inhibitors (NNRTIs): nevirapine (Viramune), delavirdine (Rescriptor), efavirenz (Sustiva), etravirine (Intelence)
5. Entry inhibitors: enfuviritide (Fuzeon) and maraviroc (Selzentry)
6. Integrase inhibitor: raltegravir (Isentress)

Due to the burden of taking multiple tablets, new combination regimens that require the person to take only one or two tablets a day have come into favor. Examples of this concept are Atripla (efavirenz + emctricitabine + tenofovir) and Truvada (emtricitabine + tenofovir) plus another agent. Combination regimens in treatment of naive patients usually contain one NNRTI plus two NRTIs. For the most current information on the advantages and disadvantages of each retroviral drug, consult the latest CDC guidelines. The health-care provider must distinguish between drug failure and drug toxicity, causing a need to change therapy. A multiplicity of factors must be considered before making a change, including viral load levels measured, CD4 cell count, treatment options, compliance and complexity of regimen, mental health issues, pharmacokinetics, patient education, and toxicity.

Follow-up: The patient should be monitored every 3 months. Yearly functional screening should be done on all patients over the age of 60 (Ruiz, Cefalu, & Ogbuokiri, 2010). If a patient's sexual contact is the source of the infection, encourage that person and any of his or her partners to undergo testing. Report the disease to the appropriate public health authorities within confidentiality guidelines and state regulations. Close monitoring of the patient for medication side effects and toxicity is especially needed with older patients. Loss of viral suppression may begin as early as 48 hours after a lapse in adherence. A lapse of 15 days confers a 50% chance of virology failure (Schackman et al., 2006). A wireless pill container (Wisepill) can be used to monitor adherence by transmitting a signal when the device is opened (Parienti et al., 2008).

Sequelae: Fatigue, anxiety, poor sleep quality, depression, pain, opportunistic infections, cognitive deficits, cardiovascular complications related to HAART, and metabolic syndrome.

Prevention/prophylaxis: Patients can prevent HIV infection through avoidance of unprotected sex and IV drug use and by considering autologous blood transfusion for any planned surgery. Health-care providers should inquire about sexual activity at each visit and target healthy older adult groups such as widow/ widower/divorce support groups for risk factor education. Immunization of HIV-positive individuals with pneumococcal and influenza vaccines is indicated, unless the patient is allergic to these vaccines. Health-care personnel should use universal precautions and proper handling and disposal of contaminated needles and blood collection equipment.

Referral: On diagnosis, refer patients to an HIV-specialty nurse practitioner or other health-care specialist in HIV. Whenever possible, management should be done by an HIV specialist. Collaborative management is indicated during stable periods. Refer patients to a nutritionist for dietary guidance for weight loss or wasting. Refer community-dwelling, older adults to home health services when appropriate. Refer to support groups, if the patient desires.

Education: Educate patients and family/caregivers about disease transmission, precautions, treatment options, self-care measures, and safe sex to prevent transmission to others. Teach patients not to take any other medications or OTC preparations without first checking with the health-care provider because of the potential for interactions with cytochrome P-450 drugs.

Research is needed regarding HIV in the older adult. Areas of suggested research include the following:

- New drug therapies in the older adult because this age group is usually excluded from drug studies
- Immune gene therapies
- New treatments for deep belly fat, caused by protease inhibitors
- Frailty syndrome in HIV-infected individuals
- HIV research on vulnerable populations such as prisoners

BOX 15-1
HIV Resources

www.aidsinfo.nih.gov
www.hivatis.org
www.iasusa.org
www.cdc.gov
www.natap.org
www.actis.org
www.niaid.nih.gov/daids/aids.htm
http://sis.nlm.nih.gov/hiv/index.php
www.avert.org
www.nlm.nih.gov/medlineplus
www.hivinsite.ucsf.edu
www.ucsf.ed/hivcntr
www.unaids.org
www.thebody.com

CLINICAL RECOMMENDATION	EVIDENCE RATING	REFERENCES
Screen everyone with risk factors for HIV; screen anyone requesting HIV testing.	A	Drayton & Grant (2011)
Antiretroviral therapy (ART) is recommended in patients >50 years of age, regardless of CD4 cell	C	AidsInfo (2012)

CLINICAL RECOMMENDATION	EVIDENCE RATING	REFERENCES
count, because the risk of non–AIDS-related complications may increase and the immunological response to ART may be reduced in older HIV-infected patients.		
HIV drug-resistance testing is recommended for persons with HIV infection when they enter into care regardless of whether ART will be initiated immediately or deferred.	C	AidsInfo (2012)
Genotypic testing is recommended as the preferred resistance testing to guide therapy in antiretroviral-naive patients.	C	AidsInfo (2012)
Conduct resistance testing in all cases of therapy failure.	A	Drayton & Grant (2011)

A = consistent, good-quality, patient-oriented evidence; B = inconsistent or limited-quality, patient-oriented evidence; C = consensus, disease-oriented evidence, usual practice, expert opinion, or case series. For information about the SORT evidence rating system, go to www.aafp.org/afpsort.xml.

IMMUNE THROMBOCYTOPENIC PURPURA (IDIOPATHIC THROMBOCYTOPENIC PURPURA)

Signal symptoms: Petechiae or ecchymoses; oral mucocutaneous bleeding. Some have no symptoms, and thrombocytopenia is an incidental finding on blood work.

Description: Immune thrombocytopenic purpura (ITP; also called idiopathic thrombocytopenic purpura) is an acquired condition manifested by thrombocytopenia from immune-mediated, accelerated platelet destruction combined with inadequate platelet production and T-cell–mediated effects (Palau, Jarque, & Sanz, 2010). Some experts define it as a platelet count $<100 \times 10^9$/L with no other cause. ITP tends to be a more chronic condition in adults and older adults, whereas it is an acute process in children. Secondary ITP occurs in association with other autoimmune diseases such as systemic lupus erythematosus, HIV, or HCV, among others. The condition has further been defined as $<100 \times 10^9$/L and divided into new diagnosis, persistent (between 3 and 12 months duration), and chronic (more than 1 year duration) (Konkle, 2012).

Etiology: Unclear but includes acquired and genetic factors.

Occurrence: Approximately 1 in 20,000; this is probably underestimated because it accounts for symptomatic disease only.

Age: Increases with age; patients more than 65 years of age have a higher risk of bleeding and mortality.

Gender: Women are affected more than men.

Ethnicity: Not significant.

Contributing factors: The condition is idiopathic or occurs after a virus in conjunction with certain drugs (e.g., heparin, salicylates, sulfonamides, quinine) or autoimmune conditions.

Signs and symptoms: Epistaxis, purpuric or ecchymotic lesions, mucocutaneous oral bleeding, possibly bleeding with aspirin use or other NSAID use. There may be no symptoms, but a routine blood test may show thrombocytopenia with no other abnormalities. The concurrent presence of an autoimmune disorder favors secondary ITP (George, 2012; Rodeghiero et al., 2009).

Diagnostic tests: CBC with peripheral blood smear. CBC will reflect thrombocytopenia but otherwise be normal. Peripheral blood smear (PBS) may show larger than normal platelets but normal RBC and white blood cell (WBC) morphology. If there are other abnormalities in the PBS, a bone marrow biopsy is required to rule out other problems. In patients over 60 years old, bone marrow biopsy is realistic due to an increase in myelodysplastic syndromes.

Differential diagnosis:
- Acute leukemia
- Thrombotic thrombocytopenic purpura
- Other autoimmune diseases
- Drug-induced thrombocytopenia
- Infection (HIV, EBV, hepatitis, CMV)
- Vasculitis
- Vitamin K deficiency
- Disseminated intravascular coagulation (DIC)
- Hemolytic uremic syndrome (HUS)
- Hypersplenism
- ITP is a diagnosis of exclusion (Smith, 2007; Snyderman & Herman, 2011).

Treatment: The goal of treatment is to sustain a safe (not normal) platelet count to avoid bleeding. This may include withholding certain drug therapy, where risks outweigh benefits. For patients with platelet counts <10,000/mm³, platelet transfusions may be indicated. Prednisone 1 mg/kg/day orally or IV immune globulin (IVIG) are used initially; a 4-day burst of dexamethasone (40 mg/day) may also be initiated or used in lieu of steroid treatment. In cases where platelet counts are <20,000/mm³ with severe mucocutaneous bleeding or any significant bleeding, hospitalization is indicated to stabilize the patient. For RhD-positive patients who have not had a splenectomy, anti-D products, such as WinRho and Rhophylac, are as effective as IVIG in refractory cases (Cines & Bussel, 2005). Splenectomy is a second-line option; the risks and benefits of surgery must be weighed. If splenectomy is planned, immunize the patient 2 to 4 weeks before the procedure against *Streptococcus pneumoniae*, *Haemophilus influenzae* type b, and *Neisseria meningi-*

tidis; these are encapsulated organisms and can be fatal if they infect an asplenic individual (Provan et al., 2010; Vesely, Perdue, Rizvi, Terrell, & George, 2004). Newer therapies include the monoclonal antibody rituximab and thrombopoietic growth factors for recalcitrant cases (Konkle, 2012; Palau et al., 2010). Other drugs that have been used successfully include cyclosporine, antifibrinolytics, and certain chemotherapy agents.

For many adult patients with ITP and a platelet count >30,000 to 40,000, watchful monitoring is all that is required if they are asymptomatic. The course of ITP in older adults tends to be chronic with initial responses to treatment but a reversal back to baseline after a few months.

Follow-up: Follow-up is variable dependent on symptoms, platelet levels, and response to treatment if needed. Patients with moderate or severe ITP will be followed by hematology.

Sequelae: Mortality rate is <1%, usually related to infections, bleeding, or refractory disease. There are some spontaneous remissions.

Prevention/prophylaxis: Unless the ITP is secondary to a known autoimmune disease, there is no prevention, because it is idiopathic.

Referral: Consultation with or referral to a hematologist is indicated in cases of severe bleeding or cases refractory to treatment. Initial hematology consultation may aid in accurate diagnosis.

Education: Patients should be instructed to avoid invasive dental procedures and other activities that could precipitate bleeding episodes. Low-impact exercise is recommended. Aspirin and NSAIDs should be avoided; alcohol intake should be limited to an occasional drink. Patients with hypertension should be encouraged to take their medications as ordered and to have frequent monitoring of their blood pressure to avoid a stroke. Periodic monitoring of platelets will be necessary.

CLINICAL RECOMMENDATION	EVIDENCE RATING	REFERENCES
Treatment decisions are influenced by platelet count and degree of bleeding; therapy is not required for platelet counts <30,000/mm³.	C	Palau et al. (2010)
The goal of treatment is to prevent bleeding, not necessarily to return platelet count to normal.	C	Cines & Bussel (2005)

CLINICAL RECOMMENDATION	EVIDENCE RATING	REFERENCES
Initial management includes treatment with oral prednisone. Other choices for treatment include high-dose dexamethasone, IVIG, and WinRho.	C	Provan et al. (2010)
Chronic refractory ITP is defined as persistence for >3 months, lack of response to splenectomy, and platelet count <50,000/mm³. Treatment options include glucocorticoids, rituximab, vincristine, cyclophosphamide, and methylprednisone.	C	Rodeghiero et al. (2009)

A = consistent, good-quality, patient-oriented evidence; B = inconsistent or limited-quality, patient-oriented evidence; C = consensus, disease-oriented evidence, usual practice, expert opinion, or case series. For information about the SORT evidence rating system, go to www.aafp.org/afpsort.xml.

LEUKEMIAS

There are four primary types of leukemia: acute lymphocytic leukemia, acute myeloid leukemia, chronic lymphocytic leukemia, and chronic myeloid leukemia.

ACUTE LYMPHOCYTIC LEUKEMIA (ALL)

Signal symptoms: Hepatosplenomegaly, fever, fatigue, lymphadenopathy, bleeding, bone or joint pain, anorexia, abdominal pain.

Description: Acute lymphocytic leukemia (ALL) is an extremely aggressive group of hematopoietic neoplasms, manifesting with an overabundance of lymphocytes or lymphoblasts manifesting in bone marrow and peripheral blood. Left untreated, there is rapid spread to lymph nodes, liver and spleen, central nervous system (CNS), and other sites.

Etiology: There are a variety of conditions that predispose an individual to ALL. The most notable condition causing increased risk for the development of ALL is trisomy 21 (Down's syndrome). With Down's syndrome, the relative risk for developing ALL is increased 15-fold. EBV infection is implicated as a predisposing factor in a minority of cases with ALL. It has been suggested that environmental exposures may increase the risk for ALL, but no clear indication of this has been found.

Occurrence: Approximately 5000 new cases of ALL are diagnosed each year in the United States. More than one-half of the newly diagnosed cases are in children; ALL is the most common malignancy in children. It accounts for approximately 25% of childhood cancers.

Age: The peak prevalence of ALL is between 2 and 9 years of age. A second peak in incidence occurs after 50 years of age. ALL accounts for a smaller proportion of adult than of pediatric malignancies, but the absolute number of adult cases is 10 times greater than the number of pediatric cases.

Gender: There is a slight male predominance.

Ethnicity: Caucasians have a twofold increased risk compared to African Americans.

Contributing factors: A variety of conditions predispose to ALL. The most notable condition that places the individual at increased risk of ALL is trisomy 21 (Down's syndrome), in which the relative risk is increased 15-fold. Other predisposing conditions include immunodeficiency and chromosomal breakage syndromes. EBV infection is implicated in a minority of cases of mature B-cell ALL. Environmental exposure risks have been suggested, but few have been shown to be a causal factor in the development of ALL.

The presence of Philadelphia chromosome occurs in about 20% of adults with ALL and only 1% to 2% of children with ALL; this abnormality constitutes a poor prognosis and is rarely curable. Karyotypes are the most important predictor of disease-free survival (DFS). In adults, cure rates are decreased with advancing age with overall DFS of approximately 40%. Patients with T-cell and mature B-cell ALL fair poorer than those with pre–B-cell types. Additional risk factors include CNS involvement. Both children and adults with ALL are at risk for CNS involvement.

Signs and symptoms: Presenting signs and symptoms are almost always caused by the blast infiltration of the bone marrow, which leads to blood count abnormalities. T-cell ALL frequently presents with bulky adenopathy, mediastinal mass, pleural effusion, and/or hyperleukocytosis.

Diagnostic tests: Diagnosis of ALL can be confirmed by the presence of lymphoblasts in the peripheral blood and/or in the bone marrow. According to the French-American-British (FAB) classification system (L1, L2, L3), L3 morphology is indicative of mature B-cell or Burkitt-type ALL, and therefore, it is of clinical and prognostic significance. Routine hematopathological staining, immunohistochemistry, flow cytometry, and cytogenetics are used to define the subtype and further identify prognostic factors. The majority of ALL is of precursor B-cell phenotype (CD10+, CD19+, CD22+, HLA-DR+, TDT+). From 10% to 20% is T-cell, and less than 5% is mature B-cell or Burkitt-type ALL. Certain cytogenetic abnormalities are not apparent on routine karyotyping. Therefore, molecular testing may be required. Lumbar puncture is required to evaluate for the possibility of meningeal leukemia.

Differential diagnosis: Precursor B-cell ALL must be differentiated from T-cell ALL, acute myeloid leukemia, and lymphomas.

Treatment: Many chemotherapy regimens have been shown to be effective for the treatment of ALL in children and adults. Treatment should be managed by pediatric or adult oncologists who are experienced in treating ALL. Treatment should be initiated as soon as possible after diagnosis. Treatment is stratified based on the phenotype and prognostic factors and includes induction, consolidation, CNS sterilization, and maintenance.

Patients with Philadelphia chromosome–positive ALL should be treated with one of the tyrosine kinase inhibitors (TKIs). Excellent early outcomes in patients treated with the TKIs have been demonstrated and are comparable to hematopoietic stem cell transplant.

The likelihood of a durable DFS decreases after relapse. Reinduction of second remission is critical. The length of the initial complete remission (CR) and the intensity of the initial therapy are important factors in determining whether prolonged DFS can be achieved after relapse. For patients with an initial CR that lasts more than 12 to 18 months with standard-risk therapy, approximately 20% to 30% will achieve prolonged DFS with high-risk disease regimens. The likelihood of durable remission is extremely low in patients with shorter complete remissions after initial therapy.

Follow-up: Patients treated with ALL will require ongoing follow-up with a medical oncologist. The follow-up evaluation will include history, physical examination, and routine laboratory studies, including CBC and chemistry panel. Patients who are in the midst of therapy for ALL will be evaluated frequently by the medical oncologist. In addition, following the completion of therapy, there will be ongoing follow-up by the medical oncologist. The importance of the follow-up evaluations is to monitor for long-term toxicity and recurrent disease for at least 5 years after the completion of therapy. The frequency of the follow-up visits is as follows:

- Every 1 to 2 months during the first year
- Every 2 to 3 months during the second year
- Every 3 to 4 months during the third year
- Every 6 months during the fourth year
- Annually thereafter

Sequelae: Nearly all patients with ALL require transfusions of packed RBCs and platelets during induction and consolidation. Blood products should be leukocyte-reduced in order to lower the risk of febrile nonhemolytic transfusion reactions. In addition, leukocyte-reduced products reduce the risk of alloimmunization to human leukocyte antigens and the subsequent development of being refractory to platelet transfusions and help to avoid the transmission of CMV. Blood products should also be gamma irradiated to reduce the risk of transfusion-related graft-versus-host disease.

Hypogammaglobulinemia is common during treatment for ALL. IgG levels should be evaluated in those with recurrent infections. If the IgG level is low, the infusion of IVIG should be considered.

Nutritional status should be monitored and recommendations for supplements should be provided if indicated. Routine folic acid use should be avoided during the administration of methotrexate, because it may counteract the therapeutic effect of folate antagonism.

Patients who have had a transplant will require reimmunizations. A schedule for the reimmunizations will be provided by the transplant team, and the primary care clinician is usually asked to provide the immunizations as indicated on the schedule. Lifelong follow-up is necessary in order to monitor for possible late complications of treatment (see Table 15-2). The most common late effects of treatment include cardiomyopathy, neurological toxicity, endocrine system dysfunction, osteonecrosis, and second cancers. Cumulative effects of anthracyclines, such as doxorubicin, increase the risk of cardiotoxicity. Therefore, the total dose of anthracyclines is limited to minimize this risk. Echocardiograms or multigated acquisition scans are performed before treatment to avoid additional impact on heart health in the event the individual already has altered left ventricular ejection fraction (LVEF). In addition, echocardiograms should be performed if there are any symptoms that question the potential impact of the prior anthracycline therapy on the LVEF and possible CHF. In the event of decreased LVEF or symptoms of CHF, the individual should be referred to a cardiologist. Neurological toxicity is an additional potential long-term effect from chemotherapy or radiation therapy. All patients should be monitored for neurological toxicity, including neurodevelopmental dysfunction. Patients should be monitored on an ongoing basis. Corticosteroids, especially dexamethasone, are associated with a high risk of osteonecrosis in survivors of ALL. Survivors of ALL who report joint or bone pain should be evaluated for the potential for osteonecrosis (Oeffinger et al., 2006).

TABLE 15-2 Long Term Effect From Cancer Therapy	
EFFECT OF TREATMENT/DIAGNOSIS	**MANAGEMENT**
1. Increased risk of influenza.	Immunize annually. May need to alter timing based on patient's ongoing therapy.
2. Increased risk of pneumonia.	Immunize at 5-year interval.
3. Increased risk of infection from live vaccines.	1. Do not use live vaccines unless cleared by medical oncologist. 2. Discuss need for live vaccine immunization of family members and risk to patient before providing immunization to family member.

4. Increased risk of cardiovascular toxicities due to prior cancer therapy.
  a. Hypertension—side effect of angiogenesis inhibitors (bevacizumab, pazopanib, sorafenib, sutinib, vandetanib)
  b. Myocardial ischemia—side effect of antimetabolites (fluorouracil, capecitabine), antimicrotubule (paclitaxel, docetaxel), monoclonal antibody-based TKIs (bevacizumab), small-molecule TKIs (erlotinib, sorafenib, pazopanib)
  c. Thromboembolism—side effect of alkylating agent (cisplatin), angiogenesis inhibitors (thalidomide, lenalidomide), histone deacetylase inhibitor (vorinostat), small-molecule TKI (erlotinib), monoclonal antibody-based TKI (bevacizumab)
  d. QTc prolongation—side effect of miscellaneous agent (arsenic), histone deacetylase inhibitors (vorinostat, romidepsin), small molecule TKIs (lapatinib, nilotinib, pazopanib, dasatinib, sunitinib)
  e. Bradycardia—side effect of antimicrotubule agent (paclitaxel) and angiogenesis inhibitor (thalidomide)
  f. Pericarditis—side effect of antimetabolite (cytarabine), anthracyclines (doxorubicin, daunorubicin), folic acid antagonist (methotrexate), small molecule tyrosine kinase inhibitor (imagine), antitumor antibiotic (bleomycin), alkylating agents (cyclophosphamide)
	1. Prevention of heart failure:
	  a. Maintain adequate blood pressure control.
	  b. Closely monitor cardiac function while receiving chemotherapy with potential cardiotoxic adverse effect.
	  c. Limit lifetime cumulative dose of anthracyclines and its analogs.
	  d. Alter the anthracycline mode of administration.
	  e. Use anthracycline analogs (e.g., liposomal anthracyclines).
	  f. Add cardioprotectants (e.g., dexrazoxane) to anthracycline therapy.
	  g. Use cardiac biomarkers for early detection of cardiotoxicity.
	  h. Initiate recommended pharmacologic heart failure regimen at initial detection of ventricular dysfunction.
	2. Evaluate for potential heart failure:
	  a. Electrocardiogram
	  b. Chest x-ray
	  c. Echocardiogram
	  d. Nuclear imaging
	  e. Coronary arteriography
	  f. Endomyocardial biopsy
	  g. Cardiovascular magnetic resonance imaging
	  h. Cardiac biomarkers (troponin I and N-terminal pro-BNP)
	  i. Thyroid function
	  j. Viral titers
	  k. Blood cultures
	  l. Iron studies
	3. Monitor and treat hyperlipidemia if appropriate.
	4. Treat heart failure.

Continued

TABLE 15-2 Long Term Effect From Cancer Therapy—cont'd	
EFFECT OF TREATMENT/DIAGNOSIS	**MANAGEMENT**
g. Cardiomyopathy—caused by anthracyclines (doxorubicin, epirubicin, idarubicin), alkylating agents (cyclophosphamide, ifosfamide), anthraquinone (mitoxantrone), antitumor antibiotic (mitomycin), antimicrotubule agent (docetaxel), proteasome inhibitor (bortezomib), monoclonal antibody-based TKs (bevacizumab, trastuzumab), small-molecule TKIs (dasatinib, imatinib, lapatinib, sunitinib, sorafenib)	
h. Heart failure—in cancer patients, heart failure is usually of nonischemic etiology secondary to chemotherapy-induced cardiomyopathy	
i. Cardiovascular complications of radiation therapy—pericardial disease including pericarditis, pericardial effusion and tamponade, coronary artery disease including premature fibrosis/atherosclerosis, valvular disease including aortic stenosis and mitral stenosis, cardiomyopathy including constrictive cardiomyopathy, diastolic dysfunction, and conduction abnormalities including A-V block, complete heart block	
5. Potential for thyroid dysfunction if received irradiation to neck.	1. Monitor thyroid function at least annually.
6. Potential for second malignancies.	1. Breast cancer-baseline mammogram between ages 35–40 years and then annually in those at increased risk. 2. Periodic CXR. 3. Colonoscopy starting at age 50 years.
7. Infertility.	1. Refer males for sperm banking prior to the initiation of therapy. 2. Refer females to gynecologist/fertility expert for discussion of potential options to enhance the likelihood of maintaining fertility during therapy.
8. Osteoporosis.	1. DEXA scan on regulary scheduld bases. 2. Manage evidence of osteopenia/osteoporosis with calcium supplements. 3. Evaluate Vitamin D level and replete if appropriate. 4. Prescribe bisphosphonate for osteoporosis.

Source: Fadol & Lech, 2011. Fulbright J, Raman S, McClelan W, & August K, 2011.

Prevention/prophylaxis: Aggressive surveillance, prophylaxis, and treatment for bacterial, fungal, viral, and opportunistic infections are essential for individuals undergoing therapy for ALL. Additional prophylaxis is needed for the prevention of other problems related to treatment for ALL. For example, patients with ALL receive corticosteroids as a component of their therapy and will need additional medications, such as a proton-pump inhibitor, to prevent gastritis. To reduce the risk of conjunctivitis that can be associated with cytarabine, corticosteroid ophthalmic solution should be administered during and for 24 to 48 hours after the completion of the cytarabine.

Referral: Patients with evidence of blasts in the peripheral blood should be referred to a medical oncologist or pediatric oncologist (based on age of patient). Because patients need rapid initiation of therapy, the referral should be completed quickly.

Education: Before referral to an oncologist, the patient will need education regarding the concerns of possible diagnosis of leukemia and the need for expedited referral. After remission is achieved, the primary care provider should continue to provide education to the patient/parent regarding the long-term effects of therapy.

CLINICAL RECOMMENDATION	EVIDENCE RATING	REFERENCES
Treatment of ALL is stratified based on phenotype and prognostic factors and includes induction, consolidation, CNS sterilization, and maintenance.	A	Rabin & Poplack (2011)
Maintenance can last 2–3 years and has been shown to improve DFS in children and adults.	A	NCCN (2012b) Rabin & Poplack (2011)
Allogeneic transplant is frequently recommended for adults due to their poorer outcome in initial treatment.	A	NCCN (2012b) Rabin & Poplack (2011)

A = consistent, good-quality, patient-oriented evidence; B = inconsistent or limited-quality, patient-oriented evidence; C = consensus, disease-oriented evidence, usual practice, expert opinion, or case series. For information about the SORT evidence rating system, go to www.aafp.org/afpsort.xml.

ACUTE MYELOID LEUKEMIA (AML)

Signal symptoms: Patients with acute myeloid leukemia (AML) usually present with symptoms related to pancytopenia (e.g., anemia, thrombocytopenia, and neutropenia). These symptoms include fatigue and weakness, infections, and bleeding such as gingival bleeding, ecchymosis, epistaxis, or menorrhagia. General fatigue is present in the majority of patients and may have been present for months before the diagnosis. Fever can be present.

Description: AML is also known as acute myelogenous leukemia. It consists of a group of hematopoietic neoplasms involving precursor cells committed to the myeloid line of cellular development. There are two major classification systems for AML: the FAB and the WHO. The FAB system consists of eight major categories based on morphology. The WHO classification was most recently updated in 2008 and includes cytogenetic abnormalities and molecular detection of mutations. Cytogenetics/karyotype is an important component in the diagnostic workup in AML. Specific cytogenetic abnormalities hold prognostic significance and are used to help determine appropriate therapy. The National Comprehensive Cancer Network (NCCN) guidelines list three groups based on the risk from the specific cytogenetic abnormalities: better risk, intermediate risk, and poor risk (see Table 15-3). The majority of patients who are older than age 60 have a poorer prognosis than those younger than age 60. Remission rates in the elderly are approximately 50% but are often short-lived. Patients over the age of 60 have a median survival of less than 1 year, and the overall survival at 5 years is only 10% (Luger, 2010). Elderly patients with AML have become the focus of current clinical trials.

Etiology: AML is characterized by clonal proliferation of myeloid precursors that have a reduced capacity to differentiate into more mature cellular elements. As a result, there is an accumulation of blasts in the bone marrow, in the peripheral blood, and occasionally in other tissues. This can cause a reduction in the production of normal RBCs, platelets, and mature granulocytes, causing anemia, thrombocytopenia, and neutropenia. The etiology and risk factors for AML are poorly understood. Risk factors that can increase the risk of developing AML include inherited genetic predisposition syndromes, such as Li-Fraumeni syndrome and familial platelet disorders; congenital factors, such as trisomy 21 and Klinefelter's syndrome (XXY); and the presence of antecedent hematological disorders, such as myelodysplastic syndrome (MDS), myeloproliferative disorders, aplastic anemia, and chronic myeloid leukemia in blast crisis (Swerdlow et al., 2008). In addition, treatment-related AML can develop after exposure to alkylating agents and topoisomerase II inhibitors. The most important prognostic indicators are cytogenetic/molecular characteristics, age, and performance status (Kantarjian, Schiffer, & Burnett, 2011).

TABLE 15-3	Prognostic Categories Based on Karyotype in AML	
RISK ASSESSMENT	**CYTOGENETICS**	
Better Risk	t(8;21)(q22;q22) t(15;17)(q22;q12-21) inv (16) or t(16;16)	Normal cytogenetics: With NPM1 mutation Isolated CEBPA mutation in absence of FLT3-ITD
Intermediate Risk	Normal cytogenetics T(9;11) +8, other non-defined	T(8;21) Inv(16) T(16;16) with c-KIT mutation
Poor Risk	Complex karyotype (≥3 clonal abnormalities) -5, -5q, -7, -7q Inv 3, t(3;3) 11q23, non t(9;11) t(6;9) t(9;22)	Normal cytogenetics: With FLT3-ITD mutation

Source: From NCCN Guidelines. Acute myelogenous leukemia. Version 2.2011. www.nccn.org. Accessed Jan 1, 2012.

Occurrence: The incidence of AML is increasing, particularly in the population of adults who are older than age 60 years. AML is the most common type of acute leukemia in adults and accounts for approximately 80% to 90% of cases of acute leukemia in adults (Kuendgen & Germing, 2009). In Europe and the United States, the incidence is 3 to 5 cases per 100,000 adult population.

Age: The incidence increases with age, and the median age at diagnosis in adults is approximately 65 years (Jemal, Siegel, Xu, & Ward, 2010). Most patients are over age 60 at diagnosis. The outcome for younger patients with AML has markedly improved over the last three decades. Advances in chemotherapy and supportive care have aided in the improved outcomes. However, little improvement has been made in the survival of older adults with AML. Older patients have more unfavorable disease characteristics, a higher frequency of comorbid conditions, and poor tolerance of therapy. The percentage of patients older than age 60 years who achieve CR is approximately 30% to 50%. The percentage who are alive at 5 years is less than 10%.

Gender: There is a male predominance, with a male-to-female ratio of 5:3.

Ethnicity: No known predominance in any specific ethnic group.

Contributing factors: AML has been associated with environmental factors such as exposure to chemicals, radiation, tobacco, or cancer chemotherapy. In addition, certain genetic abnormalities, such as trisomy 21,

Fanconi's anemia, Bloom's syndrome, and familial RUNX1 mutations, have been associated with AML. Certain benign disorders (e.g., paroxysmal nocturnal hemoglobinuria and aplastic anemia) and malignant disorders (myelodysplastic disease and myeloproliferative disorders) also have been noted to have an association with AML.

Signs and symptoms: Patients with AML usually present with symptoms related to pancytopenia (e.g., anemia, thrombocytopenia, and neutropenia). These symptoms include fatigue and weakness, infections, and bleeding such as gingival bleeding, ecchymosis, epistaxis, or menorrhagia. General fatigue is present in the majority of patients and may have been present for months before the diagnosis. Fever can be present and is usually related to infection. Fever should prompt the evaluation for an infection. Bone pain is infrequent in adults with AML, occurring in approximately 4% of patients. This can present as symmetrical or migratory polyarthritis/arthralgia. Some individuals describe sternal discomfort or tenderness with occasional reports of aching in the long bones. The discomfort in the lower extremities may be especially severe. This discomfort is associated with expansion of the medullary cavity by the leukemic process.

In patients with AML, skin conditions may change. Certain skin changes, such as pallor, petechiae, or ecchymosis, are usually related to pancytopenia. However, there may be infiltrative lesions in the skin from leukemic involvement (leukemia cutis or myeloid sarcoma) that occur in up to 13% of patients.

Diagnostic tests: A presumptive diagnosis of AML can be made by evaluation of the peripheral blood. However, definitive diagnosis usually requires a bone marrow aspirate and biopsy. Analysis of the peripheral blood at presentation indicates normocytic, normochromic anemia. The reticulocyte is normal or decreased. Most patients have platelet counts below $100 \times 10^9/L$ at diagnosis and about 25% have counts below $25 \times 10^9/L$. The median leukocyte count at diagnosis is approximately $15 \times 10^9/L$, but approximately 25% to 40% of patients have a leukocyte count that is less than $5 \times 10^9/L$. The majority of patients have circulating blasts in the peripheral blood.

Karyotype is one of the main determinants of prognosis in AML.

Multiple prognostic factors are important to the outcome in managing AML. The most powerful prognostic factors include age, cytogenetics, prior MDS, and treatment-related AML.

Differential diagnosis:
- MDS
- ALL
- Solid tumor malignancies such as small cell carcinoma of the lung
- Vitamin deficiencies such as B_{12} and folate deficiencies
- Chronic Myeloid Leukemia
- Myelodysplastic/myeloproliferative neoplasms

Treatment: Management for AML includes the use of chemotherapy; however, which specific therapy to use is based on the disease characteristics, including molecular markers, cytogenetics, and age of the patient. Therapy includes induction and postremission therapy. The gold standard for induction therapy is the combination of cytarabine with an anthracycline. The cytarabine is usually given over the course of 7 days and the anthracycline over 3 days (7 + 3) as the induction. The goal of induction is to achieve a complete response to the therapy. A complete response is defined as bone marrow blasts less than 5%, hematological recovery, and normalization of the peripheral blood smear. Nearly all patients in a complete remission, after induction therapy, will have residual disease and without further treatment will relapse. Follow-up with the medical oncologist needs to occur through treatment and in the long-term.

Sequelae: Nearly all patients with AML require transfusions of packed RBCs and platelets during induction and consolidation. Blood products should be leukocyte-reduced in order to lower the risk of febrile nonhemolytic transfusion reactions. In addition, leukocyte-reduced products reduce the risk of alloimmunization to human leukocyte antigens and the subsequent development of being refractory to platelet transfusions and avoid the transmission of CMV. Blood products also should be gamma irradiated to reduce the risk of transfusion-related graft-versus-host disease.

Prevention/prophylaxis: There is no known method to prevent AML. During and following therapy, the patient may be on prophylactic antibiotics, including antimicrobial, antifungal, and antiviral medications. For management of additional infections, consult with an oncology/transplant practitioner.

Referral: Refer the patient to a medical oncologist with notation of abnormal blood counts on CBC for work-up and management of AML.

Education: Educate the patient regarding suspicion of diagnosis of acute leukemia and rationale for referral to a medical oncologist.

CLINICAL RECOMMENDATION	EVIDENCE RATING	REFERENCES
Cytogenetics are important in the diagnostic workup and help to determine appropriate therapy.	A	NCCN (2012a)
The combination of an anthracycline along with cytarabine is standard induction therapy (7 + 3).	A	NCCN (2012a)
Demethylation agents such as azacitadine or decitabine are used to treat AML in older patients who may not tolerate the 7 + 3 regimen.	A	NCCN (2012a)

Continued

CLINICAL RECOMMENDATION	EVIDENCE RATING	REFERENCES
Post–stem cell transplant, patients need to be reimmunized. Reimmunization schedule can be obtained from the transplant team.	A	Ljungman et al. (2009)

A = consistent, good-quality, patient-oriented evidence; B = inconsistent or limited-quality, patient-oriented evidence; C = consensus, disease-oriented evidence, usual practice, expert opinion, or case series. For information about the SORT evidence rating system, go to www.aafp.org/afpsort.xml.

CHRONIC LYMPHOCYTIC LEUKEMIA (CLL)

Signal symptoms: Asymptomatic lymphadenopathy, abdominal fullness, fatigue, reduced exercise tolerance, or other constitutional symptoms. It can also be manifested as pulmonary nodules. Pleural infiltrations can lead to pleural effusions, and GI involvement can lead to GI bleeding. CNS involvement by CLL is unusual. Although night sweats or low-grade fevers can occur, it is important to evaluate the patient for infection. With advanced-stage disease, recurrent infections, weight loss, or symptoms related to anemia and thrombocytopenia may occur.

Description: Chronic lymphocytic leukemia (CLL) is one of the chronic lymphoproliferative disorders. B-cell CLL is considered to be identical to small lymphocytic lymphoma. It is characterized by a progressive accumulation of functionally incompetent lymphocytes. The survival times from initial diagnosis range from 2 to 20 years with a median survival of approximately 10 years.

Etiology: No clear environmental etiological factors have been identified. A family history of CLL is one of the strongest risk factors for the development of CLL.

Occurrence: CLL is the most common leukemia in adults of the Western world. It comprises about 11% of all hematological cancers. The incidence increases with age. Based on the SEER data, the adjusted incidence rate at diagnosis is 3.9 per 100,000, whereas it is 22.3 per 100,000 above age 65 years and higher for patients over 80 years of age (Bairey et al., 2011; Howlander et al., 2010).

Age: The median age of patients at diagnosis of CLL is 72 years. Over two-thirds of patients are over the age of 65 at diagnosis (National Cancer Institute, 2012). Age on its own can be regarded as an independent risk factor

for poorer prognosis in CLL. The level of risk based on age is dependent on the number of comorbidities and the loss of end-organ reserve that develops as one ages.

Gender: There is a slight male predominance.

Ethnicity: CLL is the most common leukemia in Western countries but is rare in Hispanics and Asians.

Contributing factors: Until recently, the prognostic factors for CLL were based on clinical parameters, such as clinical stage of disease, age, lymphocyte doubling time, and laboratory data such as serum beta-2 microglobulin and lactose dehydrogenase. However, currently, biological and molecular markers, including IgVH mutational status, CD38, ZAP-70, and CLLU1 expression, are also important in evaluating prognosis. Cytogenetics have been shown to be additional parameters for prognosis. Fluorescence in situ hybridization (FISH) analysis for chromosome 17p deletion and TP53 mutations and to some extent 11q deletion are of greatest importance with regard to the chromosomal mutations important in prognosis for CLL (Zenz, Mertens, Döhner, & Stilgenbauer, 2011). Unmutated IgVH, 11q deletion, high levels of serum beta-2 microglobulin, advanced age, and stage of disease represent poor prognostic factors. High CD38 represents a poor prognostic indicator with a shorter survival time.

Signs and symptoms: CLL is commonly diagnosed when an absolute lymphocytosis is noted on routine CBC in the asymptomatic patient. Other patients may note a painless enlarged lymph node. A minority of patients present with "B symptoms," defined as fevers, chills, night sweats, and weight loss. In addition, some patients present with infection or autoimmune hemolytic anemia or immune thrombocytopenia. In advanced-stage disease, patients may have recurrent infection, weight loss, or symptoms related to anemia (e.g., fatigue, headaches, palpitations, activity intolerance) or thrombocytopenia (bruising, petechiae, bleeding).

Diagnostic tests: According to the National Cancer Institute Working Group, the diagnosis of CLL is defined as follows:

- Absolute lymphocytosis of >5000/mcL, composed of morphologically mature-appearing cells, that is unexplained by other causes
- At least 30% lymphocytes in a normocellular or hypercellular marrow
- A monoclonal B-cell population with lymphocytes that express low levels of surface immunogobulins and express CD5, CD19, CD20, and CD23

The primary test that needs to be completed is a CBC with differential and platelets. CLL cells are predominantly small, mature-appearing lymphocytes with round nuclei, clumped chromatin, and scant cytoplasm. A classic feature is smudge cells with bare nuclei that appear squashed. Small lymphocytic lymphoma also may have circulating cells appearing as in CLL. Autoimmune hemolytic manifestations can occur with autoimmune hemolytic anemia and ITP occurring frequently in CLL.

A bone marrow biopsy is also useful in the diagnostic work-up, because the bone marrow is always involved in CLL. However, a bone marrow biopsy is not required for the diagnostic work-up, because the peripheral blood can be tested by flow cytometry to confirm the diagnosis. Flow cytometry is the single most helpful test for confirming the diagnosis of CLL. CLL cells are B cells that express D5 and CD23. They typically have weak expression of CD20, CD22, and surface immunoglobulin and are negative for FMC7, CD10, and CD103.

FISH analysis can identify abnormalities in approximately 80% of cases of CLL. Chromosome 13q deletion is present in approximately 55% of cases of CLL, deletion of 11q is present in approximately 18%, trisomy 12 in 16%, and deletion 17p in approximately 7%. Normal karyotype is noted in approximately 18% of cases. Approximately 29% of cases have two or more chromosomal abnormalities.

Computed tomography (CT) is useful in determining the extent of lymph node involvement in CLL. It also is used to evaluate the level of response to therapy. CT is generally used before the initiation of therapy to set a baseline for the extent of lymphadenopathy. However, it is not required if patients will not be treated but will be observed initially.

Positron emission tomography (PET) scans are not helpful in the diagnosis of CLL but can provide additional information in advanced-stage or relapsed disease, especially if there is a concern that the disease has transformed into high-grade lymphoma.

Prognostic factors have been identified that are independent of clinical stage. These markers can be useful in predicting the pace of disease progression in untreated patients and overall survival. Prognostic factors include the following:

- Immunoglobulin variable region heavy chain gene mutation (IgVH)—unmutated has a shorter survival than patients whose CLL cells express mutated IgVH
- ZAP-70—predicts rate of disease progression and overall survival. ZAP-70–positive patients have shorter progression-free survival than those with CLL that is ZAP-70 negative
- Cytogenetics:
  - Deletion 17p—shortened survival
  - Deletion 11q—shortened survival
  - Deletion 13q—longer survival
- CD38 expression—shorter survival
- Lymphocyte doubling time—less than 12 months indicates more rapidly progressive disease

Differential diagnosis:
- Follicular lymphoma
- Marginal zone lymphoma
- Mantle cell lymphoma
- Prolymphocytic leukemia

Treatment: At the time of diagnosis, many patients do not require treatment. Watch-and-wait is an acceptable intervention in many patients with CLL, because currently there are no therapies available that can provide a cure for CLL except for an allogeneic transplant. However, on average, patients are diagnosed with CLL in their seventies, and as a result, the majority of patients with CLL are not candidates for an allogeneic transplant. In addition, most patients with early-stage CLL are asymptomatic and have a good long-term prognosis. Patients who become symptomatic or have rapidly progressive disease warrant the initiation of therapy. In addition, if the patient exhibits either symptomatic or bulky lymphadenopathy, treatment is warranted. Symptoms of splenomegaly and significant splenomegaly are also indications to start therapy. Progressive marrow failure with worsening anemia and/or thrombocytopenia is also an indication to start therapy. Autoimmune cytopenias that are poorly responsive to corticosteroids or a rapidly progressive lymphocytosis also indicate the need for the initiation of therapy in CLL.

Treatment of CLL continues to include the use of antineoplastic chemotherapy agents alone, such as the use of bendamustine, or in combination such as fludarabine, cyclophosphamide, and rituximab (FCR). Combination therapy with FCR is considered a standard of care at many institutions and offers an overall response rate of 95%, a complete remission rate of 44%, and a median progression-free survival of 52 months (Hallek et al., 2010). Older patients frequently are treated with lower doses of this, called FCR-LITE, to decrease adverse effects and toxicity (Foon et al., 2009). There has been increasing interest in developing more targeted therapies for the management of CLL. The areas of investigation into the development of targeted therapies for the treatment of CLL include those that target the proliferation and survival of the malignant B cells directly and targeting the microenvironment. Most of the new therapies in development target signaling through the B-cell receptor (BCR). BCR signaling is known to be crucial for the proliferation and survival of B cells. A number of the major prognostic markers that are clinically useful in CLL are associated with aberrations in BCR signaling. Many treatment options are available for patients with CLL. Enrollment into a clinical trial should be considered at each interval that the patient with CLL requires therapy.

Stem cell transplantation may be a component of the patient's therapy. The majority of patients with CLL are older and are not eligible for an allogeneic transplant.

Follow-up: Because CLL is a chronic disease, patients with CLL require ongoing follow-up with the medical oncologist.

Sequelae: Autoimmune complications of CLL occur in 10% to 25% of patients during the course of their disease. Autoimmune hemolytic anemia (AIHA) is the most common, followed by ITP. Steroids usually are used front line for the management of these complications. Rituximab is one of the more active therapies for the treatment of autoimmune complications of CLL that are not responding to steroid therapy (Jaglowski, Alinari, Lapalombella, Muthusamy, & Byrd, 2010; Zecca, De Stefano, Nobili, & Locatelli, 2001).

CLL is associated with hypogammaglobulinemia. Hypogammaglobulinemia alone does not require therapy. When patients also experience recurrent infections, this is the rationale for the initiation of therapy. Not only may therapy need to be initiated to treat the CLL, but the hypogammaglobulinemia may require the administration of IVIG to replete the IgG level.

Patients with CLL are at a higher risk than the general population to develop another cancer. Lung, skin, and bone are the most common sights of second malignancies. Individuals with CLL have a twofold to fivefold increased risk of developing a second lymphoid malignancy. The most commonly reported transformations include prolymphocytic leukemia, aggressive or highly aggressive lymphoma, Hodgkin's lymphoma, and multiple myeloma.

Prevention/prophylaxis: Infections from bacterial, viral, and fungal agents are an important cause of morbidity and mortality in CLL. Primary management of patients with CLL is by oncology.

Referral: Refer patients with lymphocytosis to a medical oncologist for work-up. Bone marrow biopsies are not needed for diagnosis; peripheral blood can be sent for flow cytometry to confirm the diagnosis. CT scans are not necessary in the work-up of patients with CLL unless lymphadenopathy is present. If patients with CLL are experiencing recurrent upper respiratory infections, the medical oncologist should be notified for potential administration of IVIG.

Education: Patients with CLL need to be educated regarding the chronic nature of the disease and the need for ongoing follow-up. They need to receive immunizations regularly, especially the seasonal flu vaccine and the pneumonia vaccine to prevent illness due to the immunological suppression associated with CLL. In addition, they need to be monitored for recurrent infections, especially upper respiratory infections, that may be related to hypogammaglobulinemia.

CLINICAL RECOMMENDATION	EVIDENCE RATING	REFERENCES
Diagnosis can be made on flow cytometry analysis of the peripheral blood.	A	NCCN (2012a)
Watch and wait (observation) is an acceptable intervention in many patients who have asymptomatic disease.	A	NCCN (2012a)

CLINICAL RECOMMENDATION	EVIDENCE RATING	REFERENCES
Treatment includes the use of rituximab alone in combination with chemotherapy agents. Potential chemotherapy agents used alone or in combination include bendamustine, fludarabine, cyclophosphamide, and pentostatin. Ofatumumab can be used in recurrent disease. Alemtuzumab can also be used.	A	NCCN (2012a)
Stem cell transplant can be a component of treatment.	A	NCCN (2012a)

A = consistent, good-quality, patient-oriented evidence; B = inconsistent or limited-quality, patient-oriented evidence; C = consensus, disease-oriented evidence, usual practice, expert opinion, or case series. For information about the SORT evidence rating system, go to www.aafp.org/afpsort.xml.

CHRONIC MYELOID LEUKEMIA (CML)

Signal symptoms: Fatigue, nausea, malaise, weight loss, excessive sweating, abdominal fullness, and bleeding episodes. Anemia, WBC count >100,000/mcL, and platelet count >600,000 to 700,000/mcL. Abdominal pain and discomfort in the left upper quadrant that may be referred to the left shoulder. Early satiety, tenderness over the lower sternum. Rare presentations of chronic myeloid leukemia (CML) include chloroma, petechiae, and bruising. These features may suggest progression to accelerated or blastic phase. Because neutrophil function is preserved, CML rarely presents with bacterial or fungal infection.

Description: CML is a lymphoproliferative disorder characterized by dysregulation of the production of and uncontrolled proliferation of mature and maturing granulocytes with fairly normal differentiation. The clinical hallmark of CML is the uncontrolled production of neutrophils along with basophils and eosinophils. Untreated, the clinical course of CML progresses to accelerated and blast phases.

Etiology: CML is associated with BCR-ABL fusion oncogene, which arises from the reciprocal translocation between chromosomes 9 and 22, known as the Philadelphia chromosome (Ph). The BCR-ABL gene disrupts the regulation of downstream targets that are essential for the proliferation and survival of normal myeloid cells. The mutation results in uncontrolled growth of malignant cells.

Occurrence: CML accounts for 15% of leukemias in the adult population. It has an annual incidence of 1 to 2 cases per 100,000 people.

Age: CML can occur in all age groups, but the median age of onset of disease is 67 years (Harnicar, 2011). Incidence increases with age; it is very rare in children.

Gender: There is a slight male predominance (1.5:1)

Ethnicity: No sociogeographical preponderance.

Contributing factors: Ionizing radiation is the only known causative factor. No known genetic factors are associated with susceptibility to CML.

Signs and symptoms: Approximately 20% to 50% of patients are asymptomatic at diagnosis. Symptoms that can be present include fatigue, malaise, weight loss, excessive sweating, abdominal fullness, and bleeding. Abdominal pain and discomfort may be localized to the left upper quadrant, can radiate to the left upper shoulder, and are commonly associated with splenomegaly. Patients also can report early satiety and tenderness over the lower sternum. Patients may have symptoms of hyperuricemia such as acute gouty arthritis. Additional findings may include anemia, WBC count of >100,000/mcL, and platelet count of >600,000 to 700,000/mcL. The involvement of extramedullary tissues, such as lymph nodes, skin, and soft tissues, is usually limited to those in blast crisis.

The peripheral smear usually demonstrates leukocytosis with a median WBC count of approximately 100,000/mcL. The WBC differential includes all cells of the neutrophil series, from myeloblasts to mature neutrophils. Blasts account for less than 2% of the differential. One of the classic findings of CML is the presence of a greater percentage of myelocytes than of the more mature metamyelocytes. The granulocytes of the patients in chronic phase are morphologically normal. However, dysplasia can develop in more advanced disease, especially in an accelerated phase. Elevated absolute basophil count in the blood smear is a universal finding, and absolute eosinophil count is also elevated in more than 90% of cases. Absolute monocytosis over the level of 10,000/mcL is not uncommon; however, the percentage of monocytes is usually low (less than 3%). The platelet count can be normal or elevated over 600,000/mcL in about 15% to 30% of patients. If the platelet count is low, the diagnosis of MDS should be considered.

Diagnostic tests: CBC with differential and platelets with elevated total WBC count with basophilia and eosinophilia. Monocytosis may be present. Leukocyte alkaline phosphatase is low. Bone marrow aspiration and biopsy demonstrate granulocytic hyperplasia with a maturation pattern similar to the peripheral blood. Small megakaryocytes with hypolobulated nuclei are present. The megakaryocytes are smaller than normal megakaryocytes but not as small as those in dysplastic marrow. There are markers of increased cell turnover such as pseudo-Gaucher cells and sea-blue histiocytes. The number of blasts in the peripheral blood and bone marrow determines stage. Blast count between 10 and 19 designates accelerated phase. Blast count over 20% indicates blast crisis.

Cytogenetics are completed to determine the presence of the Philadelphia chromosome. FISH analysis can also identify BCR-ABL-1 gene rearrangements. The majority of patients with CML show the presence of t (9;22). Some of the remaining have variant translocations such as complex translocations. Quantitative PCR for BCR-ABL can quantitate evidence of oncogene BCR-ABL.

Differential diagnosis:
■ Reactive leukocytosis
■ Polycythemia vera
■ Juvenile myelomonocytic leukemia
■ Chronic myelomonocytic leukemia
■ Atypical CML
■ Chronic eosinophilic leukemia
■ Chronic neutrophilic leukemia
■ Essential thrombocythemia
■ Myelofibrosis
■ MDS

Treatment: Therapy allows regulation of the development and survival of the myeloid cells. The tyrosine kinase inhibitors that are currently available inhibit the BCR-ABL tyrosine kinase. All three agents are approved

for front-line therapy of CML: imatinib, dasatinib, and nilotinib. Currently, therapy is expected to be lifelong. All three agents are metabolized by cytochrome P450 (CYP3A4), and therefore, drug–drug interactions can occur when these agents are given concurrently with other drugs metabolized by this pathway. Toxicities among the three TKIs are similar. All three agents cause myelosuppression, including neutropenia, anemia, and thrombocytopenia. The myelosuppression is common early in therapy and is frequently associated with the death of the abnormal cells. Other toxicities include GI toxicities, rash, liver toxicity, and edema. Dose-related edema has been reported to be one of the most frequent side effects in elderly patients (Federal Drug Administration, 2013). Diuretics and a dose reduction should be considered in patients with edema.

Most patients obtain a response from the TKIs. However, some patients who develop resistance or intolerance to the TKIs may require an allogeneic stem cell transplant. Age has a major impact on outcome following a transplant. Overall, long-term follow-up indicates that approximately 65% of patients having an allogeneic transplant for CML in chronic phase will be cured of their disease.

Follow-up: When starting TKI therapy, patients with CML should be monitored to assess the response to therapy. Follow-up monitoring includes CBC, FISH, and quantitative PCR for BCR-ABL. Patients need ongoing follow-up to ensure adherence to therapy and optimal and continued response. Research has shown that patients who do not adhere to the daily dosing schedule of imatinib are more likely to have a suboptimal response to therapy. There is a strong correlation between adherence and the 6-year probability of major molecular response (MMR) and complete molecular response (CMR). Poor adherence is the principal factor contributing to the loss of cytogenetic responses and failure of therapy in patients who are on long-term therapy.

Sequelae: The response to therapy is defined as hematological response, cytogenetic response, or molecular response. Factors important in determining risk for progression include a high leukocyte count, massive splenomegaly and constitutional symptoms, patients of African origin, and a high basophil count.

Although the response rates with the three TKIs are high, patients can develop drug resistance (Apperley, 2007; Milojkovic & Apperley, 2009). Other primary reasons for decreased response level are patient nonadherence to therapy, drug oral bioavailability, and protein plasma binding. Secondary resistance, or acquired resistance, is most commonly caused by point mutations in the BCR-ABL kinase domain. Patients may develop long-term effects from therapy.

Prevention/prophylaxis: Patients who undergo an allogeneic transplant will require reimmunization. The schedule for reimmunization is provided by the transplant team.

Referral: Patients with evidence of leukocytosis should be referred to a hematologist for evaluation by the completion of a bone marrow biopsy.

Education: Patients need to be educated regarding the chronic nature of CML. Patients need to be educated about the importance of adhering to the treatment plan of daily medication to obtain optimal response.

CLINICAL RECOMMENDATION	EVIDENCE RATING	REFERENCES
Diagnosis based on presence of Philadelphia chromosome and/or presence of BCR/ABL fusion oncogene.	A	NCCN (2012a)
Treatment with any of the three FDA-approved tyrosine kinase inhibitors (imatinib, dasatinib, nilotinib) provides high response rates, high progression-free response rates, and high overall survival rates.	A	NCCN (2012a)
Stem cell transplant is reserved for patients with chronic phase CML with resistant disease or intolerance to TKIs or in patients with accelerated or blast phase CML.	A	NCCN (2012a)

A = consistent, good-quality, patient-oriented evidence; B = inconsistent or limited-quality, patient-oriented evidence; C = consensus, disease-oriented evidence, usual practice, expert opinion, or case series. For information about the SORT evidence rating system, go to www.aafp.org/afpsort.xml.

CASE STUDY

Mrs. L., a 68-year-old Caucasian woman, presents to your office today with a complaint of feeling tired all the time and now, more recently, feeling weak and like "I can't catch my breath sometimes." She has been healthy except for high cholesterol, managed by Lipitor. Her husband died 9 months ago, and she has attributed her fatigue to dealing with his death but realizes that she is feeling worse and not better as time passes.

No known drug allergies, takes only Lipitor. Past surgical history: Appendectomy in childhood; hysterectomy for uterine myoma 10 years ago. No significant medical history. Has two daughters living nearby. Blood pressure (BP) 106/70 mm Hg, heart rate (HR) 98 beats/min and regular, respiratory rate 18 breaths/min and afebrile, body mass index (BMI) 22 (10 lb weight loss since death of husband).

Slender, quiet-spoken older woman appearing tired. Conjunctiva pale, mucous membranes moist. No lymphadenopathy of neck or femoral area. Chest Computed Tomography Angiogram (CTA), good air movement. Heart tachyarrhythmic with regular rate, soft midsystolic murmur. Abdomen soft, bowel sounds ×4. Urine dipstick negative.

1. What additional subjective data are you seeking?
2. What additional objective data will you be assessing for?
3. What national guidelines are appropriate to consider?
4. What tests will you order?
5. Are there any screening tools that you want to use?
6. What are the differential diagnoses that you are considering?
7. What is your plan of care?
8. Are there any Healthy People 2020 objectives that you should consider?
9. What additional patient teaching may be needed?
10. Will you be looking for a consultation?

REFERENCES

Anemia of Chronic Disease

Bross, M. H., Soch, K., & Smith-Knuppel, T. (2010). Anemia in older persons. *American Family Physician, 82*(5), 480–487.

Chen, B. H., & Gandhi, S. (2004, August). Anemia of chronic disease. *Canadian Journal of CME*, pp. 59–62.

FDA Medwatch. (2011). Erythropoiesis-stimulating agents (ESAs) in chronic kidney disease: drug safety communication—modified dosing recommendations. Retrieved from http://www.fda.gov/Safety/MedWatch/SafetyInformation/SafetyAlertsforHuman-MedicalProducts/ucm260641.htm

National Anemia Action Council. (2009, January 7). Tracking and treating anemia in elderly patients. Retrieved from http://www.anemia.org/professionals/feature-articles/content.php?contentid=344

Ngo, K., Kotecha, D., Walters, J. A., Manzano, L., Palazzuoli, A., van Veldhuisen, D. J., & Flather, M. (2010). Erythropoiesis-stimulating agents for anaemia in chronic heart failure patients. (Cochrane Review). In *The Cochrane Library 2010*, Issue 2. Chichester, UK: John Wiley & Sons, Ltd.

Price, E. A., & Schrier, S. L. (2013). Anemia in the older adult. *UpToDate.* Retrieved from http://www.uptodate.com/contents/anemia-in-the-older-adult

Schrier, S. L., & Camaschella, C. (2011). Anemia of chronic disease. *UpToDate.* Retrieved from http://www.uptodate.com/contents/anemia-of-chronic-disease-anemia-of-chronic-inflammation

Spivak, J. (2005). Anemia in the elderly: a growing health concern. *Medscape Education,* Retrieved April 6, 2012, from www.medscape.org/viewarticle/522647

U.S. Food and Drug Administration. (2011). FDA Drug Safety Communication. Modified dosing recommendations to improve the safe use of erythropoiesis-stimulating agents (ESAs) in chronic kidney disease. Retrieved from http://www.fda.gov/drugs/drugsafety/ucm259639.htm

Weiss, G., & Goodnough, L. T. (2005). Anemia of chronic disease. *New England Journal of Medicine, 352*(10), 1011–1023.

Anemia, Iron Deficiency

Bross, M. H., Soch, K., & Smith-Knuppel, T. (2010). Anemia in older persons. *American Family Physician, 82*(5), 480–487.

Dambro, M. R. (2003). *Griffith's 5 minute consult.* Baltimore, MD: Lippincott Williams & Wilkins.

de Benoit, B., McLean, E., Egli, I., & Cogswell, M. (Eds.) (2005). Worldwide prevalence of anaemia 1993–2005: WHO global database on anaemia. Geneva, Switzerland: WHO Press.

Killip, S., Bennett, J. M., & Chambers, M. D. (2007). Iron deficiency anemia. *American Family Physician, 75*(5), 671–678.

McPhee, S. J., & Papadakis, M. A. (2010). *Lange current medical diagnosis and treatment* (49th ed.). New York City, NY: McGraw-Hill.

National Anemia Action Council. (2008, November 14). A patient's guide to oral iron supplements. Retrieved from http://www.anemia.org/patients/feature-articles/content.php?contentid=000316

National Anemia Action Council. (2009, January 7). Tracking and treating anemia in elderly patients. Retrieved from http://www.anemia.org/professionals/feature-articles/content.php?contentid=344

Ofran, A. (2011). Anemia (diagnostic approach). *Essential Evidence Plus.* Retrieved from www.essentialevidenceplus.com

Rimon, E., Kagansky, N., Kagansky, M., Mechnik, L., Mashiah, T., Namir, M., & Levy, S. (2005). Are we giving too much iron? Low-dose iron therapy is effective in octogenarians. *American Journal of Medicine, 118*(10), 1142–1147.

Van Vranken, M. (2010). Evaluation of microcytosis. *American Family Physician, 82*(9), 1117–1122.

Wadland, W., & Krishnamani, K. (2011). Anemia: iron deficiency. Retrieved April 6, 2012, from www.essentialevidenceplus.com

Zuh, A., Kaneshiro, M., & Kaunitz, J. D. (2010). Evaluation and treatment of iron deficiency anemia: a gastroenterological perspective. *Digestive Diseases & Sciences, 55*(3), 548–559. doi:10.1007/s10620-009-1108-6

Human Immunodeficiency Virus

AidsInfo. (2012, March). Guidelines for the use of antiretroviral agents in HIV-1 infected adults and adolescents. Developed by the HHS Panel on Antiretroviral Guidelines for Adults and Adolescents—a working group of the Office of AIDS Research Advisory Council (OARAC). Retrieved from http://aidsinfo.nih.gov

Anand, P., Springer, S. A., Copenhaver, M. M., & Altice, F. L. (2010). Neurocognitive impairment and HIV risk factors: a reciprocal relationship. *AIDS and Behavior, 14*(6), 1213–1226.

Barroso, J., Hammill, B. G., Leserman, J., Salahuddin, N., Harmon, J. L., & Wells Pence, B. (2010). Physiological and psychosocial factors that predict HIV-related fatigue. *AIDS and Behavior, 14*(6), 1415–1427.

Centers for Disease Control and Prevention. (2008). HIV/AIDS among persons aged 50 and older. Retrieved December 1, 2010, from www.cdc.gov/hiv

Centers for Disease Control and Prevention. (2010a). HIV in the United States. Retrieved December 1, 2010, from www.cdc.gov/hiv/topics/surveillance

Centers for Disease Control and Prevention. (2010b). Vital signs: HIV testing and diagnosis among adults—United States, 2001–2009. Retrieved December 1, 2020, from www.cdc.gov/vitalsigns/HIVTesting

Centers for Disease Control and Prevention. (2010c). HIV/AIDS among persons aged 50 and older. Resources. Retrieved December 1, 2010, from www.cdc.gov/hiv/topics/over50/resources/factsheets/print/over50.htm

Cichocki, M. (2010). HIV and the older adult—a growing population, senior citizens and HIV over 50. About.com: AIDS/HIV. Retrieved from http://aids.about.com/cs/aidsfactsheets/a/seniors.htm?p=1

Cohen, C. J., Kuritzkes, D. M., & Sax, P. E. (2011). *HIV essentials.* Boston, MA: Physicians Press.

DeCarol, P., & Linsk, N., & Center for AIDS Prevention Studies. (2010). What are HIV prevention needs of adults over 50? AIDS Research Institute. Retrieved from www.caps.ucsf.edu

Drayton, J. R., & Grant, E. P. (2011). HIV infection and AIDS. *Essential Evidence Plus.* Retrieved from www.essentialevidenceplus.com

Gaitanis, M., & Mikolich, D. J. (2011). Human immunodeficiency virus. In F. F. Ferri (Ed.), *Ferri's clinical advisor* (pp. 522–525). Philadelphia, PA: Mosby Elsevier.

Guaraldi, G., Zona, S., Alexopoulos, N., Orlando, G., Carli, F., Ligabue, G., . . . Raggi, P. (2009). Coronary aging in HIV-infected patients. *Clinical Infectious Diseases, 49*(11), 1756–1762. doi:10.1086/648080

Jacquescoley, E. (2008). Behavioral prevention study gauges HIV/AIDS and depression in the older US population. *AIDS Care, 20*(9), 1152–1153.

Katz, M. H., & Zolopa, A. R. (2011). HIV infection and AIDS. In S. J. McPhee & M. A. Papadakis (Eds.), *Current medical diagnosis and treatment 2011* (pp. 1266–1295). New York City, NY: Lange Medical Books/McGraw-Hill.

Kearney, F., Moore, A. R., Donegan, C. F., & Lambert, J. (2010). The ageing of HIV: implications for geriatric medicine. *Age and Ageing, 39*(5), 536–541.

Lundgren, J. D., & Phillips, A. N. (2010). Rescue of severely immuno-compromised HIV-positive persons. *Journal of Infectious Diseases, 202*(10), 1467–1469.

Parienti, J. J., Das-Douglas, M., Massari, V., Guzman, D., Deeks, S. G., Verdon, R., & Bangsberg, D. R. (2008). Not all missed doses are the same: sustained NNRTI treatment interruptions predict HIV rebound at low-to-moderate adherence levels. *PLoS One, 3*(7), e2783. doi:10.1371/journal.pone.0002783

Project INFORM. (2010, February). Treatment as prevention: proposed as element of the National HIV/AIDS Strategy. Retrieved from http://www.thebody.com/content/art55609.html

Ruiz, M., Cefalu, C., & Ogbuokiri, J. (2010). A dedicated screening program for geriatric HIV-infected patients integrating HIV and geriatric care. *Journal of the International Association of Physicians in AIDS Care, 9*(3), 157–161.

Schackman, B. R., Gebo, K. A., Walensky, R. P., Losina E., Muccio, T., Sax, P. E., . . . Freedberg, K. A. (2006). The lifetime cost of current human immunodeficiency virus care in the United States. *Medical Care, 44*(11), 990–997.

Sengupta, S., Lo, B., Strauss, R. P., Eron, J., & Gifford, A. L. (2010). How researchers define vulnerable populations in HIV/AIDS clinical trials. *AIDS and Behavior, 14*(6), 1313–1319.

Zelenetz, P. D., & Epstein, M. E. (1998). HIV in the elderly. *AIDS Patient Care and STDs, 12*(4), 255–262.

Immune Thrombocytopenic Purpura (Idiopathic Thrombocytopenic Purpura)

Cines, D. B., & Bussel, J. B. (2005). How I treat idiopathic thrombocytopenic purpura (ITP). *Blood, 106*(7), 2244–2251.

George, J. G. (2012). Clinical manifestations and diagnosis of immune (idiopathic) thrombocytopenic purpura in adults. *UpToDate*. Retrieved from http://www.uptodate.com/contents/clinical-manifestations-and-diagnosis-of-immune-thrombocytopenia-itp-in-adults

Konkle, B. (2012). Disorders of platelets and vessel wall. In D. L. Longo, A. S. Fauci, D. L. Kasper, S. L. Hauser, J. L. Jameson, & J. Loscalzo (Eds.), *Harrison's principles of internal medicine* (18th ed., pp. 965–973). New York City, NY: McGraw-Hill Medical.

Palau, J., Jarque, I., & Sanz, M. A. (2010). Long-term management of chronic immune thrombocytopenic purpura in adults. *International Journal of General Medicine, 3*, 305–311. doi:10.2147/IJGM.S4722

Provan, D., Stasi, R., Newland, A. C., Blanchette, V. S., Bolton-Maggs, P., Bussell, J. B., . . . Kuter, D. J. (2010). International consensus report on the investigation and management of primary immune thrombocytopenia. *Blood, 115*(2), 168–186. doi:10.1182/blood-2009-06-225565

Rodeghiero, F., Stasi, R., Gernsheimer, T., Michel, M., Provan, D., Arnold, D. M., . . . George, J. N. (2009). Standardization of terminology, definitions and outcome criteria in immune thrombocytopenic purpura of adults and children: report from an international working group. *Blood, 113*(11), 2386–2393. doi:10.1182/blood-2008-07-162503

Smith, D. S. (2007). *Field guide to bedside diagnosis* (2nd ed.). Philadelphia, PA: Lippincott Williams & Wilkins.

Snyderman, D., & Herman, J. (2013). Immune thrombocytopenia purpura. *Essential Evidence.* Retrieved from http://www.essentialevidenceplus.com

Vesely, S. K., Perdue, J. J., Rizvi, M. A., Terrell, D. R., & George, J. N. (2004). Management of adult patients with persistent idiopathic thrombocytopenic purpura following splenectomy: a systematic review. *Annals of Internal Medicine, 140*(2), 112–120.

Leukemias

Apperley, J. F. (2007). Part I: Mechanisms of resistance to imatinib in chronic myeloid leukaemia. *Lancet Oncology, 8*(11), 1018–1029.

Bairey, O., Ruchlemer, R., Rahimi-Levene, N., Herishanu, Y., Braester, A., Berrebi, A., . . . Israeli CLL Study Group (ICLLSG). (2011). Presenting features and outcome of chronic lymphocytic leukemia patients diagnosed at age 80 years or more. An ICLLSG study. *Annals of Hematology, 90*(10), 1123–1129. doi: 10.1007/s00277-011-1259-3

Foon, K. A., Boyiadzis, M., Land, S. R., Marks, S., Raptis, A., Pietragallo, L., . . . Tarhini, A. (2009). Chemoimmunotherapy with low-dose fludarabine and cyclophosphamide and high dose rituximab in previously untreated patients with chronic lymphocytic leukemia. *Journal of Clinical Oncology, 27*(4), 498–503. doi: 10.1200/JCO.2008.17.2619

Hallek, M., Fischer, K., Fingerle-Rowson, G., Fink, A. M., Busch, R., Mayer, J., . . . German Chronic Lymphocytic Leukaemia Study Group. (2010). Addition of rituximab to fludarabine and cyclophosphamide in patients with chronic lymphocytic leukaemia: a randomised, open-label, phase 3 trial. *Lancet, 376*(9747), 1164–1174. doi: 10.1016/S0140-6736(10)61381-5

Harnicar, S. (2011). Pharmacotherapy for chronic myelogenous leukemia: a case-based approach. *Journal of the National Comprehensive Cancer Network, 9*(Suppl 3), S25–S35.

Howlander, N., Krapcho, M., Garshell, J., Neyman, N., Altekruse, S. F., Kosary, C. L., . . . Cornin, K. A. (2013). SEER cancer statistics review, 1975–2010. [Based on 2013 SEER data. Bethesda, MD: National Cancer Institute.] Retrieved from http://seer.cancer.gov/csr/1975_2010/

Jaglowski, S. M., Alinari, L., Lapalombella, R., Muthusamy, N., & Byrd, J. C. (2010). The clinical application of monoclonal antibodies in chronic lymphocytic leukemia. *Blood, 116*(19), 3705–3714. doi:10.1182/blood-2010-04-001230

Jemal, A., Siegel, R., Xu, J., & Ward, E. (2010). Cancer statistics, 2010. *CA: A Cancer Journal for Clinicians, 60*(5), 277–300. doi:10.3322/caac.20073

Kantarjian, H., Schiffer, C., & Burnett, A. (2011). Hematologic malignancies: where do we stand in 2011? *Journal of Clinical Oncology, 29*(5), 473–474. doi:10.1200/JCO.2010.33.8897

Kuendgen, A., & Germing, U. (2009). Emerging treatment strategies for acute myeloid leukemia (AML) in the elderly. *Cancer Treatment Reviews, 35*(2), 97–120. doi: 10.1016/j.ctrv.2008.09.001

Ljungman, P., Cordonnier, C., Einsele, H., Englund, J., Machado, C. M., Storek, J., & Small, T. (2009). Vaccination of hematopoietic cell transplant recipients. *Bone Marrow Transplantation, 44*(8), 521–526. doi:10.1038/bmt.2009.263

Luger, S. M. (2010). Treating the elderly patient with acute myelogenous leukemia. *Hematology/the Education Program of the American Society of Hematology. American Society of Hematology Program. Education Program*, 62–69. doi: 10.1182/asheducation-2010.1.62

Milojkovic, D., & Apperley, J. (2009). Mechanisms of resistance to imatinib and second-generation tyrosine inhibitors in chronic myeloid leukemia. *Clinical Cancer Research, 15*(24), 7519–7527.

National Cancer Institute. (2012). Surveillance Epidemiology and End Results: SEER stat fact sheets: chronic lymphocytic leukemia. Retrieved from http://seer.cancer.gov/statfacts/html/clyl.html

NCCN. (2012a). Non-Hodgkin lymphoma version 2. Retrieved April 20, 2012, from www.nccn.org

NCCN. (2012b). Acute lymphoblastic leukemia. Retrieved April 21, 2012, from www.nccn.org

Oeffinger, K. C., Mertens, A. C., Sklar, C. A., Kawashima, T., Hudson, M. M., Meadows, A. T., . . . Childhood Cancer Survivor Study. (2006). Chronic health conditions in adult survivors of childhood cancer. *New England Journal of Medicine, 355*(15), 1572–1582.

Rabin, K. R., & Poplack, D. G. (2011). Management strategies in acute lymphoblastic leukemia. *Oncology (Williston Park), 25*(4), 328–335.

Swerdlow, S. H., Campo, E., Harris, N. L., Jaffe, E. S., Pileri, S. A., Stein, H., . . . Vardiman, J. W. (2008). *WHO classification of tumours of haematopoietic and lymphoid tissues* (4th ed.). Lyon, France: LARC Press.

U. S. Food and Drug Administration. (2013, August 26). *Gleevec (Imatinib Mesylate) questions and answers.* Retrieved from http://www.fda.gov/Drugs/DrugSafety/PostmarketDrugSafetyInf ormationforPatientsandProviders/ucm110505.htm

Zecca, M., De Stefano, P., Nobili, B., & Locatelli, F. (2001). Anti-CD20 monoclonal antibody for the treatment of severe, immune-mediated, pure red cell aplasia and hemolytic anemia. *Blood, 97*(12), 3995–3997.

Zenz, T., Mertens, D., Döhner, H., & Stilgenbauer, S. (2011). Importance of genetics in chronic lymphocytic leukemia. *Blood Reviews, 25*(3), 131–137. doi:10.1016/j.blre.2011.02.002

chapter 16

Psychosocial Disorders

Lori Martin-Plank

ASSESSMENT

Psychosocial assessment of the older adult is the systematic review and evaluation of patient, family, and environment. The psychosocial assessment provides the foundation for developing and implementing a comprehensive plan of care and a means for evaluating its effectiveness. The practitioner must understand what happens during the aging process, because this knowledge allows differentiation between symptoms that are normal and those considered abnormal. For the older adult, physical health, mental health, spirituality, and environmental and social problems all interact to complicate the life and function of the older patient, caregiver, and family.

The psychosocial assessment of the older adult entails evaluation of the following basic needs:

- Autonomy and independence
- Dignity, credibility, and respect
- Identity and individuality
- Communication and belonging
- Touch

An accurate psychosocial assessment is an interactive process between the practitioner and the older adult that creates an awareness of risks, limitations, and functional changes. This enables the older adult to make appropriate lifestyle changes to accommodate these changes and maintain autonomy, independence, and dignity.

The psychosocial assessment should be performed at the initial encounter and annually thereafter for all older adults. Reassessment is appropriate whenever a patient's health status changes.

Ethnicity: *Ethnicity* may be defined as affiliation with a group whose members share a common social and cultural heritage that is passed on to successive generations and provides a sense of identity. To provide culturally competent care, the nurse practitioner should perform a cultural assessment within the psychosocial assessment for a multicultural society. Specific to older adults, ethnic traditions and expectations are factors that should be addressed in the psychosocial assessment.

Contributing factors: A positive correlation exists between social supports and the use of health-care services by older adults. Older adults who are alone and lonely, depressed, or having difficulty adapting to change appear in their practitioner's office more frequently than those with adequate support systems. Social networks are an important aspect of a patient's social functions as are work, hobbies, and interests. Older adults may be reluctant to reveal social or emotional concerns and, in some cultures, may feel that it is unacceptable to share personal problems with outsiders. However, they may feel comfortable discussing a physical manifestation, such as pain or sleeplessness, with a health-care provider.

Risk factors: The older adult population is not a homogeneous group, rather, the population demonstrates a diversity in health, social and environmental supports, financial security, and cultural and personal philosophies. Some distinctive occurrences in the lives of older adults may include the following:

- Developmental milestones that have an impact on most older adults (e.g., retirement, loss of a spouse)
- Changes in financial and social resources that allow the older adult to cope effectively with age-related phenomena

Relocation, financial concerns, and lack of social supports may be the impetus for physical and mental health problems. The most common life events that place the older adult at risk for psychosocial dysfunction include the following:

- Retirement/role loss
- Loss of spouse
- Deaths of close friends
- Family problems
- Relocation
- Financial problems

Psychological Health

Because older adult patients may hesitate to discuss social or emotional problems with a health-care provider, physical symptoms may be the chief expression of underlying psychosocial dysfunction. Therefore, measurement of psychological health adds an important component to the older adult assessment. Psychological health is measured based on the two subdomains of cognition (mental status) and affect (anxiety and depression). A variety of tools, mentioned throughout this text, can be used for cognitive and emotional health assessment. Although helpful, screening tools should not replace the interactive relationship between practitioner and patient.

Socioenvironmental Tools

The heterogeneity of socioenvironmental factors precludes the use of a single tool for evaluating the older adult; however, to evaluate this domain, the environmental and safety checklist may be helpful (see Internet Home Safety Resources for Older Adults), and it may also be used for patient and family education. The information derived from this evaluation will direct the practitioner in areas of education for the patient and family.

Expected outcomes: Chronic disease, physical disability, pain and suffering, cognitive impairment, accumulated losses, and social isolation may occur when an individual is least able to cope with change. Therefore, a psychosocial assessment provides a foundation for developing and implementing a comprehensive plan of care. The expected outcome for the older adult is an enhanced quality of life.

Internet Home Safety Resources for Older Adults

www.aota.org/documentvault/documents/41878.aspx
www.cpsc.gov/cpscpub/pubs/701.pdf
www.cpsc.gov/cpscpub/pubs/older.html
http://michigan.gov/mdch/0,4612,7-132-8347-261897—,00.html
www.ces.ncsu.edu/depts/fcs/pdfs/FCS-461.pdf
http://orthoinfo.aaos.org/topic.cfm?topic<\#61>A00123
www.seniorresource.com/Senior_Home_Safety_Checklist.htm#chklst
www.choosehomecare.com/home_safety_checklist.html

AGITATION

Signal symptoms: Change in behavior.

Description: A sudden onset of restlessness, aggression, delusions, hallucinations, combativeness, threatening behavior, and/or disinhibition.

Etiology: Neurobiological changes in the brain precipitating a lower threshold to overstimulation and environmental triggers.

Occurrence: Approximately 80% of patients with Alzheimer's dementia will have episodes of agitation. Patients with Parkinson's disease, stroke, and other brain disorders occasionally experience agitation with cognitive impairment (Cohen-Mansfield, 2008; Lovheim, Sandman, Karlsson, & Gustafson, 2009).

Age: Any age but predominantly in older adults.

Gender: Both but a higher incidence in females.

Ethnicity: No data to support any increased incidence in any one group.

Contributing factors: Cognitive impairment, sensory impairment, social isolation, chronic bedrest, pain, and hunger can precipitate episodes of agitation.

Environmental triggers, such as noise, light, and visual cues from television and physical surroundings, can also lead to agitation. Psychosocial triggers, such as the approach taken by staff, interaction with other residents, and anxiety during personal care, may cause a person to become agitated.

Signs and symptoms: Restlessness, pacing, yelling, hitting, spitting, kicking, and verbal aggression can be key signs, especially if they are of new onset or increase in severity or duration in a patient who already exhibits these behaviors. Any new onset of delusions or hallucinations also should be considered suspect, because this can lead to agitation (Wetzels, Zuidema, Verhey, & Koopmans, 2010).

Diagnostic tests: Infection panel, complete metabolic panel (CMP), vitamin B_{12} level, and thyroid-stimulating hormone (TSH) to rule out medical cause of agitation.

Differential diagnosis:
- Delirium
- Psychosis
- Mania
- Infection

- Medication side effects
- Late-life delusional disorder
- Depression
- Pain
- Seizures

Treatment: There are two types of treatment for agitation: psychotropic medications and behavioral interventions. Psychotropic medications include antipsychotics, anxiolytics, and antidepressants. All three medications fall on the BEERS criteria list, where they are described as "requiring caution when prescribing for the older adult." Antipsychotics should be used only if there is evidence of psychosis. Antiseizure drugs are used for manic-like symptoms. Evidence supports the use of antiseizure medications in lieu of antipsychotics (Ballard et al., 2009; Gauthier et al., 2010). Anxiolytics treat the symptoms of anxiety that often accompany agitation. If there is evidence of depression, an antidepressant may be indicated. Behavioral interventions fall under the categories of individual approach, environmental, alternative modalities, and staff and caregiver education (Olzaran et al., 2010; Seitz et al., 2012). Tables 16-1 and 16-2 outline the most

TABLE 16-1 Psychotropic Drug Management for Agitation

Antipsychotics

DRUG	DOSE	FORM	CAUTIONS
Aripiprazole (Abilify)	2.5 mg	Tab, dissolvable	Decreased WBCs
	Max 30 mg	liquid, IM	Potentiates antihypertensives
Olanzapine (Zyprexa)	2.5–10 mg	Tab, dissolvable, IM	Weight gain, increased blood glucosez
Quetiapine (Seroquel)	25–800 mg	Tab, extended release	Potentiates antihypertensives and lorazepam
Risperidone (Risperdal)	0.25–1 mg	Tab, liquid, IM	Dose-related EPS
			Potentiated by proton inhibitors
			May be affected by Prozac, Paxil
Saphris	5–10 mg	SL	Weight gain, anxiety, depression

Antiseizure Agents

DRUG	DOSE	FORM	CAUTIONS
Carbamazepine (Tegretol)	200–1000 mg	Tab	Poor tolerability in elderly
			Monitor CBC, electrolytes, liver profile
Lamotrigine (Lamictal)	25–200 mg	Tab	Slow dose titration
			Stevens-Johnson syndrome
Divalproex sodium (Depakote)	250–2000 mg	Tab, liquid, sprinkles	Monitor CBC, platelets, liver function
			Better tolerated by the elderly

Abbreviations: CBC = complete blood count; EPS = extrapyramidal symptoms; IM = intramuscular; SL = sublingual; WBCs = white blood cells.

TABLE 16-2	Behavioral Interventions for Agitation	
Individual approach	Cognitive training	
	Redirection and reassurance	
	Validation	
	Cognitive stimulation	
	Increased activity and exercise	
	Pain management	
	Multisensory stimulation	
	Reminiscence	
	Reality orientation	
Environmental	Cuing with signage and room layout	
	Decreased noise levels	
	Ambient lighting	
	Person-centered care model	
	Availability of activities and supplies	
Alternative modalities	Music therapy	
	Pet therapy	
	Massage	
	Therapeutic touch	
	Snoezelen	
	Acupuncture	
	Aromatherapy	
	Art therapy	
Staff/caregiver education	Approach to patient	
	Behavioral intervention skills	

commonly prescribed psychotropic medications and behavioral interventions.

Follow-up: Review laboratory reports, treat any infections or acute medical conditions, and review medications. If antipsychotics were prescribed, monitor for extrapyramidal symptoms, falls, and lethargy. If indicated, attempt a gradual dose reduction of any psychotropic medications after the acute episode and further reduction at least once every 3 months.

Sequelae: Injury to the patient and/or caregivers, falls, need for specialized care, and hospitalization.

Prevention/prophylaxis: Identify antecedents, avoid triggers, educate staff and caregivers, and introduce behavior modification. Data also support the use of the person-centered care model in long-term care facilities and assisted living communities (American Psychiatric Association [APA], 2010; Whall et al., 2008).

Referral: In refractory cases, a specialist, such as a geriatric psychiatrist, a geriatrician, or a neurologist with specific expertise in pharmacological management, should be consulted.

Education: Patient safety and fall prevention, identification of triggers, reassurance and redirection techniques, simplification of activities, establishment of routine and structure, promotion of rest and sleep, and consistent caregiver assignments.

CLINICAL RECOMMENDATION	EVIDENCE RATING	REFERENCES
Assessment of symptoms	A	Wetzels et al. (2010)
Etiology and occurrence	A	Cohen-Mansfield (2008) Lovheim et al. (2009)
Identification of triggers	A	APA (2010) Whall et al. (2008)
Psychotropic drug management	A	Ballard et al. (2009) Gauthier et al. (2010)
Nonpharmacological interventions	A	Olazaran et al. (2010) Seitz & Gill (2012)

A = consistent, good-quality, patient-oriented evidence; B = inconsistent or limited-quality, patient-oriented evidence; C = consensus, disease-oriented evidence, usual practice, expert opinion, or case series. For information about the SORT evidence rating system, go to www.aafp.org/afpsort.xml.

ALCOHOL ABUSE

Signal symptoms: May be none; falls, transient confusion, insomnia, anxiety, gastrointestinal problems, alcohol odor to breath, tremulousness, recent memory loss, peripheral neuropathy.

Description: Alcohol abuse is a pathological pattern of alcohol use involving social, occupational, or functional impairment that has persisted for at least 1 month or recurred repeatedly over a long period. Older adults with alcohol problems often do not meet the American Psychiatric Association's *Diagnostic and Statistical Manual of Mental Disorders, Fourth Edition, Text Revision* (DSM-IV-TR) criteria for alcohol abuse but are impaired nonetheless. Alcohol abuse is part of a continuum of alcohol use disorders (Wilson, 2009).

Etiology: The National Institute on Alcohol Abuse and Alcoholism (NIAAA, 2005) advances several theories from biological, environmental, psychological, and sociological arenas that have been studied as etiological factors for alcohol abuse and alcoholism. Most recently, several genetic markers have been studied, and a clear case for biological heritability has been established as one factor. Neurotransmitter effects from alcohol and alterations in brain anatomy in patients with alcohol use disorders serve to reinforce the biological connection (Gold & Aronson, 2012). Consistent with the complexity of alcohol use disorders, multiple pathways appear to be involved.

Occurrence: Depending on the source and terminology, estimates of alcohol abuse in older adults vary from 1.2% to 4% (Barnes et al., 2010; Hasin, Stinson, Ogburn, & Grant, 2007; Substance Abuse and Mental Health Services Administration [SAMHSA], 2009). Approximately 16% of older adults are risky drinkers.

Age: More middle-aged adults are currently at risk for developing alcohol-related problems, because alcohol use throughout life has been greater in this cohort than in previous cohorts (Lloyd & Turner, 2008).

Ethnicity: Not significant.

Gender: Men are affected more than women (Hasin et al., 2007; Zhang et al., 2008).

Contributing factors: Male gender, major life changes, and losses are contributing factors. Concerns about alcohol consumption in the older adult are directed primarily toward the physiological changes that accompany aging and the problems posed by regular alcohol consumption. Chemical breakdown of alcohol does not seem to change with aging; however, the changes associated with aging may increase the concentration of alcohol in the blood. These age-related changes include decreased lean muscle mass, decreased amount of body water, changes in liver function, and increased nervous system sensitivity to alcohol. After drinking 1 oz. of 80-proof alcohol, a 60-year-old would have a 20% higher blood alcohol level than a 20-year-old, and a 90-year-old would have a 50% higher blood alcohol level than a 20-year-old (Gilbertson, Ceballos, Prather, & Nixon, 2009). Another major concern associated with alcohol abuse in the older adult is the increased occurrence of drug-alcohol interactions. The decreased metabolism of drugs by the liver in older adults yields significantly higher-than-normal drug levels, and alcohol increases this effect. Alcohol diminishes the effect of oral hypoglycemics, anticoagulants, and anticonvulsants and unpredictably strengthens the effects of sedatives. Six categories of alcohol-interactive (AI) drugs have been identified as being problematic: benzodiazepines, antidepressants, sleep medications, muscle relaxants, antipsychotics, and prescription narcotics (Jalbert, Quilliam, & Lapane, 2008; Pringle, Ahern, & Heller, 2006).

Patterns of alcohol dependence in older adults have been divided into two categories: early onset, which occurs before age 60, and late onset, which occurs after age 60. Early-onset alcohol abusers have a family history of alcoholism, are less well adjusted, and may have experienced alcohol-related legal problems; this category is predominantly male. It is thought that late-onset alcohol abuse is related to the stresses and losses of aging and may respond more favorably to treatment; there are more women in this category (Hasin et al., 2007). Heavy drinking has been associated with lack of social support, depression, and anxiety; binge drinking and heavy drinking were prominent in those with perceived poor health, depression, and anxiety (Kirchner et al., 2007).

Signs and symptoms: Alcohol abuse often is overlooked in older adults, because medical problems, psychosocial problems, and medication use may obscure the signs of alcoholism (Ferri, 2013). In addition, many older adults are solitary, so the drinking is hidden. One way that alcohol abuse comes to light is when older adults are brought to the emergency department due to events related to alcohol abuse. Physical signs that may be present on examination include tachycardia; peripheral neuropathy; physical trauma; tremulousness; hepatosplenomegaly; rhinophyma; inconsistent, mild hypertension; and telangiectasias (Gold & Aronson, 2012). Other symptoms possibly related to alcohol misuse include falls, confusion, anxiety, insomnia, paranoid ideation, and pancreatitis without stones.

Diagnostic and screening tests: Diagnostic assessment depends on a thorough history. The U.S. Preventive Services Task Force (USPSTF) recommends screening for alcohol misuse problems in primary care (USPSTF, 2004). Several validated screening instruments are available (Fagbemi, 2011; Wilson, 2009), including the CAGE; Alcohol Use Disorders Identification Test (AUDIT) (www.addictionsandrecovery. org/addiction-self-test.htm); Brief Michigan Alcohol Screening Test (G-MAST)–Geriatric Version (www.the-alcoholism-guide.org/michigan-alcohol-screening-test.html); and TWEAK, an alcohol screening test developed for women (http://pubs.niaaa.nih.gov/publications/AssessingAlcohol/InstrumentPDFs/74_TWEAK.pdf). The AUDIT-C, an abbreviated version of the AUDIT, has been incorporated into several electronic health record (EHR) systems (www.thenationalcouncil.org/galleries/business-practice%20files/tool_auditc.pdf). The AUDIT has been shown to have higher sensitivity than the other screening instruments and to be gender and culture neutral (Frank et al., 2008).

A psychosocial assessment that includes a mental status examination and a geriatric depression scale should be performed. Also, consider a cultural assessment if appropriate.

Table 16-3 details expected results of blood chemistry and hematology tests with patients who abuse alcohol.

Physical findings may include hepatomegaly, ascites (late stage), jaundice (with pancreatitis), and spider angiomata; men may have gynecomastia, testicular atrophy, and loss of pubic and axillary hair. A complete neurological examination that includes cranial nerves, gait, sensory, motor, reflexes, Romberg's sign, and tandem walking should be included.

Differential diagnosis:

- Abuse of other psychoactive substances such as opiates
- Use of hypnotics and sedatives, which can cause symptoms similar to those of alcohol abuse

TABLE 16-3	Potential Laboratory Test Alterations With Alcohol Abuse
TEST	**EXPECTED RESULTS WITH ALCOHOL ABUSE**
Complete blood count	Increased mean corpuscular volume (MCV) with normal hemoglobin, possible decreased hemoglobin
Aspartate aminotransferase-to-alanine aminotransferase ratio	>2 suggests alcoholic liver disease
Gamma glutamyltransferase	Increased in all liver disease, including alcoholic; may remain increased for weeks after cessation of chronic alcohol intake
Carbohydrate-deficient transferring (CDT)	Increased in heavy drinking, most accurate biomarker for alcohol abuse

- Dementia
- Cerebrovascular accident
- Urinary tract infection
- Gastritis
- Pancreatitis also should be considered

Treatment: The goal of treatment is sobriety or total abstinence from alcohol (Willenbring, Massey, & Gardner, 2009; Wilson, 2009). The level and severity of alcohol misuse determines the treatment (see under Referral). For patients who are heavy drinkers, education and brief motivational intervention by the primary care provider or cognitive-behavioral therapy may suffice (Duru et al., 2010; Fink, Elliott, Tsai, & Beck, 2005; Lin et al., 2010). Patients with symptoms of alcohol withdrawal should be hospitalized. Uncomplicated alcohol abuse can be treated in the outpatient setting. Alcoholics Anonymous (AA) is the most successful group in encouraging ongoing sobriety; however, the self-sufficient spirit, often characteristic of older adults, reduces the probability of participation. An AA volunteer of the same gender and of an age comparable to the patient's age is usually available to meet with an individual at the clinic site and can assume the role of the patient's sponsor, reducing fear and providing the support that may encourage group participation. For older adults, people who are important in their lives need to be instructed by counselors in ways to encourage the treatment process and decrease behaviors that enable the older adult to abuse alcohol. After consultation with a physician, naltrexone may be given to help maintain abstinence in healthy patients; naltrexone cannot be used if the patient is taking an opioid (Anton, 2008; Anton et al., 2006). For chronic alcoholism, the diet should be supplemented with multivitamins containing folic acid and thiamine, 100 mg/day. The patient should be evaluated for electrolyte problems and anemia.

Follow-up: Initially, the older adult should be seen weekly to provide continuity in the practitioner-patient relationship and to monitor treatment effectiveness. When the patient is participating in the treatment protocol, monthly visits should be adequate to monitor progress.

Sequelae: Alcohol abuse can lead to gastrointestinal bleeding, especially if the patient is taking aspirin or arthritis medications. More than two alcoholic drinks daily can contribute to hypertension. Gait disturbances, peripheral neuropathy, and decreased functional ability are consequences of alcohol abuse. Malnutrition, cirrhosis, urinary incontinence, decline in cognitive status, insomnia, anxiety, addiction, and tolerance with concomitant withdrawal symptoms may occur. Depression and suicide increase with alcohol use.

Prevention/prophylaxis: Taking a brief drinking history with the annual wellness visit and administering the AUDIT-C or other screening tools provides the practitioner with an opportunity for patient education. If a problem is suspected, brief interventional counseling at each visit is warranted. Although results vary in their long-term efficacy (Wutzke, Conigrave, Saunders, & Halt, 2002), brief motivational counseling is effective in some older alcohol abusers (Elliott, Tsai, & Beck, 2005; Fink et al., 2005; Lin et al., 2010). Educating patients on what constitutes "a drink" is helpful (see under Education).

Referral: A specialty physician referral is warranted for suspected complications, comorbid substance use, psychiatric diagnosis, or dependency. Consider an inpatient detoxification program for dependency. Refer the patient to a mental health professional as indicated and to a community-based, peer mentoring program such as AA.

Education: Patients must be encouraged to continue participation in a treatment program, and family members should participate in a support group. Early intervention with family members who mistakenly believe that "a few drinks can't hurt" may prevent progression. Educate patients on possible consequences of continued use. Dietary supplements should be taken as ordered. Providers and patients must be educated about what constitutes "a standard drink"; standard drinks are measured as follows: 1.5 oz. of 80-proof distilled spirits, 12 oz. of beer or wine cooler, or 5 oz. of wine. Education should include clarification about the risks and benefits of moderate drinking and specific limits in quantity, frequency, and duration for older adults (Merrick et al., 2008).

Resources:
- www.aa.org
- www.niaaa.nih.gov
- www.hazelden.org
- www.ncadd.org
- www.discus.org

CLINICAL RECOMMENDATION	EVIDENCE RATING	REFERENCES
The U.S. Preventive Services Task Force (USPSTF) recommends screening and behavioral counseling interventions to reduce alcohol misuse by adults.	B	USPSTF (2004)
Alcohol-related brief interventions and counseling are effective in the short term in reducing unsafe drinking compared to usual care. Significant long-term reductions in drinking behavior cannot be sustained without regular follow-up and reinforcement.	A	Wutzke et al. (2002)

Continued

CLINICAL RECOMMENDATION	EVIDENCE RATING	REFERENCES
Naltrexone (NTX) has some benefits for patients with alcohol dependence, but patients' adherence to treatment should be of concern. Psychosocial treatments may help patients to maintain adherence to NTX treatment.	A	World Health Organization (2009)

A = consistent, good-quality, patient-oriented evidence; B = inconsistent or limited-quality, patient-oriented evidence; C = consensus, disease-oriented evidence, usual practice, expert opinion, or case series. For information about the SORT evidence rating system, go to www.aafp.org/afpsort.xml.

ANXIETY

Description: Anxiety disorders are common in older adults and will continue to rise as this population more than doubles by 2050. In the 2000 Census, 35 million people were age 65 or older, with women outnumbering men 10 to 7 and, by age 85 and older, 10 to 4. Anxiety disorders are not normal aging, often co-occur with depression, and are more prevalent than depression. These chronic, disabling disorders can lead to suicide and are underrecognized and undertreated. Most anxious older adults are seen in primary and specialty care, rather than in mental health clinics, by providers who mistakenly attribute symptoms to normal aging or physical illness. Only about 30% of patients age 65 and older received adequate treatment (Agency for Healthcare Research and Quality, 2008; Chen et al., 2006). Compared to depression, limited research exists in assessing and treating anxiety in older adults (Cook & O'Donnell, 2005). Almost 50% of depressed older adults have anxiety disorders that are more resistant to treatment and have a higher rate of depression relapse (Cassidy, Lauderdale, & Sheikh, 2005; Cassidy & Rector, 2008; Hegel et al., 2005). Anxiety disorders are common in patients with dementia and may be a risk factor for dementia (Seignourel, Kunik, Snow, Wilson, & Stanley, 2008). A few studies found that generalized anxiety disorder (GAD) and post-traumatic stress disorder (PTSD) may predict future cognitive decline by as much as 4 times (Lenze & Wetherell, 2009; Rauch et al., 2006; Sinoff & Werner, 2003).

Etiology and contributing factors: Largely unknown. In general, risk factors include female gender, anxious personality, stress early in life, and disability. There are very few studies of structural or functional neuroimaging in older adults with anxiety disorders. Elevated cortisol levels in older adults with GAD—but not in older adults with PTSD or in healthy older adults—suggest hypothalamic-pituitary-adrenal (HPA) axis dysfunction. Research in younger adults found that higher rates of GAD were related to early-life insecure attachments where the world was perceived as dangerous, intolerance of uncertainty, poor belief in problem-solving skills, and inability to regulate anxious emotions (Garakani & Sanjay, 2006; Hall & Hall, 2000–2002).

Occurrence: Anxiety disorders' lifetime and 12-month prevalence rates for age 60 and older are 17.8% and 9%, respectively. This is higher than major depressive disorder (10.7% and 2.9%) (Harvard School of Medicine, 2005). The most prevalent anxiety disorders by rank are specific phobia, social phobia, and GAD. In nursing homes, 71% of people with dementia are anxious and 21% have anxiety disorders.

Age: Although anxiety disorders are prevalent in older adults, with the exception of GAD, they are more prevalent in age groups below age 60. Studies vary from late-age onset being rare to being as high as 50% (Kaiser et al., 2013).

Ethnicity: There are limited national data. Prevalence rates for whites are higher than African Americans. Whites are more likely to have new anxiety disorders after age 60; this tendency is related to whites being more likely to continue working and relocating in late life. But African Americans have more severe impairment, and PTSD is the most common anxiety disorder among older African Americans who experience more traumas (Ford et al., 2007; Himle, Baser, Taylor, Campbell, & Jackson, 2009).

Gender: There are no statistics on gender differences for older adults. However, the 2005 National Comorbidity Study of all ages suggests that older females' 12-month prevalence rates of anxiety disorders are more than older men's (specific phobia 12.2% vs. 5.8%; social phobia 8% vs. 6.1%; GAD 3.4% vs. 1.9%).

Signs and symptoms: These are different in older adults compared to younger adults. Up to 17% of older men and 21% of older women do not meet criteria for any anxiety disorder listed in the DSM-IV-TR. Instead of complaints of anxiety, physical complaints, such as constipation, nausea, and headache, are common as are worries about health, disability, and finances. One is more likely to learn of a patient's anxiety by asking the question "How do you feel when you are under stress?" than by asking "Are you anxious?" The same is true for the question "How do you handle stress?" rather than "Do you feel it is excessive and uncontrollable?" (American Psychiatric Association, 2000; National Institute of Mental Health, n.d.).

The most common anxiety disorders in order of lifetime prevalence are as follows (American Psychiatric Association, 2000; National Institute of Mental Health, n.d.):

- Phobic disorders: Specific phobia is anxiety from a specific feared object or situation. Social phobia is anxiety in social or performance situations. The person feels the anxiety is excessive or unreasonable. It often leads to distress or avoiding the fear. Phobias are often lifelong and are common in older adults.
- GAD is often 20 to 30 years of excessive worry about health, family, and finances with insomnia, muscle tension, restlessness, fatigue, irritability, and memory problems.
- PTSD is reexperiencing a traumatic event with increased anxiety, avoiding thoughts of the trauma, and feeling numb and uninterested and perceiving the future as short.
- Panic disorder involves recurrent, often unexpected attacks of severe anxiety with 1 month of worry about future attacks and their consequences. Panic disorder may include changes in behavior. It is rare in older adults. It is less severe and less frequent than in younger adults. Mostly, the fear keeps those who experience it from leaving home.

- Agoraphobia is avoiding places where escape is difficult or embarrassing. It is rare in older adults and usually does not occur with panic attacks.
- Obsessive-compulsive disorder is obsessions that cause anxiety or distress and/or compulsions that reduce the anxiety. It is rare in older adults and usually is lifelong.

Diagnostic tests: Take a complete history and physical examination. Laboratory tests can rule out medical conditions with anxiety symptoms, including complete blood count (CBC), CMP, and TSH. Order additional tests based on the findings of the history and physical examination.

Differential diagnosis: Medical conditions and substances that precede new-onset anxiety symptoms. Many cardiac, respiratory, endocrine, and neurological conditions may be associated with anxiety (Kim et al., 2000; Strik, Denollet, Lousberg, & Honig, 2003). Anxiety-producing medications may include anticholinergic drugs, steroids, and psychostimulants. Depression also commonly causes or co-occurs with anxiety (Calleo & Stanley, 2008; Cassidy & Rector, 2008; First, Frances, & Pincus, 2002; Hall & Hall, 2000–2002).

Treatment: Treatment for anxiety should reduce symptoms and improve functioning. Simply listening, being compassionate, and showing respect are important to improving outcomes. Treat comorbid depression and medical conditions that cause anxiety. There are no large-scale studies of pharmacotherapy for late-life anxiety disorders to guide treatment decisions. Start low and go slow with medication dosing to avoid risks from drug interactions, because older adults are more likely to take many medications and may have side effects from aging changes in absorption, metabolism, distribution, and excretion of medication. Evaluate and manage side effects, because as many as 25% of patients stop taking medication in the first 6 months due to side effects. First-line treatment is the selective serotonin reuptake inhibitors (SSRIs) citalopram (Celexa), escitalopram (Lexapro), and sertraline (Zoloft). In older adults, they have the least risk of drug interactions, side effects, or worsening existing medical conditions. Benzodiazepines, including lorazepam (Ativan), alprazolam (Xanax), and clonazepam (Klonopin), are effective according to research but are not the first choice due to the risk of falls and confusion. Research supports referral to psychotherapy for older adults, but this recommendation is limited to GAD and no other anxiety disorders (American Psychiatric Association, n.d.; Cassidy & Rector, 2008; Hollander & Simeon, 2008; Lenze et al., 2005; Lenze & Wetherell, 2009; Mohlman, 2005; National Institute of Mental Health, n.d.; Stanley et al., 2003; Wetherell, Lenze, & Stanley, 2005; Wetherell, Sorrell, Thorp, & Patterson, 2005).

Follow-up: Evaluation of the effectiveness and tolerability of treatment depends on the severity of the symptoms and impairment in functioning.

Sequelae: Higher morbidity, mortality, disability, and poor quality of life. Greater use of health services and less likely to reduce risks and follow health-care instructions (Frasure-Smith & Lespérance, 2008).

Prevention: Includes management of stress, using social supports, and maintenance of daily routines as much as possible.

Referral: Refer to a mental health professional if symptoms and impaired functioning persist. Refer to or consult with the appropriate medical specialist if necessary to evaluate and treat underlying medical conditions.

Education: Educate patients and caregivers to recognize and manage anxiety disorders. Because older adults have vision and cognitive changes due to normal aging, offer large-print handouts, explain things simply, repeat things, and ask them to repeat what was taught.

CLINICAL RECOMMENDATION	EVIDENCE RATING	REFERENCES
Practice guidelines	A	American Psychiatric Association (n.d.)
Older adults are more likely to have greater satisfaction with mental health services integrated in primary care settings than with enhanced referrals to specialty mental health and substance abuse clinics.	A	Chen et al. (2006)
Anxiety and depression predict risk of greater major adverse cardiac events in patients with stable coronary artery disease in the 2 years after baseline.	A	Frasure-Smith & Lespérance (2008)
Intensive and prolonged follow-up may be needed for depressed older adults with comorbid PTSD.	A	Hegel et al. (2005)
Somatic symptoms in older adults with anxiety disorders or anxious depression often improve with successful antidepressant treatment.	A	Lenze et al. (2005)
Cognitive-behavioral therapy improved worry and depression in primary care patients with generalized anxiety disorder in primary care compared to usual care.	A	Stanley et al. (2003)

A = consistent, good-quality, patient-oriented evidence; B = inconsistent or limited-quality, patient-oriented evidence; C = consensus, disease-oriented evidence, usual practice, expert opinion, or case series. For information about the SORT evidence rating system, go to www.aafp.org/afpsort.xml.

BIPOLAR DISORDER

Signal symptoms: Variable presentation ranging from depression to mania or hypomania, feelings of grandiosity, rapid speech. Anxiety is common in older adult bipolar disorder; cognitive deficits are also common (Sajatovic & Chen, 2012a).

Description: Bipolar disorder is a recurrent mood disorder with a broad spectrum, from mania to depression. Bipolar I disorder (BD1) is characterized by at least one episode of mania; most patients also have depressive episodes, but this is not a required component. Bipolar II disorder (BD2) includes at least one hypomanic episode and one major depressive component. Bipolar NOS (not otherwise specified) includes manifestations that do not fit either BD1 or BD2; symptoms may be too few or short in duration, but they do not represent the patient's normal behavior (DSM-IV-TR; Stovall, 2012). With the publication of the DSM-V, there is a movement to include another classification of bipolar disorder, mixed states, in which severe manic and depressive symptoms alternate in one episode (Swann et al., 2013).

Etiology: The precise etiology of bipolar disorder is unknown. Geriatric bipolar disorder has been studied only recently, and studies point to a multiplicity of possible causes and heterogeneous clinical presentations. Genetic vulnerabilities, comorbid conditions, and lifestyle, physical, and psychosocial factors are all potential contributors (Young & Shulman, 2009). Experts differ on the clinical significance of late-life emergent bipolar disorder versus the expression of bipolar disease manifesting in early adulthood and continuing into old age (Al Jurdi et al., 2012; Chu et al., 2010; Kessing, 2006; Oostervink, Boomsma, & Nolen, 2009; Van Gerpen, Johnston, & Winstead, 1999; Wylie et al., 1999).

Genetic predisposition is a common factor in most bipolar disorder patients (Sajatovic & Chen, 2011). Genetic studies show a variety of potential vulnerabilities; due to the complexities associated with genetic findings, further research is warranted (Soreff, McInnes, & Talavera, 2012).

Occurrence: Approximately 25% of bipolar disorders are found in older adults; this includes newly diagnosed adults and those who have been bipolar throughout their adult life (Sajatovic, Blow, Ignacio, & Kales, 2004). Lifetime prevalence for BD1 and BD2 ranges from 3.7% to 3.9% in the general population (Kessler et al., 2005).

Age: Bipolar disorder can occur at any age; peak age of onset is between 15 and 30 years.

Ethnicity: Bipolar disorder manifests equally in all ethnic groups (Perron, Fries, Kilbourne, Vaughn, & Bauer, 2010).

Gender: Both sexes are equally affected; women tend to have a higher incidence of mixed states and rapid cycling, whereas men tend to have more manic episodes (Merikangas et al., 2007; Soreff et al., 2012).

Contributing factors: Genetic vulnerability in families is strong. For older adults with new-onset bipolar disorder, stresses from life are postulated to be a contributing factor, including possible childhood incidents (Soreff et al., 2012). Older adults tend to have more medical illnesses, including obesity, diabetes, and cardiovascular and cerebrovascular conditions; this must be considered in initial assessment and in treatment (Soreff et al., 2012). See under Etiology.

Signs and symptoms: Elevated mood, presenting as euphoria or irritability, is common; irritability occurs more frequently in older adults. Dysphoria, manifesting with depression alone or with irritability, is another presentation. Rapid cycling includes back-and-forth shifts from mania to depression. Psychotic symptoms can present in either manic or depressed states. Cognitive impairment and medical comorbidities are also common (Sajatovic & Chen, 2012a). The acronym DIGFAST has been used to describe signs and symptoms during a manic or hypomanic phase:

- **D**istractibility
- **I**nsomnia
- **G**randiosity
- **F**light of ideas
- **A**ctivities (hyperactive, does not require rest)
- **S**peech (rapid, can be garbled)
- **T**houghtlessness (impulsivity)

Symptoms during the depressive phase are similar to those of major depression. Use the acronym SIGECAPS:

- **S**leep disturbance
- **I**nterest/pleasure reduction
- **G**uilt feelings, thoughts of worthlessness
- **E**nergy changes/fatigue
- **C**oncentration/attention impairment
- **A**ppetite/weight changes
- **P**sychomotor disturbances
- **S**uicidal thoughts

Diagnostic tests: The Mood Disorder Questionnaire (MDQ) is a validated (Hirschfeld, Holzer, et al., 2003; Hirschfeld, Williams, et al., 2000) screening tool to assess for bipolar spectrum disorder. The tool can be accessed at www.integration.samhsa.gov/images/res/MDQ.pdf and is not specific to older adults. For patients with depressive features, the Geriatric Depression Scale, regular (www.stanford.edu/~yesavage/GDS.english.long.html) or short form (www.stanford.edu/~yesavage/GDS.english.short.score.html), is recommended as a screening tool.

Diagnostic studies include a CBC and comprehensive metabolic panel, toxicology screen, urinalysis, thyroid function tests, rapid plasma reagin (RPR), HIV, electrocardiogram (ECG), and other individualized testing as indicated by the individual patient presentation and anticipation of treatment modalities (Price & Marzani-Nissen, 2012; Sajatovic & Chen, 2011). In patients with new onset of psychosis, add an electroencephalogram (EEG) and magnetic resonance imaging (MRI) or computed tomography (CT); other screening tests for cognitive disorders may be indicated (Price & Marzani-Nissen, 2012; Sajatovic & Chen, 2011).

Differential diagnosis: Substance use disorder, schizophrenia, schizoaffective disorder, major depressive disorder (unipolar), and other medical conditions, such as stroke (Huang et al., 2012), brain tumor, multiple sclerosis, hyperthyroid, mild traumatic brain injury (such as sustained in a fall), medication reaction, vascular dementia, or delirium (Sajatovic & Chen, 2011).

Treatment: Depending on the presentation and severity, inpatient treatment may be required to stabilize the patient. A collaborative care model has been successful for patients with chronic medical conditions in addition to mental health problems (Woltmann et al., 2012). Establishing a therapeutic alliance is key to management; psychotherapy is also an important part of treatment. Cognitive-behavioral therapy and treatment of the patient and family (when there are family members) are two recommended forms of psychotherapy (Soreff et al., 2012).

Mood stabilizers are first-line treatment for bipolar disorder. Lithium, valproic acid, and carbamazepine are among the most frequently used agents for adult bipolar disorder, but there are few studies specific to older adults. Because older adults are frequently on multiple medications for other comorbid conditions, monotherapy has been recommended as a starting point (Young et al., 2010) with a backup plan for adding other drugs, such as antidepressants or atypical antipsychotics, as indicated. Olanzapine is not recommended for older adults due to weight gain and metabolic consequences; quetiapine is better tolerated (Sajatovic & Chen, 2011). Patients with coexisting dementia require individualized treatment, and co-management by a geriatric psychiatrist is advised.

Drug therapy is specific to different bipolar states (Hirschfeld et al., 2002; Price & Marzani-Nissen, 2012; Sajatovic et al., 2005).

Bipolar I: Mania–Approved Drugs
- Mood stabilizers—lithium, valproic acid, divalproex, or carbamazepine
- Atypical or typical antipsychotics—risperidone, quetiapine, ziprasidone, haloperidol; aripiprazole and olanzapine are not preferred due to weight gain and metabolic load (Dhillon, 2012)
- Benzodiazepines—lorazepam only if indicated to decrease acute agitation

Bipolar II: Acute Depression/Hypomania–Approved Drugs
- Mood stabilizers—lithium, valproic acid, divalproex, carbamazepine, lamotrigine
- Atypical or typical antipsychotics—quetiapine, olanzapine, and an SSRI (not preferred due to weight gain and metabolic load) (Cipriani, Rendell, & Geddes, 2009)

Maintenance: Approved Drugs
- Mood stabilizers—lithium, valproic acid, divalproex, carbamazepine, or lamotrigine
- Atypical or typical antipsychotics—risperidone, quetiapine; olanzapine is not preferred due to weight gain and metabolic load

Dosing should begin at the lowest dose and should be slowly increased. Some sources (Hirschfeld et al., 2002) advocate cautious use of SSRIs as adjuncts for the depressive state, because they may result in hypomania or overt mania; this is less likely in BD2. APA Guideline (2002) recommends lamotrigine, bupropion, paroxetine, another SSRI, or venlafaxine as an addition for BD2 if first-line drugs are ineffective. Other sources indicate that adding an SSRI or bupropion does not improve symptoms of depression (Price & Marzani-Nissen, 2012).

Monitor lithium levels at recommended intervals. Concurrent use of NSAIDs, thiazide or loop diuretics, and angiotensin-converting enzyme (ACE) inhibitors may adversely affect lithium levels (Rej, Herrmann, & Shulman, 2012; Shulman, 2010; Taylor & Laraia, 2009). Electroconvulsive therapy (ECT) should be considered if drug therapy is ineffective for bipolar disorder depression (Hirschfeld et al., 2002; Price &

Marzani-Nissen, 2012; Sajatovic & Chen, 2011; Soreff et al., 2012).

Follow-up: Regular follow-up, particularly during active periods of mania or depression, is essential. Family members are usually included when feasible, because bipolar disorder affects the entire family. Patients on lithium require initial evaluation of renal, cardiac, and thyroid function before initiating therapy and then periodically during therapy. Lithium levels also need close monitoring during the initial period and periodic monitoring once stabilized. Patients being treated with valproic acid also require close monitoring; drug levels, liver function tests (LFTs), and CBC should be checked. Adverse effects include hepatotoxicity, pancreatitis, and thrombocytopenia.

Prevention/prophylaxis: Teach patients, caregivers, and families to avoid stress that could precipitate an acute manic episode. Also, educate caregivers and families to recognize early signs of mania such as decreased sleep or pressured speech, so they can act to obtain intervention before a full-blown episode occurs. Work with the patient and his or her family to develop an emergency strategy if the patient demonstrates injurious behavior that is directed toward self or others (Sherrod, Quinlan-Colwell, Lattimore, Shattell, & Kennedy-Malone, 2010). Educate the patient and his or her family on the importance of medication adherence and regular follow-up with a designated health-care provider.

Sequelae: Bipolar disorder is a chronic health condition with both physical and mental health sequelae. Some studies have demonstrated that older adults with bipolar disorder do not achieve a sustained level of recovery or stability (Gildengers et al., 2005). Medications used to treat bipolar disorder cause weight gain and metabolic issues as well as potential liver and kidney damage. Concurrent substance abuse or sexual hyperactivity can result in legal consequences and can complicate bipolar disorder.

Referral: Initial referral to a psychiatrist skilled in the assessment and management of bipolar disorder is important, particularly in older adults with cognitive deficits or medical comorbidities. Referral of the patient and his or her family to support services is important.

Education: Patients who have had bipolar disorder from early adulthood may require reinforcement or reeducation. Those with new-onset bipolar disorder will require extensive education on the disease. Poor insight is part of the clinical picture, so frequent reeducation is indicated. For patients who are in a group living setting, education of caregiving staff is also essential so that manic and hypomanic episodes in particular are not misinterpreted as deliberate aggression. Spouse and family, if present, also require education in the disease process, the chronic nature of the disorder, and the importance of medication adherence. Avoidance of alcohol and other addictive substances is an important part of the education of the patient and his or her family and friends.

Resources:
- National Institute of Mental Health: www.nimh.nih.gov
- Depression and Bipolar Support Alliance: www.dbsalliance.org
- National Alliance on Mental Illness: www.nami.org
- Mental Health America: www.nmha.org
- Association for Behavioral and Cognitive Therapies: www.aabt.org
- American Psychiatric Association: www.psych.org

CLINICAL RECOMMENDATION	EVIDENCE RATING	REFERENCES
Social support in recognizing early warning signs of mood relapse improves outcomes in patients with bipolar disorders.	A	Morriss et al. (2007)
Screen patients with symptoms of depression, irritability, or impulsivity for bipolar disorder using a validated instrument.	C	Brennan & Rapport (2011)
Assess the safety of patients and others, and determine the need for hospitalization, intensive outpatient therapy, and/or close monitoring.	A	Brennan & Rapport (2011)

Continued

CLINICAL RECOMMENDATION	EVIDENCE RATING	REFERENCES
Drug therapy is essential during acute episodes and in the maintenance phase to reduce symptoms and improve functioning.	A	Brennan & Rapport (2011)
Lithium, valproate, and some antipsychotics are effective treatments for acute mania in bipolar disorders.	A	Parikh, LeBlanc, & Ovanessian (2010) Yatham et al. (2009)
Lithium, valproate, lamotrigine, and some antipsychotics are effective treatments for acute depression in bipolar disorders.	A	Van Lieshout & MacQueen (2010) Yatham et al. (2009)
Lithium, valproate, lamotrigine, and some atypical antipsychotics are effective for maintenance therapy of bipolar disorders.	A	Burgess et al. (2001) Cipriani, Rendell, & Geddes (2009) Yatham et al. (2009)
Currently, there is no compelling evidence to suggest that lithium should be avoided in elderly patients for fear of renal side effects.	A	Rej et al. (2012)

A = consistent, good-quality, patient-oriented evidence; B = inconsistent or limited-quality, patient-oriented evidence; C = consensus, disease-oriented evidence, usual practice, expert opinion, or case series. For information about the SORT evidence rating system, go to www.aafp.org/afpsort.xml.

DELIRIUM

Signal symptoms: Change in mental status, confusion, disorientation (time, place, person), agitation.

Description: Delirium presents as a disturbance of consciousness (decreased awareness of the environment) with a reduced ability to focus, sustain, or shift attention (DSM-IV-TR Criterion A). Cognitive changes (poor memory, disorientation, speech disturbance) and/or perceptual disturbances are distinct from a pre-existing, established, or evolving dementia (DSM-IV-TR Criterion B). The onset of the disturbance is rapid (hours to days) and typically fluctuates over the course of the day (DSM-IV-TR Criterion C). Delirium frequently represents a sudden and significant decline from a previous level of functioning, and there is usually evidence from the history, physical examination, or laboratory tests of a direct physiological etiology of a general medical condition, substance intoxication or withdrawal, use of a medication, toxin exposure, or a combination of these factors (DSM-IV-TR Criterion D) (Neufeld et al., 2011).

The DSM-IV-TR differentiates delirium by etiology:

1. Delirium due to a general medical condition
2. Substance-induced delirium
3. Delirium due to multiple etiologies
4. Delirium NOS

Etiology: Causes of delirium are numerous, and in elderly hospitalized patients there are often multiple etiologies:

- *Metabolic:* renal failure, hepatic failure, anemia, hypoxia, hypoglycemia, thiamine deficiency, electrolyte abnormalities
- *Infection:* meningitis, encephalitis, sepsis, urinary tract infection (UTI), respiratory infection
- *Cardiac:* myocardial infarction, congestive heart failure, arrhythmia

- *Neurological:* stroke, intracranial hemorrhage, head trauma, seizures, undiagnosed pain
- *Pulmonary:* respiratory failure, chronic obstructive pulmonary disease (COPD) causing hypoxia
- *Sensory impairment:* visual and/or hearing deficits
- *Medications:* benzodiazepines, sedative-hypnotics, opioids, anticholinergics, antihypertensives, corticosteroids, lithium
- *Toxins:* alcohol, amphetamines, cocaine, substance intoxication or withdrawal

Regardless of cause, a consistent finding is significant reduction in regional cerebral perfusion during periods of delirium in comparison with blood flow patterns after recovery. A possible neurological common pathway may involve acetylcholine and dopamine, and the disruption in the sleep-wake cycle in delirium indicates melatonin as a possible factor (Lemstra et al., 2008; Maldonado, 2008). A recent clinical review of studies on biomarkers for delirium was inconclusive but implicated inflammatory markers including cytokines along with insulin-like growth factor and the presence of S-100 β, a substance expressed by astrocytes and found in traumatic brain injury and stroke; S-100 β was also found in high levels in patients with delirium (Khan, Zawahiri, Campbell, & Boustani, 2011).

Changes in brain function, multiple general medical problems, polypharmacy, reduced hepatic metabolism of medications, multisensory declines, and brain disorders, such as dementia, make the elderly particularly vulnerable to delirium. A careful medical evaluation that includes attention to level of oxygenation, possible occult infection (e.g., UTI), and the role of medications is essential. Although many medications can be a causative factor, those with anticholinergic effects are frequently responsible (Flacker, 2010; Tullmann, Fletcher, & Foreman, 2012).

Occurrence: Prevalence in the general population is 0.4% in adults age 18 years and older and rises with age to 1.1% in those age 55 and older. In the hospitalized medically ill, the prevalence of delirium ranges from 14% to 56% (Pandharipande, Jackson, & Ely, 2005). The prevalence of delirium in long-term care residents ages 75 and older may be as high as 60% at any given time. In the hospitalized elderly, approximately 10% to 15% exhibit delirium on admission, and 10% to 40% may develop delirium during their hospital stay. Prevalence varies depending on the underlying condition(s), procedures and surgeries performed, and other medical interventions provided. Hospital mortality rate from delirium ranges from 25% to 33%.

It is not uncommon for hospitalized cancer patients (25%) and hospitalized AIDS patients (30% to 40%) to develop delirium. Approximately half of postoperative patients develop delirium, and the majority of those with terminal illness (up to 80%) develop delirium as they approach death (Breitbart & Alici, 2012). Symptoms of subclinical delirium, such as restlessness, anxiety, irritability, distractibility, or sleep disturbance, may be manifested in the days before the onset of overt delirium and may progress to full-blown delirium over the course of a few days. The duration of delirium can range from less than 1 week to more than 2 months but typically resolves within 10 to 12 days (Flacker, 2010).

Age: Any medically ill patient can develop delirium; however, older adults are more prone to delirium due to preexisting conditions, aging processes, and greater vulnerability to acute opportunistic disease processes (Eeles, White, O'Mahony, Bayer, & Hubbard, 2012).

Ethnicity: Culture and ethnicity should be taken into consideration when evaluating an individual's mental status and capacity. Some patients may not be familiar with information used in cognitive rating scales (general knowledge, geographical information, memory, and orientation/location), and many scales adjust for these factors as well as educational level in the interpretation of scores.

Gender: Males tend to have a higher incidence rate, and the male gender appears to be an independent risk factor for delirium.

Contributing factors: (See under Etiology, Occurrence, and Age.) Quinlan et al. (2011) have proposed that frailty and delirium are related entities.

Signs and symptoms: The clinical presentation may include confusion; difficulty sustaining and shifting attention; extreme distractibility; disorganized thinking; rambling, irrelevant, pressured, and incoherent speech; impaired reasoning ability and goal-directed behavior; disorientation to time and place; impairment of recent memory; misperceptions about the environment, including illusions and hallucinations; emotional instability; and psychomotor activity that fluctuates between agitation, purposeless movements, and a vegetative state (Borja, Borja, & Gade, 2007; Lundström, Stenvall, & Olofsson, 2012). Disorientation to other persons occurs commonly, but disorientation to self is rare. Dysarthria is a frequent speech and language disturbance, and dysnomia (impaired ability to name objects), dysgraphia (impaired ability to write), or aphasia may be observed. Commonly associated features of delirium include disturbances in the sleep-wake cycle such as daytime sleepiness, nighttime agitation, and disturbances in sleep continuity. Complete reversal of the sleep-wake cycle or fragmentation of the circadian sleep-wake pattern can occur. Emotional disturbances may include anxiety, fear, depression, irritability, anger, euphoria, and apathy. Affective lability (rapid and unpredictable shifts from one emotional state to another) may occur (Flacker, 2010). Possible autonomic signs associated with delirium include tachycardia, sweating, flushed face, dilated pupils, and elevated blood pressure (Tullmann et al., 2012). A small study comparing postoperative delirium in patients diagnosed with dementia and those without dementia found that dementia patients were more hyperactive, manifesting with restlessness and aggression, and had communicative difficulties and irritability. Patients without dementia were more hypoactive (Lundström et al., 2012).

Diagnostic and screening tests: Laboratory work will assist in identifying potential causative factors as will rating scales that measure cognition and establish diagnostic data such as Folstein's Mini-Mental State Examination (MMSE), the Confusion Assessment Method (CAM), the Delirium Rating Scale–Revised, or the Delirium Observation Screening Scale. These scales assist in tracking progress and in the patient's return to baseline functioning (Flacker, 2010; Tullmann et al., 2012). However, because of fluctuating levels of consciousness and cognition, it may be difficult to assess mental status and cognitive function. When possible, obtain information from the medical record, medical staff, and others, especially family members.

Differential diagnosis: (See under Etiology.) The most common differential diagnostic challenge is whether the patient has dementia or delirium, has delirium alone, or has a delirium superimposed on a preexisting dementia. Although there are common cognitive disturbances in delirium and dementia, a primary difference is that the patient with dementia usually is alert, whereas the patient with delirium manifests overt disturbances of consciousness or arousal. The rapid onset and course of cognitive impairments and the reversibility of symptoms are helpful in distinguishing between delirium and dementia. The severity of delirium symptoms typically fluctuates over the course of a day, whereas dementia symptoms generally do not fluctuate (Lundström

et al., 2012). Information from medical records, caregivers, and family members may help determine whether dementia was present before the onset of delirium. Depression is another differential diagnosis, because patients often manifest cognitive and psychomotor symptoms common to dementia and delirium.

Treatment: Appropriate treatment for delirium involves discovering the causes, many of which are reversible, and preventing complications through prompt treatment of specific, identified disorders. A thorough, comprehensive assessment; evaluation of medications, interactions, and contraindications; and ordering of laboratory work will assist in ruling out/in the many etiologies of delirium. While assessing for probable etiology and definitive treatment, management should focus on ensuring safety from behavioral disturbances by combining environmental, behavioral, and pharmacological therapies. A recent trend is the introduction of acute care for the elderly units in the hospital setting and the designation of delirium beds within these units (Rubin, Neal, Fenlon, Hassan, & Inouye, 2011). Specially trained nursing staff assess and monitor patients with delirium. Further research is needed to determine the efficacy and cost-effectiveness of this model.

Nonpharmacological Interventions: A therapeutic environment would include frequent reassurance and reality orientation; clear communication; caregiver consistency; decreased stimuli (noise reduction, adequate lighting, sufficient time to perform tasks); decreased stress and anxiety through frequent reassurance and provision of a daily routine; comfort maintenance (eyeglasses, hearing aids, personal belongings); reestablishment of a sleep-wake cycle by controlling nighttime noise and unnecessary disruptions; guarantee of adequate daily fluid intake; assurance that elimination needs are met; provision of space and programs for physical activity, ambulation, and range of motion; and avoidance of chemical or physical restraint. Medication should be used as a last resort (Tullmann et al., 2012).

Pharmacotherapy: Data support the use of first-generation (e.g. haloperidol) and second-generation (e.g. olanzapine, risperidone, ziprasidone, and quetiapine) antipsychotic medications to control behavioral symptoms of delirium and prevent injury to self or others (Flaherty, Gonzales, & Dong, 2011; Siddiqi, Stockdale, Britton, & Holmes, 2007). Cholinesterase inhibitors (e.g., donazepil) were not found more effective than placebo in managing the symptoms of delirium in a very small study; further study is needed (Overshott, Karim, & Burns, 2009). The avoidance of benzodiazepines except for specific indications (e.g., alcohol or γ-hydroxybutyric acid [GHA] withdrawal delirium, delirium related to seizures) continues to be a recommendation.

Patients in critical care settings who are receiving high doses of parenteral lorazepam should be monitored closely for toxicity (e.g., renal dysfunction, hyperosmolar metabolic acidosis). Dexmedetomidine, when used in intensive care unit (ICU) settings for sedation, has shown less association with delirium than midazolam and propofol and more cost-effectiveness (Maldonado et al., 2009). It is important to periodically reassess the patient's mental status and other psychiatric symptoms and behaviors such as depression, suicidal ideation or behavior, hallucinations, delusions, aggression, agitation, anxiety, disinhibition, affective lability, cognitive deficits, and sleep disturbances, because these symptoms can fluctuate rapidly. Regular monitoring and serial assessments of mental status and symptoms will allow for the adjustment of treatment strategies and may indicate the effectiveness of interventions and new or worsening medical conditions (Tullman et al., 2012).

Follow-up: Close follow-up for treatment efficacy, appropriate laboratory and diagnostic studies to monitor resolution of the underlying cause, and monitoring of mental status and cognitive functioning are essential to ensure full recovery.

Sequelae: During overt periods of delirium, there is risk of injury to self or others due to confusion, altered perception, and impaired insight and judgment. Fear is often a precipitant to injury in patients with delirium and may result in attacking others, falling out of bed, or pulling on IV lines, oxygen tubing, tracheotomy or gastrointestinal tubes, urinary catheters, or other medical equipment. Although the majority of patients recover fully, delirium may progress to stupor, coma, seizures, or death. Full recovery is less likely in the elderly, and persistent cognitive deficits are common (Girard et al., 2010; McAvay et al., 2006; Witlox et al., 2010). Such deficits may be due to preexisting dementia that was not clearly established. The elderly have a significantly increased risk of developing complications, such as pneumonia and decubitus ulcers, which may result in longer hospital stays. In postoperative patients, delirium may limit recovery and contribute to poorer long-term outcomes. Increased risk for postoperative complications, longer postoperative recuperation periods, longer hospital stays, and long-term disability are associated with delirium. Delirious patients with alcohol or sedative-hypnotic withdrawal, cocaine intoxication, head trauma, hypoglycemia, strokes, or extensive burns are at increased risk for seizures. Delirium in the medically ill is associated with an increased mortality rate, and patients who develop delirium during a hospitalization also have a very high rate of death during the months following discharge (Robinson et al., 2009).

Prevention/prophylaxis: Preventive measures to lessen the likelihood of delirium include elimination or minimization of risk factors. These measures include judicious use of high-risk medications (BEERS List; STOPP/START), timely management and good control of acute and chronic medical disease processes, correction of sensory deficits (eyeglasses, magnifying glasses, adequate lighting, hearing aids, cerumen removal), promotion of normal sleep patterns through good sleep hygiene measures, provision of adequate nutrition and hydration with oral/parenteral supplementation as necessary, prompt attention to elimination needs, participation in activities that maintain and stimulate cognitive and physical functioning, and provision of general supportive measures (environmental modifications, reality orientation, control of external stimuli) (Francis, 2012). For hospitalized elders and long-term care residents, encourage frequent visits by family members to provide familiarity, reality orientation, reassurance, and comfort.

Referral: Patients with delirium should be hospitalized so that diagnostic testing, identification of underlying causes, and management can occur in a rapid, coordinated manner during concurrent treatment of acute symptoms to ensure patient safety and comfort. Care of the patient with delirium should be coordinated by the primary care provider and managed jointly with internal medicine, psychiatry, neurology, and other specialty physicians to ensure appropriate comprehensive evaluation and care.

Education: Patients and families should be educated about the etiology of delirium and the expected course of illness while being provided reassurance that delirium is usually temporary and that the symptoms are part of a medical condition. The American Delirium Society (www.americandeliriumsociety.org) is a multidisciplinary professional group dedicated to delirium research and the education of professionals and families of patients with delirium.

CLINICAL RECOMMENDATION	EVIDENCE RATING	REFERENCES
Assessment of predisposing/vulnerability factors includes findings from the patient's history and physical assessment. Preexisting cognitive impairment, severity of presenting illness, and age are the most consistent risk factors identified for the development of delirium.	B	Sendelbach & Guthrie (2009)
Nurses' recognition and assessment of delirium can be enhanced with education on assessing cognition, cognitive impairment, features of delirium, and factors associated with poor recognition of delirium.	B	Sendelbach & Guthrie (2009)
Nursing admission and daily assessment processes should incorporate the use of standardized instruments for assessing cognition and the presence of delirium.	B	Sendelbach & Guthrie (2009)
Clinicians' implementation or adherence to multicomponent intervention strategies is essential to improve patient outcomes.	B	Sendelbach & Guthrie (2009)
Intervention strategies aimed at prevention for patients at high risk is the most effective approach.	A	Sendelbach & Guthrie (2009)

A = consistent, good-quality, patient-oriented evidence; B = inconsistent or limited-quality, patient-oriented evidence; C = consensus, disease-oriented evidence, usual practice, expert opinion, or case series. For information about the SORT evidence rating system, go to www.aafp.org/afpsort.xml.

DEMENTIA

Alzheimer's disease (AD) is the most common cause of dementia and is the primary focus of this section. *Dementia* is defined as a syndrome of acquired persistent intellectual impairment with compromised function in multiple spheres of mental activity (Fong, 2013). In the differential diagnosis, it is important to ascertain whether an individual has an illness with similar or overlapping signs and symptoms, a reversible "dementia" (secondary to treatable systemic disorders), or irreversible dementia (primarily caused by progressive systemic or neurological disorders whereby individuals deteriorate over time, regardless of treatment). Once dementia is ruled in, the type of dementia can then be determined (DeSilets & Bryant, 2010; Kalapatapu, 2010).

Signal symptoms: Confusion, disorientation (as to time, place, person), impaired short-term memory, and cognitive dysfunction.

Description: Clinicians must consider normal aging processes and factors that may contribute to the overall clinical picture when assessing a patient who presents with signs or symptoms of dementia. *Dementia* is defined as a syndrome of acquired persistent intellectual impairment with compromised function in multiple spheres of mental activity (APA, 2007). AD has a gradual onset, and the course of illness and progression is typically slow (Gebretsadik & Grossberg, 2008). The duration of AD ranges from 3 to 20 years and averages 10 years as comorbidities complicate the course of illness. Symptoms vary from person to person, and cognitive deficits cause significant impairment in social and occupational functioning, impaired ability to care for oneself, and altered behavioral patterns. Signs and symptoms progress from memory loss to impaired executive functioning, aphasia, apraxia, and agnosia (total or partial loss of the ability to recognize familiar people or objects). A hallmark of dementia is anosognosia, whereby the individual is unaware of impairment and denies illness (APA, 2007).

The National Institute on Aging and the Alzheimer's Association workgroup have recently introduced new diagnostic staging for Alzheimer's including preclinical, mild cognitive impairment due to AD, and dementia due to AD (Albert et al., 2011; McKhann et al., 2011; Sperling et al., 2011).

Etiology: The etiology of dementia includes numerous systemic disorders. In many cases, treating the underlying disease process resolves the correlating dementia. However, most cases of dementia are irreversible, because dementia is a progressive disease process unto itself.

- *Central nervous system (CNS) disorders:* mild cognitive impairment (MCI), AD (most common type of dementia, 60% to 80%), Lewy body dementia–Parkinson's disease (15% to 30%), vascular dementia (4% to 22%), primary degenerative dementia, frontotemporal dementia or Pick's disease (20% to 50%), mass lesions, Huntington's disease
- *Cardiovascular disease:* cerebral hypoxia/anoxia, vascular insults to brain, cardiac arrhythmias, inflammatory blood vessel disease
- *Infectious processes:* AIDS, Creutzfeldt-Jakob syndrome, neurosyphilis
- *Liver disease:* chronic progressive hepatic encephalopathy
- *Neoplastic conditions:* intracranial lesions, primary or metastasis
- *Pulmonary disease:* respiratory encephalopathy, COPD/CO_2 toxicity
- *Urinary tract disease:* UTI, chronic or progressive uremic encephalopathy

Occurrence: Currently, 5.4 million Americans are living with AD, and one in eight people ages 65 and older (13%) have AD (Alzheimer's Association, 2012). For every 5-year age group after 65, the percentage of AD doubles. The annual number of new AD cases is predicted to rise sharply by 2040 when all baby boomers will be 65 or older. The estimated number of AD cases by 2050 will be 959,000 new cases and 11 to 16 million total cases (Alzheimer's Association, 2012).

Age: Early-onset AD affects those 65 years old or younger, is usually familial, and represents less than 5% of AD cases. Late-onset AD affects those 65 years old and older and may or may not be related to family history (National Institute on Aging, 2012).

Ethnicity: Blacks and Hispanics are at highest risk of developing AD. African Americans are approximately 2 times more likely to develop AD than whites, and Hispanics have approximately 1.5 times the risk of their white counterparts.

Gender: More women than men have dementia, primarily because women live longer.

Contributing factors: Risk factors for AD are designated as actual and probable.

Actual Risk Factors
- Age
- Genetics/family history (Mihaescu et al., 2010; National Institute on Aging, 2012)
  - Gene mutations chromosomes 1, 14, 21
  - A 50/50 chance of developing early-onset AD if one parent had AD
  - Apolipoprotein E (ApoE) gene on chromosome 19
  - ApoE alleles $\epsilon2$, $\epsilon3$, $\epsilon4$
  - Possibly chromosomes 9, 10, 12
  - Down's syndrome
- Less than 5% of AD cases are caused by rare genetic variations found in a small number of families worldwide. In these inherited forms of AD, the disease tends to develop before age 65, sometimes in people as young as 30. The genetic mutations involve the following chromosomes:
  - Chromosome 21 on the gene for the amyloid precursor protein
  - Chromosome 14 on the gene for the presenilin 1 protein
  - Chromosome 1 on the gene for presenilin 2 (National Institute on Aging, 2012).

Probable Risk Factors
- Low educational level, low lifetime achievements
  - More years of education (vs. fewer years) provides a "cognitive reserve" that enables compensation for symptoms of AD/other dementia
  - Differences in education and dementia risk may reflect increased risk for disease in general and less access to medical care in lower socioeconomic groups
- Female gender, low estrogen levels
  - Framingham Study: lifetime risk for any dementia in females who reached age 55 = 21% and for males = 14%
- Depression, brain injury
- Cardiovascular disease, hypertension, type 2 diabetes mellitus, smoking, obesity

Signs and symptoms: Signs and symptoms vary according to the stage of dementia and disease progression. AD is a multiyear brain disease; it is thought to begin well before clinical manifestations appear. Preclinical changes in the brain can begin 10 to 20 years before symptoms present. These changes include diffuse cerebral plaques, neuritic plaques and tangles, neuron and synapse loss, and some cognitive impairment (Ariga, Miyatake, & Yu, 2010; Sperling et al., 2011). The onset of clinical symptoms typically begins with memory loss. The duration of each stage varies, and functional changes usually occur late in the disease process (Table 16-4).

TABLE 16-4	Stages of Alzheimer's Disease and Associated Symptoms	
STAGE	**ASSOCIATED SYMPTOMS**	**DURATION**
Preclinical	Impaired memory, excused or covered	2–4 years or longer
	Insidious instrumental activities of daily living (ADL) losses (money handling, bills)	
	Preserved basic ADLs	
	Poor judgment and decisions	
	Subtle personality changes	
	Decreased spontaneity, sense of initiative	
	Increased anxiety, socially normal	
Mild–moderate	Obvious memory impairment	2–10 years
	Overt instrumental ADL impairment	
	Basic ADLs failing	
	Prominent behavioral difficulties	
	Shortened attention span	
	Language difficulty	
	Variable social skills	
	Supervision required	
Severe	Memory fragments only	1–2 years or longer
	No recognition of familiar people	
	Assistance with basic ADLs required	
	Fewer troublesome behaviors	
	Reduced mobility	
	Weight loss, infections	
	Seizures, dysphagia	
	Incontinence	
	Groaning, moaning, grunting	

Many patients manifest noncognitive behavioral symptoms (NCBS) years before being diagnosed with dementia (Box 16-1). Once dementia is diagnosed, NCBS may continue to manifest similarly or progress to symptoms more difficult to manage.

Differential diagnosis: Numerous disorders and disease processes have similar or overlapping symptoms to dementia (see under Etiology), and a comprehensive assessment is necessary for accurate diagnosis. The primary focus of differential diagnoses for dementia is depression and delirium, because symptoms may be very difficult to differentiate in an acutely ill patient (Table 16-5). Additional differential diagnoses include the following:

- *Psychiatric:* depression, delirium, mild cognitive impairment, vascular cognitive impairment, amnesic disorder
- *Neurological:* multiple sclerosis, normal-pressure hydrocephalus, intracranial tumors, subdural hematoma, dementia pugilistica
- *Infection:* HIV, neurosyphilis
- *Inflammatory:* rheumatoid cerebrovasculitis, lupus cerebrovasculitis, neurosarcoidosis
- *Endocrine:* hypothyroidism, hypoparathyroidism, Cushing's disease, Addison's disease, hyperthyroidism, hyperparathyroidism
- *Metabolic:* vitamin B deficiency
- *Toxins:* alcohol/substance abuse/dependence

Once depression, delirium, and systemic causes of dementia are eliminated from the differential, it is important to differentiate the type of dementia manifested by the patient. Dementia that is primarily caused

BOX 16-1
Noncognitive Behavioral Symptoms of Dementia
Apathy
Agitation, aggression
Combativeness
Delusions, hallucinations
Depression, anxiety
Disinhibition/sexual behaviors
Emotional lability
Irritability
Wandering
Sleep disturbances
Sundowning

TABLE 16-5	Differential Diagnosis of Dementia, Delirium, and Depression		
CLINICAL FEATURES	**DEMENTIA**	**DELIRIUM**	**DEPRESSION**
Onset	Insidious	Rapid	May be abrupt, with life changes
Course	Long, progressive	Short, diurnal variation	Situational
Duration	Months to years	Hours to 1 month	2 weeks, months, years
Awareness	Clear	Reduced	Clear
Alertness	Normal	Impaired	Normal
Orientation	Impaired	Impaired	Selective
Thought process	Poor, abstract thinking; diminished thoughts; poor judgment; difficulty with word finding/verbalizing	Disorganized, distorted, fragmented, diminished or expansive thoughts, incoherence	Intact, linear; themes of hopelessness, helplessness, poor self-esteem
Perception	Frequent misperceptions	Distorted with illusions, delusions, hallucinations	Intact
Psychomotor behavior	Normal, apraxia	Varies/mixed; hypokinetic, hyperkinetic	Varies with restlessness, agitation, retardation
Sleep-wake cycle	Fragmented, disturbed, reversed	Disturbed, reversed	Disturbed sleep patterns (increased/decreased); early, mid, late insomnia; napping
Associated features	Affect superficial, labile, inappropriate; may be in attempt to conceal deficits	Variable affective changes, increased arousal, personality exaggeration	Affect and mood depressed, increased somatic complaints, preoccupation, rumination
Mental status testing	Increased effort to find appropriate replies, frequent near-miss answers, word searching	Distracted from task, inability to focus	Inability to focus/concentrate; makes little effort; gives up; shows indifference, apathy

by degenerative CNS processes or sequelae includes vascular dementia, Lewy body dementia (associated with Parkinson's disease), frontotemporal lobe dementia (Pick's disease), AD, and mixed dementia. There are similar/overlapping symptoms and distinct symptoms of each type, which help with the differential diagnosis.

Differentiation of dementia: Dementia can be classified as vascular, Lewy body/Parkinson's, frontotemporal lobe/Pick's disease, or mixed (Shaik & Varma, 2012).

Vascular Dementia
■ Sequelae from transient ischemic attacks, ministrokes, cerebrovascular accidents
■ No or little cortical shrinkage
■ Cognitive, behavioral, and functional losses defined by area of infarct
■ Stepwise deterioration over time

Clinical presentation:

■ Abnormal executive functioning
■ Impaired psychomotor performance
■ Changes in personality and mood
■ Disturbances in gait (slow and unsteady)
■ Hyperreflexia, extensor plantar response
■ Urinary incontinence
■ Hemiparesis, including lower facial weakness
■ Hemisensory deficits
■ Visual problems (field defect, diplopia)
■ Pseudobulbar syndrome (e.g., dysarthria, dysphagia, emotional incontinence)
■ Focal deficits

Lewy Body/Parkinson's Dementia
■ Diffuse presence of Lewy body proteins in brain, including cerebral cortex
■ Lewy bodies deplete dopamine

- Acetylcholine is depleted, causing disruption of perception, thinking, and behavior
- Resultant parkinsonian symptoms: stiff, shuffling gait, stiffness in arms and legs, tremors, frequent falls, mask-like facies with blank stare, flat affect, stooped posture, drooling, runny nose

Clinical presentation:

- Parkinsonian signs
- Symptoms may fluctuate as often as moment to moment, hour to hour, or day-to-day
- Fluctuating cognition, varying degrees of alertness and attention
- Progressive memory loss
- Visual hallucinations
- Rapid eye movement (REM) sleep difficulties

Frontotemporal Lobe Dementia/Pick's Disease
- Gradual and progressive changes in behavior—socially inappropriate, disinhibition, easily frustrated, impulsive, compulsive behaviors; or
- Gradual and progressive language dysfunction—problems with expression of language, incorrect words, naming objects
- Difficulties with reading and writing

Mixed Dementia
- More than one type of dementia (e.g., combination of AD and vascular dementia)

Assessment of dementia: A thorough diagnostic evaluation aimed at identifying the specific etiology of dementia is necessary and will guide treatment decisions. The evaluation should determine if any treatable psychiatric or general medical conditions might be causing or exacerbating the symptoms manifested by the patient. The clinician must obtain a comprehensive history, and because of questionable reliability secondary to cognitive deficits, a family member or caregiver should be present to validate and obtain collateral information. Take care to note the patient's attitude toward the family member (e.g., friendly, positive, suspicious, paranoid, angry, hostile) who is answering the examiner's questions; if the family member is frequently "correcting" the patient's answer to a question, consider patient and/or family denial, compensation, inconsistency, and fabrication of information (Fletcher, 2012). The history should include the following:

- Family history, past medical history, occupation, current health status
- Onset and frequency of memory and cognitive lapses
- Word-finding difficulties

- Ability to perform activities of daily living (ADLs), instrumental ADLs
- Sleep patterns
- Ability to drive without getting lost
- Recognition of known others and recall of names
- Wandering

Diagnostic and Screening Tests: Evidence-based studies support the following routine laboratory studies: CBC, electrolytes, glucose, blood urea nitrogen (BUN), creatinine, LFTs, TSH, serum B_{12}, folate, syphilis serology, and urinalysis (Gebretsadik & Grossberg, 2008; Kalapatapu, 2010). A noncontrast CT scan will detect vascular insults (infarcts, stroke), and based on history and physical findings and clinical suspicion, an MRI may assist in ruling out medical/neurological processes and assist in differential diagnosis. Tests for early diagnosis of AD are in investigative stages and include a positron emission tomography (PET) scan and biological markers (Albert et al., 2011).

Mental Status Examination and Cognitive Testing: A full mental status examination may uncover mood and neurovegetative symptoms that indicate treatable comorbid psychiatric conditions (e.g., depression, anxiety) that may contribute to cognitive difficulties. Instruments that assess orientation, attention, calculation, and memory should be initiated early to assist in diagnosis and establish baseline and should be routinely repeated to objectively document and measure changes over time.

Although readily available and commonly used, the MMSE has poor specificity for dementia and may exhibit poor sensitivity in highly intelligent or well-educated patients; copyright limitations also apply. Additionally, sensory loss and physical frailty may lower scores.

Other cognitive instruments may unmask deficits in executive function, abstraction, praxis, and visuospatial performance and test clock-drawing ability, word fluency, proverb interpretation, and praxis (e.g., ability to brush teeth or comb hair). The Montreal Cognitive Assessment (MoCA) and the St. Louis University Mental Status Exam (SLUMS) are well-validated instruments that may be used in the assessment of dementia. The MoCA is a screening test to detect MCI and has greater sensitivity and specificity in distinguishing normal controls from MCI when compared to the MMSE. The MoCA assesses attention and concentration, executive functions, memory, language, visuoconstructional skills, conceptual thinking, calculations, and orientation

(Nasreddine et al., 2005). The SLUMS is useful for detecting MCI and dementia, is more sensitive than the MMSE, and tests orientation, short-term memory, word fluency, attention, concentration and recall, clock drawing, and identification (Tariq, Tumosa, Chibnall, Perry, & Morley, 2006).

The Clock Drawing Test (CDT) can be administered alone or within other cognitive screening instruments (e.g., SLUMS) and screens for Alzheimer's and other types of dementia. The CDT offers clues regarding areas of cognitive change or damage and provides information about general cognitive and adaptive functioning (memory, information processing, vision, visual-spatial skills). Of note, the CDT lacks sensitivity for MCI. The patient is asked to draw a clock with all of the numbers and set the hands to read a certain time (e.g., 10 past 8). Certain errors, such as grossly distorted contour or erroneous markings, are rarely produced by intact cognition (Ehreke et al., 2009).

Physical Examination: A general medical assessment should be completed with emphasis on the cardiovascular, respiratory, neurological, and musculoskeletal systems. Assess for endocrine, inflammatory, and infectious processes that may contribute to cognitive symptoms, and note focal motor or sensory signs and altered reflexes, gait, or coordination. The presence of tremor, rigidity, or cogwheeling may indicate a parkinsonian process and vertical gaze paralysis may suggest supranuclear palsy. Look for funduscopic changes that may indicate vascular damage or intracranial pressure and vision and hearing loss that can mimic or worsen cognitive decline. Unless there are comorbid medical disease processes, the physical examination does not typically reveal many findings.

Diagnosis: Definitive diagnosis of AD is only possible on autopsy and upon finding disease-specific pathology in the brain. As such, the diagnosis of AD is presumptive and based upon the following diagnostic criteria:

DSM-IV-TR Diagnostic Criteria for Alzheimer's Disease (usually indicates severe AD):
Memory impairment (learning new information, recall of previously learned information) PLUS one or more of the following:
  ■ Aphasia (language disturbance)
  ■ Apraxia (inability to carry out motor activities)
  ■ Agnosia (inability to recognize objects, persons, sounds, shapes, despite intact sensory function)
  ■ Executive function disturbance (planning, organization, sequencing)

■ Cognitive deficits cause significant social/occupational dysfunction
■ Significant decline from previous level of functioning
■ Gradual onset, continuous decline
■ Cognitive deficits
  ■ Not due to other CNS, systemic, or substance-induced conditions
  ■ Not occurring during delirium
  ■ Not accounted for by another psychiatric disorder such as major depression or schizophrenia

Treatment: A comprehensive, multidimensional treatment plan for dementia includes biological, psychotherapeutic, social, family, and pharmacological interventions (APA, 2007).

Biological Interventions: Treat underlying medical disorders with medications, medical or surgical procedures, and ongoing evaluation and management as indicated.

Psychotherapeutic Interventions: Include behavioral management, reminiscence therapy, validation therapy, supportive psychotherapy, sensory integration, simulated presence therapy, reality orientation, skills training, recreation and art therapy, exercise, and aromatherapy.

Social Interventions: Include a functional and safety assessment, environmental modifications, assessment for abuse and neglect, provision of supervision and home health care, cleaning and meal services, assessment for appropriate level of care, financial and estate planning, and legal provisions for power of attorney.

Family Interventions: Include caregiver education, training and support, respite care, and support groups.

Pharmacotherapy: Cholinesterase inhibitors (ChEIs) are the cornerstone of pharmacological therapy with the aim to enhance or preserve cognitive and behavioral status. Acetylcholine is important for the functioning of brain cells involved in memory, thought, and judgment, and brain levels are significantly decreased in those with AD. ChEIs inhibit breakdown of acetylcholine, which increases levels within the brain; this mechanism of action may improve or delay a decline in memory. ChEIs are effective in approximately 30% of patients and are not curative, preventive, or disease-reversing agents. The choice of ChEI is based on the patient's clinical presentation and comorbid conditions.

The three commonly prescribed ChEIs are donepezil, rivastigmine, and galantamine (APA, 2007; Desilets & Bryant, 2010; Fong, 2013). Clinical and safety issues for ChEIs include medical and psychosocial factors before drug initiation, consideration of when to initiate the medication, and side effects, which are fewer with slower dose titration. Careful monitoring for efficacy and side effects is necessary. Common side effects of ChEIs are nausea, vomiting, dyspepsia, anorexia, diarrhea, insomnia, vivid dreams, fatigue, increased urination, and cramps. Uncommon side effects of ChEIs are syncope, bradycardia, confusion, depression, and agitation. Use cautiously in patients with liver or gastric disease, COPD, bradycardia, and inadequate supervision.

Considerations regarding when to stop ChEIs may include intolerable side effects, new medical contraindications, poor compliance, lack of supervision, and rapid cognitive and/or functional decline. Any benefits of treatment are rapidly lost upon discontinuation. Long-term treatment may continue to offer advantages such as slowing of cognitive decline, continued ability to perform ADLs, fewer noncognitive behavioral symptoms, and decreased caregiver burden.

Another medication approved to treat dementia is memantine (Namenda), an *N*-methyl-D-aspartate (NMDA) receptor antagonist. Memantine assists in regulating high levels of glutamate in the brain, typically found in AD. Common side effects include headache and constipation, and an uncommon side effect is confusion. Memantine is excreted through the kidneys, and caution is advised in patients with renal impairment. Combination therapy of memantine with a ChEI is a good strategy, because these medications work differently (APA, 2007). Usually medications are started when AD severity is moderate, but they can be initiated earlier depending on individual patient clinical presentations (Table 16-6).

TABLE 16-6	FDA-Approved Medications for Alzheimer's Disease			
	DONEPEZIL (ARICEPT) CHEI	**RIVASTIGMINE (EXCELON) CHEI**	**GALANTAMINE (REMINYL) AND EXTENDED RELEASE (RAZADYNE) CHEI**	**MEMANTINE (NAMENDA) (NMDA RECEPTOR AGONIST)**
FDA approval	1996; mild, moderate, severe AD	2000; mild, moderate AD	2001; mild, moderate AD	2004; moderate, severe AD
Benefit	Typically well tolerated; improves cognitive and behavioral status, caregiver burden, and capacity for ADLs	Improves cognitive, behavioral, and functional impairments; is more selective for central processes and regions critical for cognition and memory	Significantly improves cognitive, behavioral, and functional symptoms of AD	Delays loss of daily functions, cognition, and global performance; decreases agitation
Dosage strengths (mg)	5, 10	1.5, 3, 4.5, 6	4, 8, 12 Extended Release: 8, 16, 24	Titrate to 10 mg bid over 4 wk
Oral solution	1 mg/mL	2 mg/mL	4 mg/mL	
Starting dose	5 mg qd	1.5 mg bid	4 mg bid	
Maximum recommended dose	10 mg qd	6 mg bid	8–10 mg bid Extended Release: 16–24 mg qd	10 mg bid
T1/2 (hours)	73	5	6–8	60–80
Plasma protein binding	96%	40%	18%	
CYP450 substrate of	2D63A4	NA	2D63A4	
CYP450 inhibitor of	NA	NA	NA	NA

Management of Noncognitive Behavioral Symptoms (NCBS) of Dementia: Includes determination and management of other potential or influencing factors, including the following:

- Environmental: external (noise) or internal (UTI, constipation)
- Situational: time of day, unknown trigger
- Psychiatric: depression, anxiety, panic, fear
- Medical: medication, pain, metabolic, infection, sensory deficits, cardiopulmonary

Nonpharmacologic Approaches for NCBS: Include the following (Carnahan, 2010):

- Ensure safety and provision of adequate supervision
- Analyze behavior(s) for clues to potential causes
- Environmental interventions
- Provide structure—usual routines and predictability are important to allay anxiety
- Provide pleasurable experiences
- Do not rely on learning or memory
- Educate caregivers and other support systems
- Use of physical or chemical restraint discouraged and may be used as last resort only, in order to ensure safety to self and/or others (APA, 2007; Grimes & Hatch, 2010).
- Caregiver education for managing agitation (Table 16-7)

Treatment Strategies and Pharmacotherapy for Noncognitive Behavioral Symptoms and Psychiatric Comorbidities: It is estimated that up to 90% of patients with dementia have psychiatric comorbidities (Shub & Kunik, 2009). Depression affects 20% to 32% of persons with dementia, and prevalence is higher in vascular dementia than in AD. Depressive symptoms may present as initial manifestations of dementia and may fluctuate over time. There are more reports of decreased ability to concentrate and indecisiveness and fewer reports of insomnia or hypersomnia, feelings of worthlessness and guilt, or thoughts of suicide and death. Diagnostic criteria for comorbid depression in dementia include the addition of irritability, social withdrawal, and isolation with frequent, concurrent apathy and anxiety. The Cornell Scale for Depression in Dementia (CSDD) is a validated screening tool designed for use in the assessment of those who can communicate basic needs. The CSDD differentiates between the diagnostic categories and severity of depression (Alexopoulos, Abrams, Young, & Shamoian, 1988). Other diagnostic instruments include the MADRS, PHQ-9, QIDS-SR, BDI, and the GDS (see under Depression). First-line treatment strategies for comorbid depression include supportive psychotherapy and an SSRI such as citalopram (Celexa), fluoxetine (Prozac), or sertraline (Zoloft). If interventions are ineffective and/or suffering is severe and persistent, patients may be referred to psychiatry for consideration of ECT, a well-established and effective treatment option.

The prevalence of anxiety in those with dementia is approximately 20%. GAD occurs in 5% of patients with AD. There is a higher percentage of anxiety with vascular and frontotemporal dementia, which is reflected in estimates of clinically significant anxiety as high as 70%. Notably, there is a high comorbidity of

---

TABLE 16-7 | **Managing Agitation: Caregiver Education**

DO	DON'T	PREVENTION	SAFETY
Ask permission to approach/provide assistance	Raise voice	Create a calm environment	Use alarms and/or locks on doors and gates
Use a calm approach	Take offense	Follow a routine with set structure and tasks	Remove or secure firearms
Slow down (do not rush patient or self)	Corner or crowd	Use verbal cueing	
	Rush or pressure	Redirect attention	
Use visual and verbal cues	Criticize or condescend	Use a clock and calendar	
Provide time and space	Argue or attempt reason	Monitor heat, cold, hunger, sleep, elimination, and comfort	
	Shame or ignore		
Limit stimuli	Demand, force		
	Make sudden movements		
	Restrain		

anxiety with major depression in AD (more than 75%). Manifestations of anxiety in dementia include restlessness, irritability, muscle tension, and fear. Respiratory symptoms, such as hyperventilation or difficulty catching one's breath, correlate with excessive anxiety and worry. Diagnostic instruments to assist in diagnosing anxiety in those with dementia include the Worry Scale and the Rating Anxiety in Dementia Scale. First-line treatment options include psychosocial interventions and an SSRI or buspirone (Buspar). Use of benzodiazepines (e.g., lorazepam) is discouraged due to sedating side effects and increased risk for falls. However, individualized treatment strategies that include benzodiazepines continue to be an option when other interventions have been ineffective.

Psychosis in AD is frequently present with other cognitive symptoms (global deficits, anosognosia), affective symptoms (depression, elevated mood), and behavioral symptoms (agitation and overt aggression). Approximately 18% of dementia patients present with delusions that typically manifest as persecutory and misidentification delusions. Hallucinations are present in approximately 14% of dementia patients with the occurrence of visual hallucinations more than twice that of auditory hallucinations. Capgras syndrome (belief that a close relative or friend has been replaced by an impostor) and "phantom boarder syndrome" (belief that strangers are living in the home) may be associated with agnosia. Instruments to assist in diagnosing psychosis in dementia include the Behavioral Pathology in Alzheimer's Disease (BEHAVE-AD) scale and the Dementia Psychosis Scale. Behavioral and environmental interventions are first-line treatment strategies.

Before initiating pharmacological treatment with antipsychotic medications, the clinician should carefully analyze the risks and benefits of the use of such medications for each patient. Based on studies demonstrating increased risk for stroke and mortality in the elderly, the U.S. Food and Drug Administration (FDA) has issued a black box warning for use of antipsychotic medications in this population. Judicial and cautious use of antipsychotic medication should be reserved for hallucinations, delusions, aggression, agitation, hostility, and uncooperative behavior that significantly interferes with care. Antipsychotics effective at low doses include aripiprazole (Abilify), haloperidol (Haldol), olanzapine (Zyprexa), quetiapine (Seroquel), risperidone (Risperdal), and ziprasidone (Geodon). Research evidence, FDA warnings, and clinical guidelines recommend use of antipsychotic medication only when (1) behavioral symptoms are due to mania or psychosis, (2) symptoms present a danger to the patient or others, or (3) the patient is experiencing inconsolable or persistent distress, a significant decline in function, or substantial difficulty receiving needed care (Ballard & Waite, 2006; Steinberg & Lyketsos, 2012; Wulsin, 2005).

Antipsychotic medication should not be used for sedation or restraint and should be used at the minimum dosage for the minimum amount of time possible. Careful monitoring for efficacy and side effects is required. Patients, caregivers, and those with power of attorney (POA) should be educated and informed about the risks and benefits of antipsychotic use, and the clinician may wish to consider obtaining written informed consent before initiating treatment with this type of medication.

Approximately 27% of dementia patients exhibit agitation and/or aggression. Prevalence increases as dementia progresses (13% in mild dementia, 24% in moderate dementia, and 29% in severe dementia). *Agitation* is defined as intermittent psychomotor hyperactivity, disinhibition, screaming, physical aggression, and combativeness. There are many potential causes for agitation, including the underlying pathophysiology of dementia (e.g., serotonergic deficiency) and an inability to communicate needs (e.g., hunger) or physical discomfort (e.g., pain, constipation). Psychosocial stressors that may induce agitation include changes in one's living situation, caregiver(s), or environment. Medical evaluation is needed to rule out occult medical problems, medication side effects, and delirium. Instruments that may assist in accurate diagnosis are the Abbey pain scale for those who cannot verbalize discomfort (Abbey et al., 2004), the BEHAVE-AD scale, and the Cohen-Mansfield Agitation Inventory (Kalapatapu, 2010). Interventions include evaluation and management of antecedents and/or causes of agitation, behavioral approaches (e.g., distraction, pleasurable activities), and calming activities or gentle sensory stimulation (e.g., music, art, routine/known physical activities such as folding towels). Pharmacotherapy options might include off-label use of mood stabilizers, such as carbamazepine or Depakote, to effectively manage agitation. Antipsychotic medications are not considered to be first-line treatment, because they are less effective than first believed; however, they should be considered when behaviors present a safety risk to self or others (Ballard & Waite, 2006). For sleep problems, low-dose doxepin may be effective and is FDA approved for insomnia.

Follow-up: After the presumptive diagnosis of AD is made, the patient should be followed closely upon pharmacotherapy initiation and following any adjustments for efficacy and side effects. Thereafter, follow-up visits every 3 to 6 months to assess physical, mental, and emotional status should be individualized to the patient. Reevaluation of cognitive function with the same scale used at diagnosis/baseline (e.g., Folstein's MMSE) is useful to track cognitive stability or decline. The patient's functional status, ability to perform ADLs and instrumental ADLs, behavior, sleep, appetite, weight, elimination, communication, and signs of anxiety or depression should routinely be evaluated at follow-up visits. The physical examination is individualized to the patient and any episodic or chronic illnesses should be well managed to maintain optimum quality of life and avoid complications or worsening of cognitive function.

The ability to drive competently and safely is a frequent concern of family members, and clinicians are often asked to assist in making the difficult decision to revoke the patient's driver's license. Dementia exacerbates age-related changes in driving ability and poses a substantial risk to safe driving. The American Medical Association (AMA) National Highway Safety Administration guidelines state that a dementia diagnosis is not sufficient to withdraw driving privileges and recommend basing decisions on an individual's driving ability. Determining whether a patient with mild dementia is fit to drive presents a challenge to the clinician and begins with discussion of driving history, safety, and cessation with the patient. Data from physical and cognitive assessments, family and caregiver reports, and when available, on-road testing will assist in the decision-making process. For patients deemed to be safe, discuss the necessity of future driving cessation and suggest driving training and self-limitation. A history of significant traffic problems, inability to find the way home, inattention, and psychosis are indications of progressive cognitive decline and driving skill deterioration. When driving safety is uncertain and the patient wishes to continue driving, a referral for on-road driving evaluation is needed. Those with mild dementia who pass an on-road driving test should be reevaluated and retested at least every 6 months. If driving safety is uncertain and the patient decides to stop driving or if the patient is deemed unsafe to drive, the department of motor vehicles and the patient should be notified by letter, and a copy of the letter should be placed in the patient's medical record. International consensus groups agree that a diagnosis of moderate-to-severe dementia precludes driving, and the driver's license should be revoked. Driving is essential to autonomy, and the vast majority of older adults rely on driving as their primary mode of transportation. Although the clinician's recommendation for driving cessation is distressing to patients and families, it is critical to the patient and to public safety (AMA, 2010; Rapoport, Sarracini, Molnar, & Herrmann, 2008).

Caregiver burden regarding patient care, household and financial responsibilities, and ability to provide adequate supervision and care at home should be determined at each follow-up visit. When the patient loses bowel and/or bladder control, his or her behavior becomes too difficult to manage, or the patient's or caregiver's safety is compromised, institutional care should be discussed.

Sequelae: Complications from severe dementia include immobility, swallowing disorders, malnutrition, and significantly increased risk of developing pneumonia, which is the most commonly identified cause of death among the elderly with AD and other dementias. Although there is a blurred distinction between death *with dementia* and death *from dementia*, the AD mortality rate is on the rise (46.1% rise from 2000 to 2006), and in 2006, AD was the seventh leading cause of death in the United States and the fifth leading cause of death among those 65 years of age and older.

Prevention/prophylaxis: A recent comprehensive evidence review commissioned by the Agency for Healthcare Research and Quality (AHRQ) was undertaken by the Duke Center for Evidence-Based Practice to identify factors associated with prevention of cognitive decline and AD. Factors, such as nutrition, medical conditions, social/economic/behavioral factors, prescription and nonprescription medications, genetics, and environment, were studied. The project included 25 systematic reviews and 250 primary research studies, both observational and randomized clinical trials (RCTs). The primary conclusion was that there was a dearth of evidence for any strong recommendations for preventive interventions for AD (Williams, Plassman, Burke, Holsinger, & Benjamin, 2010). Physical activity and cognitive engagement were factors that demonstrated fairly constant association with prevention of cognitive decline and AD; diabetes, depression, smoking, and APOE e4 were associated with increased risk of cognitive impairment and AD.

Referral: Neurology, geriatric psychiatrist, geriatric nurse practitioner, psychiatric mental health nurse practitioner or clinical nurse specialist, psychology, support groups for patients and caregivers.

Education: The impact of AD on caregivers expands as the course of illness progresses. Caregivers, family, and friends of those with AD experience new or changing responsibilities such as shopping, meal preparation, cleaning, financial management, provision of ADLs, and managing behavioral issues. Caregivers also experience financial burden, physical and emotional stress, fatigue, and depression. It is estimated that 60% of caregivers are women, 46% are 50 to 64 years old, many are within the "sandwich" generation, and most average 69 to 100 hours per week providing care.

Patient and caregiver education and support needs include the following:

- Disease process, course of illness, staging
- Anticipatory guidance, life planning, advance directives, POA

Preservation of the following:

- Safety at all times
- Dignity, respect, and self-esteem
- Independence and autonomy for as long as possible/practical/safe
- Daily schedules and routines
- Least restrictive environment
- Cognitive, behavioral, and pharmacological therapies

CLINICAL RECOMMENDATION	EVIDENCE RATING	REFERENCES
Dementia with Lewy bodies should be suspected in patients presenting with dementia accompanied by hallucinations, fluctuating cognition, and parkinsonism.	C	Neef (2011)
The diagnosis rests on clinical criteria, but evaluation should include a validated brief cognitive test and laboratory tests focused on treatable causes.	C	Hagen (2009)
Laboratory evaluation should include complete blood count, thyroid-stimulating hormone, serum calcium and electrolytes, B12, and fasting glucose levels to examine for treatable causes of cognitive decline. Consider serum folate, tests for syphilis, and HIV serology if patient is at risk for those conditions.	C	Feldman et al. (2008)
There is currently no adequate, robust evidence to recommend the use of any nonpharmacological intervention to reduce wandering in dementia.	A	Robinson et al. (2010)
No evidence has been found of any significant general improvement in manifestations of agitation, other than aggression, among demented patients treated with haloperidol, compared with controls.	A	Lonergan, Luxenberg, Colford, & Birks (2002)
Memantine has a small, clinically detectable effect on cognitive function and clinical decline measured at 6 months in patients with moderate-to-severe Alzheimer's disease.	A	McShane, Areosa Sastre, & Minakaran (2006)

CLINICAL RECOMMENDATION	EVIDENCE RATING	REFERENCES
Donepezil is beneficial for people with mild, moderate, and severe dementia due to Alzheimer's disease.	A	Birks & Harvey (2002)
Clinicians should base the decision to initiate a trial of therapy with a cholinesterase inhibitor or memantine on individualized assessment.	B	Qaseem et al. (2008)

A = consistent, good-quality, patient-oriented evidence; B = inconsistent or limited-quality, patient-oriented evidence; C = consensus, disease-oriented evidence, usual practice, expert opinion, or case series. For information about the SORT evidence rating system, go to www.aafp.org/afpsort.xml.

DEPRESSION

Signal symptoms: Feeling sad, discouraged, lack of pleasure in usual activities, unmotivated, low energy, and sleep and/or appetite disturbances.

Description: Transient symptoms of depression are normal, healthy responses to life stressors and disappointments. Pathological depression manifests when a patient's coping skills are inadequate and adaptation to stressful life events or loss is ineffective. Depression is described as a pervasive feeling of sadness or a lack of interest or pleasure in previously enjoyed or usual activities. Feelings of guilt, low self-esteem, sleep and appetite disturbances, low energy, and poor concentration are common. *Depression* may be defined as an initial or single episode, recurrent or chronic and may be qualified as mild, moderate, or severe, with or without melancholic or psychotic features and/or a seasonal pattern. Common categories in geriatric depression include major depressive disorder (MDD), vascular depression, dysthymia, and depression that manifests as a comorbid condition in dementia, bipolar disorder, and executive dysfunction (Zizza & Shteinlukht, 2010).

Etiology: Causative factors for depression include physiological influences such as medication side effects, neurological disorders, cardiac disease, neuroendocrine disturbances, electrolyte and hormonal disturbances, and nutritional deficiencies in vitamins D and B_{12}. Psychosocial and cognitive theories postulate internalized loss with ego dysfunction, learned helplessness, early separation from a significant other, and cognitive distortions with negative attitudes and thoughts as contributors to depression (Dozois, Seeds, & Collins, 2009). Difficulty accomplishing developmental tasks associated with life stages may contribute to and/or be a consequence of depression. Environmental and social factors contribute to depression when major stressors occur and social support systems are inadequate. Depression can be triggered by a single major life event or a combination of events and stressors. Loss of any kind may contribute to depression and in the older adult may include loss of a spouse/loved one or loss of mobility, independence, one's home, and financial security along with deterioration of physical health and social isolation. Biological theories point to impaired synthesis, deficiencies, increased uptake, and increased metabolism or breakdown of the neurotransmitters serotonin, norepinephrine, and dopamine as causative factors in depression (Hariri & Brown, 2006). The comorbidity of depression, vascular disease, vascular risk factors, and the association of ischemic cerebral lesions with distinctive behavioral symptoms supports the "vascular depression" hypothesis. This hypothesis proposes that cerebrovascular disease may predispose, precipitate, or perpetuate some geriatric depressive syndromes. Neurogenetic studies suggest that there may be a genetic variant in the serotonin transporter protein gene associated with differences in human mood, temperament, and response to stress; the variant may influence human behavior and depression (Gelenberg, 2009).

Occurrence: Late-life depression is not uncommon, and the overall prevalence is similar to that of younger adults.

There is a 10% to 44% prevalence of *depressive symptoms* in the elderly, and the percentage is higher in those with disabilities. Approximately 2% to 16% of elders have *major depressive disorder*, and there is an increase in recurrence with increased age. The prevalence of depression in older adults varies depending on the setting in which they live: 2% to 4% in the community, 13% to 24% in assisted living or residential care facilities, and 12% to 20% in nursing home residents. Nursing home residents are 3 to 4 times more likely to suffer from depression compared to older adults living in the community (Zizza & Shteinlukht, 2010). Unfortunately, up to 85% of older adults with depression remain untreated, because it is often underdiagnosed, misdiagnosed, or obscured by comorbidities or somatic complaints that are considered to be physical problems (Park & Unützer, 2011). Additionally, older adults and some cultural groups are unwilling to discuss emotional distress and suffering due to social stigmas attached to mental illness (Raue & Sirey, 2011). An environmental barrier to accurate diagnosis and treatment of depression is ineffective communication among the treatment team in residential care facilities, where residents who are more vocal or agitated are more likely to receive psychiatric consultation than those who may be depressed.

Age: Age 65 and older.

Ethnicity: Studies demonstrate that Hispanics and African Americans have higher rates of late-life depression than whites, possibly due to greater health burdens and lack of health insurance.

Gender: Statistics reveal that depression is more common in women than men. However, it is thought that although men experience and suffer from depression, they either do not report or underreport their depressive symptoms, therefore skewing the epidemiological data.

Contributing factors:

Psychosocial: single or multiple losses: loved ones, independence, mobility, function, financial security, autonomy, privacy, social network; changes in environment, admission to health-care facility, limited social support, loneliness, negative life events

Physical Illnesses: diabetes, cancer, Parkinson's disease, AD, cerebrovascular accident, vascular brain lesions, heart disease, arthritis, hypothyroidism, vitamin deficiencies, anemia, COPD, any chronic illness/pain syndromes, disabilities

Psychiatric Illnesses: alcohol, substance abuse, family or personal history of psychiatric illness or depression

Medications: anxiolytics, sedatives/hypnotics, antipsychotics, cardiac medications, antihypertensives, beta blockers, H_2 blockers, narcotic analgesics, and steroids, either alone or in combination with other medications (monotherapy, polypharmacy, drug-drug interactions) can cause behavioral, affective, and cognitive changes; the BEERS list and the Centers for Medicare and Medicaid Services (CMS) unnecessary medications list indicate medications to avoid prescribing for the elderly (Lotrich & Pollock, 2005; Pham & Dickman, 2007)

Signs and symptoms: Symptoms of depression may encompass four domains: affect/mood, cognition, physiological, and behavior. Sadness, anhedonia, apathy, helplessness, hopelessness, worthlessness, and loneliness are common affective symptoms. Ambivalence, uncertainty, inability to concentrate, confusion, poor memory, slowed speech, lack of motivation, a pessimistic outlook, negative thoughts, self-criticism, and poor self-esteem are common cognitive symptoms. Assess for perceptual disturbances, such as hallucinations, illusions, and delusions, to determine if psychotic features of an agitated depressive episode are present. Sleep, appetite, and energy disturbances, weight change, constipation, pain, headache, decreased libido, sexual nonresponsiveness, and exaggerated concerns over bodily functions are common physiological presentations in depression. Note behavioral symptoms such as psychomotor retardation or agitation, irritability, poor personal hygiene, tearfulness, and social withdrawal. It is of paramount importance to question the patient about suicidal ideation and/or plans and assess accessibility to lethal weapons. Some patients experience excessive worry, preoccupation, and generalized anxiety. Clinical presentation may include inattention to personal appearance, poor hygiene, poor eye contact, and a blunted or flat affect (Dozois et al., 2009; Kotbi, Mahgoub, & Odom, 2010).

The *DSM-IV-TR* (APA, 2000) diagnostic criteria for MDD include depressed mood or anhedonia and at least five of the following symptoms, which must coexist during the same 2-week period, most of the day, nearly every day.

- Obsessive rumination or worry over physical health and pain
- Change in appetite and weight
- Change in sleep pattern: insomnia (difficulty falling asleep or staying asleep, waking earlier than necessary, inability to fall back asleep), hypersomnia, frequent napping

- Psychomotor agitation or retardation
- Fatigue and loss of energy
- Feelings of worthlessness, excessive guilt
- Diminished concentration, indecisiveness
- Recurrent thoughts of death, suicidal ideation or gestures, suicide attempt, suicide plan

Distinct clinical manifestations in older adults include the following:

- Report of lack of emotions (versus depressed mood)
- Excessive concern with bodily functions
- Seeking reassurance and support
- Isolative, withdrawn behavior
- Change in previous level of function, decline in ADLs
- Feeling overwhelmed, easily frustrated, excessive crying
- Irritability, fearfulness, agitation
- Transient, recurring symptoms, diurnal fluctuations or pattern
- Minimizing expressed death wishes or passive suicidal behavior

Assessment should include a comprehensive physical examination to look for secondary causes of depressive symptoms, a full mental health assessment, and a mental status examination if confusion or cognitive impairment is manifested.

Diagnostic and screening tests: Diagnostics to assess for underlying or undiagnosed medical causes of depressive symptoms should be ordered. Standard blood work includes CBC with differential, comprehensive metabolic panel, lipid panel, thyroid function studies (TSH with reflex T_4), and serum vitamin B_{12} and vitamin D levels. Clinical evaluation instruments and scales are useful in assessing symptoms and severity of depression, cognitive impairment, and disability. Such instruments provide objective measures of signs and symptoms of illness and help in establishing baseline information with which future assessments can be compared in evaluating efficacy of treatment and interventions.

Depression Scales:
- Beck Depression Inventory (BDI)
- Patient Health Questionnaire (PHQ)–9
- Quick Inventory of Depressive Symptomology—Self-Report (QIDS-SR)
- Geriatric Depression Scale (GDS, long and short forms)
- Scale for Suicide Ideation

Overall Cognitive Functioning:
- Folstein's Mini-Mental Status Exam (MMSE)

Differential diagnosis:
- Mood disorder due to general medical condition such as diabetes, cancer, epilepsy, stroke, multiple sclerosis, Parkinson's disease, cardiac disease, acute prolonged illness, or injury
- Substance-induced mood disorder from alcohol, illicit drugs, prescription drug abuse, or side effects
- Dysthymic disorder that manifests symptoms of mild depression and may have an early or late onset and is chronic in nature, lasting more than 2 years
- Bipolar affective disorder in which bipolar depression is often misdiagnosed as unipolar depression
- Delirium
- Dementia
- Grief and bereavement
- Somatization disorder
- Sleep disorder, sleep apnea

Treatment: The treatment goal for depression is full remission and recovery. Additional goals of treating late-life depression include the following: prevent or reduce relapse or recurrence, improve quality of life and functioning, improve medical health, and reduce mortality. The initial step in treating depression in older adults is to evaluate the present medication regimen and remove or change any medications that may contribute to symptoms. Treat any systemic disorder that may have predisposed the patient to depression. Ensure adequate nutrition, elimination, sleep, and physical comfort (Andreescu et al., 2009; Kiosses & Ravdin, 2010).

Pharmacotherapy: There are many types of antidepressants; however, SSRIs are considered first-line treatment for depression (Bezchlibnyk-Butler & Jeffries, 2006; Stahl, 2011). In older adults, it is generally best to start with a low dose and titrate upward slowly, depending on the patient's response (efficacy and side effects). Other types of antidepressants include serotonin-norepinephrine reuptake inhibitors (SNRIs), norepinephrine-dopamine reuptake inhibitors (NDRIs), serotonin modulators, norepinephrine-serotonin modulators, tricyclic antidepressants (TCAs), and monoamine oxidase inhibitors (MAOIs) (Table 16-8). Choice of antidepressant medication depends on primary symptoms, symptom clusters, past history of

TABLE 16-8 Types of Antidepressant Medication	
TYPE OF ANTIDEPRESSANT	**MEDICATION—GENERIC/TRADE NAMES**
Selective serotonin reuptake inhibitor (SSRI)	fluoxetine/Prozac, sertraline/Zoloft, paroxetine/Paxil, citalopram/Celexa, escitalopram/Lexapro, fluvoxamine/Luvox
Serotonin-norepinephrine reuptake inhibitor (SNRI)	venlafaxine/Effexor/Pristiq (extended release), duloxetine/Cymbalta
Norepinephrine-dopamine reuptake inhibitor (NDRI)	bupropion/Wellbutrin
Serotonin modulator	trazodone/Desyrel
Norepinephrine-serotonin modulator	mirtazapine/Remeron
Tricyclic antidepressant (TCA)	amitriptyline/Elavil, clomipramine/Anafranil, desipramine/Norpramin, nortriptyline/Pamelor, imipramine/Tofranil, doxepin/Sinequan
Monoamine oxidase inhibitor (MAOI)	phenelzine/Nardil, isocarboxazid/Marplan, tranylcypromine/Parnate, moclobemide/Manerix, selegiline/Emsam (patch)

medications used, efficacy and side effect tolerance, and family history of effective medication use. If possible, avoid use of TCAs in the geriatric patient to avoid anticholinergic and cardiovascular side effects. MAOIs are usually prescribed by a psychiatrist.

It is very important to maximize the dose of an antidepressant for an adequate period of time to attain efficacy and full remission. Monitor and evaluate therapeutic response to antidepressant therapy, and observe for side effects, tolerance, and unremitting symptoms of depression. Studies show that the majority of patients on a single agent (monotherapy) do not tolerate it, have limited or no response, stop the medication within the first 3 months, or never receive an adequate dose or trial of medication. Consequently, monotherapy is effective in approximately one-third of patients, and the rest do not reach remission. For those patients who do not respond adequately to monotherapy, other treatment strategies may be employed. Switching agents within the same class or combining different types of antidepressants (e.g., a combination of sertraline and bupropion) may result in symptom remission. With multiple failed trials of monotherapy or combination therapy, the patient may be considered to have treatment-resistant depression. Two second-generation antipsychotic agents are FDA approved for augmentation to antidepressant therapy in treatment resistant depression: aripiprizole (Abilify) and quetiapine extended release (Seroquel XR). Symbyax, a combination of fluoxetine and olanzepine, is also FDA approved for augmenting treatment-resistant depression as is L-methylfolate (Deplin). Providers who are not familiar or comfortable with switching, combination, and augmentation strategies or off-label use of mood stabilizers, other second-generation antipsychotics, or stimulant medications to augment antidepressants should refer patients to a psychiatric mental health nurse practitioner or a psychiatrist (Dew et al., 2007).

Promoting adherence is important to achieve full recovery. Partnering with the patient through inquiry into prior antidepressant use, shared decision making, and education regarding expected therapeutic response time will positively affect patient adherence to the therapeutic regimen. Discussion regarding common and potentially bothersome side effects and the likelihood that they will wane over time promotes adherence. The sexual side effects of SSRIs may not wane over time and should be addressed as depressive symptoms remit and the patient expresses concern about and/or regains desire for sexual activity. Educate patients about serious or potentially dangerous effects of antidepressant medication and instruct them when it is necessary to notify their prescriber (Table 16-9). As patients begin to feel better, advise them to continue the medication and explain the risk of stopping medication abruptly or too soon.

Length of Pharmacotherapy Treatment and Follow-Up: When initiating or changing the dose of antidepressant medication, it is critical to monitor the patient closely for efficacy and side effects. Observe for worsening of

TABLE 16-9 Common Side Effects and Potentially Serious/Dangerous Side Effects of Antidepressants

SSRIs, NDRIs, SNRIs: common side effects	Mild nausea, loose bowel movements, anxiety, headache, insomnia, increased sweating, weight gain/loss, sexual dysfunction, vivid dreams, rash, syndrome of inappropriate SIADH
TCAs: side effects	Anticholinergic effects—dry mouth, constipation, blurred vision, urinary retention; cardiovascular effects—tachycardia and orthostatic hypotension; sedation, weight gain, seizures
Serotonin modulators: side effects	Sedation, weight gain, mild anticholinergic symptoms; priapism, a side effect of trazodone, is a medical emergency
Serotonin syndrome (excessive serotonin)	Lethargy, restlessness, confusion, flushing, diaphoresis, tremor, myoclonic jerks
SSRI discontinuation syndrome	Dizziness, headache, paresthesia, nausea, diarrhea, insomnia, and irritability; seen with missed doses and abrupt discontinuation of antidepressants with a short half-life
SSRI apathy syndrome	Loss of motivation, increased passivity, lethargy, and a "flat" feeling; not to be confused with a relapse/recurrence of depression (absence of other depressive symptoms)

Abbreviations: NDRIs = norepinephrine-dopamine reuptake inhibitors; SIADH = secretion of antidiuretic hormone; SSRIs = selective serotonin reuptake inhibitors; TCAs = tricyclic antidepressants

depression, suicidal thoughts or actions, unusual changes in behavior, agitation, and irritability. Educate patients, families, and caregivers to pay close attention to sudden changes in mood, behaviors, thoughts, or feelings as well as suicidal thoughts and to report these concerns immediately to the provider. It is well established that as depression begins to remit patients may become more energized and may be able to follow through on prevailing suicidal ideation and plans. Factors that increase risk for suicide include severe insomnia, homosexuality, chronic pain or disability, a family history of suicide (especially in the same-sex parent), previous suicide attempts, loss of a loved one, lack of employment, and increased financial burden. The March 2004 FDA Public Health Advisory regarding the possible risk of worsening depression and suicidality in patients taking antidepressants supports close monitoring during initiation and dosing phases of treatment. A return office visit every 2 to 4 weeks is strongly recommended.

Length of antidepressant treatment varies depending on whether it is a first or recurrent episode. With each recurrence, there is an increased risk of future recurrence if medication is discontinued, and as a result, antidepressant therapy must be maintained for longer periods of time if not indefinitely. The *acute phase* of treatment lasts up to 3 months after the start of medication with the goal to achieve remission. Close follow-up is critical and highly individualized; however,

there should be patient contact within the first month and additional contact every 4 weeks or sooner with dosage adjustments, switching, combination, or augmentation. The *continuation phase* of treatment begins once remission is achieved, and medication should be continued for at least another 4 to 12 months. With one lifetime episode of MDD, a trial discontinuation of medication is optional if the patient has remained asymptomatic for the duration of the continuation phase of treatment. Patients in the continuation phase of treatment should be seen every 5 or 6 months or sooner. The *maintenance phase* of antidepressant therapy is specifically for patients with two or more lifetime episodes of MDD. These patients should be maintained on medication at the same dosage for another 15 months to 5 years. Patients in the maintenance phase of treatment should be seen every 6 to 12 months or sooner.

Psychotherapy: Research studies demonstrate that supportive counseling, psychotherapy, cognitive-behavioral therapy, problem-solving therapy, interpersonal psychotherapy, reminiscence therapy, group therapy, and support groups improve remission and recovery rates when patients actively participate (Kiosses, Leon, & Areán, 2011). For patients with mild depression, therapy alone may be sufficient as a treatment strategy. Those with moderate-to-severe depression experience significantly better outcomes with concurrent psychotherapy and pharmacotherapy.

Other Therapies: Patients should be encouraged to engage in relaxation exercises, meditation, yoga, and visual imagery to assist in developing healthy coping skills. Evidence supports dietary or supplemental intake of omega-3 fatty acids and exercise in treating depression. Symptom severity in elders residing in long-term care facilities may decrease if they are engaged in a physical or cognitive activity, involved in group activities, exposed to bright light therapy, and provided with emotional support (Wright, 2010). Studies suggest significant improvement in depressive symptoms when long-term care facility treatment teams provide simple psychosocial interventions.

Biological Therapies: Should SSRIs and counseling/psychotherapy be ineffective in achieving full recovery, phototherapy (intermittent bright light therapy), trans-magnetic stimulation (TMS), vagus nerve stimulation (VNS), and ECT are often effective for severe, refractory, or psychotic depression.

General Follow-Up Guidelines:
- Use diagnostic scales/instruments (symptom and severity tools) to objectively assess progress compared to baseline evaluation
- Assess for therapy and medication adherence, response, and side effects
- Assess suicidal ideation
- Titrate medication dose for total remission
- If trial discontinuation, taper over 2 to 4 weeks
- Monitor for early signs of recurrence

Sequelae: There are many potential negative outcomes if depression is not identified and treated appropriately, and full remission and recovery is not reached. Complications of depression include impaired interpersonal relationships, interpersonal problems, increased medical comorbidity and medical risk factors over time, worsening of cognitive impairment, self-neglect, decreased mobility, increased disability, and increased mortality from suicide and interactions with medical conditions such as cardiovascular and cerebrovascular disease. Additionally, there is an increased risk of homicide/suicide (murder of loved one/spouse before suicide). Depression diminishes health and overall life span.

Prevention/prophylaxis: Prevention of depression encompasses the initial episode, recurrent episodes, and protection from complications. Studies show that minimizing risk factors has demonstrated a reduction in the incidence of depression (Hindi, Dew,

Albert, Lotrich, & Reynolds, 2011; Miller, 2005; Reynolds, 2009). Major risk factors for depression include stress, stressful life events, responses to stress, and unhealthy coping styles. Stress management, relaxation exercises, and problem-solving and decision-making skills can be taught and maintained as a prevention strategy. Another major risk factor for depression is persistent negative thinking, which can be modified with cognitive restructuring, self-monitoring of thought processes, and strategies such as increased awareness and mindfulness. Poor health, loss of independence, and physical disability place elders at high risk for depression. Self-care strategies, such as a nutritious diet, exercise, weight management, social interaction, cognitive stimulation, counseling, and a positive attitude toward life and aging, aid in maximizing physical and mental health. Prevention of vascular causes of late-life depression may be accomplished through identification and modification of shared risk factors, which include vascular inflammation, atherosclerosis, dyslipidemia, hypertension, diabetes, alcohol consumption, obesity, and smoking. Tertiary prevention of depression in patients with established vascular disease includes intensive management of risk factors and active disease processes (Lavretsy & Meeks, 2009). The goals of prevention are to decrease complications of late-life depression, thereby increasing overall health and quality of life and prolonging the life span (Kiosses & Ravdin, 2010).

Referral: Patients who should be referred to psychiatry are those who have prominent suicide/self-harm thoughts or previous suicide attempts, a questionable diagnosis, possible bipolar disorder or comorbid psychiatric conditions (especially Axis 2), persistent residual symptoms, and partial or no response to monotherapy, combination, augmentation, or adjunctive medications. For counseling, refer the patient to a psychiatric nurse practitioner, a psychiatric clinical nurse specialist, or a licensed clinical psychologist, and provide resources for support groups and appropriate service professionals and agencies.

Education: Patient and family education should include information about the disease process, causative factors, heritability, risk of relapse or recurrence, suicide risk, treatment strategies and recommendations, psychotropic medication use, side effects, and length of time for medication efficacy.

CLINICAL RECOMMENDATION	EVIDENCE RATING	REFERENCES
No significant difference in performance of screening instruments, so choose a tool most practical for the clinical setting.	B	Rubin (2011)
Best diagnostic tool is a detailed history performed by the practitioner in context of *Diagnostic and Statistical Manual of Mental Disorders, Fourth Edition* (DSM-IV) criteria and clinical judgment.	C	Rubin (2011)
Antidepressant medications and psychotherapy are equally effective.	A	Rubin (2011)
Only half of patients respond to the first medication used regardless of class selected, so reevaluate effectiveness at least monthly until symptom remission.	A	Rubin (2011)
Risk factors for depression in older adults include chronic diseases, poor self-perceived health, functional disability, personality traits, inadequate coping strategies, previous psychopathology, small network size, being unmarried, qualitative aspects of social network, stressful life events, and female gender.	A	Vink, Aartsen, & Schoevers (2008)

A = consistent, good-quality, patient-oriented evidence; B = inconsistent or limited-quality, patient-oriented evidence; C = consensus, disease-oriented evidence, usual practice, expert opinion, or case series. For information about the SORT evidence rating system, go to www.aafp.org/afpsort.xml.

ELDER ABUSE

Signal symptoms: Elder abuse can be difficult to detect. A pattern of missed appointments, health-care provider shopping, oversolicitousness by caregiver, bruises, and financial mismanagement are potential clues (Bonnel, 2012).

Description: Elder abuse is doing something or failing to do something that results in harm to an elderly person or puts a helpless older person at risk of harm as described by the National Institutes of Health. The Department of Health and Human Services Administration on Aging states that the term *elder abuse* is any knowing, intentional, or negligent act performed by a caregiver or another person that may cause harm or risk of harm to an older adult who is vulnerable (Administration on Aging, 2012).

Types of abuse include the following:

■ Physical abuse—causing physical pain or injuring a vulnerable elder
■ Sexual abuse—sexual contact with a vulnerable elder without his or her consent
■ Neglect—failing to provide food, shelter, health care, or protection for a vulnerable elder
■ Exploitation—the taking of funds, property, or any assets of a vulnerable elder without legal consent and not for the benefit of the elder
■ Emotional abuse—using verbal or nonverbal means to cause mental pain, anguish, or distress in an elder
■ Abandonment—leaving the vulnerable elder once someone has assumed responsibility for that individual

■ Self-neglect—the elder has not performed the needed activities to protect his or her own health and safety (lacks food/utilities, refuses medications, hoardes, lives in unsafe conditions, neglects his or her grooming/appearance, is unable to handle finances, isolation, is disoriented, develops a dependence on drugs and/or alcohol) (Elder abuse, 2012)

In a report from the National Center on Elder Abuse, about 55% of all of these types of abuse involve neglect. This report did not differentiate whether this was perpetrator neglect or self-neglect situations (Elder abuse prevalence and incidence: fact sheet, 2005).

Etiology: Abuse of vulnerable elders can happen in many settings, from their private home environment to that of a community nursing home or even a hospital setting. The days when the family lived close by and took responsibility for its members are fading. Families are spread out and lack the close communication of past years. This leaves the one member residing close to the elder adult to be fully responsible. This is a stress to the responsible family member, and little support is generally provided for this individual's efforts. Conflict can arise between the family members, leaving the one actually providing care with mixed messages and little support. This can become a volatile situation, increasing the opportunity for abuse. When the elder moves into an already stressed and overcrowded household, the stress level of juggling the multiple responsibilities may become overwhelming for the caregiver. Preparation for this responsibility is usually minimal or nonexistent. For the 4% of older adults living in skilled or long-term care facilities, the risk for abuse is still present, though much less common. Again, adequate training to provide care for the older adult can lessen this risk (*Lippincott's Nursing Guide to Expert Elder Care*, 2011). Touhy and Jett (2009) suggest that the abused elder is more likely female and age 80 or older. She generally has a physical and/or mental disability and may live alone or with the abuser. The abuser is generally found to be a middle-aged male who has a history of substance abuse and/or mental health issues. He may be financially dependent on the elder and have a history of inflicting abuse or of being abused himself. The Patient Page on Elder Abuse in *JAMA* (Hildreth, Burke, & Glass, 2009) states that in 90% of cases of abuse of an adult age 60 or older, the culprit is a family member. These cases result in an increased risk of death for the vulnerable elder involved in the abusive situation.

Occurrence: The actual numbers of cases of elder abuse are difficult to quantify due to the variance in mandatory state reporting laws. A variance in reporting goes from 2.7 per 1000 to 8.6 per 1000. The higher numbers were from states with penalties issued for failure to report. This variance in reporting also includes whether the state reports only physical abuse or the other defined forms of abuse. The National Center on Elder Abuse Fact Sheet (Elder abuse prevalence and incidence: Fact sheet, 2005) states that for every reported case of abuse there are about five that go unreported. It also states that about only 1 of every 14 incidents of self-neglect cases and 1 in 25 cases of financial abuse are ever investigated. An estimated 1 to 2 million elders are thought to be in an abusive situation, with only 1 in 14 of the situations being investigated. These numbers are expected to increase with the increase in the elder population.

Signs and symptoms: The National Center on Elder Abuse offers some ideas on things to observe in older patients. Physical signs include slap marks and unexplained burns or blisters, especially circular as from a cigarette. Unusual bruising in areas that are not usually thought to be accidental can raise suspicion of possible abuse. Any bruising around breasts or genital area and/or unexplained sexually transmitted diseases might indicate sexual abuse. Emotional abuse can be suspected if a patient withdraws from his or her normal activities or has an unusual change in his or her level of alertness or any other change in behavior that has not been previously observed. The National Institute of Justice adds warnings for changes in finances and accounts, unexplained changes to wills or trusts, unexplained bank withdrawals, and loss of propert; such incidents may indicate a problem of exploitation of an elder. Signs of neglect can be decubitus that is untreated, missing medical appointments or lack of medical or dental care, unkempt appearance, and unusual weight loss. These are all concerns that need to be followed up as possible signs of self-neglect or abuse from someone else (Lachs, 2000).

Diagnostic tests: The basis to establishing a baseline of health is a head-to-toe examination of the patient in question. The baseline examination will dictate the needed laboratory tests and any imaging required to establish a diagnosis. If memory or alertness is suspected, perform a mental test to establish the current level of the patient's cognitive ability. Chen and Koval (2002) suggest that the health-care provider listen carefully to both the elder and the caregiver during the visit. The health-care provider may need to separate the elder and his or her caregiver to see if their stories match. This may help determine any other examinations or tests that may need to be performed. *Lippincott's Nursing Guide to Expert Elder Care* (2011) discusses some tools to assist health-care providers in collecting information to support suspicion of abuse.

Treatment: If elder abuse is suspected, it is the health-care professional's responsibility—and in most cases his or her legal obligation—to report this to either 911 or the state elder abuse hotline, according to the National Center on Elder Abuse. Carefully collect information regarding the patient, using physical findings, testing results, and verbal information from the patient and his or her caregivers. Use the interdisciplinary team, and speak with social workers, nursing staff, and others who may have interacted with the patient and caregiver. Document all findings, because they may be required to be presented in court later. Especially document any differences in verbal accounts between the patient and his or her caregiver (Cooper, Selwood, & Livingston, 2009). When a patient has dementia, a history can be difficult to evaluate. This collection of information will assist the adult protective services case workers in their case investigation. The information may protect the patient from further exploitation, neglect, or abuse. Be sure to follow up with the case workers to determine the outcome of the case. It sometimes takes several reports before the true picture of neglect, exploitation, or abuse can be investigated thoroughly, and the elder individual moved to a safe environment.

Sequelae: The elder may need to be moved to a safe environment such as a long-term care setting or the residence of another family member. There may be legal proceedings that can involve the health-care professional's testimony based on the observations and findings that have been carefully documented. The abuser may be incarcerated for his or her acts. Sometimes what is required is an evaluation of support in resources to assist the caregiver in improving his or her knowledge of the caregiving role. This requires education and counseling from community resources (Reuben, 2013).

Prevention/prophylaxis: Prevention can come in the form of education at multiple levels. The caregiver especially requires education on the care of the elderly charge. This can be done in part on regular clinical visits with the primary care provider, in community offerings, at Area Agency on Aging seminars, and with other local resources. In some communities, there are social workers and nurses who provide support services to families through private agencies. Respite programs can be accessed to lessen the stress on the caregiver by providing much-needed time for themselves. Adult day-care services are available in larger communities as are meal services and other resources that can assist the caregiver in lessening the burden of providing care. Education of health-care professionals is also needed so that there is an understanding of those responsible for the care of elder adults. Providing education on normal aging body expectations found in the older patient and what to do when there are red flags that require further investigation can help professionals provide better care for elders.

Referral: See under Treatment.

Education: See under Prevention.

CLINICAL RECOMMENDATION	EVIDENCE RATING	REFERENCES
One in four vulnerable elders are at risk of abuse, and only a small proportion of this is currently detected. Elders, family, and professional caregivers are willing to report abuse and should be asked about it routinely. Valid, reliable measures and consensus on what constitutes an adequate standard for validity of abuse measures are needed.	A	Cooper, Selwood, & Livingston (2008)

Continued

CLINICAL RECOMMENDATION	EVIDENCE RATING	REFERENCES
Findings of this systematic review of elder abuse interventions suggest that there is currently insufficient evidence to support any particular intervention related to elder abuse targeting clients, perpetrators, or health-care professionals. Although elder abuse is an increasingly important issue internationally, there is little high-quality research on the effectiveness of interventions. Further, the review suggests that there may be both positive and negative consequences of elder- abuse interventions.	A	Ploeg, Fear, Hutchison, MacMillan, & Bolan (2009)
The state of current elder-abuse research is comprised primarily of descriptive, observational case studies, no meta-analyses, and a few intervention trials. Little evidence is available that supports any intervention to prevent elder abuse. More rigorous elder-abuse research and more investigators are needed.	A	Daly, Merchant, & Jogerst (2011)

A = consistent, good-quality, patient-oriented evidence; B = inconsistent or limited-quality, patient-oriented evidence; C = consensus, disease-oriented evidence, usual practice, expert opinion, or case series. For information about the SORT evidence rating system, go to www.aafp.org/afpsort.xml.

GRIEF AND BEREAVEMENT

Signal symptoms: May be none; may have feelings of depression with associated symptoms, crying, insomnia, fatigue, anger, sadness, withdrawal (Baier & Buechsel, 2012).

Description: Grief is a normal emotional response to loss; grieving, bereavement, or mourning is the process of dealing with loss. Complicated grief refers to the inability to cope with the loss or becoming "stuck"; when the patient is unable to work through his or her grief, physical or psychological illness may occur (Boelen & van den Bout, 2008; Hefren & Thyer, 2012; Sorrell, 2012).

Etiology: Loss or change perceived as loss; for older adults, the loss of a spouse or life partner is the most common and significant event (Utz, Caserta, & Lund, 2012). Other losses include loss of a parent, child, sibling, or close friend.

Occurrence: Approximately 50% of women over the age of 65 are widows; 13% of men over the age of 65 are widowers.

Age: Grief may occur at any age.

Ethnicity: Not significant.

Gender: Grief affects more women than men.

Contributing factors: Length of illness, amount of suffering, relationship quality, survivor guilt, financial burden of illness, caregiver burden, personality attributes of deceased and survivor, and cultural expectations all may be related to the variety of grief responses. A recent systematic review examined factors deemed predictive of complicated grief (Lobb et al., 2010). Factors present in the anticipatory grieving stage include attachment style, relationship to the departed, prior loss, previous psychiatric problems, or traumatic exposure. Being unprepared for the death, violent death, marital intimacy, and caregiving quality were features associated with the actual death that foretold complicated grieving (Lobb et al., 2010). Widows and widowers with recent disabilities (Utz et al., 2012), few friends, and poor relationships with their children were more apt to require counseling (Pai & Carr, 2010). Current studies have questioned the validity of the "grief work" theory and demonstrate that there is great variability in individual responses to grief as well as differences in the timeline for bereavement (Chan & Chan, 2011; Stroebe & Schut, 1999).

Signs and symptoms: Grief is characterized by feelings of depression with associated symptoms of poor appetite and weight loss or compulsive eating and weight gain, sleep disturbance, tearfulness, lack of interest, withdrawal and isolation, emptiness, indecisiveness, and guilt feelings; some grieving individuals may respond by making dramatic changes in a short time to avoid dealing with feelings. Somatic symptoms are common in the early months of bereavement and may require referrals outside of the primary care arena (Stroebe, Schut, & Stroebe, 2007; Utz et al., 2012).

Diagnostic tests: None.

Differential diagnosis:
- Social phobia
- Depression
- Adjustment reaction

Treatment: Provide emotional support, allowing the older adult to express feelings. Contact close family members who were not present at the bedside of the deceased immediately after the event and offer condolences, answer any questions, and allow them to view the body if feasible. A card or letter from professionals who cared for the patient is also recommended. Reaching out to the surviving spouse in the early bereavement period is also helpful. Sleep disruptions are common in the first 2 weeks and a sedative/hypnotic may be needed (Block, 2009). Reminiscence is helpful to many. Encourage patients to return to their normal routine as soon as possible. Daily physical exercise can help patients cope with the depression that accompanies grief. Referral to a bereavement support group may help some individuals but not all. In cases of complicated grief, psychotherapy and/or antidepressant medication may be indicated.

Follow-up: Guidelines from palliative care and other sources speak of a need for bereavement visits or follow-up, but specifics are lacking (Griffin, Koch, Nelson, & Cooley, 2007; Hudson, et al., 2010; Institute for Clinical Systems Improvement, 2011; National Consensus Project for Quality Palliative Care, 2009; Truog et al., 2008; Zhang, El-Jawahri, & Prigerson, 2006).

Prevention/prophylaxis: The goal is to encourage and support the patient in the normal grieving process and prevent dysfunctional grieving. Bereavement groups, activation of social and spiritual support networks, discussion of anticipated loss by participants, and involvement in group activities or volunteerism may be helpful (Chan & Chan, 2011).

Sequelae: In the first 3 months after the death of a spouse for adults over 65, the mortality rate increases 48% in men and 22% in women; this increase in mortality is across the board and is unrelated to prior health status and socioeconomic level (Moon, Kondo, Glymour, & Subramanian, 2011; Shah et al., 2012). Practitioners must be alert to older adults who do not improve in 3 months after the loss. Additionally, a major depressive syndrome that occurs for 2 or more weeks early in the course of bereavement should be taken seriously and managed accordingly.

Referral: Older adults experiencing abnormal grieving may benefit from a mental health referral. Referral to support groups, such as Widow-to-Widow, may be helpful in the grieving process. It is most desirable if the survivor self-initiates contact with a resource.

Education: Make patients and their support networks aware of the variability of normal grieving; alert them to signs of dysfunctional grieving and resources for help. A helpful resource for survivors and families is www.nlm.nih.gov/medlineplus/bereavement.html.

CLINICAL RECOMMENDATION	EVIDENCE RATING	REFERENCES
For all patients with advanced lung cancer (and their families), it is recommended that palliative care be integrated into their treatment, including those pursuing curative or life-prolonging therapies.	C	Griffin et al. (2007)

Continued

CLINICAL RECOMMENDATION	EVIDENCE RATING	REFERENCES
Following the death of the patient, it is essential to allow the patient's loved ones to perform any customs or rituals that are important to them, within the policy guidelines of the facility. Clinicians should be available to answer questions and offer support.	C	ICSI (2011)
Bereavement services and follow-up are made available to the family for at least 12 months or for as long as is needed after the death of the patient.	C	National Consensus Project for Quality Palliative Care (2009)
Clinical assessment is used to identify people at risk for complicated grief and bereavement and associated depression and comorbid complications, particularly among the elderly.	C	National Consensus Project for Quality Palliative Care (2009)
A postdeath bereavement plan is activated. An interdisciplinary team member is assigned to the family in the postdeath period to help with religious practices, funeral arrangements, and burial planning.	C	National Consensus Project for Quality Palliative Care (2009)

A = consistent, good-quality, patient-oriented evidence; B = inconsistent or limited-quality, patient-oriented evidence; C = consensus, disease-oriented evidence, usual practice, expert opinion, or case series. For information about the SORT evidence rating system, go to www.aafp.org/afpsort.xml.

INSOMNIA

Signal symptoms: Patient report of not sleeping, excessive daytime sleepiness, loud snoring (sleep apnea), complaint of restless legs, difficulty falling asleep and staying asleep, irritability, difficulty concentrating, sleep that is not refreshing and restful (Schutte-Rodin, Broch, Buysse, Dorsey, & Sateia, 2008).

Description: Insomnia is difficulty falling asleep or staying asleep despite the desire to do so and regardless of adequate conditions to promote sleep; poor-quality sleep and difficulty with daytime functioning are also part of insomnia (Bloom et al., 2009; Buysse, 2008).

Etiology: Insomnia can have several etiologies, including medical, behavioral, circadian, or psychiatric. Sleeping states and sleep schedules change with age. Sleep efficiency (time actually sleeping versus time in bed) is less than 80% in older adults, and time to fall asleep is extended. The most important age-related changes in sleep include the following:

- Decreased continuity of sleep with an increase in the number of arousals
- Tendency for the major period of sleep and rapid eye movement (REM) sleep to occur earlier in the night
- A decrease in the deepest parts of non–rapid eye movement (NREM) sleep
- Increased napping during the day
- Tendency to spend more time in bed

Several classifications are in use including primary versus comorbid. In primary, there is no identified cause; comorbid includes psychiatric, medical, somatic, or other sleep disorders (Bloom et al., 2009).

Transient Insomnia: Lasts a few nights, is related to situational stress, and usually resolves without medical intervention when the older adult adapts to the change or removes it.

Short-Term Insomnia: Is similar to transient insomnia, lasts less than 1 month, and is related to an acute medical or psychological condition or to persistent situational stress.

Chronic Insomnia: Lasts more than 1 month and results from age-related changes in sleep and chronic stressors (Bonnet & Arand, 2012c; Krishnan & Hawranik, 2008).

Occurrence: Approximately 42% of people more than 65 years of age experience and regularly complain of poor sleep quality. Poor health confounds this problem, with older adults with respiratory problems reporting 40% greater difficulty with insomnia, and those with psychiatric problems being 2.5 times more likely to experience insomnia (Bloom et al., 2009).

Age: Insomnia can occur at any age; however, older adults have greater difficulty falling asleep and staying asleep.

Ethnicity: Not significant.

Gender: Women who are widowed, separated, or divorced have more insomnia up to age 85 years; men have more insomnia in the over-85-years age group (Doghramji, 2006).

Contributing factors: Factors that may contribute to insomnia include the following:

- Restless legs syndrome
- Periodic limb movement disorder
- Sleep apnea
- Dementia
- Depression
- Anxiety (Brenes et al., 2009)
- Drugs, including caffeine, alcohol, nicotine, antipsychotics, beta blockers, stimulant decongestants, sedative-hypnotics, sympathomimetic bronchodilators, diuretics, carbidopa-levodopa, H_2 blockers, and centrally acting α-agonist antihypertensives, stimulant antidepressants, corticosteroids, calcium channel blockers, anticholinergics (Schutte-Rodin et al., 2008)

Many chronic medical conditions can cause insomnia, including musculoskeletal, cardiac, respiratory, gastrointestinal, renal, endocrine, and neurological (Schutte-Rodin et al., 2008). Insomnia is associated with an increase in hypertension (Fernandez-Mendoza et al., 2012) and atherosclerosis (Nakazaki et al., 2012).

Hospitalization with acute onset of illness can also induce insomnia in susceptible patients (Young, Bourgeois, Hilty, & Hardin, 2008). The few studies that have been done focused on ICU patients and found that acuity of illness, delirium, pain, and hospital environment all were contributing factors for insomnia or sleep disorders. An assessment of sleep and a sleep history is recommended as part of initial and ongoing patient management. Point of intervention would include alleviation of suspected causes by nonpharmacological measures whenever possible before considering drug intervention (Young, Bourgeois, Hilty, & Hardin, 2009).

Signs and symptoms: A complete history should reveal a full description of the problems. Patients may complain about difficulty falling asleep and staying asleep, frequent awakenings, early morning awakening and inability to return to sleep, daytime fatigue with unwanted naps, irritability, or difficulty concentrating. Additionally, an older adult may spend 10 to 12 hours in bed at night trying to sleep. A pertinent physical examination should evaluate the systems associated with any medical conditions listed here. Falling may be a sign of insomnia. A mental status examination is useful in detecting cognitive or psychiatric disease (Bloom et al., 2009; Bonnet & Arand, 2012a; Krishnan & Hawranik, 2008).

Diagnostic tests: None, unless indicated by history and physical examination.

Differential diagnosis:
- Anxiety
- Inadequate sleep hygiene
- Medical problems
- Medication-related sleep disorder
- Depression
- Alcohol-related sleep disorder or primary sleep disorder

Treatment: For transient insomnia, patients should avoid caffeine for 12 hours before bedtime and discontinue alcohol and unnecessary sleep-interrupting drugs. Over-the-counter (OTC) melatonin or prescription ramelteon can be tried. If ineffective, initiate a short-acting sedative-hypnotic, such as zolpidem (Ambien) or zaleplon (Sonata), at lowest dosage before desired bedtime for 1 week or less. Suggest spacing dosing to every other day to avoid side effects.

If a benzodiazepine is used, temazepam (Restoril) is relatively short-acting. If this is ineffective, reevaluate the diagnosis and restructure the treatment modalities.

For chronic insomnia, the treatment is more complex. A complete medical and psychiatric history is indicated, including any family history of sleep problems. A validated self-administered instrument, such as the Epworth Sleepiness Scale (www.stanford.edu/~dement/epworth.html) or Stanford Sleepiness Scale (www.stanford.edu/~dement/sss.html), can be used to focus on specific aspects of the problem. The University of Pittsburgh Sleep Center also has several instruments that require permission for use (www.sleep.pitt.edu). The patient should keep a sleep diary and bring it to the next office visit. If the patient has a bed partner, this person should be interviewed as well. If sleep apnea is suspected, refer for polysomnography. Review sleep hygiene tips. Cognitive-behavioral therapy focused on reducing time in bed, correcting false beliefs and expectations regarding sleep, and decreasing exposure to stimuli that deter sleep has been shown to be superior and long-lasting compared with short-term sedative-hypnotic use (Morin et al., 2009). Combined, sleep hygiene instruction and cognitive-behavioral therapy are more effective than either modality alone or usual treatment (Montgomery & Dennis, 2008a; Morgan, Gregory, Tomeny, David, & Gascoigne, 2012). Medications should be evaluated in light of ability to interfere with sleep, and modifications should be made where possible. Gradual increase from sedentary to moderate aerobic exercise combined with sleep hygiene is also an effective intervention (Montgomery & Dennis, 2008b; Reid et al., 2010; Yang, Ho, Chen, & Chien, 2012). Mindfulness meditation is a successful treatment in motivated patients, and results have been sustained over a long period (Ong, Shapiro, & Manber, 2008, 2009; Ong & Sholtes, 2010). An RCT comparing training in tai chi chih versus health education for older adults with moderate sleep problems found tai chi chih to be more effective in resolving sleep problems (Irwin, Olmstead, & Motivala, 2008). Treat underlying or coexisting disorders. De Niet, Tiemens, Kloos, and Hutschemaekers (2009) found music to be a successful nonpharmacological intervention to induce relaxation to sleep.

Approved pharmacological therapy includes temazepam (Restoril) for sleep onset insomnia, eszopiclone (Lunesta) for sleep onset and sleep maintenance, zolpidem CR and zolpidem (AmbienCR and Ambien) and zolpidem sublingual (Intermezzo) for sleep maintenance, and zaleplon (Sonata) and ramelteon (Rozerem) for sleep onset insomnia. The FDA (U.S. FDA, 2013) has issued a drug safety communication requiring lower doses of zolpidem products to avoid risk of next-day impairment. Intermezzo was not included in this warning.

Follow-up: Patients should return in 2 weeks. Examine the patient's sleep diary, and evaluate the effectiveness of the treatment. If indicated, reevaluate the diagnosis and restructure the treatment. Sedative-hypnotics should be considered a last choice and every effort should be made to wean the patient from these or avoid long-term use.

Sequelae: Includes reduced quality of life, depression, increased risk for falls/injury, and potential for drug dependence or drug interactions resulting from use of OTC sleep aids.

Prevention/prophylaxis: Sleep hygiene suggestions may include the following:

- Establish a regular bedtime and wake-up time.
- Set aside a time each evening for relaxation and thinking.
- Avoid caffeine, alcohol, and nicotine, because they all interrupt sleep.
- Minimize awake time in bed, reserving bed for sleep and sexual activity.
- Create an optimal sleep environment.
- Establish regular eating habits, because hunger can interrupt sleep.
- Avoid napping.
- Exercise daily to extent possible, but avoid exercise just before bedtime.
- Maximize daytime exposure to bright light.

Referral: If therapy brings no improvement and other underlying causes have been eliminated, refer the patient to a sleep laboratory for evaluation.

Education: Explain age-related sleep changes to the patient and his or her family. Teach the patient to follow the guidelines listed under Prevention/prophylaxis. Educate the patient to avoid OTC antihistamines, because they can have dangerous side effects, including dry mouth and a "hangover" effect. Teach the patient to avoid alcohol use with prescribed sleep medication to prevent accidental overdose. Provider education is also needed, because many providers do not recognize insomnia in the older adult as a problem.

CLINICAL RECOMMENDATION	EVIDENCE RATING	REFERENCES
Cognitive-behavioral therapy is an effective treatment for insomnia in older adults.	A	Montgomery & Dennis (2008) National Institutes of Health (2005)
Sedative-hypnotics (zolpidem, ramelteon, zaleplon, and eszopiclone) are effective but also have adverse effects such as depression and rebound insomnia.	A	Sontheimer (2011)
Most patients do not require diagnostic testing; the practitioner should consider performing a polysomnography if obstructive sleep apnea or periodic limb movement disorder is suspected.	C	Sontheimer (2011)
A single study found exercise to benefit insomnia in older adults with insomnia; further research is indicated.	B	Montgomery & Dennis (2008)

A = consistent, good-quality, patient-oriented evidence; B = inconsistent or limited-quality, patient-oriented evidence; C = consensus, disease-oriented evidence, usual practice, expert opinion, or case series. For information about the SORT evidence rating system, go to www.aafp.org/afpsort.xml.

PRESCRIPTION DRUG ABUSE

Signal symptoms: Variable depending on abused substance. Opioids and benzodiazipines are among the most frequent categories. Pinpoint pupils, constipation, confusion, memory loss, depression, behavioral changes, drowsiness, difficulty breathing, other behavioral symptoms including personality changes.

Description: Prescription drug abuse or misuse includes the willful use of prescribed drugs for non-medical purposes, accidental misuse due to inaccurate dosing, sharing prescribed drugs with another person, or accepting drugs prescribed for another person for one's own use (Sehgal, Manchikanti, & Smith, 2012). Willful or accidental mixing of prescription drugs with other psychoactive substances, such as alcohol, is another form of prescription drug abuse. Deliberate diversion of prescription drugs for personal gain is another form of prescription drug abuse (Manchikanti, 2006; Office of National Drug Control Policy, n.d.).

Etiology: Multiple factors are involved: genetic predisposition to addiction, unrealistic expectations for pain relief, coexisting mental health problem (often undiagnosed) or substance use problem, undiagnosed cognitive impairment, socioeconomic hardship. Recent evidence shows that family and friends are the primary source for opiate diversion, and most prescriptions are obtained from a single source as opposed to shopping around to multiple providers (SAMHSA, 2009).

Age: Multiple studies show a higher rate of prescription drug abuse in the 50 to 64 year age group (Blazer & Wu, 2009; Gossop & Moos, 2008; Wu & Blazer, 2011).

Ethnicity: All are affected.

Occurrence: The United States consumes 80% of the world's opioids and 99% of the hydrocodone supply globally, despite comprising only 4.6% of the population worldwide (Manchikanti & Singh, 2008).

Gender: A national survey found that overall more men have prescription drug abuse problems, but women who abuse prescription drugs are less likely to receive treatment (Back, Payne, Simpson, & Brady, 2010). In two studies specific to older adults (Culberson & Ziska, 2008; Simoni-Wastila & Yang, 2006), female gender was cited as a risk factor for prescription drug abuse.

Contributing factors: Lack of perception by the patient that prescription drug abuse is problematic (Wu & Blazer, 2011), unmet need for chronic pain relief (Sjøgren, Ekholm, Peuckmann, & Grønbaek, 2009), coexisting mental health problems or substance use disorder (Lofwall, Schuster, & Strain, 2008; Sehgal et al., 2012), genetic predisposition to addiction, availability of abused substances from trusted sources such as family and friends (Hernandez & Nelson, 2010).

Signs and symptoms: Vary depending on class of drug. Can often be mistaken for a medical or cognitive problem in an older adult. Drug-seeking behavior may be the initial sign. Reporting lost prescriptions or unmanageable pain despite being given an appropriate dose. Pinpoint pupils, constipation, confusion or disorientation in familiar surroundings, memory loss, slurred speech, ataxia, depression, behavioral changes, drowsiness, difficulty breathing, irritability, personality changes.

Diagnostic tests: Urine drug screening at random intervals to detect presence of prescribed drug and any other illicit drugs. Use of a screening tool before prescribing an opioid drug may be helpful, although most tools have not been validated (Sehgal et al., 2012; Tinsley, 2011). Screening, Brief Intervention, and Referral to Treatment (SBIRT) is another approach that can be used in alcohol and substance use disorders (Babor et al., 2007).

Differential diagnosis:
- Dementia
- Delirium
- Constipation
- Inadequate pain management
- Neurological problem
- Depression
- Alcohol use disorder

Treatment: Treatment depends on the extent of the abuse and the particular class of drug abused, patient comorbidities, and presentation. The possibility of multiple substances being abused simultaneously must be assessed. The two most commonly abused classes are addressed.

Acute Opioid Intoxication: An acute care setting is required. Discontinue all opioids, and remove any transdermal patches. Obtain a comprehensive toxicology screen, monitor patient, and provide supportive care, including management of any medical comorbidities. Administer naloxone, an opioid antagonist, with dosage determined by patient's respiratory status. Management of opioid dependency is usually done on an outpatient basis. Methadone maintenance, naltrexone, and most recently buprenorphine (Suboxone) in an outpatient setting with regular monitoring, urine drug screening, and a patient contract are all options (Maldonado, 2010).

Acute Benzodiazepine Intoxication: This is more likely to occur in the presence of concurrent alcohol use or abuse. Offer supportive care and close monitoring in the acute care setting; discontinue all benzodiazipines; and obtain a comprehensive toxicology screen to check for other substances. Treat medical comorbidities. Flumazenil, a benzodiazepine antagonist, may be used in severe cases. Management of benzodiazepine dependency is controversial, with some providers using a long-acting benzodiazepine, slowly withdrawing the agent over time. Other substitutes include carbamazepine, topirimate, gabapentin, or valproate (Maldonado, 2010). In addition to pharmacological management, psychotherapy or counseling is indicated. A meta-analysis of current treatment approaches to discontinuation of benzodiazepines found that gradual dose reduction (GDR) combined with a psychological modality was more effective than either of those alone. There was insufficient evidence to support other pharmacological substitutes (Parr, Kavanagh, Cahill, Mitchell, & McD. Young, 2008). The SBIRT approach is also recommended (Babor et al., 2007).

Follow-up: Patients with prescription drug abuse may require individualized follow-up in an outpatient treatment program and should also be monitored by their primary care provider.

Sequelae: Deaths from prescription drug abuse and misuse have risen steadily. Alcohol and drug interactions are common in older adults, leading to significant morbidity and mortality (Pringle, Ahern, Heller, Gold, & Brown, 2005). Legal and criminal prosecution can result from drug diversion.

Prevention/prophylaxis: Educate providers, pharmacists, patients, families, and the public about the use and misuse of prescription drugs. Make an assessment of pain and abuse potential of patients when prescribing and allow for the ongoing monitoring of patients' medication use, using patient contracts and random drug testing as indicated. The FDA and the Department of Justice Drug Enforcement Administration (DEA) have collaborated to develop a Risk Evaluation and Mitigation Strategy (REMS) for extended-release and long-acting opioid analgesics. This REMS program will require education of providers and pharmacists, education of patients/families by the provider, and continued education at site of prescription dispensing by the pharmacist (www.ER-LA-opioidREMS.com). Prescription drug monitoring programs are also in place in many states, and the programs allow prescribers and dispensers to access records of controlled substance for a particular patient in live time. These safety measures are a beginning step, but the responsibility rests with the provider and the patient for ongoing monitoring and reevaluation of a continued need for the prescribed drug. To date, there is insufficient evidence on the efficacy of opioids for noncancer chronic pain (Manchikanti, Fellows, Ailinani, & Pampati, 2010) but the preponderance of prescriptions are for that purpose. Providers should regularly monitor for clinical guideline updates on prescription drug abuse and safe prescribing of commonly abused drugs (Manchikanti et al., 2012a, 2012b).

Referral: Older adults who regularly abuse or misuse prescription drugs should be referred to an addictions specialist or treatment program for co-management and follow-up. Refer addicted adults to community-based support groups, such as Narcotics Anonymous, for mentoring.

Education: Educate providers, patients, families, and the public (see under Prevention/prophylaxis). For patients, families, and the public, education on the dangers of using or sharing drugs that are not prescribed for the individual is essential.

CLINICAL RECOMMENDATION	EVIDENCE RATING	REFERENCES
Primary attention in opioid overdose is airway and ventilation management.	C	Kraft (2011)
The use of naloxone is a key diagnostic and therapeutic intervention; naloxone reversal should be titrated to ventilation, rather than to the level of arousal, to prevent withdrawal symptomatology.	C	Kraft (2011)
Intoxication with longer-acting opioids predicts recurrence of respiratory depression after naloxone reversal.	B	Kraft (2011)
There is current evidence supporting that case management can enhance linkage with other services. However, evidence that case management reduces drug use or produces other beneficial outcome is not conclusive.	A	Hesse, Vanderplasschen, Rapp, Broekaert, & Fridell (2007)
Psychosocial treatments offered in addition to pharmacological detoxification treatments are effective in terms of completion of treatment, use of opiate, participants abstinent at follow-up, and clinical attendance.	A	Amato, Minozzi, Davoli, & Vecchi (2011)

Continued

CLINICAL RECOMMENDATION	EVIDENCE RATING	REFERENCES
Currently, there is not enough evidence to conclude that psychosocial treatments alone are adequate to treat people with opiate abuse and dependence.	A	Mayet, Farrell, Ferri, Amato, & Davoli (2004)
SBIRT yields short-term improvements in individuals' health; long-term effects on population health have not yet been demonstrated, but simulation models suggest that the benefits could be substantial.	B	Babor et al. (2007)

A = consistent, good-quality, patient-oriented evidence; B = inconsistent or limited-quality, patient-oriented evidence; C = consensus, disease-oriented evidence, usual practice, expert opinion, or case series. For information about the SORT evidence rating system, go to www.aafp.org/afpsort.xml.

CASE STUDY

Mrs. C. is a 69-year-old married woman who presents to your practice with a chief complaint of fatigue. She tells you that she is tired all the time despite sleeping through the night. She is concerned she may be coming down with something. You ask her about other symptoms, and she confesses that she is under a lot of stress. Her husband has terminal cancer and is also depressed. He is still functional but has refused all interventions. Mrs. C. relates that she quit her job to take care of him, but it is "dragging her down," because he is so depressed. She has four children, three of whom are close by, but she feels like she is bearing the burden herself, and the children do not realize what is happening. She tells you tearfully, "I want to have a life, too, before it is all over."

Review of her chart shows recent CBC and chemistry profiles that are normal, normal TSH, and normal ECG. There is a family history of alcohol abuse (her father) and suicide (a sibling).

1. What additional subjective data are you seeking?
2. What additional objective data will you be assessing for?

3. What national guidelines are appropriate to consider?
4. What tests will you order?
5. Are there any screening tools that you want to use?
6. What are the differential diagnoses that you are considering?
7. What is your plan of care?
8. Are there any Healthy People 2020 objectives that you should consider?
9. What additional patient teaching may be needed?
10. Will you be looking for a consultation?

REFERENCES

Agitation

American Psychiatric Association. (2010). *Practice guidelines for the treatment of patients with Alzheimer's disease and other dementias* (2nd ed.). Arlington, VA: American Psychiatric Association.

Ballard, C. G., Gauthier, S., Cummings, J. L., Brodaty, H., Grossberg, G. T., Robert, P., & Lyketsos, C. G. (2009). Management of agitation and aggression associated with Alzheimer disease. *National Review of Neurology, 5*(5), 245–255.

Cohen-Mansfield, J. (2008). Agitated behavior in persons with dementia: the relationship between type of behavior, its frequency, and its disruptiveness. *Journal of Psychiatric Research, 43*(1), 64–69.

Gauthier, S., Juby, A., Dalziel, W., Réhel, B., Schecter, R., & EXPLORE investigators. (2010). Effects of rivastigmine on common symptomatology of Alzheimer's disease (EXPLORE). *Current Medical Research and Opinion, 26*(5), 1149–1160.

Lovheim, H., Sandman, P. O., Karlsson, S., & Gustafson, Y. (2009). Sex differences in the prevalence of behavioral and psychological symptoms of dementia. *International Psychogeriatrics, 21*(3), 469–475.

Olazarán, J., Reisberg, B., Clare, L., Cruz, I., Peña-Casanova, J., Del Ser, T., . . . Muñiz, R. (2010). Nonpharmacological therapies in Alzheimer's disease: a systematic review of efficacy. *Dementia and Geriatric Cognitive Disorders, 30*(2) 161–178.

Seitz, D. P., Brisbin, S., Hermann, N., Rapoport, M. J., Wilson, K., Rines, J., . . . Conn, D. (2012). Efficacy and feasibility of nonpharmacological interventions for neuropsychiatric symptoms of dementia in long term care: a systematic review. *Journal of the American Medical Directors, 13*(6), 503–506.

Wetzels, R., Zuidema, S., Verhey, F., & Koopmans, R. (2010). Course of neuropsychiatric symptoms in residents with dementia in long-term care institutions: a systematic review. *International Psychogeriatrics, 22*(7), 1040–1053.

Whall, A. L., Colling, K. B., Kolanowski, A., Kim, H., Son Hong, G. R., DiCicco, B., . . . Beck, C. (2008). Factors associated with aggressive behavior among nursing home residents with dementia. *Gerontologist, 48*(6), 721–731.

Alcohol Abuse

American Psychiatric Association. (2000). *Diagnostic and statistical manual of mental disorders* (4th ed., text rev., pp. 213–214). Washington, DC: American Psychiatric Association.

Anton, R. F. (2008). Naltrexone for the management of alcohol dependence. *New England Journal of Medicine, 359*(7), 715–721. doi:10.1056/NEJMct0801733

Anton, R. F., O'Malley, S. S., Ciraulo, D. A., Cisler, R. A., Couper, D., Donovan, D. M., . . . COMBINE Study Research Group. (2006). Combined pharmacotherapies and behavioral interventions for alcohol dependence: the COMBINE study: a randomized controlled trial. *Journal of the American Medical Association, 295*(17), 2003–2017.

Barnes, A. J., Moore, A. A., Xu, H., Ang, A., Tallen, L., Mirkin, M., & Ettner, S. L. (2010). Prevalence and correlates of at-risk drinking among older adults: the project SHARE study. *Journal of General Internal Medicine, 25*(8), 840–846. doi:10.1007/s11606-010-1341-x

Duru, O. K., Xu, H., Tseng, C.-H., Mirkin, M., Ang, A., Tallen, L., . . . Ettner, S. L. (2010). Correlates of alcohol-related discussions between older adults and their physicians. *Journal of the American Geriatrics Society, 58*(12), 2369–2374. doi:10.1111/j.1532-5415.2010.03176.x

Fagbemi, K. (2011). Q: What is the best questionnaire to screen for alcohol use disorder in an office practice? *Cleveland Clinic Journal of Medicine, 78*(10), 649–651. doi:10.3949/ccjm.78a.10186

Ferri, F. (2013). Alcoholism. In F. Ferri (Ed.), *Ferri's clinical advisor 2013* (pp. 46–48). Philadelphia, PA: Elsevier Mosby.

Fink, A., Elliott, M. N., Tsai, M., & Beck, J. C. (2005). An evaluation of an intervention to assist primary care physicians in screening and educating older patients who use alcohol. *Journal of the American Geriatrics Society, 53*(11), 1937–1943. doi:10.1111/j.1532-5415.2005.00476.x

Frank, D., DeBenedetti, A. F., Volk, R. J., Williams, E. C., Kivlahan, D. R., & Bradley, K. A. (2008). Effectiveness of the AUDIT-C as a screening test for alcohol misuse in three race/ethnic groups. *Journal of General Internal Medicine, 23*(6), 781–787.

Gilbertson, R., Ceballos, N. A., Prather, R., & Nixon, S. J. (2009). Effects of acute alcohol consumption in older and younger adults: perceived impairment versus psychomotor performance. *Journal on Studies of Alcohol and Drugs, 70*(2), 242–252.

Gold, M., & Aronson, M. D. (2012). Alcohol abuse and dependence: epidemiology, clinical manifestations, and diagnosis. *UpToDate.* Retrieved from http://www.uptodate.com/contents/alcohol-abuse-and-dependence-epidemiology-clinical-manifestations-and-diagnosis?detectedLanguage=en&source=search_result&search=Alcohol+abuse+and+dependence%3A+Epidemiology%2C+clinical+manifestations%2C+and+diagnosis.&selectedTitle=1%7E150&provider=noProvider

Hasin, D. S., Stinson, F. S., Ogburn, E., & Grant, B. F. (2007). Prevalence, correlates, disability, and comorbidity of DSM-IV alcohol abuse and dependence in the United States: results from the National Epidemiologic Survey on Alcohol and Related Conditions. *Archives of General Psychiatry, 64*(7), 830–842.

Jalbert, J. J., Quilliam, B. J., & Lapane, K. L. (2008). A profile of concurrent alcohol and alcohol interactive prescription drug use in the US population. *Journal of General Internal Medicine, 23*(9), 1318–1323. doi:10.1007/s11606-008-0639-4

Kirchner, J. E., Zubritsky, C., Cody, M., Coakley, E., Chen, H., Ware, J. H., . . . Levkoff, S. (2007). Alcohol consumption among older adults in primary care. *Journal of General Internal Medicine, 22*(1), 92–97. doi: 10.1007/sl-1606-006-0017-z

Lin, J. C., Karno, M. P., Barry, K. L., Blow, F. C., Davis, J. W., Tang, L., & Moore, A. A. (2010). Determinants of early reductions in drinking among older at-risk drinkers participating in the intervention arm of a trial to reduce at-risk drinking in primary care. *Journal of the American Geriatrics Society, 58*(2), 227–233. doi:10.1111/j.1532-5415.2009.02676.x

Lloyd, D. A., & Turner, R. J. (2008). Cumulative lifetime adversities and alcohol dependence in adolescence and young adulthood. *Drug and Alcohol Dependence, 93*(3), 217–226.

Merrick, E. L., Horgan, C. M., Hodgkin, D., Garnick, D. W., Houghton, S. F., Panas, L., . . . Blow, F. C. (2008). Unhealthy drinking patterns in older adults: prevalence and associated characteristics. *Journal of the American Geriatrics Society, 56*(2), 214–223. doi:10.1111/j.1532-5415.2007.01539.x

National Institute on Alcohol Abuse and Alcoholism (NIAAA). (2005). Social work education for the prevention and treatment of alcohol use disorders. Module 2: etiology and natural history of alcoholism. Retrieved from http://pubs.niaaa.nih.gov/publications/Social/Module2Etiology%26NaturalHistory/Module2.html

Pringle, K., Ahern, F., & Heller, D. (2006). Alcohol and prescription drug interactions among aging adults. *Geriatrics and Aging, 9,* 635–641.

Substance Abuse and Mental Health Services Administration (SAMHSA). (2009). *Results from the 2008 National Survey on Drug Use and Health: national findings* (Office of Applied Studies, Substance NSDUH Series H-36, HHS Publication No. SMA 09-4434). Rockville, MD: SAMHSA.

U.S. Preventive Services Task Force. (2004). Screening and behavioral counseling interventions in primary care to reduce alcohol misuse: recommendation statement. *Annals of Internal Medicine, 140*(7), 554–556.

Willenbring, M. L., Massey, S. H., & Gardner, M. B. (2009). Helping patients who drink too much: an evidence-based guide for primary care clinicians. *American Family Physician, 80*(1), 44–50.

Wilson, J. F. (2009). In the clinic: alcohol use. *Annals of Internal Medicine, 150*(5), ITC3-1, ITC3-13.

World Health Organization (WHO). (2009). *Pharmacological treatment of mental disorders in primary health care.* Retrieved from http://www.who.int/mental_health/management/psychotropic/en/index.html

Wutzke, S. E., Conigrave, K. M., Saunders, J. B., & Halt, W. D. (2002). The long-term effectiveness of brief interventions for unsafe alcohol consumption: a 10-year follow-up. *Addiction, 97*(6), 665–675.

Zhang, Y., Guo, X., Saitz, R., Levy, D., Sartini, E., Niu, J., & Ellison, R. C. (2008). Secular trends in alcohol consumption over 50 years: the Framingham Study. *American Journal of Medicine, 121*(8), 695–701. doi:10.1016/j.amjmed.2008.03.013

Anxiety

Agency for Healthcare Research and Quality (AHRQ). (2008). National healthcare disparities report. Retrieved November 7, 2010, from www.ahrq.gov/qual/nhdr08/chap2b.htm

American Psychiatric Association. (2000). *Diagnostic and statistical manual of mental disorders, fourth edition, text revision (DSM-IV-TR).* Arlington, VA: American Psychiatric Association.

American Psychiatric Association. (n.d.). Practice guidelines.

Calleo, J., & Stanley, M. (2008). Anxiety disorders in later life: differentiated diagnosis and treatment strategies. *Psychiatric Times, 25*(8).

Cassidy, E. L., Lauderdale, S., & Sheikh, J. I. (2005). Mixed anxiety and depression in older adults: clinical characteristics and management. *Journal of Geriatric Psychiatry and Neurology, 18*(2), 83–88.

Cassidy, K., & Rector, N. A. (2008). The silent geriatric giant: anxiety disorders in late life. *Geriatrics and Aging, 11*(3), 150–156.

Chen, H., Coakley, E. H., Cheal, K., Maxwell, J., Costantino, G., Krahn, D. D., . . . Levkoff, S. E. (2006). Satisfaction with mental health services in older primary care patients. *American Journal of Geriatric Psychiatry, 14*(4), 371–379.

Cook, J. M., & O'Donnell, C. (2005). Assessment and psychological treatment of posttraumatic stress disorder in older adults. *Journal of Geriatric Psychiatry and Neurology, 18*(2), 61–71.

First, M. B., Frances, A., & Pincus, H. A. (2002). *DSM-IV-TR handbook of differential diagnosis.* Arlington, VA: American Psychiatric Publishing.

Ford, B. C., Bullard, K. M., Taylor, R. J., Toler, A. K., Neighbors, H. W., & Jackson, J. S. (2007). Lifetime and 12-month prevalence of DSM-IV disorders among older African Americans: findings from the National Survey of American Life (NSAL). *American Journal of Geriatric Psychiatry, 15*(8), 652–659.

Frasure-Smith, N., & Lespérance, F. (2008). Depression and anxiety as predictors of 2-year cardiac events in patients with stable coronary artery disease. *Archives of General Psychiatry, 65*(1), 62–71.

Garakani, A., & Sanjay, J. M. (2006). Neurobiology of anxiety disorders and implications for treatment. *Mount Sinai Journal of Medicine, 73*(7), 941–949.

Hall, Richard C. W., & Hall, Ryan C. W. (2000–2002). Anxiety and endocrine disease. Retrieved April 26, 2012, from www.drrichardhall.com/anxiety.htm

Harvard School of Medicine. (2005). National Comorbidity Survey Replication (NCS-R). Retrieved April 26, 2012, from www.hcp.med.harvard.edu/ncs/index.php

Hegel, M. T., Unützer, J., Tang, L., Arean, P. A., Katon, W., Noel, P. H., . . . Lin, E. H. (2005). Impact of comorbid panic and posttraumatic stress disorder in outcomes of collaborative care for late-life depression in primary care. *American Journal of Geriatric Psychiatry, 13*(1), 48–58.

Himle, J. A., Baser, R. E., Taylor, R. J., Campbell, R. D., & Jackson, J. S. (2009). Anxiety disorders among African Americans, blacks of Caribbean descent, and non-Hispanic whites in the United States. *Journal of Anxiety Disorders, 23*(5), 578–590.

Hollander, E., & Simeon, D. (2008). Anxiety disorders. In R. E. Hales, S. C. Yudofsky, & G. O. Gabbard (Eds.), *The American Psychiatric Publishing textbook of psychiatry* (5th ed., chap. 12). Philadelphia, PA: Mosby.

Kaiser, A. P., Wachen, J. S., Potter, C., Moye, J., & Davison, E. (with the Stress, Health, and Aging Research Program (SHARP)). (2013). Posttraumatic stress symptoms among older adults: a review. Washington, D.C.: U.S. Department of Veterans Affairs. Retrieved from http://www.ptsd.va.gov/professional/pages/ptsd_symptoms_older_adults.asp

Kim, H. F., Kunik, M. E., Molinari, V. A., Hillman, S. L., Lalani, S., Orengo, C. A., . . . Goodnight-White, S. (2000). Functional impairment in COPD patients: the impact of anxiety and depression. *Psychosomatics, 41*(6), 465–471.

Lenze, E. J., Karp, J. F., Mulsant, B. H., Blank, S., Shear, M. K., Houck, P. R., & Reynolds, C. F. (2005). Somatic symptoms in late-life anxiety: treatment issues. *Journal of Geriatric Psychiatry and Neurology, 18*(2), 89–96.

Lenze, E. J., & Wetherell, J. L. (2009). Anxiety disorders. In D. G. Blazer & D. C. Steffens (Eds.), *The American Psychiatric Publishing textbook of geriatric psychiatry* (4th ed., chap. 18). Arlington, VA: American Psychiatric Publishing, Inc.

Mohlman, J. (2005). Does executive dysfunction affect treatment outcome in late-life mood and anxiety disorders? *Journal of Geriatric Psychiatry and Neurology, 18*(2), 97–108.

National Institute of Mental Health. (n.d.). Anxiety disorders. Retrieved from http://www.nimh.nih.gov/health/topics/anxiety-disorders/index.shtml

Rauch, S. A., Morales, M., Knashawn, H., Zubritsky, C., Knott, K., & Oslin, D. (2006). Posttraumatic stress, depression, and health among older adults in primary care. *American Journal of Geriatric Psychiatry, 14*(4), 316–324.

Seignourel, P. J., Kunik, M. E., Snow, L., Wilson, N., & Stanley, M. (2008). Anxiety in dementia: a critical review. *Clinical Psychology Review, 28*(7), 1071–1082.

Sinoff, G., & Werner, P. (2003). Anxiety disorder and accompanying subjective memory loss in the elderly as a predictor of future cognitive decline. *International Journal of Geriatric Psychiatry, 18*(10), 951–959.

Stanley, M. A., Hopko, D. R., Diefenbach, G. J., Bourland, S. L., Rodriguez, H., & Wagener, P. (2003). Cognitive-behavior therapy for late-life generalized anxiety disorder in primary care: preliminary findings. *American Journal of Geriatric Psychiatry, 11*(1), 92–96.

Strik, J. J., Denollet, J., Lousberg, R., & Honig, A. (2003). Comparing symptoms of depression and anxiety as predictors of cardiac events and increased health care consumption after myocardial infarction. *Journal of the American College of Cardiology, 42*(10), 1801–1807.

Wetherell, J. L., Lenze, E. J., & Stanley, M. A. (2005). Evidence-based treatment of geriatric anxiety disorders. *Psychiatric Clinics of North America, 28*(4), 871–896.

Wetherell, J. L., Sorrell, J. T., Thorp, S. R., & Patterson, T. L. (2005). Psychological interventions for late-life anxiety: a review and early lessons from the CALM study. *Journal of Geriatric Psychiatry and Neurology, 18*(2), 72–82.

Bipolar Disorder

Al Jurdi, R. K., Nguyen, Q. X., Petersen, N. J., Pilgrim, P., Gyulai, L., & Sajatovic, M. (2012). Acute bipolar I affective episode presentation across life span. *Journal of Geriatric Psychiatry and Neurology, 25*(1), 6–14. doi:10.1177/0891988712436686

Brennan, J. A., & Rapport, D.(2011). Bipolar disorder. *Essential Evidence Plus.* Retrieved from http://www.essentialevidenceplus.com/search/?query=bipolar+disorder&source=&searchbutton.x=47&searchbutton.y=18

Burgess, S., Geddes, J., Hawton, K., Townsend, E., Jamison, K., & Goodwin, G. (2001). Lithium for maintenance treatment of mood disorders. *Cochrane Database Syst Rev,* (3):CD003013.

Chu, D., Gildengers, A. G., Houck, P. R., Anderson, S. J., Mulsant, B. H., Reynolds, C. F., III, & Kupfer, D. J. (2010). Does age at onset have clinical significance in older adults with bipolar disorder? *International Journal of Geriatric Psychiatry, 25*(12), 1266–1271.

Cipriani, A., Rendell, J. M., & Geddes, J. (2009). Olanzapine in long-term treatment for bipolar disorder. *Cochrane Database of Systematic Reviews* (1):CD004367.

Dhillon, S. (2012). Aripiprazole: a review of its use in the management of mania in adults with bipolar I disorder. *Drugs, 72*(1), 133–162.

Gildengers, A. G., Butters, M. A., Chisholm, D., Rogers, J. C., Holm, M. B., Bhalla, R. K., . . . Mulsant, B. H. (2007). Cognitive functioning and instrumental activities of daily living in late-life bipolar disorder. *American Journal of Geriatric Psychiatry, 15*(2), 174–179.

Gildengers, A. G., Mulsant, B. H., Begley, A. E., McShea, M., Stack, J. A., Miller, M. D., . . . Reynolds, C. F., III. (2005). A pilot study of standardized treatment in geriatric bipolar disorder. *American Journal of Geriatric Psychiatry, 13*(4), 319–323.

Hirschfeld, R. M. A., Bowden, C. L., Gitlin, M. J., Keck, P. E., Suppes, T., Thase, M. E., . . . Workgroup on Bipolar Disorder. (2002). Practice guideline for the treatment of patients with bipolar disorder (2nd ed.). doi: 10.1176/appi.books.9780890423363.50051

Hirschfeld, R. M. A., Holzer, C., Calabrese, J. R., Weissman, M., Reed, M., Davies, M., . . . Hazard, E. (2003). Validity of the mood disorder questionnaire: a general population study. *American Journal of Psychiatry, 160*(1), 178–180.

Hirschfeld, R. M. A., Williams, J. B., Spitzer, R. L., Calabrese, J. R., Flynn, L., Keck, P. E., Jr., . . . Zajecka, J. (2000). Development and validation of a screening instrument for bipolar spectrum disorder: the Mood Disorder Questionnaire. *American Journal of Psychiatry, 157*(11), 1873–1875.

Huang, S.-H., Chung, K.-H., Hsu, J.-L., Wu, J.-Y., Huang, Y.-L., & Tsai, S.-Y. (2012). The risk factors for elderly patients with bipolar disorder having cerebral infarction. *Journal of Geriatric Psychiatry and Neurology, 25*(1), 15–19. doi:10.1177/0891988712436689

Kessing, L. V. (2006). Diagnostic subtypes of bipolar disorder in older versus younger adults. *Bipolar Disorders, 8*(1), 56–64.

Kessler, R. C., Berglund, P., Demler, O., Jin, R., Merikangas, K. R., & Walters, E. E. (2005). Lifetime prevalence and age-of-onset distributions of DSM-IV disorders in the National Comorbidity Survey Replication. *Archives of General Psychiatry, 62*(6), 593–602.

Merikangas, K. R., Akiskal, H. S., Angst, J., Greenberg, P. E., Hirschfeld, R. M., Petukhova, M., & Kessler, R. C. (2007). Lifetime and 12-month prevalence of bipolar spectrum disorder in the National Comorbidity Survey replication. *Archives of General Psychiatry, 64*(5), 543–552.

Morriss, R. K., Faizal, M. A., Jones, A. P., Williamson, P. R., Bolton, C., & McCarthy, J. P. (2007). Interventions for helping people recognise early signs of recurrence in bipolar disorder. *Cochrane Database of Systematic Reviews* (1):CD004854.

Oostervink, F., Boomsma, M. M., Nolen, W. A., & EMBLEM Advisory Board. (2009). Bipolar disorder in the elderly; different effects of age and of age of onset. *Journal of Affective Disorders, 116*(3), 176–183. doi:10.1016/j.jad.2008.11.012

Parikh, S. V., LeBlanc, S. R., & Ovanessian, M. M. (2010). Advancing bipolar disorder: key lessons from the Systematic Treatment Enhancement Program for Bipolar Disorder (STEP-BD). *Canadian Journal of Psychiatry, 55*(3), 136–143.

Perron, B. E., Fries, L. E., Kilbourne, A. M., Vaughn, M. G., & Bauer, M. S. (2010). Racial/ethnic group differences in bipolar symptomatology in a community sample of persons with bipolar I disorder. *Journal of Nervous and Mental Disease, 198*(1), 16–21. doi:10.1097/NMD.0b013e3181c818c5

Price, A. L., & Marzani-Nissen, G. R. (2012). Bipolar disorders: a review. *American Family Physician, 85*(5), 483–493.

Rej, S., Herrmann, N., & Shulman, K. (2012). The effects of lithium on renal function in older adults—a systematic review. *Journal of Geriatric Psychiatry and Neurology, 25*(1), 51–61. doi:10.1177/0891988712436690

Sajatovic, M., Blow, F. C., Ignacio, R. V., & Kales, H. C. (2004). Age-related modifiers of clinical presentation and health service use among veterans with bipolar disorder. *Psychiatric Services (Washington, D.C.), 55*(9), 1014–1021.

Sajatovic, M., & Chen, P. (2011). Geriatric bipolar disorder. *Psychiatric Clinics of North America, 34*(2), 319–333. doi:10.1016/j.psc.2011.02.007

Sajatovic, M., & Chen, P. (2012a). Geriatric bipolar disorder: epidemiology, clinical features, assessment, and diagnosis. *Essential Evidence Plus.* Retrieved from http://www.essentialevidenceplus.com/search/?query=bipolar+disorder&source=&searchbutton.x=47&searchbutton.y=18

Sajatovic, M., & Chen, P. (2012b). Geriatric bipolar disorder: acute treatment. *Essential Evidence Plus.* Retrieved from http://www.essentialevidenceplus.com/search/?query=bipolar+disorder&source=&searchbutton.x=47&searchbutton.y=18

Sajatovic, M., & Chen, P. (2012c). Geriatric bipolar disorder: maintenance treatment and prognosis. *Essential Evidence Plus.* Retrieved from http://www.essentialevidenceplus.com/search/?query=bipolar+disorder&source=&searchbutton.x=47&searchbutton.y=18

Sajatovic, M., Gyulai, L., Calabrese, J. R., Thompson, T. R., Wilson, B. G., White, R., & Evoniuk, G. (2005). Maintenance treatment outcomes in older patients with bipolar I disorder. *American Journal of Geriatric Psychiatry, 13*(4), 305–311

Sherrod, T., Quinlan-Colwell, A., Lattimore, T. B., Shattell, M. M., & Kennedy-Malone, L. (2010). Older adults with bipolar disorder: guidelines for primary care providers. *Journal of Gerontological Nursing, 36*(5), 20–27; quiz 28–29. doi:10.3928/00989134-20100108-05

Shulman, K. I. (2010). Lithium for older adults with bipolar disorder: should it still be considered a first-line agent? *Drugs & Aging, 27*(8), 607–615.

Soreff, S., McInnes, L. A., & Talavera, F. (2012). Bipolar affective disorder treatment and management. *Medscape Reference.* Retrieved from http://emedicine.medscape.com/article/286342

Stovall, J. (2012). Bipolar disorder in adults: epidemiology and diagnosis. *Essential Evidence Plus.* Retrieved from http://www.essentialevidenceplus.com/search/?query=bipolar+disorder&source=&searchbutton.x=47&searchbutton.y=18

Swann, A. C., Lafer, B., Perugi, G., Frye, M. A., Bauer, M., Bahk, W.-M., . . . Suppes, T. (2013). Bipolar mixed states: an International Society for Bipolar Disorders task force report of symptom structure, course of illness, and diagnosis. *American Journal of Psychiatry, 170*(1), 31–42. doi:10.1176/appi.ajp.2012.12030301

Taylor, D. L., & Laraia, M. T. (2009). Psychopharmacology. In G. W. Stuart (Ed.), *Principles and practices of psychiatric nursing* (9th ed., pp. 500–534). St. Louis, MO: Mosby.

Van Gerpen, M. W., Johnson, J. E., & Winstead, D. K. (1999). Mania in the geriatric patient population: a review of the literature. *American Journal of Geriatric Psychiatry, 7*(3), 188–202.

Van Lieshout, R. J., & MacQueen, G. M. (2010). Efficacy and acceptability of mood stabilisers in the treatment of acute bipolar depression: systematic review. *British Journal of Psychiatry, 196*(4), 266–273.

Woltmann, E., Grogan-Kaylor, A., Perron, B., Georges, H., Kilbourne, A. M., & Bauer, M. S. (2012). Comparative effectiveness of collaborative chronic care models for mental health conditions across primary, specialty, and behavioral health care settings: systematic review and meta-analysis. *American Journal of Psychiatry, 169*(8), 790–804.

Wylie, M. E., Mulsant, B. H., Pollock, B. G., Sweet, R. A., Zubenko, G. S., Begley, A. E., . . . Kupfer, D. J. (1999). Age at onset in geriatric bipolar disorder: effects on clinical presentation and treatment outcomes in an inpatient sample. *American Journal of Geriatric Psychiatry, 7*(1), 77–83.

Yatham, L. N., Kennedy, S. H., Schaffer, A., Parikh, S. V., Beaulieu, S., O'Donovan, C., . . . Kapczinski, F. (2009). Canadian Network for Mood and Anxiety Treatments (CANMAT) and International Society for Bipolar Disorders (ISBD) collaborative update of CANMAT guidelines for the management of patients with bipolar disorder: update 2009. *Bipolar Disorders, 11*(3), 225–255. doi:10.1111/j.1399-5618.2009.00672.x

Young, R. C., Schulberg, H. C., Gildengers, A. G., Sajatovic, M., Mulsant, B. H., Gyulai, L., . . . Alexopoulos, G. S. (2010). Conceptual and methodological issues in designing a randomized, controlled treatment trial for geriatric bipolar disorder: GERI-BD. *Bipolar Disorders, 12*(1), 56–67.

Young, R. C., & Shulman, K. I. (2009). Bipolar disorders in late life: early days, gradual progress. *American Journal of Geriatric Psychiatry, 17*(12), 1001–1003.

Delirium

Borja, B., Borja, C. S., & Gade, S. (2007). Psychiatric emergencies in the geriatric population. *Clinics in Geriatric Medicine, 23*(2), 391–400.

Breitbart, W., & Alici, Y. (2012). Evidence-based treatment of delirium in patients with cancer. *Journal of Clinical Oncology, 30*(11), 1206–1214. doi:10.1200/JCO.2011.39.8784

Eeles, E. M., White, S. V., O'Mahony, S. M., Bayer, A. J., & Hubbard, R. E. (2012). The impact of frailty and delirium on mortality in older inpatients. *Age and Ageing, 41*(3), 412–416. doi:10.1093/ageing/afs021

Flacker, J. M. (2010). Delirium. In F. J. Domino (Editor-in-Chief), *The 5-minute clinical consult* (5th ed., pp. 352–353). Philadelphia, PA: Wolters Kluwer/Lippincott Williams & Wilkins.

Flaherty, J. H., Gonzales, J. P., & Dong, B. (2011). Antipsychotics in the treatment of delirium in older hospitalized adults: a systematic review. *Journal of the American Geriatrics Society, 59*(Suppl. 2), S269–S276. doi:10.1111/j.1532-5415.2011.03675.x

Francis, J. (2012). Prevention and treatment of delirium and confusional states. *Essential Evidence Plus.* Retrieved from http://www.essentialevidenceplus.com/search/?query=delirium&source=&searchbutton.x=0&searchbutton.y=0

Girard, T. D., Jackson, J. C., Pandharipande, P. P., Pun, B. T., Thompson, J. L., Shintani, A. K., . . . Ely, E. W. (2010). Delirium as a predictor of long-term cognitive impairment in survivors of critical illness. *Critical Care Medicine, 38*(7), 1513–1520.

Khan, B. A., Zawahiri, M., Campbell, N. L., & Boustani, M. A. (2011). Biomarkers for delirium—a review. *Journal of the American Geriatrics Society, 59*(Suppl. 2), S256–S261. doi:10.1111/j.1532-5415.2011.03702.x

Lemstra, A. W., Kalisvaart, K. J., Vreeswijk, R., van Gool, W. A., & Eikelenboom, P. (2008). Pre-operative inflammatory markers and the risk of postoperative delirium in elderly patients. *International Journal of Geriatric Psychiatry, 23*(9), 943–948.

Lundström, M., Stenvall, M., & Olofsson, B. (2012). Symptom profile of postoperative delirium in patients with and without dementia. *Journal of Geriatric Psychiatry and Neurology, 25*(3), 162–169. doi:10.1177/0891988712455221

Maldonado, J. R. (2008). Pathoetiological model of delirium: a comprehensive understanding of the neurobiology of delirium and an evidence-based approach to prevention and treatment. *Critical Care Clinics, 24*(4), 789–856. doi:10.1016/j.ccc.2008.06.004

Maldonado, J. R., Wysong, A., van der Starre, P. J., Block, T., Miller, C., & Reitz, B. A. (2009). Dexmedetomidine and the reduction of postoperative delirium after cardiac surgery. *Psychosomatics, 50*(3), 206–217.

McAvay, G. J., Van Ness, P. H., Bogardus, S. T., Jr., Zhang, Y., Leslie, D. J., Leo-Summers, L. S., & Inouye, S. K. (2006). Older adults discharged from the hospital with delirium: 1-year outcomes. *Journal of the American Geriatrics Society, 54*(8), 1245–1250.

Neufeld, K. J., Joseph Bienvenu, O., Rosenberg, P. B., Mears, S. C., Lee, H. B., Kamdar, B. B., . . . Needham, D. M. (2011). The John Hopkins Delirium Consortium: a model for collaborating across disciplines and departments for delirium prevention and treatment. *Journal of the American Geriatrics Society, 59*(Suppl. 2), S244–S248.

Overshott, R., Karim, S., & Burns, A. (2009). Cholinesterase inhibitors for delirium (Cochrane review). In *The Cochrane Library 2009*, Issue 1. Chichester, UK: John Wiley & Sons, Ltd.

Pandharipande, P., Jackson, J., & Ely, E. W. (2005). Delirium: acute cognitive dysfunction in the critically ill. *Current Opinion in Critical Care, 11*(4), 360–368.

Quinlan, N., Marcantonio, E. R., Inouye, S. K., Gill, T. M., Kamholz, B., & Rudolph, J. L. (2011). Vulnerability: the crossroads of frailty and delirium. *Journal of the American Geriatrics Society, 59*(Suppl. 2), S262–S268. doi:10.1111/j.1532-5415.2011.03674.x

Robinson, T. N., Raeburn, C. D., Tran, Z. V., Angles, E. M., Brenner, L. A., & Moss, M. (2009). Postoperative delirium in the elderly: risk factors and outcomes. *Annals of Surgery, 249*(1), 173–178. doi:10.1097/SLA.0b013e31818e4776

Rubin, F. H., Neal, K., Fenlon, K., Hassan, S., & Inouye, S. K. (2011). Sustainability and scalability of the Hospital Elder Life Program (HELP) at a community hospital. *Journal of the American Geriatrics Society, 59*(2), 359–365. doi:10.1111/j.1532-5415.2010.03243.x

Sendelbach, S., & Guthrie, P. F. (2009, March). *Acute confusion/ delirium.* Iowa City, IA: University of Iowa Gerontological Nursing Interventions Research Center, Research Translation and Dissemination Core.

Siddiqi, N., Stockdale, R., Britton, A. M., & Holmes, J. (2007). Interventions for preventing delirium in hospitalised patients. *Cochrane Database of Systematic Reviews* (2):CD005563.

Tullmann, D. F., Fletcher, K., & Foreman, M. D. (2012). Delirium. In M. Boltz, E. Capezuti, T. Fulmer, & D. Zwicker (Eds.), *Evidence-based geriatric nursing protocols for best practice* (4th ed., pp. 186–199). New York City, NY: Springer.

Witlox, J., Eurelings, L. S., de Jonghe, J. F., Kalisvaart, K. J., Eikelenboom, P., & van Gool, W. A. (2010). Delirium in elderly patients and the risk of postdischarge mortality, institutionalization, and dementia: a meta-analysis. *Journal of the American Medical Association, 304*(4), 443–451. doi:10.1001/jama.2010.1013

Dementia

Abbey, J., Piller, N., De Bellis, A., Esterman, A., Parker, D., Giles, L., & Lowcay, B. (2004). The Abbey pain scale: a 1-minute numerical indicator for people with end-stage dementia. *International Journal of Palliative Nursing, 10*(1), 6–13.

Albert, M. S., DeKosky, S. T., Dickson, D., Dubois, B., Feldman, H. H., Fox, N. C., . . . Phelps, C. H. (2011). The diagnosis of mild cognitive impairment due to Alzheimer's disease: recommendations from the National Institutes on Aging–Alzheimer's Association workgroups on diagnostic guidelines for Alzheimer's disease. *Alzheimer's & Dementia, 7*(3), 270–279.

Alexopoulos, G. S., Abrams, R. C., Young, R. C., & Shamoian, C. A. (1988). Cornell scale for depression in dementia. *Biological Psychiatry, 23*(3), 271–284.

Alzheimer's Association. (2012). 2012 Alzheimer's disease facts and figures. *Alzheimer's & Dementia, 8*(2), 131–168. doi:10.1016/j.jalz.2012.02.001

American Medical Association. (2010). AMA physician's guide to assessing and counseling older drivers. Retrieved from www.ama-assn.org/ama/pub/physician-resources/public-health/promoting-healthy-lifestyles/geriatric-health/older-driver-safety/assessing-counseling-older-drivers.page

American Psychiatric Association. (2007). Practice guidelines: treatment of patients with Alzheimer's disease and other dementias, second edition. *Psychiatry Online.* doi:10.1176/appi.books.9780890423967.152139

Ariga, T., Miyatake, T., & Yu, R .K. (2010). Role of proteoglycans and glycosaminoglycans in the pathogenesis of Alzheimer's disease and related disorders: amyloidogenesis and therapeutic strategies—a review. *Journal of Neuroscience Research, 88*(11), 2303–2315.

Ballard, C., & Waite, J. (2006). The effectiveness of atypical antipsychotics for the treatment of aggression and psychosis in Alzheimer's disease. *Cochrane Database of Systematic Reviews* (1):CD003476.

Birks, J., & Harvey, M. J. (2002). Donepezil for dementia due to Alzheimer's disease. *Cochrane Database of Systematic Reviews 2002,* Issue 1, Art. No.: CD001190. doi:10.1002/14651858. CD 1190pub2

Carnahan, R. M. (2010). How to manage your patient's dementia by discontinuing medications. *Current Psychiatry, 9*(7), 34–37.

DeSilets, A. R., & Bryant, K. (2010). Dementia. In F. J. Domino (Editor-in-Chief), *The 5-minute clinical consult* (5th ed., pp. 354–355). Philadelphia, PA: Wolters Kluwer/Lippincott Williams & Wilkins.

Ehreke, L., Luppa, M., Luck, T., Wiese, B., Weyerer, S., Eifflaender-Gorfer, S., . . . AgeCoDe group. (2009). Is the clock drawing test appropriate for screening for mild cognitive impairment?—Results of the German study on Ageing, Cognition and Dementia in Primary Care Patients (AgeCoDe). *Dementia and Geriatric Cognitive Disorders, 28*(4), 365–372. doi:10.1159/000253484

Feldman, H. H., Jacova, C., Robillard, A., Garcia, A., Chow, T., Borrie, M., . . . Chertkow, H. (2008). Diagnosis and treatment of dementia: 2. Diagnosis. *Canadian Medical Association Journal, 178*(7), 825–836. doi:10.1503/cmaj.070798

Fletcher, K. (2012). Geriatric nursing protocol: recognition and management of dementia. In M. Boltz, E. Capezuti, T. T. Fulmer, D. Zwicker, & A. O'Meara (Eds.), *Evidence-based geriatric nursing protocols for best practice* (4th ed.). Retrieved from http://consultgerirn.org/topics/dementia/want_to_know_more

Fong, T. G. (2013). Dementia. In F. Ferri (Ed.), *Ferri's clinical advisor 2013* (pp. 302–303). Philadelphia, PA: Elsevier Mosby.

Gauthier, S., Cummings, J., Ballard, C., Brodaty, H., Grossberg, G., Robert, P., & Lyketsos, C. (2010). Management of behavioral problems in Alzheimer's disease. *International Psychogeriatrics/ IPA, 22*(3), 346–372.

Gebretsadik, M., & Grossberg, G. T. (2008). Is it Alzheimer's? How to pare down the possibilities. *Current Psychiatry, 7*(1), 53–62.

Grimes, J. A. & Hatch, L. H. (2010). Alzheimer's disease. In F. J. Domino (Editor in-Chief), *The 5-minute clinical consult* (5th ed., pp. 32–33). Philadelphia, PA: Wolters Kluwer/Lippincott Williams & Wilkins.

Hagen, M. D. (2009). Dementia (diagnosis). *Essential Evidence Plus.* Retrieved from http://www.essentialevidenceplus.com/search/ ?query=dementia&source=&searchbutton.x=11&searchbutton.y=18

Kalapatapu, R. K. (2010, February 9). Dementia: a focused review. *Psychiatric Times.* Retrieved from www.psychiatrictimes.com/articles/dementia-focused-review

Lonergan, E., Luxenberg, J., Colford, J. M., & Birks, J. (2002). Haloperidol for agitation in dementia. *Cochrane Database of Systematic Reviews 2002,* Issue 2, Art. No.: CD002852. doi:10.1002/14651858

McKhann, G. M., Knopman, D. S., Chertkow, H., Hyman, B. T., Jack, C. R., Jr., Kawas, C. H., . . . Phelps, C. H. (2011). The diagnosis of dementia due to Alzheimer's disease: recommendations from the National Institutes on Aging–Alzheimer's Association workgroups on diagnostic guidelines for Alzheimer's disease. *Alzheimer's & Dementia, 7*(3), 263–269.

McShane, R., Areosa Sastre, A., & Minakaran, N. (2006). Memantine for dementia. *Cochrane Database of Systematic Reviews 2006,* Issue 2, Art. No.: CD003154. doi:10.1002/14651858

Mihaescu, R., Detmar, S. B., Cornel, M. C., van der Flier, W. M., Heutink, P., Hol, E. M., . . . Janssens, A. C. (2010). Translational research in genomics of Alzheimer's disease: a review of current practice and future perspectives. *Journal of Alzheimer's Disease, 20*(4), 967–980. doi:10.3233/JAD-2010-1410

Nasreddine, Z. S., Phillips, N. A., Bédirian, V., Charbonneau, S., Whitehead, V., Collin, I., . . . Chertkow, H. (2005). The Montreal Cognitive Assessment, MoCA: a brief screening tool for mild cognitive impairment. *Journal of the American Geriatrics Society, 53*(4), 695–699.

National Institute on Aging. (2012). Alzheimer's disease genetics fact sheet. Retrieved from www.nia.nih.gov/alzheimers/publication/alzheimers-disease-genetics-fact-sheet

Neef, D. (2011). Dementia: Lewy body dementia. *Essential Evidence Plus.* Retrieved from http://www.essentialevidenceplus.com/search/?query=dementia&source=&searchbutton.x=11&searchbutton.y=18

Qaseem, A., Snow, V., Cross, J. T., Jr., Forciea, M. A., Hopkins, R., Jr., Shekelle, P., . . . American College of Physicians/American Academy of Family Physicians Panel on Dementia. (2008). Current pharmacologic treatment of dementia: a clinical practice guideline from the American College of Physicians and the American Academy of Family Physicians. *Annals of Internal Medicine, 148*(5), 370–378.

Rapoport, M., Sarracini, C. Z., Molnar, F., & Herrmann, N. (2008). Driving with dementia: how to assess safety behind the wheel. *Current Psychiatry, 7*(12), 37–48.

Robinson, L., Hutchings, D., Dickinson, H. O., Corner, L., Beyer, F., Finch, T., . . . Bond, J. (2007). Effectiveness and acceptability of non-pharmacological interventions to reduce wandering in dementia: a systematic review. *International Journal of Geriatric Psychiatry, 22*(1), 9–22.

Seitz, D. P., & Gill, S. S. (2012). Review: non-pharmacological interventions delivered by family caregivers improve symptoms in people with dementia. *Evidence Based Mental Health, 16*(1), 22. doi: 10.1136/eb-2012-101095

Shaik, S. S., & Varma, A. R. (2012, January/February). Differentiating the dementias: a neurological approach. *Progress in Neurology and Psychiatry,* pp. 11–18. Retrieved from www.progressnp.com

Shub, D., & Kunik, M. E. (2009). Psychiatric comorbidity in persons with dementia: assessment and treatment strategies. *Psychiatric Times, 26*(4). Retrieved from http://www.psychiatrictimes.com/articles/comorbidity-psychiatric-comorbidity-persons-dementia

Sperling, R. A., Aisen, P. S., Beckett, L. A., Bennett, D. A., Craft, T., Fagan, A. M., . . . Phelps, C. H. (2011). Toward defining the preclinical stages of Alzheimer's disease: recommendations from the National Institute on Aging–Alzheimer's Association workgroups on diagnostic guidelines for Alzheimer's disease. *Alzheimer's & Dementia, 7*(3), 280–292.

Steinberg, M., & Lyketsos, C. G. (2012). Atypical antipsychotic use in patients with dementia: managing safety concerns. *American Journal of Psychiatry, 169*(9), 900–906. doi:10.1176/appi.ajp.2012.12030342

Tariq, S. H., Tumosa, N., Chibnall, J. T., Perry, M. H., III, & Morley, J. E. (2006). Comparison of the Saint Louis University mental status examination and the mini-mental state examination for detecting dementia and mild neurocognitive disorder—a pilot study. *American Journal of Geriatric Psychiatry, 14*(11), 900–910.

Williams, J. W., Plassman, B. L., Burke, J., Holsinger, T., & Benjamin, S. (2010, April). *Preventing Alzheimer's disease and cognitive decline.* Evidence Report/Technology Assessment No. 193. (Prepared by the Duke Evidence-based Practice Center under Contract No. HHSA 290-2007-10066-I.) AHRQ Publication No. 10-E005. Rockville, MD: Agency for Healthcare Research and Quality.

Wulsin, L. R. (2005). Antipsychotics in the elderly: reducing risks of stroke and death. *Current Psychiatry, 4*(11), 75–78.

Depression

American Psychiatric Association. (2000). *Diagnostic and statistical manual of mental disorders, fourth edition, text revision.* Washington, DC: American Psychiatric Association.

Andreescu, C., Mulsant, B. H., Houck, P. R., Whyte, E. M., Mazumdar, S., Dombrovski, A. Y., . . . Reynolds, C. F. (2009, Winter). Empirically derived decision trees for the treatment of late-life depression. *Focus, 7*(1), 79–87.

Bezchlibnyk-Butler, K. Z., & Jeffries, J. J. (2006). *Clinical handbook of psychotropic drugs* (16th ed.). Ashland, OH: Hogrefe & Huber Publications.

Dew, M. A., Whyte, E. M., Lenze, E. J., Houck, P. R., Mulsant, B. H., Pollock, B. G., . . . Reynolds, C. F. (2007). Recovery from major depression in older adults receiving augmentation of antidepressant pharmacotherapy. *American Journal of Psychiatry, 164*(6), 892–899. doi:10.1176/appi.ajp.164.892

Dozois, D. J. A., Seeds, P. M., & Collins, K. A. (2009). Transdiagnostic approaches to the prevention of depression and anxiety. *Journal of Cognitive Psychotherapy, 23*(1), 44–59. doi:10.1891/0889-8391.23.1.44

Gelenberg, A. J. (2009). *Depression symptomatology and neurobiology.* Memphis, TN: Physicians Postgraduate Press, Inc.

Hariri, A. R., & Brown, S. M. (2006). Serotonin. *American Journal of Psychiatry, 163,* 12. doi:10.1176/appi.ajp.163.1.12

Hindi, F., Dew, M. A., Albert, S. M., Lotrich, F. E., & Reynolds, C. F. (2011). Preventing depression in later life: state of the art and science circa 2011. *Psychiatric Clinics of North America, 34*(1), 67–78. doi:10.1016/j.psc.2010.11.008

Kiosses, D. N., Leon, A. C., & Arean, P. A. (2011). Psychosocial interventions for late-life major depression. *Psychiatric Clinics North America, 34*(2), 377–401.

Kiosses, D. N. & Ravdin, L. D. (2010). Psychosocial interventions for depressed older adults with cognitive impairment and disability: improving functionality and quality of life. *Psychiatric Times, 27*(9). Retrieved from http://www.psychiatrictimes.com/articles/psychosocial-interventions-depressed-older-adults-cognitive-impairment-and-disability

Kotbi, N., Mahgoub, N., & Odom, A. (2010). Depression in older adults: how to treat its distinct clinical manifestations. *Current Psychiatry, 9*(8), 39–46.

Lavretsky, H., & Meeks, T. (2009). Late-life depression: managing mood in patients with vascular disease. *Current Psychiatry, 8*(12), 20–38.

Lotrich, F. E., & Pollock, B. G. (2005). Aging and clinical pharmacology: implications for antidepressants. *Journal of Clinical Pharmacology, 45*(10), 1106–1122. doi:10.1177/0091270005280297

Miller, M. D. (2005). Late-life depression: focused IPT eases loss and role changes. *Current Psychiatry, 4*(11), 40–50.

Park, M., & Unützer, J. (2011). Geriatric depression in primary care *Psychiatric Clinics of North America, 34*(2), 469–487. doi:10.1016/j.psc.2011.02.009

Pham, C. B., & Dickman, R. L. (2007). Minimizing adverse drug events in older patients. *American Family Physician, 76*(12), 1837–1844. Retrieved December 5, 2010, from www.aafp.org/afp/2007/1215/p1837.html

Raue, P. J., & Sirey, J. A. (2011). Designing personalized treatment engagement interventions for depressed older adults. *Psychiatric Clinics of North America, 34*(2), 489–500. doi:10.1016/j.psc.2011.02.011

Reynolds, C. F. (2009). Prevention of depressive disorders: a brave new world. *Depression and Anxiety, 26*(12), 1062–1065. doi:10.1002/da.20644

Rubin, S. R. (2011). Depression. *Essential Evidence Plus*. Retrieved from http://www.essentialevidenceplus.com/search/?query=depression&source=&searchbutton.x=0&searchbutton.y=0

Stahl, S. M. (2011). *The prescriber's guide (Stahl's essential psychopharmacology)* (4th ed.). New York City, New York: Cambridge University Press.

Vink, D., Aartsen, M. J., & Schoevers, R. A. (2008). Risk factors for anxiety and depression in the elderly: a review. *Journal of Affective Disorders, 106*(1–2), 29–44.

Wright, K. (2010). Prevention and treatment of depression in care homes. *Nursing & Residential Care, 12*(4), 188–191.

Zizza, A. M., & Shteinlukht, T. P. (2010). Geriatric depression. In F. J. Domino (Editor-in-Chief), *The 5-minute clinical consult* (5th ed., pp. 366–367). Philadelphia, PA: Wolters Kluwer/Lippincott Williams & Wilkins.

Elder Abuse

Administration on Aging. (2012). What is elder abuse? Retrieved April 18, 2012, from www.aoa.gov/aoaroot/aoa_programs/elder_rights/ea_prevention/whatisea.aspx

Bonnel, W. (2012, March 15). Elder abuse: primary care strategies for screening. *Clinical Advisor*. Retrieved March 21, 2012, from www.clinicaladvisor.com/elder-abuse-primary-care-strategies-for-screening/article/232204/#

Chen, A., & Koval, K. J. (2002). Elder abuse: the role of the orthopaedic surgeon in diagnosis and management. *Journal of the American Academy of Orthopedic Surgeons, 10*(1), 25–31.

Cooper, C., Selwood, A., & Livingston, G. (2008). The prevalence of elder abuse and neglect: a systematic review. *Age and Ageing, 37*(2), 151–160. doi:10.1093/ageing/afm194

Cooper, C., Selwood, A., & Livingston, G. (2009). Knowledge, detection, and reporting of abuse by health and social care professionals: a systematic review. *American Journal of Geriatric Psychiatry, 17*(10), 826–838.

Daly, J. M., Merchant, M. L., & Jogerst, G. J. (2011). Elder abuse research: a systematic review. *Journal of Elder Abuse & Neglect, 23*(4), 348–365.

Elder abuse. (2012). U.S. National Library of Medicine, National Institutes of Health. Retrieved April 18, 2012, from www.nlm.nih.gov/medlineplus/elderabuse.html

Elder abuse prevalence and incidence: Fact sheet. (2005). Washington, DC: National Center on Elder Abuse.

Hildreth, C. J., Burke, A. E., & Glass, R. M. (2009). Elder abuse. *Journal of the American Medical Association, 302*(5), 588. doi:10.1001/jama.302.5.588

Lachs, M. (2000). Elder abuse roundtable: detection and diagnosis. U.S. Department of Justice, Office of Justice Programs. National Institute of Justice. Retrieved April 18, 2012, from www.nij.gov/topics/crime/elder-abuse/roundtable/detection-diagnosis.htm

Lippincott's nursing guide to expert elder care. (2011). Ambler, PA: Wolters Kluwer/Lippincott Williams & Wilkins Health.

Ploeg, J., Fear, J., Hutchison, B., MacMillan, H., & Bolan, G. (2009). A systematic review of interventions for elder abuse. *Journal of Elder Abuse & Neglect, 21*(3), 187–210.

Reuben, D. (2013). *Geriatrics at your fingertips* (13th ed.). New York City, NY: American Geriatrics Society.

State Elder Abuse Hotlines. (2012). National Council on Child Abuse and Family Violence. Retrieved April 18, 2012, from www.nccafv.org/state_elder_abuse_hotlines.htm

Touhy, T., & Jett, K. (Eds.) (2011). *Ebersole and Hess' toward healthy aging: human needs and nursing response* (8th ed.). St. Louis, MO: Elsevier Health Sciences.

Grief and Bereavement

Baier, M., & Buechsel, R. (2012). A model to help bereaved individuals understand the grief process. *Mental Health Practice, 16*(1), 28–32.

Block, S. D. (2009). Grief and bereavement. *UpToDate*. Retrieved from http://www.uptodate.com/contents/grief-and-bereavement?detectedLanguage=en&source=search_result&search=grief+and+bereavement&selectedTitle=1%7E84&provider=noProvider

Boelen, P. A., & van den Bout, J. (2008). Complicated grief and uncomplicated grief are distinguishable constructs. *Psychiatry Research, 157*(1–3), 311–314.

Chan, W. C. H., & Chan, C. L. W. (2011). Acceptance of spousal death: the factor of time in bereaved older adults' search for meaning. *Death Studies, 35*(2), 147–162.

Griffin, J. P., Koch, K. A., Nelson, J. E., Cooley, M. E.; & American College of Chest Physicians. (2007). Palliative care consultation, quality-of life measurements, and bereavement for end-of-life care in patients with lung cancer: ACCP evidence-based clinical practice guidelines (2nd edition). *Chest, 132*(3 Suppl.), 404S–422S.

Hefren, J. E., & Thyer, B. A. (2012). The effectiveness of guided mourning for adults with complicated mourning. *Journal of Human Behavior in the Social Environment, 22*(8), 988–1002. doi:10.1080/10911359.2012.707946

Hudson, P., Remedios, C., Zordan, R., Thomas, K., Clifton, D., Crewdson, M., . . . Clarke, D. (2010). *Clinical practice guidelines for the psychosocial and bereavement support of family caregivers of palliative care patients*. Melbourne, Australia: Centre for Palliative Care, St Vincent's Hospital Melbourne.

Institute for Clinical Systems Improvement (ICSI). (2011, November). *Palliative care*. Bloomington, MN: ICSI.

Lobb, E. A., Kristjanson, L. J., Aoun, S. M., Monterosso, L., Halkett, G. K. B., & Davies, A. (2010). Predictors of complicated grief: a systematic review of empirical studies. *Death Studies, 34*(8), 673–698. doi: 10.1080/07481187.2010.496686

Moon, J. R., Kondo, N., Glymour, M. M., & Subramanian, S. V. (2011). Widowhood and mortality: a meta-analysis. *PLoS ONE, 6*(8), e23465. doi:10.1371/journal.pone.0023465

National Consensus Project for Quality Palliative Care. (2009). *Clinical practice guidelines for quality palliative care* (2nd ed.). Pittsburgh, PA: National Consensus Project for Quality Palliative Care.

Pai, M., & Carr, D. (2010). Do personality traits moderate the effects of late-life spousal loss on psychological distress? *Journal of Health and Social Behavior, 51*(2), 183–199.

Shah, S. M., Carey, I. M., Harris, T., DeWilde, S., Victor, C. R., & Cook, D. G. (2012). Do good health and material circumstances protect older people from the increased risk of death after bereavement? *American Journal of Epidemiology, 176*(8), 689–698.

Sorrell, J. M. (2012). Widows and widowers in today's society. *Journal of Psychosocial Nursing and Mental Health Services, 50*(9), 14–18. doi:10.3928/02793695-20120807-04

Stroebe, M., & Schut, H. (1999). The dual process model of coping with bereavement: rationale and description. *Death Studies, 23*(3), 197–224. doi: 10.1080/074811899201046

Stroebe, M., Schut, H., & Stroebe, W. (2007). Health outcomes of bereavement. *Lancet, 370*(9603), 1960–1973.

Truog, R. D., Campbell, M. L., Curtis, J. R., Haas, C. E., Luce, J. M., Rubenfeld, G. D., . . . American Academy of Critical Care Medicine. (2008). Recommendations for end-of-life care in the intensive care unit: a consensus statement by the American College of Critical Care Medicine. *Critical Care Medicine, 36*(3), 953–963.

Utz, R. L., Caserta, M., & Lund, D. (2012). Grief, depressive symptoms, and physical health among recently bereaved spouses. *Gerontologist, 52*(4), 460–471. doi:10.1093/geront/gnr110

Zhang, B., El-Jawahri, A., & Prigerson, H. G. (2006). Update on bereavement research: evidence-based guidelines for the diagnosis and treatment of complicated bereavement. *Journal of Palliative Medicine, 9*(5), 1188–1203.

Insomnia

Bloom, H. G., Ahmed, I., Alessi, C. A., Ancoli-Israel, S., Buysse, D. J., Kryger, M. H., . . . Zee, P. C. (2009). Evidence-based recommendations for the assessment and management of sleep disorders in older persons. *Journal of the American Geriatrics Society, 57*(5), 761–789. doi:10.1111/j.1532-5415.2009.02220.x

Bonnet, M. H., & Arand, D. L. (2012a). Overview of insomnia. *UpToDate.* Retrieved from http://www.uptodate.com/contents/overview-of-insomnia?detectedLanguage=en&source=search_result&search=overview+of+insomnia&selectedTitle=1%7E150&provider=noProvider

Bonnet, M. H., & Arand, D. L. (2012b). Treatment of insomnia. *UpToDate.* Retrieved from http://www.uptodate.com/contents/treatment-of-insomnia?detectedLanguage=en&source=search_result&search=overview+of+insomnia&selectedTitle=3%7E150&provider=noProvider

Bonnet, M. H., & Arand, D. L. (2012c). Types of insomnia. *UpToDate.* Retrieved from http://www.uptodate.com/contents/types-of-insomnia?detectedLanguage=en&source=search_result&search=overview+of+insomnia&selectedTitle=4%7E150&provider=noProvider

Brenes, G. A., Miller, M. E., Stanley, M. A., Williamson, J. D., Knudson, M., & McCall, W. V. (2009). Insomnia in older adults with generalized anxiety disorder. *American Journal of Geriatric Psychiatry, 17*(6), 465–472.

Buysse, D. J. (2008). Chronic insomnia. *American Journal of Psychiatry, 165*(6), 678–686.

De Niet G. J., Tiemens, B. G., Kloos, M. W., & Hutschemaekers, G. J. (2009). Review of systematic reviews about the efficacy of non-pharmacological interventions to improve sleep quality in insomnia. *International Journal of Evidence-Based Healthcare, 7*(4), 233–242. doi:10.1111/j.1744-1609.2009.00142.x

Doghramji, K. (2006). The epidemiology and diagnosis of insomnia. *American Journal of Managed Care, 12*(Suppl. 8), S214–S220.

Fernandez-Mendoza, J., Vgontzas, A. N., Liao, D., Shaffer, M. L., Vela-Bueno, A., Basta, M., & Bixler, E. O. (2012). Insomnia with objective short sleep duration and incident hypertension: the Penn State cohort. *Hypertension, 60*(4), 929–935.

Irwin, M. R., Olmstead, R., & Motivala, S. J. (2008). Improving sleep quality in older adults with moderate sleep complaints: a randomized controlled trial of tai chi chih. *Sleep, 31*(7), 1001–1008.

Krishnan, P., & Hawranik, P. (2008). Diagnosis and management of geriatric insomnia: a guide for nurse practitioners. *Journal of the American Academy of Nurse Practitioners, 20*(12), 590–599. doi:10.1111/j.1745-7599.2008.00366.x

Montgomery, P., & Dennis, J. (2008a). Cognitive behavioural interventions for sleep problems in adults aged 60+ (Cochrane review). In *The Cochrane Library 2008*, Issue 2. Chichester, UK: John Wiley & Sons, Ltd.

Montgomery, P., & Dennis, J. (2008b). Physical exercise for sleep problems in adults aged 60+ (Cochrane review). In *The Cochrane Library 2008*, Issue 2. Chichester, UK: John Wiley & Sons, Ltd.

Morgan, M., Gregory, P., Tomeny, M., David, B. M., & Gascoigne, C. (2012). Self-help treatment for insomnia symptoms associated with chronic conditions in older adults: a randomized controlled trial. *Journal of the American Geriatrics Society, 60*(10), 1803–1810. doi:10.1111/j.1532-5415.2012.04175.x

Morin, C. M., Vallières, A., Guay, B., Ivers, H., Savard, J., Mérette, C., . . . Baillargeon, L. (2009). Cognitive-behavior therapy, singly and combined with medication, for persistent insomnia: acute and maintenance therapeutic effects. *Journal of the American Medical Association, 301*(19), 2005–2015. doi:10.1001/jama.2009.682

Nakazaki, C., Noda, A., Koike, Y., Yamada, S., Murohara, T., & Ozaki, N. (2012). Association of insomnia and short sleep duration with atherosclerosis risk in the elderly. *American Journal of Hypertension, 25*(11), 1149–1155. doi:10.1038/ajh.2012.107

National Institutes of Health. (2005). State of the science conference statement on manifestations and management of chronic insomnia in adults. *Sleep, 28*(9), 1049–1057.

Ong, J. C., Shapiro, S. L., & Manber, R. (2008). Combining mindfulness meditation with cognitive-behavior therapy for insomnia: a treatment-development study. *Behavior Therapy, 39*(2), 171–182.

Ong, J. C., Shapiro, S. L., & Manber, R. (2009). Mindfulness meditation and cognitive behavioral therapy for insomnia: a naturalistic 12-month follow-up. *Explore, 5*(1), 30–36.

Ong, J., & Sholtes, D. (2010). A mindfulness-based approach to the treatment of insomnia. *Journal of Clinical Psychology, 66*(11), 1175–1184. doi:10.1002/jclp.20736

Reid, K. J., Baron, K. G., Lu, B., Naylor, E., Wolfe, L., & Zee, P. C. (2010). Aerobic exercise improves self-reported sleep and quality of life in older adults with insomnia. *Sleep Medicine, 11*(9), 934–940. doi:10.1016/j.sleep.2010.04.014

Schutte-Rodin, S., Broch, L., Buysse, D., Dorsey, C., & Sateia, M. (2008). Clinical guideline for the evaluation and management of chronic insomnia in adults. *Journal of Clinical Sleep Medicine, 4*(5), 487–504.

Sontheimer, D. (2011). Insomnia and sleep disorders. *Essential Evidence Plus.* Retrieved from http://www.essentialevidenceplus.com/search/?query=insomnia+and+sleep+disorders&source=&searchbutton.x=0&searchbutton.y=0

U.S. Food and Drug Administration. (2013, January 10). FDA Drug Safety Communication: risk of next-morning impairment after use of insomnia drugs; FDA requires lower recommended doses for certain drugs containing zolpidem (Ambien, Ambien CR, Edluar, and Zolpimist). Retrieved from www.fda.gov/Drugs/DrugSafety/ucm334033.htm

Yang, P. Y., Ho, K. H., Chen, H. C., & Chien, M. Y. (2012). Exercise training improves sleep quality in middle-aged and older adults with sleep problems: a systematic review. *Journal of Physiotherapy, 58*(3), 157–163. doi:10.1016/S1836-9553(12)70106-6

Young, J. S., Bourgeois, J. A., Hilty, D. M., & Hardin, K. A. (2008). Sleep in hospitalized medical patients, part 1: Factors affecting sleep. *Journal of Hospital Medicine, 3*(6), 473–482. doi:10.1002/jhm.372

Young, J. S., Bourgeois, J. A., Hilty, D. M., & Hardin, K. A. (2009). Sleep in hospitalized medical patients, part 2: Behavioral and pharmacological management of sleep disturbances. *Journal of Hospital Medicine, 4*(1), 50–59. doi:10.1002/jhm.397

Prescription Drug Abuse

Amato, L., Minozzi, S., Davoli, M., & Vecchi, S. (2011). Psychosocial and pharmacological treatments versus pharmacological treatments for opioid detoxification. *Cochrane Database of Systematic Reviews 2011*, Issue 9. Art. No.: CD005031. doi:10.1002/14651858.CD005031.pub4

Babor, T. F., McRee, B. G., Kassebaum, P. A., Grimaldi, P. L., Ahmed, K., & Bray, J. (2007). Screening, Brief Intervention, and Referral to Treatment (SBIRT): toward a public health approach to the management of substance abuse. *Substance Abuse, 28*(3), 7–30.

Back, S. E., Payne, R. L., Simpson, A. N., & Brady, K. T. (2010). Gender and prescription opioids: findings from the National Survey on Drug Use and Health. *Addictive Behaviors, 35*(11), 1001–1007. doi:10.1016/j.addbeh.2010.06.018

Blazer, D. G., & Wu, L.-T. (2009). Nonprescription use of pain relievers by middle-aged and elderly community-living adults: National Survey on Drug Use and Health. *Journal of the American Geriatrics Society, 57*(7), 1252–1257. doi:10.1111/j.1532-5415.2009.02306.x

Culberson, J. W., & Ziska, M. (2008). Prescription drug misuse/abuse in the elderly. *Geriatrics, 63*(9), 22–31.

Gossop, M., & Moos, R. (2008). Substance misuse among older adults: a neglected but treatable problem. *Addiction, 103*(3), 347–348.

Hernandez, S. H., & Nelson, L. S. (2010). Prescription drug abuse: insight into the epidemic. *Clinical Pharmacology & Therapeutics, 88*(3), 307–317. Retrieved from www.nature.com/doifinder/10.1038/clpt.2010.154

Hesse, M., Vanderplasschen, W., Rapp, R., Broekaert, E., & Fridell, M. (2007). Case management for persons with substance use disorders. *Cochrane Database of Systematic Reviews 2007*, Issue 4. Art. No.: CD006265. doi:10.1002/14651858.CD006265.pub2

Kraft, W. K. (2011). Opioid toxicity. *Essential Evidence Plus.* Retrieved from http://www.essentialevidenceplus.com/search/?query=Opioid+toxicity&source=&searchbutton.x=0&searchbutton.y=0

Lofwall, M. R., Schuster, A., & Strain, E. C. (2008). Changing profile of abused substances by older persons entering treatment. *Journal of Nervous and Mental Disease, 196*(12), 898–905.

Maldonado, J. R. (2010). An approach to the patient with substance use and abuse. *Medical Clinics of North America, 94*(6), 1169–1205. doi:10.1016/j.mcna.2010.08.010

Manchikanti, L. (2006). Prescription drug abuse: what is being done to address this new drug epidemic? Testimony before the Subcommittee on Criminal Justice, Drug Policy and Human Resources. *Pain Physician, 9*(4), 287–321.

Manchikanti, L., Abdi, S., Atluri, S., Balog, C. C., Benyamin, R. M., Boswell, M. V., . . . American Society of Interventional Pain Physicians. (2012a). American Society of Interventional Pain Physicians (ASIPP) guidelines for responsible opioid prescribing in chronic non-cancer pain: Part I—evidence assessment. *Pain Physician, 15*(3 Suppl.), S1–S65.

Manchikanti, L., Abdi, S., Atluri, S., Balog, C. C., Benyamin, R. M., Boswell, M. V., . . . American Society of Interventional Pain

Physicians. (2012b). American Society of Interventional Pain Physicians (ASIPP) guidelines for responsible opioid prescribing in chronic non-cancer Pain: Part 2—guidance. *Pain Physician, 15*(3 Suppl.), S67–S116.

Manchikanti, L., Fellows, B., Ailinani, H., & Pampati, V. (2010). Therapeutic use, abuse, and nonmedical use of opioids: a ten-year perspective. *Pain Physician, 13*(5), 401–435.

Manchikanti, L., & Singh, A. (2008). Therapeutic opioids: a ten-year perspective on the complexities and complications of the escalating use, abuse, and nonmedical use of opioids. *Pain Physician, 11*(2 Suppl.), S63–S88.

Mayet, S., Farrell, M., Ferri, M., Amato, L., & Davoli, M. (2004). Psychosocial treatment for opiate abuse and dependence. *Cochrane Database of Systematic Reviews 2004*, Issue 4. Art. No.: CD004330. doi:10.1002/14651858.CD004330.pub2

Office of National Drug Control Policy. (n.d.). Prescription drug abuse. Retrieved from www.whitehouse.gov/ondcp/prescription-drug-abuse

Parr, J. M., Kavanagh, D. J., Cahill, L., Mitchell, G., & McD. Young, R. (2009). Effectiveness of current treatment approaches for benzodiazepine discontinuation: a meta-analysis. *Addiction, 104*(1), 13–24. doi:10.1111/j.1360-0443.2008.02364.x

Pringle, K. E., Ahern, F. K., Heller, D. A., Gold, C. H., & Brown, T. V. (2005). Potential for alcohol and prescription drug interactions in older people. *Journal of the American Geriatrics Society, 53*(11), 1930–1936.

Sehgal, N., Manchikanti, L., & Smith, H. S. (2012). Prescription opioid abuse in chronic pain: a review of opioid abuse predictors and strategies to curb opioid abuse. *Pain Physician, 15*(3 Suppl.), ES67–ES92.

Simoni-Wastila, L., & Yang, H. K. (2006). Psychoactive drug abuse in older adults. *American Journal of Geriatric Pharmacotherapy, 4*(4), 380–394.

Sjøgren, P., Ekholm, O., Peuckmann, V., & Grønbaek, M. (2009). Epidemiology of chronic pain in Denmark: an update. *European Journal of Pain, 13*(3), 287–292. doi:10.1016/j.ejpain.2008.04.007

Substance Abuse and Mental Health Services Administration. (2009). *Results from the 2008 National Survey on Drug Use and Health: national findings.* Rockville, MD: Substance Abuse and Mental Health Services Administration.

Tinsley, J. A. (2011, Winter). Assessment and treatment of substance use disorders. *Focus, IX*(1), 3–14.

Wu, L.-T., & Blazer, D. G. (2011). Illicit and nonmedical drug use among older adults: a review. *Journal of Aging and Health 23*(3), 481–504. doi:10.1177/0898264310386224

unit IV

Complex Illness

chapter 17

Nutritional Support in the Older Adult

LaTroy Navaroli and Lori Martin-Plank

Nutritional issues in older adults are common, and the risks for developing undernutrition and overnutrition malnutrition are multifactorial, with both intrinsic and extrinsic factors contributing to these two prevalent conditions (Loreck, Chimakurthi, & Steinle, 2012). Thus, malnutrition has been defined as a "state of nutrition in which a deficiency or excess of energy, protein and other nutrients causes measurable adverse effects on the tissue/body form (overall body shop, size and composition) and function, and clinical outcomes" (Nieuwenhuizen, Weenen, Rigby, & Hetherington, 2009, p. 160). People are considered undernourished if they have not consumed adequate amounts of food and/or the body fails to absorb or improperly absorbs required nutrients (Reuben, 2007). The National Institute for Health and Clinical Excellence (2012) indicates that patients with a body mass index (BMI) of less than 18.5 kg/m^2, an unintentional weight loss greater than 10% in the last 3 to 6 months, or a BMI of less than 20 kg/m^2 accompanied by unintentional weight loss greater than 5% within the last 3 to 6 months are suffering from undernutrition, a form of malnutrition. Additionally, people who meet the following criteria are at risk of undernutrition: they have eaten little or nothing for more than 5 days and/or are likely to eat little or nothing for 5 days or longer, or they possess a poor absorptive capacity and/or high nutrient losses and/or increased nutritional needs from causes such as catabolism (National Institute for Health and Clinical Excellence, 2012). Overnutrition, a condition that is defined in terms of excess nutrient and caloric energy intake over time, is another form of malnutrition; it contributes to obesity or possibly micronutrient poisoning (Villareal, Apovian, Kushner, & Klein, 2005). The most common type of overnutrition in the United States is due to the regular consumption of excess calories, fats, saturated fats, and cholesterol. However, nutrition should be assessed and addressed by the nurse practitioner whenever there is a suspected deficit of nutrient and/or calorie intake. Such a deficit can result in suboptimal resources for resumption and maintenance of good health at any time, including following illness or stress.

FINANCIAL CAUSES OF MALNUTRITION IN THE ELDERLY

If a patient's nutritional intake is poor due to financial difficulty or the lack of food in the residence, involve family members, with the patient's permission, who may be able to provide or prepare food for their loved one and may be unaware of their loved one's difficulty. Educate the patient on high-quality, calorie-dense food. Offer a consultation with a nutritionist if

For "Nutritional Assessment," refer to Chapters 2 and 4. For "Malnutrition," "Obesity," and "Failure to Thrive," refer to Chapter 14.

the patient's educational needs are more extensive than can be addressed in the nurse practitioner's practice setting.

Evaluate the availability of community support. In many areas programs exist that assist the elderly and/or poor in obtaining food, such as food stamps. The Supplemental Nutrition Assistance Program (SNAP) is a federal program administered by state or local agencies that provides a monthly allotment of food stamp benefits issued via electronic benefit transfer cards (Food Research and Action Center, 2010). As part of Title III C of the Older Americans Act (OAA), adults age 60 and over can attend congregate meal sites for a nutritious meal. If the patient is unable to prepare food, ready-to-eat food is available from a local Meals on Wheels Association of America (2012) branch or other services that are widely available to provide free or low-cost prepared foods delivered to the home. Eligibility based on income is not a prerequisite for receiving the benefit of this program (Kamp, Wellman, & Russell, 2010). Title VI OAA specifically provides nutritional support for Native American, Native Alaskans, and Native Hawaiian older adults (Kamp et al., 2010).

Further information on available resources can be obtained by contacting local elder service providers, assistance agencies, and local social work offices. Food banks can provide information about the criteria used to determine who qualifies for their food. If the patient is a church member, ask the patient if he or she would accept food donations from the church, which are often available for free or at reduced charge to members in need. Additional information on community nutrition programs is delineated in Table 17-1.

FACTORS INFLUENCING MALNUTRITION

Current practice encourages the use of oral food intake to meet the nutritional needs of older adults, in all settings, in patients with the ability to consume food orally. Support this goal by consulting speech therapists when you suspect any patient is not meeting his or her nutritional needs. Work with the speech therapist to determine if adequate intake can be achieved with therapy or diet and food texture modification (Loreck et al., 2012). Illness, disease, and normal sequelae of aging can predispose the elderly patient to a poor appetite or physical disability that affects usual meal consumption. Flavor-enhanced foods have been shown to increase nutritional intake in older adults with decreased taste and smell perception (Henry et al., 2003). Studies have also shown that presenting palatable food to older adults can enhance the desire to eat in patients with loss of appetite (Sørensen, Møller, Flint, Martens, & Raben, 2003).

TABLE 17-1 Community-Based Nutritional Assistance Programs Benefiting Older Adults

PROGRAM	PURPOSE	SERVICE
OAA Title III	Nutrition services for older adults ≥60 years, not based on financial qualifications	Congregate and home-delivered meals; nutrition screening, assessment, and counseling
OAA Title VI	Nutrition and caregiver support services distributed through Tribal organizations or Native Hawaiian Program	Congregate and home-delivered meals; nutrition screening, assessment, and counseling. Additional caregiver and support services are available.
Supplemental Nutrition Assistance Program (SNAP)	Financial assistance for low-income individuals and families to purchase food items	Electronic card benefits to purchase food items
Senior's Farmers Market Nutrition Program	Older adults ≥ age 60 with household incomes not >18.5% of federal poverty limit qualify to use a voucher to obtain produce	Availability of vouchers that can be exchanged for fresh produce at local farmers markets
Feeding America	Nationwide nonprofit organization that consists of a network of >200 food banks and food rescue organizations	Food items for meal preparation are available from local food banks. Home delivery of food items may be available in individual counties.

A complete physical examination of the patient is warranted to determine if there is a physical and treatable cause. A multidisciplinary team evaluation can help determine if there are means, such as therapy or utensil modification, that could ameliorate the problem without the use of nutritional supplementation. Consider the possible benefit of adding an appetite stimulant to the patients' regimen temporarily. If the patient is unable to meet his or her caloric or nutritional needs despite these measures, nurse practitioners must identify the least invasive intervention to increase the patient's intake to meet his or her needs.

ORAL FOOD SUPPLEMENTS

If a patient is unable to meet his or her nutritional needs with the current dietary intake, oral nutritional supplements (ONS) can be recommended. Generally, these are not covered by insurance, but occasionally, a patient will have a plan that will cover these with a diagnosis of malnutrition or protein-calorie malnutrition.

Most oral supplements contain from 240 to 360 calories. Depending on the patient's needs, one to three cans daily can be recommended, with or between meals. See Table 17-2 for a brief comparison of commonly used nutritional supplements. There are subtle differences among products, and most are available in sugar-free versions for use in diabetic patients. Formulas to help with diabetic nutrition while protecting blood glucose control are sold as Boost Glucose Control (Boost, 2012) and Ensure's

Glucerna (Abbott Nutrition, 2012). Nutritional beverages, such as Ensure and Boost, contain a base of calories from carbohydrates, fats, and proteins, with added vitamins and minerals. You will find only subtle differences between these products, and each brand has available specially designed nutritional supplements that have higher levels of particular nutrients, such as protein, to meet a patient's individual needs (see Table 17-2). These products are generally palatable and come in a variety of flavors.

Originally offered only in hospitals, the makers of these products also make nutritionally enhanced shakes and snack bars, and they can be found at most retail food suppliers. Determine what your patients need to help choose the best product for them. For homebound older adults, arrangements can be made with many of the manufacturers to ship products directly to the home (often with free shipping when meeting a minimum purchase).

NUTRITIONAL SUPPLEMENTS AND THE HOSPITALIZED PATIENT

Poor oral food intake is an independent risk factor for mortality in inpatients (Hiesmayr et al., 2009). Add ONS to your patients' diets when appropriate. Add 240 mL of your facility's preferred ONS to your hospitalized patients' diets 2 to 3 times daily to increase caloric and nutritional intake when poor appetite has been identified and lasts longer than

TABLE 17-2	Nutritional Comparison of Common Nutritional Supplements						
	MANUFACTURER	CALORIES	PROTEIN (G)	FAT (G)	SODIUM (MG)	CARBS (G)	SUGAR (G)
Boost	Nestle	240	10	4	150	41	25
Boost Plus	Nestle	360	14	14	200	45	22
Carnation Instant Breakfast (in 1 cup skim milk)	Nestle	220	13	0.05	190	39	31
Ensure	Abbott	250	9	6	200	40	23
Ensure Plus	Abbott	350	13	11	220	50	20
Glucerna	Abbott	237	9.9	12.9	220	22.8	6

3 days. Check with your facility's dietitian to see if he or she can supplement the patients' diets with calorie- and nutrient-enhanced foods. Consult a speech therapist to determine if dysphagia or aspiration risks are present and affecting oral intake (Loreck et al., 2012).

A systemic review of 36 articles on oral nutrition supplements in adults, across settings, with a mean age of 74 years found benefits in those given a high-protein supplement (Cawood, Elia, & Stratton, 2012). These benefits included increased weight, improved grip strength, reduced complications, reduced readmissions to hospital, and little reduction in normal food intake. Clear clinical and economic benefits result. There was insufficient evidence to determine if ONS *not* containing high levels of protein afforded the same benefits.

The rate of postoperative complications appears to be higher in patients who are malnourished (Karl et al., 2011). A review of 21 relevant studies of supplements used in surgical patients found that an immunomodulating enteral diet containing increased amounts of arginine and fish oil used in high-risk patients undergoing major surgery appears to reduce infections, wound complications, and length of stay (Marik & Zaloga, 2010). Supportive nutritional therapy may help optimize clinical outcomes of malnourished surgical patients, although more research is needed to determine optimal supplementation in this subgroup.

NUTRITION AND WOUND HEALING

Although malnutrition was identified as a risk factor for poor healing as long ago as the 1980s, the assessment of nutrition and interventions related to correction of inadequate nutrition has developed more recently (Posthauer, 2012). Malnutrition, inadequate protein intake, and unintended weight loss have been identified as independently increasing the risk of developing pressure ulcers (Banks, Bauer, Graves, & Ash, 2009; Shahin et al., 2010).

Patients given ONS develop fewer pressure ulcers, and their existing pressure ulcers heal faster (Anholt et al., 2010; Ohura, Nakajo, Okada, & Adachi, 2011). These effects are seen in patients on oral as well as enteral supplemental feedings, even if the patient is not considered malnourished (Anholt et al., 2010). Although there are no specific, evidence-based guidelines to direct the supplementation of wounded patients, providing ONS in addition to regular food intake corrects deficiencies of macronutrients and micronutrients and provides nutrients for safeguarding and strengthening tissue and supporting tissue repair.

The 2009 National Pressure Ulcer Advisory Panel (NPUAP) guidelines recommend assessment of patients at risk of malnutrition and pressure ulcers and referral to an interdisciplinary team including a registered dietitian. Assessment of nutrition in relation to healing is addressed along with other factors affecting pressure ulcer development, with a recommendation of the Braden Scale (www.bradenscale.com), a validated scale commonly used in the United States to assess for pressure ulcer risk (Kottner, Halfens, & Dassen, 2009).

Many nutritional supplements available over the counter, such as Ensure and Boost, can be recommended for enhancement of wound healing in those with calorie and protein malnutrition. When extra calories are not desirable for the enhancement of healing in the normal-weight or overweight adult, consider the use of whey protein supplements, which are low in calories in the powder form, widely available, and inexpensive. A role for specific addition of arginine to healing patients' diets has been discussed and examined for benefit, but to date, the therapeutic effect of arginine supplementation on healing wounds and its possible role in enhancing the healing of acute and chronic wounds in humans is undetermined as is how much arginine is recommended to meet metabolic needs during wound healing (Anholt et al., 2010; Brewer et al., 2010; Debats et al., 2009; Stechmiller, Childress, & Cowan, 2005). There are many ONS available that have been designed specifically to meet the needs of the healing patient, with protein, some including arginine, and other nutrients. See Table 17-3 for a comparison of ONS designed to optimize wound healing. Some recent studies suggest there is a benefit to the healing patient in adding a fish oil supplement to the patient's diet. Benefits measured include improvement in inflammation markers in wounds and faster healing (McDaniel, Belury, Ahijevych, & Blakely, 2008; McDaniel, Massey, & Nicolaou, 2011; Theila et al., 2012). Current research is not adequate to create evidence-based recommendations for optimal micronutrient intake in the healing patient. It is interesting to note that research to date has not found a benefit to patients with dementia in terms of pressure sore prevention or healing when receiving enteral feedings (Teno et al., 2012).

TABLE 17-3	Comparison of Common Nutritional Supplements Used to Enhance Wound Healing							
	PROSTAT AWC	JUVEN (UNFLAVORED)	PROSOURCE POWDER	PROSOURCE ZAC	LPS 15/30	ARGINAID	ARGINAID EXTRA	BENEPROTEIN
Manufacturer	Medical Nutrition USA, Inc. (a division of Nutricia, North America)	Abbott Nutrition	National Nutrition	National Nutrition	ND Labs	Nestle Nutrition	Nestle Nutrition	Nestle Nutrition
Calories/serving	108	70	30	70	100	45	250	25
Serving size	30 mL	24 g powder	1 scoop/7.5 g	30 mL	30 mL	9.2 g powder	237 mL/brik pak	1 scoop/7 gram packet
Total protein (g)	17	0	6	17	15		10.5	6
Arginine (g)	2.5	7	0	3.2	0	4.5	4.5	0
Vitamin C (mg)	175	0	0	175	0	156	250	0
Zinc (mg)	10	0	0	10	0	0	15	0
Phosphorus (mg)	5.9	0	23	55	10	0	850	15
Potassium (mg)	3.9	0	18.9	25	23	5	<22	35
Carbohydrates (g)	10.2	4	0	0	8	2	52	0
Sugar (g)	10.2	0	0	0		0	52	0
Sodium (mg)	13	0	30	40	14	30	<70	15

ENTERAL NUTRITION IN THE HOSPITALIZED PATIENT

When the hospitalized patient is unable to consume enough to meet his or her metabolic needs orally and the patient or his or her health-care proxy desires, refeeding, enteral nutrition (EN) is appropriate. Consider enteral feedings if the hospitalized patient is malnourished or at risk of malnutrition.

In a patient in whom a long-term solution to inadequate oral feeding is desired, gastrostomy tube insertion can be considered. In some cases, such as anticipated short-term inadequate oral intake in which the patient cannot use oral supplements, a nasogastric tube is more appropriate. Common reasons to consider gastrostomy tube insertion include dysphagia following stroke, malignancy with accompanying dysphagia, dementia, and neurological disease (Malmgren et al., 2011).

Enteral nutrition consists of delivery of enteral products as feedings through an enteral access device into a functioning gastrointestinal (GI) tract. For EN to be effective and safe, the patient must have a GI tract with sufficient length and absorptive capacity to obtain nutritional benefit (Bankhead et al., 2009). Enteral feeding via gastrostomy tube placement should be considered for patients whose need for supplemental feedings exceeds 4 weeks or is likely to be permanent. Patients with upper GI dysfunction or an inaccessible upper GI tract should be considered for placement of a postpyloric, duodenal, or jejunal access feeding device (National Institute for Health and Clinical Excellence, 2006). Consider the risks and benefits before placing a permanent feeding device.

A.S.P.E.N., the American Society for Parenteral and Enteral Nutrition, recommends that enteral feedings begin postoperatively in most surgical patients within 24 to 48 hours; feedings via percutaneous endoscopic gastrostomy (PEG) tube may begin within 2 hours of placement in adult patients (Bankhead et al., 2009).

Early initiation of EN in those patients unable to eat on admission may have a positive effect on patient outcome. In critically ill patients, a small study ($n = 36$) found fewer episodes of pneumonia, faster wean from ventilator, and reduced mortality rate in patients in whom enteral nutrition was started within 24 hours of admission (Woo et al., 2010).

A formulary should be available to the nurse practitioner that lists available EN formulas specific to the institution. The EN must be chosen based on patient population and estimated nutritional needs (Bankhead et al., 2009). It is appropriate to enlist the support of a nutritionist to help determine patients' energy and nutrition needs in their current state of health. Enteral tube feeding should be stopped when the patient has established an adequate oral intake.

COMPLICATIONS

Although gastrostomy insertion is relatively straightforward, it is not without the possibility of complications in the elderly as well as in other vulnerable groups of patients. A multidisciplinary approach is necessary to ensure that the procedure is appropriate for the patient. Predictors of increased risk of postgastrostomy tube insertion mortality include advanced age, diabetes, and low BMI (less than 18.5) (Janes, Price, & Khan, 2005; Zopf et al., 2011).

Enteral feedings in the hospitalized patient can contribute to GI motility disorders. The most commonly seen problems are constipation and diarrhea. Assess your patients daily for signs and symptoms of these disorders, and provide the appropriate interventions as needed. Hospitalized patients with delayed gastric emptying who are not tolerating enteral tube feeding should be given a pro-motility agent unless there is a pharmacological cause that can be corrected or a question of bowel obstruction (National Institute for Health and Clinical Excellence, 2006). If delayed gastric emptying continues to limit feeding into the stomach despite pro-motility medication, postpyloric enteral tube feeding or parenteral nutrition should be considered (National Institute for Health and Clinical Excellence, 2006).

REFEEDING SYNDROME

Patients entering the hospital with diagnoses of cachexia and malnutrition present a special challenge in terms of improving nutritional status while preventing refeeding syndrome. Risk factors for developing this condition include patients with a BMI of less than 18.5, unintentional weight loss of more than 10% within the last 3 to 6 months, and limited or no nutritional intake for more than 5 days. Additionally, patients who also have a history of alcohol abuse or are on diuretics, antacids, or chemotherapeutic agents experiencing any of the above nutritional abnormalities are at increased risk. Refeeding syndrome, though potentially fatal, is preventable. This problem, with its hallmark hypophosphatemia, hypomagnesemia, hypokalemia, and thiamine deficiency, presents most commonly in severely cachectic patients who receive rapid refeeding after a period of undernutrition (Sunnoqrot, Kant, May, & Gambert, 2012). Consider ordering baseline laboratory measures for malnourished older adults at risk for refeeding syndrome, including phosphorus, magnesium, calcium, sodium, prealbumin, glucose, renal and liver function, serum vitamin B_{12}, and serum folate levels (Sunnoqrot et al., 2012).

Refeeding syndrome is most commonly seen in patients receiving enteral feedings by nasogastric or PEG tube and in patients receiving parenteral feeding (Ormerod, Farrer, Harper, & Lal, 2010; Zeki, Culkin, Gabe, & Nightingale, 2011). A decrease in serum phosphate to less than 0.6 mmol/L is indicative of refeeding syndrome characterized by hypophosphatemia and electrolyte shifts. Patients to monitor for this risk include those with dysphagia, those who are chronically undernourished, and those with little or no food intake for more than 10 days (Mehanna, Nankivell, Moledina, & Travis, 2009). It is appropriate to check serum phosphate levels daily in patients at risk of refeeding syndrome (National Institute for Health and Clinical Excellence, 2006).

Consult with experts trained in nutritional support of older adults to be involved in the care of these vulnerable patients (Sunnoqrot et al., 2012). Refeeding should be ordered at the rate of 10 kcal/kg per day in patients at risk and increased slowly over days; smaller amounts are recommended in extreme cases. Thiamine, vitamin B complex, and multivitamin supplements should be started with refeeding. New guidelines state that prefeeding correction of electrolyte and fluid deficits is unnecessary but should be done concurrently with refeeding (National Institute for Health and Clinical Excellence, 2006).

NUTRITION IN PALLIATIVE CARE

Patients in palliative care often are unable to meet their nutritional needs with oral diet alone. Management of this can involve oral nutritional supplements, enteral feeding, or parenteral feeding. The information included in this chapter addresses oral and enteral supplementation.

In curative treatment, nutritional care is intended to enhance response to treatment while minimizing complications and morbidity. In contrast, in palliative care, the goal of nutritional intervention is to improve the patient's quality of life (Caro, Laviano, & Pichard, 2007). Ethical care is provided in cases involving end-of-life care by including the patient in decisions about adding alternate forms of nutrition. Nurse practitioners make recommendations regarding supplemental nutrition in palliative care after considering the wishes and goals of the patient and his or her family. One study of palliative care in colorectal cancer patients found that early addition of parenteral nutrition to oral diet including ONS resulted in less weight loss and improved quality of life as compared to patients simply given ONS in addition to oral diet (Hasenberg, Essenbreis, Herold, Post, & Shang, 2010). The effect of supplemental nutrition on mortality, morbidity, and quality of life in palliative care patients warrants more study before definitive recommendations can be provided.

Consider risks and benefits of the type and route of supplementation used. Although some studies suggest that patients in palliative care may benefit from nutritional supplementation with improved quality and length of life, more research is needed to strengthen the evidence in this area (Good, Cavenaugh, Mather, & Ravenscroft, 2008).

ORAL NUTRITIONAL SUPPLEMENTATION IN PALLIATIVE CARE

Request that speech therapy evaluate the patient to assess the need for physical assistance with feeding, which can ameliorate early fatiguing during mealtime. Dysphagia therapy or adaptive equipment may improve patients' ability to consume adequate food orally. To increase patients' oral intake, adding ONS is a simple and noninvasive strategy (Caro et al., 2007). Supplementation can lead to increased body weight accompanied by improvement in quality of life in patients in palliative care. If the patient is unable to maintain a safe and adequate oral intake with the addition of ONS, consider enteral nutritional therapy.

ENTERAL FEEDING IN PALLIATIVE CARE

Malnutrition and cachexia adversely affect cancer patients' quality of life at many points during the course of their care. During noncurative phases of cancer treatment, improved nutrition via enteral feeding can improve the patient's quality of life by decreasing nausea, vomiting, and pain related to eating. It can also postpone loss of autonomy (Caro et al., 2007).

Oral feeding problems and weight loss in dementia patients are expected in the late course of the disease, at a point where it is not possible to determine the patient's desires (Cullen, 2011). In addition, oral feeding may actually increase the risk of developing pneumonia due to aspiration (Good et al., 2008). In view of conflicting results from recent research about whether enteral feeding improves nutrition and length of life, particular care should be taken in deciding whether patients with dementia should have a gastrostomy (Attanasio et al., 2009; Freeman, Ricevuto, & DeLegge, 2010; Higaki, Yokota, & Ohishi, 2008; Regnard, Leslie, Crawford, Mathews, & Gibson, 2010; Sampson & Jones, 2009).

There is no strong evidence to indicate that enteral feeding in patients with dementia improves nutrition or is effective in prolonging survival, improving quality of life, or lessening the risk of pressure sores. In addition, enteral feeding may increase the risk of developing pneumonia due to aspiration (Good et al., 2008). Decisions regarding EN during end-of-life care or where patients are not lucid enough to make an informed judgment are particularly challenging and must be made on a case-by-case basis, considering the patient's wishes, if known.

A multidisciplinary approach is appropriate to determine if all of the patient's needs have been assessed. Request a consultation from a speech and language therapist to evaluate for dysphagia, which is common in late dementia (Freeman et al., 2010), as well as other neurological disorders, including Parkinson's disease, and head and neck malignancies (Lin, Lin, & Liou, 2011). Educate the family about the possible complications and the possibility that the patient may need to be restrained, should a feeding tube be inserted, to prevent unintentional removal (Teno et al., 2011). Query the family regarding their feelings about how enteral feeding may affect their perception of their loved one's end-of-life experience. Offer the alternative of comfort feeding, in which the patient is offered safe and preferred foods in a supported and assisted environment as desired (Palecek et al., 2010).

PARENTERAL NUTRITION

Oral and enteral nutrition should be the first feeding alternative choice for any geriatric patient. However, in patients unable to meet their nutritional needs orally and for whom enteral nutrition is contraindicated, parenteral nutrition is a generally safe method of nutritional support. It should be considered in any patient facing a period of 3 days of no oral or enteral nutritional intake (Sobotka et al., 2009). Parenteral nutrition carries its own set of risk factors and complications, not to mention a higher level of nursing involvement for safe care. It should be reserved for those patients for whom parenteral nutrition is indicated, considering individual factors such as probable survival, rehabilitation potential, and risk of complication (Sobotka et al., 2009) as well as the patient's desires.

CLINICAL RECOMMENDATION	EVIDENCE RATING	REFERENCES
In older adult patients unable to meet their nutritional needs with their current oral dietary intake, high-protein oral nutritional supplements (ONS) provide benefits.	A	Cawood et al. (2012)
Enteral nutrition containing fish oil and arginine reduces infections, wound complications, and length of stay in malnourished surgical patients.	A	Marik & Zaloga (2010)
Malnutrition, inadequate protein intake, and unintended weight loss are independent risk factors for the development of pressure ulcers.	A	Banks et al. (2009) Cowan, Stechmiller, Rowe, & Kairalla (2012) Shahin et al. (2010)
Early initiation of enteral nutrition in critically ill patents unable to eat on admission to the hospital has a positive effect on patient outcomes, including reduced mortality.	B	Woo et al. (2010)
Risk factors for increased mortality after gastrostomy tube insertion include advanced age, low BMI (<18.5), and diabetes mellitus.	B	Janes et al. (2005) Zopf et al. (2011)
Enteral feedings in patients with dementia may not improve nutrition, prolong survival, improve quality of life, or lessen the risk of pressure sores.	C	Good et al. (2008)

A = consistent, good-quality, patient-oriented evidence; B = inconsistent or limited-quality, patient-oriented evidence; C = consensus, disease-oriented evidence, usual practice, expert opinion, or case series. For information about the SORT evidence rating system, go to www.aafp.org/afpsort.xml.

CASE STUDY

A. D., an 80-year-old widow, is brought to see you by her concerned daughter, who reports that her mother is not eating and has lost 15 lb in the past 8 months—"her clothes just hang on her now." A. D. lives alone in an apartment in low-income senior housing. She has been independent in activities of daily living (ADLs), and her daughter takes her shopping or shops for her. Recently her daughter has noticed spoiled food in the refrigerator, and A. D. seems to be tired all the time, despite her claim that she sleeps well at night. When asked about eating, A. D. responds, "I just don't have an appetite like I used to. It seems like so much trouble to cook a meal just for me."

Past medical history: coronary artery disease, currently stable—has prescription for Nitrostat 0.4 mg SL as needed for chest pain but has never had to use the medication. Hypertension, currently stable—takes Vaseretic 10 to 25 mg once daily. Hyperlipidemia—stable—takes simvastatin 20 mg PO daily in evening. The patient also takes vitamin D_3 2000 IU PO daily and omega-3 Fish oil daily at bedtime. The patient has no known drug allergies.

A.D. is a retired homemaker and high school graduate. Her husband has been deceased for 5 years. She has three children, all alive and well; her oldest daughter lives nearby, and her other two children live far away but keep in touch by phone.

A.D. likes to play Bingo at senior housing. She participates in no other activities but has friends in the building. A.D. denies any change in status or any acute health problems outside of feeling more tired than usual and having a poor appetite.

Objective: Petite, slender older woman, using a cane for support, appears her stated age; well-groomed but clothing is too large.

Blood pressure (BP) 134/78 mm Hg, pulse 84 and regular, respiratory rate 16 breaths/min and afebrile. Height 58 inches, weight 88 lb, BMI 18.4. Last visit 6 months ago, weight was 100 lb, BMI was 22. Physical examination unremarkable.

1. What additional subjective data are you seeking?
2. What additional objective data will you be assessing for?
3. What national guidelines are appropriate to consider?
4. What tests will you order?
5. What are the differential diagnoses that you are considering?
6. What is your plan of care?
7. Are there any Healthy People 2020 objectives that you should consider?
8. What additional patient education may be needed?
9. Will you be looking for a consultation?

REFERENCES

Abbott Nutrition. (2012). Adult oral nutrition. Retrieved from http://abbottnutrition.com/Adult/Adult-Oral-Nutrition-Products.aspx

Anholt, R. D., Sobotka, L., Meijer, E. P., Heyman, H., Groen, H. W., Topinkova, E., . . . Schols, J. M. (2010). Specific nutritional support accelerates pressure ulcer healing and reduces wound care intensity in non-malnourished patients. *Nutrition, 26*(9), 867–872.

Attanasio, A., Bedin, M., Stocco, S., Negrin, V., Biancon, A., Cecchetto, G., & Tagliapietra, M. (2009). Clinical outcomes and complications of enteral nutrition among older adults. *Minerva Medica, 100*(2), 159–166.

Bankhead, R., Boullata, J., Brantley, S., Corkins, M., Guenter, P., Krenitsky, J., . . . A.S.P.E.N. Board of Directors. (2009). A.S.P.E.N. enteral nutrition practice recommendations. *Journal of Parenteral and Enteral Nutrition, 33*(2), 122–167. doi:10.1177/0148607108330314

Banks, M., Bauer, J., Graves, N., & Ash, S. (2009). Malnutrition and pressure ulcer risk in adults in Australian health care facilities. *Nutrition, 26*(9), 896–901.

Boost. (2012). Which BOOST is right for my patients? Retrieved from http://www.boost.com/healthcare-professionals

Brewer, S., Desneves, K., Pearce, L., Mills, K., Dunn, L., Brown, D., & Crowe, T. (2010). Effect of an arginine-containing nutritional supplement on pressure ulcer healing in community spinal patients. *Journal of Wound Care, 19*(7), 311–116.

Caro, M., Laviano, A., & Pichard, C. (2007). Impact of nutrition on quality of life during cancer. *Current Opinion in Clinical Nutrition and Metabolic Care, 10*(4), 480–487.

Cawood, A. L., Elia, M., & Stratton, R. J. (2012). Systematic review and meta-analysis of the effects of high protein oral nutritional supplements. *Ageing Research Reviews, 11*(2), 278–296.

Centers for Medicare and Medicaid Services. (2010). National health expenditure projections 2010–2020. Retrieved from https://www.cms.gov/Research-Statistics-Data-and-Systems/Statistics-Trends-and-Reports/NationalHealthExpendData/downloads/proj2010.pdf

Coleman, K., Austin, B., Brach, C., & Wagner, E. (2009). Evidence on the chronic care model in the new millennium. *Health Affairs, 28*(1), 75–85.

Conwell, L., & Boult, C. (2008). The effects of complications and comorbidities on the quality of preventive diabetes care: a literature review. *Population Health Management, 11*(4), 217–228.

Cowan, L. J., Stechmiller, J. K., Rowe, M., & Kairalla, J. A. (2012). Enhancing Braden pressure ulcer risk assessment in acutely ill adult veterans. *Wound Repair and Regeneration, 20*(2), 137–148. doi:10.1111/j.1524-475X.2011.00761.x

Cullen, S. (2011). Symposium 1: gastrostomy tube feeding in adults: the risks, benefits, and alternatives. *Proceedings of the Nutrition Society, 70*(3), 293–298.

Debats, I. B., Wolfs, T. G., Gotoh, T., Cleutiens, J. P., Peutz-Kootstra, C. J., & van der Hulst, R. R. (2009). Role of arginine in superficial wound healing in man. *Nitric Oxide: Biology and Chemistry, 21* (3–4), 175–183.

European Pressure Ulcer Advisory Panel and National Pressure Ulcer Advisory Panel. (2009). *Prevention and treatment of pressure ulcers: quick reference guide.* Retrieved from http://www.npuap.org/wp-%09content/uploads/2012/03/Final_Quick_Prevention_for_web_2010.pdf

Food Research and Action Center. (2010). SNAP/food stamps. Retrieved from http://frac.org/federal-foodnutrition-programs/snapfood-stamps

Freeman, C., Ricevuto, A., & DeLegge, M. H. (2010). Enteral nutrition in patients with dementia and stroke. *Current Opinion in Gastroenterology, 26*(2), 156–159.

Good, P., Cavanagh, J., Mather, M., & Ravenscroft, P. (2008). Medically assisted nutrition for palliative care in adult patients. *Cochrane Database of Systemic Reviews, 2008* (4). doi:10.1002/14651858.CD006274.pub2

Hasenberg, T., Essenbreis, M., Herold, A., Post, S., & Shang, E. (2010). Early supplementation of parenteral nutrition is capable of improving quality of life, chemotherapy-related toxicity and body composition in patients with advanced colorectal carcinoma undergoing palliative treatment: results from a prospective, randomized clinical trial. *Colorectal Disease, 12*(10), 190–199. doi:10.1111/j.1463-1318.2009.02111.x

Henry, C. J., Woo, J., Lightowler, H. J., Yip, R., Lee, R., Hui, E., . . . Seyoum, T. A. (2003). Use of natural food flavours to increase food and nutrient intakes in hospitalized elderly in Hong Kong. *International Journal of Food Sciences and Nutrition, 54*(4), 321–327.

Hiesmayr, M., Schindler, K., Pernicka, E., Schuh, C., Schoeniger-Hekele, A., Bauer, P., . . . Ljungqvist, O. (2009). Decreased food intake is a risk factor for mortality in hospitalised patients: the NutritionDay survey 2006. *Clinical Nutrition, 28*(5), 484–491.

Higaki, F., Yokota, O., & Ohishi, M. (2008). Factors predictive of survival after percutaneous endoscopic gastrostomy in the elderly: is dementia really a risk factor? *American Journal of Gastroenterology, 103*(4), 1011–1016.

Janes, S. E., Price, C. S., & Khan, S. (2005). Percutaneous endoscopic gastrostomy: 30-day mortality trends and risk factors. *Journal of Postgraduate Medicine, 51*(1), 23–29.

Kamp, B., Wellman, N. S., & Russell, C. (2010). Position of the American Dietetic Association, American Society for Nutrition, and Society for Nutrition Education: food and nutrition programs for community-residing older adults. *Journal of Nutrition Education and Behavior, 42*(2), 72–82.

Karl, A., Staehler, M., Bauer, R., Tritschler, S., Hocaoglu, Y., Buchner, A., . . . Rittler, P. (2011). Malnutrition and clinical outcome in urological patients. *European Journal of Medical Research, 16*(10), 469–472.

Kottner, J., Halfens, R., & Dassen, T. (2009). An interrater reliability study of the assessment of pressure ulcer risk using the Braden scale and the classification of pressure ulcers in a home care setting. *International Journal of Nursing Studies, 46*(10), 1307–1312.

Lawton, M., & Brody, E. (1969). Assessment of older people: self-maintaining and instrumental activities of daily living. *The Gerontologist, 9*(3), 179–186.

Lin, Y. L., Lin, I. C., & Liou, J. C. (2011). Symptom patterns of patients with head and neck cancer in a palliative care unit. *Journal of Palliative Medicine, 14*(5), 556–559.

Loreck, E., Chimakurthi, R., & Steinle, N.I. (2012). Nutritional assessment of the geriatric patient: a comprehensive approach toward evaluating and managing nutrition. *Clinical Geriatrics, 20*(4), 20–26.

Lorig, K., Ritter, P., Laurent, D., Plant, K., Green, M., Jernigan, V., & Case, S. (2010). Online diabetes self-management program: a randomized study. *Diabetes Care, 33*(6), 1275–1281.

Malmgren, A., Wärn Hede, G., Karlström, B., Cederholm, T., Lundquist, P., Wirén, M., & Faxén-Irving, G. (2011). Indications for percutaneous endoscopic gastrostomy and survival in old adults. *Food & Nutrition Research, 55*(10). doi:10.3402/fnr.v55i0.6037

Marik, P. E., & Zaloga, G. P. (2010). Immunonutrition in high-risk surgical patients: a systematic review and analysis of the literature. *Journal of Parenteral and Enteral Nutrition, 34*(4), 378–386.

Maslow, M., & Mezey, M. (2008). Recognition of dementia in hospitalized older adults. *American Journal of Nursing, 108*(1), 40–50.

McDaniel, J. C., Belury, M., Ahijevych, K., & Blakely, W. (2008). Omega-3 fatty acids effect on wound healing. *Wound Repair and Regeneration, 16*(3), 337–345. doi:10.1111/j.1524-475X.2008.00388.x

McDaniel, J. C., Massey, K., & Nicolaou, A. (2011). Fish oil supplementation alters levels of lipid mediators of inflammation in microenvironment of acute human wounds. *Wound Repair and Regeneration, 19*(2), 189–200. doi:10.1111/j.1524-475X.2010.00659.x

Meals on Wheels Association of America. (2012). Retrieved from http://www.mowaa.org

Mehanna, H., Nankivell, P. C., Moledina, J., & Travis, J. (2009). Refeeding syndrome—awareness, prevention, and management. *Head & Neck Oncology, 1*(4). doi:10.1186/1758-3284-1-4

Moore, J., Von Korff, M., Cherkin, D., Saunders, K., & Lorig, K. (2000). A randomized controlled trial of a cognitive-behavioral program for enhancing back pain self care in a primary care setting. *Pain, 88*(2), 145–153.

Murtaugh, C., Spillman, B., & Wang, X. (2011). Lifetime risk and duration of chronic disease and disability. *Journal of Aging and Health, 23*(3), 554–577.

National Institute for Health and Clinical Excellence. (2006). *Nutrition support in adults: oral nutrition support, enteral tube feeding and parenteral nutrition.* London: National Institute for Health and Clinical Excellence.

National Institute for Health and Clinical Excellence. (2012). *Prescribing of adult oral nutritional supplements: guiding principles for improving the systems and processes for ONS use.* Retrieved from http://www.npc.nhs.uk/quality/ONS/resources/borderline_substances_final.pdf

Nieuwenhuizen, W., Weenen, H., Rigby, P., & Hetherington, M. M. (2009). Older adults and patients in need of nutritional support: review of current treatment options and factors influencing nutritional intake. *Clinical Nutrition, 29*(2), 160–169.

Ohura, T., Nakajo, T., Okada, K., & Adachi, K. (2011). Evaluation of effects of nutrition intervention on healing of pressure ulcers and nutritional states (randomized controlled trial). *Wound Repair and*

Regeneration, 19(3), 330–336. doi:10.1111/j.1524-475X.2011.00691.x

Ormerod, C., Farrer, K., Harper, L., & Lal, S. (2010). Refeeding syndrome: a clinical review. *British Journal of Hospital Medicine, 71*(12), 686–690.

Palecek, E. J., Teno, J. M., Casarett, D. J., Hanson, L. C., Rhodes, R. L., & Mitchell, S. L. (2010). Comfort feeding only: a proposal to bring clarity to decision-making regarding difficulty with eating for persons with advanced dementia. *Journal of the American Geriatrics Society, 58*(3), 580–584. doi:10.1111/j.1532-5415.2010.02740.x

Posthauer, M. E. (2012). The role of nutrition in wound care. *Advances in Skin & Wound Care, 25*(2), 62–63.

Regnard, C., Leslie, P., Crawford, H., Mathews, D., & Gibson, L. (2010). Gastrostomies in dementia: bad practice or bad evidence? *Age and Ageing, 39*(3), 282–284. doi:10.1093/ageing/afq012

Reuben, D. B. (2007). Quality indicators for the care of undernutrition in vulnerable elders. *Journal of the American Geriatrics Society, 55*(Suppl. 2), S438–S442.

Sampson, E., Blanchard, M., Jones, L., Tookman, A., & King, M. (2009). Dementia in the acute hospital: prospective cohort study of prevalence and mortality. *British Journal of Psychiatry, 195*(1), 61–66.

Sampson, E. L., & Jones, C. B. (2009). Enteral tube feeding for older people with advanced dementia. *Cochrane Database of Systemic Reviews, 15*(2). doi:10.1002/14651858.CD007209.pub2

Shahin, E. S., Meijers, J. M., Schols, J. M., Tannen, A., Halfens, R. J., & Dassen, T. (2010). The relationship between malnutrition parameters and pressure ulcers in hospitals and nursing homes. *Nutrition, 26*(9), 886–889.

Sobotka, L., Schneider, S. M., Berner, Y. N., Cederholm, T., Krznaric, Z., Shenkin, A., . . . Volkert, D. (2009). ESPEN guidelines on parenteral nutrition. *Clinical Nutrition, 28*(4), 461–466. doi:10.1016/j.clnu.2009.04.004

Sørensen, L. B., Møller, P., Flint, A., Martens, M., & Raben, A. (2003). Effect of sensory perception of foods on appetite and food intake: a review of studies on humans. *International Journal of Obesity, 27*(10), 1152–1166.

Stechmiller, J. K., Childress, B., & Cowan, L. (2005). Arginine supplementation and wound healing. *Nutrition in Clinical Practice, 20*(1), 52–61.

Steinbrook, R. (2009). Healthcare and the American Recovery and Reinvestment Act. *New England Journal of Medicine, 360*(11), 1057–1060.

Sunnoqrot, N., Kant, R., May, C., & Gambert, S. R. (2012). Diagnosing and management of refeeding syndrome in older adults. *Clinical Geriatrics, 20*(12), 24–27.

Teno, J. M., Gozalo, P., Mitchell, S. L., Kuo, S., Fulton, A. T., & Mor, V. (2012). Feeding tubes and the prevention or healing of pressure ulcers. *Archives of Internal Medicine, 172*(9), 697–701.

Teno, J. M., Mitchell, S. L., Kuo, S. K., Gozalo, P. L., Rhodes, R. L., Lima, J. C., & Mor, V. (2011). Decision-making and outcomes of feeding tube insertion: a five-state study. *Journal of the American Geriatrics Society, 59*(5), 881–886. doi:10.1111/j.1532-5415.2011.03385.x

Theila, M., Schwartz, B., Cohen, J., Shapiro, H., Anbar, R., & Singer, P. (2012). Impact of a nutritional formula enriched in fish oil and micronutrients on pressure ulcers in critical care patients. *American Journal of Critical Care, 21*(4), 102–109.

Villareal, D. T., Apovian, C. M., Kushner, R. F., & Klein, S. (2005). Obesity in older adults: technical review and position statement of the American Society for Nutrition and NAASO, the Obesity Society. *Obesity Research, 13*(11), 1849–1863.

Warsi, A., Wong, P., LaValley, M., Avorn, J., & Soloman, D. (2004). Self-management education programs in chronic disease: a systematic review and methodological critique of the literature. *Archives of Internal Medicine, 164*(15), 1641–1649.

Woo, S. H., Finch, C. K., Broyles, J. E., Wan, J., Boswell, R., & Hurdle, A. (2010). Early versus delayed enteral nutrition in critically ill medical patients. *Nutrition in Clinical Practice, 25*(2), 205–211.

Zeki, S., Culkin, A., Gabe, S. M., & Nightingale, J. M. (2011). Refeeding hypophosphataemia is more common in enteral than parenteral feeding in adult inpatients. *Clinical Nutrition, 30*(3), 365–368.

Zopf, Y., Maiss, J., Konturek, P., Rabe, C., Hahn E. G., & Schwab, D. (2011). Predictive factors of mortality after PEG insertion: guidance for clinical practice. *Journal of Parenteral and Enteral Nutrition, 35*(1), 50–55.

chapter 18

Chronic Illness and the Advanced Practice Registered Nurse (APRN)

M. Catherine Wollman

Evidence-based management of common chronic diseases is an essential skill for advanced practice nurses. It is also essential to understand and manage complex challenges that exist across systems of care in order to provide quality care for patients with chronic disease. This chapter reviews the effect of chronic illness on older patients, their families, providers, and the overall health-care system. Specific topics include the demographics of chronic disease, the significance of multiple comorbid conditions, new models of care that reorganize health care in an effort to improve outcomes for complex patients with chronic disease, and the role of the advanced practice registered nurse (APRN) in chronic illness.

DEFINITIONS OF CHRONIC DISEASE AND CHRONIC ILLNESS

Definitions of chronic disease reflect the pathophysiology of disease and, more importantly, consider the meaning of chronic illness and include the experience of the patient, family, and provider as they struggle to cope with the range of mildly complicated to extreme challenges. Anderson and Horvath (2004) define *chronic conditions* as conditions lasting 1 year or more and requiring ongoing medical attention and/or the limiting of activities of daily (ADLs) living. *Chronic disease* or a *chronic condition* is also defined as any condition that requires ongoing modification by the affected person and requires periodic interaction with the health-care system (Improving Chronic Illness Care, 2012). Curtin and Lubkin defined *chronic illness* as "the irreversible presence, accumulation, or latency of disease states or impairments that involve the total human environment for supportive-care and self-care, maintenance of function, and prevention of further disability" (1995, pp. 6–7).

DEMOGRAPHICS OF CHRONIC ILLNESS

Increased life expectancy and health-care advances are the main reasons for the overwhelming increase in numbers of patients with chronic illness. The population of individuals ages 65 years and older increased by 18% between 2000 and 2011, from 35 million to 41.4 million. That growth is projected to increase to 79.7 million in 2040. The population of individuals ages 85 years and older is projected to increase from 5.7 million in 2011 to 14.1 million in 2040 (Administration on Aging [AOA], Administration for Community

Living [ACL], U.S. Department for Health and Human Services [DHHS], 2012).

One-half of adults, or 133 million individuals, were living with at least one chronic condition in the United States in 2005. By 2020, that number is expected to grow to 157 million (Bodenheimer, Chen, & Bennett, 2009). The most common chronic diseases in the population of individuals age 65 years and older include hypertension (60%), dyslipidemia (41%), arthritis (28%), cardiac disease (25%), and eye disease (23%) (Robert Wood Johnson Foundation [RWJF], 2010). The prevalence of diabetes for those older than 65 years is approximately 20% (Centers for Disease Control and Prevention [CDC], 2010).

The health-care system was initially created to deal with acute, episodic care and has not evolved to deal with a population for whom numerous and complex issues of chronic disease are the pervasive concern. The prevalence and cost of chronic health conditions in the United States have significant consequences for patients, their families, and the health-care system. Although individual clinical needs may differ, patients with one or multiple chronic conditions share common problems related to access to and quality of appropriate and coordinated treatments and services and the cost of that care.

Minority populations have increased from 5.7 million in 2000 (16.3% of older adults) to 8.1 million in 2010 (20%) and are projected to increase to 13.1 million in 2020 (24%). Between 2010 and 2030, the white population age 65 years and older is projected to increase by 59% compared with 160% for older minorities (AOA, DHHS, 2011). The U.S. burden of chronic illness is increasing; compellingly, many of the increases are in minority and low-income populations.

DISABILITY AND DEATH WITH CHRONIC ILLNESS

Seven of every 10 deaths in the United States are caused by chronic conditions. Heart disease, cancer, chronic obstructive pulmonary disease (COPD), and stroke are the leading causes of death, with heart disease as the number one cause of death among both men and women. Other major diseases that contribute to the 70% death rate from chronic disease include diabetes and Alzheimer's disease (CDC, 2010).

It is important to understand how the duration of an illness and the disabilities related to each common chronic illness affect the complexity of the plan of care. For women, arthritis is the most common chronic condition, followed by diabetes and COPD. Among men, diabetes has the longest duration of illness, followed by COPD. Individuals with obesity have the greatest risk of disability. It is known that women who have been very overweight most of their lives lose approximately 3 years of life (Murtaugh, Spillman, & Wang, 2011).

The individual and systemic requirements of care for specific chronic diseases, such as heart failure or HIV, have changed dramatically in the last two decades. HIV has evolved from an untreatable and usually fatal disease to a chronic illness with a life expectancy of several decades (Losina & Freedberg, 2011). In the United States, the incidence of heart failure has not declined over the last two decades, but there has been an overall increase in survival. Many patients with heart failure are very old with increasing debility and very complex health-care regimens (Roger et al., 2004).

Programs of research are carefully examining the mechanisms by which disability occurs in chronic illness as well as specific risk factors that lead to severe disability and the treatments that are most effective in prevention and restoration of function (George Mason University, 2011). Recognition of the burden of disease and the risk of disability assists providers in the development of management plans that will minimize risk factors and prevent progression of disease.

A medical diagnosis is necessary to communicate information about diseases and disorders to other providers and to determine payment mechanisms. Documentation and consideration of functional status is at least equally important in the care of older adults with chronic disease. ADLs and instrumental ADLs (IADLs) are used to measure functional status. ADLs are measures of functions that people perform on a daily basis and include feeding, bathing, dressing, grooming, toileting, ambulating, and transferring (Katz et al., 1963). IADLs are indicators of more complex functions required on a regular basis, including use of the telephone, shopping, housekeeping, laundry, transportation, management of medications, and handling of finances (Lawton & Brody, 1969).

In 2000, 34.5% of all noninstitutionalized individuals older than 65 reported limitations in activity due to a chronic condition, and this increased to 44.7% for those over 75 (Weierbach & Glick, 2009). Many of those with functional limitations will eventually require more personal care and coordination of formal home care or long-term care services.

COST BURDEN OF CHRONIC DISEASE

The current hospital-focused system of acute care and reimbursement does not address the effect of chronic disease. Medicare spending clearly demonstrates the influence of chronic disease. About 10% of chronically ill Medicare beneficiaries account for three-fourths of program expenditures each year. Medical spending is 3 to 10 times higher for older adults with one or more chronic conditions than for those with none (Joyce, Keeler, Shang, & Goldman, 2005). These trends have resulted in national health-care expenditures that reached more than $2.6 trillion in 2009, which surpassed rates for inflation (Centers for Medicare and Medicaid Services, 2009).

In a 2004 study, almost one-fifth of Medicare patients had unplanned rehospitalizations within 30 days of release, with a cost of $17.4 billion (Jencks, Williams, & Coleman, 2009). It is essential to identify high-risk populations who are most at risk for lack of coordinated care. Cost and complexity of care are greater for individuals with multiple chronic diseases, who account for 75% of overall health care spending (Thorpe, Ogden, & Galactionova, 2010).

Heart failure is the highest cause of hospital readmission. The increased prevalence and life expectancy of heart failure is expected to contribute to an increase in annual direct medical costs from the present estimate of $24.7 billion to approximately $77.7 billion over the next two decades. Indirect costs due to reduced productivity are expected to increase from $9.7 to $17.4 billion (Konstam, 2012). The medical care costs of obesity in the United States are overwhelming. In 2008, those costs totaled about $147 billion dollars (Finkelstein, Trogdon, Cohen, & Dietz, 2009).

THE CHALLENGE OF MULTIPLE COMORBIDITIES

When considering the increasing number of people with chronic disease, it is necessary to take into account the fact that almost one-half of them have multiple chronic conditions or comorbidities. There are presently 48% of Medicare beneficiaries with at least three chronic conditions, 21% with five or more conditions, and approximately 60 million Americans with multiple comorbidities. The number of those with multiple comorbidities will grow to 81 million in less than 10 years or by 2020 (Anderson & Horvath, 2004).

The challenge is more difficult, because most chronic illnesses increase in prevalence and severity with aging. Besides multiple providers, individuals with multiple chronic problems also have multiple prescriptions and increased hospitalizations (RWJF, 2010). There is subsequently a mandate to closely monitor those high-risk patients and their families. Older adults with multiple comorbidities require a comprehensive and holistic approach to care that includes support for complex medication and treatment regimens, counseling for family issues related to caregiving and finances, access to community resources, use of advance care planning, and the vigilant management of other comorbid conditions.

Medicare patients are typically seen by two primary care providers and five specialty providers across four different sites of care (Pham, Schrag, O'Malley, Wu, & Bach, 2007). Certain chronic diseases will offer additional challenges and increase the risk for poor outcomes because of the inherent complexity of care. Patients with chronic kidney disease (CKD) may have 2 to 9 providers, 5 to 14 prescriptions, and an additional 5 to 11 comorbid conditions (Rifkin et al., 2010).

The number of people with type 2 diabetes is expected to double in the next 25 years, from 24 million to 48 million. More than one-half of patients with type 2 diabetes mellitus also have hypertension, and another one-third have coronary artery disease (CAD) (Rothman & Wagner, 2003). Disabilities among those with diabetes are multifactorial, and research has suggested that the presence of depression and the macrovascular and microvascular complications of diabetes are highly associated with increased risk of disability (Conwell & Boult, 2008).

By 2023, the number of people with chronic mental disorders will increase from 30 to 47 million individuals (Bodenheimer et al., 2009). The literature identifies a significantly greater risk of medical comorbidity in those with mental health diagnoses. The number of older adults who require management of addictions is projected to double from 1.7 to 2.8 million in 2000 to 4.4 to 5.6 million in 2020 (Han, Gfroerer, Colliver, & Penne, 2009). Community-dwelling older adults with comorbid substance abuse disorders and mental illness have a much greater risk of chronic physical conditions and increased complexity of medical care (Lin, Zhang, Leung, & Clark, 2011).

Dementia

One in eight people age 65 and older has Alzheimer's disease and nearly half of people age 85 and older have Alzheimer's disease. The presence of cognitive impairment clearly affects other comorbid conditions. Maslow & Mezey (2008) reported that, based on Medicare data, about 25% of all hospital patients ages 65 and over have a diagnosis of dementia. In a study of 600 hospitalized individuals over 70 years of age, it was determined that 42% had cognitive impairment, and only one-half of that number had been diagnosed before hospitalization. The patients with dementia had a higher mortality rate during hospitalization, and 24% with severe dementia died during a hospital admission (Sampson, Blanchard, Jones, Tookman, & King, 2009).

Most people with Alzheimer's and other dementias have at least one other serious physical comorbidity, and Alzheimer's exponentially increases costs for other chronic diseases (Alzheimer's Association, 2012). Medicaid payments are 19 times higher for older adults with Alzheimer's disease and other dementias, and Medicare payments for the same chronic diseases are almost 3 times higher. An older adult with diabetes and Alzheimer's costs Medicare 81% more than an older adult with diabetes alone, and an older adult with cancer and Alzheimer's costs an additional 53% (Bynum, 2011).

Cognitive impairment and related behavioral symptoms complicate the management of care and result in additional and longer hospital stays (Alzheimer's Association, 2012). The lack of awareness of baseline cognitive function can prevent the implementation of an appropriate plan of care and may contribute to morbidity and other poor outcomes.

Frailty

Frailty is not synonymous with comorbidity or disability, but comorbidity is a risk factor for frailty, and disability is an outcome of frailty. Frailty has been defined as a clinical syndrome when three or more of the following criteria are present: unintentional weight loss of 10 lb in the past year, self-reported exhaustion, weakness based on grip strength, slow walking speed, and low physical activity (Fried et al., 2001). It is important to understand frailty in order to develop accurate assessments, help patients and families with anticipatory planning, and make appropriate decisions about interventions and treatment.

Obesity

Obesity is one of the negative health trends facing older adults in the United States. In 2008, 37% of men and 34% of women ages 60 and older were considered obese. Some ethnic groups show significantly higher levels of obesity, with 50% of non-Hispanic black women ages 60 and older considered to be obese (Himes & Reynolds, 2012). Health consequences of obesity include hypertension; dyslipidemia; coronary heart disease and cerebrovascular disease; type 2 diabetes; endometrial, breast, or colon cancer; liver and gallbladder disease; sleep apnea; osteoarthritis; and infertility (CDC, 2011). Although obesity is no longer a major factor related to the mortality of aging, it plays a major role in disability (Himes & Reynolds, 2012).

The literature related to older adults and multiple comorbid conditions identifies the foremost need for integration of holistic health care and mental health services. Resources for high-risk patients and coordination of care must be available to individuals with dementia, multiple comorbidities, functional impairment, and complex health-care regimens.

EVIDENCE-BASED PRACTICE AND COMPLEX OLDER ADULTS

There is wide diversity in the older adult population in life expectancy, functional status, and individual priorities and preferences related to health care. Available evidence for individual chronic diseases is available within clinical practice guidelines (CPGs). It is essential to evaluate those guidelines, however, to determine if they are appropriate for frail, older adults with multiple comorbidities. Several characteristics of older populations may limit the use of specific disease-oriented models of care. Complex comorbid conditions and geriatric syndromes are common, and usual signs and symptoms, such as fatigue, may be due to one or several chronic diseases, problems, or syndromes and require different or multiple interventions.

When CPGs have been evaluated for content that considers unique issues of complex older adults with multiple comorbidities, it has been determined that only a few CPGs address those issues. The neglected content includes identifying patient and caregiver concerns, setting clinical priorities based on life expectancy, managing expectations around prognosis, maintaining communication, and considering patient, provider, or system barriers to implementation (Mutasingwa, Ge, & Upshur, 2011).

There is limited information about the safety and effectiveness of CPG recommendations as they relate to the diverse older populations. Older adults with multiple medical conditions have poorer outcomes when treated according to disease-specific guidelines. Those outcomes may be due to decreased benefit from therapy directed at any one chronic disease, the presence of polypharmacy, or the increased likelihood that the high-risk older adult will have a poor response to any recommended intervention (Fried, Tinetti, & Iannone, 2011). To improve decision making, clinicians require unique data about the frail older adult, specific alternative guidelines, approaches that include patient and family values, support of specialty providers and other members of the team, and a restructured reimbursement system (Fried et al., 2011). There continues to be an imperative to improve the evidence base that supports the care of frail older adults with multiple comorbidities.

Person-Centered Care

Geriatric experts have always favored an individualized, patient-centered approach to care over traditional, disease-specific approaches. An individualized approach prioritizes patient preferences and embraces the concept that signs and symptoms may not reflect a single disease process but are likely the complex interaction between multiple biopsychosocial factors.

Treatment interventions are related to prognosis and to unique patient and family values and are used to suggest, rather than to mandate, treatment decisions. Research has consistently demonstrated that an individualized, patient-centered approach to care has much more to offer the older adult and his or her family than a traditional, disease-based approach (Bowling & O'Hare, 2012).

The Institute of Medicine (IOM) Committee on Quality of Health Care in America (2001) originally defined the dimensions of person-centered care (PCC) and included as part of the definition the importance of coordination and integration of care across conditions and settings as well as over time. The IOM (2011) recently reiterated the need for nursing professionals to rethink approaches to care and to develop and implement person-centered models of care.

Interprofessional Care

Prevention and management of complex older adults with chronic illness are best implemented by multidisciplinary teams in primary care and in most other sites of care. It is suggested that a larger interdisciplinary workforce is needed, and payment for primary care should reward practices that incorporate multidisciplinary teams (Bodenheimer et al., 2009).

The passage of the Recovery and Reinvestment Act of 2009 (Steinbrook, 2009) and the Patient Protection and Affordable Care Act of 2010 (Josiah Macy Jr. Foundation, 2013) has stimulated new approaches or models of care to achieve better outcomes in primary care, especially for the high-risk and chronically ill and other at-risk populations. Improved interprofessional teamwork and team-based care play critical roles in many of the new primary care approaches.

Interprofessional, collaborative practice core competency domains have been established, and those competencies need to be incorporated and evaluated within clinical practice models for older adults with multiple chronic conditions (Interprofessional Education Collaborative Expert Panel, 2011).

CHRONIC CARE MODEL OF QUALITY IMPROVEMENT

A majority of Americans with major chronic illnesses are not receiving appropriate or effective management. The consequences of inadequate care are poor disease control, exacerbations, and complications that far exceed those seen with appropriate care. The IOM (2001) has described this difference between usual and appropriate care as the "quality chasm."

Extensive evidence exists about the dismal quality of care and health-care economics of our present system of care, which has prompted the agenda for new models of care. The Chronic Care Model (CCM) (Fig. 18-1) was developed through funds from the Robert Wood Johnson Foundation to improve care for people who suffer from chronic illness. Although clinical and interventional advancements in hypertension, diabetes, and congestive heart failure have increased, the number of patients receiving evidence-based care is declining (Wagner et al., 2001). The CCM is an evidence-based policy response to reduce the problems inherent in a health-care system that is currently not designed to meet the needs of chronically ill patients and their families. The CCM is also used to direct quality improvement and overall systems change for patients with chronic illnesses.

The CCM approaches care of the chronically ill away from the reactive acute care visit to a planned patient-centered encounter. The CCM involves six elements considered essential to effective chronic care management and depicted in the model. Those

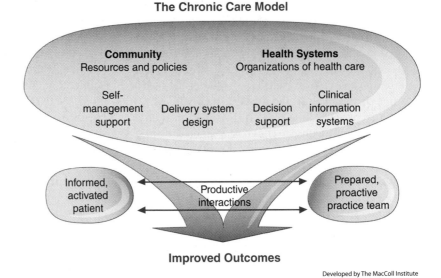

FIGURE 18-1. The chronic care model (CCM). *(Wagner, E. H. (1998). Chronic disease management: What will it take to improve care for chronic illness?* Effective Clinical Practice, 1, *2–4, Figure 1. With permission from the American College of Physicians.)*

elements are community resources and policies, organization of health-care systems, self-management support, delivery system design, decision support, and clinical information systems.

APRNs are ideally suited to incorporate elements of the CCM into practice. The typical functions of the APRN depicted in the CCM include identification of resources for unique populations and involvement in key policy decisions that affect those populations. APRNs excel in patient education and patient empowerment, with the goal of supporting the patient's self-management skills. APRNs are involved in technology and clinical information systems with shared medical appointments, telehealth, electronic documentation, and developing and maintaining data for quality improvement. APRNs embrace evidence-based care that is maximized with decision support tools and algorithms.

Self-Management Support

The body of research on self-management programs comes from Lorig and others from Stanford University. Their Chronic Disease Self-Management Program (CDSMP) includes five core skills: problem solving, decision making, resource utilization, formation of a patient–health-care provider partnership, and taking action (Lorig & Holman, 2003). Lorig and her colleagues found modest but encouraging benefits related to health behaviors and health status in several studies (Lorig et al., 2010; Moore, Von Korff, Cherkin, Saunders, & Lorig, 2000). In another systematic review of self-care management, a few promising results were

noted, but many results were not statistically significant, and there was a large number of study limitations (Warsi, Wang, LaValley, Avorn, & Solomon, 2004).

At this time and in the immediate future, patient and family self-care will continue to be the primary means by which chronic diseases are managed. Patients' infrequent contact with their health-care providers is inadequate to deal with the complexity of self-care problems, and coordinated programs to provide reasonable quality support systems are limited. On a daily basis, individuals, families, and informal caregivers are largely on their own in dealing with symptoms, taking medications, and managing evolving changes in their disease. New models of care are essential to provide tools to improve self-management and quality support systems.

NEW LEGISLATION AND CHRONIC DISEASE

In March 2010, the Patient Protection and Affordable Care Act (PPACA or the ACA) was signed into law with provisions that recognize and address the enormity of chronic disease. The ACA includes incentives for the creation of accountable care organizations (ACOs). Beginning in 2012, the law authorized Medicare to contract with ACOs in a Medicare Shared Savings Program. ACOs provide financial incentives to improve the coordination and quality of care for Medicare beneficiaries while reducing costs. The Centers for

Medicare and Medicaid Services (CMS) has released a proposed rule for implementing the new program, laying out requirements for groups of providers to qualify as ACOs and methods for monitoring and assessing ACO performance and dispensing shared savings (Josiah Macy Jr. Foundation, 2013).

A key element of ACOs will relate to the effective discharge of patients from acute care settings and initiatives to reduce admissions. All members of the ACO are incentivized to coordinate care of patients across the continuum in order to achieve savings. Long-term care and home care facilities will be part of ACOs (Turner, 2012). An additional provision of the ACA is the Hospital Readmissions Reduction Program that financially penalizes hospitals for excess readmissions within 30 days of discharge (Turner, 2012).

Patient-Centered Medical Home

The 2011 National Committee for Quality Assurance (NCQA) has defined standards for the patient-centered medical home (PCMH), which reinforce the central components of primary care. Those core components include an ongoing relationship with a provider, person-centered care, enhanced access to care, coordinated care, quality and safety, and a payment structure (NCQA, n.d.). Additional requirements for PCMH designation include patient tracking and registry, a care management component, patient self-management support, advanced electronic communication (including electronic prescribing), and performance reporting and improvement. Outcome measures include patient and family satisfaction, decreased emergency department use, decreased hospitalization, improved health parameters (e.g., blood pressure, hemoglobin A1C), provider satisfaction, decreased cost, improved preventive care, and patient language preference.

Initial demonstration projects are reporting evidence that indicates improved outcomes for the PCMH, including reduction in emergency department visits and hospitalizations, improved patient satisfaction, and increased use of measures such as recommended diabetes services (Schram, 2012). Advanced practice nurses are involved in providing primary care as well as care coordination, health system navigation, and community team members.

Primary Care at Home

The health-care reform law also includes the Independence at Home Act, funding a demonstration project in which physician and nurse practitioner teams will provide home-based primary care. In addition to the medical home and independence-at-home concepts, the health reform law also promotes ACOs and changes the funding to Medicare Advantage private insurance plans. Both of these initiatives will likely require primary care providers to redesign how they deliver chronic care to older patients with limited mobility and multiple comorbid illnesses. The emergence of the medical home, independence-at-home, and related concepts makes it a good time for APRNs to explore how they can collaborate across levels of care to better meet the needs of complex older adults (Landers, Suter, & Hennessey, 2010).

Transitional Care

Transitional care is defined as a set of actions necessary to ensure the coordination and continuity of care as patients transfer between different sites of care or from one level of care to another within the same site (Coleman & Berenson, 2004). Health-care services for older adults in the United States are a complex and fragmented mix of acute care, post–acute care, long-term care, home health care, and community-based services (Coleman, Berenson, & American Geriatrics Society Health Care Systems Committee, 2004). Health-care transitions occur as patients receive an extensive range of services across multiple providers, payers, and settings for different acute episodes or for the same episode of care.

Because of the dramatic costs involved in readmissions, a growing importance is placed on transitions across providers and sites of care (Jencks et al., 2009). Frequent changes in health status among frail older adults increase the numbers of those transitions, especially between long-term care and acute care. The National Transitions of Care Coalition (2008) states that there is significant evidence to conclude that poor transitions compromise patient safety and quality of care; place significant burden on patients, families, and caregivers; and increase costs to patients, providers, and payers.

SUMMARY

The effect of the PPACA of 2010, the obesity epidemic, the rise in complex chronic diseases, and the continuing growth of the aging population are combining to create a huge demand for health-care services. A perfect storm is brewing and will have a major effect on the U.S. health-care system.

National attention has been placed on the removal of all scope-of-practice restrictions on APRNs as a way to drive down costs, while increasing high-quality access to primary health care. Numerous studies have shown the importance of APRNs in delivering care to frail older adults. The importance of APRNs has been cited as a key component of an overall health-care system strategy to address chronic disease (Greenberg & Greenberg, 2007).

The involvement of APRNs at all levels of care positively affects the chronic illness experience of the patient and family and improves outcomes. Nurse practitioners are committed to providing affordable, accessible, and high-quality primary care through partnerships with patients, families, communities, and other health-care professionals.

CLINICAL RECOMMENDATION	EVIDENCE RATING	REFERENCES
Develops and operationalizes a phenotype of frailty in older adults and assesses concurrent and predictive validity.	B	Fried et al. (2001)
Systematic review of the Chronic Care Model (CCM). Examines articles published since 2000 that use one of five key CCM papers as a reference. Evidence supports that the CCM leads to improved patient care and better health outcomes.	B	Coleman, Austin, Brach, & Wagner (2009)
Analysis of Medicare claims data from 2003–2004 to describe the patterns of rehospitalization and the relation of rehospitalization to demographic characteristics of the patients and characteristics of hospitals.	B	Jencks et al. (2009)
Systematic review on the quality of diabetes preventive care. Assesses trends in the reports of complications and comorbidities of diabetes and the limitations of current measures.	B	Conwell & Boult (2008)
Case study approach. Supports individualized approach to patient preferences and suggests that observed signs and symptoms reflect a complex interplay between multiple factors.	C	Bowling & O'Hare (2012)

A = consistent, good-quality, patient-oriented evidence; B = inconsistent or limited-quality, patient-oriented evidence; C = consensus, disease-oriented evidence, usual practice, expert opinion, or case series. For information about the SORT evidence rating system, go to www.aafp.org/afpsort.xml.

CASE STUDY

Mrs. A. is an 82-year-old Caucasian woman. She lives with her 86-year-old husband, who has mild-to-moderate dementia. Mrs. A. has a primary care provider, endocrinologist, cardiologist, ophthalmologist, and podiatrist. She has a daughter nearby who assists with shopping and housekeeping. Mrs. A. is overweight and has hypertension, type 2 diabetes, CKD, macular degeneration, incontinence, and peripheral neuropathy with chronic pain. She has trouble sleeping, complains of chronic fatigue, and has fallen twice in the

CASE STUDY—cont'd

past 2 months. She is on nine prescription medications. Her self-care regimen includes monitoring her glucose, weighing herself daily, taking medications twice daily, and managing her nutrition and exercise. She is also responsible for managing her husband's meals and medications.

Additional comprehensive assessment is critical to developing a person-centered plan of care for Mrs. A. A multidisciplinary and continuity-of-care focus will prevent poor outcomes.

1. What multiple factors place Mrs. A. at high risk for poor outcomes?

2. What additional assessment data are essential to determine if Mrs. A. can safely manage her complex health-care regimen at home?

3. How do Mrs. A.'s multiple chronic diseases contribute to the complexity of her care?

4. What communication is necessary to provide ongoing coordination of care?

5. What community resources may be available to support Mrs. A.?

6. What additional team members would be appropriate to contribute to a safe and person-centered plan of care?

7. What new models of care can potentially contribute to Mrs. A.'s quality of care while she is at home or in the event of her hospitalization?

REFERENCES

Administration on Aging, Administration for Community Living, U.S. Department of Health and Human Services. (2012). *A profile of older Americans: 2012.* Retrieved from http://www.aoa.gov/Aging_Statistics/Profile/2012/docs/2012profile.pdf

Administration on Aging, U.S. Department of Health and Human Services. (2011). *A profile of older Americans: 2011.* Retrieved from http://www.aoa.gov/aoaroot/aging_statistics/Profile/2011/docs/2011profile.pdf

Alzheimer's Association. (2012). Alzheimer's disease facts and figures. *Alzheimer's & Dementia, 8*(2), 131–168.

Anderson, G., & Horvath, J. (2004). The growing burden of chronic disease in America. *Public Health Reports, 119*(3), 263–270.

Bodenheimer, T., Chen, E., & Bennett, H. D. (2009). Confronting the growing burden of chronic disease: can the US health care workforce do the job? *Health Affairs, 28*(1), 64–74.

Bowling, C. B., & O'Hare, A. M. (2012). Managing older adults with CKD: individualized versus disease-based approaches. *American Journal of Kidney Diseases, 59*(2), 293–302.

Bynum, J. (2011). [Tabulations based on data from the National 20% Sample Medicare Fee-for-Service Beneficiaries for 2009]. Unpublished raw data.

Centers for Disease Control and Prevention. (2010). Chronic disease overview. Retrieved from http://www.cdc.gov/chronicdisease/overview/index.htm

Centers for Disease Control and Prevention. (2011). *Percentage of civilian, noninstitutionalized population with diagnosed diabetes, by age, United States, 1980–2011.* Retrieved from http://www.cdc.gov/diabetes/statistics/prev/national/figbyage.htm

Centers for Medicare and Medicaid Services. (2010). *National Health Expenditure Projections 2010-2020.* Retrieved from https://www.cms.gov/Research-Statistics-Data-and-Systems/Statistics-Trends-and-Reports/NationalHealthExpendData/downloads/proj2010.pdf

Coleman, E., & Berenson, M., American Geriatrics Society Health Care Systems Committee (2004). Lost in transition: challenges and opportunities for improving the quality of transitional care. *Annals of Internal Medicine, 141*(7), 533–535.

Coleman, K., Austin, B., Brach, C., & Wagner, E. (2009). Evidence on the chronic care model in the new millennium. *Health Affairs, 28*(1), 75–85. doi:10.1377/hlthaff.28.1.75

Conwell, L. J., & Boult, C. (2008). The effects of complications and comorbidities on the quality of preventive diabetes care: a literature review. *Population Health Management, 11*(4), 217–228. doi:10.1089/pop.2007.0017

Curtin, M., & Lubkin, I. (1995). What is chronicity? In I. Lubkin (Ed.), *Chronic illness: impact and interventions* (3rd ed., pp. 3–25) Sudbury, MA: Jones & Bartlett.

Finkelstein, E., Trogdon, J., Cohen, J., & Dietz, W. (2009). Annual medical spending attributable to obesity: payer- and service-specific estimates. *Health Affairs, 228*(5), w822–w831.

Fried, L. P., Tangen, C. M., Walston, J., Newman, A. B., Hirsch, C., Gottdiener, J., . . . McBurnie, M. A. (2001). Frailty in older adults: evidence for a phenotype. *Journals of Gerontology Series A: Biological Sciences & Medical Sciences, 56*(3), M146–M156.

Fried, T. R., Tinetti, M. E., & Iannone, L. (2011). Primary care clinicians' experiences with treatment decision making for older persons with multiple conditions. *Archives of Internal Medicine, 171*(1), 75–80.

George Mason University College of Health and Human Services. (2011). *The center for study of chronic illness and disability (CCID).* Retrieved from http://chhs.gmu.edu/ccid/index.html

Greenberg, J., & Greenberg, H. (2007). More physicians are not the answer. *American Journal of Cardiology, 99*(10), 1476–1478.

Han, B., Gfroerer, J. C., Colliver, J. D., & Penne, M. A. (2009). Substance use disorder among older adults in the United States in 2020. *Addiction, 104*(1), 88–96. doi:10.1111/j.1360-0443.2008.02411.x

Himes, C. L., & Reynolds, S. L. (2012). Effect of obesity on falls, injury, and disability. *Journal of the American Geriatrics Society, 60*(1), 124–129.

Improving Chronic Illness Care. (2012). *The Chronic Care Model.* Retrieved from http://www.improvingchroniccare.org/index.php?p=the_chronic_care_model&s=2

Institute of Medicine. (2011). *The future of nursing: leading change, advancing health.* Washington, DC: National Academies Press.

Institute of Medicine, Committee on Quality of Health Care in America. (2001). *Crossing the quality chasm: a new health system for the 21st century.* Washington, DC: National Academies Press.

Interprofessional Education Collaborative Expert Panel. (2011). *Core competencies for interprofessional collaborative practice: report of an expert panel.* Retrieved from http://www.aacn.nche.edu/education-resources/ipecreport.pdf

Jencks, S., Williams, M., & Coleman, E. A. (2009). Rehospitalizations among patients in the Medicare fee-for-service program. *New England Journal of Medicine, 360*(14), 1418–1428.

Josiah Macy Jr. Foundation. (2013). *Transforming patient care: aligning interprofessional education with clinical practice redesign.* Retrieved from http://macyfoundation.org/docs/macy_pubs/TransformingPatientCare_ConferenceRec.pdf

Joyce, G. F., Keeler, E. B., Shang, B., & Goldman, D. P. (2005). The lifetime burden of chronic disease among the elderly. *Health Affairs, 25*(Suppl. 2), R18–R29. doi:10.1377/hlthaff.w5.r18

Katz, S., Ford, A., Moskowitz, R., Jackson, B., Jaffe, M., & Cleveland, M. (1963). The index of ADL: a standardized measure of biological and psychosocial function. *Journal of the American Medical Association, 185*(12), 914–919.

Konstam, M. A. (2012). Home monitoring should be the central element in an effective program of heart failure disease management. *Circulation, 125*(6), 820–827.

Landers, S. H., Suter, P., & Hennessey, B. (2010). Bringing home the "medical home" for older adults [Case Reports]. *Cleveland Clinic Journal of Medicine, 77*(10), 661–675.

Lawton, M. P., & Brody, E. M. (1969). Assessment of older people: self-maintaining and instrumental activities of daily living. *The Gerontologist, 9*(3), 179–186. doi:10.1093/geront/9.3_Part_1.179

Lin, W. C., Zhang, J., Leung, G. Y., & Clark, R. E. (2011). Chronic physical conditions in older adults with mental illness and/or substance use disorders. *Journal of the American Geriatrics Society, 59*(10), 1913–1921.

Lorig, K., & Holman, H. (2003). Self-management education: history, definition, outcomes and mechanisms. *Annals of Behavioral Medicine, 26*(1), 1–7.

Lorig, K., Ritter, P. L., Laurent, D. D., Plant, K., Green, M., Jernigan, V. B. B., & Case, S. (2010). Online diabetes self-management program: a randomized study. *Diabetes Care, 33*(6), 1275–1281. doi:10.2337/dc09-2153

Losina, E., & Freedberg, K. A. (2011). Life expectancy in HIV. *British Medical Journal, 343*, d6015. doi:10.1136/bmj.d6015

Maslow, K., & Mezey, M. (2008). Recognition of dementia in hospitalized older adults. *American Journal of Nursing, 108*(1), 40–50. doi:10.1097/01.NAJ.0000304475.80530.a6

Moore, J., Von Korff, M., Cherkin, D., Saunders, K., & Lorig, K. (2000). A randomized trial of a cognitive-behavioral program for enhancing back pain self care in a primary care setting. *Pain, 88*(2), 145–153. doi: 10.1016/S0304-3959(00)00314-6

Murtaugh, C. M., Spillman, B. C., & Wang, X. (2011). Lifetime risk and duration of chronic disease and disability. *Journal of Aging and Health, 23*(3), 554–577. doi:10.1177/0898264310389491

Mutasingwa, D., Ge, H., & Upshur, R. (2011). How applicable are clinical practice guidelines to elderly patients with comorbidities? *Canadian Family Physician, 57*(7), e253–e262.

National Committee for Quality Assurance. (n.d.). *The patient-centered medical home.* Retrieved from http://www.ncqa.org/tabid/631/default.aspx

National Transitions of Care Coalition. (2008). *Improving on transitions of care: how to implement and evaluate a plan.* Retrieved from http://www.ntocc.org/Portals/0/ImplementationPlan.pdf

Patient Protection and Affordable Care Act, Pub. L. No. 111–148, §2702, 124 Stat. 119, 318–319 (2010).

Pham, H., Schrag, D., O'Malley, A., Wu, B., & Bach, P. (2007). Care patterns in Medicare and their implications for pay for performance. *New England Journal of Medicine, 356*(11), 1130–1139.

Rifkin, D. E., Laws, M. B., Rao, M., Balakrishnan, V. S., Sarnak, M. J., & Wilson, I. B. (2010). Medication adherence behavior and priorities among older adults with CKD: a semistructured interview study. *American Journal of Kidney Diseases, 56*(3), 439–446.

Robert Wood Johnson Foundation. (2010). *Chronic care: making the case for ongoing care.* Retrieved from http://www.rwjf.org/content/dam/farm/reports/reports/2010/rwjf54583

Roger, V. L., Weston, S. A., Redfield, M. M., Hellermann-Homan, J. P., Killian, J., Yawn, B. P., & Jacobsen, S. J. (2004). Trends in heart failure incidence and survival in a community-based population. *Journal of the American Medical Association, 292*(3), 344–350.

Rothman, A., & Wagner, E. H. (2003). Chronic illness management: what is the role of primary care? *Annals of Internal Medicine, 138*(3), 256–261.

Sampson, E. L., Blanchard, M. R., Jones, L., Tookman, A., & King, M. (2009). Dementia in the acute hospital: prospective cohort study of prevalence and mortality. *British Journal of Psychiatry, 195*(1), 61–66. doi:10.1192/bjp.bp.108.055335

Schram, A. P. (2012). The patient-centered medical home: transforming primary care. *The Nurse Practitioner, 37*(4), 33–39.

Steinbrook, R. (2009). Health care and the American Recovery and Reinvestment Act. *New England Journal of Medicine, 360*(11), 1057–1060. doi:10.1056/NEJMp0900665

Thorpe, K. E., Ogden, L. L., & Galactionova, K. (2010). Chronic conditions account for rise in Medicare spending from 1987 to 2006. *Health Affairs, 29*(4), 718–724.

Turner, S. (2012). What's new for 2012? *Geriatric Nursing, 33*(1), 54–55.

Wagner, E., Austin, B., Davis, C., Hindmark, M., Schaefer, J., & Bonomi, A. (2001). Improving chronic illness care: translating evidence into action. *Health Affairs, 20*(6), 64–87.

Warsi, A., Wong, P. S., LaValley, M. P., Avorn, J., & Soloman, D. H. (2004). Self-management education programs in chronic disease: a systematic review and methodological critique of the literature. *Archives of Internal Medicine, 164*(15), 1641–1649. doi:10.1001/archinte.164.15.1641

Weierbach, F., & Glick, D. (2009). Community resources for older adults with chronic illness. *Holistic Nursing Practice, 23*(6), 355–360.

chapter 19

Palliative Care and End-of-Life Care

M. Jane Griffith and Norma K. Branham

OVERVIEW OF PALLIATIVE CARE

Description: The goals of palliative care are to relieve pain and other distressing symptoms using an interdisciplinary approach that addresses not only the physical but also the psychosocial and spiritual aspects of patient care (World Health Organization [WHO], 2010). Families are included in the care planning. Patients and families benefit from the availability of palliative care services early in the disease process, particularly when symptoms affect their quality of life. As the disease advances, hospice care becomes an option. Hospice is a program of care designed for the last 6 months of a person's life (Beach, 2007). Hospice care uses the principles of palliative care to support patients and their families through the dying process and includes bereavement services. Hospice services are covered by Medicare, Medicaid, and most private insurance providers.

Etiology: According to Murphy, Xu, and Kochanek (2012), the five leading causes of death in the elderly are heart disease, malignant neoplasms, chronic respiratory disease, cerebrovascular disease, and accidents (Box 19-1).

Numerous medical advances in the management of these illnesses have led to people living longer with chronic health conditions. Accurate prognostication of chronic illnesses is difficult, and the difficulty of prognostication can result in overuse of acute care interventions at the end of life and delays in referral to hospice care. Of those who died in 2011, 44.6% were cared for in a hospice program (National Hospice and Palliative Care Organization [NHPCO], 2012). However, 35.7% of those admitted to hospice programs died within 7 days. The median length of stay was 21.1 days, meaning one-half of patients died within 3 weeks of enrollment in a hospice program. The average length of stay in a hospice program was 69.1 days. Thus, most people are not benefiting fully from the Hospice Medicare Benefit, which is designed to provide care for patients in the last 6 months of life. There are several obstacles to implementing palliative care in the geriatric setting. These include inadequate communication among decision makers and lack of agreement on goals of care, failure to recognize futile treatments, and lack of advance directives guiding end-of-life care plans (Derby & O'Mahony, 2006). Failure to acknowledge the limits of medicine, lack of health-care provider training, poor understanding of hospice and palliative care services, denial of death, and rules and regulations are all barriers that affect quality care at the end of life (Glare et al., 2003; NHPCO, 2009).

Occurrence: According to the National Institute on Aging data, 45% of the elderly die in a hospital,

24% die in a nursing home, and 30% die at home (National Institute on Aging, 2005). Of those 75 and older, 33% die in a nursing home, and of those 85 and older, 42% die in a nursing home (Ferrell, Ersek, Virani, Malloy, & Kelly, 2011). It is important to provide access to hospice and palliative care services in all settings. The goal is to ensure a peaceful, dignified death with symptoms well managed and support for the family and caregivers.

Age: Average life expectancy is 77.9 years according to 2007 Census data (U.S. National Center for Health Statistics, 2010). The fastest growing segment of the population is the 85 and older age group (Federal Interagency Forum on Aging-Related Statistics, 2002). Palliative care is beneficial for frail elderly with functional limitations, cognitive impairment, symptom burden, and lack of family or social support (Derby, 2007).

Caregiving needs increase with advanced age and are typically met by the family. As caregivers, frail, elderly spouses face challenges in meeting both the patient's needs and the caregiver's own needs. Caregivers are at risk for physical and psychological illness, including depression, insomnia, fatigue, and anxiety (Derby, 2007).

Gender: The average overall life expectancy for females is 80.4 years, and the average life expectancy for males is 75.4 years (U.S. National Center for Health Statistics, 2010).

Contributing factors: Contributing factors include advanced age and multiple comorbidities.

Ethnicity: The average life expectancy for Caucasian females is 80.8 years, and the average life expectancy for Caucasian males is 75.9 years. The average life expectancy for black females is 76.8 years, and the average life expectancy for black males is 70 years (U.S. National Center for Health Statistics, 2010). Cultural influences affect how people define health and illness and shape their beliefs and practices in end-of-life care. The medical practitioner should avoid stereotyping and making assumptions and judgments (Wilson, 2007).

Signs and symptoms: See Symptom Management.

Differential diagnosis: Not applicable.

SYMPTOM MANAGEMENT

The most prevalent symptoms in end-of-life care in the geriatric population are delirium, dyspnea, and pain (Derby & O'Mahony, 2006). Additional symptoms such as nausea and vomiting, constipation, diarrhea, depression, anxiety, and insomnia are also common. These latter symptoms are described in detail elsewhere in this book.

DELIRIUM

Description: Delirium is an acute and fluctuating change in mental status, characterized by disturbances in attention, level of consciousness, and cognition, including alterations in thinking, perception, and memory (American Psychiatric Association, 1994). Delirium can be hyper or hypo depending on the level of psychomotor activity (Heidrich & English, 2010).

Etiology: There are numerous potential causes of delirium in the dying patient related to the terminal disease itself, treatment of the disease, metabolic effects of organ failure, electrolyte imbalance including hypoglycemia, infection, hematological disorders, nutritional deficiencies, dehydration, hypoxia, uncontrolled pain, sensory deprivation, insomnia, alcohol or drug withdrawal, diarrhea, constipation, and urinary retention. Many medications, particularly those with anticholinergic properties, can cause delirium (Derby, O'Mahony, & Tickoo, 2010).

Occurrence: Delirium is common at end of life and can be very distressing to the family as well as to the patient. Delirium occurs in as much as 80% of the terminally ill (Perley, 2007b).

Age: The risk for delirium increases with advancing age, particularly in those over 70 years of age (Kennedy-Malone, Fletcher, & Plank, 2004).

Gender: No significance.

Ethnicity: Delirium can affect all people.

Contributing factors: The frail elderly with less physiological reserve, multiple comorbidities, polypharmacy, preexisting dementia, previous history of delirium, sensory impairment, and in an unfamiliar environment are more vulnerable to delirium. Patients admitted to the hospital, in particular to an intensive care unit, are at increased risk for delirium (Kennedy-Malone et al., 2004).

Signs and symptoms: Acute onset and fluctuating course of inattention, altered level of consciousness, and disorganized thinking are signs of delirium.

Diagnostic tests: Taking a patient history and assessment, including a review of patient's medications, is the first step in diagnosing delirium. Disorientation, memory impairment, perceptual disturbances, psychomotor agitation or retardation, and impaired sleep-wake cycle are common findings. The Confusion Assessment Method (CAM) has been validated as an effective tool to diagnose delirium (Inouye et al., 1990). CAM assesses for the presence of acute onset and fluctuating course as well as inattention and either disorganized thinking or altered levels of consciousness. These findings are diagnostic of delirium. Other tools include the Memorial Delirium Assessment Scale, which has been validated in the inpatient palliative care setting, and the Bedside Confusion Scale, which has been validated in advanced cancer palliative patients (Breitbart et al., 1997; Lawlor et al., 2000; Sarhill, Walsh, Nelson, LeGrand, & Davis, 2001).

More invasive diagnostic tools may be indicated to determine etiology if further evaluation is consistent with goals of care.

Differential diagnosis: Consider the possibility of dementia, depression, or the coexistence of either of these with delirium.

Treatment: The first step in treating delirium is to identify the cause(s) if possible. Make appropriate changes to the plan of care based on the etiology. Interventions include attention to fluid and electrolyte imbalances, elimination, and the provision of a supportive and safe environment. Music therapy can be effective (McCaffrey & Locsin, 2004). Regular review of medications to eliminate unnecessary agents is beneficial. Consider inadequate pain control, but remember that opiates can cause delirium, and dose reduction may be necessary (Zimmerman, Rudolph, Salow, & Skarf, 2011). Pharmacological intervention with haloperidol may be necessary. Haloperidol is considered the mainstay of delirium management, beginning with low doses, such as 0.5 mg, and titrating slowly (Zimmerman et al., 2011). Atypical antipsychotics, such as olanzapine, risperidone, or quetiapine, also can be considered for the agitated patient (Perley, 2007b). However, these agents carry an increased risk of cardiovascular events and death in the elderly with dementia (Zimmerman et al., 2011). Benzodiazepines, such as lorazepam, may lead to paradoxical agitation, causing symptoms of delirium to worsen. Therefore, these agents should be used cautiously. Benzodiazepines may benefit patients with a seizure disorder or alcohol withdrawal and those who cannot tolerate antipsychotic medications (Quill et al., 2010).

Follow-up: Provide adequate treatment of underlying cause. Due to multimodal causes, an interdisciplinary approach is preferred.

Sequelae: Prompt evaluation and treatment can improve outcomes. Delirium is distressing to patients, their families, and health-care providers. Delirium contributes to increased morbidity and mortality (Derby et al., 2010). Patients are at risk for falls and potential injury. In end-of-life care, the goal is supportive care to promote a peaceful death.

Prevention/prophylaxis: Avoid polypharmacy, maintain adequate hydration and nutrition as appropriate, minimize invasive devices such as catheters, avoid physical restraints, and use music, massage, and appropriate environmental stimulation.

Referral: Refer the patient to a geriatric psychiatrist, geriatrician, geriatric nurse practitioner, and/or palliative medicine practitioner as needed.

Education: Teach the patient's family signs of delirium, and ask that they report the signs promptly to the medical team. Teach nonpharmacological methods of providing a supportive environment. Avoid over-the-counter medications.

DYSPNEA

Description: Dyspnea is a sensation of breathlessness, with labored or difficult breathing (Derby et al., 2010). It is a distressing symptom at end of life and affects quality of life (Dudgeon, 2010).

Etiology: Dyspnea can have multiple causes such as infection, cancer, heart failure, chronic obstructive pulmonary disease (COPD), asthma, pulmonary fibrosis, pneumothorax, pleural effusion, anemia, and amyotrophic lateral sclerosis.

Occurrence: Occurrence of dyspnea ranges from 10% to 95% depending on the underlying disease. Dyspnea can have as much as a 70% occurrence in cancer patients, an 88% occurrence in those with heart disease, and a 90% to 95% occurrence in those with COPD (Dudgeon, 2010).

Age: Certain causes, such as heart failure, cancer, and chronic lung disease, are more common in the elderly.

Gender: No gender-specific differences.

Ethnicity: Not applicable.

Contributing factors: Smoking and comorbidities can contribute to the development of dyspnea.

Signs and symptoms: Shortness of breath at rest and/or exertion, tachypnea, use of accessory muscles, hypoxia, adventitious breath sounds, cyanosis, pursed-lip breathing are all signs of dyspnea.

Diagnostic tests: Diagnostic tools should be used as appropriate, considering the patient's goals of care. Consider oxygen saturation testing to determine the need for supplemental oxygen. Other diagnostic tests include laboratory tests, such as complete blood count to determine anemia, basic metabolic panel to evaluate renal function, chest x-ray, and electrocardiogram (ECG). Computed tomography (CT) scan to evaluate for malignancy and/or pulmonary embolism may be indicated.

Differential diagnosis: Consider all etiologies as outlined above. If cough is present consider pneumonia; pleural effusion; side effects of medications, such as angiotensin-converting enzyme inhibitors; and gastroesophageal reflux disease.

Treatment: Treatments should be aimed at the underlying etiology. Interventions might include diuretics, bronchodilators, vasodilators, steroids, antibiotics, opioids, and/or sedatives (Ferrell et al., 2011). Nonpharmacological interventions include the use of compressed air or a fan for comfort, oxygen if hypoxic, the elevation of the head of the patient's bed, relaxation, and breathing exercises. Specific pharmacological interventions include nonopioid antitussives, such as dextromethorphan and benzonatate; opioids; and inhaled anesthetics, such as lidocaine or bupivicaine (Dudgeon, 2006). In addition, anxiolytics can be considered (Dudgeon, 2010) (See DiSalvo, Joyce, Culkin, Tyson, & MacKay, 2007, in Appendix 19-1).

Follow-up: Follow up is dependent on etiology. Ongoing assessment, reevaluation, and adjustment of plan of care should be used as needed. Monitor for therapeutic effect as well as adverse effects from interventions.

Sequelae: Dependent on etiology and goals of care. Dyspnea should improve when the cause is treated. However, dyspnea is also common in the dying person, and the goal is comfort measures when death is an anticipated outcome.

Prevention/prophylaxis: Preventive measures are dependent on the cause. Smoking cessation is beneficial as is the avoidance of smoke exposure. Use energy conservation and durable medical equipment for the severely dyspneic patient with advanced illness.

Referral: Referral may be indicated based on etiology and goals of care. Appropriate referrals may include visits to a palliative care specialist, cardiologist, pulmonologist, and/or oncologist.

Education: Smoking cessation; the proper use of medications, including inhalers and nebulizers; the use of fans; energy conservation; and potential adverse effects of medications.

PAIN

Description: According to McCaffery (1968), pain is whatever the person says it is. The patient's own report is the best indicator of pain (American Geriatrics Society [AGS], 2009). (See Appendix 19-2.) Most elderly, including those with dementia, can effectively communicate pain, but a more detailed assessment of pain can be challenging. Several pain assessment tools are available, including the Visual Analogue Scale (VAS), the Numerical Analogue Scale (NAS), the Wong-Baker FACES pain rating scale, and the Pain Assessment in Advanced Dementia (PAIN-AD) scale (Quill et al., 2010).

Etiology: Pain is a common end-of-life symptom in the elderly. Pain is often due to musculoskeletal disorders such as degenerative spine disease and arthritis. Cancer and/or its treatment is another common cause of pain. Neuropathic pain is a common sequela of diabetes, herpes zoster, and peripheral vascular disease as well as postsurgical pain syndromes (AGS, 2009).

Occurrence: Pain is common in the elderly. About 80% of cancer patients experience pain (International Association for the Study of Pain, 2009), and about 45% to 80% of nursing home residents experience pain (Ferrell, 1995). Over 40% of nursing home residents who experienced pain at initial assessment were in severe pain 60 to 180 days later (Teno, Weitze, Wetle, & Mor, 2001).

Age: The comorbidities experienced with aging make pain more likely. The elderly, particularly those with cognitive impairment, are at risk for undertreatment of pain (Ferrell et al., 2011). Many of the interventions to treat these challenging symptoms are pharmacological interventions. It is important to consider geriatric pharmacology when formulating treatment plans. Several physiological factors affect drug distribution, including cardiac output, regional blood flow, body mass and composition (which affect hydrophilic and lipophilic drug distribution), and plasma protein concentration. These changes make an elderly person more susceptible to adverse drug effects. Drug metabolism and clearance in the elderly is often slowed due to declining renal and liver function. Drug interactions, particularly with drugs metabolized through the P-450 enzyme system, also put an elderly person at risk. The health-care provider needs to be mindful of these effects when prescribing. Begin with low doses and titrate carefully, with frequent reassessment, to optimize pain relief and minimize adverse effects (AGS, 2009; Derby & O'Mahoney, 2006).

Gender: Women and men are at equal risk for undertreatment of pain (Ferrell et al., 2011).

Ethnicity: Culture affects how a person experiences and communicates pain. Patients of nondominant cultures are at risk for undertreatment of pain (Ferrell et al., 2011).

Contributing factors: Multiple comorbidities.

Signs and symptoms: Complete a thorough pain assessment, including history, location, intensity (using a VAS as appropriate), quality, pattern, aggravating/relieving factors, temporal pattern medication history, and cultural influences (Ferrell et al., 2011).

Diagnostic tests: Patient history and physical examination should direct appropriate diagnostic testing to assess the underlying cause.

Differential diagnosis: Determine somatic, visceral, and/or neuropathic pain.

Treatment: The WHO Step Ladder (WHO, 2011) provides a framework for pharmacological interventions. The first step is NSAIDs and acetaminophen for mild pain. Acetaminophen is still considered an effective agent for pain associated with osteoarthritis and low back pain. Caution must be used to limit total acetaminophen dose from all sources to 4000 mg/day to avoid liver toxicity (moderate quality of evidence, strong recommendation; AGS, 2009). In those with hepatic insufficiency or alcohol abuse, acetaminophen dose should be reduced by 50% to 75% (moderate quality of evidence, strong recommendation; AGS, 2009). Liver failure is an absolute contraindication (high quality of evidence, strong recommendation; AGS, 2009). Recent guidelines from the American Geriatrics Society advise against the routine use of NSAIDs in the elderly due to the significant potential for adverse effects. The guidelines recommend that NSAIDs be used with extreme caution in highly selected patients (high level of evidence, strong recommendation; AGS, 2009). These include gastrointestinal toxicity, with the risk of gastrointestinal bleeding increasing with the addition of daily aspirin; renal toxicity; and platelet dysfunction, including interference with the antiplatelet effect of aspirin therapy, particularly with ibuprofen. NSAIDs also may have adverse effects on blood pressure control and heart failure management. The COX-2 inhibitors may place a person at greater risk for cardiovascular events, including myocardial infarction. Absolute contraindications for NSAIDs include current, active peptic ulcer disease (low quality of evidence, strong recommendation); chronic kidney disease (moderate level of evidence, strong recommendation); and heart failure (moderate level of evidence, weak recommendation). Relative contraindications and cautions include hypertension, *Helicobacter pylori*, history of peptic ulcer disease, and concomitant use of corticosteroids or selective serotonin reuptake inhibitors (SSRIs) (moderate quality of evidence, strong recommendation; AGS, 2009).

Patients with moderate-to-severe pain with functional impairment and/or decreased quality of life due to pain should be considered for opioid therapy (low quality of evidence, strong recommendation; AGS, 2009). Step 2 of the WHO ladder adds opioids, typically in combination with acetaminophen, which limits the amount of total opioid given. Examples include hydrocodone with acetaminophen and oxycodone with acetaminophen. These are used for moderate pain.

For severe pain, advance to step 3, which includes opioid pain medications. Opioids with a short half-life are recommended in the elderly (Derby et al., 2010). Common opioids include morphine, oxycodone, and hydromorphone. Monitor the patient on short-acting pain medication, and if the patient requires regular dosing every 4 to 6 hours, consider a long-acting formulation, but monitor closely for adverse effects (including altered mental status). Patients with continuous pain may be treated with around-the-clock dosing to achieve steady state (low quality of evidence, weak recommendation; AGS, 2009). Adjust the dose as needed. Controlled-release opiates are appropriate for chronic pain (Derby et al., 2010). Long-acting opioids for pain control include morphine sulfate sustained release, oxycodone sustained release, and fentanyl patch. A long-acting hydromorphone preparation, Exalgo, recently has been released on the market (Epocrates, 2011). Methadone is another long-acting pain medication, but it requires careful dosing and monitoring due to its variable half-life, potential prolongation of QT interval, and numerous drug interactions (AGS, 2009; McPherson, 2010). Be cautious with opioid rotation, and use an appropriate equianalgesic dosing chart (McPherson, 2010). Pay attention to renal and hepatic function due to the risk of altered drug metabolism and elimination with renal and hepatic impairment. Monitor for signs of drug accumulation, which can include delirium, sedation, and myoclonus. Also monitor polypharmacy due to potential for drug interactions. Opiates should not be stopped abruptly, because this could potentiate withdrawal symptoms.

Anticipate, assess for, and identify potential adverse effects (moderate quality of evidence, strong recommendation; AGS, 2009). Common adverse effects include constipation, nausea, and sedation. Sedation precedes respiratory depression, so monitor closely,

particularly in the opioid-naive patient. Begin with short-acting medications before adding a long-acting formulation (AGS, 2009). Most people develop a tolerance to all of the adverse effects with the exception of constipation, which typically requires an aggressive bowel regimen with regular dosing of a laxative and stool softener and/or osmotic agent. Methylnaltrexone is a newer agent approved for severe opioid-induced constipation, and naloxone given orally has also demonstrated effectiveness (Economou, 2010). In addition, the FDA recently approved lubiprostone for treating opioid-induced constipation (International Foundation for Functional Gastrointestinal Disorders [IFFGD], 2013). If fecal impaction is suspected, administer a lubricant, such as a glycerin suppository or mineral oil enema, and disimpact manually. Suppositories and enemas should be avoided in patients with neutropenia and thrombocytopenia. Because disimpaction can be a painful procedure, the patient may require premedication with an appropriate analgesic (Economou, 2010; Sigler, Kelly, & Dahlin, 2007).

Adjuvant medications may improve pain control and can be added at any step of the WHO Step Ladder (WHO, 2011). Tricyclic antidepressants may improve neuropathic pain. Adverse effects due to anticholinergic activity need to be considered. Nortriptyline and desipramine may be better tolerated in the elderly (Derby et al., 2010). Duloxetine, an inhibitor of norepinephrine and serotonin reuptake, is another option, indicated for diabetic neuropathy and chronic musculoskeletal pain as well as for fibromyalgia (Epocrates, 2013). Anticonvulsants can be beneficial for lancinating neuropathic pain, which is often described as burning, shooting, and electrical. Gabapentin and pregabalin are commonly used (Paice, 2010). Topical analgesics, such as lidocaine 5% patch, can be beneficial for postherpetic neuropathy. Capsaicin cream has shown benefit in neuropathic and nonneuropathic pain syndromes; however, about 30% of people do not tolerate the adverse burning sensation when treatment is initiated (AGS, 2009). Corticosteroids improve the pain of nerve or spinal cord compression. They also reduce edema and inflammation, resulting in improved pain (Derby et al., 2010). Corticosteroids also may improve pain management related to bowel obstruction and headaches caused by increased intracranial pressure (AGS, 2009). Caution is advised due to the adverse effects of corticosteroids. Calcitonin may be beneficial for bone pain due to vertebral compression fracture, pelvic fractures, and pain due to bony metastatic disease (AGS, 2009). Baclofen, a muscle relaxant, can be used for spasticity due to central nervous system injury and neuromuscular disorders. Start with a low dose and increase slowly to minimize dizziness, sedation, and gastrointestinal disorders. Baclofen should be tapered slowly to avoid potential delirium and seizure (AGS, 2009).

Nonpharmacological approaches include behavioral therapies such as relaxation, mindfulness, distraction, imagery, prayer, and cognitive reframing (Ferrell et al., 2011). Physical measures include heat and/or cold application, repositioning, massage, and other complementary therapies such as acupuncture (Ferrell et al., 2011).

Follow-up: Ongoing assessment, reevaluation, and adjustment of plan of care as needed. Monitor for therapeutic effect as well as adverse effects. The elderly are more susceptible to the adverse effects of opioids and other nonopioid analgesics and adjuvant medications and thus require close follow-up (AGS, 2009).

Sequelae: Unrelieved pain is associated with functional impairment, falls, mood disorders (including depression and anxiety), sleep and appetite disturbances, and decreased socialization (AGS, 2009). Improved pain control improves function and quality of life. Potential negative outcomes of opioids can include sedation, respiratory depression, coma, and death. These adverse events can typically be avoided by choosing the appropriate medication for the patient, starting at a low dose, and titrating slowly to effect while monitoring for adverse effects. Addiction, though rare, can occur and should be monitored.

Prevention/prophylaxis: Dependent on etiology. Pain escalation may indicate advancing disease, particularly in the cancer patient. Monitor with ongoing assessment. Anticipate painful procedures, such as wound care, and treat appropriately.

Referral: Refer the patient to a palliative care specialist or pain management team for complicated pain syndromes or intolerance to common analgesics.

Education: Explain causes of pain syndromes, treatment strategies, and importance of regular follow-up for reassessment of pain and possible adverse effects. Educate patient/family about the risks of opioids and appropriate interventions for common adverse effects such as nausea and constipation. Advise patient, family, and staff that sedation precedes respiratory depression and to report excessive sedation promptly.

THE DYING PATIENT

Description: Hospice care is mostly considered a medical event in today's society, but the growing acceptance of hospice care is creating a more natural dying experience. Of the patients enrolled in hospice care in 2009, 40.1% died in their own home, 18.9% died in a nursing home, 9.6% died in a residential facility, 21.2% died in a hospice inpatient facility, and 10.1% died in the hospital (NHPCO, 2010).

Etiology: Multiple comorbidities with influence of the aging process.

Occurrence: Mortality rate is 100%. All hospice patients will die.

Age: Risk of death increases with advancing age.

Gender: No gender differences.

Ethnicity: The meaning and experience of death are often influenced by one's culture and ethnicity. Honor the patient's cultural beliefs, traditions, rights, and rituals (Ferrell et al., 2011).

Contributing factors: Advancing age, terminal illness, and comorbidities.

Signs and symptoms: A person typically experiences the following physical symptoms in varying degrees: disorientation, agitation, restlessness, delirium, generalized weakness, drowsiness, sleeping more, decreased oral intake, dysphagia, fever, bowel changes, and incontinence. People sleep more as death approaches with only brief periods of interactions. However, many experience a surge of energy. Patients may experience near-death awareness (Ferrell et al., 2011; Quill et al., 2010).

During the last 48 hours of life, the most prevalent physical symptoms are decreased urine output, cold and mottled extremities, changes to vital signs, and an irregular shallow breathing pattern and periods of apnea. Respiratory congestion, often termed *death rattle*, is common, as are breathlessness, fever, and diaphoresis. Myoclonus also may occur (Ferrell et al., 2011; Quill et al., 2010).

Diagnostic tests: Usually not appropriate in the dying patient.

Differential diagnosis: Not applicable.

Treatment: Assess the dying person frequently for objective signs of distress, such as grimacing and moaning, and treat distressing symptoms as follows: morphine intensol or oxycodone intensol for pain and/or shortness of breath/air hunger; lorazepam intensol for restlessness and anxiety; haloperidol intensol for agitation/delirium or nausea; atropine ophthalmic drops, scopolamine patch, glycopyrulate, or hyoscyamine for upper airway secretions; acetaminophen suppository for fever; and compazine suppository for nausea and vomiting. Focus on comfort measures such as oral care, skin care, continence care, and repositioning as appropriate; provide a calm environment (Ferrell et al., 2011; Quill et al., 2007).

Include the interdisciplinary team when addressing the spiritual, psychosocial, and emotional needs of the patient and the family. For most people, being "fully present" with the dying person is important. When death is inevitable, the dying person's attention shifts to the spiritual process of withdrawing from life. This process can create fear of abandonment, fear of the unknown, and fear of the dying process itself. Thus, it is essential for active involvement of the interdisciplinary team to support the patient and family through this process (Ferrell et al., 2011).

Follow-up: Ensure 24-hour access to care for the dying patient and his or her family. Provide bereavement care for the family.

Sequelae: Death of the patient; bereavement follow-up for the family.

Prevention/prophylaxis: An important consideration for dying persons is to be able to communicate their end-of-life wishes to their family and to their medical team if they are able to do so ahead of time. These discussions are best had when the person is not actively dying and should be had at a time in the person's life when he or she can clearly express his or her wishes. A useful tool for providers is Buckman's S-P-I-K-E-S protocol with its focus on setting, perception, invitation, knowledge, empathy, and strategy/summary (Baile et al., 2000; Buckman, 1992, 2005). Ensuring a private setting for the discussion of goals of care is important as is inviting patients and family members to participate. Before discussing the plan of care, assess what the patient already understands about his or her condition and in how much detail the patient would like to know about his or her illness and prognosis. Before delivering bad news, give a warning that bad news is coming, and respond to emotions. It is also important to summarize the meeting and agreed-upon goals of care (Buckman, 2005).

Referral: Timely referral to hospice care. Refer to palliative care if end-of-life symptoms are difficult to manage such as intractable pain or terminal delirium.

Education: Teach the patient's family the signs of impending death, and ask them to notify the medical team of distressing symptoms. Educate on comfort measures such as oral care, repositioning, and incontinence care. Prepare the family for the patient's possible near-death experience. Educate the patient's family on the signs of death and care at the time of death. Educate on bereavement resources (Ferrell et al., 2011).

CLINICAL RECOMMENDATION	EVIDENCE RATING	REFERENCES
Opioids should be used for dyspnea at the end of life. Multiple studies have shown that nebulized opioids have no benefit over systemic administration in terms of effect or adverse effects.	A	Abernethy et al. (2003) Jennings, Davies, Higgins, & Broadley (2001)
Opioids should be used for pain at the end of life. The ethical limitations of withholding opioids have limited the study of opioids versus placebo, except in neuropathic pain.	C	Eisenberg, McNicol, & Carr (2005)

CLINICAL RECOMMENDATION	EVIDENCE RATING	REFERENCES
Stimulant laxatives are effective for prevention and treatment of constipation in persons on opioids. There is no clear benefit of one regimen over another.	C	Cherny et al. (2001) Miles, Fellowes, Goodman, & Wilkinson (2006)
Methylnaltrexone (Relistor) can be used for treatment of opioid bowel dysfunction. It has recently been added as a treatment option.	B	McNicol, Boyce, Schumann, & Carr (2008) Thomas et al. (2008)
Corticosteroids can be used for malignant bowel obstruction.	B	Feuer & Broadley (2000)
Haloperidol (formerly Haldol) is effective for nausea and vomiting.	B	Büttner, Walder, von Elm, & Tramèr (2004) Markowitz & Rabow (2008)
Hyoscyamine (Levsin) should be used for the "death rattle" (excessive respiratory secretions).	C	Wee & Hillier (2008)

A = consistent, good-quality, patient-oriented evidence; B = inconsistent or limited-quality, patient-oriented evidence; C = consensus, disease-oriented evidence, usual practice, expert opinion, or case series.
Source: Clary, P., & Lawson, P. (2009). Pharmacologic pearls for end of life care. American Family Physician, 79(12), 1059–1065.

GRIEF AND BEREAVEMENT

Description: Bereavement is the state of experiencing the death of a loved one, and it includes grief and mourning. It is a process that involves adjusting to a world without the deceased. Grief is the emotional response to a loss. Mourning is the outward, social expression of the loss (Corless, 2010; Ferrell et al., 2011). Grief is a normal reaction to loss and is affected by the circumstances at the time of death (Quill et al., 2010). It affects the patient's loved ones and anyone who was involved in the patient's care. There are three different types of grief: anticipatory, normal, and complicated grief. Anticipatory grief is experienced before the death and can be experienced by everyone involved, including the patient. Normal grief encompasses the typical emotional, physical, cognitive, and spiritual reactions to a loss. Complicated grief is described as chronic, delayed, exaggerated, masked, or disenfranchised (Perley, 2007a). Stages of grief include notification and shock, followed by experiencing the loss emotionally and cognitively, and finally, reintegration (Corless, 2010). The tasks of grieving include acknowledging the reality of death, sharing in the process of working through the pain of grief, reorganizing the family system, restructuring the relationship with the deceased, and reinvesting in other relationships and life pursuits (Corr & Doka, 1994).

Etiology: Death of a loved one as experienced by family and caregivers.

Occurrence: Loss of relationships and role identity culminating in death, the ultimate loss experience. Complicated grief occurs in 10% to 20% of survivors (Quill et al., 2010).

Age: Affects people of all ages. Consider developmental stages of children in bereavement care.

Gender: Men and women express grief differently, with women typically more expressive and men more restrained (Fullerton.edu, 2011).

Ethnicity: Grief is influenced by one's culture and religion (Corless, 2010).

Contributing factors: Death of a loved one. Contributing factors for complicated grief include a sudden or untimely death, a violent death, death of a child, multiple losses, difficult terminal illness and/or lack of social support, preexisting mental health issues, or substance abuse (Ferrell et al., 2011; Quill et al., 2010).

Signs and symptoms: Normal grieving includes physical, emotional, cognitive, and behavioral responses. Physical responses may include chest tightness, breathlessness, headaches, insomnia, exhaustion, weakness, and oversensitivity to noise. Emotional symptoms may include sadness, anxiety, guilt, shame, and anger as well as relief and a sense of peace. Cognitive responses may include confusion, poor concentration, a sense that the deceased is present, and a search for meaning in the loss. Behavioral symptoms may include crying, withdrawal, impaired work performance, and overreactivity (Corless, 2010; Ferrell et al., 2011).

Complicated grieving typically includes intense shock, anger and denial, feelings of numbness or hopelessness, a blunted emotional expression, anxiety and panic, and chronic depression as well as a risk for self-harm such as suicide or substance abuse (Perley, 2007a).

Differential diagnosis: Depression.

Treatment: Support grieving as a normal experience. Provide emotional and spiritual support. Consider referral for bereavement support groups and pastoral counseling. For complicated grief, refer to a bereavement specialist, physician, and/or psychologist/psychiatrist. Encourage expression of feelings, and encourage reminiscence and life review. Journal writing, letter writing, and drawing pictures can be beneficial. Caregivers can support the bereaved by sending a note, attending the funeral or memorial service, or making a supportive phone call. Use active listening skills, and allow the bereaved to tell their story. Staff bereavement may include encouraging staff to express their grief, reviewing deaths and their effects on staff, enabling staff to attend memorial services, creating staff mourning rituals, and encouraging self-care (Ferrell et al., 2011; Perley, 2007a).

Due to the paucity of rigorous studies among the bereaved, there is a lack of evidence to support current practice (Eberl, 2008). Interventions are guided by expert opinion.

Follow-up: Ensure regular health-care appointments with primary provider.

Sequelae: Complicated grief. About 17% to 27% of patients experience clinical depression during the first year after a loved one's death, with suicidal ideation present in up to 54% in the first 6 months (Casarett, Kuter, & Abrahm, 2001).

Prevention: Allowing expression of grief with appropriate support.

Referral: Refer surviving family and friends to bereavement support groups, bereavement counseling, and psychiatric care if indicated.

Education: Instruct on normal grief reactions, bereavement resources in the community, awareness of signs of complicated grief and depression.

CASE STUDY

Mrs. M. is an 85-year-old woman with breast cancer with metastasis to the lungs. She is receiving palliative chemotherapy. Her husband died 5 years ago, and she is currently living with her daughter, who works outside the home. A private caregiver has been hired through a community agency. Mrs. M. enjoys visits from her family and fellow church members. Mrs. M. is seen by the geriatric nurse practitioner when she comes to her follow-up appointment in the oncology clinic. She is experiencing moderate-to-severe right chest wall pain. She also is experiencing dyspnea on exertion, nausea, constipation, and fatigue. A recent CT scan revealed disease progression on third-line chemotherapy.

Her past medical history is noncontributory. Current medications: hydrochlorothiazide 12.5 mg PO daily and levothyroxine 50 mcg PO daily; and senna PO bid for constipation/APAP. She has no known allergies.

Exploring her symptoms: She rates her right chest wall pain at 7/10. It is a dull, aching pain and worsens with activity. The pain has been present for 2 weeks. Hydrocodone/APAP had initially helped but is no longer effective. Because of the pain and dyspnea, she spends most of her time sitting in a reclining chair or lying in bed. Her appetite has decreased. She has not moved her bowels in 2 days. She complains of fatigue and insomnia.

Focused physical examination: temperature 98.2°F, heart rate (HR) 75 beats/min, respiratory rate (RR) 22 breaths/min, blood pressure (BP) 120/80 mm Hg, oxygen saturation 94%, weight

CASE STUDY—cont'd

105 lb, height 5 feet 4 inches, body mass index (BMI) 18 kg/m².

Mrs. M. is in moderate distress. She appears thin and frail. Her color is sallow, and her heart sounds reveal regular rate and rhythm, no murmur, rub, or gallop. Her lungs have bibasilar crackles, greater on the right, no wheezing. Her abdomen is soft with active bowel sounds, nontender to palpation.

What would you recommend for her symptom management?

Putting Evidence into Practice® Card on Dyspnea

The optimal treatment of dyspnea includes using specific therapies as appropriate to reverse the causes along with using palliative therapies to treat irreversible causes for symptomatic relief. The interventions discussed in this document are palliative and are a result of a review of the literature focused solely on cancer-related dyspnea. Evidence from research that considers dyspnea attributed to other etiologies may be beneficial in cancer-related dyspnea but is beyond the scope of this document.

RECOMMENDED FOR PRACTICE

Interventions for which effectiveness has been demonstrated by strong evidence from rigorously designed studies, meta-analyses, or systematic reviews and for which expectation of harm is small compared with the benefits.

Immediate-Release Oral or Parenteral Opioids

Evidence supports the use of oral and parenteral opioids for management of dyspnea in patients with terminal or advanced cancer, because opioids reduce ventilatory demand by decreasing the central respiratory drive. In a systematic review and several smaller studies, patients reported dyspnea relief with opioids (Allard, Lamontagne, Bernard, & Tremblay, 1999; Bruera, Macmillan, Pither, & MacDonald, 1990; Jennings, Davies, Higgins, Gibbs, & Broadley, 2002; Mazzocato, Buclin, & Rapin, 1999).

- Morphine was the predominant opioid evaluated in the studies, but other opioids also were included.

- In general, those patients who were opioid-naive were given smaller doses of opioid than those who were opioid-tolerant. A wide range of doses were used in the studies.
- In patients already receiving opioids on a regular basis, supplemental oral and parenteral doses consisting of either 25% or 50% of the equivalent 4-hour opioid dose (e.g., total 24-hour opioid dose divided into 4-hour portions) have been assessed. One study found that supplemental opioid doses at 25% of the regular 4-hour dose can reduce dyspnea for as many as 4 hours (Allard et al., 1999).
- Overall, the opioids were well tolerated, with the exception of nausea and vomiting.
- More research is needed to define the most effective doses of oral and parenteral opioids and to determine those patients who are most likely to benefit from the use of opioids.

LIKELY TO BE EFFECTIVE

Interventions for which there is evidence from a single rigorously conducted, controlled trial; consistent evidence from well-designed, controlled trials using small samples or from meta-analyses/systematic reviews using small samples; or evidence from guidelines developed from evidence and supported by expert opinion are likely to be effective in treating dyspnea.

Expert consensus recommends the following palliative interventions to relieve cancer-related dyspnea (National Comprehensive Cancer Network, 2006). The consensus guidelines for dyspnea are categorized by estimated life expectancy.

The life expectancy category labeled years to months to weeks includes the following measures to relieve symptoms.

■ Temporary ventilator support if clinically indicated for severe reversible conditions
■ Oxygen therapy (see also supplemental oxygen evidence listed in the Effectiveness-Not-Established category) (Bruera, de Stoutz, Velasco-Leiva, Schoeller, & Stoutz, 1993; Bruera et al., 2003)
■ Benzodiazepines for anxiety
■ Increasing ambient air flow directed at the face or nose such as generated by a fan
■ Provision of cooler temperatures
■ Promotion of relaxation and stress reduction
■ Educational, emotional, and psychosocial support for patients and family caregivers and referral to other disciplines as appropriate

Interventions recommended for a dying patient experiencing dyspnea include the previous measures and the following.

■ Reduce excessive secretions with scopolamine, hyoscyamine, or atropine.
■ Implement oxygen therapy, if subjective report of relief (see supplemental oxygen evidence listed later in the Effectiveness-Not-Established category) (Bruera et al., 1993; Bruera et al., 2003).
■ Institute sedation as needed.
■ Discontinue fluid support, and consider low-dose diuretics if fluid overload may be a contributing factor.

EFFECTIVENESS NOT ESTABLISHED

Interventions for which effectiveness has not been established include treatments that are currently insufficient or around which there are conflicting data or data of inadequate quality.

Pharmacological

EXTENDED-RELEASE MORPHINE

One small study testing the regular administration of extended-release morphine failed to show a significant reduction in dyspnea for those who completed the study (Boyd & Kelly, 1997). In addition, out of 15 patients entered in the study, 3 withdrew because of sedation, and 3 died without showing a reduction in dyspnea. The high incidence of sedation and

dizziness at 48 hours after initiation should raise concern, especially in opioid-naive patients, and emphasizes the need to monitor patients carefully (Boyd & Kelly, 1997).

MIDAZOLAM PLUS MORPHINE

Only one trial has been reported to support the use of the combination of midazolam* plus morphine in patients with severe dyspnea in the last week of their lives (Navigante, Cerchietti, Castro, Lutteral, & Cabalar, 2006). This regimen cannot be recommended without more research.

NEBULIZED FENTANYL

Evidence is insufficient to recommend the use of nebulized fentanyl.* One small study reported a perceived benefit by the majority of patients (Coyne, Viswanathan, & Smith, 2002). However, there were limitations to this study. Further research is needed before nebulized fentanyl can be recommended.

NEBULIZED FUROSEMIDE

Evidence is insufficient to support the use of nebulized furosemide* in the treatment of dyspnea. As reported by one uncontrolled study (Shimoyama & Shimoyama, 2002) and three case reports (Kohara et al., 2013), the majority of patients reported that inhalation of furosemide decreased the sensation of dyspnea. However, further rigorous research is required before this regimen can be recommended.

NEBULIZED LIGNOCAINE (LIDOCAINE HYDROCHLORIDE)*

One small study evaluated nebulized lignocaine* in people with cancer experiencing breathlessness at rest (Wilcock, Corcoran, & Tattersfield, 1994). No benefit was seen with the inhaled lignocaine. In fact, the distress of breathing increased after nebulized lignocaine.

NEBULIZED OPIOIDS[†]

At this point, insufficient evidence exists to recommend the use of nebulized opioids in the treatment of dyspnea. Investigation into the use of inhaled nebulized opioids has yielded mixed results. Although some individual studies indicate the potential for efficacy (Bruera et al., 2005; Joyce, McSweeney,

---

*The use of this drug in the treatment of dyspnea has not been approved by the U.S. Food and Drug Administration and is considered off-label use.
†The use of the nebulized form of this drug in the treatment of dyspnea has not been approved by the U.S. Food and Drug Administration and is considered off-label use.

Carrieri-Kohlnman, & Hawkins, 2004; Quigley, Joel, Patel, Baksh, & Slevin, 2002; Tanaka et al., 1999), higher-level reviews have failed to show positive effects of nebulized opioids for the treatment of dyspnea and recommend further research with rigorous designs and larger samples (Jennings et al., 2002; Zeppetella, 1997).

SUPPLEMENTAL OXYGEN

- In hypoxic patients experiencing dyspnea at rest, one small trial demonstrated that oxygen (which can reduce ventilatory demand) is beneficial (Bruera et al., 1993).
- For nonhypoxic dyspneic patients, the routine use of supplemental oxygen did not demonstrate benefit (Bruera et al., 2003). A study looking at the use of a different gas mixture (heliox 28%) in nonhypoxic dyspneic patients undergoing exercise indicated that there may be some benefit of this gas mixture (American Thoracic Society, 1999).

Nonpharmacological

ACUPUNCTURE

One study evaluated 20 patients with cancer-related breathlessness who received acupuncture (Ahmedzai, Laude, Robertson, Troy, & Vora, 2004). The patients acknowledged an improvement in their breathlessness after the acupuncture, but these results may have been contaminated by the nurse remaining with the patient for 90 minutes after the intervention. Further evaluation of acupuncture for cancer-related breathlessness is indicated.

COGNITIVE-BEHAVIORAL APPROACH

One multicenter and two smaller studies examined the effect of specialized nursing interventions on the quality of life of patients with lung cancer who are experiencing breathlessness (Bredin et al., 1999; Corner, Plant, A'Hern, & Bailey, 1996; Filshie, Penn, Ashley, & Davis, 1996). Interventions offered in the studies included the following.

- Assessment of breathlessness—what improves and what hinders
- Provision of information and support for patients and families in the management of breathlessness
- Exploration of the significance of breathlessness with patients, their disease, and their future

- Instruction in breathing control, relaxation, and distraction techniques
- Goal setting to enhance breathing and relaxation techniques as well as to enhance function, enable participation in social activities, and develop coping skills
- Identification of early signs of problems that need medical or pharmacotherapy intervention

Patients receiving these interventions reported a significant improvement in breathlessness, emotional and physical well-being, and performance status. Further trials are needed to pinpoint which interventions are essential to improve the dyspnea outcome.

EXPERT OPINION

Low-risk interventions are those (1) that are consistent with sound clinical practice, (2) that are suggested by an expert in a peer-reviewed publication (journal or book chapter), and (3) for which limited evidence exists. An expert is an individual who has authored articles published in a peer-reviewed journal in the domain of interest.

Although limited evidence exists, experts recommend the following supportive interventions in patients experiencing cancer-related dyspnea (Campbell, 2004; Dudgeon, 2002; Gallo-Silver & Pollack, 2000; Hately, Laurence, Scott, Baker, & Thomas, 2003).

- Maximize treatments that have proven beneficial to individual patients, such as avoiding volume overload and using oxygen and nebulized bronchodilators.
- Use upright positioning that affords patients optimal lung capacity, especially with a coexisting diagnosis of chronic obstructive pulmonary disease.
- Educate patients about breathing exercises such as diaphragmatic breathing, altering breathing rhythm, and pursed-lip breathing to optimize lung function (Dudgeon, 2002).
- Educate patients to recognize physical maneuvers that precipitate dyspnea. Employ interventions, such as cognitive-behavioral techniques (e.g., relaxation, imaging therapy), to decrease the anticipatory component associated with exertional dyspnea.

- Consider the use of assistive devices, such as a wheelchair and portable oxygen, to decrease physical activities that precipitate dyspnea.
- Expert opinion is conflicted regarding the use of benzodiazepines.* Some recommend it to treat anxiety associated with dyspnea (Hately et al., 2003; National Comprehensive Cancer Network, 2006).

Authors: Wendye M. Disalvo, RN, ARNP, MS, AOCN; Margaret M. Joyce, PhD, RN, AOCN; Ann E. Culkin, RN, OCN; Leslie B. Tyson, MS, APRN, BC, OCN; and Kathleen Mackay, RN, BSN, OCN.

Oncology Nursing Society

125 Enterprise Drive, Pittsburgh, PA 15275

412-859-6100

Definitions of the interventions and full citations: www.ons.org/outcomes

Literature search completed through September 2006.

This content, published by the Oncology Nursing Society (ONS), reflects a scientific literature review. There is no representation nor guarantee that the practices described herein will, if followed, ensure safe and effective patient care. The descriptions reflect the state of general knowledge and practice in the field as described in the literature as of the date of the scientific literature review. The descriptions may not be appropriate for use in all circumstances. Those who use this card should make their own determinations regarding safe and appropriate patient-care practices, taking into account the personnel, equipment, and practices available at their health-care facility. ONS does not endorse the practices described herein. The editors and publisher cannot be held responsible for any liability incurred as a consequence of the use or application of any of the contents of this text.

Copyright 2007 by Oncology Nursing Society

REFERENCES

Ahmedzai, S. H., Laude, E., Robertson, A., Troy, G., & Vora, V. (2004). A double blind, randomized, controlled phase II trial of heliox 28 gas mixture in lung cancer patients with dyspnoea on exertion. *British Journal of Cancer, 90*(2), 366–371.

Allard, P., Lamontagne, C., Bernard, P., & Tremblay, C. (1999). How effective are supplementary doses of opioids for dyspnea in terminally ill cancer patients? A randomized continuous sequential clinical trial. *Journal of Pain and Symptom Management, 17*(4), 256–265.

American Thoracic Society. (1999). Dyspnea: mechanisms, assessment, and management: a consensus statement. *American Journal of Respiratory and Critical Care Medicine, 159*(1), 321–340.

Boyd, K. J., & Kelly, M. (1997). Oral morphine as symptomatic treatment of dyspnea in patients with advanced cancer. *Palliative Medicine, 11*(4), 277–281.

Bredin, M., Corner, J., Krishnasamy, M., Plant, H., Bailey, C., & A'Hern, R. (1999). Multicenter randomized controlled trial of nursing intervention for breathlessness in patients with lung cancer. *BMJ, 318*(7188), 901–904.

Bruera, E., de Stoutz, N., Velasco-Leiva, A., Schoeller, T., & Hanson, J. (1993). Effects of oxygen on dyspnea in hypoxaemic terminal-cancer patients. *Lancet, 342*(8862), 13–14.

Bruera, E., Macmillan, K., Pither, J., & MacDonald, R. N. (1990). Effects of morphine on the dyspnea of terminal cancer patients. *Journal of Pain and Symptom Management, 5*(6), 341–344.

Bruera, E., Sala, R., Spruyt, O., Palmer, J. L., Zhang, T., & Willey, J. (2005). Nebulized versus subcutaneous morphine for patients with cancer dyspnea: a preliminary study. *Journal of Pain and Symptom Management, 29*(6), 613–618.

Bruera, E., Sweeney, C., Willey, J., Palmer, J. L., Strasser, F., Morice, R. C., & Pisters, K. (2003). Randomized controlled trial of supplemental oxygen versus air in cancer patients with dyspnea. *Palliative Medicine, 17*(8), 659–663.

Campbell, M. L. (2004). Terminal dyspnea and respiratory distress. *Critical Care Clinics, 20*(3), 403–417.

Corner, J., Plant, H., A'Hern, R., & Bailey, C. (1996). Non-pharmacological intervention for breathlessness in lung cancer. *Palliative Medicine, 10*(4), 299–305.

Coyne, P. J., Viswanathan, R., & Smith, T. J. (2002). Nebulized fentanyl citrate improves patients' perception of breathing, respiratory rate, and oxygen saturation in dyspnea. *Journal of Pain and Symptom Management, 23*(2), 157–160.

Dudgeon, D. J. (2002). Managing dyspnea and cough. *Hematology/Oncology Clinics of North America, 16*(3), 557–577.

Filshie, J., Penn, K., Ashley, S., & Davis, C. L. (1996). Acupuncture for the relief of cancer related breathlessness. *Palliative Medicine, 10*(2), 145–150.

Gallo-Silver, L., & Pollack, B. (2000). Behavioral interventions for lung cancer–related breathlessness. *Cancer Practice, 8*(6), 268–273.

Hately, J., Laurence, V., Scott, A., Baker, R., & Thomas, P. (2003). Breathlessness clinics within specialist palliative care settings can improve the quality of life and functional capacity of patients with lung cancer. *Palliative Medicine, 17*(5), 410–417.

Jennings, A. L., Davies, A. N., Higgins, J. P., Gibbs, J. S., & Broadley, K. E. (2002). A systematic review of the use of opioids in the management of dyspnoea. *Thorax, 57*(11), 939–944.

Joyce, M., McSweeney, M., Carrieri-Kohlnman, K. L., & Hawkins, J. (2004). The use of nebulized opioids in the management of dyspnea: evidence synthesis. *Oncology Nursing Forum, 31*(3), 551–561.

Kohara, H., Ueoka, H., Aoe, K., Maeda, T., Takeyama, H., Saito, R., . . . Uchitomi, Y. (2003). Effect of nebulized furosemide in terminally ill cancer patients with dyspnea. *Journal of Pain and Symptom Management, 26*(4), 962–967.

Mazzocato, C., Buclin, T., & Rapin, C. H. (1999). The effects of morphine on dyspnea and ventilatory function in elderly patients

---

*The use of this drug in the treatment of dyspnea has not been approved by the U.S. Food and Drug Administration and is considered off-label use.

with advanced cancer: a randomized double-blind controlled trial. *Annals of Oncology, 10*(12), 1511–1514.

National Comprehensive Cancer Network. (2006). *Clinical practice guidelines in oncology: palliative care, version 1.* Retrieved from http://www.nccn.org/professionals/physician_gls/PDF/palliative.pdf

Navigante, A. H., Cerchietti, L. C., Castro, M. A., Lutteral, M. A., & Cabalar, M. E. (2006). Midazolam as adjunct therapy to morphine in the alleviation of severe dyspnea perception in patients with advanced cancer. *Journal of Pain and Symptom Management, 31*(1), 38–47.

Quigley, C., Joel, S., Patel, N., Baksh, A., & Slevin, M. (2002). A phase I/II study of nebulized morphine-6-glucuronide in patients with cancer related breathlessness. *Journal of Pain and Symptom Management, 23*(1), 7–9.

Shimoyama, N., & Shimoyama, M. (2002). Nebulized furosemide as a novel treatment for dyspnea in terminal cancer patients. *Journal of Pain and Symptom Management, 23*(1), 73–76.

Tanaka, K., Shima, Y., Kakinuma, R., Kubota, K., Ohe, Y., Hojo, F., . . . Nishiwaki, Y. (1999). Effect of nebulized morphine in cancer patients with dyspnea: a pilot study. *Japanese Journal of Clinical Oncology, 29*(12), 600–603.

Wilcock, A., Corcoran, R., & Tattersfield, A. E. (1994). Safety and efficacy of nebulized lignocaine in patients with cancer and breathlessness. *Palliative Medicine, 8*(1), 35–38.

Zeppetella, G. (1997). Nebulized morphine in the palliation of dyspnoea. *Palliative Medicine, 11*(4), 267–275.

Guideline Recommendations for Pharmacological Management of Persistent Pain in Older Persons

NONOPIOIDS

(I) Acetaminophen should be considered as initial and ongoing pharmacotherapy in the treatment of persistent pain, particularly musculoskeletal pain, owing to its demonstrated effectiveness and good safety profile (high quality of evidence; strong recommendation).

   (A) Absolute contraindications: liver failure (high quality of evidence, strong recommendation).

   (B) Relative contraindications and cautions: hepatic insufficiency, chronic alcohol abuse or dependence (moderate quality of evidence, strong recommendation).

   (C) Maximum daily recommended dosages of 4 g per 24 hours should not be exceeded and must include "hidden sources" such as from combination pills (moderate quality of evidence, strong recommendation).

(II) Nonselective NSAIDs and COX-2 selective inhibitors may be considered rarely, and with extreme caution, in highly selected individuals (high quality of evidence, strong recommendation).

   (A) Patient selection: other (safer) therapies have failed, evidence of continuing therapeutic goals not met, ongoing assessment of risks and complications outweighed by therapeutic benefits (low quality of evidence, strong recommendation).

   (B) Absolute contraindications: current active peptic ulcer disease (low quality of evidence, strong recommendation), chronic kidney disease (moderate level of evidence, strong recommendation), heart failure (moderate level of evidence, weak recommendation).

   (C) Relative contraindications and cautions: hypertension, *Helicobacter pylori*, history of peptic ulcer disease, concomitant use of corticosteroids or SSRIs (moderate quality of evidence, strong recommendation).

(III) Older persons taking nonselective NSAIDs should use a proton pump inhibitor or misoprostol for gastrointestinal protection (high quality of evidence, strong recommendation).

(IV) Patients taking a COX-2 selective inhibitor with aspirin should use a proton pump inhibitor or misoprostol for gastrointestinal protection (high quality of evidence, strong recommendation).

(V) Patients should not take more than one nonselective NSAID or COX-2 selective inhibitor for pain control (low quality of evidence, strong recommendation).

(VI) Patients taking aspirin for cardioprophylaxis should not use ibuprofen (moderate quality of evidence, weak recommendation).

(VII) All patients taking nonselective NSAIDs and COX-2 selective inhibitors should be routinely assessed for gastrointestinal and renal toxicity, hypertension, heart failure, and other drug-drug and drug-disease interactions (weak quality of evidence, strong recommendation).

OPIOIDS

(VIII) All patients with moderate-to-severe pain, pain-related functional impairment, or diminished quality of life due to pain should be considered for opioid therapy (low quality of evidence, strong recommendation).

(IX) Patients with frequent or continuous pain on a daily basis may be treated with around-the-clock, time-contingent dosing aimed at achieving steady-state opioid therapy (low quality of evidence, weak recommendation).

(X) Clinicians should anticipate, assess for, and identify potential opioid-associated adverse effects (moderate quality of evidence, strong recommendation).

(XI) Maximal safe doses of acetaminophen or NSAIDs should not be exceeded when using fixed-dose opioid combination agents as part of an analgesic regimen (moderate quality of evidence, strong recommendation).

(XII) When long-acting opioid preparations are prescribed, breakthrough pain should be anticipated, assessed, and prevented or treated using short-acting immediate-release opioid medications (moderate quality of evidence, strong recommendation).

(XIII) Only clinicians well versed in the use and risks of methadone should initiate it and should titrate it cautiously (moderate quality of evidence, strong recommendation).

(XIV) Patients taking opioid analgesics should be reassessed for ongoing attainment of therapeutic goals, adverse effects, and safe and responsible medication use (moderate quality of evidence, strong recommendation).

ADJUVANT ANALGESIC DRUGS

(XV) All patients with neuropathic pain are candidates for adjuvant analgesics (strong quality of evidence, strong recommendation).

(XVI) Patients with fibromyalgia are candidates for a trial of approved adjuvant analgesics (moderate quality of evidence, strong recommendation).

(XVII) Patients with other types of refractory persistent pain may be candidates for certain adjuvant analgesics (e.g., back pain, headache, diffuse bone pain, temporomandibular disorder) (low quality of evidence, weak recommendation).

(XVIII) Tertiary tricyclic antidepressants (amitriptyline, imipramine, doxepin) should be avoided because of high risk for adverse effects (e.g., anticholinergic effects, cognitive impairment) (moderate quality of evidence, strong recommendation).

(XIX) Agents may be used alone, but often the effects are enhanced when used in combination with other pain analgesics and nondrug strategies (moderate quality of evidence, strong recommendation).

(XX) Therapy should begin with the lowest possible dose and increase slowly based on response and side effects, with the caveat that some agents have a delayed onset of action and therapeutic benefits are slow to develop. For example, gabapentin may require 2 to 3 weeks for onset of efficacy (moderate quality of evidence, strong recommendation).

(XXI) An adequate therapeutic trial should be conducted before discontinuation of a seemingly ineffective treatment (weak quality of evidence, strong recommendation).

OTHER DRUGS

(XXII) Long-term systemic corticosteroids should be reserved for patients with pain-associated inflammatory disorders or metastatic bone pain. Osteoarthritis should not be considered an inflammatory disorder (moderate quality of evidence, strong recommendation).

(XXIII) All patients with localized neuropathic pain are candidates for topical lidocaine (moderate quality of evidence, strong recommendation).

(XXIV) Patients with localized nonneuropathic pain may be candidates for topical lidocaine (low quality of evidence, weak recommendation).

(XXV) All patients with other localized nonneuropathic persistent pain may be candidates for topical NSAIDs (moderate quality of evidence, weak recommendation).

(XXVI) Other topical agents, including capsaicin or menthol, may be considered for regional pain syndromes (moderate quality of evidence, weak recommendation).

(XXVII) Many other agents for specific pain syndromes may require caution in older persons and merit further research (e.g., glucosamine, chondroitin, cannabinoids, botulinum toxin, alpha-2 adrenergic agonists, calcitonin, vitamin D, bisphosphonates, ketamine) (low quality of evidence, weak recommendation).

American Geriatrics Society. (2009). Pharmacological management of persistent pain in older persons. *Journal of the American Geriatrics Society, 57*(8), 1331–1346. Reprinted with permission from American Geriatrics Society, www.americangeriatrics.org.

REFERENCES

Abernethy, A. P., Currow, D. C., Frith, P., Fazekas, B. S., McHugh, A., & Bui, C. (2003). Randomised, double blind, placebo controlled crossover trial of sustained release morphine for the management of refractory dyspnea. *British Medical Journal, 327*(7414), 523–528.

American Geriatrics Society. (2009). Pharmacological management of persistent pain in older persons. *Journal of the American Geriatrics Society, 57*(8), 1331–1346. Retrieved from http://www.americangeriatrics.org/files/documents/2009_Guideline.pdf

American Psychiatric Association. (1994). *Diagnostic and statistical manual of mental disorders* (4th ed.). Washington, DC: American Psychiatric Association.

Baile, W. F., Buckman, R., Lenzi, R., Glober, G., Beale, E. A., & Kudelka, A. P. (2000). SPIKES—A six-step protocol for delivering bad news: application to the patient with cancer. *Oncologist, 5,* 302–311.

Beach, P. (2007). The evolution of hospice and palliative nursing. In M. J. Perley & C. M. Dahlin (Eds.), *Core curriculum for the advanced practice hospice and palliative nurse* (pp. 3–11). Pittsburgh, PA: Hospice and Palliative Nurses Association.

Breitbart, W., Rosenfeld, B., Roth, A., Smith, M. J., Cohen, K., & Passik, S. (1997). The memorial delirium assessment scale. *Journal of Pain and Symptom Management, 13*(3), 128–137.

Buck, C. (2010). *ICD-9 CM for physicians, volumes 1 & 2, professional edition.* St. Louis, MO: American Medical Association, Saunders/Elsevier.

Buckman, R. (1992). *How to break bad news: a guide for health care professionals.* Baltimore, MD: Johns Hopkins Press.

Buckman, R. (2005). Breaking bad news: the S-P-I-K-E-S strategy. *Community Oncology, 2*(2), 138–142.

Büttner, M., Walder, B., von Elm, E., & Tramèr, M. R. (2004). Is low-dose haloperidol a useful antiemetic? A meta-analysis of published and unpublished randomized trials. *Anesthesiology, 101*(6), 1454–1463.

Casarett, D., Kuter, J. S., & Abrahm, J. (2001). Life after death: a practical approach to grief and bereavement. *Annals of Internal Medicine, 134*(3), 208–215.

Cherny, N., Ripamonti, C., Pereira, J., Davis, C., Fallon, M., McQuay, H., . . . Ventafridda, V. (2001). Strategies to manage the adverse effects of oral morphine: an evidence-based report. *Journal of Clinical Oncology, 19*(9), 2542–2554.

Clary, P., & Lawson, P. (2009). Pharmacologic pearls for end of life care. *American Family Physician, 79*(12), 1059–1065.

Corless, I. B. (2010). Bereavement. In B. R. Ferrell & N. Coyle (Eds.), *Oxford textbook of palliative nursing* (3rd ed., pp. 597–611). New York, NY: Oxford University Press.

Corr, C. A., & Doka, K. J. (1994). Current models of death, dying and bereavement. *Critical Care Nursing Clinics of North America, 6*(3), 545–552.

Derby, S. A. (2007). Geriatric populations. In M. J. Perley & C. M. Dahlin (Eds.), *Core curriculum for the advanced practice hospice and palliative nurse* (pp. 363–382). Pittsburgh, PA: Hospice and Palliative Nurses Association.

Derby, S., & O'Mahoney, S. (2006). Elderly patients. In B. R. Ferrell & N. Coyle (Eds.), *Textbook of palliative nursing* (2nd ed., pp. 635–660). New York, NY: Oxford University Press.

Derby, S., O'Mahoney, S., & Tickoo, R. (2010). Elderly patients. In B. R. Ferrell & N. Coyle (Eds.), *Oxford textbook of palliative nursing* (3rd ed., pp. 713–743). New York, NY: Oxford University Press.

Dudgeon, D. (2006). Dyspnea, death rattle and cough. In B. R. Ferrell & N. Coyle (Eds.), *Textbook of palliative nursing care* (2nd ed., pp. 249–264). New York, NY: Oxford University Press.

Dudgeon, D. (2010). Dyspnea, death rattle and cough. In B. R. Ferrell & N. Coyle (Eds.), *Oxford textbook of palliative nursing* (3rd ed., pp. 303–319). New York, NY: Oxford University Press.

Eberl, M. (2008). *Bereavement interventions: evidence and ethics* [PowerPoint presentation]. Retrieved from http://www.bioethics.buffalo.edu/bereavement.ppt

Economou, D. (2010). Bowel management: constipation, diarrhea, obstruction, and ascites. In B. R. Ferrell & N. Coyle (Eds.), *Oxford textbook of palliative nursing* (3rd ed., pp. 269–289). New York, NY: Oxford University Press.

Eisenberg, E., McNicol, E. D., & Carr, D. B. (2005). Efficacy and safety of opioid agonists in the treatment of neuropathic pain of nonmalignant origin. *Journal of the American Medical Association, 293*(24), 3043–3052.

Epocrates. (2011). Retrieved from http://www.epocrates.com

Epocrates. (2013). Retrieved from http://epocrates.com

Federal Interagency Forum on Aging-Related Statistics. (2002). *Older Americans 2000: key indicators of well-being.* Washington, DC: Federal Interagency Forum on Aging-Related Statistics.

Ferrell, B. (1995). Pain evaluation and management in the nursing home. *Annals of Internal Medicine, 123*(9), 681–687.

Ferrell, B., Ersek, M., Virani, R., Malloy, P., & Kelly, K. (2007, revised 2011). *End-of-life nursing education consortium (ELNEC): geriatric curriculum.* Washington, DC: City of Hope National Medical Center and American Association of Colleges of Nursing (AACN).

Feuer, D. J., & Broadley, K. E. (1999). Corticosteroids for the resolution of malignant bowel obstruction in advanced gynaecological and gastrointestinal cancer. *Cochrane Database of Systematic Reviews,* (3). doi:10.1002/14651858.CD001219

Fullerton.edu. (2011). *The difference between normal grief and clinical depression.* Retrieved from http://www.fullerton.edu/universityblues depression/depression_grievance.htm

Glare, P., Virik, K., Jones, M., Hudson, M., Eychmuller, S., Simes, J., & Christakis, N. (2003). A systematic review of physicians' survival predictions in terminally ill cancer patients. *British Medical Journal, 327*(7408), 195–198.

Heidrich, D., & English, N. (2010). Delirium, confusion, agitation and restlessness. In B. R. Ferrell & N. Coyle (Eds.), *Oxford textbook of palliative nursing* (3rd ed., pp. 449–467). New York, NY: Oxford University Press.

Inouye, S., van Dyck, C., Alessi, C., Balkin, S., Siegal, A., & Horwitz, R. (1990). Clarifying confusion: the Confusion Assessment Method. A new method for detection of delirium. *Annals of Internal Medicine, 113*(12), 941–948.

International Association for the Study of Pain. (2009). *Global year against cancer pain: cancer pain in older people.* Retrieved from http://www.iasp-pain.org/AM/Template.cfm?Section=Fact_Sheets1&Template=/CM/ContentDisplay.cfm&ContentID=7195

International Foundation for Functional Gastrointestinal Disorders. (2013). Treatment news. *Digestive Health Matters, 22*(1). Retrieved from http://www.iffgd.org/site/learning-center/digestive-health-matters-magazine/treatment-news

Jennings, A. L., Davies, A. N., Higgins, J. P., & Broadley, K. E. (2001). Opioids for the palliation of breathlessness in advanced disease and terminal illness. *Cochrane Database of Systematic Reviews,* (3). doi:10.1002/14651858.CD002066

Kennedy-Malone, L., Fletcher, K. R., & Plank, L. M. (2004). *Management guidelines for nurse practitioners working with older adults* (2nd ed.). Philadelphia, PA: F. A. Davis Co.

Lawlor, P. G., Nekolaichuk, C., Gagnon, B., Mancini, I. L., Pereira, J. L., & Bruera, E. D. (2000). Clinical utility, factor analysis, and further validation of the Memorial Delirium Assessment Scale in patients with advanced cancer: assessing delirium in advanced cancer. *Cancer, 88*(12), 2859–2867.

Markowitz, A. J., & Rabow, M. W. (2008). Management of intractable nausea and vomiting in patients at the end of life: "I was feeling nauseous all of the time . . . nothing was working." *Journal of the American Medical Association, 299*(15), 1826.

McCaffery, M. (1968). *Nursing practice theories related to cognition, bodily pain, and man-environment interactions.* Los Angeles, CA: UCLA Press.

McCaffrey, R., & Locsin, R. (2004). The effect of music listening on acute confusion and delirium in elders undergoing elective hip and knee surgery. *Journal of Clinical Nursing, 13*(s2), 91–96. doi:10.1111/j.1365-2702.2004.01048.x

McNicol, E. D., Boyce, D., Schumann, R., & Carr, D. B. (2008). Mu-opioid antagonists for opioid-induced bowel dysfunction. *Cochrane Database of Systematic Reviews,* (2). doi:10.1002/14651858.CD006332.pub2

McPherson, M. L. (2010). *Demystifying opioid conversion calculations: a guide for effective dosing.* Bethesda, MD: American Society of Health-System Pharmacist, Inc.

Miles, C. L., Fellowes, D., Goodman, M. L., & Wilkinson, S. (2006). Laxatives for the management of constipation in palliative care patients. *Cochrane Database of Systematic Reviews,* (4). doi:10.1002/14651858.CD003448

Murphy, S., Xu, J., & Kochanek, K. (2012). Deaths: preliminary data for 2010. *National Vital Statistics Reports, 60*(4), 1–51.

National Hospice and Palliative Care Organization. (2009). *NHPCO facts and figures sheet.* Retrieved from http://www.NHPCO.org

National Hospice and Palliative Care Organization. (2010). *NHPCO facts and figures on hospice care.* Retrieved from http://www.NHPCO.org

National Hospice and Palliative Care Organization. (2012). NHPCO facts and figures: hospice care in America. Retrieved from http://www.nhpco.org/sites/default/files/public/Statistics_Research/2012_Facts_Figures.pdf

National Institute on Aging. (2005). The health and retirement study. Retrieved from http://hrsonline.isr.umich.edu

Paice, J. (2010). Pain at the end of life. In B. R. Ferrell & N. Coyle (Eds.), *Oxford textbook of palliative nursing* (3rd ed., pp. 161–185). New York, NY: Oxford University Press.

Perley, M. J. (2007a). Psychiatric issues in palliative care. In M. J. Perley & C. M. Dahlin (Eds.), *Core curriculum for the advanced practice hospice and palliative nurse* (pp. 439–480). Pittsburgh, PA: Hospice and Palliative Nurses Association.

Perley, M. J. (2007b). Psychosocial, emotional and spiritual issues. In M. J. Perley & C. M. Dahlin (Eds.), *Core curriculum for the advanced practice hospice and palliative nurse* (pp. 417–438). Pittsburgh, PA: Hospice and Palliative Nurses Association.

Quill, T., Holloway, R., Shah, M., Caprio, T., Olden, A., & Storey, P. (2010). *Primer of palliative care* (5th ed.). Glenview, IL: American Academy of Hospice and Palliative Medicine.

Sarhill, N., Walsh, D., Nelson, K. A., LeGrand, S., & Davis, M. P. (2001). Assessment of delirium in advanced cancer: the use of the bedside confusion scale. *American Journal of Hospice and Palliative Medicine, 18*(5), 335–341.

Sigler, J. M., Kelly, D. H., & Dahlin, C. M. (2007). Gastrointestinal conditions. In M. J. Perley & C. M. Dahlin (Eds.), *Core curriculum for the advanced practice hospice and palliative nurse* (pp. 259–292). Pittsburgh, PA: Hospice and Palliative Nurses Association.

Teno, J., Weitze, S., Wetle, T., & Mor, V. (2001). Persistent pain in nursing home residents. *Journal of the American Medical Association, 285*(16), 2081.

Thomas, J., Karver, S., Cooney, G. A., Chamberlain, B. H., Watt, C. K., Slatkin, N. E., . . . Israel, R. J. (2008). Methylnaltrexone for opioid-induced constipation in advanced illness. *New England Journal of Medicine, 358*(22), 2332–2343. doi:10.1056/NEJMoa0707377

U.S. National Center for Health Statistics. (2010). Deaths: final data for 2007. *National Vital Statistics Reports, 58*(19), 1–135.

Wee, B., & Hillier, R. (2008). Interventions for noisy breathing in patients near to death. *Cochrane Database of Systematic Reviews,* (1). doi:10.1002/14651858.CD005177.pub2

Wilson, S. A. (2007). Cultural Issues. In M. J. Perley & C. M. Dahlin (Eds.), *Core curriculum for the advanced practice hospice and palliative nurse* (pp. 347–362). Pittsburgh, PA: Hospice and Palliative Nurses Association.

World Health Organization. (2010). *WHO definition of palliative care.* Retrieved from http://www.who.int/cancer/palliative/definition

World Health Organization. (2011). *WHO's pain ladder for adults.* Retrieved from http://www.who.int/cancer/palliative/painladder/en

Zimmerman, K., Rudolph, J., Salow, M., & Skarf, L. M. (2011). Delirium in palliative care patients: focus on pharmacotherapy. *American Journal of Hospice and Palliative Medicine.* Advance online publication. doi:10.1177/1049909111403732

Physiological Influences of the Aging Process

AGE-RELATED CHANGE	APPEARANCE OR FUNCTIONAL CHANGE	IMPLICATION
Integumentary System		
Loss of dermal and epidermal thickness	Paper-thin skin	Prone to skin tears
Flattening of papillae	Shearing and friction force more readily peels off the epidermis Diminished cell-mediated immunity in the skin	Prone to skin breakdown and injury
Atrophy of the sebaceous glands	Decreased production of oil and cerumen	Frequent pruritus and xerosis
Atrophy of the eccrine glands	Decreased sweating ability	Impaired thermoregulation
Decreased vascularity	Slower recruitment of sweat glands by thermal stimulation	Alteration in thermoregularity response; diminished ability to adapt to temperature changes Fluid requirements may change seasonally
	Decreased body odor Decreased heat loss Dryness	Loss of skin water Increased risk of heat stroke
Collagen cross-linking	Increased wrinkling	Potential effect on one's morale and feeling of self-worth
Elastin regression	Laxity of skin	
Loss of subcutaneous fat	Intraosseous atrophy, especially to the back of hands and to the face	Loss of fat tissue on soles of feet—trauma of walking increases foot problems
Decreased elasticity		Difficulty assessing skin turgor
Loss of subcutaneous tissue	Purpuric patches after minor surgery	Reduced insulation against cold temperatures; *prone to hypothermia* Check why injury is occurring; be alert for potential abuse or falls
Decreased number of melanocytes	Loss of pigment	Teach the importance of using sun block creams; refer to a dermatologist as needed
	Pigment plaque appears	

Continued

AGE-RELATED CHANGE	APPEARANCE OR FUNCTIONAL CHANGE	IMPLICATION
Integumentary System—cont'd		
Decreased turnover rate of keratinocytes	Increased exposure of the epidermal cells to the environment to include UV radiation	Increased risk of nonmalignant skin cancers and malignant melanoma
Decline in fibroblast proliferation	Decreased epidermal growth rate Slower reepithelialization	Decreased tissue repair response
	Decreased vitamin D production and synthesis	Increased risk for developing osteoporosis and other conditions associated with vitamin D deficiency
Decreased hair follicle density	Loss of body hair	
Decreased growth phase of individual fibers	Thin, short villus hairs predominate	
	Slower hair growth	
Loss of melanocytes from the hair bulb	Graying of the hair	Potential effect on self-esteem
Alternating hyperplasia and hypoplasia of nail matrix	Longitudinal ridges	Nails prone to splitting
	Thinner nails of the fingers	Advise patient to wear gloves, keep nails short, and avoid nail polish remover (causes dryness); refer patient to podiatrist
	Thickened, curled toenails or clawlike nails known as onychogryphosis	May cause discomfort
Respiratory System		
Decreased lung tissue elasticity	Decreased vital capacity	Reduced overall efficiency of ventilatory exchange
	Increased residual volume Decreased maximum breath capacity	
Thoracic wall calcification	Increased anteroposterior diameter of chest Displacement of apical impulse	Obscuration of heart and lung sounds
Cilia atrophy	Change in mucociliary transport; mucous-producing cells increase	Increased susceptibility to infection
Decreased respiratory muscle strength	Reduced ability to handle secretions and reduced effectiveness against noxious foreign particles Partial inflation of lungs at rest	Prone to atelectasis
Less sensitivity to hypoxia; impaired ability to recognize bronchoconstriction	Increased respiratory distress	Increased risk of mortality from acute respiratory conditions
Cardiovascular System		
Heart valves fibrose and thicken	Reduced stroke volume; cardiac output may be altered	Decreased responsiveness to stress; heart rate and blood pressure take longer to return to normal resting rate following exertion
	Slight left ventricular hypertrophy	Increased incidence of murmurs, *particularly aortic stenosis and mitral regurgitation*

AGE-RELATED CHANGE	APPEARANCE OR FUNCTIONAL CHANGE	IMPLICATION
Cardiovascular System—cont'd		
Mucoid degeneration of mitral valve	S_4 sound commonly heard Valve less dense; mitral leaflet stretches with intrathoracic pressure	
Fibroelastic thickening of the sinoatrial node; decreased number of pace-maker cells	Slower heart rate Irregular heart rate	Increased prevalence of arrhythmias and extra heart beats become more common
Increased subpericardial fat		
Collagen accumulation around heart muscle		
Elongation of tortuosity and calcification of arteries	Increased rigidity of arterial wall	Aneurysms may form
Elastin and collagen cause progressive thickening and loss of arterial wall resiliency	Increased peripheral vascular resistance	Decreased blood flow to body organs Altered distribution of blood flow
Loss of elasticity of the aorta dilation		Increased systolic blood pressure, contributing to coronary artery disease
Increased lipid content in artery wall	Lipid deposits form	Increased incidence of atherosclerotic events such as *angina pectoris*, stroke, gangrene
Decreased baroreceptor sensitivity (stretch receptors)	Decreased sensitivity to change in blood pressure	Prone to loss of balance—potential for falls
	Decreased baroreceptor mediation to straining	Valsalva maneuver may cause sudden drop in blood pressure, orthostatic hypotension, and dizziness when the patient changes from a lying or sitting position to standing
Gastrointestinal System		
Liver becomes smaller	Decreased storage capacity; decreased efficiency in metabolizing drugs that pass through the liver	
Less efficient cholesterol stabilization absorption	Increased evidence of gallstones	
Atrophy of muscles and bones of the jaw	Difficulty with mastication	Ability to thoroughly chew food is impaired and can contribute to dysphagia with solid foods
Dental enamel thins	Staining of tooth surface occurs	Tooth and gum decay; tooth loss
Gums recede	Teeth deprived of nutrients	
Fibrosis and atrophy of salivary glands	Prone to dry mucous membranes	Shift to mouth breathing is common; frequent complaints of dry mouth are expressed
	Decreased salivary ptyalin	Membrane more susceptible to injury and infection May interfere with breakdown of starches

Continued

AGE-RELATED CHANGE	APPEARANCE OR FUNCTIONAL CHANGE	IMPLICATION
Gastrointestinal System—cont'd		
Atrophy and decrease in number of taste buds	Decreased taste sensation	Altered ability to taste sweet, sour, and bitter Change in nutritional intake Excessive seasoning of foods
Delay in esophageal emptying	Decline in esophageal peristalsis Stiffening of the esophageal wall	Occasional discomfort as food stays in esophagus longer
Decreased hydrochloric acid secretion	Reduction in amount of iron and vitamin B_{12} that can be absorbed	Possible delay in vitamin and drug absorption, *especially calcium and iron*
Decrease in gastric acid secretion		Altered drug effect
Decreased muscle tone	Altered motility Decreased colonic peristalsis	Prone to constipation, functional bowel syndrome, esophageal spasm, diverticular disease
Atrophy of mucosal lining	Decreased hunger sensations and emptying time	
Decreased proportion of dietary calcium absorbed	Altered bone formation, muscle contractility, hormone activity, enzyme activation, clotting time, immune response	Symptoms more marked in women than in men
Decreased basal metabolic rate (rate at which fuel is converted into energy)		May need fewer calories Possible effect on life span
Genitourinary and Reproductive Systems		
Reduced renal mass	Decreased sodium-conserving ability	Administration and dosage of drugs may need to be modified
Loss of glomeruli	Decreased glomerular filtration rate Decreased creatinine clearance Increased blood urea nitrogen concentration	
Histological changes in small vessel walls	Decreased renal blood flow	
Sclerosis of supportive circulatory system		
Decline in number of functioning nephrons	Decreased ability to dilute urine concentrate	Altered response to reduced fluid load or increased fluid volume
Reduced bladder muscular tone	Decreased bladder capacity or increased residual urine	Sensation of urge to urinate may not occur until bladder is full
Atrophy and fibrosis of cervical and uterine walls	Menopause; decline in fertility	Urination at night may increase
Reduced number and viability of oocytes in the aging ovary	Narrowing of cervical canal	
Decreased vaginal wall elasticity	Vaginal lining thin, pale, friable Narrowing of vaginal canal	Potential for discomfort in sexual intercourse

AGE-RELATED CHANGE	APPEARANCE OR FUNCTIONAL CHANGE	IMPLICATION
Genitourinary and Reproductive Systems—cont'd		
Decreased levels of circulating hormones	Reduced lubrication during arousal state	Increased frequency of sexual dysfunction
Degeneration of seminiferous tubules	Decreased seminal fluid volume Decreased force of ejaculation Reduced elevation of testes	
Proliferation of stromal and glandular tissue	Prostatic hypertrophy	Potentially compromised genitourinary function; *urinary frequency and increased risk of malignancy*
Involution of mammary gland tissue	Connective tissue replaced by adipose tissue	Easier to assess breast lesions
Neuromuscular System		
Decreased muscle mass	Decreased muscle strength	Increased muscle cramping
	Tendons shrink and sclerose	Decreased tendon jerks
Decreased myosin adenosine triphosphatase activity	Prolonged contraction time, latency period, relaxation period	Decreased motor function and overall strength
Deterioration of joint cartilage	Bone makes contact with bone	Potential for pain, crepitation, and limitation of movement
Loss of water from the cartilage	Narrowing of joint spaces	Loss of height
Decreased bone mass	Decreased bone formation and increased bone resorption, leading to osteoporosis	More rapid and earlier changes in women
Decreased osteoblastic activity		Greater risk of fractures
Osteoclasts resorb bone	Hormonal changes	Gait and posture accommodate to changes
Increased proportion of body fat	Centripetal distribution of fat and invasion of fat in large muscle groups	Anthropometric measurements required
Regional changes in fat distribution		Increased relative adiposity
Thickened leptomeninges in spinal cord	Loss of anterior horn cells in the lumbosacral area	Leg weakness may be correlated
Accumulation of lipofuscin	Altered RNA function and resultant cell death	
Loss of neurons and nerve fibers	Decreased processing speed and vibration sense	Increased time to perform and learn
	Altered pain response Decreased deep tendon, Achilles tendon	Possible postural hypotension
		Safety hazard
Decreased conduction of nerve fibers	Decreased psychomotor performance	Alteration in pain response
Few neuritic plaques		Possible cognitive and memory changes
Neurofibrillary tangles in hippocampal neurons		Heavy tangle formation and neuritic plaques in cortex of patients with Alzheimer's disease

Continued

AGE-RELATED CHANGE	APPEARANCE OR FUNCTIONAL CHANGE	IMPLICATION
Neuromuscular System—cont'd		
Changes in sleep-wake cycle	Decreased stage 4, stage 3, and rapid eye movement phases	Increased or decreased time spent sleeping
	Deterioration of circadian organization	Increased nighttime awakenings
		Changed hormonal activity
Slower stimulus identification and registration	Delayed reaction time	Prone to falls
Decreased brain weight and volume		May be present in absence of mental impairments
Sensory System		
Morphological changes in choroid, epithelium, retina	Decreased visual acuity	Corrective lenses required
	Visual field narrows	Increased possibility of disorientation and social isolation
Decreased rod and cone function		Slower light and dark adaptation
Pigment accumulation		
Decreased speed of eye movements	Difficulty in gazing upward and maintaining convergence	
Sclerosis of pupil sphincter	Difficulty in adapting to lighting changes	Glare may pose an environmental hazard
	Increased threshold for light perception	Dark rooms may be hazardous
Increased intraocular pressure	Increased incidence of glaucoma	
Distorted depth perception		Incorrect assessment of height of curbs and steps; potential for falls
Ciliary muscle atrophy	Altered refractive powers	Corrective lenses often required
Nuclear sclerosis (*lens*)	Presbyopia	Near work and reading may become difficult
Reduced accommodation	Hyperopia	
Increased lens size	Myopia	
Accumulation of lens fibers		
Lens yellows	Color vision may be impaired	Less able to differentiate low color tones: blues, greens, violets
Diminished tear secretion	Dullness and dryness of the eyes	Irritation and discomfort may result
		Intactness of corneal surface jeopardized
Loss of auditory neurons	Decreased tone discrimination and voice localization	Suspiciousness may be increased because of paranoid dimensions secondary to hearing loss
	High-frequency sounds lost first	Social isolation
Angiosclerosis calcification of inner ear membrane	Progressive hearing loss, especially at high frequency	Difficulty hearing, particularly under certain conditions such as *background noise, rapid speech, poor acoustics*
	Presbycusis	

AGE-RELATED CHANGE	APPEARANCE OR FUNCTIONAL CHANGE	IMPLICATION
Sensory System—cont'd		
Decreased number of olfactory nerve fibers	Decreased sensitivity to odors	May not detect harmful odors
		Potential safety hazard
Alteration in taste sensation		Possible changes in food preferences and eating patterns
Reduced tactile sensation	Decreased ability to sense pressure, pain, temperature	Misperceptions of environment and safety risk
Endocrine System		
Decline in secretion of testosterone, growth hormone, insulin, adrenal androgens, aldosterone, thyroid hormone	Decreased hormone clearance rates	Increased mortality associated with certain stresses (burns, surgery); increased prevalence of hormonal disease
Defects in thermoregulation	Shivering less intense	Susceptibility to temperature extremes (*hypothermia/hyperthermia*)
Reduction of febrile responses	Poor perceptions of changes in ambient temperature Reduced sweating; increased threshold for the onset of sweating Fever not always present with infectious process	Unrecognized infectious process operative
Alteration in tissue sensitivity to hormones	Decreased insulin response, glucose tolerance, and sensitivity of renal tubules to antidiuretic hormone	
Enhanced sympathetic responsivity		
Increased nodularity and fibrosis of thyroid		Increased frequency of thyroid disease
Decreased basal metabolic rate	Alteration in carbohydrate tolerance	Increased incidence of obesity
Hematological System		
Decreased percentage of marrow space occupied by hematopoietic tissue	Ineffective erythropoiesis	Risky for patients who lose blood
Immune System		
Thymic involution and decreased serum thymic hormone activity	Decreased number of T cells	Less vigorous and/or delayed hypersensitivity reactions
	Production of anti-self reactive T cells	
Decreased T-cell function	Impairment in cell-mediated immune responses	Increased risk of mortality
Appearance of autoantibodies	Decreased cyclic adenosine monophosphate and glucose monophosphate	Increased incidence of infection
	Decreased ability to reject foreign tissue	Reactivation of latent infectious diseases
	Increased laboratory autoimmune parameters	Increased prevalence of autoimmune disorders

Continued

AGE-RELATED CHANGE	APPEARANCE OR FUNCTIONAL CHANGE	IMPLICATION
Immune System—cont'd		
Redistribution of lymphocytes	Impaired immune reactivity	
Changes in serum immunoglobulin	Increased immunoglobulin A levels Decreased immunoglobulin G levels	Increased prevalence of infection

REFERENCES

Mauk, K. (2013). *Gerontological nursing: competencies for care* (3rd ed.). Boston, MA: Jones and Bartlett.

Smith, C. M. & Cotter, V. T. (2012). Age-related changes in health. In M. Boltz, E. Capezuti, D. T. T. Fulmer, D. Zwicker, & A. O'Meara (Eds.), *Evidence-based geriatric nursing protocols for best practice* (4th ed., pp. 23–47). New York, NY: Springer Publishing.

Laboratory Values in the Older Adult

LABORATORY TEST	NORMAL VALUES	CHANGES WITH AGE	COMMENTS
Urinalysis			
Protein	0–5 mg/100 mL	Rises slightly	May be due to kidney changes with age, urinary tract infection, or renal pathology
Glucose	0–15 mg/100 mL	Declines slightly	Glycosuria appears after high plasma level; unreliable
Specific gravity	1.005–1.020	Lower maximum in elderly, 1.016–1.022	Decline in nephrons impairs ability to concentrate urine
Hematology			
Erythrocyte sedimentation rate	Male: 0–20 mm/hour Female: 0–30 mm/hour	Significant increase	Neither sensitive nor specific in the aged
Iron Iron binding	50–160 mcg/dL 230–410 mcg/dL	Slight decrease Decrease	
Hemoglobin	Male: 13 gm/dL Female: 11.0 gm/dL	Male: 11.5 gm/dL Female: 11.0 gm/dL	Anemia common in the elderly
Hematocrit	Male: 40%–54% Female: 36%–46%	Slight decrease speculated	Decrease in anemias, multiple myeloma, protein malnutrition, CDK, rheumatoid arthritis, increased dehydration, severe diarrhea
Leukocytes	4300–10,800/mm^3	Drop to 3100–9000/mm^3	Decrease may be due to drugs or sepsis and should not be attributed immediately to age
Lymphocytes	500–2400 T cells/mm^3 50–200 B cells/mm^3	T-cell and B-cell levels fall	Risk of infection is higher; immunization is encouraged
Platelets	150,000–350,000/mm^3	No change in number	
Blood Chemistry			
Albumin	3.5–5.0 gm/dL	Decline	Related to decrease in liver size and enzymes; protein-energy malnutrition common

Continued

LABORATORY TEST	NORMAL VALUES	CHANGES WITH AGE	COMMENTS
Blood Chemistry—cont'd			
Globulin	2.3–3.5 g/100 mL	Slight increase	
Total serum protein	6.0–8.4 g/100 mL	No change in number	Decreases may indicate malnutrition, infection, liver disease
Blood urea nitrogen	Men: 10–25 mg/100 mL Women: 8–20 mg/100 mL	Increases significantly up to 69 mg/100 mL	Decline in glomerular filtration rate; decreased cardiac output
Creatinine	0.6–1.5 mg/100 mL	Increases to 1.9 mg/100 mL seen	Related to decreases in lean body mass
Creatinine clearance	104–124 mL/min	Decreases 10%/decade after 40 years of age	Decreased renal impairment, hyperthyroidism, thiazides, increased hypothyroidism
Glucose tolerance	62–110 mg/dL after fasting; <120 mg/dL after 2 hours postprandial	Slight increase of 10 mg/dL/decade after 30 years of age	Diabetes increasingly prevalent; drugs may cause glucose intolerance
Triglycerides	40–150 mg/100 mL	20–200 mg/100 mL	Risk of coronary artery disease
Cholesterol	120–220 mg/100 mL	Males: increase to 50 mg/100 mL, then decrease Females: increase postmenopausally	Risk of cardiovascular disease
Thyroxine	4.5–13.5 mcg/dL	3.3–8.6 mcg/dL	Changes suggest thyroid disease; may be seen in euthyroid patients with acute or chronic illness or caloric deficiencies
Triiodothyronine	90–220 ng/dL	Decrease 25%	May impact metabolism, body temperature, or heart rate
Thyroid-stimulating hormone	0.5–5.0 mcg/mL	Slight increase	Sensitive indicator for diagnosing thyroid disease
Alkaline phosphatase	13–39 IU/L	Increase by 8–10 IU/L	Elevations (20% usually due to disease; elevations may be found with bone abnormalities, drugs (e.g., narcotics), and consumption of a fatty meal. For best results, this test should be ordered during fasting (Edwards & Baird, 2005; Toughy & Jeff, 2012).

REFERENCES

Edwards, N.,& Baird, C. (2005). Interpreting laboratory values in older adults. *Medsurg Nursing, 14*(4) 220–229.

Jett, K. F. (2012). Laboratory values and diagnostics. In T. A. Toughy & K. F. Jett (Eds.), *Toward healthy aging: human needs and nursing responses* (8th ed., pp. 118–113). St. Louis, MO: Mosby.

INDEX

Note: Page references with f, t, and b indicate figures, tables, and boxes respectively.